Atlas of
Advanced Operative Surgery

Atlas of Advanced Operative Surgery

Vijay P. Khatri, MBChB, FACS
Professor of Surgery
University of California, Davis School of Medicine
Sacramento, California

SAUNDERS
ELSEVIER

ELSEVIER
SAUNDERS

1600 John F. Kennedy Blvd.
Ste 1800
Philadelphia, PA 19103-2899

ATLAS OF ADVANCED OPERATIVE SURGERY ISBN: 978-1-4160-4109-2

Notices

Knowledge and best practice in this field are constantly changing. As new research and experience broaden our understanding, changes in research methods, professional practices, or medical treatment may become necessary.

Practitioners and researchers must always rely on their own experience and knowledge in evaluating and using any information, methods, compounds, or experiments described herein. In using such information or methods they should be mindful of their own safety and the safety of others, including parties for whom they have a professional responsibility.

With respect to any drug or pharmaceutical products identified, readers are advised to check the most current information provided (i) on procedures featured or (ii) by the manufacturer of each product to be administered, to verify the recommended dose or formula, the method and duration of administration, and contraindications. It is the responsibility of practitioners, relying on their own experience and knowledge of their patients, to make diagnoses, to determine dosages and the best treatment for each individual patient, and to take all appropriate safety precautions.

To the fullest extent of the law, neither the Publisher nor the authors, contributors, or editors assume any liability for any injury and/or damage to persons or property as a matter of products liability, negligence or otherwise, or from any use or operation of any methods, products, instructions, or ideas contained in the material herein.

Library of Congress Cataloging-in-Publication Data
Atlas of advanced operative surgery / [edited by] Vijay P. Khatri.
p. ; cm.
Includes bibliographical references and index.
ISBN 978-1-4160-4109-2 (hardcover : alk. paper)
I. Khatri, Vijay P.
[DNLM: 1. Surgical Procedures, Operative—methods—Atlases. WO 517]
617.9022′3—dc23
2012030451

Executive Content Strategist: Michael Houston
Content Development Specialist: Roxanne Halpine Ward
Publishing Services Manager: Anne Altepeter
Project Manager: Louise King
Design Manager: Steven Stave

Printed in China

Last digit is the print number: 9 8 7 6 5 4 3 2 1

To my wife, Anjana, and my children, Amit and Shevani

Contributors

Anders Albäck, MD, PhD
Associate Professor and Head, Department of Vascular Surgery, Helsinki University Hospital, Helsinki, Finland
Femorodistal (Peroneal/Dorsalis Pedis) Bypass for Occlusive Disease

Mohamed Ali, MD
Associate Professor, Department of Surgery, Chief, Bariatric Surgery, Director, Minimally Invasive and Robotic Surgery, University of California, Davis, Davis, California
Laparoscopic Roux-en-Y Gastric Bypass Surgery

Fady K. Balaa, MD
Assistant Professor, Department of Surgery, University of Ottawa, The Ottawa Hospital–Civic Campus, Ottawa, Ontario, Canada
Laparoscopic Approach to Hepatic Cysts
Laparoscopic Radiofrequency Ablation of Liver Tumors

Hans G. Beger, MD, MD(Hon), FACS(Hon), JSS(Hon)
Professor Emeritus, Department of General and Visceral Surgery, Klinikum University of Ulm; Senior Surgeon, Department of Oncological, Endocrinological, and Minimally Invasive Surgery, Donau-Klinikum, Neu-Ulm, Germany
Beger and Frey Procedure for Chronic Pancreatitis

Jacques Belghiti, MD
Department of HepatoBilioPancreatic Surgery, University of Denis Diderot, Hospital Beaujon, Clichy, France
Right and Left Trisectionectomies

Lana Bijelic, MD, FACS
Attending Surgeon, Department of Surgery, Washington Hospital Center; Assistant Professor of Clinical Surgery, Georgetown University, Washington, District of Columbia
Surgical Procedures for Peritoneal Surface Malignancy

Henri Bismuth, MD, FACS(Hon)
Director, Henri Bismuth Hepatobiliary Institute, Villejuif, France
Liver Segmentectomies
Resection Hilar Cholangiocarcinoma with En Bloc Hepatectomy

Jan D. Blankensteijn, MD, PhD
Associate Professor of Vascular Surgery, Department of Surgery, Vrije Universiteit (VU) Medical Center, Amsterdam, The Netherlands
Endovascular Repair of Abdominal Aortic Aneurysms

Antonio Briccoli, MD
Associate Professor of Surgery, General and Thoracic Surgical Oncology, University of Bologna, Istituto Ortopedico Rizzoli, Bologna, Italy
Chest Wall Resection/Reconstruction

Henry Buchwald, MD, PhD
Professor of Surgery and Biomedical Engineering, Owen H. and Sarah Davidson Wangensteen Chair in Experimental Surgery Emeritus, Department of Surgery, University of Minnesota, Minneapolis, Minnesota
Laparoscopic Roux-en-Y Gastric Bypass Surgery

Guy Bernard Cadière, MD, PhD
Professor of Surgery, Chief, Department of Gastrointestinal Surgery, Director, European School of Laparoscopic Surgery, Saint-Pierre University Hospital, Brussels, Belgium
Esophagectomy by Thoracoscopy in Prone Position Followed by Laparoscopy and Cervicotomy
Laparoscopic Adjustable Gastric Banding

Mitchell A. Cahan, MD, FACS
Associate Professor of Surgery, University of Massachusetts Medical School, Worcester, Massachusetts
Laparoscopic Adrenalectomy (Right and Left)

Laura Campanacci, MD, PhD
Orthopaedic Surgeon, Clinica Ortopedica IV, Oncological Orthopaedics, Istituto Ortopedico Rizzoli, Bologna, Italy
Scapular Resections

Grant W. Carlson, MD
Wadley R. Glenn Professor, Department of Surgery, Chief of Plastic Surgery, Division of Plastic Surgery, Emory University, Atlanta, Georgia
Skin-Sparing Mastectomy and Sentinel Lymph Node Biopsy

Daniel Cherqui, MD
Professor, Department of Surgery, Henri Mondor Hospital, Paris, France
Resection Hilar Cholangiocarcinoma with En Bloc Hepatectomy

Gaetano Ciancio, MD, MBA, FACS
Brandon and Kyle Simonsen Professor of Surgery and Urology, Miami Transplant Institute; Department of Surgery, Division of Kidney and Kidney/Pancreas Transplantation, and Department of Urology, University of Miami Miller School of Medicine, Miami, Florida
Radical Nephrectomy with Inferior Vena Cava Tumor Thrombectomy

Robert R. Cima, MD, MA
Associate Professor, Department of Surgery, Mayo Clinic College of Medicine; Consultant, Colon and Rectal Surgery, Mayo Clinic, Rochester, Minnesota
Laparoscopic Colon Resection (Right, Left, Sigmoid)

Orlo H. Clark, MD, FACS
Professor, Department of Surgery, University of California, San Francisco, San Francisco, California
Total Thyroidectomy with Central Neck Dissection

Marc Coggia, MD
Professor, Department of Vascular Surgery, Ambroise Pare University Hospital, Boulogne-Billancourt, France
Laparoscopic Abdominal Aortic Aneurysm Repair

Alvin H. Crawford, MD, FACS
Founding Director, Crawford Spine Center; Professor, Division of Pediatric Surgery, Cincinnati Children's Hospital, Cincinnati, Ohio
Thoracoscopic First Rib Resection for Thoracic Outlet Syndrome

Giovanni Dapri, MD, FACS, FASMBS
Assistant Professor of Surgery, Department of Gastrointestinal Surgery, European School of Laparoscopic Surgery, Saint-Pierre University Hospital, Brussels, Belgium
Esophagectomy by Thoracoscopy in Prone Position Followed by Laparoscopy and Cervicotomy
Laparoscopic Adjustable Gastric Banding

Ara Darzi, PC, KBE, HonFREng, FMedSci
Professor, Division of Surgery, Imperial College London; Honorary Consultant Surgeon, Division of Surgery, Imperial College Healthcare National Health Service Trust and the Royal Marsden Hospital NHS Foundation Trust, London, United Kingdom
Laparoscopic Splenectomy

Francesca De Lorenzi, MD, PhD
Department of Plastic and Reconstructive Surgery, European Institute of Oncology, Milan, Italy
Nipple- and Areola-Sparing Mastectomy

Herbert Decaluwe, MD
Department of Thoracic Surgery, Leuven Lung Cancer Group, University Hospital Leuven, Leuven, Belgium
Radical Esophagectomy with Two- or Three-Field Lymphadenectomy

Samer S. Deeba, MD, MD(res), MRCS(Eng)
Academic Clinical Fellow, Department of Surgery and Cancer, Faculty of Medicine, Imperial College London, London, United Kingdom
Laparoscopic Splenectomy

Leigh Delbridge, MD, FRCS, FACS
Professor and Head, Department of Surgery, The University of Sydney, Sydney, Australia
Minimally Invasive Parathyroidectomy

Antonino Ditto, MD
Attending Surgeon, Division of Gynecological Oncology, Fondazione IRCCS, Istituto Dei Tumori, Milan, Italy
Nerve-Sparing Radical Abdominal Hysterectomy with Regional Lymphadenectomy

Quan-Yang Duh, MD, FACS
Professor in Residence, Department of Surgery, University of California, San Francisco; Attending Surgeon, Surgical Service, Veterans Affairs Medical Center, San Francisco, California
Revision Parathyroidectomy

Frederick R. Eilber, MD, FACS
Professor Emeritus, Department of Surgery, Division of Surgical Oncology, University of California, Los Angeles, Los Angeles, California
Anterior Thigh Tumor Resection
Resection of Flexor Fossa (Axilla and Groin) Sarcoma

Fritz C. Eilber, MD
Associate Professor, Departments of Surgery and Molecular and Medical Pharmacology, Division of Surgical Oncology, University of California, Los Angeles, Los Angeles, California
Anterior Thigh Tumor Resection
Resection of Flexor Fossa (Axilla and Groin) Sarcoma

Dina M. Elaraj, MD, FACS
Assistant Professor, Section of Endocrine Surgery, Department of Surgery, Northwestern University Feinberg School of Medicine, Chicago, Illinois
Revision Parathyroidectomy

Costantino Errani, MD, PhD
Orthopaedic Surgeon, Orthopaedic Service, Rizzoli-Sicilia, Bagheria, Italy
Hip Disarticulation

José Carlos Marques de Faria, MD, PhD
Plastic and Reconstructive Surgery, Hospital A.C. Camargo, Antonio Prudente Foundation, São Paulo, Brazil
External Hemipelvectomy

Diana Farmer, MD, FACS, FRCS
Pearl Stamps Stewart Professor and Chair, Chair, Department of Surgery, UC Davis School of Medicine; Surgeon-in-Chief, UC Davis Children's Hospital, UC Davis Health System, Davis, California
Foreword

Laureano Fernández-Cruz, MD, FRCS Ed(Hon), FCRSI(Hon)
Professor, Chairman of Surgery, Department of Surgery, Hospital Clínic Barcelona, University of Barcelona, Barcelona, Spain
Distal Subtotal Pancreatectomy with and without Spleen Preservation

Philip Fransen, MD
Consultant, Laparoscopic and Endo-Urological Urology, Department of Urology, Maria Hospital Overpelt, Overpelt; Consultant, Laparoscopic and Endo-Urological Urology, Department of Urology, ZMK Hospital, Maaseik, Belgium
Laparoscopic Retroperitoneal Lymph Node Dissection for Low-Stage Nonseminomatous Testis Cancer

Anthony J. Froix, MD
General Surgeon, United Memorial Medical Center, Surgical Associates, Jerome Center, United Memorial Medical Center, Batavia, New York
Hepatic Artery Infusion Pump Placement

Takeo Fukagawa, MD, PhD
Head Surgeon, Gastrointestinal Oncology, Gastric Surgery Division, National Cancer Center Hospital, Tokyo, Japan
Total Gastrectomy with D2 Lymph Node Dissection

Michel Gagner, MD, FRCSC, FACS
Clinical Professor of Surgery, Herbert Wertheim College of Medicine, Florida International University, Miami, Florida; Attending Surgeon (Associate Member), Department of Surgery, Hopital du Sacre Coeur, Montreal, Quebec, Canada; Senior Consultant, Chief, Bariatric and Metabolic Surgery, Department of Surgery, Hamad General Hospital, Doha, Qatar; Senior Consultant, Department of Surgery, Al-Seef Hospital, Kuwait City, Kuwait
Laparoscopic Gastric Sleeve Resection with Duodenal Switch
Laparoscopic Nissen Fundoplication

Jeffrey M. Gauvin, MD, MSc
Director, Department of Surgical Education, Santa Barbara Cottage Hospital, Santa Barbara, California
Forequarter Amputation

David A. Geller, MD
Richard L. Simmons Professor of Surgery, Chief, Division of Hepatobiliary and Pancreatic Surgery, Co-Director, University of Pittsburgh Medical Center Liver Cancer Center, University of Pittsburgh, Pittsburgh, Pennsylvania
Laparoscopic Approach to Hepatic Cysts
Laparoscopic Radiofrequency Ablation of Liver Tumors

David M. Gershenson, MD
Professor and Chairman, Department of Gynecologic Oncology and Reproductive Medicine, The University of Texas MD Anderson Cancer Center, Houston, Texas
Surgical Management of Ovarian Cancer

Bruce L. Gewertz, MD
Surgeon-in-Chief, Chair, Department of Surgery, Vice President, Interventional Services, Vice Dean, Academic Affairs, Cedars-Sinai Medical Center, Los Angeles, California
Carotid Endarterectomy/Stent Placement
Axillofemoral Bypass
Renal Artery Revascularization
Celiac and Mesenteric Artery Revascularization

Jean-François Gigot, MD, PhD, FRCS
Professor and Chairman, Department of Abdominal Surgery and Transplantation, Cliniques Universitaires Saint-Luc, Brussels, Belgium
Resection of Congenital Bile Duct Cysts
Laparoscopic Left Lateral Hepatic Lobectomy

Olivier Goëau-Brissonnière, MD, PhD
Professor of Vascular Surgery and Chair, Department of Vascular Surgery, Ambroise Paré University Hospital, Boulogne-Billancourt; Faculté de Médecine Paris-Ile de France-Ouest, Versailles Saint Quentin en Yvelines University, Versailles, France
Laparoscopic Abdominal Aortic Aneurysm Repair

Ziya L. Gokaslan, MD, FACS
Professor, Vice Chairman, Director, Department of Neurosurgery–Spine, Johns Hopkins University School of Medicine, Baltimore, Maryland
Total and Subtotal Sacrectomy for En Bloc Resections of Primary Tumors of the Sacrum

Ho-Seong Han, MD, PhD
Chairman, Department of Surgery, Seoul National University College of Medicine, Seoul National University Bundang Hospital, Seoul, Korea
Resection of the Caudate Lobe

Francesco Hanozet, MD
Attending Surgeon, Division of Gynecological Oncology, National Cancer Institute, Milan, Italy
Radical Vulvectomy with Groin Dissection

Richard J. Heald, OBE, MChir, FRCS
Director of Surgery, Pelican Cancer Foundation, Basingstoke, Hampshire, United Kingdom
Total Mesorectal Excision with Colonic J-Pouch Coloanal Reconstruction for Rectal Cancer

Alan W. Hemming, MD, MSc, FRCSC, FACS
Professor and Chief, Division of Hepatobiliary Surgery and Transplantation, Department of Surgery, University of California, San Diego, San Diego, California
Hepatectomy with Inferior Vena Cava Resection and Reconstruction

J. Michael Henderson, MBChB, FRCS
Chief Quality Officer/Staff, General Surgery, Quality and Patient Safety Institute, Cleveland Clinic, Cleveland, Ohio
Variceal Decompression: Distal Splenorenal, Portocaval, and Mesocaval Shunts

Harald J.J. Hoekstra, MD, PhD
Professor, Department of Surgical Oncology, University Medical Center Groningen, Groningen, The Netherlands
Radical Superficial and Deep Groin Dissection
Composite Axillary and Supraclavicular Lymph Node Dissection

Michael K.Y. Hsin, MBBChir(Cantab), MA(Cantab), FRCS CTh, FHKCS, FHKAM
Honorary Assistant Professor, Department of Surgery, The Chinese University of Hong Kong, Shatin, Hong Kong; Research Fellow, Latner Thoracic Surgical Research Laboratories, University of Toronto, Toronto, Ontario, Canada
Lung Volume Reduction Surgery

Catherine Hubert, MD
HepatoBilioPancreatic Surgery, Digestive Surgery and Abdominal Transplantation Unit, St. Luc University Hospital, Brussels, Belgium
Laparoscopic Left Lateral Hepatic Lobectomy

Seiji Ishiguro, MD, PhD
Department of Gastroenterological Surgery, Aichi Cancer Center Hospital, Nagoya, Japan
Pelvic Exenteration: Total/Anterior/Posterior

Ferenc Jakab, MD, PhD, DMSc
Professor, Department of Surgery and Vascular Surgery, Uzsoki Teaching Hospital/Semmelweis University, Budapest, Hungary
Transverse Hepatectomy

Guenter Janetschek, MD
Professor of Urology, Krankenhaus der Elisabethinen, Linz, Austria
Laparoscopic Retroperitoneal Lymph Node Dissection for Low-Stage Nonseminomatous Testis Cancer

Eliad Karin, MD
Senior Surgeon, General Surgery Division, Sourasky Medical Center, Tel Aviv, Israel
Popliteal Lymph Node Dissection
Radical Axillary Dissection

Namir Katkhouda, MD, FACS
Professor of Surgery, Vice Chairman of Clinical Affairs, Director, University of Southern California Bariatric Surgery Program, Department of Surgery, Keck School of Medicine of the University of Southern California, Los Angeles, California
Laparoscopic Vagotomy and Seromyotomy with Antrectomy
Laparoscopic Paraesophageal Hernia Repair

Stephen M. Kavic, MD, FACS
Assistant Professor, Department of Surgery, University of Maryland School of Medicine, Baltimore, Maryland
Laparoscopic Pancreatic Pseudocyst Drainage

M. Margaret Kemeny, MD, FACS
Professor, Department of Surgery, Mount Sinai School of Medicine, New York, New York; Director, Queens Cancer Center, Queens Hospital Center, Queens, New York
Hepatic Artery Infusion Pump Placement

Vijay P. Khatri, MBChB, FACS
Professor of Surgery, University of California, Davis School of Medicine, Sacramento, California
Transverse Hepatectomy
Mesohepatectomy
Forequarter Amputation
Posterior Thigh Tumor Resection

Seigo Kitano, MD, PhD, FACS
President, Oita University, Oita-city, Oita, Japan
Laparoscopy-Assisted Distal Gastrectomy with Lymphadenectomy

H. Christoph Klingler, MD, FEBU
Suppl Head and Chair, Department of Urology, Medical University of Vienna, Vienna, Austria
Laparoscopic Nephrectomy

Ferdinand Köckerling, MD, PhD
Department of Surgery, Centre for Minimally Invasive Surgery, Vivantes Hospital Spandau, Berlin, Germany
Laparoscopic Abdominoperineal Resection of the Rectum
Laparoscopic Rectopexy for Rectal Prolapse

Sang W. Lee, MD, FACS, FASCRS
Associate Professor of Surgery, Division of Colon and Rectal Surgery, New York-Presbyterian Hospital, Weill Cornell Medical College, New York, New York
Restorative Proctocolectomy with J-Pouch Ileoanal Anastomosis

Francesco Leo, MD, PhD
Thoracic Surgeon, Thoracic Surgery Department, National Cancer Institute, Milan, Italy
Radical Pneumonectomy

Mauri Lepäntalo, MD, PhD
Emeritus Professor of Vascular Surgery, Institute of Clinical Medicine, Helsinki University; Former Head, Department of Vascular Surgery, Helsinki University Central Hospital, Helsinki, Finland
Femorodistal (Peroneal/Dorsalis Pedis) Bypass for Occlusive Disease

Toni Lerut, MD, PhD
Emeritus Professor and Chairman, Department of Thoracic Surgery, University Hospital Gasthuisberg, Leuven, Belgium
Radical Esophagectomy with Two- or Three-Field Lymphadenectomy

Demetrius E.M. Litwin, MD, MBA
Harry M. Haidak Distinguished Professor and Chairman, Department of Surgery, University of Massachusetts Medical School, Worcester, Massachusetts
Laparoscopic Common Bile Duct Exploration
Laparoscopic Adrenalectomy (Right and Left)

Ademar Lopes, MD, PhD
Head, Department of Pelvic Surgery, A.C. Camargo Hospital; Associate Professor, Department of Oncology Discipline, Mogi Das Cruzes University, Mogi Das Cruzes; President, Brazilian Society of Surgical Oncology, São Paulo, Brazil
External Hemipelvectomy
Total Internal Hemipelvectomy

James D. Luketich, MD, FACS
Henry T. Bahnson Professor of Cardiothoracic Surgery, Chairman, Department of Cardiothoracic Surgery, University of Pittsburgh, Pittsburgh, Pennsylvania
Laparothoracoscopic Esophagectomy
Transthoracic Fundoplication: Belsey Fundoplication

Catharina Ihre Lundgren, MD, PhD
Senior Consultant, Department of Breast and Endocrine Surgery, Karolinska University Hospital, Institution for Molecular Medicine and Surgery, Karolinska Institutet, Stockholm, Sweden
Minimally Invasive Parathyroidectomy

N.J. Lygidakis, MD, PhD, FRCST(H), FJSS(H)
Chairman and Head, Department of Surgical Oncology, Athens Medical Centre, Athens, Greece
Pancreaticoduodenectomy with Superior Mesentericoportal Venous Resection

Jean-Yves Mabrut, MD, PhD
Professor of Surgery, Digestive and Liver Transplant Unit, Croix-Rousse University Hospital, Lyon, France
Resection of Congenital Bile Duct Cysts

Ali Mahtabifard, MD
Attending Surgeon, Cedars-Sinai Center for Chest Diseases; Clinical Chief, Thoracic Surgery, Cedars-Sinai Medical Center, Los Angeles, California
Video-Assisted Thoracoscopic Lobectomy
Thoracoscopic Lung Biopsy

Masatoshi Makuuchi, MD, PhD
President, Japanese Red Cross Medical Center; Professor Emeritus, University of Tokyo, Tokyo, Japan
Radical Cholecystectomy/Liver Bed Resection with Regional Lymph Node Dissection

Martin M. Malawer, MD, FACS
Director of Orthopedic Oncology, Professor of Orthopedic Surgery, George Washington University School of Medicine, Washington, District of Columbia; Professor of Orthopedics, Professor of Pediatrics (Hematology and Oncology), Georgetown University School of Medicine, Washington, District of Columbia; Consultant, Pediatric and Surgery Branch, National Cancer Institute, National Institutes of Health, Bethesda, Maryland
Tikhoff-Linberg Procedure and Modifications for Shoulder Girdle Resections

Michael Marberger, MD, FRCS
Professor and Chairman, Department of Urology, Medical University of Vienna, Vienna, Austria
Laparoscopic Nephrectomy

Robert J. McKenna, Jr., MD
Head, Division of Thoracic Surgery, Cedars-Sinai Medical Center, Los Angeles, California
Video-Assisted Thoracoscopic Lobectomy
Thoracoscopic Lung Biopsy

Jesus E. Medina, MD, FACS
Professor, Department of Otorhinolaryngology, University of Oklahoma Health Sciences Center, Oklahoma City, Oklahoma
Radical Neck Dissection
Excision of Submandibular Gland and Submandibular Triangle Dissection

Reza John Mehran, MD, SBStJ, MDCM, MSc, FRCSC, FACS
Professor, Department of Thoracic and Cardiovascular Surgery, The University of Texas MD Anderson Cancer Center, Houston, Texas
Resection of Pulmonary Metastases

Kristin L. Mekeel, MD, FACS
Associate Professor of Surgery, Transplantation and Hepatobiliary Surgery, University of California, San Diego, San Diego, California
Hepatectomy with Inferior Vena Cava Resection and Reconstruction

†Mario Mercuri, MD
Chief of Orthopaedic Service, Musculoskeletal Oncology Department, Istituto Ortopedico Rizzoli, Bologna, Italy
Hip Disarticulation
Scapular Resections

Fabrizio Michelassi, MD, FACS
Lewis Atterbury Stimson Professor and Chairman, Department of Surgery, Weill Cornell Medical College; Surgeon in Chief, Department of Surgery, New York-Presbyterian Hospital/Weill Cornell Medical Center, New York, New York
Restorative Proctocolectomy with J-Pouch Ileoanal Anastomosis

K. Thomas Moesta, MD, PhD
Head, Department of General and Visceral Surgery, Center for Minimally Invasive Surgery, Siloah Hospital, Hannover, Germany
Laparoscopic Abdominoperineal Resection of the Rectum
Laparoscopic Rectopexy for Rectal Prolapse

A.R. Moossa, MD, FACS, FRCS
Emeritus Chair and Distinguished Professor, Department of Surgery, University of California, San Diego School of Medicine, San Diego, California
Total Pancreatectomy

Brendan J. Moran, FRCSI, MCh, FRCS
Consultant Colorectal Surgeon, Colorectal Department, Basingstoke and North Hampshire NHS Foundation Trust, Basingstoke, Hampshire, United Kingdom
Total Mesorectal Excision with Colonic J-Pouch Coloanal Reconstruction for Rectal Cancer

Yoshihiro Moriya, MD
Colorectal Surgery Division, Japanese Red Cross Medical Center, Tokyo, Japan
Total Pelvic Exenteration with Distal Sacrectomy for Fixed Locally Recurrent Rectal Cancer
Pelvic Exenteration: Total/Anterior/Posterior

Alexander P. Nagle, MD, FACS
Associate Professor, Department of Surgery, Northwestern University, Chicago, Illinois
Laparoscopic Ventral Hernia Repair
Laparoscopic Transabdominal Preperitoneal Repair of Inguinofemoral Hernia

Calvin S.H. Ng, BSc(Hon), MBBS(Hon)(Lond), MD(Res), FRCSEd(CTh)
Associate Consultant, Department of Cardiothoracic Surgery, Prince of Wales Hospital; Clinical Associate Professor, Department of Cardiothoracic Surgery, The Chinese University of Hong Kong, Shatin, Hong Kong
Videothoracoscopic Thymectomy

†Deceased

Manish Parikh, MD
Assistant Professor of Surgery, Director of Bariatric and Minimally Invasive Surgery, Bellevue Hospital Center, New York University School of Medicine, New York, New York
Laparoscopic Gastric Sleeve Resection with Duodenal Switch
Laparoscopic Nissen Fundoplication

Adrian E. Park, MD, FRCSC, FACS, FCS (ECSA)
Chairman, Department of Surgery, Anne Arundel Medical Center, Annapolis, Maryland
Laparoscopic Pancreatic Pseudocyst Drainage

John H. Pemberton, MD
Professor of Surgery, Mayo Clinic College of Medicine; Consultant, Colon and Rectal Surgery, Mayo Clinic, Rochester, Minnesota
Laparoscopic Colon Resection (Right, Left, Sigmoid)

Arjun Pennathur, MD, FACS
Assistant Professor, Department of Cardiothoracic Surgery, University of Pittsburgh, Pittsburgh, Pennsylvania
Transthoracic Fundoplication: Belsey Fundoplication

Alberto Peracchia, MD, FACS
Emeritus Professor, Department of Surgery, University of Milan; Senior Consultant, General and Minimally Invasive Surgery, Istituto Clinico Humanitas IRCCS, Rozzano (Milan), Milan, Italy
Transhiatal Esophagectomy via Laparoscopy and Transmediastinal Endodissection
Laparoscopic Approach for Achalasia and Epiphrenic Diverticulum

Jean Yves Petit, MD
Department of Plastic and Reconstructive Surgery, European Institute of Oncology, Milan, Italy
Nipple- and Areola-Sparing Mastectomy

Bertram Poch, MD
Assistant Professor and Head, Centre of Oncological, Endocrine, and Minimally Invasive Surgery, Neu-Ulm, Germany
Beger and Frey Procedure for Chronic Pancreatitis

Claire Pomeroy, MD, MBA
Vice Chancellor for Human Health Sciences, Dean, School of Medicine, University of California, Davis, Sacramento, California
Foreword

Irinel Popescu, MD
Professor of General Surgery, University of Medicine and Pharmacy "Carol Davila"; Department Head, General Surgery and Liver Transplantation, Fundeni Clinical Institute, Bucharest, Romania
Central Pancreatectomy
Extended Pancreatectomy with Resection of the Celiac Axis (Appleby Operation)

Zeno I. Popovici, MD, PhD
Professor and Doctorship Coordinator in Surgery, First Department of Surgery; Medical Science Academy (ASM), Department of Surgery, University of "Lucian Blaga"; ISDE Federation Governor of East Europe, Surgery, Sibiu, Romania
Esophageal Reconstruction with Colonic Interposition

Pedro T. Ramirez, MD
Professor, Department of Gynecologic Oncology and Reproductive Medicine, The University of Texas MD Anderson Cancer Center, Houston, Texas
Surgical Management of Ovarian Cancer

Francesco Raspagliesi, MD
Director, Gynaecologic Oncology Unit, Department of Surgery, Fondazione IRCCS Istituto Nazionale Tumori, Milan, Italy
Nerve-Sparing Radical Abdominal Hysterectomy with Regional Lymphadenectomy
Radical Vulvectomy with Groin Dissection

Mark S. Roh, MD, MMM
Chair, Department of Surgery, MD Anderson Cancer Center Orlando, Orlando, Florida
Mesohepatectomy

Riccardo Rosati, MD, FACS
Head, General and Minimally Invasive Surgery, Istituto Clinico Humanitas IRCCS, Rozzano (Milan); Professor of Surgery, Translational Medicine, University of Milan, Milan, Italy
Transhiatal Esophagectomy via Laparoscopy and Transmediastinal Endodissection
Laparoscopic Approach for Achalasia and Epiphrenic Diverticulum

Ernest L. Rosato, MD
Chief, Division of General Surgery, Thomas Jefferson University, Philadelphia, Pennsylvania
Pancreaticoduodenectomy with or without Distal Gastrectomy and Radical Lymphadenectomy

Jack A. Roth, MD
Professor, Department of Thoracic and Cardiovascular Surgery, The University of Texas MD Anderson Cancer Center, Houston, Texas
Resection of Pulmonary Metastases

Keiji Sano, MD
Professor, Department of Surgery, Teikyo University School of Medicine, Tokyo, Japan
Radical Cholecystectomy/Liver Bed Resection with Regional Lymph Node Dissection

Mitsuru Sasako, MD, PhD
Professor and Chairman, Department of Surgery, Division of Upper Gastrointestinal Surgery, Hyogo College of Medicine, Nishinomiya, Japan
Total Gastrectomy with D2 Lymph Node Dissection

Olivier Scatton, MD, PhD
Professor of Surgery, Department of Hepatobiliary Surgery and Liver Transplantation, Université Pierre et Marie Curie, Assistance Publique–Hôpitaux de Paris, Paris, France
Right and Left Trisectionectomies

Richard L. Scher, MD, FACS
Professor and Associate Chief, Otolaryngology–Head and Neck Surgery, Associate Vice Chair for Ambulatory Services, Department of Surgery, Duke University Health System, Durham, North Carolina
Operative Approach to Zenker Diverticulum

Schlomo Schneebaum, MD
Head, Radio Guided Surgery Unit, Head, Breast Health Center, Department of Surgery, Tel Aviv Sourasky Medical Center; Associate Professor of Surgery, Sackler Faculty of Medicine, Tel Aviv University, Tel Aviv, Israel
Popliteal Lymph Node Dissection
Radical Axillary Dissection

Leo J. Schultze Kool, MD, PhD
Professor of Interventional Radiology, Department of Radiology, Radboud University Nijmegen Medical Center, Nijmegen, The Netherlands
Endovascular Repair of Abdominal Aortic Aneurysms

Ashok R. Shaha, MD, FACS
Jatin P. Shah Chair in Head and Neck Surgery, Head and Neck Service, Memorial Sloan-Kettering Cancer Center; Professor of Surgery, Department of Surgery, Weill Cornell Medical College, New York, New York
Modified Neck Dissection
Superficial Parotidectomy

Sandesh Kumar Sharma, MS
IASG Fellow and Assistant Professor, Department of Surgical Gastroenterology, Bhopal Memorial Hospital and Research Centre, Bhopal, Madhya Pradesh, India
Pancreaticoduodenectomy with Superior Mesentericoportal Venous Resection

Manisha Shende, MBBS, MS, FACS
Assistant Professor, Department of Cardiothoracic Surgery, University of Pittsburgh, Pittsburgh, Pennsylvania
Laparothoracoscopic Esophagectomy

Norio Shiraishi, MD, PhD
Professor, Surgical Division, Center for Community Medicine, Oita University Faculty of Medicine, Yufu-city, Oita, Japan
Laparoscopy-Assisted Distal Gastrectomy with Lymphadenectomy

Rebecca S. Sippel, MD, FACS
Associate Professor; Chief of Endocrine Surgery, Department of Surgery, University of Wisconsin, Madison, Wisconsin
Total Thyroidectomy with Central Neck Dissection

Donald G. Skinner, MD, FACS
Emeritus Professor and Chairman, Department of Urology, Keck School of Medicine of the University of Southern California, Los Angeles, California
Radical Cystectomy

Helen J. Sohn, MD
Department of Surgery, Sharp Grossmont Hospital, La Mesa, California
Laparoscopic Paraesophageal Hernia Repair

Mark S. Soloway, MD
Professor and Chairman Emeritus, Department of Urology, Miller School of Medicine, University of Miami, Miami, Florida
Radical Nephrectomy with Inferior Vena Cava Tumor Thrombectomy

Nathaniel J. Soper, MD
Loyal and Edith Davis Professor and Chair, Department of Surgery, Northwestern University Feinberg School of Medicine; Surgeon-in-Chief, Northwestern Memorial Hospital, Chicago, Illinois
Laparoscopic Ventral Hernia Repair
Laparoscopic Transabdominal Preperitoneal Repair of Inguinofemoral Hernia

Lorenzo Spaggiari, MD, PhD
Director, Department of Thoracic Surgery, European Institute of Oncology; Professor, Department of Thoracic Surgery, University of Milan, Milan, Italy
Radical Pneumonectomy

†John P. Stein, MD, FACS
Professor, Department of Urology, Keck School of Medicine of the University of Southern California, Los Angeles, California
Radical Cystectomy

†Deceased

[†]René Stoppa, MD, PhD, FACS
Professor Emeritus, Faculty of Medicine, University of Picardy–Jules Verne, Amiens, Picardy, France
Preperitoneal Repair of Recurrent Hernia with Giant Prosthesis (Stoppa Repair)

Paul H. Sugarbaker, MD, FACS, FRCS
Section Director, Program in Peritoneal Surface Malignancy, MedStar Washington Hospital Center, Washington, District of Columbia
Surgical Procedures for Peritoneal Surface Malignancy
Tikhoff-Linberg Procedure and Modifications for Shoulder Girdle Resections
Abdominoinguinal Incision for Resection of Pelvic Tumors

Guido Torzilli, MD, PhD
Director, Liver Surgery Unit, Department of Surgery, Istituto Clinico Humanitas IRCCS–Humanitas Cancer Center Rozzano–Milano; Associate Professor of Surgery, Department of Translational Medicine, School of Medicine, University of Milan, Milan, Italy
Liver Segmentectomies

Jacqueline Y. Tracey, MD, FACS
Attending Surgeon, Department of Surgery, Florida Medical Clinic, Tampa, Florida
Total Pancreatectomy

Keisuke Uehara, MD
Assistant Professor, Division of Surgical Oncology, Department of Surgery, Nagoya University Graduate School of Medicine, Nagoya, Japan
Total Pelvic Exenteration with Distal Sacrectomy for Fixed Locally Recurrent Rectal Cancer

Pierre Verhaeghe, MD, PhD, FACS
Digestive and Metabolic Surgery, Centre Hospitalier Universitaire d'Amiens; Faculty of Medicine, University of Picardy–Jules Verne, Amiens, Picardy, France
Preperitoneal Repair of Recurrent Hernia with Giant Prosthesis (Stoppa Repair)

Theo Wobbes, MD, PhD
Professor, Department of Surgery, Division of Surgical Oncology, Radboud University Medical Center, Nijmegen, The Netherlands
Radical Superficial and Deep Groin Dissection
Composite Axillary and Supraclavicular Lymph Node Dissection

Randall K. Wolf, MD, FACS, FACC
Co-Director, International Atrial Fibrillation Center, Department of Cardiothoracic Surgery, The Indiana Heart Hospital, Indianapolis, Indiana
Thoracoscopic First Rib Resection for Thoracic Outlet Syndrome

[†]Deceased

Jean-Paul Wolinsky, MD
Associate Professor and Clinical Director, Johns Hopkins Spine Program, Department of Neurosurgery, Johns Hopkins University School of Medicine, Baltimore, Maryland
Total and Subtotal Sacrectomy for En Bloc Resections of Primary Tumors of the Sacrum

Jason T. Wong, MD, FRCSC
South Orange County Surgical Medical Group, Inc., Laguna Hills, California
Laparoscopic Common Bile Duct Exploration

Tristan D. Yan, BSc(Med), MBBS, MS, MD, PhD
The Baird Institute and Department of Cardiothoracic Surgery, Royal Prince Alfred Hospital, Sydney, Australia
Abdominoinguinal Incision for Resection of Pelvic Tumors

Charles J. Yeo, MD
Samuel D. Gross Professor and Chair, Department of Surgery, Thomas Jefferson University, Philadelphia, Pennsylvania
Pancreaticoduodenectomy with or without Distal Gastrectomy and Radical Lymphadenectomy

Anthony P.C. Yim, MD, FRCS, FACS
Honorary Professor, Division of Cardiothoracic Surgery, The Chinese University of Hong Kong, Shatin, Hong Kong
Lung Volume Reduction Surgery
Videothoracoscopic Thymectomy

Claudio Zanon, MD
Chief, Oncological Surgery Division, Department of Surgery, San Giovanni Battista Hospital, Torino, Italy
Insertion of the Denver Peritoneovenous Shunt

Christopher K. Zarins, MD
Chidester Professor Emeritus, Department of Surgery, Stanford University, Stanford, California
Carotid Endarterectomy/Stent Placement
Axillofemoral Bypass
Renal Artery Revascularization
Celiac and Mesenteric Artery Revascularization

Ricardo Zorron, MD, MSC, PhD
Professor of Surgery and Director, Innovative Surgery Division, Klinikum Bremerhaven Reinkenheide, Bremerhaven, Germany
Natural Orifice Transluminal Endoscopic Cholecystectomy

Foreword

The *Atlas of Advanced Operative Surgery,* edited by Vijay Khatri, MBChB, FACS, is an exciting, comprehensive resource for practical guidance on complex surgical techniques as well as on handling challenges that may arise during more common procedures. Its easily accessible format is optimal for busy surgeons at all levels of experience. The content will be of great interest to surgeons in their senior years of training, yet advanced enough to serve as a useful resource to experienced general surgeons.

This book offers 100 chapters on general and specialty surgeries, including head and neck, thoracic, abdominal, urologic, gynecologic, endocrine, soft tissue, bone, and vascular operations. The standardized format of the chapters is well designed, allowing for efficiently finding critical information. Each chapter features a specific operation and provides clear, step-by-step bulleted guidance on preoperative preparation, incision, exposure and operative technique, closure, and postoperative care.

Accompanying the text is a wealth of color images that provides instant clarity to the points made in the text, including clinical imaging studies (often comparing normal and abnormal diagnostic images), illustrations highlighting the anatomy of interest, and close-up photographs of the operative field.

The *Atlas of Advanced Operative Surgery* follows Dr. Khatri's *Operative Surgery Manual*, an enormously popular one-stop reference for students and residents since it was published. Expanding on the *Manual* by covering more advanced surgeries, the *Atlas* retains the same concise, clear style that has facilitated rapid acquisition of detailed information.

Dr. Khatri has taken great care to select contributors who are leading international experts in their specialty. Each chapter provides pearls from their experience in the operating room, including pros and cons of alternative technical approaches, the use of new specialty devices, and frequently encountered anatomic variations.

In a time when surgical techniques are rapidly advancing, the book emphasizes cutting-edge methods, including accessing the surgical target via a natural orifice and using laparoscopic procedures if applicable. More than a third of the procedures described use minimally invasive techniques.

This book automatically provides the reader with access to the online service, Expert Consult. There, the entire content of the *Atlas* is available from any computer with access to the Internet, offering full-search functionality and downloadable images to facilitate teaching.

Dr. Khatri is an active surgeon and teacher with more than 20 years of surgical experience. In his practice, he manages a broad spectrum of cancers and has special interests in complex soft tissue sarcoma, rectal carcinoma, melanoma, and primary and metastatic liver cancers. He also is a researcher, currently investigating the role of radiofrequency ablation for early breast cancer and colorectal liver metastases.

It is my great pleasure to be a colleague of Dr. Khatri's for nearly 10 years. He is a true exemplar of a surgeon who provides the highest quality of patient care. His commitment to excellence, both in the operating room and in disseminating his expertise to new surgeons, is indeed evident throughout this *Atlas*.

Claire Pomeroy, MD, MBA
Vice Chancellor for Human Health Sciences, Dean, School of Medicine,
University of California, Davis, Sacramento, California

Foreword

The field of surgery is rapidly changing. As I often tell medical students and residents, more than half of what I do now did not exist when I finished my surgical training. The same is true for many practicing surgeons. Laparoscopic duodeno-pancreatectomies, proctocolectomies, intraoperative ultrasound guided tumor resections, and radiofrequency ablation of hepatic metastases are all examples of rapidly changing advances in surgery.

The *Atlas of Advanced Operative Surgery* is a logical and necessary continuation of *Operative Surgery Manual*, an excellent guidebook for the journeyman surgeon. With this new atlas, Dr. Khatri and his colleagues extend their reach to provide a reference for experienced surgeons on the advanced procedures in use today.

Dr. Khatri's experience on both sides of the Atlantic as a surgeon and a teacher, and the experience of his international team of expert surgeons and contributors, results in a truly useful surgical guide that has global reach. As complex surgical procedures increasingly find their way to all corners of the world, this excellent, clear, and concise atlas continues to serve as a valued companion.

Diana Farmer, MD, FACS, FRCS
Pearl Stamps Stewart Professor and Chair, Chair, Department of Surgery,
UC Davis School of Medicine; Surgeon-in-Chief, UC Davis Children's Hospital,
UC Davis Health System, Davis, California

Preface

"I do the very best I know how, the very best I can, and I mean to keep doing so until the end."

Abraham Lincoln

As we as surgeons prepare to wield the scapel, Metzebaum scissors, cautery, or any of the vast array of energy devices, let us not forget the enormous responsibility bestowed upon our shoulders; the profound trust conferred in us alone is, in itself, deserving of no less than our very best.

Arriving at this moment has been a long journey, enriched by the opportunity to work with numerous talented individuals and concluding with a product that we hope the readers will find a valuable reference. As always, the inspiration for such an endeavor was derived from the enthusiasm of countless medical students, residents, fellows, and junior faculty. The constant contact with surgeons at various trajectories in their training or practice provided a unique perspective in understanding the need for such a reference book.

This atlas was developed as a natural follow-up to *Operative Surgery Manual,* also published by Elsevier, which was written to serve as an easy reference for medical students during their surgical rotation and junior surgical residents as they learn the essential surgical procedures. During their senior years in training, surgical residents are exposed to a higher level of sophisticated surgical procedures. Senior and chief residents often must refer to several atlases covering various subspecialties to obtain information regarding these high-index operative cases; hence the need to develop a book that consolidates some of these operative procedures under one title.

This atlas is divided into the major components of general surgery and other surgical specialties. Not surprisingly, with increasing application of laparoscopic approaches to various operative procedures, well over a third of the content deals with minimally invasive techniques. We also included the concept of natural orifice transluminal endoscopic surgery. Some of the techniques covered in this book are primarily undertaken in a tertiary center; thus community surgeons might not perform them. Nevertheless, these chapters will be valuable to junior faculty in academic institutions.

Each chapter is formatted using a simple but effective outline that includes the subheadings Position, Incision, Main Dissection, and Closure. Maintaining this consistent format allows the reader to browse the chapters with ease and develop a methodical approach to performing the operative procedure. Where relevant, the chapters are accompanied by computed tomography or magnetic resonance imaging scans or angiograms that help the reader understand the importance of imaging studies in preparation for the advanced operative procedure. At the end of each chapter, specific complications are outlined in a bulleted format, aiding the reader's awareness of them and facilitating discussions with patients.

In preparing the content for this book, we solicited contributions from leading national and international authorities based in the United States, Europe, Asia, South America, and Australia to provide a truly global perspective. I would like to express my appreciation to all the contributors for their quality submissions, and to Rob Flewell for his outstanding color illustrations and the ability to edit them in real time with the use of the latest digital technology in graphics and communication. Scott Scheidt, Jean Nevius, Kristine Oberle, Roxanne Ward, and Rebecca Gruliow are the dedicated content development professionals, and Louise King, the project manager, whose tireless efforts aided in completing this atlas. Thanks is also extended to Peggy Firth for her contributions to the illustrations in the book. It was a remarkable feat. I am indebted to Judith Fletcher, publishing director, and her successor, Mary Gatsch, as well as Michael Houston, publishing manager, for their unrelenting support through the undulating journey undertaken in producing this atlas. My sincere gratitude is also extended to Dean Pomeroy and Dr. Farmer for graciously providing the forewords to this edition. Finally, none of this would have been possible without the support of my family as we strive to balance the various responsibilities of an academic life and a personal life.

Vijay P. Khatri, MBChB, FACS

Contents

SECTION I

Head and Neck

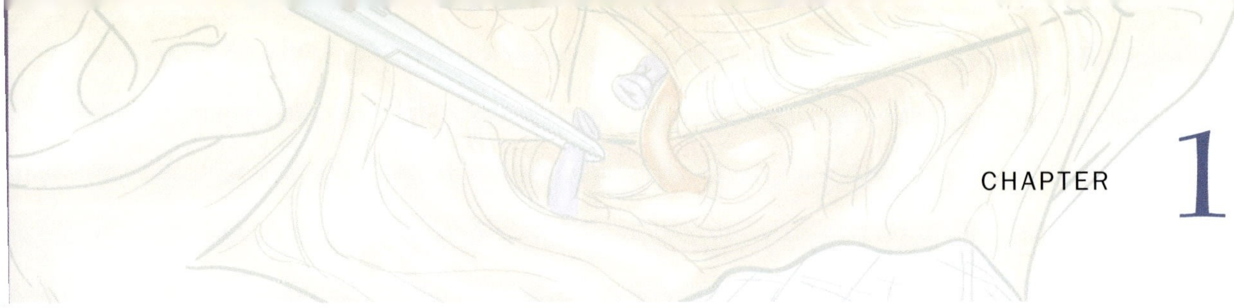

CHAPTER 1

Radical Neck Dissection

Jesus E. Medina, MD, FACS

Background and History

- The first description of a systematic en bloc removal of the lymphatics of the neck was published by Crile in 1906. The operation he described has come to be known as the radical neck dissection. Even though the radical neck dissection, as it is conceptualized today, removes the lymph node–bearing tissues of one side of the neck in conjunction with the sternocleidomastoid muscle, the internal jugular vein, and the spinal accessory nerve, the drawings that illustrate Crile's publication depict the spinal accessory nerve and the ansa hypoglossi being preserved.
- Removal of the spinal accessory nerve during cervical lymphadenectomy was actually advocated by Blair and Brown in 1933. These surgeons believed that removal of the nerve decreased operating time and, more important, ensured complete removal of the cervical lymph nodes. The latter concept was championed and popularized in the 1950s by Martin, whom I quote: "Any technique that is designed to preserve the spinal accessory nerve should be condemned unequivocally." Because of Martin's influence, the radical neck dissection was considered for many years the only acceptable operation for the treatment of the neck in patients with cancer.
- Currently, head and neck surgeons throughout the world use a number of different cervical lymph node dissections for the surgical treatment of the neck in patients with cancer of the head and neck region. The purpose of this chapter is to present a description of the radical neck dissections and an outline of the current indications for this operation.

I. SPECIAL PREOPERATIVE PREPARATION

- The radical neck dissection consists of the removal of the lymph node–bearing tissues of one side of the neck, from the inferior border of the mandible to the clavicle and from the lateral border of the strap muscles to the anterior border of the trapezius, including in the resection the spinal accessory nerve, the internal jugular vein, and the sternocleidomastoid muscle.

Indications

- This operation is indicated in the following situations:
  - ▲ When there are multiple palpable cervical lymph node metastases, particularly when they involve the lymph nodes of the posterior triangle of the neck and are located in close proximity to the spinal accessory nerve;
  - ▲ When there is a large metastatic tumor mass or there are multiple matted nodes in the upper portion of the neck;
  - ▲ When an ill-advised open incisional biopsy of a neck node has been performed. In some cases, a radical neck dissection is performed because extensive undermining and postoperative inflammation, scarring, or tumor dissemination obscure the relationship of the tumor to structures that may have been preserved otherwise.
- It must be emphasized that it is not currently warranted to perform a radical neck dissection in the absence of palpable cervical metastases (i.e., in the treatment of the N0 neck).

II. OPERATIVE TECHNIQUE

Position

- The patient is placed in the supine position. The operating table is usually rotated 90 degrees with the side to be operated on opposite the anesthesia machine. In some instances the table is rotated 180 degrees. In either case, a small shoulder roll is placed under the patient and the head is rotated toward the side opposite to the dissection.

Incision

- The incisions most commonly used to perform a radical neck dissection are shown in Figure 1-1. Skin flaps are usually developed by sharp dissection in a subplatysmal plane. However, if a large tumor mass is present, it may be advisable to leave the platysma attached to it as the skin flaps are elevated.

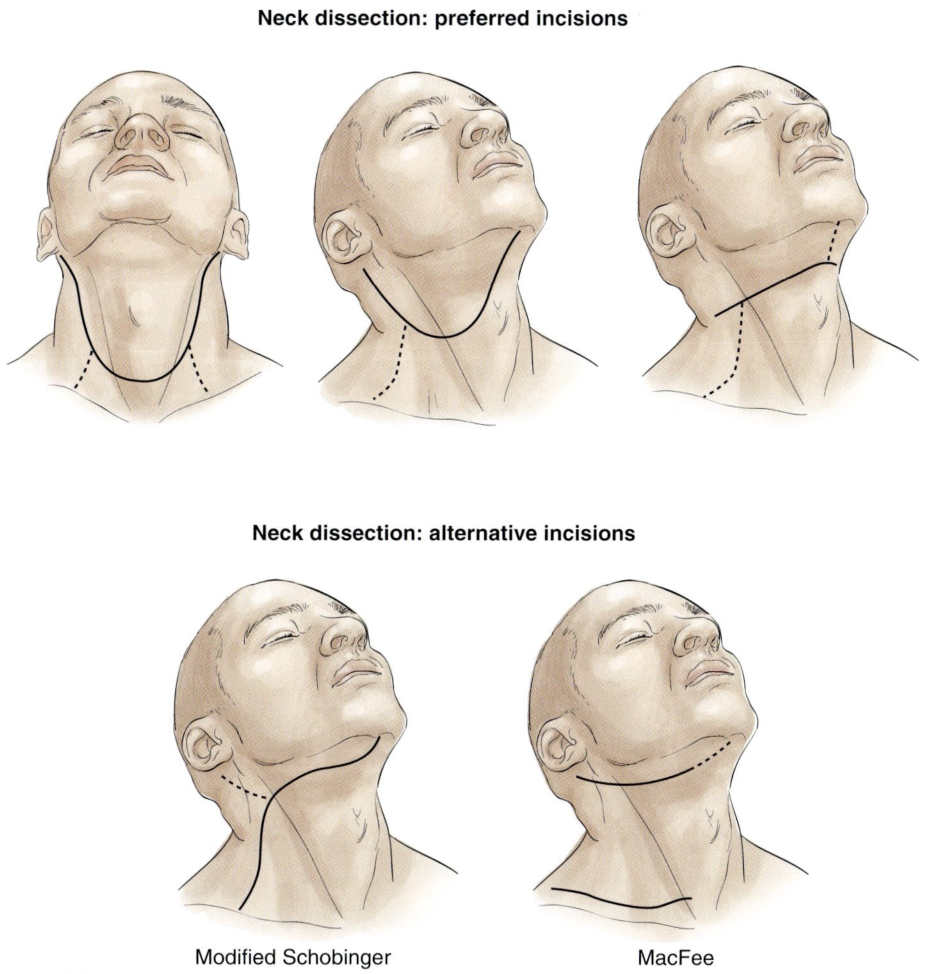

Figure 1-1.

Main Dissection

- As the superior neck flap is elevated, the ramus mandibularis is exposed and preserved if possible (Fig. 1-2).
- The submandibular prevascular and retrovascular lymph nodes, which are usually in close proximity to the nerve, are carefully dissected away from the nerve. In doing so, the facial vessels are exposed and divided (see Fig. 1-2).
- The fibrous fatty tissue of the submental triangle is dissected off the anterior bellies of the digastric muscles and the mylohyoid. The fascia is then dissected off the anterior belly of the digastric muscle and the specimen is retracted posteriorly, removing the fibrous fatty tissue containing lymph nodes lateral to the mylohyoid muscle. When the dissection reaches the posterior border of the mylohyoid, this is retracted anteriorly, exposing the lingual nerve and the submandibular gland duct, which are divided. The hypoglossal nerve and the veins that usually accompany the nerve are left undisturbed as the dissection continues in a posterior direction. Finally, the facial artery is ligated as it crosses forward, under the posterior belly of the digastric muscle (see Fig. 1-2).
- The tail of the parotid gland is transected, and the posterior facial vein and the greater auricular nerve are divided. The sternocleidomastoid muscle is then incised close to its insertion in the mastoid process. The fibrofatty tissue medial to the muscle is incised, exposing the splenius capitis and the levator scapulae muscles. Depending on the location and the extent of the tumor in the neck, it may be necessary to include the posterior belly of the digastric muscle in the dissected specimen. Otherwise, incising the fascia below the digastric muscle and gentle inferior traction of the specimen allows identification of the hypoglossal nerve, the upper end of the internal jugular vein, and the spinal accessory nerve. At this point in the dissection, the internal jugular vein and the spinal accessory nerve are divided if the location and extent of the tumor permit it (Figs. 1-3 and 1-4).

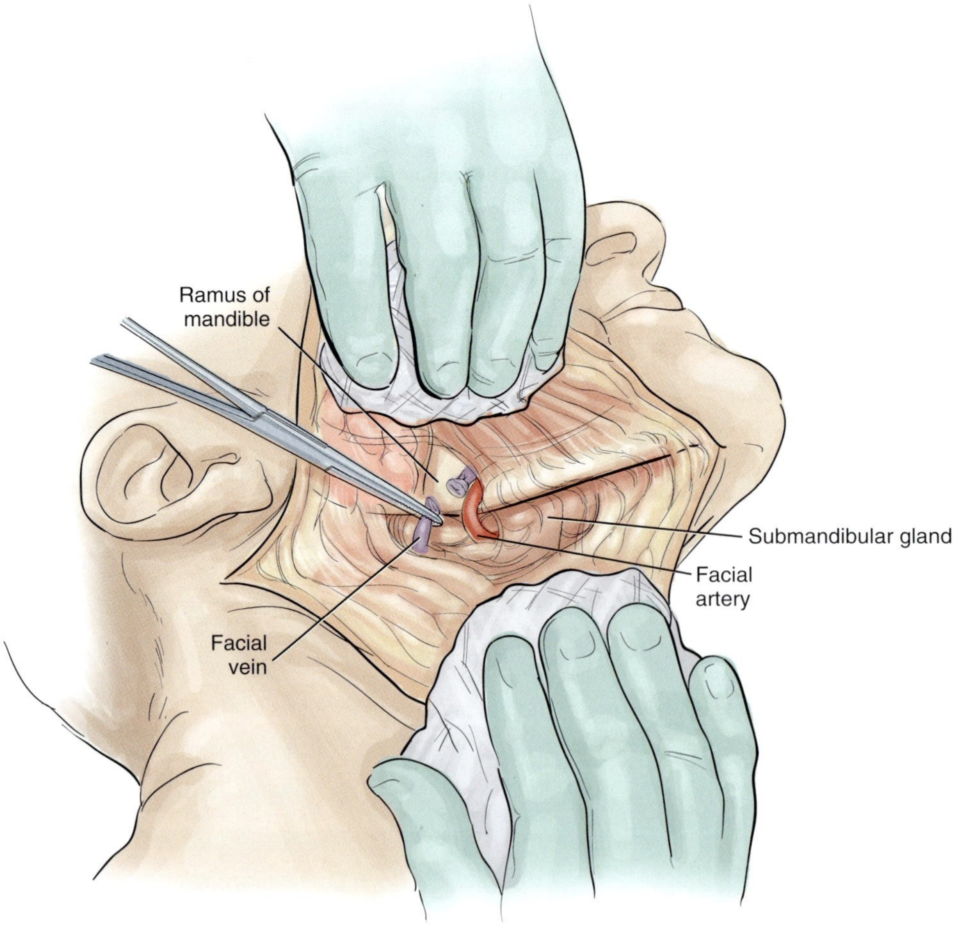

Figure 1-2.

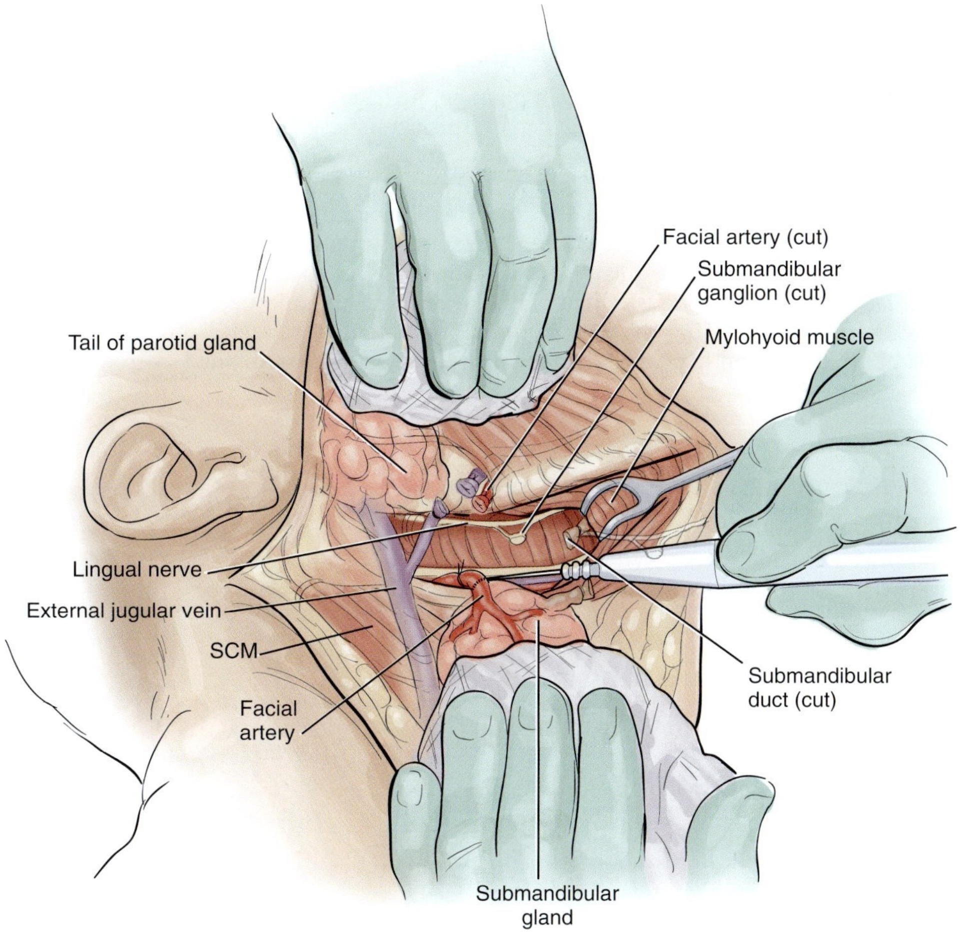

Figure 1-3. *SCM*, Sternocleidomastoid.

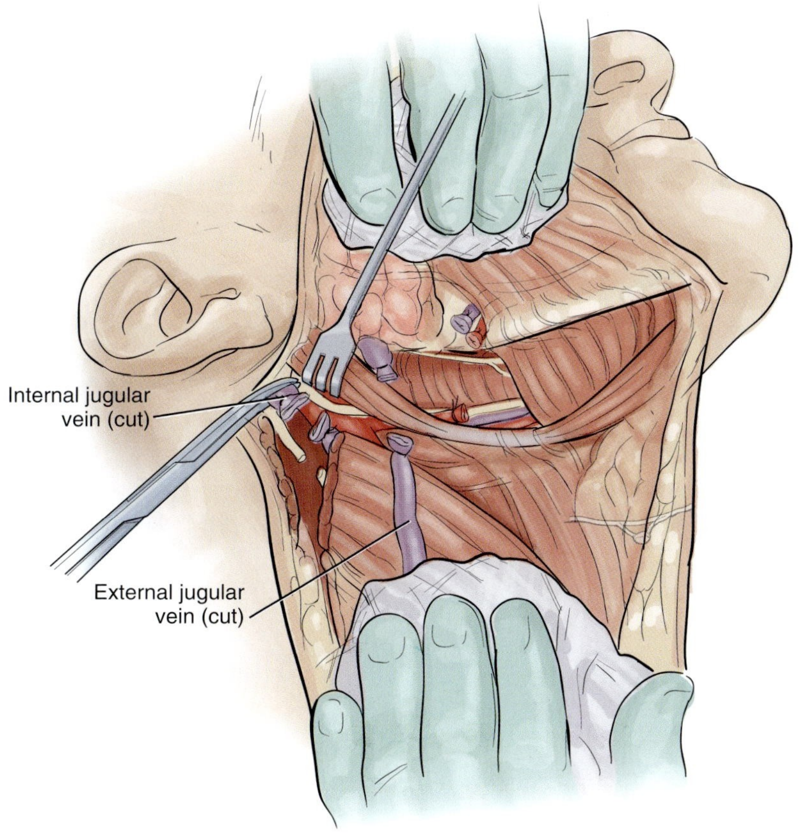

Figure 1-4.

- The dissection is continued posteriorly and inferiorly along the anterior border of the trapezius muscle. The spinal accessory nerve and the transverse cervical vessels are divided as they cross the anterior border of the trapezius muscle (Fig. 1-5). The fibrofatty tissue of the posterior triangle of the neck is then dissected forward and downward in a plane immediately lateral to the fascia of the splenius and the levator scapulae muscles. During this step of the operation, it is important to preserve the branches of the cervical plexus that innervate the levator scapulae muscle, unless the extent of the disease in the neck precludes it.
- The sternocleidomastoid muscle and the superficial layer of the deep cervical fascia are incised above the superior border of the clavicle. The external jugular vein and the omohyoid muscle are divided. The fibrofatty tissue in this region is then gently pushed in an upward direction, exposing the brachial plexus, the scalenus anticus muscle, and the phrenic nerve (Fig. 1-6). Posteriorly, the dissection is continued to join the previous dissection along the anterior border of the trapezius. In this area of the neck, multiple veins must be diligently ligated and divided.

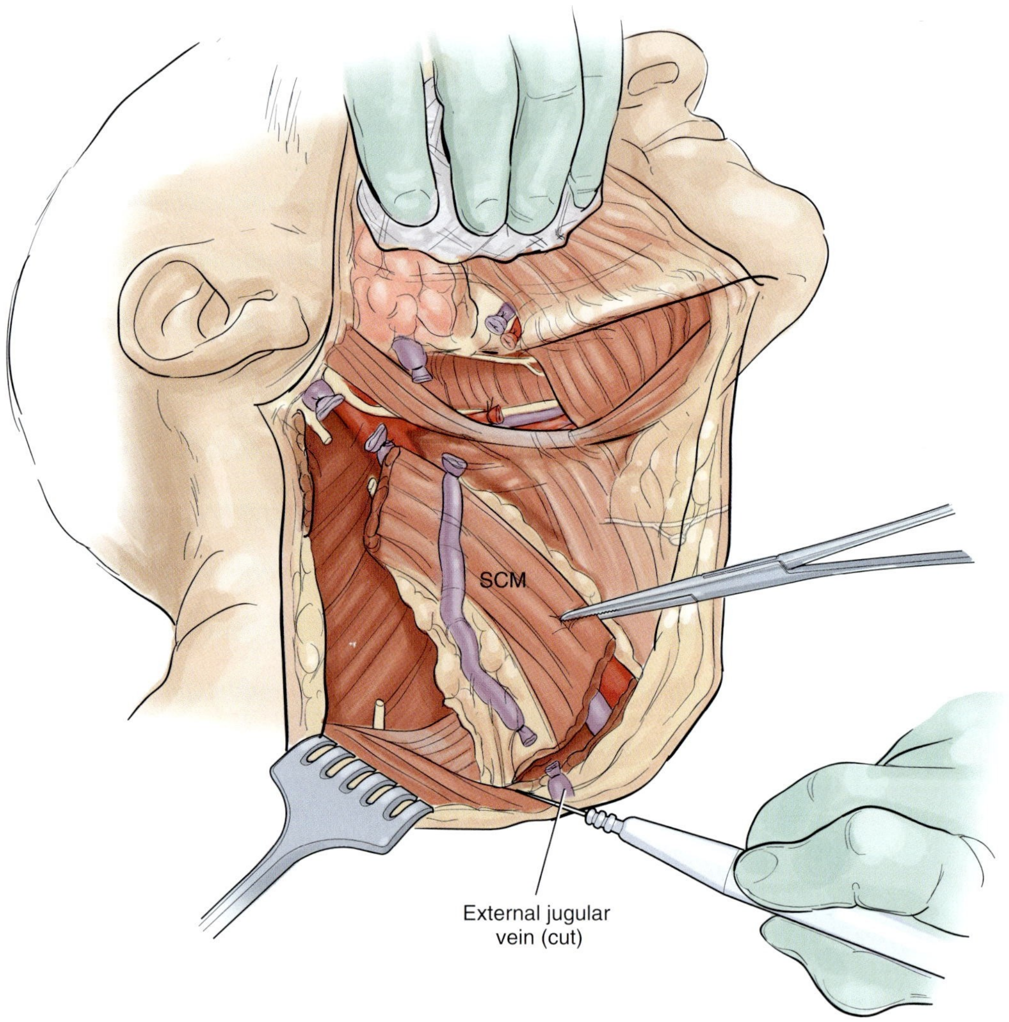

Figure 1-5. *SCM*, Sternocleidomastoid.

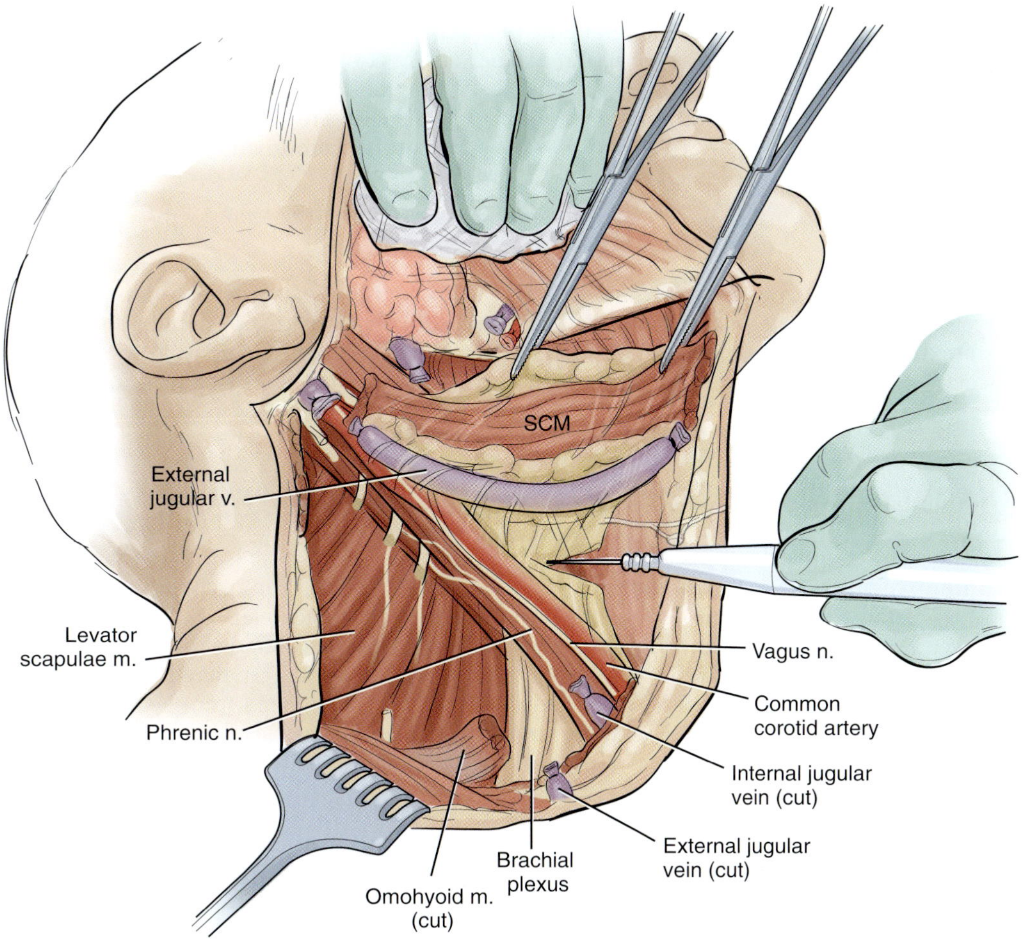

Figure 1-6. *SCM*, Sternocleidomastoid.

- The dissection is then carried forward as the specimen is dissected off of the scalenus medius, the brachial plexus, and the scalenus anticus. At this point, the cutaneous branches of the cervical plexus are exposed and divided. Once this is done, care must be taken as the dissection is continued medially because there is only a relatively thin layer of tissue that needs to be incised to expose the vagus nerve, the common carotid artery, and the internal jugular vein. Inferiorly, the phrenic nerve must be identified and protected. This is best done by conducting the dissection in a plane that is superficial to the fascia of the scalenus anticus muscle. In this area of the neck, the surgeon must also deal with the thoracic duct, which arches downward and forward from behind the common carotid to open into the internal jugular vein, the subclavian vein, or the angle formed by the junction of these two vessels. In its short course through this region of the neck, the duct is located anterior or superficial to the anterior scalene muscle and the phrenic nerve. To prevent a chyle leak, the surgeon must also remember that the thoracic duct may be multiple in its upper end and that at the base of the neck it usually receives a jugular, a subclavian, and perhaps other minor lymphatic trunks, which must be individually ligated or clipped.
- The internal jugular vein can be divided either superiorly or inferiorly, depending on the location of the disease in the neck. If the tumor mass is located low in the jugulodigastric region or in the midjugular region, the internal jugular vein is first ligated and divided superiorly. The dissection then continues in an inferior direction, separating the specimen from the vagus nerve, the carotid artery, and the superior thyroid vessels. The medial limit of the dissection is marked by the strap muscles. If, on the other hand, the disease is located high in the jugulodigastric region, the internal jugular vein is divided inferiorly, and the dissection is carried in a superior direction along the common carotid artery. This is especially useful when the tumor is extensive and may require removal of the external carotid artery or the hypoglossal nerve. Mobilization of the surgical specimen from below allows easier dissection from the internal carotid artery and, if possible, the external carotid and the hypoglossal nerve.

Closure

- The completed dissection is shown in Figure 1-7. The incision is usually closed in two layers: the first layer approximates the platysma anteriorly and the subcutaneous tissue laterally, and the second layer approximates the skin. One or two suction drains are left in place. The drain(s) should not rest immediately over the carotid artery or in the area of the thoracic duct. Bulky or pressure dressings are not necessary.

III. ALTERNATIVE TECHNICAL APPROACHES (PRO/CON) AND PEARLS

- An alternative surgical approach is to begin the dissection inferiorly, ligating the internal jugular vein and proceeding with the dissection in a cephalad direction. This approach is preferred when there is a large volume of tumor in the upper portion of the neck, which can make it difficult to begin the dissection superiorly as described here. In such cases, adequate removal of the tumor may require resection of the external carotid, the hypoglossal nerve, or both. This may be easier and safer if the internal carotid and the vagus nerve have been identified and isolated from below.
- A comprehensive knowledge of anatomy and physiology is necessary to understand the nuances of surgical planning and technique as well as the prevention and management of the sequelae and complications of neck dissection.

IV. SPECIAL POSTOPERATIVE CARE

- The postoperative care following radical neck dissection focuses on ensuring proper functioning of the wound drains to prevent seroma and on early detection and management of sequelae and complications.
- The most notable sequelae observed in patients who have undergone a radical neck dissection are related to removal of the spinal accessory nerve. The resulting denervation of the trapezius muscle causes destabilization of the scapula with progressive flaring at the vertebral border, drooping, and lateral and anterior rotation. The loss of trapezius function decreases the patient's ability to abduct the shoulder above 90 degrees at the shoulder. These physical changes result in a syndrome of pain, weakness, and deformity of the shoulder girdle commonly associated with the radical neck dissection.

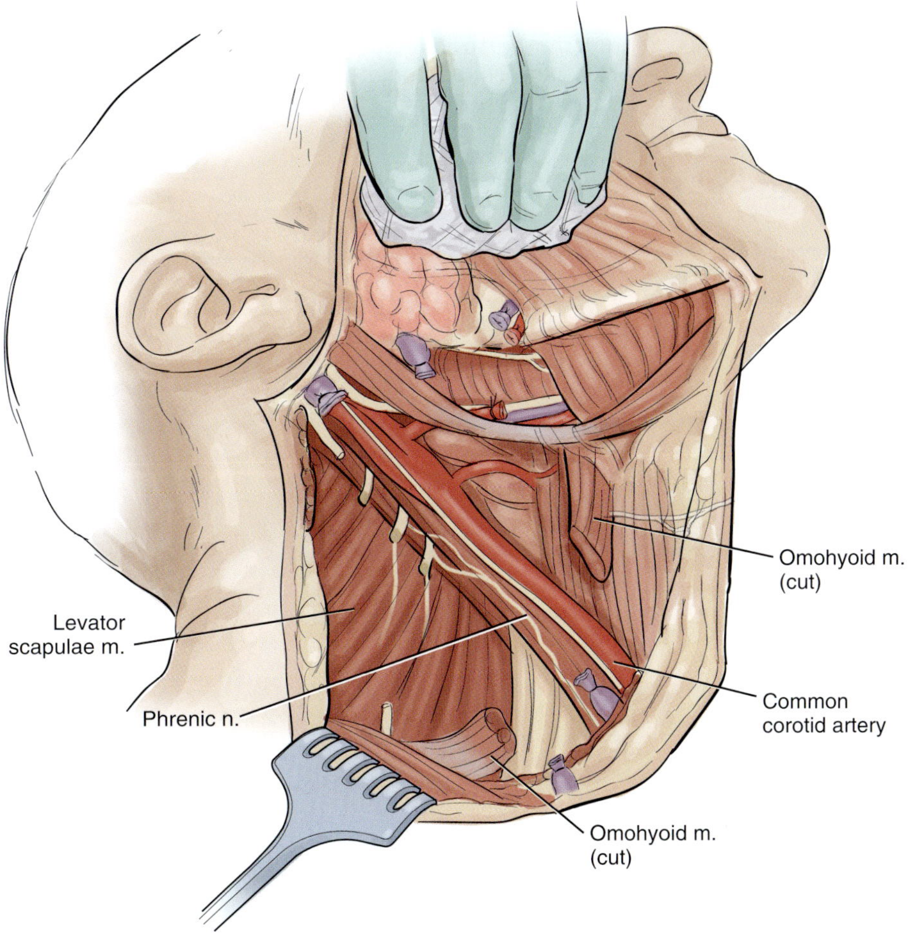
Omohyoid m.
(cut)
Levator
scapulae m.
Phrenic n.
Common
corotid artery
Omohyoid m.
(cut)

Figure 1-7.

- Every patient who undergoes radical neck dissection must be evaluated by a physical therapist early in the postoperative period and should be properly counseled and coached to ensure proper rehabilitation of the shoulder.
- Complications after radical neck dissection include:
  - Infection.
  - Air leaks as a result of improper sealing of the wound or a drain that leads to circulation of air through a wound drain.
  - Postoperative bleeding.
  - Chylous fistula. The reported incidence varies between 1% and 2.5%. Management depends on the time of onset of the fistula, on the amount of chyle drainage in a 24-hour period, and on the presence or absence of accumulation of chyle under the skin flaps. When the daily output of chyle exceeds 600 mL in a day or 200 to 300 mL per day for 3 days, especially when the chyle fistula becomes apparent immediately after surgery, conservative closed wound management is unlikely to succeed, and surgical exploration is indicated.
  - Synchronous bilateral radical neck dissections, in which both internal jugular veins are ligated, can result in the development of facial edema, cerebral edema, or both; blindness; and hypoxia.
  - Carotid artery rupture. The most feared and often lethal complication after neck surgery is exposure and rupture of the carotid artery. Therefore, every effort must be made to prevent it. If the skin incisions have been designed properly, the carotid seldom becomes exposed in the absence of a salivary fistula. If the carotid becomes exposed, it should be covered promptly with well-vascularized tissue.

SUGGESTED READINGS

Blair VP, Brown JP: The treatment of the cancerous or potentially cancerous cervical lymph nodes, *Ann Surg* 98:650–651, 1933.
Crile G: Excision of cancer of the head and neck, *JAMA* 47:1780–1786, 1906.
Martin H, DelValle B, Erhlich H, Cahan WG: Neck dissection, *Cancer* 4:441–449, 1951.

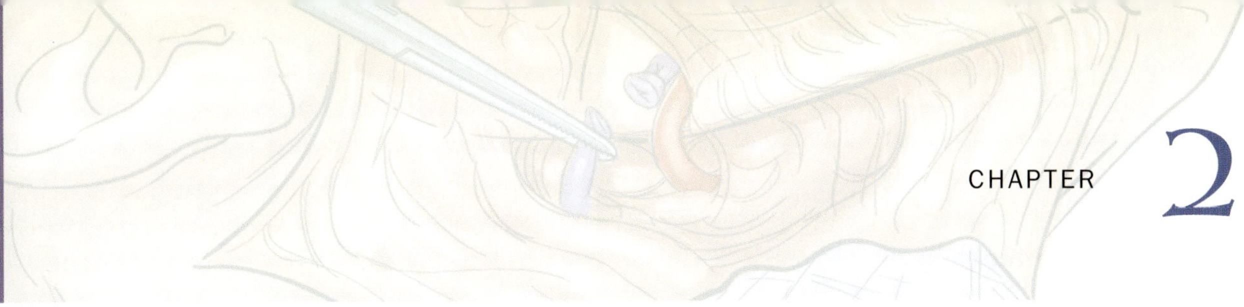

CHAPTER 2

Modified Neck Dissection

Ashok R. Shaha, MD, FACS

Radical neck dissection was considered to be the standard of care for metastatic disease in the neck for almost 75 years. George Crile, Sr., reported an experience of 132 radical neck dissections in *JAMA* in 1906, and since then it has been considered the gold standard for surgical management of metastatic disease in the neck. The concept was a monobloc resection of the metastatic disease along with three important structures in the neck: the sternomastoid muscle, accessory nerve, and jugular vein. For the past quarter century, various surgeons have challenged the philosophy of radical neck dissection, especially sacrifice of the accessory nerve, which leads to considerable functional disability and issues related to quality of life. Understanding of patterns of nodal metastasis has grown, as well as that of the compartment-based orientation of metastatic disease. Oswaldo Suarez from Argentina was the first to popularize functional neck dissection based on facial compartments in the neck and preservation of the accessory nerve. This operation became very popular in Europe in the early 1970s, and subsequently in the United States after 1980. Radical neck dissection is rarely performed today because of shoulder dysfunction and cosmetic considerations.

The major problem with a modified neck dissection is the considerable difficulty in nomenclature and standardization of the surgical technique and extent of neck dissection. The American Academy of Otolaryngology—Head and Neck Surgery has made genuine efforts to standardize the nomenclature and surgical procedure. A variety of modified neck dissections are quite popular; however, modified neck dissection type 1, which preserves the accessory nerve, is described here. A comprehensive neck dissection includes removal of all lymph nodes in the neck with preservation of the accessory nerve, sternomastoid muscle, and jugular vein. Other modified neck dissections include supraomohyoid neck dissection (commonly performed as a staging procedure—elective neck dissection—in patients with cancer of the oral cavity or oropharynx), the jugular neck dissection or anterolateral neck dissection (commonly performed for patients with tumors of the oropharynx and laryngopharyngeal area), and lateral neck dissection (mainly performed for patients presenting with metastatic melanoma or skin cancer posterior to the sternomastoid muscle).

I. SPECIAL PREOPERATIVE PREPARATION

- The exact extent of the disease in the neck should be evaluated with appropriate imaging studies. The common studies are computed tomography scan or magnetic resonance imaging, and a positron emission tomography scan may be of some help in estimating the extent of disease and to rule out other metastatic foci. The extent of disease, the possibility of extranodal spread, and the proximity of the disease to the carotid artery should be evaluated.
- Clinical evaluation is extremely important to ascertain whether the tumor is fixed to the deeper structures and to determine surgical resectability. If the tumor is very close to the accessory nerve, obviously the accessory nerve may need to be sacrificed.
- The elective nodal dissection is performed in patients presenting with no clinically apparent metastatic disease in the neck. The extent of the primary disease should be fully evaluated, and a combined decision should be made regarding treatment of the primary and the neck.
- Shoulder function should be evaluated preoperatively to rule out frozen shoulder or arthritis, which may have a direct relation to postoperative recovery and shoulder function.

II. OPERATIVE TECHNIQUE

Position

- The position is supine in the operating room with a shoulder bolster and a donut to hold the head. The head is turned away from the surgical site, approximately 45 degrees to the midline. This will help expose the posterior region of the neck.
- The neck is prepared as usual with exposure of the ear, which is quite helpful in neck dissection as an anatomical landmark.
- The endotracheal tube is well secured on the other side of the surgical procedure, and the table is positioned in a 15- to 20-degree reverse Trendelenburg position to diminish venous congestion and blood loss. Venodynes are routinely used.

Incision

- For a standard modified neck dissection, even though a variety of incisions are well described, the classic incision used starts from the mastoid process in a curvilinear fashion approximately three finger breadths below the angle of the mandible up to the tip of the hyoid and extending to the midline of the chin (Fig. 2-1).
- A vertical limb is placed behind the carotid artery. The vertical incision is placed in a lazy S fashion to avoid scar contracture in the future.
- The skin is infiltrated with lidocaine and epinephrine to avoid annoying skin bleeding.
- The posterior incision begins from the mastoid process and goes almost to the tip of the hyoid. In the beginning there is no need to extend the incision to the chin area, which is done at a later time.

Main Dissection

- Skin and subcutaneous tissue are incised in the horizontal fashion initially up to the level of the platysma. The vertical incision is then completed as planned. Every attempt should be made to avoid injury to the external jugular vein. After incision of the platysma, the posterior flap is raised until the trapezius can be visualized.
- The dissection continues on the posterior flap, which is quite thin. There is very little platysma in the posterior portion, and every effort should be made to avoid a buttonhole in the skin as the posterior flap is raised.
- After visualizing the trapezius muscle, the anterior flap is raised and the superior flap is raised until the angle of the mandible and the submandibular salivary gland can be seen (Fig. 2-2). The dissection is done here against the platysma to avoid any injury to the ramus mandibularis.
- The inferior flap is raised up to the clavicle. Again, every effort should be made to avoid injury to the external and anterior jugular vein. There is no need to raise the flap beyond the midline.
- The dissection proceeds in the posterior triangle. The greater auricular nerve is transected near the tail of the parotid. There are two different ways to find the accessory nerve near the insertion of the nerve in the anterior border of the trapezius. A gentle dissection should be done anterior to the trapezius, where the nerve can be found in the posterior triangle against the fibrofatty tissue. There are multiple small venous channels that may cause bleeding in this region. Alternatively, the nerve may be found 1 cm above the exit of the greater auricular nerve in the posterior portion of the sternomastoid muscle (Fig. 2-3).

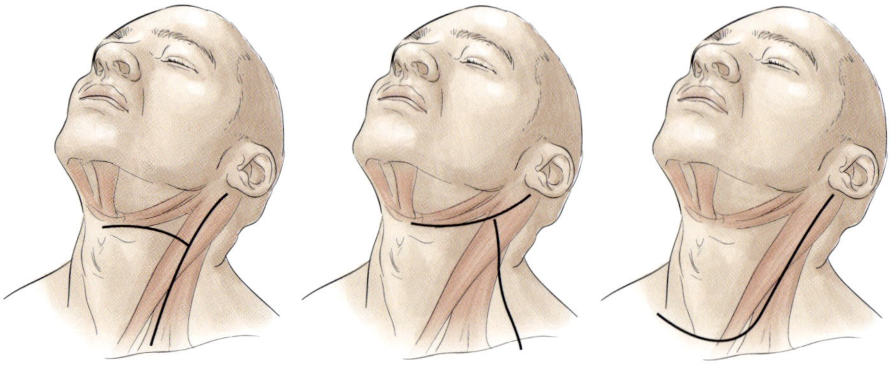

Figure 2-1.

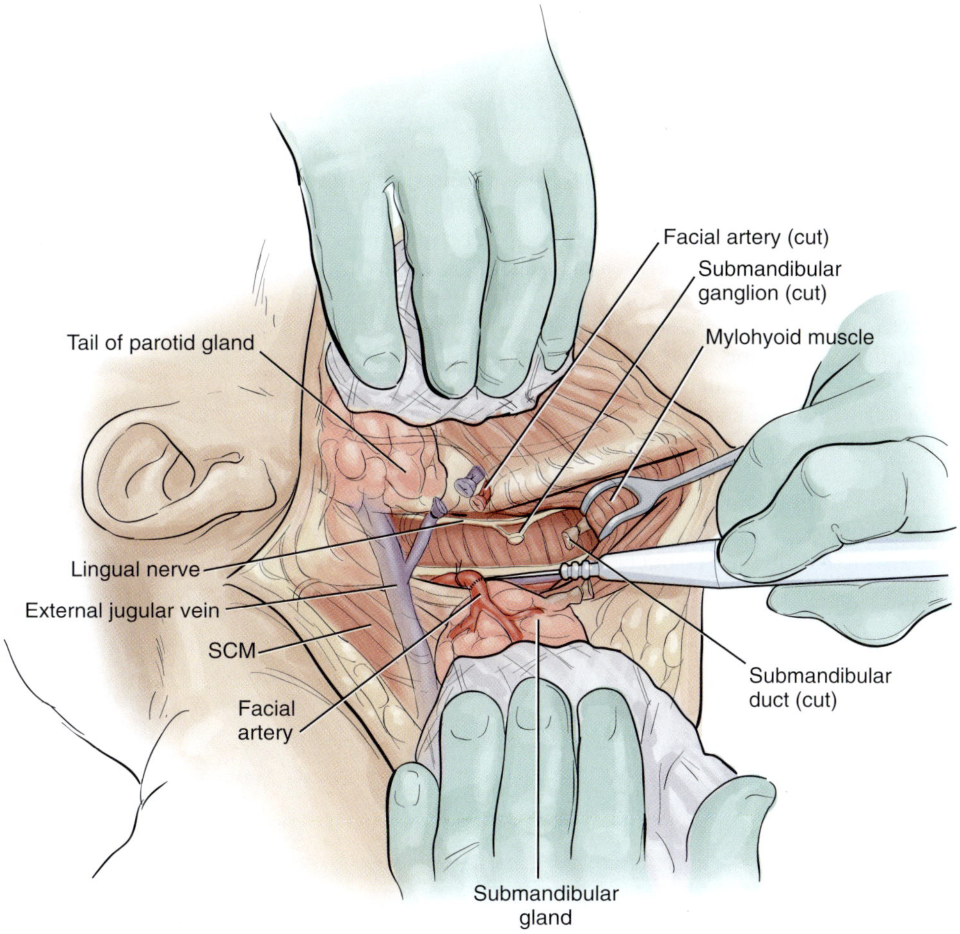

Figure 2-2.

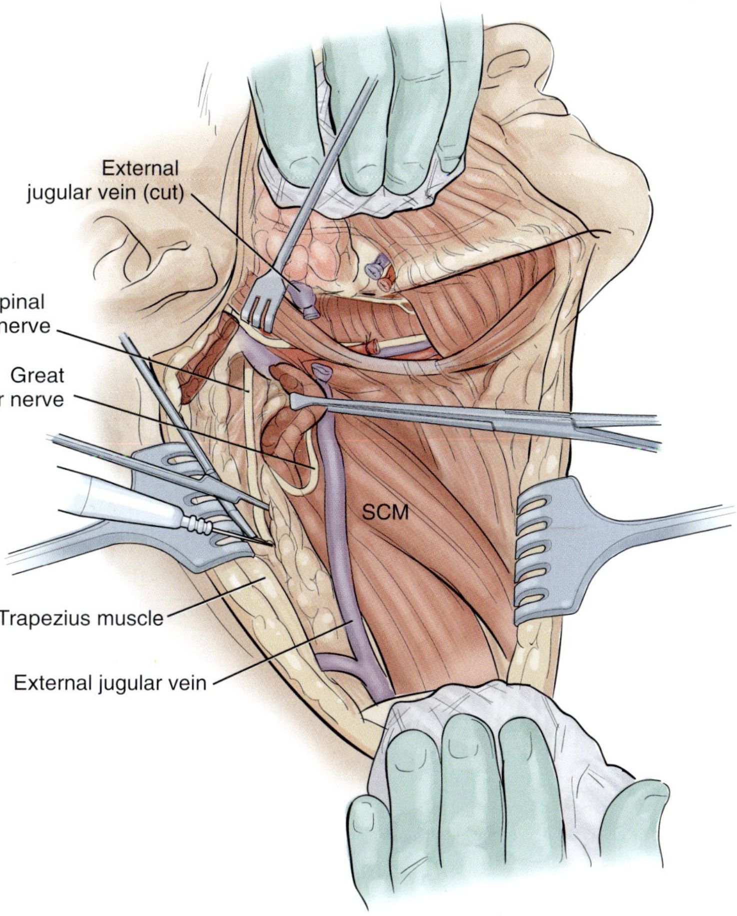

Figure 2-3. *SCM*, Sternocleidomastoid.

- Once the accessory nerve is identified, it is dissected in its entire length from insertion into the trapezius to the posterior portion of the sternomastoid muscle. The portion of the sternomastoid is cut in this region anterior to the accessory nerve. There may be a branch of the accessory nerve going to the sternomastoid, which needs to be sacrificed.
- After full exposure of the accessory nerve, dissection continues in the posterior triangle above the accessory nerve up to the mastoid process. As the mastoid process is exposed, the origin of the sternomastoid is transected against the mastoid region. This continues anteriorly until the entire sternomastoid is cut and peeled inferiorly, preserving the accessory nerve. Dissection is done above the accessory nerve, and all the lymphoid and fibrofatty tissue is peeled behind the accessory nerve, along with the portion of the sternomastoid muscle that has already been cut.
- The dissection now continues against the sternomastoid muscle, and the inferior belly of the omohyoid is identified and is transected close to the clavicle. As the omohyoid is cut, the brachial plexus and the internal jugular veins should be identified (Figs. 2-4 through 2-6).
- The dissection continues in the supraclavicular fossa. Every effort should be made to ligate all the lymphatic channels. On the left-hand side, use the utmost care to avoid injury to the thoracic duct. If one of the major lymphatic channels is identified, ligate with nonabsorbable suture material, such as silk. Hemoclips may be used in this area as well. The Harmonic scalpel may be used, if available, and is supposed to be a good sealant for the lymphatic channels.
- The inferior portion of the sternomastoid is then transected, and the medial head is generally tendinous. As the sternomastoid is transected near the sternoclavicular area, the internal jugular vein is again exposed. Careful dissection is done in the carotid sheath to avoid injury to the vagus nerve (see Figs. 2-4 through 2-6).

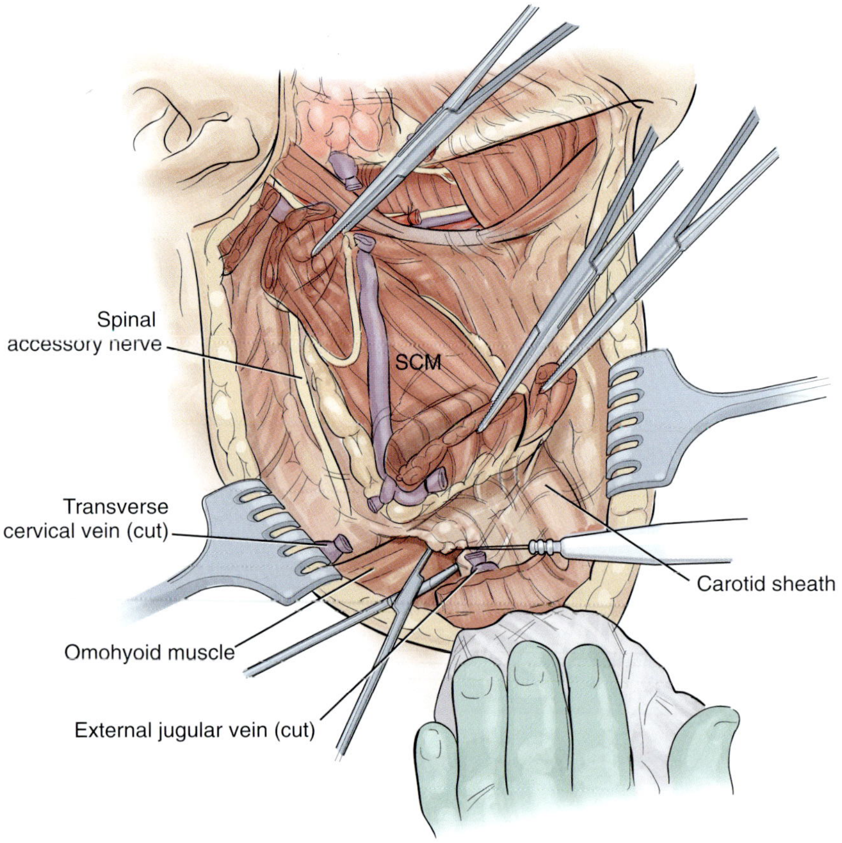

Figure 2-4. *SCM*, Sternocleidomastoid.

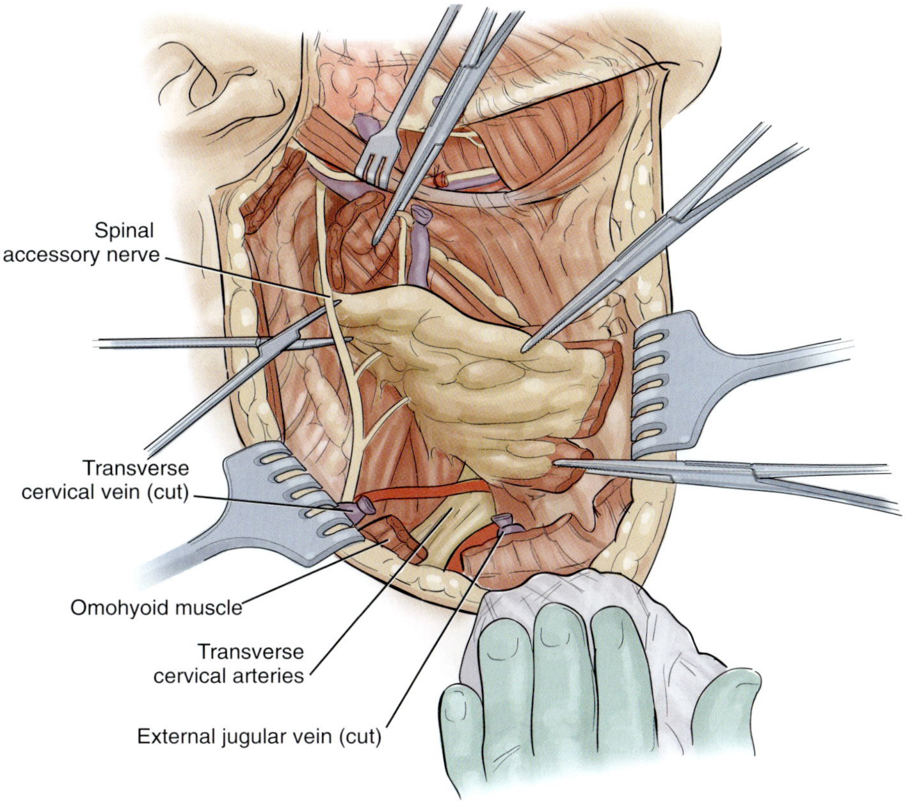

Figure 2-5.

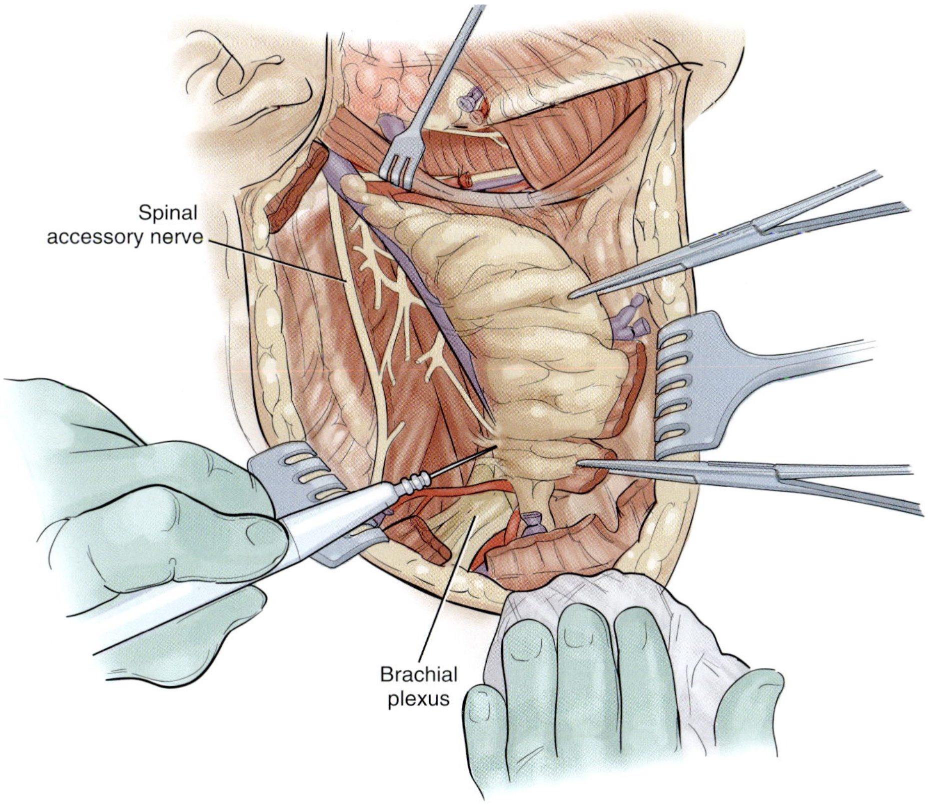

Figure 2-6.

- The internal jugular vein is dissected all around. There may be a tiny tributary to the internal jugular vein posteriorly that needs to be ligated carefully; otherwise, bleeding may begin in this area. A curved right-angle clamp is passed around the internal jugular vein and is clamped, ligated, and cut. A suture ligature is helpful to avoid any untoward slipping of the ligature (see Figs. 2-4 through 2-6).
- Once the internal jugular vein is ligated, the dissection continues between the internal jugular vein, the carotid artery and the vagus nerve. This area is essentially avascular, and the dissection can be done lateral to the internal jugular vein. All the fibrofatty tissue and the lymphoid contents of the posterior triangle are pulled anteriorly.
- This is the time when the anterior skin flap is extended up to the midchin area. As the anterior flap is raised, the submandibular salivary gland is exposed. The dissection continues superiorly. There may be troublesome bleeding in the tail of the parotid that is best left alone or controlled by bipolar cautery.
- As dissection continues on the tail of the parotid, the posterior facial vein may be identified and may require ligation. The posterior belly of the digastric is exposed (Fig. 2-7).
- The dissection continues anteriorly to the midline of the chin area. The anterior belly of the digastric is exposed, and the submental region is dissected. There are multiple tiny venous tributaries in this area that require bipolar coagulation. The submental triangle is exposed, and tiny submental lymph nodes and fibrofatty tissue are peeled toward the submandibular salivary gland. The geniohyoid is exposed, and the dissection continues on the surface of the digastric (Fig. 2-8, and see Fig. 2-2).
- The tendon of the digastric is identified, and mylohyoid muscle is exposed lateral to the anterior belly of the digastric muscle. The submandibular salivary gland is exposed. The mylohyoid is pulled anteriorly. There may be nerves to the mylohyoid that again will require appropriate coagulation. The mylohyoid muscle is retracted anteriorly, and the deeper portion of the submandibular salivary gland and the duct of the submandibular salivary gland is exposed.
- As dissection continues in this area superior to the submandibular salivary gland, the lingual nerve is identified, and the chorda tympani is also identified and is transected.
- Below the level of the submandibular salivary gland and superomedial to the angle of the digastric muscle, the hypoglossal nerve is exposed. This is carefully dissected off the digastric muscle. There are always tiny veins alongside the hypoglossal nerve that need to be carefully ligated or preserved.
- As the mylohyoid muscle is pulled anteriorly, the submandibular salivary gland duct is exposed, which is ligated with clamps. The submandibular salivary gland is retracted laterally and posteriorly. The dissection is now done on the hyoglossus muscle.
- As dissection continues superiorly, the facial artery and vein are exposed. Dissection is done on the surface of the facial artery to identify the ramus mandibularis. There may be tiny prevascular and postvascular facial lymph nodes that will require careful dissection and preservation of the ramus mandibularis. As the facial artery is ligated, the tie is pulled superiorly, which will protect the ramus mandibularis.
- Dissection is now done on the surface of the submandibular salivary gland by opening the fascia covering the submandibular salivary gland. The entire gland is peeled posteriorly off the hyoglossus muscle. The facial artery is again identified posterior to the submandibular salivary gland and medial to the posterior belly of the digastric. A double ligature is required. The posterior facial vein is also ligated in this area.
- Now that the entire submandibular salivary gland is pulled posteriorly, the digastric muscle is fully exposed, along with muscles covering the digastric (styloid group of muscles: styloglossus, stylopharyngeus, and stylohyoid). The posterior belly of the digastric is pulled superiorly, and the internal jugular vein is identified. There may be a posterior occipital artery in this region crossing the internal jugular vein, which will require appropriate ligation.

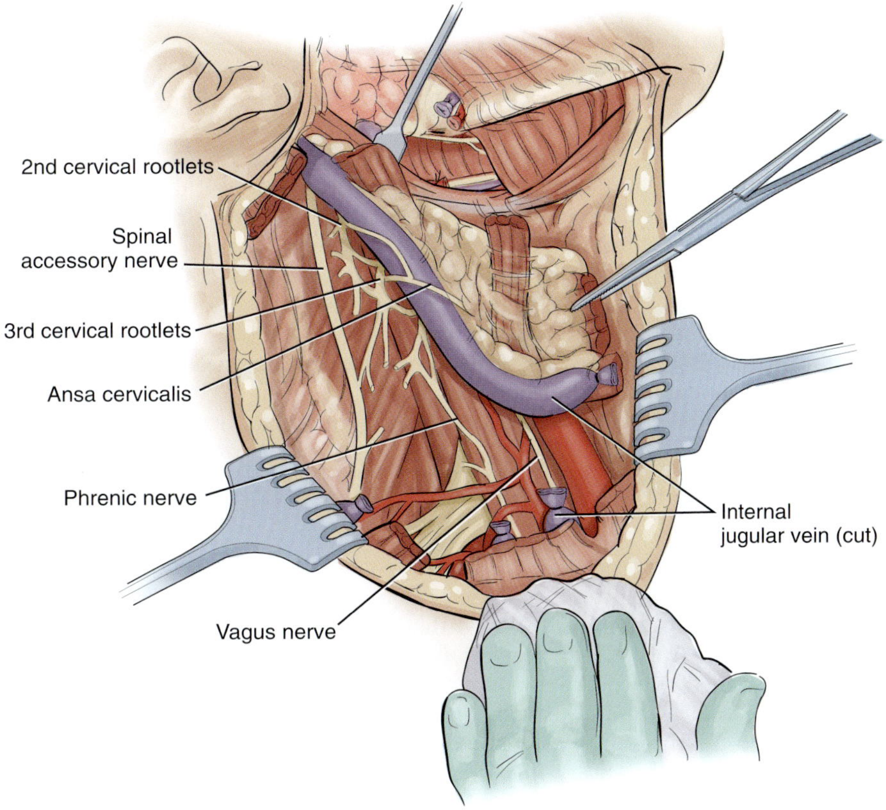

Figure 2-7.

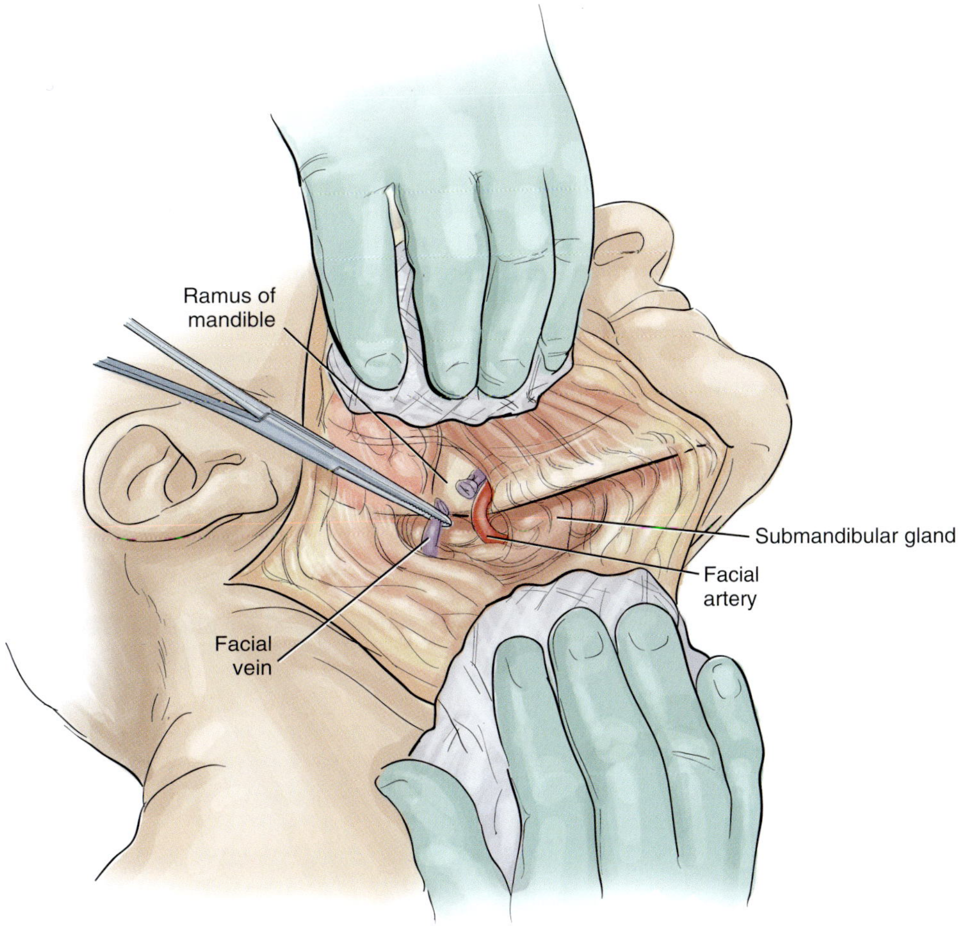

Figure 2-8.

- The dissection continues on the surface of the internal jugular vein, carefully preserving the accessory nerve, which has been identified previously.
- As the dissection continues on the anterior portion of the internal jugular vein, the entire specimen is pulled inferiorly, and the internal jugular vein is clamped and ligated. Suture ligation of the proximal end is preferred (Fig. 2-9). If the decision was made previously to preserve the internal jugular vein and it was preserved in the lower portion, then a decision should be made at this time to preserve or sacrifice the internal jugular vein, depending on the extent of disease. If there is no tumor adherence to the internal jugular vein, it can be easily preserved or ligated, as required.
- The entire neck dissection specimen is now separated, along with lymph nodes at levels I, II, III, IV, and V, and the sternomastoid muscle, submandibular salivary gland, and jugular vein. The jugular vein may need to be preserved, and it should be planned in advance if the patient is undergoing microvascular free-flap reconstruction.
- After removal of the specimen, hemostasis is achieved. Bipolar electrocautery is used to control any bleeding from the muscle bellies. Careful attention should be given to the fibrofatty tissue in the posterior triangle to control any bleeding vessels that may get retracted in the posterior triangle against the trapezius muscle.

Closure

- A Jackson-Pratt or Reliavac drain is used, and the wound should be closed in layers with Vicryl stitches on the platysma and staples or nylon stitches on the skin.
- The vertical incision needs to be closed very carefully against the transverse incision, and this area of the skin should be handled very delicately to avoid any skin necrosis or devascularization caused by pulling the skin. The drains are placed to self-suction. The patient should be observed carefully in the recovery room for any bleeding. Every attempt should be made to smoothly extubate to avoid any coughing or bucking against the endotracheal tube.

III. ALTERNATIVE TECHNICAL APPROACHES (PRO/CON) AND PEARLS

A variety of modified neck dissections are well recognized, and specific names have been applied, such as supraomohyoid neck dissection, central neck dissection, jugular neck dissection, posterolateral neck dissection, and extended neck dissection.

Supraomohyoid Neck Dissection

- This operation is performed mainly as a staging procedure for cancer of the oral cavity or oropharynx. The groups of lymph nodes to be removed are level I, II, and III. Occasionally level IV lymph nodes are removed, specifically in patients with cancer of the oral tongue, as there is an approximately 9% to 11% risk of nodal disease at level IV.
- A horizontal or curvilinear incision is taken in the upper skin crease, approximately two finger breadths below the angle of the mandible. For supraomohyoid neck dissection alone, a transverse skin-crease incision is much better than a curvilinear incision.
- The flaps are raised as usual under the platysma. The greater auricular nerve may be preserved as the dissection is done on the anterior and medial aspect of the sternomastoid muscle.
- The sternomastoid muscle is exposed. The fascia on the surface of the sternomastoid muscle is released, and the dissection continues on the medial aspect of the sternomastoid muscle.
- The accessory nerve is identified and carefully preserved. The dissection is performed at level IIB above the accessory nerve. This dissection should be done carefully to avoid any bleeding or injury to the accessory nerve.
- The dissection continues on the surface of the digastric muscle, and the digastric is completely exposed.

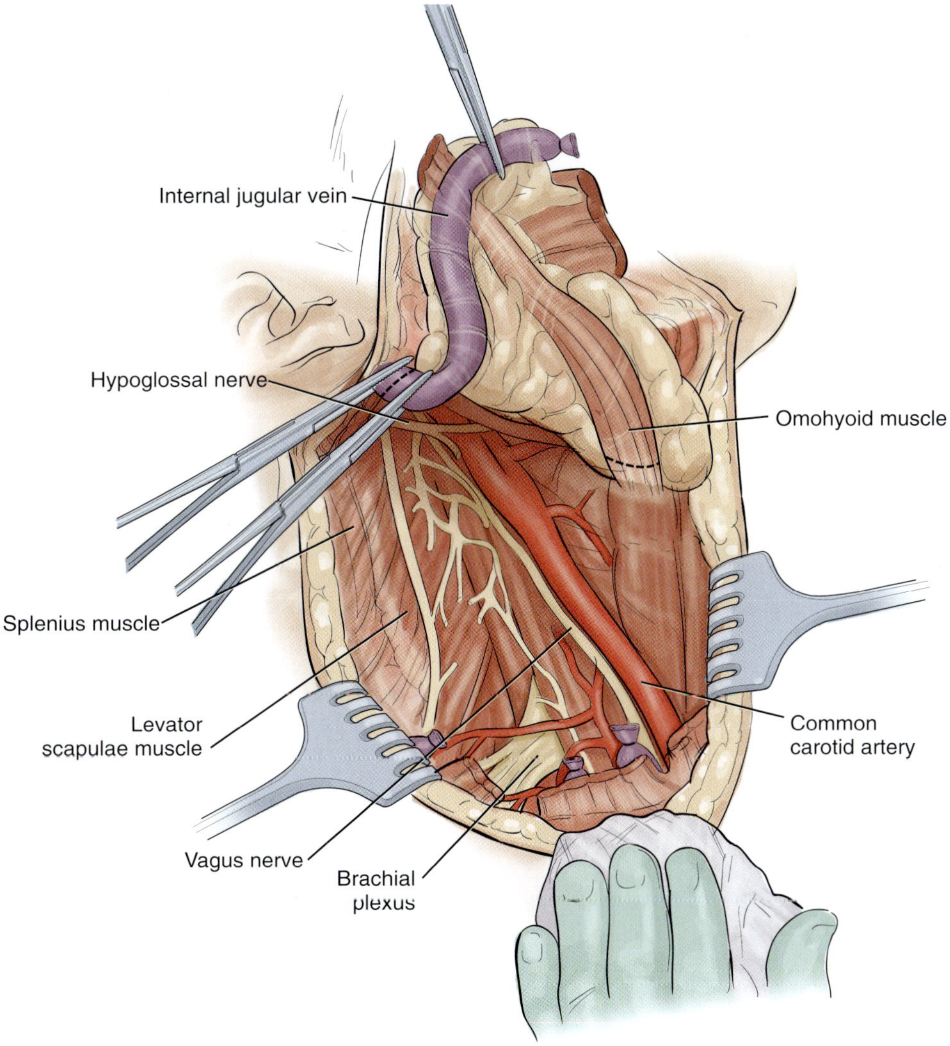
Internal jugular vein
Hypoglossal nerve
Omohyoid muscle
Splenius muscle
Levator
scapulae muscle
Common
carotid artery
Vagus nerve
Brachial
plexus

Figure 2-9.

- At this time, the dissection is done inferior to the accessory nerve and lateral to the jugular vein. The submandibular salivary gland is exposed, and the dissection continues between the submandibular salivary gland and the mandible. The ramus mandibularis is identified under the platysma and carefully preserved. The facial vessels are clamped and ligated, and as the facial vessels are pulled superiorly, the ramus mandibularis is carefully preserved.
- As the submental dissection is performed, the entire submental triangle is exposed with exposure of the geniohyoid muscle, and the specimen is pulled inferiorly. As the specimen is released in the submental triangle, the mylohyoid muscle is exposed.
- The dissection continues on the surface of the mylohyoid muscle to identify a deeper portion of the submandibular salivary gland. In this region, the hypoglossal nerve and the lingual nerves are identified. A branch of the lingual (chorda tympani) going to the submandibular salivary gland is clamped and ligated.
- The under aspect of the mylohyoid muscle is exposed, and the deeper portion of the submandibular salivary gland is carefully dissected. A clamp is placed on the deeper portion of the submandibular salivary gland along with the Wharton duct. The specimen is retracted posteriorly.
- The dissection continues on the hyoglossus muscle. The facial artery is clamped and ligated medial to the posterior belly of the digastric muscle.
- Now the dissection continues posteriorly behind the jugular vein in the posterior triangle. The cervical plexus is identified. The lymphoid structures are pulled anteriorly, and the dissection continues on the surface of the internal jugular vein.
- The lowermost dissection is done at the junction of the internal jugular vein and the omohyoid muscle. Occasionally, level IV lymph nodes are removed in selected patients with cancer of the oral cavity, by pulling the omohyoid anteriorly and dissecting in the supraclavicular region. In this area, utmost care is taken to avoid any injury to the lymphatic channels or thoracic duct.
- After the specimen is removed, the specimen is oriented by multiple sections to the pathologist, and levels I, II, and III lymph nodes are sent separately to the pathologist.
- A Reliavac drain is placed, and the wound is closed in layers. Monocryl subcuticular stitches may be placed for best cosmetic results.

Central Neck Dissection

- This surgical procedure is performed mainly for patients with carcinoma of the thyroid. Occasionally it is also performed for patients with laryngeal cancer or subglottic cancer, but generally those patients will undergo jugular neck dissection with central compartment dissection.
- The lymph nodes at level VI are removed after completing the total thyroidectomy, or as the total thyroidectomy is progressing.
- The recurrent laryngeal nerve is identified. Utmost care is taken to identify the parathyroid glands, separate them from the thyroid and the lymphoid tissue, and preserve them with their own blood supply. If, for any reason, a parathyroid gland appears to be devascularized, a small portion of the parathyroid should be sent for frozen section to confirm the gland to be parathyroid, and the remaining portion is minced into multiple small pieces and autotransplanted in the sternomastoid muscle on the contralateral side of the cancer.
- The dissection continues in the paratracheal area. Delphian and pretracheal lymph nodes are also removed. Hemostasis is generally achieved with bipolar cautery. Occasionally there may be extensive disease along the tracheoesophageal groove at level VII, which also may be cleared along with the central neck dissection.

Jugular Neck Dissection

- This surgical procedure is mainly performed for cancer of the oropharynx or the laryngopharyngeal area.
- The dissection is generally performed by retracting the sternomastoid muscle laterally, identifying the accessory nerve, clearing the lymph nodes below the accessory nerve, and clearing the jugular vein at levels II, III, and IV.
- Utmost care is taken to avoid any injury to the lymphatic channels at level IV.

Posterolateral Neck Dissection

- This surgical procedure is performed mainly for patients with melanoma or skin cancer in the scalp or occipital region.
- The trapezius muscle is identified, the dissection is done behind the sternomastoid muscle in the posterior triangle, and the accessory nerve is identified approximately 1 cm about the Erb point or in front of the trapezius muscle.

- The accessory nerve is dissected from all angles, preserving it carefully and dissecting the lymphoid tissue under the accessory nerve.
- The lymphoid structures in front of the trapezius muscle and occasionally between the trapezius and splenius are also removed by retracting the trapezius carefully or transecting a portion of the trapezius below the nuchal line.

Pearls and Pitfalls

- Neck dissection is an anatomically very sound surgical procedure with minimal blood loss. It is performed mainly for patients undergoing elective nodal dissection or therapeutic neck dissection for clinically palpable disease.
- For cancers of the oral cavity, the classical operation is supraomohyoid neck dissection, whereas patients with palpable disease from the upper aerodigestive tract generally undergo a modified neck dissection preserving the accessory nerve.
- Utmost care should be taken to avoid bleeding in the posterior triangle of the neck or injury to the transverse cervical vessels, and careful dissection should be undertaken along the accessory nerve to avoid devascularization.
- Avoid injury to the ramus mandibularis.
- The blood loss should be minimal.

IV. SPECIAL POSTOPERATIVE CARE

Wound Hematoma

- The overall incidence of wound hematoma is approximately 2%. This may be related to excessive coughing or bucking during extubation due to increased intrathoracic pressure and a rise in venous pressure. It may also be related to slipping of a ligature.
- Generally the hematoma is recognized by collection of blood under the flaps and tenting of the skin flaps. It may be recognized if there is a large amount of drainage through the Reliavac drain.
- These patients need to be brought back to the operating room as soon as possible, the wound reopened, the drains replaced, and the bleeding point ligated. Quite often no specific bleeding point can be identified, and there is a diffuse ooze that requires a conservative approach and close follow-up.

Chyle Leak

- Another concerning complication of neck dissection is persistent chyle leak. A minor chyle leak is fairly common. However, a persistent chyle leak may occur in 2% to 5% of patients.
- The drain is generally left in place for an extended period of time until the drainage slows down. Very rarely, the wound may need to be reexplored if there is more than 500 to 700 mL of drainage every day.
- The patient is generally placed on a low-fat diet or medium-chain triglyceride diet.
- The chyle leak usually slows down over the next 5 to 7 days, and the drains can then be removed. Occasionally the patient may continue to have a chyle leak, and the drains may have to stay in place for an extended period of time. The best approach in this case is to send the patient home with drains with regular follow-up in the outpatient setting.
- A medium-chain triglyceride diet is helpful to slow down the chyle leak.

Miscellaneous Complications

- Accessory nerve weakness may occur because of excessive traction or devascularization of the accessory nerve, which may lead to frozen shoulder or inability to abduct the arm fully. Physiotherapy is quite helpful under these circumstances.
- Injury to the ramus mandibularis may lead to lower lip weakness. Quite often it is a temporary event. However, in 2% to 5% of patients, it may be permanent. There is no specific definitive treatment available. A plastic surgery consultation for facial reanimation may be considered if the patient's cancer is well controlled.
- Long-term complications include stump neuroma or numbness of the face and ear area.
- The skin edges may necrose and the wound may separate at the trifurcation. This is more likely to occur in patients who have received previous radiation therapy. Conservative wound care will help further healing of the wound.

SUGGESTED READINGS

Ferlito A, Rinaldo A, Silver CE, et al: Neck dissection: then and now, *Auris Nasus Larynx* 33:365–374, 2006.
Ferlito A, Robbins KT, Shah JP, et al: Proposal for a rational classification of neck dissections, *Head Neck* 33:445–450, 2011.
Shah JP, Andersen PE: The impact of patterns of nodal metastasis on modifications of neck dissection, *Ann Surg Oncol* 1:521–532, 1994. Review.

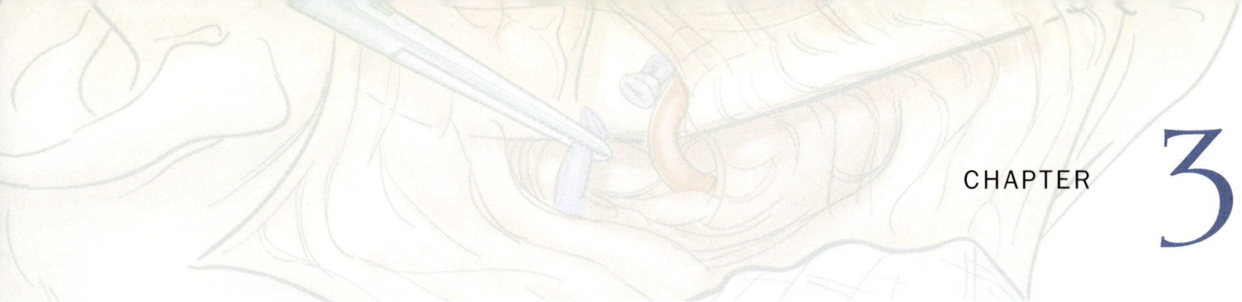

CHAPTER 3

Superficial Parotidectomy

Ashok R. Shaha, MD, FACS

I. SPECIAL PREOPERATIVE PREPARATION

- Even though parotid tumors are rare, the most common salivary tumors are located in the parotid, 80% of which are benign. Tumors involving the submandibular salivary gland and the minor salivary gland have an incidence of malignancy of approximately 50% and 80%, respectively. The most common benign tumor of the parotid gland is pleomorphic adenoma, followed by Warthin tumor and oncocytoma.
- The most common presentation is a mass in the parotid region. The mass might have been present for a long time, and there may be a recent and rapid increase in the size of the mass. The clinical signs of malignancy include skin involvement, facial nerve palsy, fixation of the tumor to the surrounding structures, and presence of nodal metastasis.
- Special preoperative preparation includes a thorough clinical evaluation, including evaluation of the location of the tumor, facial nerve function, and status of the lymph nodes.
- For a standard benign mixed tumor or parotid tumor, imaging studies are not very helpful. However, imaging will indicate the location of the tumor and whether the margins are irregular. Imaging is helpful for the patient presenting with an aggressive parotid tumor, such as facial nerve palsy or a long-standing deep-lobe parotid tumor. Tumors in the tail of the parotid are usually Warthin tumors, and a preoperative fine-needle aspiration biopsy (FNA) is quite helpful. Even though there continues to be considerable controversy about the role of FNA, in select circumstances it is quite helpful. FNA will distinguish between salivary and nonsalivary pathology. FNA is also quite helpful in identifying suspected lymphoma or cystic lesions of the parotid, such as a benign parotid cyst or lymphoepithelial lesions of the parotid. The major concern in using FNA is the inability to distinguish between benign and malignant parotid tumors. However, it does help to confirm that one is dealing with a salivary pathology.
- The patient should be well informed about the surgical procedure, the need for identification of the facial nerve and its branches, and the potential for temporary or permanent injury to the peripheral branches or main trunk of the facial nerve, which can lead to complete facial paralysis. Even though total facial palsy is rare in patients undergoing superficial parotidectomy, the peripheral branches of the facial nerve may become weak, and it is not uncommon for a patient to have weakness of the lower lip, cheek, or eye. Most of the temporary weakness will improve over a period of 4 to 6 weeks.

II. OPERATIVE TECHNIQUE

Position

- The position on the operating table is supine, with preparation of the ipsilateral face. The ear is kept in the field, as most of the dissection is performed in the pretragal area. The eye should be kept under observation. The eyelids may be sutured together, or a corneal shield may be used to cover the eye. I generally prefer a piece of tape placed on the eye with preparation including the face and the eye, with the eye region covered with a transparent drape. The transparent drape is helpful to evaluate eye movements and to clearly visualize the face, cheek, and lip. The entire ipsilateral neck is prepared up to the clavicle, as the dissection is performed in the upper part of the neck with a curvilinear incision.
- The patient should be intubated in a nontraumatic fashion, generally with a no. 6 or 7 endotracheal tube. The tube should be secured to the contralateral side of the commissure with tape and the

ipsilateral cheek and face completely exposed without any tape. The endotracheal tube should be inserted slightly more deeply, as there is a likelihood of tube withdrawal during neck manipulation and positioning of the head to the contralateral side. The head should rest on a donut throughout the surgical procedure. For the induction of anesthesia, it is appropriate to paralyze the patient. However, after the initial paralysis, any further anesthetic paralysis should be avoided so that facial nerve function can be tested during surgery. At the conclusion of the procedure, the patient should be extubated smoothly to avoid coughing or strenuous movements.

Incision

- The incision for a parotidectomy begins in the pretragal area along the crease in front of the tragus with a curvilinear extension along the ear lobe and mastoid process to the upper portion of the neck. This is a long S-shaped curvilinear incision, also known as a *modified Blair incision* (Fig. 3-1). The incision can be extended in the neck if the tumor is lodged in the tail of the parotid, or superiorly along the hairline if the tumor is high up near the zygoma. The cervical incision can be extended anteriorly with a vertical limb in the middle if neck dissection is contemplated.

Main Dissection

- The skin is infiltrated with lidocaine and epinephrine. This is helpful to avoid annoying bleeding from the skin incision.
- The skin and subcutaneous tissue are incised with a scalpel, and the dissection is done with a point electrocautery. The entire length of the skin is incised, and the anterior flap is raised just above the platysma. In the neck, the platysma is well-visualized. This is incised along the incision line.
- The anterior flap is raised almost up to the masseter muscle. This may vary, however, depending on the location of the tumor. Every effort should be made to avoid perforation of the anterior flap, because most of the time it is quite thin. As the anterior flap is raised, it is important to stay very close to the skin to avoid any injury to the peripheral branches of the facial nerve.
- The dissection continues in the neck until the sternomastoid muscle is visualized. The posterior flap needs to be raised until the mastoid process is exposed and the posterior portion of the sternomastoid is also exposed.
- The sternomastoid fascia is incised, and the dissection continues along the sternomastoid muscle. Here the deep cervical fascia is exposed and the posterior belly of the digastric is also seen.
- The dissection is done on the surface of the digastric muscle as the posterior facial layer of the parotid gland is exposed. At this time, a retractor is placed to pull the parotid gland anteriorly, and the dissection continues in the deep jugulodigastric area. This area is inspected, and dissection may be done there to see if there are any enlarged lymph nodes. There are always reactive lymph nodes in this region, which may be removed and sent for frozen section or permanent section.
- As the dissection continues on the surface of the digastric muscle, the entire tumor and the parotid gland become mobilized (Fig. 3-2).
- The anterior facial vein may be seen in this region, and this should be ligated. The greater auricular nerve may need to be transected off the sternomastoid muscle, because it will get in the way of dissection and invariably the nerve will be very close to the parotid tumor.
- The dissection continues superiorly in the pretragal area (see Fig. 3-2). The external auditory canal is exposed, and the dissection is done very close to cartilage to avoid any bleeding from the substance of the parotid gland. Any dissection in the parotid gland leads to a considerable amount of bleeding; therefore bipolar electrocautery will be helpful in this situation.
- The dissection continues on the anterior surface of the external auditory canal until the fingertip feels the junction of the external auditory canal and bony canal. At this time the dissection continues inferiorly, and the area between the mastoid process, the sternomastoid muscle, and the external auditory canal is dissected carefully. The dissection continues until the bony canal is felt or seen.
- At this juncture, one has to be concerned about identifying and preserving the main trunk of the facial nerve. A nerve stimulator may be helpful from this point onward. It is important to make sure that the patient is not paralyzed at this stage. However, some surgeons do prefer the patient to be completely paralyzed.
- As the dissection continues anterior to the external auditory canal, a tragal pointer should be noted at the junction of the mastoid process and the external auditory canal. Blunt dissection with the curved portion of the clamp continues in this area until the posterior portion of the digastric muscle is exposed.
- Once the digastric muscle is seen, the nerve should be anterior to this region, just below the external auditory canal. Dissection is performed with a blunt clamp, teasing the soft tissue above the nerve in the direction of the facial nerve. There is a small arterial branch, which is approximately 4 to 5 mm superficial to the facial nerve, which may cause troublesome bleeding in this area. It is best to identify this artery and clamp and ligate it. It is important to be absolutely sure that the structure that is being ligated is the artery and not a branch of the facial nerve (Fig. 3-3).

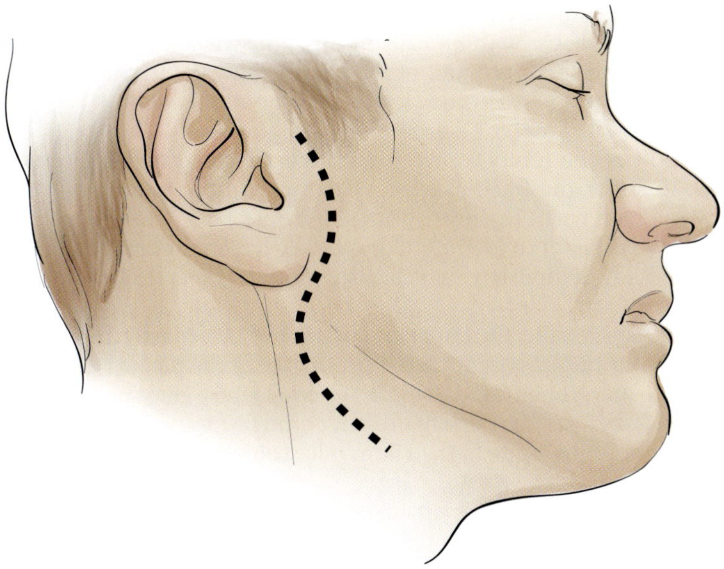

Figure 3-1.

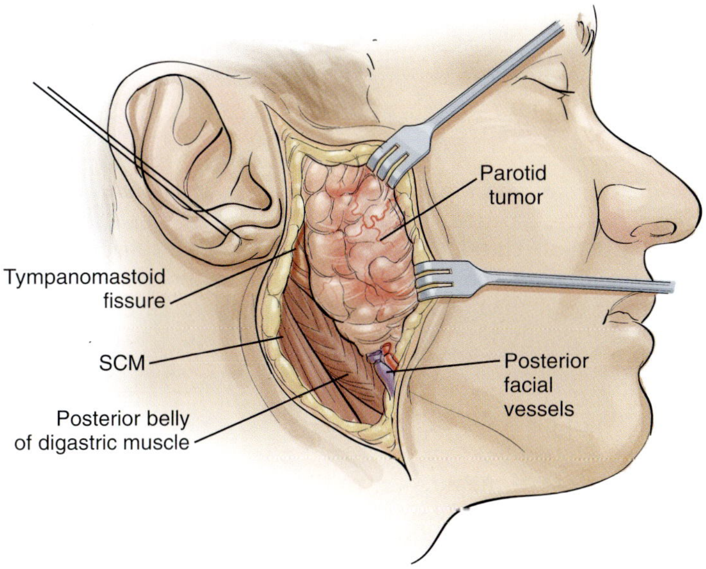

Figure 3-2. *SCM*, Sternocleidomastoid.

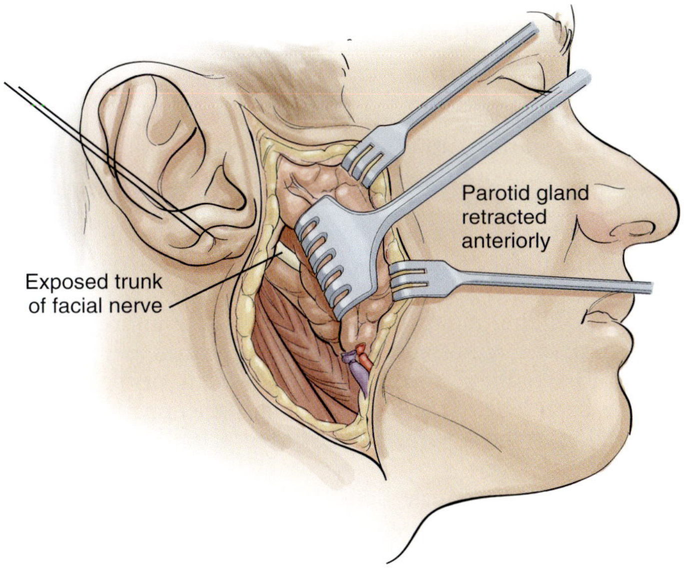

Figure 3-3.

- Once the facial nerve is tentatively identified, it can be stimulated to confirm that it is a facial nerve. The dissection now continues on the surface of the facial nerve without causing any injury to the vasa nervorum or perineurium. The dissection continues with the blunt end of the clamp, with the tip of the clamp pointing to the surface. The division and two branches of the facial nerve should be identified to confirm that the structure being dealt with is a facial nerve (Fig. 3-4).
- The dissection continues, depending on the location of the tumor, onto either the upper division or the lower division. Every effort should be made to avoid any traction or surface injury to the ramus mandibularis, which is an extremely sensitive nerve. Similarly, the orbital branch should be carefully dissected. The buccal branch is quite thin and may be difficult to identify. Occasionally a communicating branch may be noted between the upper and lower division, which also should be carefully preserved.
- The dissection should continue up to the masseter muscle, and the entire tumor should be separated from the surrounding parotid tissue. There can be a continuous ooze from the cut surface of the parotid substance, which invariably will stop after the specimen is removed. Bipolar electrocautery may be quite helpful in this region. A Harmonic scalpel may be used in this area to cut through the parotid tissue. However, it is important to recognize that the anterior blade of the Harmonic scalpel may cause surrounding tissue injury.
- As the dissection is done anteriorly, the surface of the masseter muscle is exposed. The parotid duct may be noted in this region and should be clamped and ligated. Approximately 20% of the parotid tissue deep to the facial nerve is generally left in situ unless the tumor involves the deep lobe of the parotid gland.
- After the entire specimen is removed, the parotid bed is visualized for any bleeding, and the branches of the facial nerve may be stimulated to confirm the functionality of the facial nerve (Fig. 3-5). The specimen may be sent for frozen section; however, the frozen section may not be completely accurate in evaluation of parotid tumors.

Closure

- The wound is irrigated, hemostasis achieved, and the wound is closed in layers. A Reliavac or closed suction (Jackson-Pratt) drain may be used (Fig. 3-6). A Penrose drain may be used in this area also. The subcutaneous tissue is approximated with 3-0 Vicryl. Skin stitches may be taken in interrupted fashion with 5-0 nylon, or continuous subcuticular Monocryl may be used. With the use of a suction drain, there is generally no need for extensive dressing. However, if a Penrose drain is used, a mastoid type of dressing should be used.

III. ALTERNATIVE TECHNICAL APPROACHES (PRO/CON) AND PEARLS

- If the tumor is in the tail of the parotid and it appears more likely to be a benign or Warthin tumor, an entire superficial parotidectomy is generally not necessary. A satisfactory margin of soft tissue in the parotid should be achieved, and the tumor can be resected with a partial parotidectomy. However, it is extremely important to identify the main trunk of the facial nerve and at least the lower division of the facial nerve. It may not be absolutely necessary to dissect the upper trunk fully.
- If the jugulodigastric node is suspicious or positive on frozen section for metastatic tumor, appropriate modified neck dissection should be considered, including removal of the lymph nodes at levels II, III, and V. Utmost care should be taken in this region to avoid injury to the accessory nerve, which is medial to the sternomastoid muscle. This may require anterior extension of the skin incision up to the mental area.
- If there is clinical or radiologic evidence that the tumor involves the deep lobe of the parotid tissue, a similar dissection should be entertained. The facial nerve should be identified, the facial nerve carefully preserved, and the tumor removed from the deeper portion of the parotid gland by dissection on the surface of the facial nerve. There is a higher incidence of temporary injury to the marginal branch under these circumstances.
- If the tumor entirely involves the deep lobe of the parotid tissue and presents mainly as a parapharyngeal mass, the dissection may be done on the surface of the digastric muscle, transecting the digastric and the styloid group of muscles (stylohyoid, styloglossus, and stylopharyngeus), opening the stylohyoid window and resecting the tumor medial to the ascending ramus of the mandible. The entire dissection of the facial nerve is generally not necessary in these circumstances. The styloid process may need to be resected, and utmost care should be taken to avoid any injury to the main trunk of the facial nerve. Patients with a benign mixed tumor of the deep lobe of the parotid gland, presenting as a parapharyngeal mass, do not necessarily require resection of the superficial lobe of the parotid. The nerve can be retracted along with the angle of the mandible.
- The majority of deep lobe parotid tumor resections are generally enucleations. If the tumor is very close to the lower division of the facial nerve, then the nerve should be identified and carefully dissected off the parotid tumor. If the tumor involves the anterior portion of the parotid gland, it may be

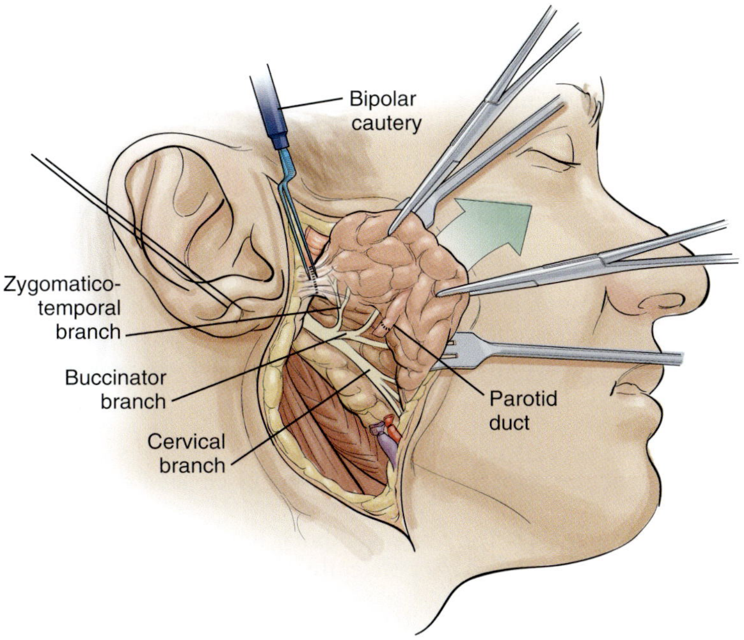

Figure 3-4.

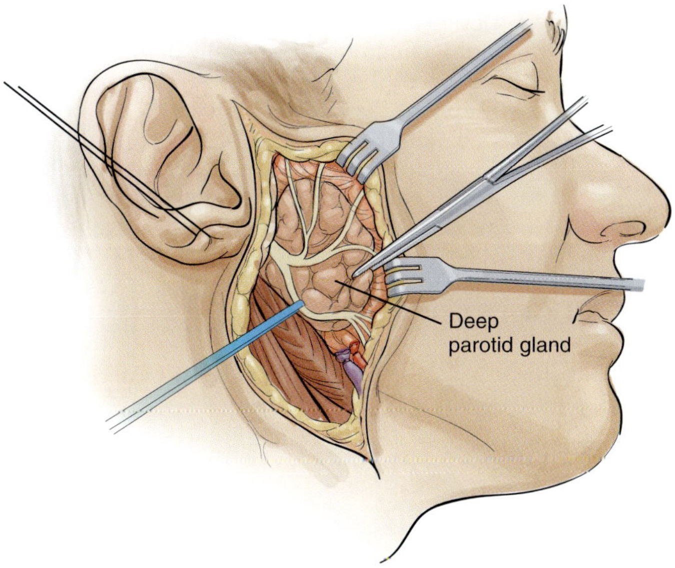

Figure 3-5.

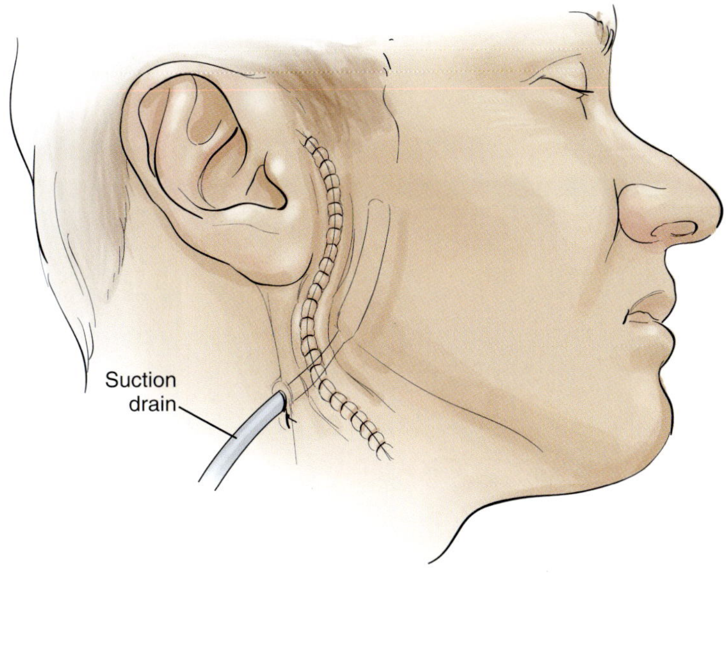

Figure 3-6.

an accessory parotid tumor. This requires careful dissection along the branches of the facial nerve, identifying and preserving the lower and upper divisions of the facial nerve, carefully dissecting the accessory parotid tumor off the masseter muscle. The chances of injuring the buccal branch in this situation are quite high. However, it may not have a major functional impact.

- An accessory parotid tumor may present as a cheek mass, and the best approach is the preparotid skin incision approach, rather than incision into the cheek mucosa using a transmucosal approach.

IV. SPECIAL POSTOPERATIVE CARE

- The drains should be kept in place until drainage is minimal. Generally, 10 mL or less per day is preferred before removal of the drain. The usual wound care is offered. The patient is usually discharged from the hospital within 48 to 72 hours, depending on the drainage levels. The patient may be sent home with the drain in place, having the drain removed after a few days depending on the amount of drainage in the outpatient setting.
- The stitches are removed within 1 week. However, the subcuticular stitches will dissolve, and the scar will have a minimal impact on appearance. Most of the scar, especially in women, can be covered with the patient's hair.
- There may be a slight indentation in the retromandibular area. The retromandibular indentation may be filled in with sternomastoid muscle or a fat graft. Most surgeons do not prefer this, because follow-up evaluation of the parotid bed might be made quite difficult.
- The ramus mandibularis is an extremely sensitive nerve, and surgery may lead to temporary weakness of the lip. This should improve in 4 to 6 weeks.
- Rarely, the patient may have a salivary leak through the wound, which may require multiple aspirations and careful observation.
- Delayed complications include Frey syndrome. Even though there is no definite or specific explanation of this syndrome, it generally occurs 6 to 9 months after surgery and is thought to be related to regeneration of the nerves and aberrant nerve supply from the facial nerve to the parasympathetic nerve supply to the sweat glands in the region of the parotidectomy. Most patients handle Frey syndrome well. Rarely, however, they may require additional procedures such as insertion of fascia lata or a Gore-Tex graft under the skin. Some surgeons have used Alloderm or the fascia covering the sternomastoid muscle to intervene between the skin and the facial nerve. However, long-term follow-up data for these methods are not available at this time.

SUGGESTED READINGS

Klintworth N, Zenk J, Koch M, Iro H: Postoperative complications after extracapsular dissection of benign parotid lesions with particular reference to facial nerve function, *Laryngoscope* 120:484–490, 2010.

Rodino W, Shaha AR: Surgical management of accessory parotid tumors, *J Surg Oncol* 54:153–156, 1993.

Wang RC, Barber AE, Ditmyer M, Vantine P: Distal facial nerve exposure: a key to partial parotidectomy, *Otolaryngol Head Neck Surg* 140:875–879, 2009.

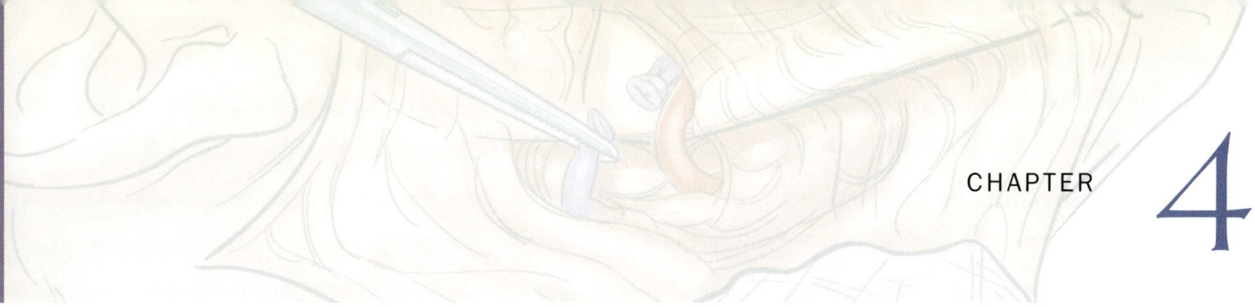

CHAPTER 4

Excision of Submandibular Gland and Submandibular Triangle Dissection

Jesus E. Medina, MD, FACS

I. SPECIAL PREOPERATIVE PREPARATION

Indications

This operation is indicated in the following situations:

- Chronic submandibular sialadenitis, most commonly due to sialolithiasis. When the stone or stones are lodged in the duct, close to the "hilum" of the gland, it is usually not possible to remove the stones through the mouth, making it necessary to remove the gland.
- A mass in the submandibular gland. In this case we prefer to perform a dissection of the submandibular triangle, including the various lymph node groups in the area. The reason is that about 50% of submandibular tumors are malignant.
- Metastatic tumor in a submandibular lymph node. There are four distinct groups of nodes in the submandibular triangle: the prevascular nodes located medially and anterior to the facial artery and vein as they pass over the inferior border of the mandible; the retrovascular nodes located medially and posterior to these vessels; the preglandular nodes located between the anterior border of the submandibular gland and the anterior belly of the digastric muscle, and lateral to the mylohyoid muscle; and a node located close to the inferior portion of the anterior facial vein near the lower border of the submandibular gland. Metastases to the lymph nodes in this region can occur from a primary tumor in the skin of the face, nasal vestibule, maxillary sinus, the lips, or the oral cavity. A dissection of the submandibular triangle may be necessary for diagnostic purposes: for instance, when repeated fine-needle aspiration biopsies of a mass in a submandibular node yield inconclusive results and the clinician's index of suspicion for metastasis is high. It may also be necessary for therapeutic purposes in patients who have had previous neck dissection sparing this area of the neck. This situation occurs, for example, in patients treated previously for cancer of the larynx (in whom this area of the neck is usually not included in the neck dissection) or who present with a new primary tumor in the previously mentioned areas of the head and neck.

II. OPERATIVE TECHNIQUE

Position

- The patient is placed in the supine position. The operating table is rotated 90 degrees with the operative side away from the anesthesia machine. A small shoulder roll is placed under the patient, and the head is rotated toward the side opposite to the dissection.

Incision

- The incision used varies depending on the indication. In the case of chronic sialadenitis, the incision used commonly is about 3 to 4 cm in length, and it is placed on or parallel to a natural crease in the skin overlying the inferior portion of the gland or slightly below the gland.
- If a submandibular triangle dissection is planned and the possibility exists that the operation may have to be extended to perform some type of cervical lymphadenectomy, it is best to outline the incision the surgeon will use to do the neck dissection and select a portion of that incision that is close to the submandibular area (Fig. 4-1, *A* and *B*).
- Skin flaps are usually developed by sharp dissection in a subplatysmal plane. However, if a large tumor mass is present, it may be advisable to leave the platysma attached to it as the skin flaps are elevated.

Main Dissection

- As the superior neck flap is elevated, the ramus mandibularis is exposed and preserved if possible (Fig. 4-2). If the operation is being done for an adenoid cystic carcinoma of the submandibular gland, a tumor known for its propensity for perineural spread, the surgeon should pay attention to the appearance of the ramus mandibularis. If the nerve appears enlarged, a segment is removed and examined by frozen section. Needless to say, the patient should be counseled preoperatively about such possibility.
- The submandibular prevascular and retrovascular lymph nodes, which are usually in close proximity to the nerve, are carefully dissected away from it. In doing so, the facial vessels are exposed and divided (see Fig. 4-2).
- The fibrous fatty tissue containing lymph nodes lateral to the mylohyoid muscle is dissected off the mylohyoid in a posterior and inferior direction. When the dissection reaches the posterior border of the mylohyoid, the fatty tissue is retracted anteriorly, exposing the lingual nerve and the submandibular gland duct, which are divided (Fig. 4-3).

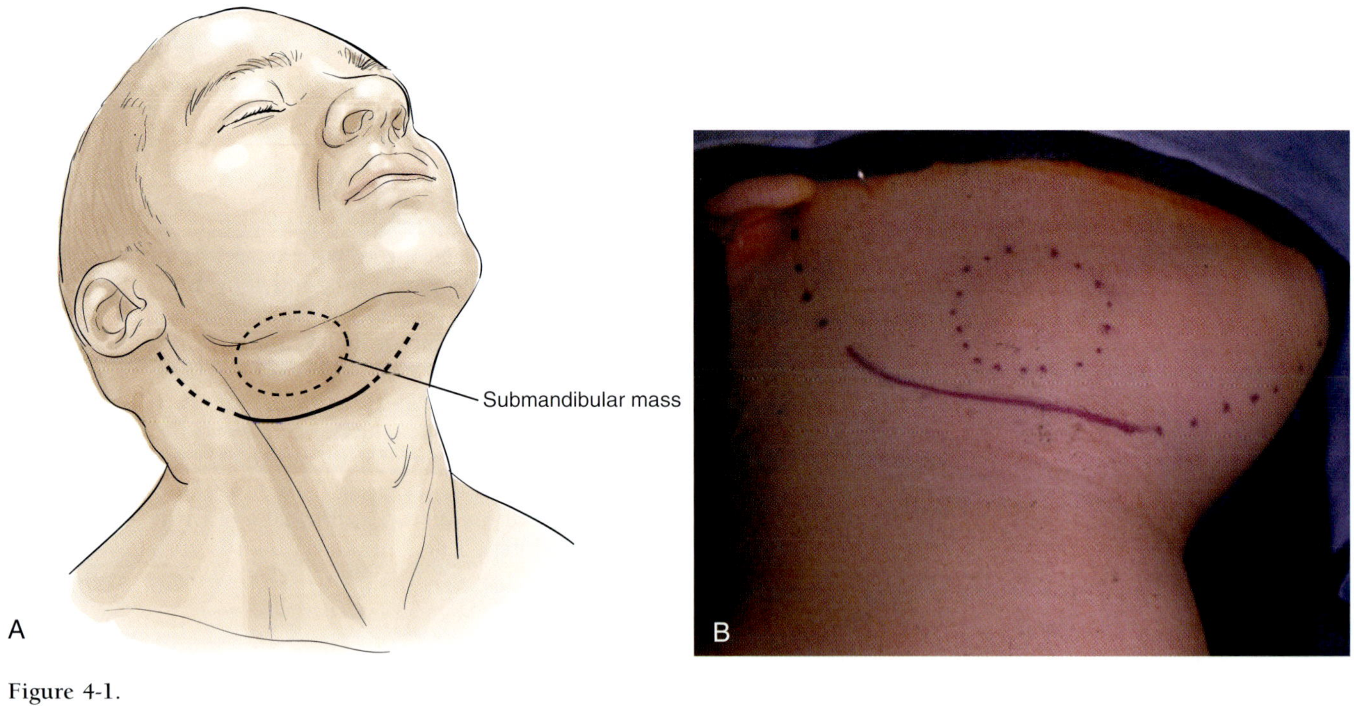

Figure 4-1.

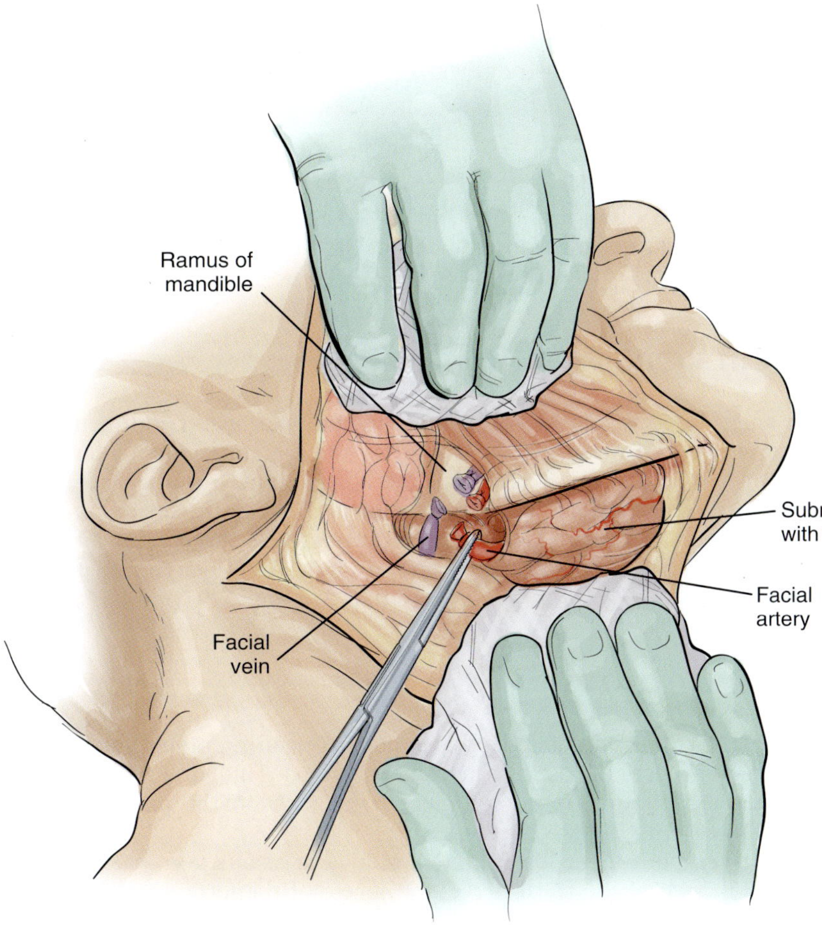

Figure 4-2.

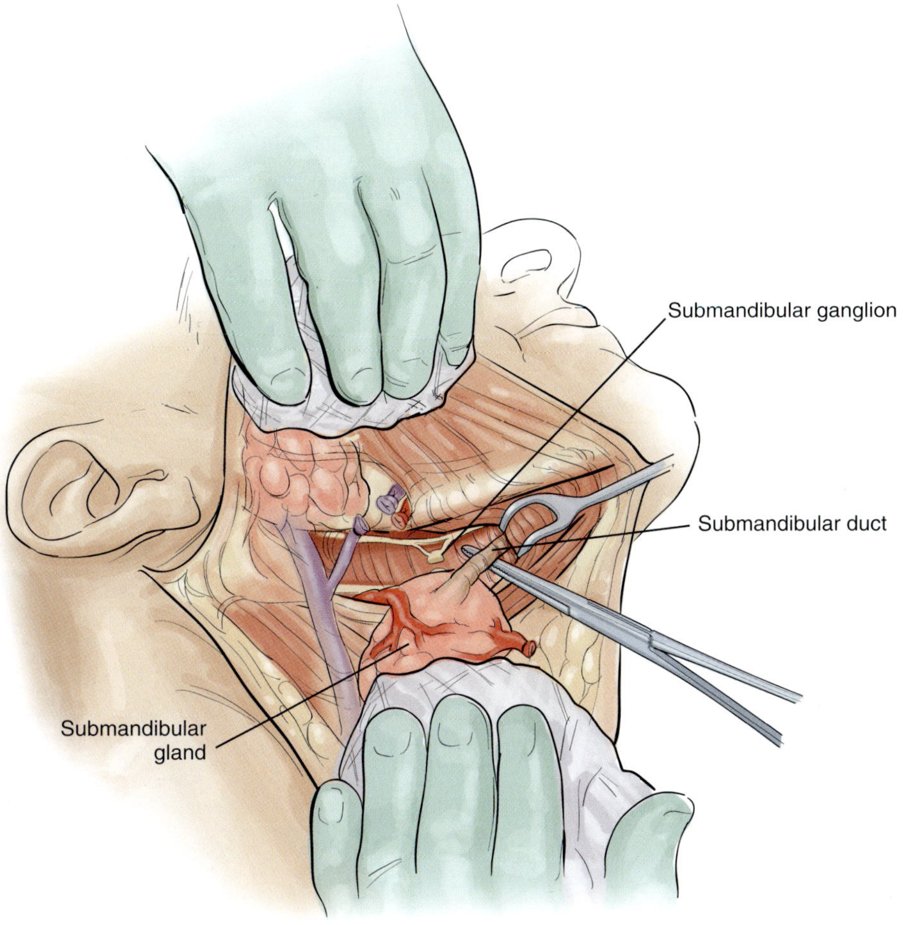

Figure 4-3.

- Once these structures are divided, the hypoglossal nerve and the veins that usually accompany it are left undisturbed as the dissection continues in a posterior direction. Finally, the facial artery is ligated as it crosses forward, under the posterior belly of the digastric (Figs. 4-4 and 4-5).

Closure

- The platysma is then approximated with either continuous or interrupted 3-0 absorbable sutures. The skin can be closed with either 4-0 absorbable sutures placed in the dermis or with 5-0 monofilament nylon.

III. ALTERNATIVE TECHNICAL APPROACHES (PRO/CON) AND PEARLS

- Some surgeons advocate ligating the anterior facial vein low over the submandibular gland and then retracting the superior portion of it upward, as a means to avoid injuring the marginal mandibular branch of the facial nerve, which is always located lateral to the vein. This approach may be appropriate when the submandibular gland is resected for chronic sialadenitis. However, when the operation is performed for primary neoplasm of the submandibular gland or for metastasis to the submandibular nodes, ligating and retracting the vein in this manner can obscure one or more of the lymph nodes that need to be removed.

IV. SPECIAL POSTOPERATIVE CARE (COMPLICATIONS)

- Postoperative care following resection of the submandibular gland is limited to ensuring proper functioning of the wound drain(s). Premature removal of the drains can result in seroma. This complication can be cumbersome, often requiring multiple aspirations or reinsertion of drains. To avoid this problem, it is usually necessary to drain the wound for 5 to 7 days.
- The most notable complication of these operations is the lower lip deformity that results from paresis or paralysis of the marginal mandibular branch of the facial nerve. Awareness of the location of the nerve is paramount when only the submandibular gland is resected. On the other hand, identification and sometimes appropriate isolation of the nerve are necessary when the lymph nodes of the submandibular triangle are included in the dissection.

SUGGESTED READINGS

Byers RM, Jesse R, Luna M: Malignant tumors of the submaxillary gland, *Am J Surg* 126:458–463, 1973.
Hsu AK, Kutler DI: Indications, techniques, and complications of major salivary gland extirpation, *Oral Maxillofac Surg Clin North Am* 21:313–321, 2009.
Isa AY, Hilmi OJ: An evidence based approach to the management of salivary masses, *Clin Otolaryngol* 34:470–473, 2009. Review.

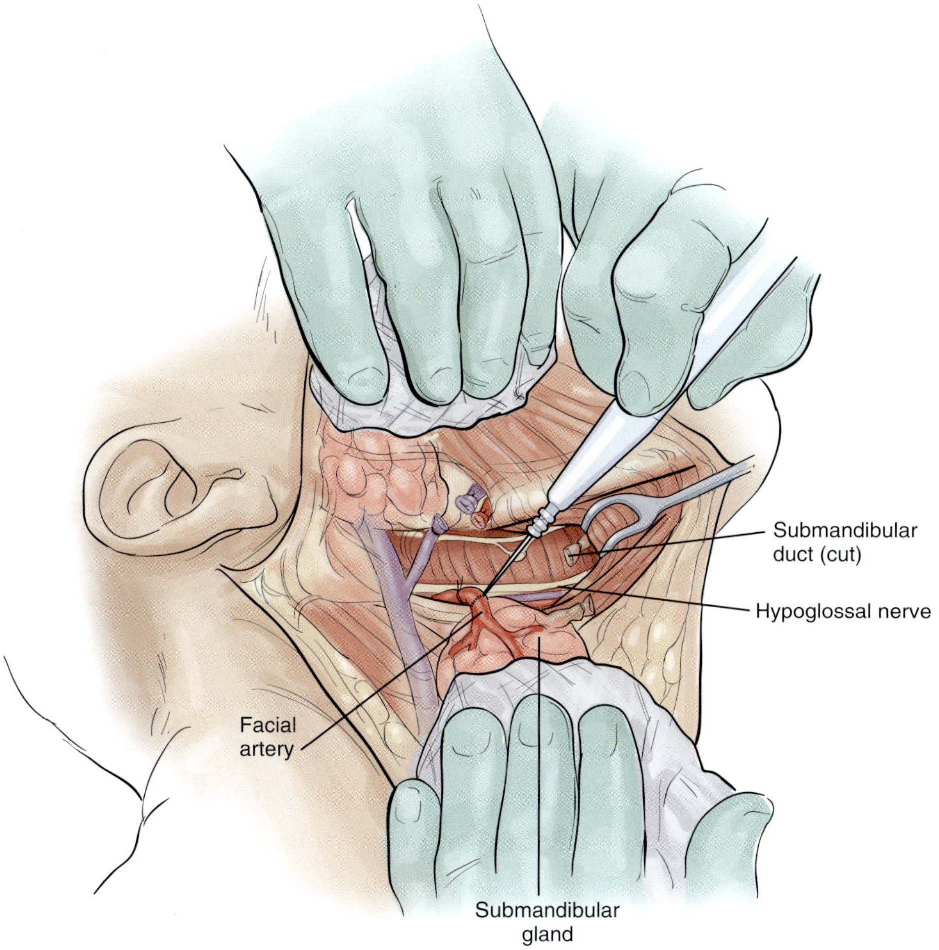

Figure 4-4.

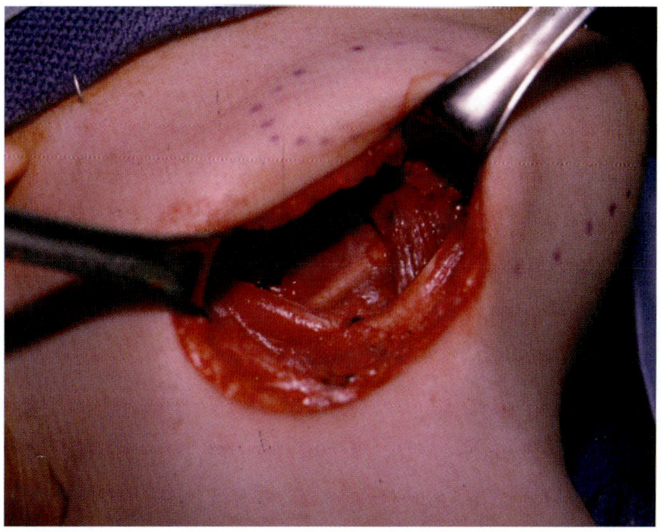

Figure 4-5.

SECTION II

Thoracic

CHAPTER 5

Radical Pneumonectomy

Francesco Leo, MD, PhD, and Lorenzo Spaggiari, MD, PhD

I. SPECIAL PREOPERATIVE PREPARATION

Indications

- Pneumonectomy is usually required in case of central non–small-cell lung cancer or carcinoid. The reason can be bronchial (involvement of the main bronchus), vascular (pulmonary artery and/or pulmonary vein), transfissural, lymph nodal (interbronchial or upper lobe nodal metastases in lower lobe tumors), or mixed. Pneumonectomy may be required for primary mediastinal tumors (thymoma, sarcoma) infiltrating the pulmonary hilum.
- In the case of pulmonary metastases requiring pneumonectomy, the indication is controversial and the decision should be made in the context of multidisciplinary discussion.
- Pneumonectomy may be considered the last resort in case of destroyed lung tissue owing to benign diseases (mainly tuberculosis), keeping in mind that morbidity and mortality are higher as compared to elective pneumonectomy for cancer.

Preoperative Workup

- Key points in preoperative staging are spiral chest/upper abdomen computed tomography (CT) scan, bronchoscopy, and positron emission tomography scan. Relationships between the tumor and pulmonary vessels may predict the type of dissection needed (Fig. 5-1). A brain CT scan is desirable in clinical stage III candidates for pneumonectomy, even in the absence of neurologic symptoms.
- Respiratory function is assessed by blood gas analysis, spirometry (possibly with evaluation of carbon monoxide lung diffusing capacity [DLCO]), and lung perfusion scan. We consider pneumonectomy contraindicated in patients with a predicted postoperative forced expiratory volume 1 or DLCO less than 30% of the predicted value. Exercise tests can be useful in improving risk assessment in doubtful cases, as patients with oxygen consumption during maximum exercise (VO_2max) between 10 and 15 mL/kg/min are considered at high risk, and in those with VO_2max less than 10, the risk is prohibitive. Preoperative cardiac echography should be performed in every case, because pulmonary hypertension drastically increases the risk.
- An increased mortality is expected for pneumonectomy in patients aged 70 years or more, in those with a previous history of cardiac ischemic disease, and when the affected lung is well perfused.
- Preoperative chemotherapy probably increases the risk of respiratory complications.
- When informed consent is discussed, patients should be informed of the expected postoperative mortality (5% to 8%) and possible impact on quality of life.

II. OPERATIVE TECHNIQUE

Position

- The patient is placed in the lateral decubitus position with a pillow at the level of the tip of the scapula, with the arm abducted at 90 degrees and gently fixed, avoiding tension at the level of the brachial plexus (Fig. 5-2, *A*).

Incision

- Our preferred access is lateral thoracotomy because of the absence of definitive injuries to the chest wall element. This incision permits all types of extension of the resection, such as superior vena cava (SVC) replacement, tracheal sleeve pneumonectomy, or left atrial resection. The muscles encountered during the thoracotomy incision are shown in Figure 5-2, *B*.
- The incision line is at the level of the fifth intercostal space, which is entered after separating the serratus anterior muscle fibers.

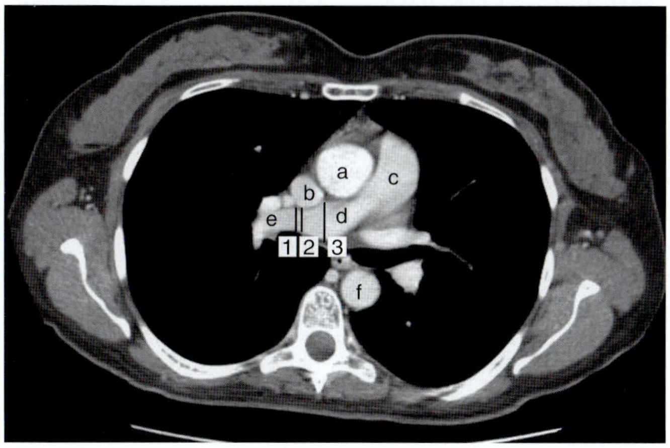

Figure 5-1. The position of the tumor on computed tomography scan may anticipate the type of pulmonary artery isolation needed. The right pulmonary artery can be isolated extrapericardially (*1*), intrapericardially (*2*), or in the Theile sinus (*3*). *a,* Ascending aorta; *b,* superior vena cava, *c,* pulmonary artery common trunk; *d,* right main pulmonary artery; *e,* intermediate artery; *f,* descending aorta.

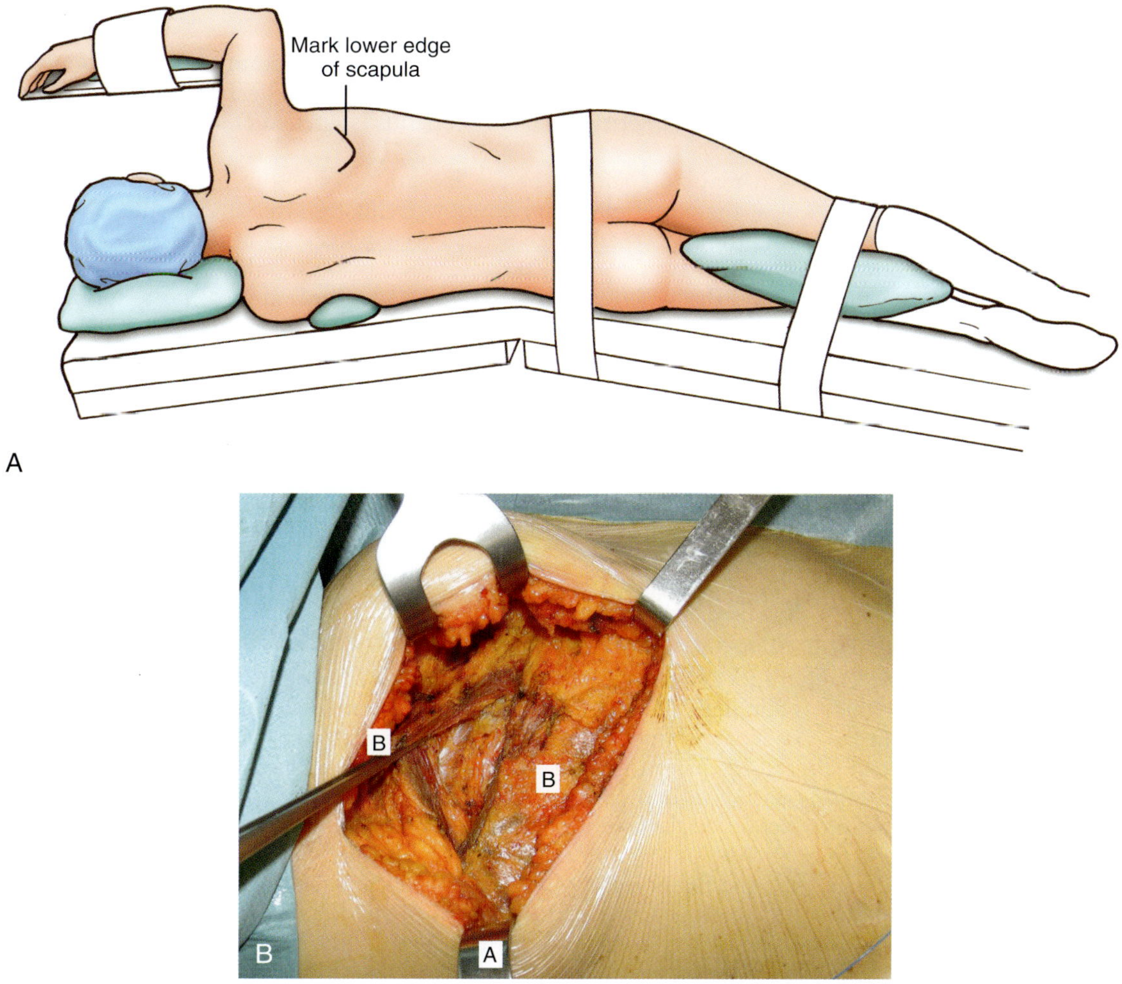

Figure 5-2.

- In case of large paramediastinal masses or involvement of the jugulo-subclavian confluence, sterno-thoracotomy (hemi-clamshell) or anterolateral thoracotomy combine with transmanubrial approach can be used.
- Sternotomy may be the choice in case of mediastinal tumors.

Main Dissection

- Four aspects should be considered intraoperatively before starting resection:
  - ▲ Diagnosis of malignancy should be established when not available preoperatively.
  - ▲ Any suspicion of pleural metastases should be ruled out by frozen section.
  - ▲ Any definitive damage (phrenic nerve, vascular ligation) should be avoided until feasibility of the resection is confirmed by complete exploration.
  - ▲ In case of lung cancer, complete mediastinal dissection should precede lung resection.

Right Hilar Dissection

- After dividing the pulmonary ligament, the inferior pulmonary vein is encircled. The lung is retracted anteriorly, the mediastinal pleura is incised and subcarinal nodal dissection is completed (Fig. 5-3). After ligation of one or more bronchial arteries, the posterior part of the bronchus is exposed.
- At this time, the lung is retracted posteriorly and the anterior hilum dissected. The pulmonary artery (PA) portion visible above the superior pulmonary vein is the mediastinal trunk (the "Boyden" artery) for the upper lobe. The isolation of the entire trunk of the right PA requires the "Price-Thomas maneuver," the section of the pericardial extension (Fig. 5-4) connecting the SVC with the space between the Boyden trunk and the intermediate artery, which is underneath the pulmonary vein. Once this ligament sectioned, the SVC is separated from the main trunk of the artery and an adequate space for isolation is obtained.
- At this time, the superior vein is encircled and retracted downward to further facilitate exposition of the artery, which is now isolated (dissecting it in the subadventitial plane and by the use of a large clamp with a smooth tip).

Left Hilar Dissection

- The first part of the dissection is similar to the case of right pneumonectomy. After division of the pulmonary branches of the vagus nerve and usually one bronchial artery ligation, the space between the descending aorta, esophagus, and inferior left main bronchus is opened and the subcarinal region is exposed.
- The superior pulmonary vein may be encircled before the artery, once the plane between them is identified. Nodal dissection of the aortopulmonary window facilitates arterial exposure at this level. Care should be taken to avoid injury to the left recurrent nerve, which lies at this level.
- The left PA is shorter than the right artery, and its subadventitial plane should be discovered (a) anteriorly to reach the space behind the superior vein (retracted downward) and (b) posteriorly to reach the upper border of the left main bronchus. These two points are the entry and the exit of the dissector when it encircles the blind inferior portion of the artery. In this zone a straight vascular clamp should be positioned in case of PA injury during dissection.

Intrapericardial Dissection

- When tumor extension does not allow a safe preparation of the vessels, the pericardium should be opened and vessels isolated at this level. The pericardial sac is opened in front of the superior pulmonary vein, avoiding phrenic nerve damage.
- **Pulmonary veins:** Pulmonary vein isolation usually is easy because these veins have a portion that is almost completely intrapericardial. After isolating the right inferior pulmonary vein, the pericardial reflection connecting it with the inferior vena cava should be divided.
- **Pulmonary artery:** The right PA can be isolated intrapericardially at two different levels, on the lateral side of the SVC (which is simpler), or in the space between the medial border of the SVC and the ascending aorta, in the Theile sinus (more demanding). In the first case, after separating the artery from the SVC, a large dissector is passed in the subadventitial plane under the guide of the left index finger inserted posteriorly. In the second case, the Theile sinus is opened by gentle retraction on the SVC and more intense retraction on the ascending aorta. At this time, posterior pericardium is incised along the upper and lower border of the artery, and the vessel is encircled.
- On the left side, usually only the inferior part of the artery is intrapericardial. Once the initial part of its extrapericardial portion is identified, the pericardium is divided, and the dissection is continued on its inferior part between the artery and the bronchus. Then, a dissector is passed and the vessel encircled. The section of the ligamentum arteriosum may facilitate this step.

Vascular Ligation

- The timing of vascular ligation is not important in terms of spillage of neoplastic cells or in terms of pulmonary engorgement. In standard cases, we prefer to start with the inferior pulmonary vein, then passing to the superior pulmonary vein and finally to the PA. As for ligation, our preference is for the use of a stapling device (Endo GIA Universal Roticulator 30-2.5, Autosuture, Norwalk, Conn.) both for PA and pulmonary veins. The advantage is the possibility of suturing both sides. The use of a thoracoabdominal (TA) stapler remains a valid alternative, given the favorable angle of the machine. When the ligation of the vessel is preferred, effort should be made to avoid the slipping of the ligature by the use of a transfixed ligature. For the PA, we prefer its section after clamping and subsequent running suture with Prolene 4-0. The distal section is controlled with a second running suture. When this technique is used, it is better to maintain the final ends of the suture, in case clamp repositioning is needed. When suturing the left PA intrapericardially, a generous proximal clamping should be avoided, as the common pulmonary trunk can be restricted, with a consequent impaired blood flow to the right lung, and subsequent right heart failure.

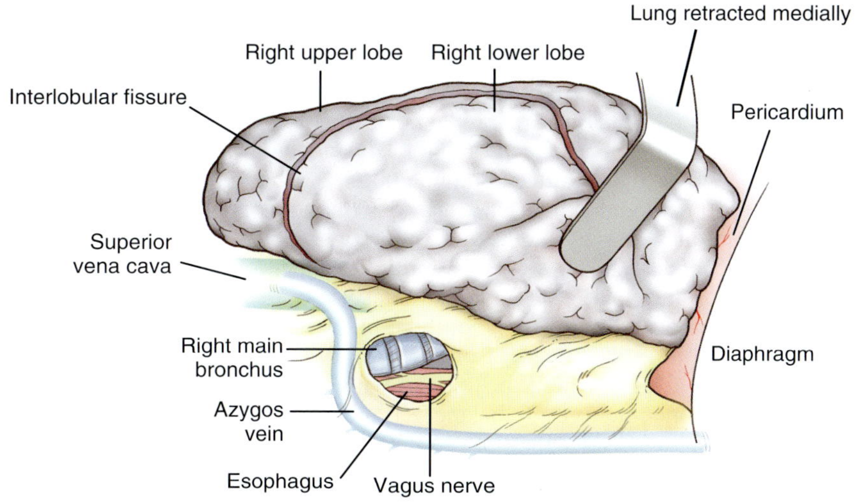

Figure 5-3.

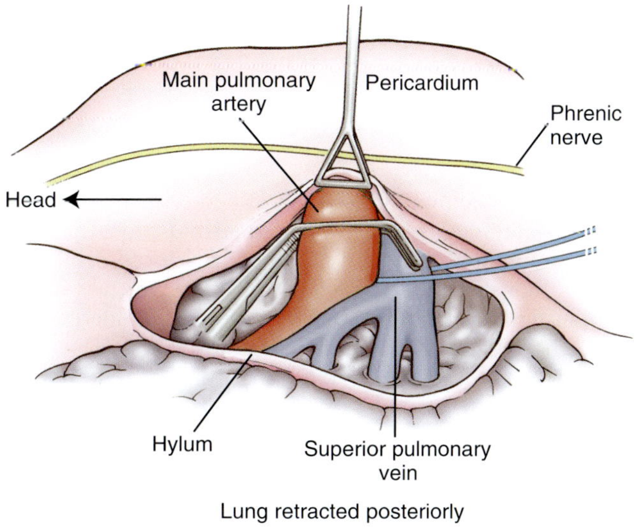

Figure 5-4.

Bronchial Dissection and Suture

- Once the PA is sectioned, dissection continues, separating the bronchus from the pericardium. On the right side, the subcarinal region and the tracheobronchial angle are reached. On the left side, the main bronchus is long, and dissection should be continued until the tracheobronchial angle is reached. Care should be taken to avoid rupture of the membranous bronchial wall. The bronchus is sutured, by placing a TA 30 as close as possible to the carina, and then sectioned. On the left side, upward traction of the lung facilitates positioning the stapler close to the carina (Fig. 5-5). At this time, the lung is removed. The view after completion of the pneumonectomy is seen in Figure 5-6.
- The bronchial suture should be checked for the presence of air leak with an endobronchial pressure greater than 25 cm H_2O. In case of air leak, the bronchial suture should be doubled using the technique of manual bronchial closure. Four to six U stitches are passed and knotted on the cartilaginous part; then a running suture completes the suture.
  - The bronchial stump should be covered to reduce the risk of fistula, especially after right pneumonectomy. The advantage of the use of a pediculated flap (intercostal muscle, pericardial fat) over an autologous nonpediculated flap (pleura, pericardium) remains controversial.

Closure

- **Pericardial closure:** In the case of pericardial resection, the pericardium should be always repaired on the right side, to avoid cardiac herniation. Integrity can be restored by the use of prosthetic material. Reconstruction should be large enough to avoid cardiac constriction (two fingers should be easily able to enter the pericardial sac once the reconstruction is completed) and not watertight to avoid the development of pericardial effusion. Our preference is the use of a Vicryl or bovine pericardium prosthesis fixed by separate 3-0 Prolene stitches. On the left side, pericardial openings can be left unrepaired if they are large enough to avoid cardiac strangulation.
- **Hemostasis:** The postpneumonectomy space is at risk of bleeding by definition, because of its negative pressure and the presence of multiple sites of potential delayed bleeding (site of nodal dissection, pleurectomy, mediastinal fat). All sites of active bleeding, even if minimal, should be controlled before closure. In the case of diffuse parietal bleeding, systematic ligature of intercostal arteries can be useful. Once hemostasis is completed, the cavity should be filled with saline, and the surgeon should wait for 5 to 10 minutes to confirm the absence of new sites of bleeding before definitive closing.
- **Drainage:** We use a 32 Ch chest drain positioned with the tip below the bronchial stump line, connected to a Pleur-Evac pneumonectomy balanced double-valve collecting system.
- **Closure:** Thoracotomy is closed by the use of two Maxon loop "X" stitches.

III. ALTERNATIVE TECHNICAL APPROACHES (PRO/CON) AND PEARLS

The "Sandwich" Technique for Bronchial Protection

- The technique we developed for bronchial stump protection is the "sandwich" technique. The stump is covered by 2.5 mL of fibrin glue (Tissucol) (Fig. 5-7). Then a large flap of parietal pleura is prepared and positioned on the stump, separating the mediastinum from the pleural cavity. Finally, an additional 2.5 mL of fibrin glue is instilled on the border of the flap to fix its position.

Extended Pneumonectomy

- In very selected cases, pneumonectomy may be associated with resection of structures contiguous to the lung (in order of technical difficulty: chest wall, left atrium, SVC, tracheal carina). These operations are defined as extended pneumonectomy and require experienced centers and skilled surgeons.
- **Left atrium:** When the tumor infiltrates the left atrium through the pulmonary vein, atrial resection can be performed by an intrapericardial approach. Before starting the resection, the atrial clamp should be positioned to verify the absence of hemodynamic instability. Then, pneumonectomy is begun, leaving the atrial resection as the last step. If additional space is required, the Sondergaard maneuver (preparation of the interatrial sulcus) can be carefully performed. Atrial clamp positioning should avoid tumor squeezing that can cause tumoral embolism. After atrial section, a double running suture is performed using 3-0 Prolene.
- **Superior vena cava:** Surgical strategy depends on the degree of SVC infiltration. Direct repair is the simplest reconstruction but it is acceptable when the caliber of the repaired SVC is 50% or more of the original value. When this is not the case, the SVC can be repaired by an autologous pericardial patch or replaced by a prosthesis (Teflon or bovine pericardium; we prefer the latter) (Fig. 5-8). SVC replacement is performed using temporary cross-clamping of the vessel. It requires different fluid management before cross-clamping as compared to the other types of pneumonectomy to reduce the risk of cerebral edema. In some cases, SVC resection is combined with carinal resection; in this case it represents the first step of the procedure.

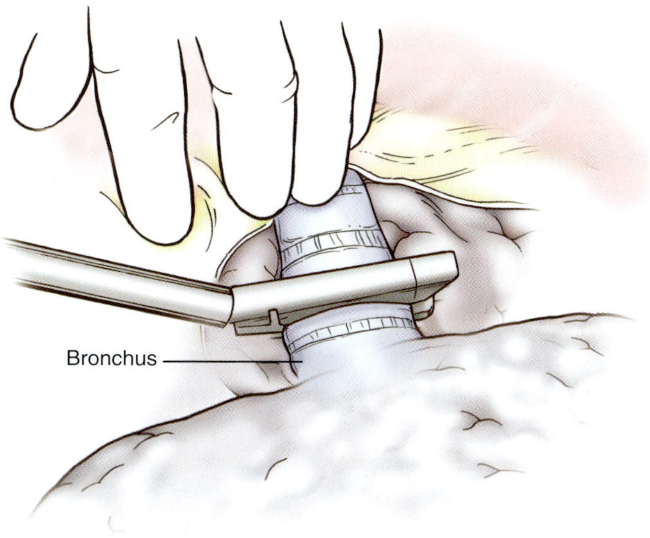

Figure 5-5.

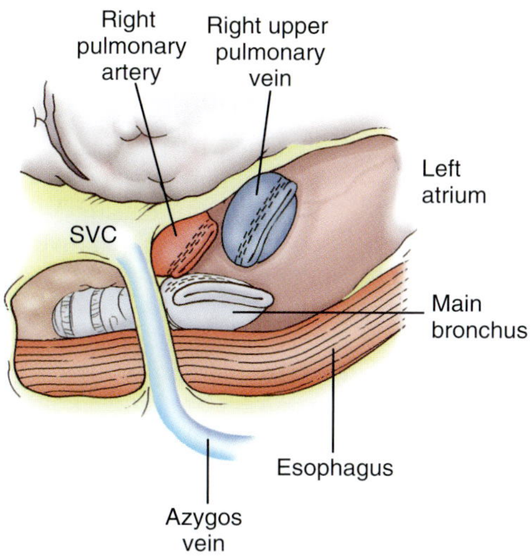

Figure 5-6. *SVC,* Superior vena cava.

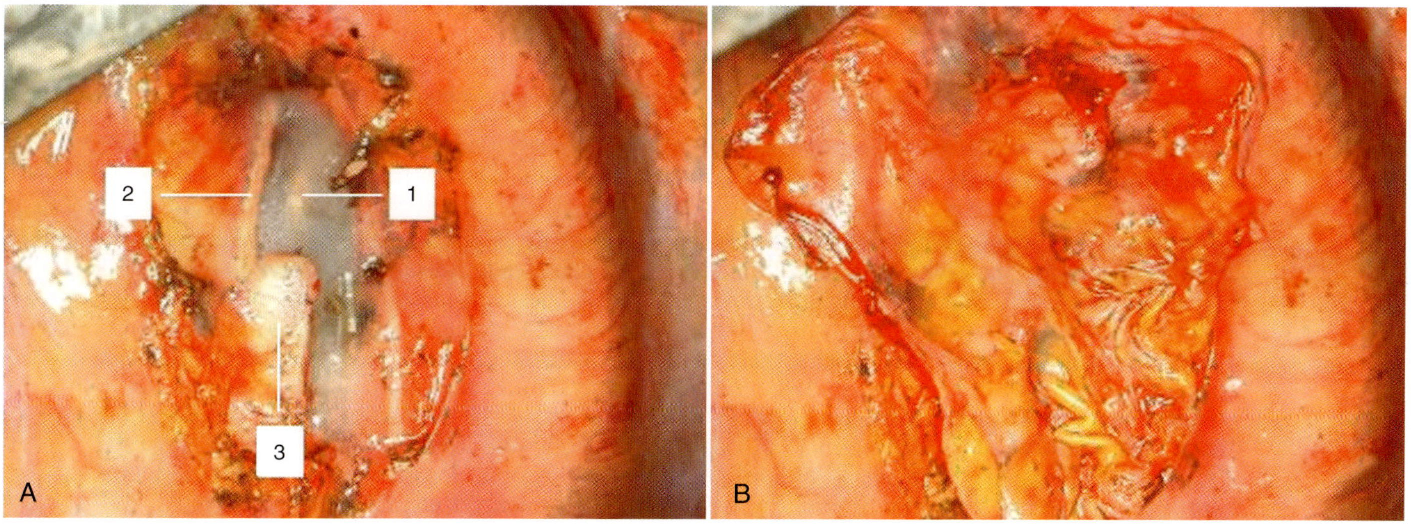

Figure 5-7. The "sandwich" technique for the bronchial stump protection. A, Bronchial stump (*1*) is covered by 2.5 mL of fibrin glue (Tissucol) (*2*) pulmonary artery stump; (*3*) superior pulmonary vein stump.). **B,** Large flap of parietal pleura is prepared and positioned on the stump, separating the mediastinum from the pleural cavity. Then an additional 2.5 mL of fibrin glue is instilled on the border of the flap to fix its position.

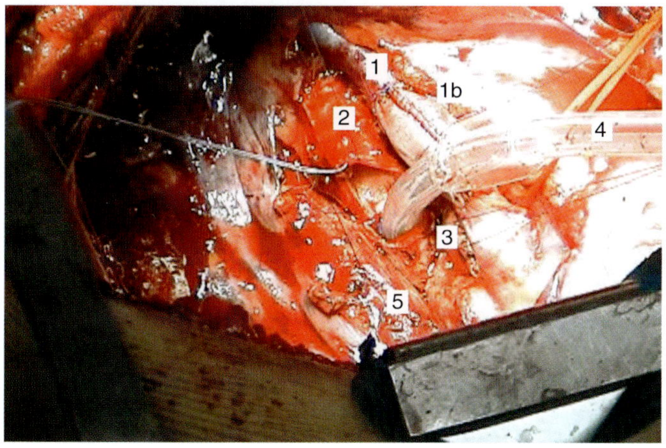

Figure 5-8. Right tracheal sleeve pneumonectomy associated to superior vena cava resection. After replacement of the superior vena cava (*1*) using a bovine pericardium prosthesis (*1b*), airways are sectioned at the level of the trachea (*2*) and the left main bronchus origin (*3*). Once the right lung is removed en bloc with the carina, the lung is ventilated through the operative field (*4*) and the airway reconstructed by a continuous anastomosis (*5,* esophagus).

- **Tracheal sleeve pneumonectomy:** Infiltration of the tracheobronchial carina may require its resection to obtain a radical resection. This situation is rare on the right side, exceptional on the left side. After vascular steps, section of the azygos vein, and adequate preparation, the trachea and the left main bronchus are sectioned and the right lung removed en bloc with the carina. Left lung oxygenation is obtained by the mean of left intubation through the operative field (see Fig. 5-8) or jet ventilation. Meanwhile, the suture between the trachea and the left main bronchus is performed (continuous running suture using 3-0 Prolene). To reduce the tension on the anastomosis, the pericardium is widely opened. If postoperative fistula occurs, there is no effective repair procedure to overcome the problem, and this represents the main risk of the procedure (5% to 10%).

Pearls

- In case of difficult dissection, do not hesitate to open the pericardium and isolate vessels intrapericardially.
- The dissection of the PA should be done in the subadventitial plane.
- Maximal care should be taken with bronchial closure and protection.
- Meticulous hemostasis is mandatory, particularly after chemotherapy.
- Minimize intravenous fluid intake intraoperatively and for the first 3 postoperative days.

IV. SPECIAL POSTOPERATIVE CARE

Perioperative Management

- Perioperative management should be devoted to minimizing the damage to the remaining lung. The key points are intravenous fluid restriction (on the order of 5-7 mL/kg/hr crystalloid infusion, not exceeding a total of 1500 mL in 24 hours) and a protective-ventilation strategy (a tidal volume at or below 6 mL/kg, a driving pressure less than 20 cm H_2O above the positive end-expiratory pressure value, permissive hypercapnia, and the preferential use of pressure-limited ventilatory modes).

Bronchopleural Fistula

- Pleural space is progressively filled by fluid during the first 7 to 10 postoperative days. Over a period of several months, the cavity retracts, and fluid is almost completely substituted by fibrous tissue.
- The early persistent incomplete filling of the cavity or the late reappearance of air in the cavity are radiologic signs of bronchopleural fistula, even in asymptomatic patients, and require bronchoscopy. The main symptom of fistula is cough, at rest or evoked by decubitus on the nonoperated side. Other signs are respiratory (due to fluid spillage on the contralateral lung) and infectious (fever, weight loss, purulent cough). Once the diagnosis is obtained, the cavity should be drained (under CT guidance in case of mediastinal shift). Early fistula (<15 days) is generally due to technical causes, and surgical repair is advisable. In case of small (<5 mm) late fistula, endoscopic closure with multiple fibrin glue instillations may be successful, eventually associated with prolonged pleural lavage if tolerated. In the case of a large, late fistula, thoracostomy should be performed once general conditions are stabilized.

SUGGESTED READINGS

Goldstraw P: Pneumonectomy and its modifications. In Shields TW, LoCicero J, Ponn RB, editors: *General thoracic surgery*, ed 5, Philadelphia, 2000, Lippincott Williams & Wilkins, pp 411–421.

Jougon J, Dubois G, Velly JF: Les techniques de pneumonectomie. In *Encyclopedie medico-chirurgicale*. Chirurgie thoracique [vol I], pp 142–300.

Le Brigand H: Les pneumonectomies. In Le Brigand H, editor: *Nouveau traité de technique*, Paris, 1973, Masson & C Editeurs, pp 245–261.

CHAPTER 6

Resection of Pulmonary Metastases

Reza Mehran, MD SBStJ, MDCM, MSc, FRCSC, FACS, and Jack A. Roth, MD

I. SPECIAL PREOPERATIVE PREPARATION

- The primary lesion must be controlled locally with no evidence of residual disease. Any suspicion of residual or recurrent disease must be evaluated before the resection of pulmonary metastases.
- There must be no evidence of metastatic disease elsewhere, particularly to such sites as the liver or the brain, which can be occult unless specifically looked for. Usual evaluation of the liver is by computed tomography (CT) scan and the brain by magnetic resonance imaging. A positron emission tomography scan may be useful for evaluating other sites.
- Review of previous radiographs of the patient gives an insight into the doubling time of the tumor. Patients with tumor doubling times less than 20 days usually do not do well, often recur shortly after resection, and have a median survival of less than 1 year. Patients with a tumor doubling time of more than 40 days have a 65% 5-year survival. An exception can be made for those patients requiring a palliative resection for a tumor not amenable to less invasive palliative measures such as stereotactic radiation therapy or selective bronchial artery embolization.
- Other poor risk factors in relation to outcome after surgery include disease-free interval of less than 6 months, and histology of breast cancer or melanoma, which tend to metastasize to other viscera before they invade the lung.
- Although there is no threshold to the limit of metastases that can be removed in one patient, most studies show that patients with more than four metastases tend to have a markedly shortened survival.
- In some cases synchronous extrapulmonary metastases can be resected before the pulmonary metastasectomy. An example is a patient with colorectal metastases to the liver and lung. The extrathoracic sites should be dealt with first in order for the patient to have full lung function during the extrathoracic surgery.
- All pulmonary metastases must be resectable by multiple wedges, segmentectomy, or lobectomy. Only in special circumstances should a pneumonectomy be considered in the management of patients with metastases.
- The patient must have an adequate pulmonary reserve to be able to tolerate the planned procedure. Pulmonary reserve is evaluated by: (1) an office determination of the Zubrod performance status obtained from an adequate history and physical examination and a walk test, and (2) a flow loop study. If the patient shows borderline function, then further evaluation by a ventilation perfusion scan and a calculation of oxygen consumption should be done.
- Some primary tumors, when metastatic to the lung, can also spread to local and regional lymph nodes. Typical examples are colon cancer and renal cell carcinoma. In these patients, the preoperative evaluation should include also a search for such nodes in the hilum or the mediastinum. Enlarged lymph nodes can be biopsied by mediastinoscopy or by endobronchial ultrasound–guided biopsy. The indication for surgery in patients with lymph node involvement is not clear because these patients generally have a poor prognosis. If a patient has a single metastatic lesion with lymph nodes in one station only, a case can be made to resect all visible disease.
- With standard CT scanning techniques using collimations of 1 cm, the risk of underestimating the number of metastases is 35% to 40%. The risk of overestimating the lesions is 25% to 30%. Therefore, accurate information is only obtained in about 70% to 75% of patients. When CT is used to look for

metastatic disease, collimations of 5 mm or less should be used, because this increases the accuracy of the preoperative evaluation.

- A single pulmonary lesion in a patient with a previous history of malignancy cannot be assumed to be metastatic unless properly investigated. This requires a tissue diagnosis. A solitary pulmonary nodule is likely to be a metastasis in 60% to 80% of patients with a history of sarcoma or melanoma, in 50% of patients with prior adenocarcinoma, and in less than 20% of patients with prior squamous cell or prostatic carcinoma.
- Unless contraindicated, patients should have a trial of systemic therapy before resection (Fig. 6-1). This is particularly true for osteosarcomas and germ cell tumors metastatic to the chest. Leaving the metastases in situ during the administration of systemic chemotherapy offers a window into the therapeutic efficacy of the first-line chemotherapy chosen. The period in which the patient is on chemotherapy is also an excellent opportunity to assess the progression of the disease. For patients with renal cell carcinoma, effective chemotherapy is not available, and the primary treatment of pulmonary metastases is surgery.
- In patients with many small metastases, the chances of missing a lesion is increased as the size of the lesions decreases. Metastasectomy should not be attempted for lesions less than 5 mm in size unless tissue is needed for diagnostic or experimental therapeutic reasons such as the determination of genetic makeups. Small lesions of indeterminate etiology can be followed by serial CT scans.
- All patients treated surgically for metastatic disease need a careful follow-up after resection to detect recurrence (Fig. 6-2). About 50% of patients will eventually recur after an initial resection and require more surgery, an argument for using lung-sparing maneuvers at the time of each resection.
- Other modalities to treat patients with fewer than four metastases include stereotactic radiation therapy and radiofrequency ablation. These techniques can be used in combination with surgery in patients with bilateral disease, or in those cases where the patient refuses or is not a candidate for surgery (Fig. 6-3).

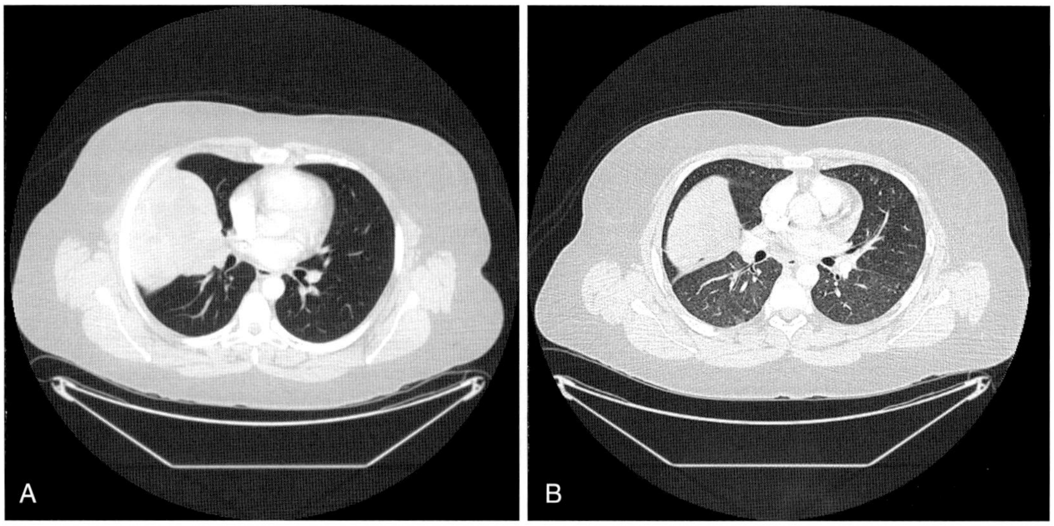

Figure 6-1.

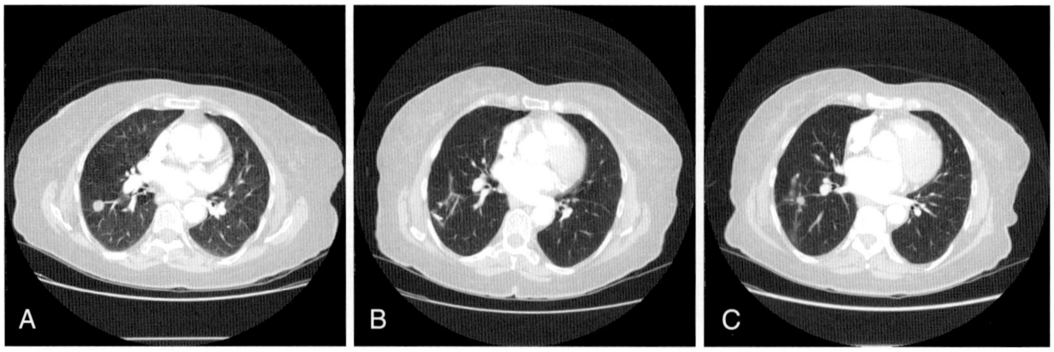

Figure 6-2.

II. OPERATIVE TECHNIQUE

Position

- The position of the patient is based on the planned procedure. For unilateral metastases, patients are usually positioned in the lateral decubitus position and prepared for a posterolateral thoracotomy or video-assisted thoracoscopic surgery (VATS) (Fig. 6-4). Bilateral lesions are approached by either sequential thoracotomies, or by sternotomy which can be done midline or transverse (clamshell incision).

Incision

- The first part of the procedure consists in localizing all metastases as indicated by the CT scan which should be displayed in the operating room at the time of the surgery. The CT scan is used as a road map. The lung must be palpated to detect any other disease not picked up by the CT scan. This is the reason some surgeons do not perform VATS, where a complete palpation of the lung is difficult.

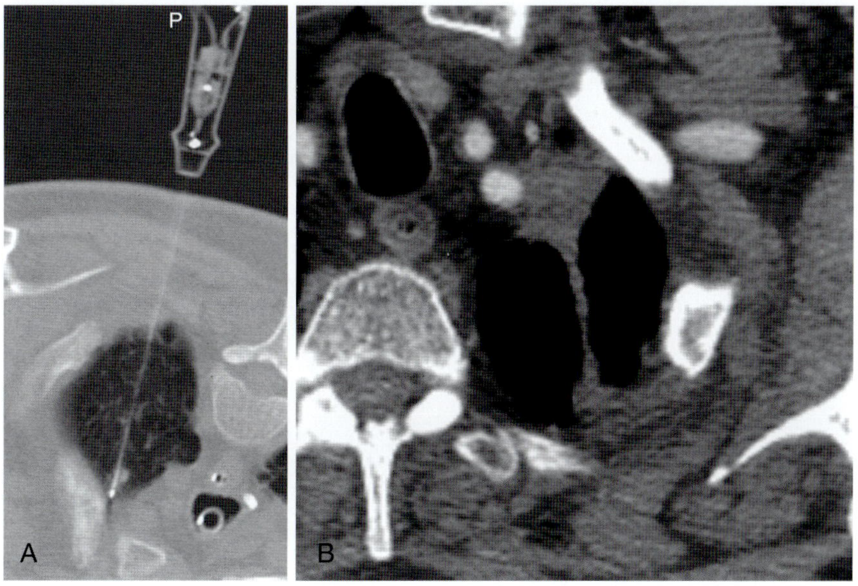

Figure 6-3.

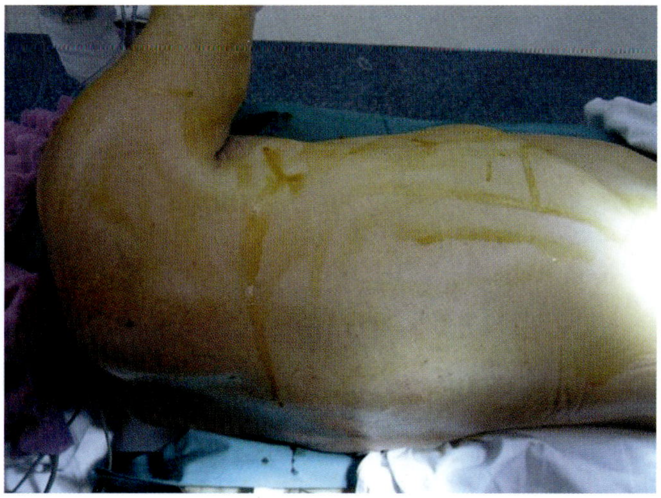
Figure 6-4.

- The placement of the trocar for VATS can be done in a standard fashion for every case (Fig. 6-5, *A*). The thoracoscope trocar is place about four finger breadths below the tip of the scapula. This is followed by a 5-mm trocar inserted posterior to the scapula. The utility incision should be the size of the tumor or the lung to be removed (see Fig. 6-5, *B*). An entire lobe can be resected through a 5-cm incision. Tumors of up to 4 cm can be removed without rib spreading.

Main Dissection

- The index finger of the surgeon must be inserted through the anterior access incision and a careful exploration of the entire lung done. The surface of the lung can be palpated using a forceps to bring the inaccessible lung to the tip of the finger (Fig. 6-6). Care must be taken to avoid injuring the lung with the forceps. A parenchymal hematoma can mimic a mass, and in patients with many small metastases this can confuse the exploration. To prevent this problem, the lung should be grasped on its sharp edges rather than on its flat surface.
- Once the metastases have all been accounted for, the resections can be planned.

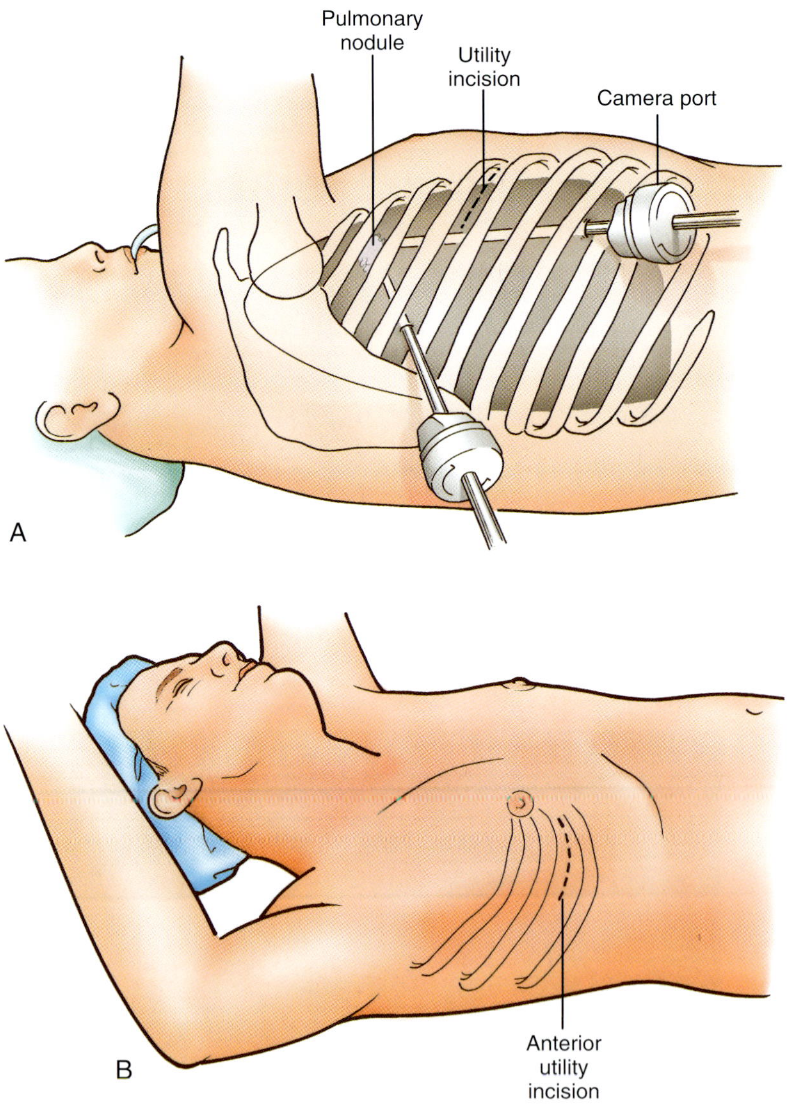

Figure 6-5.

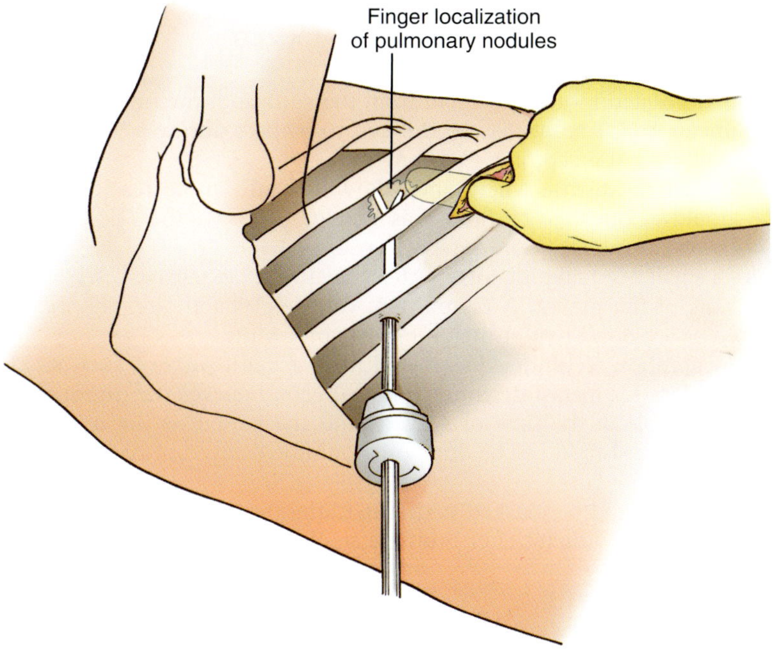

Figure 6-6.

- Metastasectomy is performed with staple applicators (Fig. 6-7). The thickness of the staple is based on the health and thickness of the lung surrounding the metastasis. Usually a cartridge containing the thickest staples (green load with all manufacturers) is appropriate in normal lung. To prevent air leak after resection in patients with emphysema, a thinner staple or reinforcement of the thickest one with Dacron or bovine pericardium should be used.
- If a lobectomy or segmentectomy is necessary to remove a centrally located tumor, the procedure can be done in either an anatomic or nonanatomic fashion.
- With colon, breast, and renal-cell carcinomas, lymph nodes should be sampled at the time of resection of the metastases.
- In patients with single metastatic deposits where the tumor involves the chest wall, diaphragm, or mediastinal structures, the type of resection must be dictated by the type of tumor-host relationship. Tumors with slow doubling time and long disease-free interval can be candidates for a more aggressive resection.

Closure

- When a metastasis is passed through the chest wall, especially when the incision is small, such as in thoracoscopic procedures, the wound must be protected from tumor spillage, because tumor implantation can occur.
- The wound must be then irrigated copiously with saline or water.
- Pleural drainage is established, and the wounds are closed in layers.

III. ALTERNATIVE APPROACHES (PRO/CON) AND PEARLS

- In general, lesions situated more than 3 cm from the surface of the inflated lung, or those less than 5 to 8 mm in diameter on CT scan, may be difficult to palpate during a VATS procedure. These lesions should be removed by a thoracotomy incision.
- In patients with bilateral disease where one side will require more resection than the other, the less involved side should be operated on first. This strategy will leave the side with more residual lung for one-lung ventilation during the more extensive resection.
- The problem of a small residual lung for the chest cavity after extensive resection should be anticipated before the opening of the pleura. A pleural tent can be elevated after the incision of the intercostal muscle and used as a pleural tent at the end of the procedure.
- Intraoperative localization techniques borrowed from general surgery, such as radiologically inserted wire, are not necessary for metastasectomy. If the surgeon believes the tumor, or one of the tumors, is too small to be palpable at the time of surgery, and the patient is not a candidate for an anatomic resection, the procedure should not be done or should be delayed until the tumor becomes larger and more palpable.
- All identified lesions should be marked with a marking pen or suture before resection. Identification of nodules becomes more difficult after multiple staple lines are present.

IV. SPECIAL POSTOPERATIVE CARE

- The immediate postoperative care of patients after metastasectomy is similar to that of patients who have had any type of pulmonary resection. Chest tubes are used to drain fluid and air under suction until ready to be removed.
- In patients with a small residual lung, airway mucus mobilization should be encouraged aggressively. In patients with continuous leak of air beyond 3 days, pneumoperitoneum, blood patch, or talc sclero therapy can be used to collapse any residual pleural space.
- Serum tumor markers, when appropriate, should be repeated immediately after the surgery.
- Patients should have a baseline CT scan repeated once the lung has healed, at about 3 months after the resection, and then every 6 months thereafter. The length of the follow-up must be tailored to the tumor-host relationship.
- Results of pulmonary metastasectomy are histology dependent. Soft tissue sarcoma has a 5-year survival of 30% to 60%, colorectal carcinoma 25% to 30%, renal cell carcinoma 20% to 50%, testicular carcinoma 60% to 80%, and head and neck carcinoma 20% to 30%. The prognosis for patients with melanoma and breast carcinoma metastatic to the lung is poor, although selected patients with lung as the first and only site of metastases that can be completely resected can achieve long-term survival.

SUGGESTED READINGS

Casiraghi M, De Pas T, Maisonneuve P, et al: A 10-year single-center experience on 708 lung metastasectomies: the evidence of the "International Registry of Lung Metastases", *J Thorac Oncol* 6:1373–1378, 2011.

Mehran RJ: Assessment of the patient with pulmonary metastases. In Deslauriers J, Mehran R, editors: *Handbook of perioperative care in general thoracic surgery*, Philadelphia, 2005, Mosby, p 129.

Putnam JB Jr: New and evolving treatment methods for pulmonary metastases, *Semin Thorac Cardiovasc Surg* 14:49–56, 2002.

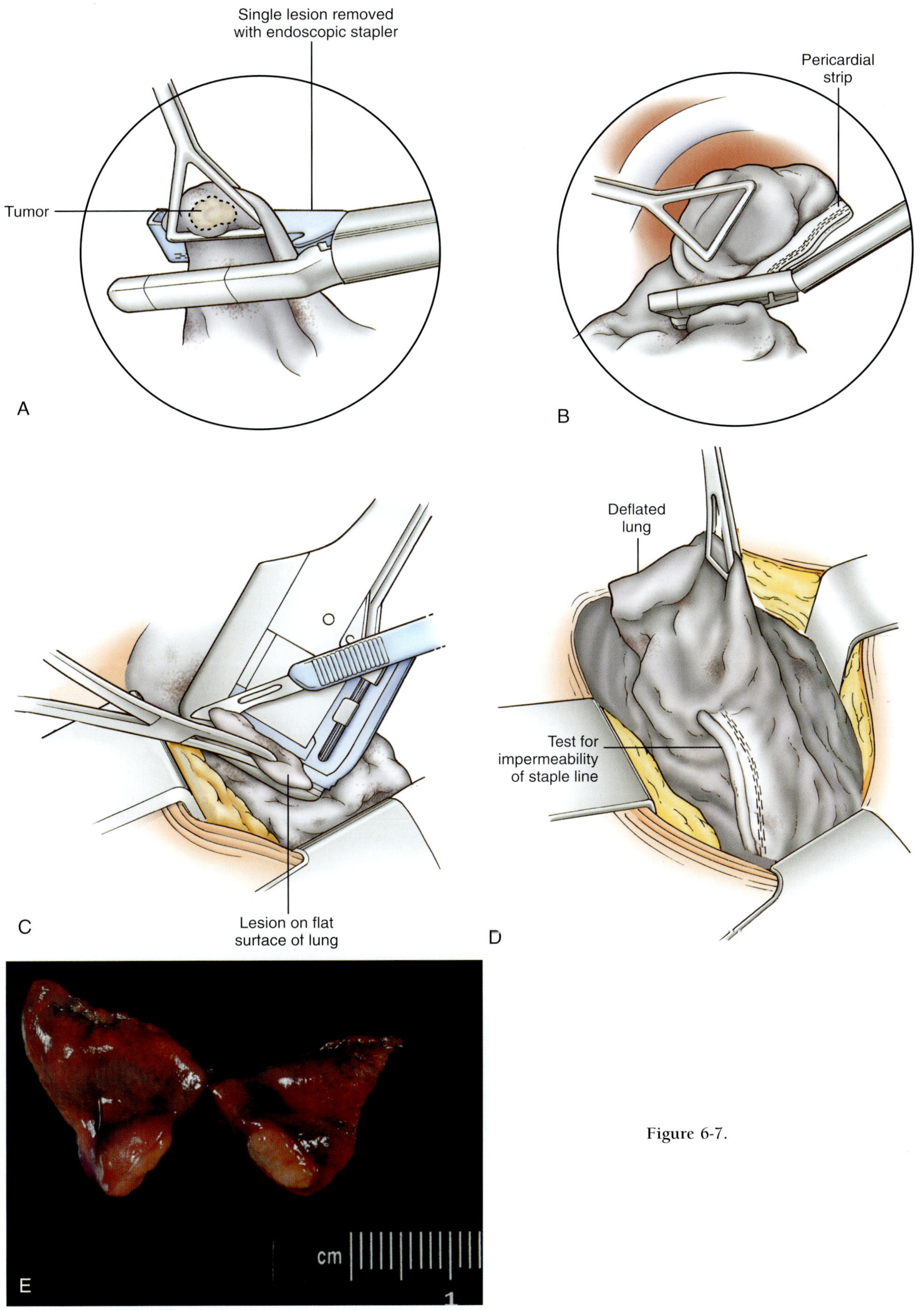
Single lesion removed
with endoscopic stapler
Tumor
A
Pericardial
strip
B
Deflated
lung
Test for
impermeability
of staple line
C
Lesion on flat
surface of lung
D
cm
E

Figure 6-7.

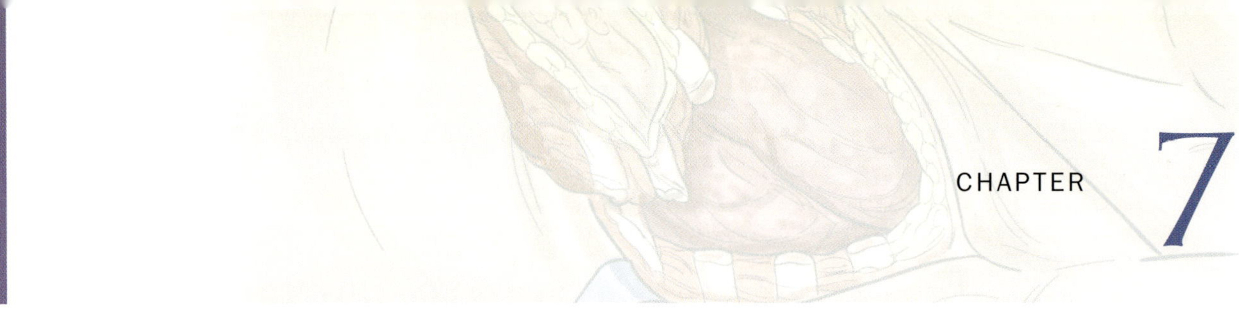

CHAPTER 7

Video-Assisted Thoracoscopic Lobectomy

Robert J. McKenna, Jr., MD, and Ali Mahtabifard, MD

I. SPECIAL PREOPERATIVE PREPARATION

- Almost all patients with stage I non-small cell lung carcinoma (NSCLC) are candidates for lobectomy by video-assisted thoracoscopic surgery (VATS).
- The workup includes a physiologic evaluation to ensure that there are no medical contraindications, such as poor pulmonary function or severe cardiac disease.
- We do not routinely obtain cardiac stress testing unless the electrocardiogram is abnormal or unless there is a history of cardiac disease.
- Pulmonary function tests should predict that the postoperative forced expiratory volume 1 (FEV_1) will be at least 40% of predicted. If the pulmonary function test is borderline, the patient may need a quantitative pulmonary perfusion test to determine if the area to be resected has minimal function, so that it can be resected.
- Patients are also evaluated to rule out metastatic disease.
- Specific tests are ordered based upon the patients' symptoms. For example, a brain MRI is only ordered if the patient has headaches or neurologic symptoms.
- Positron emission tomography (PET) scans are currently used to look for nodal or distant metastases.
- Mediastinoscopy is performed unless the tumor is clinical stage IA by preoperative PET and computed tomography (CT) scans.
- Almost all lobectomies for stage I disease can be done with VATS. Table 7-1 lists the indications and relative contraindications for VATS lobectomy. Except for inability to tolerate single-lung ventilation, most limitations are due to anatomical considerations.

II. OPERATIVE TECHNIQUE

Position

- VATS lobectomy is performed under general anesthesia with one-lung ventilation.
- After intubation with a double-lumen tube, perform fiberoptic bronchoscopy to ensure proper placement of the tube and to rule out any endobronchial lesions.
- Intraoperative hypoxia, even in patients with very severe emphysema ($FEV_1 < 30\%$), is usually due to poor placement of the double-lumen endotracheal tube and can be corrected by simple adjustment of the tube using bronchoscopy.
- Place the patient in lateral decubitus position with a slight posterior tilt.
- Flex the bed to help get the hip out of the way of the trocar and thoracoscope. This also helps to open the intercostal spaces.
- The surgeon stands on the anterior side of the patient and the assistant stands posteriorly.

Incision

- The *first incision* is a 2-cm incision for most firings of the stapler (Fig. 7-1). Make it in the sixth intercostal space in the midclavicular line. This is usually one intercostal space below the mammary crease or halfway between the mammary crease and the costal margin. Make the incision in the middle of the interspace and tunnel it posteriorly through the tissues of the chest wall. Make the incision perpendicular to the skin because there may be bleeding from smaller branches of the mammary artery, and instruments passing through this incision will bump into the pericardium.

- For preemptive analgesia, inject local anesthetic (0.5% bupivacaine with epinephrine) close to the spine into the intercostal spaces from about T4 to T10. Be careful to infiltrate the inferior border of ribs without injecting into the intravascular space. This can be done under visualization by the thoracoscope. The goal is to "raise a pleural wheal" just superficial to the endothoracic fascia. This provides an effective intercostal nerve block, which can reduce postoperative pain.
- Make a *second incision* for the trocar and thoracoscope. Place it through a 5-mm incision in the eighth or ninth intercostal space in the midaxillary line or the posterior axillary line. Make the incision 1 cm below a rib and angle it superiorly to reduce the pressure on the intercostal nerve.
- A 5- or 10-mm thoracoscope can be used. We use a 5-mm scope because it requires a smaller incision and places less torque on the intercostal nerve. Place this incision low in the chest to achieve the best panoramic view of the thoracic cavity. In addition, the 30-degree lens allows much greater flexibility for the surgeon to see around the hilar structures. Make all other incisions directly through the middle of an intercostal space.
- A ring forceps through the midclavicular incision pushes the lung posteriorly to expose the superior pulmonary vein. Make the *third* 4- to 6-cm utility *incision* directly up from the superior pulmonary vein (generally the fourth intercostal space) for upper lobectomies, or one intercostal space lower for middle or lower lobectomies.

TABLE 7-1 Indications and Contraindications for Video-Assisted Thoracoscopic Surgery Lobectomy

INDICATIONS	CONTRAINDICATIONS
Stage 1 lung cancer	Chest wall invasion
Tumor ≦ 6 cm	Tumor > 6 cm
? Sleeve resection	Preoperative radiation
Benign disease (bullae, sequestration, etc.)	? Sleeve resection
	Abnormal nodes
	Surgeon's technical ability

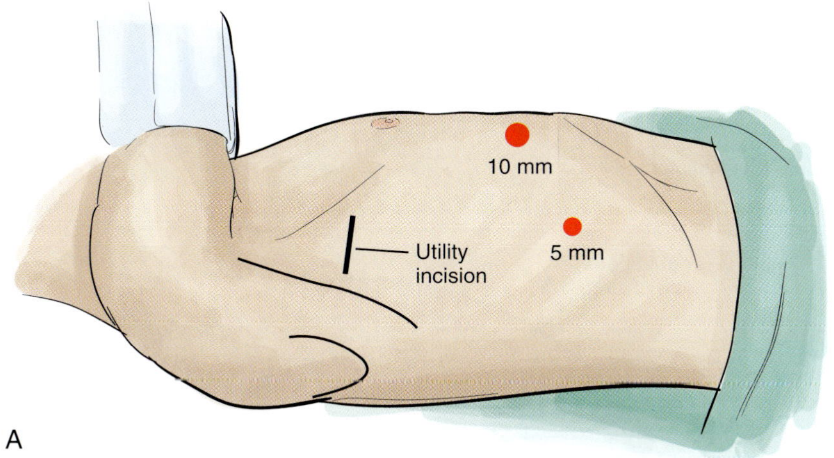

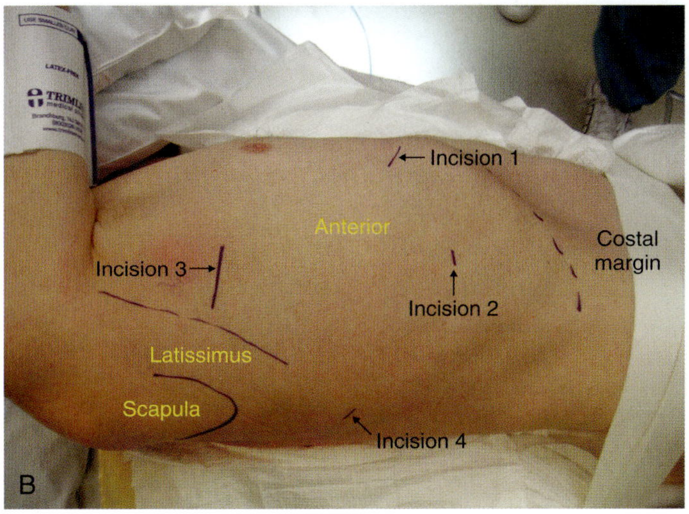

Figure 7-1. (*B from McKenna RJ, Mahtabifard A, Swanson S, editors:* Atlas of minimally invasive thoracic surgery [VATS], *Philadelphia, 2010, Saunders.*)

- Through this incision, a finger first palpates the lung to find the lung nodule; we rarely perform transthoracic needle biopsies of suspicious masses. A VATS wedge resection of the mass is performed through these same incisions and sent to pathology. If the mass proves to be an NSCLC on frozen section, extend this third incision to about 4 to 5 cm and perform a VATS lobectomy.
- Do not spread the ribs, but a Weitlaner retractor or an Alexis wound protector may be used to hold the soft tissues of the chest wall open, because the lung would expand if no air could enter the chest through the incision while suctioning in the chest and because the open incision allows easier passage of instruments into the chest. The hilar structures are easily accessible for dissection through this incision.
- The *fourth incision* is a 1-cm incision made posteriorly in the auscultatory triangle to facilitate dissection and provide further control of the operation, especially when teaching.

Main Dissection

- Because the lung is very mobile, almost all aspects of the lung, and therefore all lesions, can be directly palpated through the utility incision.

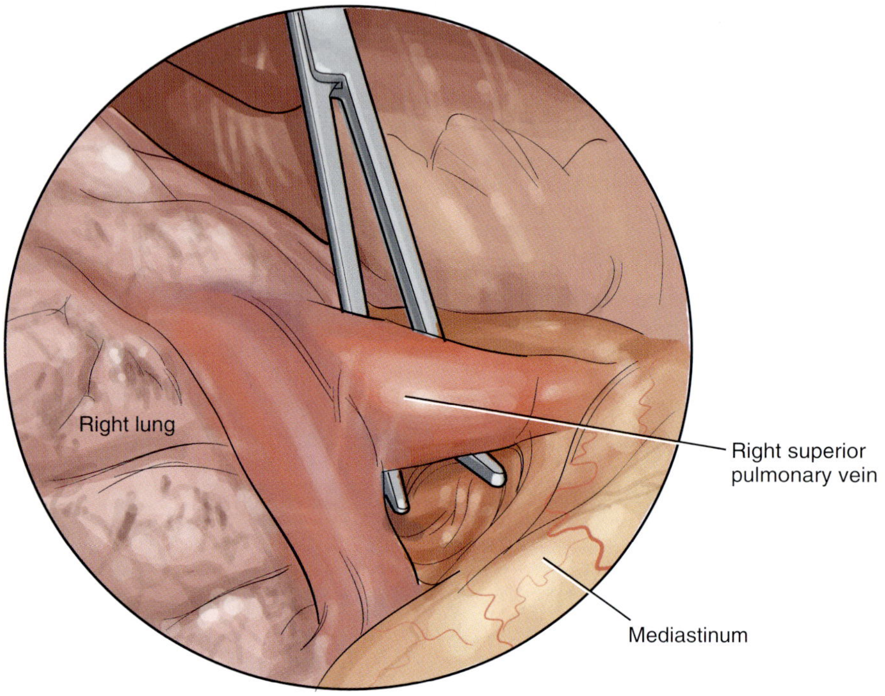

Figure 7-2.

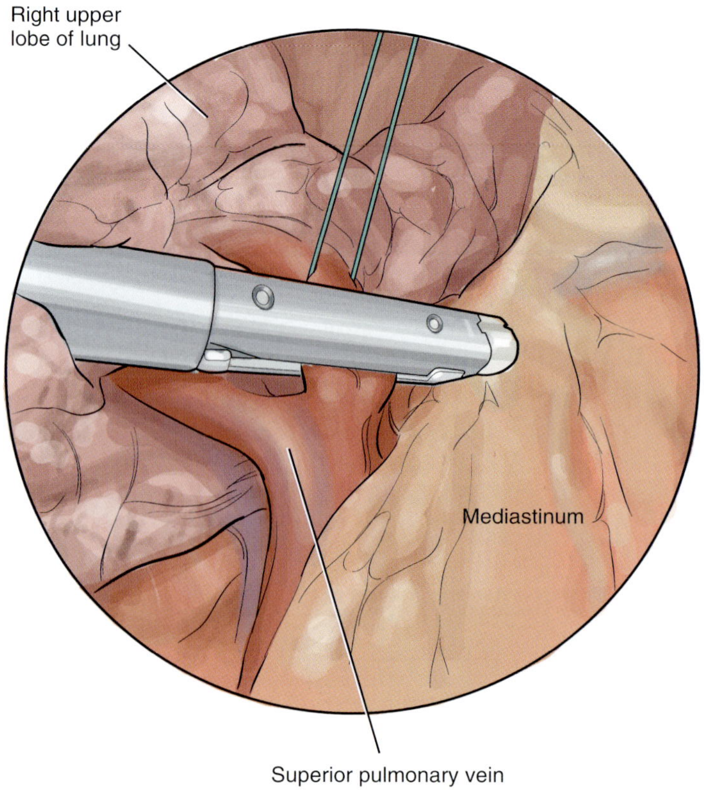

Figure 7-3.

- Trocars are not used except for the camera.
- Perform the entire operation with conventional long instruments that are available in any operating room and are familiar to the thoracic surgeon.
- Visualization of the chest cavity and the hilum is on the monitor and not through the incision.
- Next, begin the dissection of the hilar structures with visualization on the monitor. The clarity and magnification that is afforded by modern day optics provides a comprehensive view of the hilar structures.
- We have previously noted the technical details of how to perform the various lobectomies.
- The general concept is that the pulmonary vein, artery, and bronchus are individually identified, dissected, isolated, and stapled (Ethicon, Cincinnati). Articulation of the stapler is unnecessary as proper placement of the incisions at the outset provides optimal angles. A VATS lobectomy should be a standard anatomic dissection. Simultaneous ligation of hilar structures should be discouraged.
- In general, the pulmonary vein is the first structure to be dissected and stapled with a vascular stapler (Figs. 7-2 and 7-3).
- Next, dissect and staple the branches of the pulmonary artery (Figs. 7-4 and 7-5).

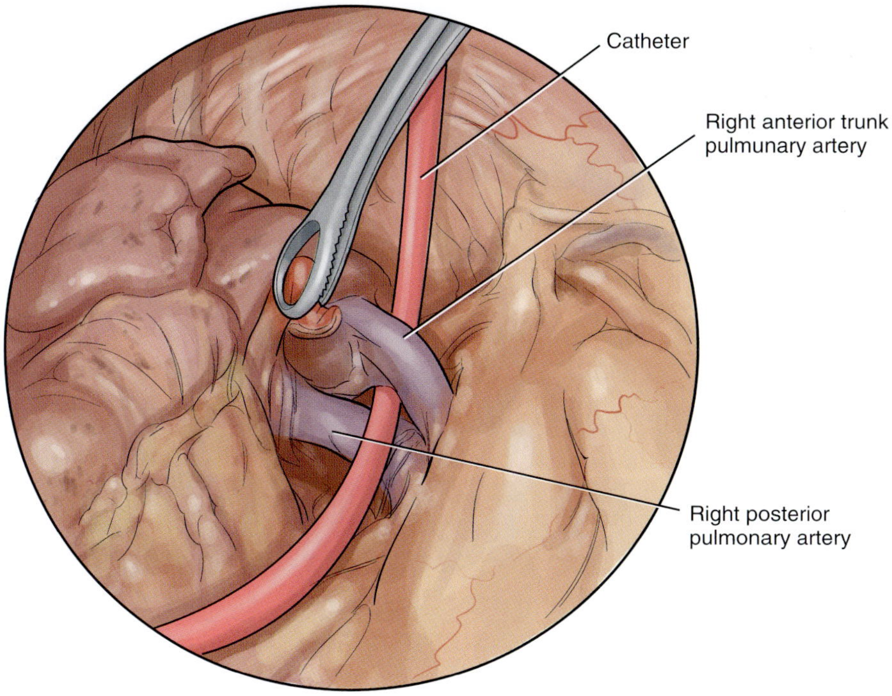

Figure 7-4.

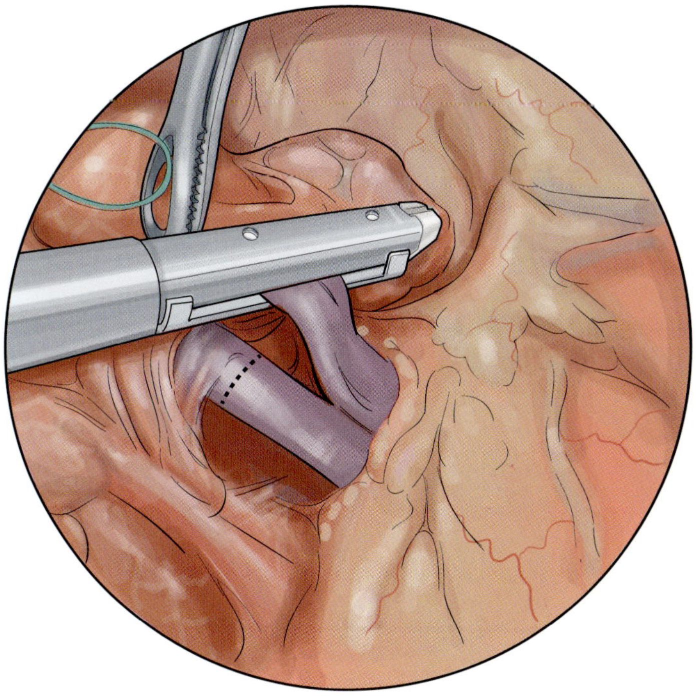

Figure 7-5.

- Last, isolate and staple the bronchus with a tissue (4.8-mm) stapler (Fig. 7-6).
- Complete the fissure (Fig. 7-7) and place the lobe in a LapSac (Cook Urological, Spencer, Ind.) for removal through the utility incision (Figs. 7-8 and 7-9).
- Although the fissure is usually completed after the vessels and the bronchus are transected, do not hesitate to complete the fissure earlier if this maneuver provides better access to the vessels or the bronchus.
- A largely fused fissure is not a contraindication to VATS lobectomy and, in fact, should not alter the conduct of the operation in any way.
- Perform a complete mediastinal lymph node dissection thoracoscopically, as outlined in prior publications.
- Irrigate the chest and check the bronchial stump for an air leak.

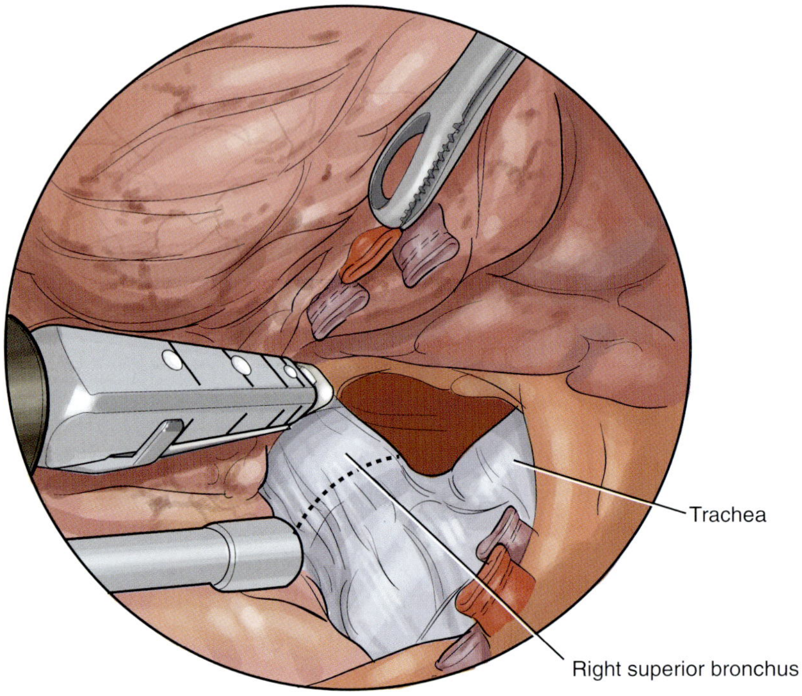

Figure 7-6.

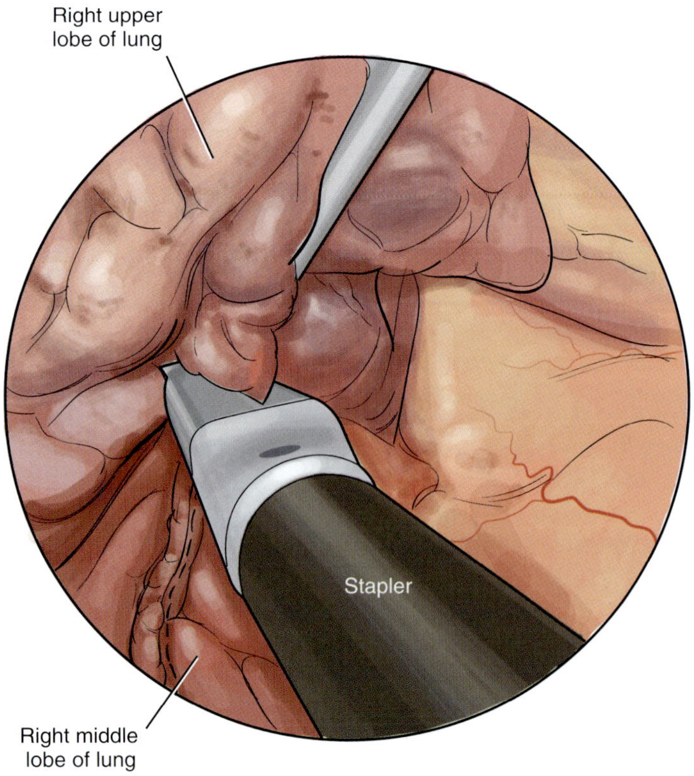

Figure 7-7.

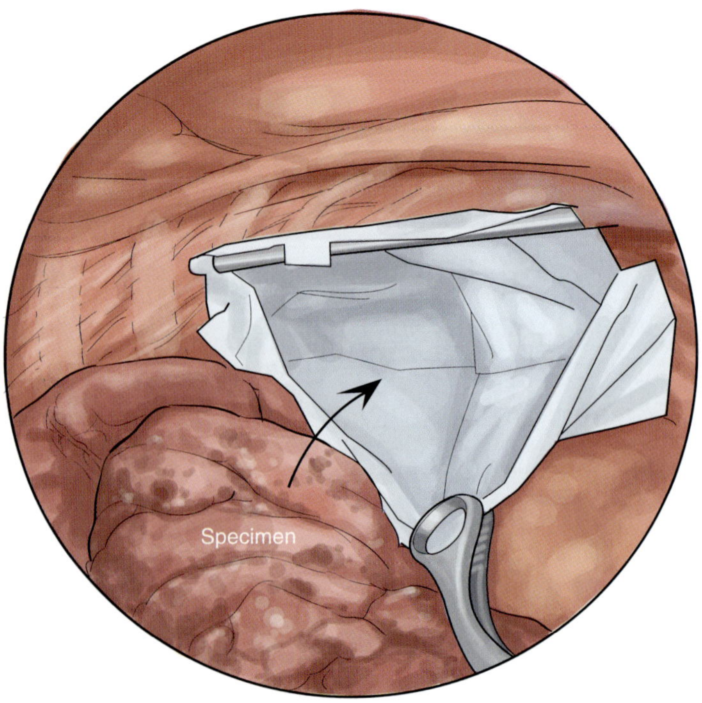

Figure 7-8.

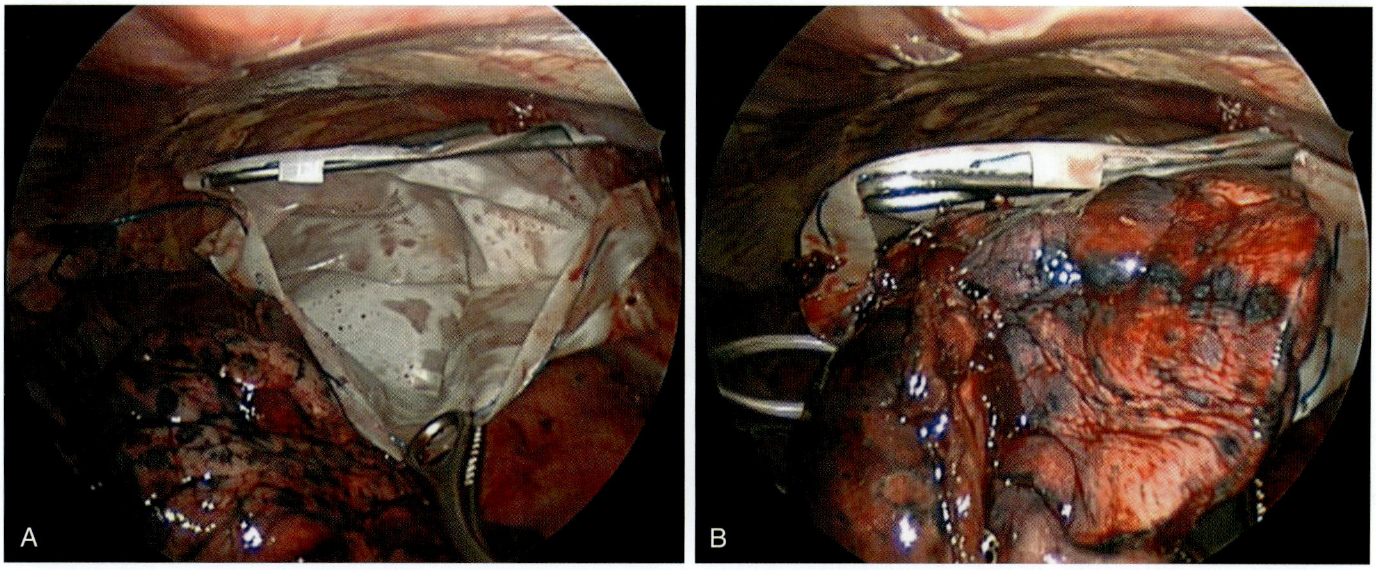

Figure 7-9. *(From McKenna RJ, Mahtabifard A, Swanson S, editors:* Atlas of minimally invasive thoracic surgery (VATS), *Philadelphia, 2010, Saunders.)*

Closure

- Drain the chest with two 28-Fr chest tubes—one straight tube to the apex of the chest and one right-angled tube to the diaphragm.
- Place the straight chest tube through the same skin incision as for the camera port and direct it posteriorly in the chest to the apex.
- A separate skin incision is made for the angled chest tube, which is directed posteriorly over the diaphragm.
- The incisions are then closed in three layers, including the skin.

III. ALTERNATIVE TECHNICAL APPROACHES (PRO/CON) AND PEARLS

- Eventually, major lung surgery will be performed through a single instrument with very different instruments directed by remote control. We are not there yet.
- Lobectomy can be performed with the aid of a robot. There are surgeons who will never perform a minimally invasive lobectomy for philosophical reasons or because they have a small volume of lobectomies. There are those who are very facile with minimally invasive surgery, so they use VATS. There are others who find the robot helpful to be able to offer minimally invasive surgery.
- There are different locations for the incisions. Some surgeons place their incisions lower. We prefer the utility incision higher in the chest because it provides access to feel more of the chest, gives better access for full nodal dissection, and is in a better location for sleeve lobectomies.

IV. SPECIAL POSTOPERATIVE CARE

- Unless the patient has severe respiratory compromise preoperatively, it is uncommon for the patient to go to the intensive care unit postoperatively.
- Most patients are sent to the recovery room and then to the thoracic surgery ward.
- The chest drainage system is not attached to suction unless the patient develops significant subcutaneous emphysema.
- Postoperative pain management is usually subcutaneous hydromorphone (Dilaudid) and oral hydrocodone/acetaminophen (Vicodin).
- Patients have no dietary restrictions and are ambulated as soon as possible.
- No routine labs or chest radiographs are ordered unless clinically indicated.
- Criteria for chest tube removal are the absence of an air leak and minimal drainage (<300 mL in 24 hours).
- The median chest tube duration and length of stay for our recent 300 VATS lobectomies is 3 days; 46% are discharged on postoperative day 1 or 2.

SUGGESTED READINGS

Burfeind WR, D'Amico T: Thoracoscopic lobectomy, *Operat Tech Thorac Cardiovasc Surg* 9:98–114, 2004.

McKenna RJ Jr: VATS for anatomic pulmonary resections by VATS. In Franco KL, Putnam JB, editors: *Advanced therapy in thoracic surgery*, Hamilton, Ontario, Canada, 2004, BC Decker.

McKenna RJ Jr, Houck W, Fuller CB: Video-assisted thoracic surgery lobectomy: experience with 1,100 cases, *Ann Thorac Surg* 81:421–426, 2006.

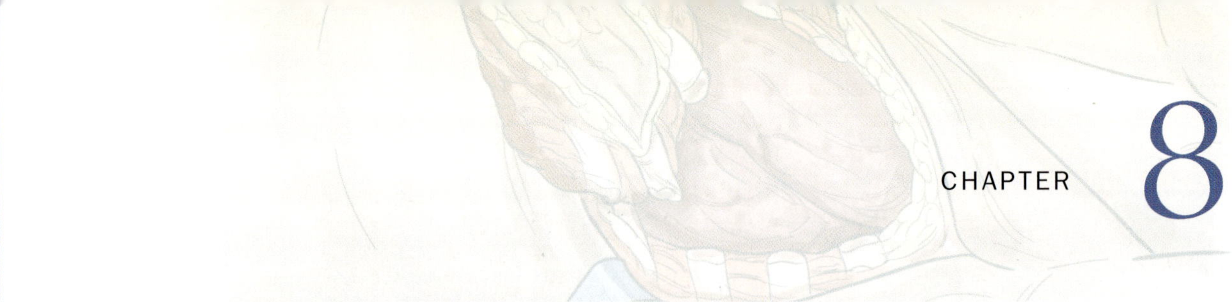

CHAPTER 8

Thoracoscopic Lung Biopsy

Robert J. McKenna, Jr., MD, and Ali Mahtabifard, MD

I. SPECIAL PREOPERATIVE PREPARATION

- Video-assisted thoracoscopic surgery (VATS) is the most common and simplest method for lung biopsy. The biopsy can be requested for diagnosis of a mass or interstitial lung disease.
- A computed tomography (CT) scan of the chest is the standard for visualization of the lung. An excellent understanding of lung anatomy and its correlation with CT images is critical to obtaining a biopsy of the desired area of the lung. Unless a mass is on the surface of the lung and visible, a finger through the incision in the fourth intercostal space can palpate the nodule.
- Pulmonary function testing is usually not necessary.
- Very small nodules deep in the lung parenchyma that may be difficult to palpate can be located with wire localization placed under CT guidance by an interventional radiologist. This is the hook wire used for localization of a breast mass. The wire is cut flush with the chest wall, the site marked and taped, and the patient is transferred to the preoperative holding area.

II. OPERATIVE TECHNIQUE

Position

- Lung biopsies are usually performed under general anesthesia with one-lung ventilation. A double-lumen tube allows better decompression and isolation of the lung to be biopsied than a single-lumen tube with a bronchial blocker.
- Place the patient in the lateral decubitus position with a slight posterior tilt (Fig. 8-1).
- Flex the bed to help get the hip out of the way of the trocar and thoracoscope. It may also help to widen the intercostal spaces.

Incision

- A lung biopsy usually is performed with three incisions—one each for the camera, a stapler, and a clamp to hold the lung (Fig. 8-2). Many thoracic surgeons place their incisions with the concept of a baseball diamond: The camera is home plate, the target tissue inside the chest is at second base, and the incisions to perform the operation are at first and third base. However, we prefer to not place an incision at the third-base position. Make an incision at home plate for the camera and at first and second base for incisions that allow the surgeon to perform the operation. Because an incision at third base would be posterior where the intercostal spaces are smaller, this incision is less functional than an incision anteriorly where the spaces are wider.
- The first incision is a 2-cm incision for the stapler. Make it in the sixth intercostal space in the midclavicular line. This is usually one intercostal space below the mammary crease or halfway between the mammary crease and the costal margin. Make the incision in the middle of the interspace and tunnel posteriorly through the tissues of the chest wall. If the incision is made perpendicular to the skin, there may be bleeding from smaller branches of the mammary artery, and instruments passing through this incision will bump into the pericardium.
- Make a second incision for the trocar and thoracoscope. This 5-mm incision is in the eighth or ninth intercostal space in the midaxillary line or the posterior axillary line. Make the incision 1 cm below a rib and angle it superiorly to reduce the pressure on the intercostal nerve.
- Use a 5- or 10-mm thoracoscope. We use a 5-mm scope because it requires a smaller incision and places less torque on the intercostal nerve.

- The third incision is 2 cm and is made in the fourth intercostal space. It begins at the border of the latissimus muscle and extends anteriorly. Through this incision, first a finger palpates the lung, and later a ring forceps holds the lung for the biopsy.

Main Dissection

- The lung is very mobile, so most of it can be palpated through the incision in the fourth intercostal space. Ring forceps through the midclavicular (first) incision can pull the lung close to a finger through this incision (Fig. 8-3). Care should be taken to not crush lung tissue with the ring forceps until the area of concern has been palpated and clearly identified. It is possible to crush a small mass so that it can no longer be palpated.
- A thorough understanding of pulmonary anatomy and its correlation with the chest CT scan is important for the surgeon to find a mass and biopsy the proper area of the lung. It is rarely necessary to convert to a thoracotomy to perform a biopsy.
- Rarely, localization techniques are used to find the mass. Place a hook wire (used for breast biopsies) under CT guidance on the day of the biopsy. The patient then goes to the operating room for resection

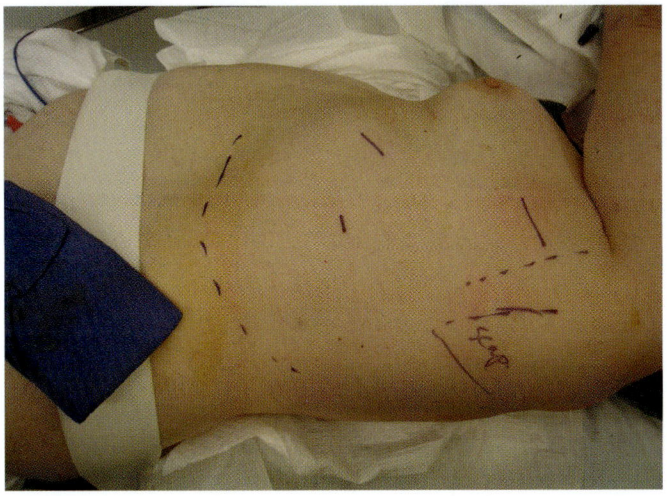

Figure 8-1.

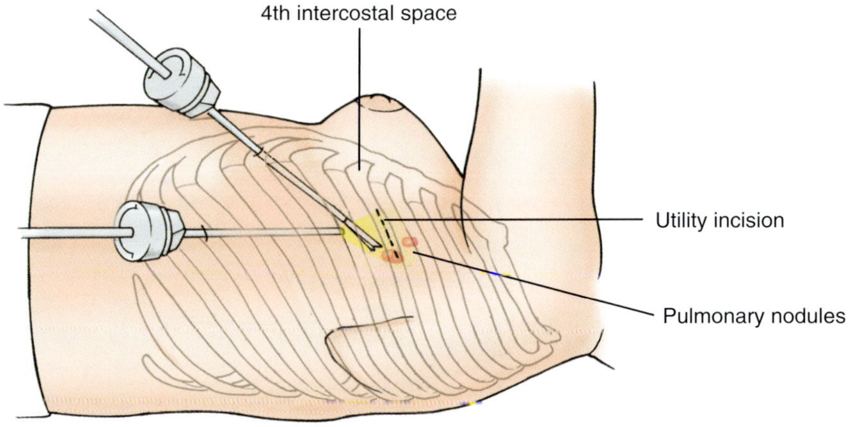

Figure 8-2. This figure depicts the use of pericardial strips, which are rarely needed, and only when the patient has severe emphysema.

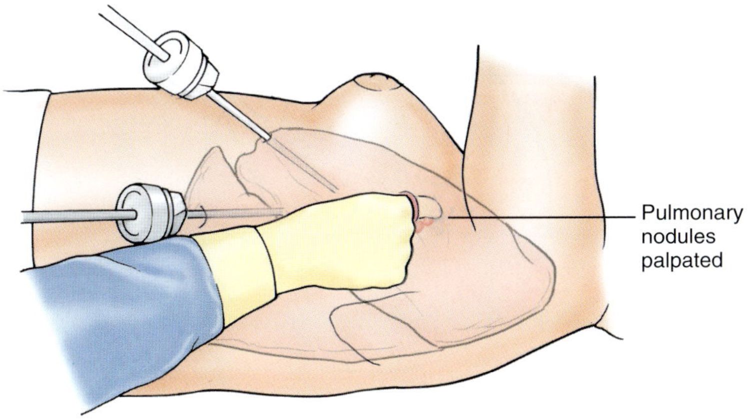

Figure 8-3.

of the area of lung identified by the wire. This is helpful for small masses below the surface, especially for small ground-glass opacities less than 1 cm or 2 cm below the surface of the pleura, because they may be difficult to palpate.

- Palpate the lung through the incision at the second-base position (Fig. 8-3). A ring forceps through that incision holds the area of lung to be biopsied (Fig. 8-4). Pass the stapler through the incision at the first-base position (Fig. 8-5). At times, the stapler can be passed through the incision at the second-base position to place the stapler perpendicular to the staple line that has been created.
- If there is a possibility that the mass is malignant, place the specimen in a standard Endocatch bag (United States Surgical Corp., Norwalk, Conn) for removal. This is the same bag that is used for laparoscopic cholecystectomy (Fig. 8-6).

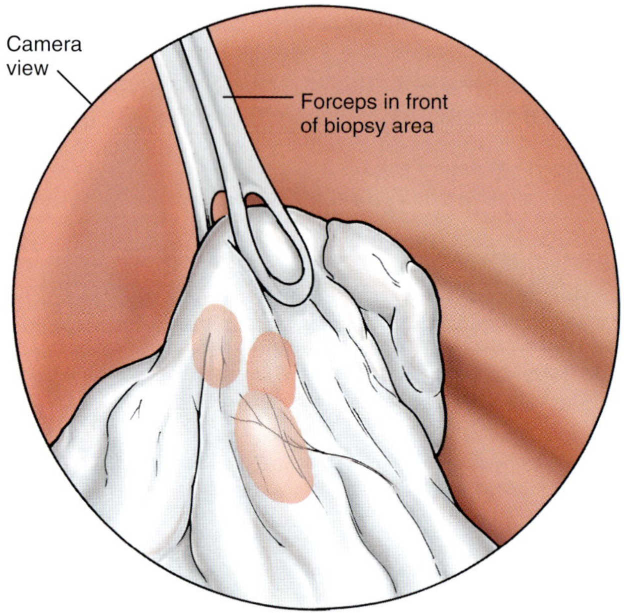

Figure 8-4.

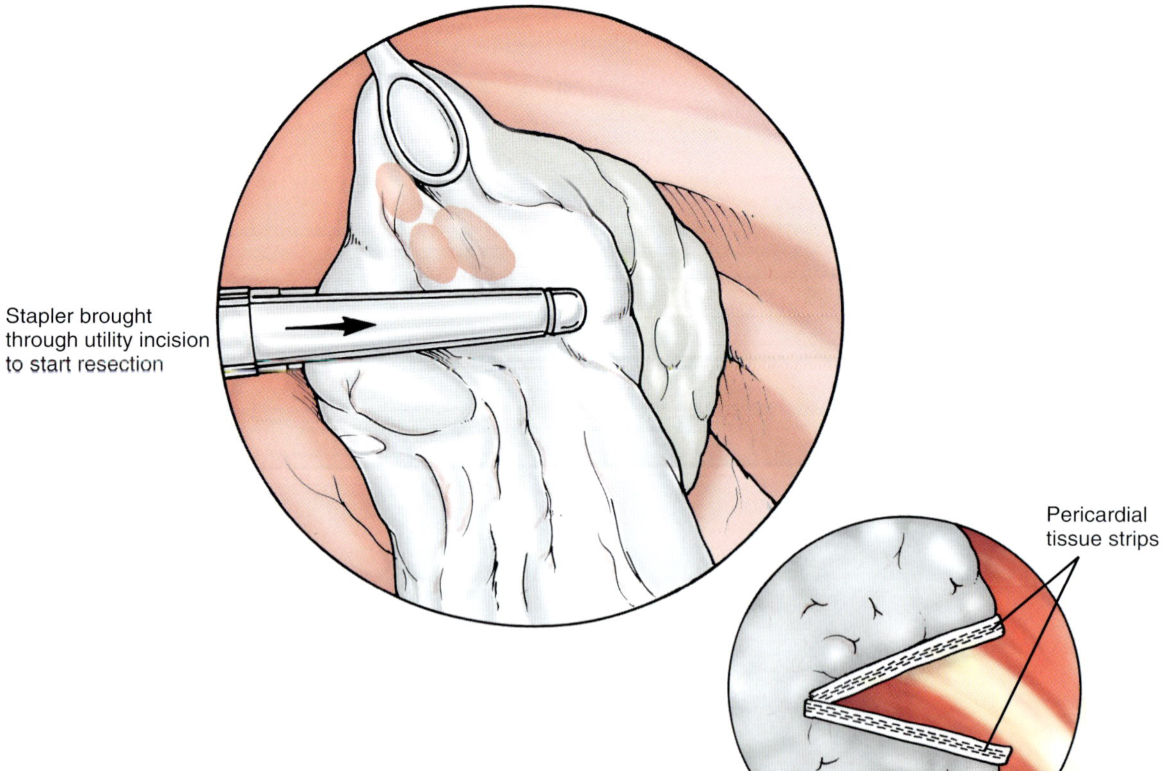

Figure 8-5. This figure depicts the use of pericardial strips, which are rarely needed, and only when the patient has severe emphysema.

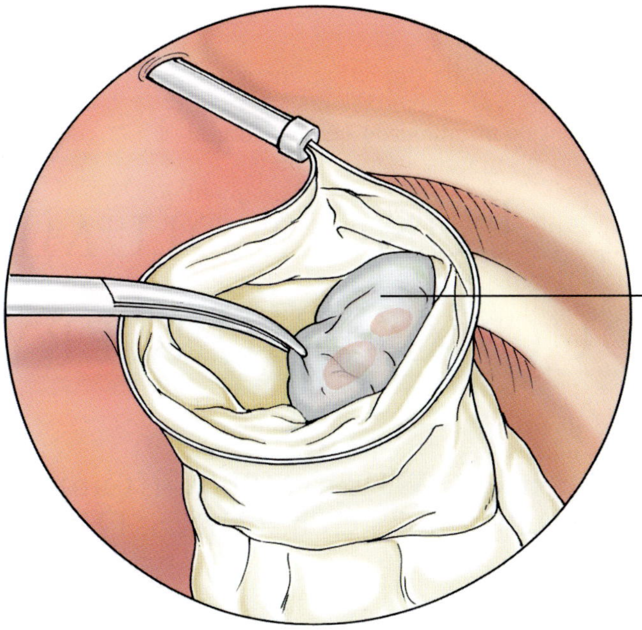

Figure 8-6.

- We obtain a frozen section for diagnosis to make sure that a diagnostic sample has been obtained. If an inflammatory process is suspected, cultures of the specimen are sent. If the mass proves to be a lung cancer, we then proceed with a VATS lobectomy.

Closure

- The chest is then drained with a single 28-Fr straight chest tube. It is placed through the same skin incision as for the camera port and should course posteriorly in the chest to the apex.
- The incisions are then closed in three layers.

III. ALTERNATIVE TECHNICAL APPROACHES (PRO/CON) AND PEARLS

- An alternative approach for localization of a mass is transthoracic percutaneous radiotracer injection with thoracoscopic radioprobe localization and excision of small pulmonary nodules. Using this technique, a CT-guided injection of radiotracer solution is made into or adjacent to the nodule the day of surgery. Next, an intraoperative gamma probe is used to localize the lesion, followed by thoracoscopic excision of the lesion.
- Ultrasound for identification of lung masses has been tried. This has not been very successful because unless the lung is totally atelectatic, the air in the lung prevents good visualization of the mass.

IV. SPECIAL POSTOPERATIVE CARE

- Unless the patient has severe respiratory compromise preoperatively, it is uncommon for the patient to go to the intensive care unit postoperatively.
- Although there are reports of outpatient lung biopsies, the procedure is usually an inpatient procedure.
- Do not attach the chest drainage system to suction, unless the patient develops significant subcutaneous emphysema.
- Postoperative pain management is usually subcutaneous hydromorphone (Dilaudid) and oral hydrocodone/acetaminophen (Vicodin).
- The patients have no dietary restriction and are ambulated immediately.
- No routine labs or chest x-rays are necessary unless clinically indicated.
- As long as there is no air leak and the chest tube drainage is minimal (<300 mL in 24 hours), the chest tube is removed on the first postoperative day, and the patient is discharged the same day.

SUGGESTED READINGS

Bensard DD, McIntyre RC, Waring BJ: Comparison of video thoracoscopic lung biopsy to open lung biopsy in the diagnosis of interstitial lung disease, *Chest* 103:765–770, 1993.

Daniel TM: A proposed diagnostic approach to the patient with the subcentimeter pulmonary nodule: techniques that facilitate video-assisted thoracic surgery excision, *Semin Thorac Cardiovasc Surg* 17:115–122, 2005.

Stiles BM, Altes TA, Jones DR, et al: Clinical experience with radiotracer-guided thoracoscopic biopsy of small, indeterminate lung nodules, *Ann Thorac Surg* 82:1191–1196, 2006.

CHAPTER 9

Lung Volume Reduction Surgery

Anthony P.C. Yim, MD, FRCS, FACS, and Michael K.Y. Hsin, MBBChir(Cantab), MA(Cantab), FRCS CTh, FHKCS, FHKAM

I. SPECIAL PREOPERATIVE PREPARATION

- The key to success in lung volume reduction surgery (LVRS) rests on a multidisciplinary approach, with appropriate patient selection through rigorous preoperative evaluation, optimization of medical treatment, and enrollment into an intensive pulmonary rehabilitation program.

Patient Selection Criteria/Exclusion Criteria

- See Box 9-1A for inclusion criteria and Box 9-1B for exclusion criteria according to the National Emphysema Treatment Trial (NETT).

Special Investigations

- Full lung function
- High-resolution computed tomography (CT) (Fig. 9-1)
- Perfusion scan (Fig. 9-2)
- 6-minute walk/shuttle walk test

Importance of Preoperative Intensive Pulmonary Rehabilitation Program plus Maximal Medical Therapy

- There should be strict smoking abstinence.
- The medications for chronic obstructive pulmonary disease should be optimized.
- Patients receiving oral steroid should have the dosage tapered to the lowest possible level before surgery.
- The pulmonary rehabilitation program involves a period of 4 to 6 weeks preoperatively, where the patient is taught the use of incentive spirometry, breathing exercises, sputum clearance and nutritional repletion. There are supervised aerobic exercises, usually on a stationary bicycle, and weight exercises that strengthen the upper limbs and chest musculature. The goal is to perform uninterrupted exercises on a bicycle for 30 minutes.

Anesthetic Considerations

- Standard anesthetic monitoring should include arterial line, central venous line, Foley catheter, pulse oximetry, and exhaled gas capnography.
- Intubation:
  - ▲ Double-lumen endotracheal tube to achieve one-lung ventilation
  - ▲ Routine flexible bronchoscopy to assess airway anatomy

II. OPERATIVE TECHNIQUE

Position

- For unilateral LVRS, the patient is placed in the lateral decubitus position, with the surgical side uppermost.
- For bilateral disease, LVRS can be performed sequentially during the same anesthesia, with the more severe side operated on first. The patient is then turned, prepped, and draped again for the operation on the remaining side.
- Alternatively, the procedure can be staged at 4 to 6 week intervals, if the patient's condition after having the unilateral procedure is assessed as being unsuitable to proceed to an operation on the other side.
- In the standard lateral decubitus thoracotomy position, the patient is secured with sand bag and straps, and the table is flexed to open the intercostal spaces.
- One-lung ventilation is commenced, and the video-assisted thoracoscopic surgery (VATS) ports are created.

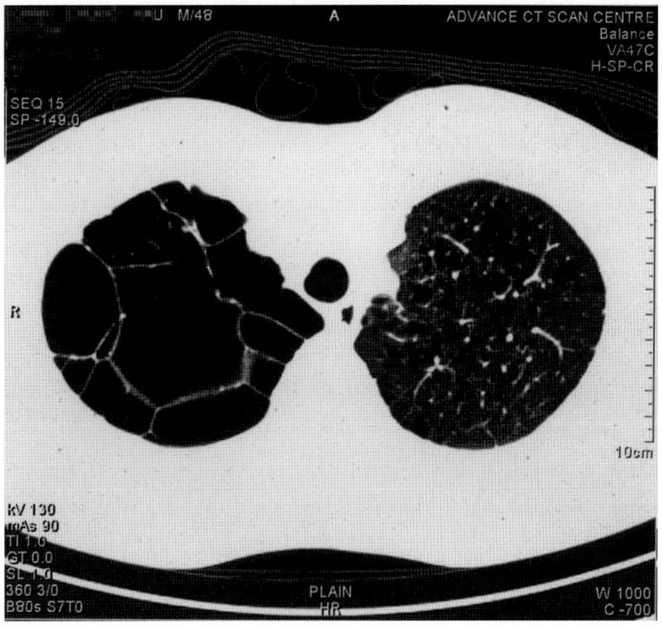

Figure 9-1.

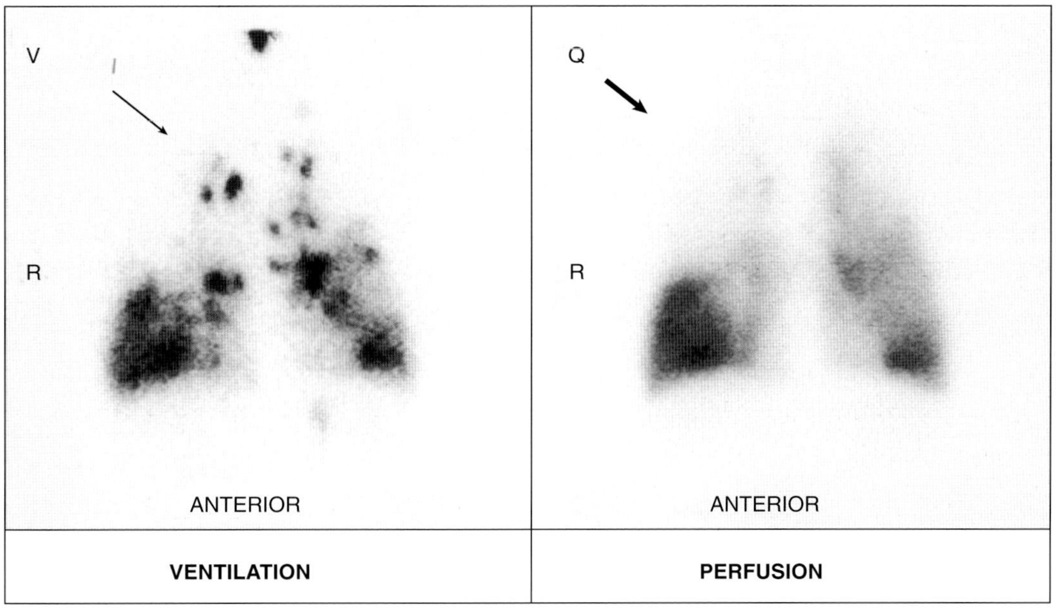

Figure 9-2. *R,* Right side; *Q,* perfusion scan; *V,* ventilation scan.

BOX 9-1A. Inclusion Criteria

History and physical exam consistent with emphysema
CT scan evidence of bilateral emphysema
Prerehabilitation postbronchodilator TLC ≥ 100% predicted
Prerehabilitation postbronchodilator RV ≥ 150% predicted
Prerehabilitation FEV_1 (maximum of pre- and postbronchodilator values) ≤ 45% of predicted and, if age ≥ 70 years prerehabilitation, FEV_1 (maximum of pre- and postbronchodilator values) ≥ 15% of predicted
Prerehabilitation room air, resting $PaCO_2$ ≤ 60 mm Hg (≤55 mm Hg in Denver)
Prerehabilitation room air, resting PaO_2 ≥ 45 mm Hg (≥30 mm Hg in Denver)
Prerehabilitation plasma cotinine ≤ 13.7 ng/ml (if not using nicotine products)
or prerehabilitation arterial carboxyhemoglobin ≤ 2.5% (if using nicotine products)
Body mass index* ≤ 31.1 (males) or ≤ 32.3 (females) as of randomization
Nonsmoker (tobacco products) for 4 months before initial interview and patient remains a nonsmoker throughout screening (by history)
Approval for surgery by cardiologist if any of the following findings are noted before randomization (approval must be obtained before randomization):
Unstable angina
Left ventricular ejection fraction cannot be estimated from the echocardiogram
Left ventricular ejection fraction < 45%
Dobutamine-radionuclide cardiac scan indicates coronary artery disease or ventricular dysfunction
More than five premature ventricular beats/minute (does not apply during exercise testing)
Cardiac rhythm other than sinus or premature atrial contractions noted during resting electrocardiogram
S_3 gallop on physical examination
Completion of all prerehabilitation assessments
Judgment by study physician that patient is likely to be approved for surgery on completion of the rehabilitation program
Completion of NETT rehabilitation program
Completion of all postrehabilitation and all randomization assessments
Approval for surgery by pulmonary physician and thoracic surgeon in consultation with the anesthesiologist, postrehabilitation and just before randomization
Consent

From Supplement to National Emphysema Treatment Trial Research Group: A randomized trial comparing lung-volume-reduction surgery with medical therapy for severe emphysema, *N Engl J Med* 348:2059–2073, 2003.
CT, Computed tomography; *FEV_1*, forced expiratory volume in 1 second; *NETT*, National Emphysema Treatment Trial; *$PaCO_2$*, partial pressure of arterial carbon dioxide; *PaO_2*, partial pressure of arterial oxygen; *RV*, residual volume; *TLC*, total lung capacity.
*Body mass index is the weight in kilograms divided by the square of the height in meters.

BOX 9-1B. Exclusion Criteria

Postrehabilitation, postbronchodilator FEV_1 ≤ 20% predicted and either nonheterogeneous emphysema on CT scan or DLCO ≤ 20% predicted (enacted May 2001)
Inability to provide a valid DLCO measurement (enacted May 2001)
CT scan evidence of diffuse emphysema judged unsuitable for LVRS
Previous LVRS (laser or excision)
Pleural or interstitial disease that precludes surgery
Giant bulla (≥ ⅓ of the volume of the lung in which the bulla is located)
Clinically significant bronchiectasis
Pulmonary nodule requiring surgery
Previous sternotomy or lobectomy
Myocardial infarction within 6 months of interview and ejection fraction < 45%
Congestive heart failure within 6 months of interview and ejection fraction < 45%
Uncontrolled hypertension (systolic > 200 mm Hg or diastolic > 110 mm Hg)
Pulmonary hypertension: mean P_{PA} on right heart catheterization ≥ 35 mm Hg (≥38 mm Hg in Denver) or peak systolic P_{PA} on right heart catheterization ≥ 45 mm Hg (≥50 mm Hg in Denver); right heart catheterization is required to rule out pulmonary hypertension if peak systolic P_{PA} on echocardiogram > 45 mm Hg
Unplanned, unexplained weight loss > 10% usual weight in 90 days before interview or unplanned, explained weight loss > 10% usual weight in 90 days before interview that is judged likely to interfere with completion of the trial
History of recurrent infections with daily sputum production judged clinically significant
Daily use of more than 20 mg of prednisone or its equivalent as of randomization
History of exercise-related syncope
Resting bradycardia (<50 beats/min), frequent multifocal PVCs, or complex ventricular arrhythmia or sustained SVT
Other cardiac dysrhythmia that, in the judgment of the supervising physician, might pose a risk to the patient during exercise testing or training
Oxygen requirement during resting or Part 1 oxygen titration exceeding 6 L/min to keep saturation ≥ 90%
Evidence of systemic disease or neoplasia that is expected to compromise survival over the duration of the trial
Any disease or condition that may interfere with completion of tests, therapy, or follow-up
Six-minute walk distance ≤140 m postrehabilitation
Inability to complete successfully any of the screening or baseline data collection procedures (e.g., hypoxemia to SpO_2 < 80% within 2 minutes of unloaded pedaling despite supplemental oxygen, inability to coordinate a regular cadence of > 40 cpm, inability to complete 3 minutes unloaded pedaling, claudication, lower extremity or back orthopedic problems that prohibit sustained pedaling)

From Supplement to National Emphysema Treatment Trial Research Group: A randomized trial comparing lung-volume-reduction surgery with medical therapy for severe emphysema, *N Engl J Med* 348:2059–2073, 2003.
CT, Computed tomography; *DLCO*, carbon monoxide lung diffusing capacity; *FEV_1*, forced expiratory volume in 1 second; *LVRS*, lung volume reduction surgery; *P_{PA}*, pulmonary artery pressure; *PVC*, premature ventricular contraction; *SVT*, supraventricular tachycardia; *SpO_2*, oxygen saturation by pulse oximetry.

Incision

- Typically, three incisions are placed in the following positions (Fig. 9-3):
  1. The first incision, 1.5 cm in length, is in the midaxillary line in the sixth or seventh intercostal space. The 30-degree thoracoscope is placed through this space via a camera port once digital palpation has confirmed the absence of adhesions (Fig. 9-4).
  2. The second incision is placed after inspection of the intrathoracic anatomy, avoiding areas of adhesions. The anterior utility incision is 1 to 2 cm long and placed in the fifth intercostal space starting at the anterior axillary line.
  3. The posterior incision is placed one or two intercostal spaces below and posterior to the tip of the scapula.
- The 30-degree thoracoscope gives excellent visualization of practically the entire thoracic cavity.
- The operating surgeon stands facing the front of the patient, as does the assistant holding the camera, with the scrub nurse standing facing the back of the patient.

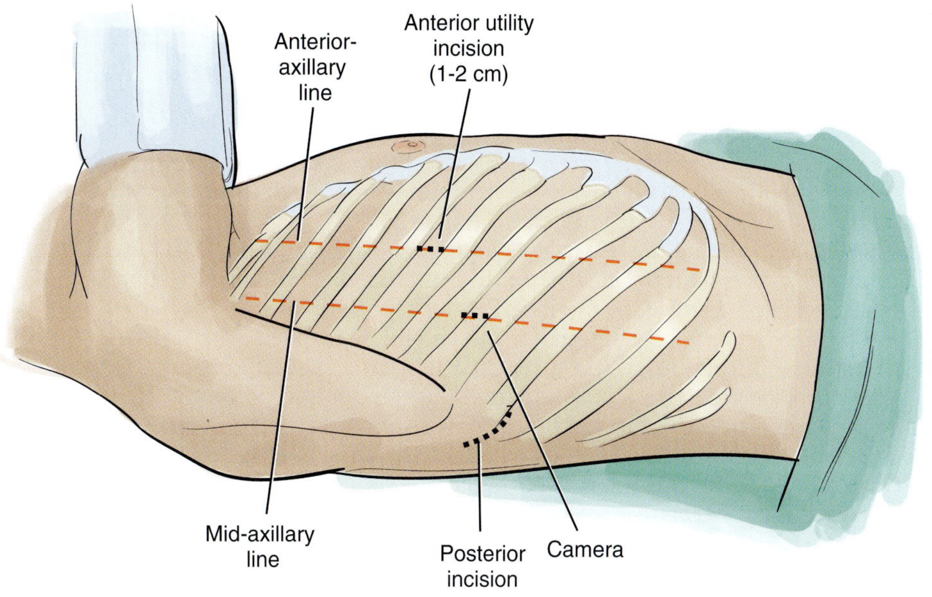

Figure 9-3.

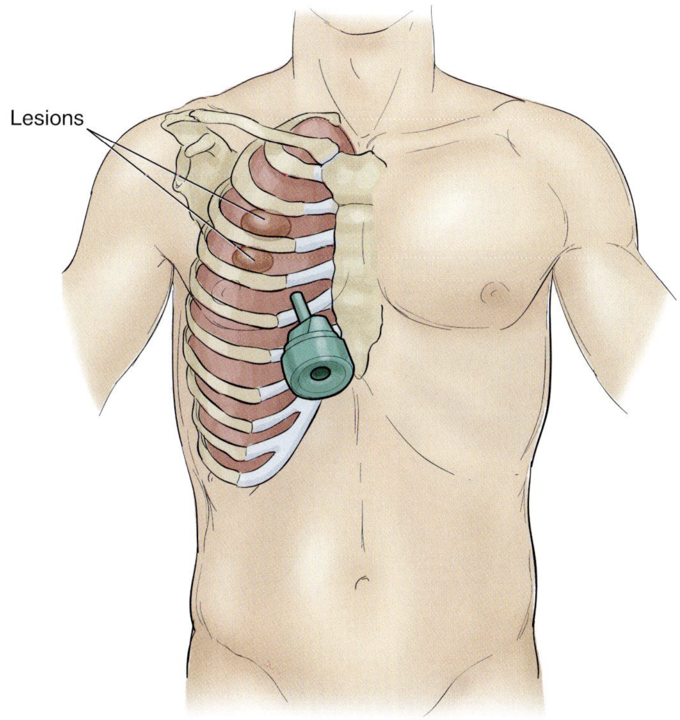

Figure 9-4.

Main Dissection

- The goal of LVRS is to resect about 25% to 35% of the lung volume. The targeted area should be identified on the preoperative CT and perfusion scan.
- Adhesions are frequently present, especially over the apex and the mediastinal aspect. These should be released with cautery, with care taken not to damage important neighboring structures. This allows the lung to collapse completely and permits full reexpansion of the lung at the end of the procedure. It also allows manipulation of the instruments to grasp the targeted area for resection.
- During adhesiolysis on the mediastinal side, care is taken not to damage the phrenic nerve.
- Visual inspection of the lung during absorptive atelectasis, as well as intermittent partial reinflation, helps the surgeon to confirm the area of lung targeted for resection. Indeed, one advantage of the lateral VATS approach over the median sternotomy is the relative ease of adhesiolysis, especially in the posterior aspect, which may not be easily accessible from the anterior approach.
- Two sponge holders (without the sponge) are inserted via the anterior and posterior ports. Bear in mind that emphysematous lung tissue is often fragile, and minimal handling of lung parenchyma reduces the amount of air leak from rough handling of lung. Every effort should be made to use the sponge holders to grasp only areas of lung that are intended for resection.
- The first maneuver is to use the sponge holder from the anterior incision to grasp the upper lobe close to the apex. This is then retracted superiorly and laterally, which allows the surgeon to assess the extent of resection (Fig. 9-5).
- Once the targeted area has been identified, with one sponge holder grasping the lung by the edge, the other sponge holder is used to clamp the lung along the line of intended resection to form a "track" of thinned lung. This is then released, and an endoscopic stapler, such as the Ethicon EZ 45 stapling device (4.8-mm staples; Ethicon, Cincinnati) buttressed with bovine pericardium (Peristrips, Biovascular, Minneapolis), is inserted via the anterior utility port, to begin the resection (Fig. 9-6).
- This is then repeated in a gradual fashion, alternating between clamping the lung parenchyma followed by resection with the stapler, as one proceeds from an anterior-to-posterior direction. The resultant line of resection should follow an inverted J shape, or the inverted hockey stick.
- Crossed staple lines tend to cause more air leak at the junction and should be avoided. The posterior sponge holder is readjusted from time to time to grasp on resected lung to achieve the appropriate traction. It is important to assess the progress of the staple line from the anterior and posterior aspect, so as not to cut too deep into the lung or too close to the hilum (Fig. 9-7).
- The correct amount of lung that should be resected is not always easy to determine: resecting too little diseased lung reduces the effectiveness of the operation, whereas removing too much "functioning" lung tissue compromises postoperative gas exchange.
- The resected lung specimen is retrieved via the larger anterior port.
- Tissue glue maybe added at the end of the procedure along the staple lines.
- The pulmonary ligament is routinely released to optimize reexpansion of the lower lobe (Fig. 9-8).

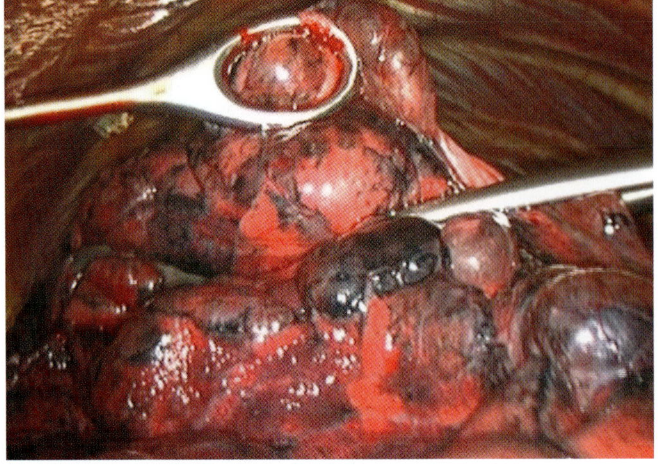

Figure 9-5.

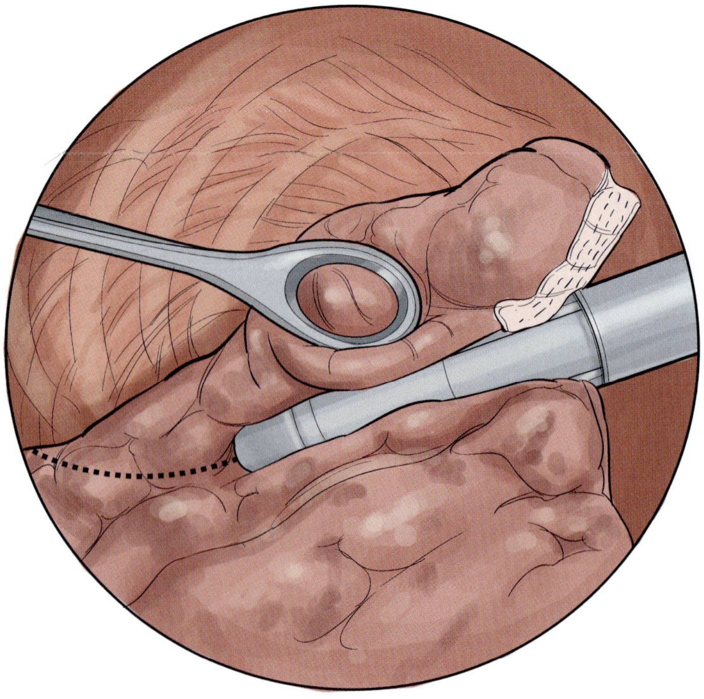

Figure 9-6.

Closure

- At the end of the procedure, the hemithorax is filled with warm saline, and gentle reinflation of the lung by hand ventilation (using the lowest pressure possible that achieves reexpansion) allows identification of areas of significant air leaks. These can then be dealt with by extra staples, suturing, or glue.
- If a significant apical space is encountered, the creation of a pleural tent may be indicated.
- Intercostal infiltration with 0.5% bupivacaine to the appropriate spaces is performed.
- One or two large-bore chest drains (28 Fr or more) are inserted, typically using the inferior port for one of the drains, and connected to a standard underwater seal bottle without suction. Lung reexpansion is confirmed by videoscopy. The other port sites are closed.
- In the case of bilateral disease, the patient is turned to the other side, reprepped, and redraped for the same procedure. Care is taken when turning the patient to ensure that the chest drains do not become kinked or obstructed. A short period of two-lung ventilation may be beneficial for these patients, and if the arterial blood gas demonstrates hypercapnia, then it may be necessary to prolong this period of two-lung ventilation to normalize the blood gas before attempting one-lung ventilation again. The same procedure is then performed as described on the remaining chest. During one-lung ventilation of the side that underwent the initial LVRS, care is taken to keep the pressures to a minimum to reduce stress on the staple lines.

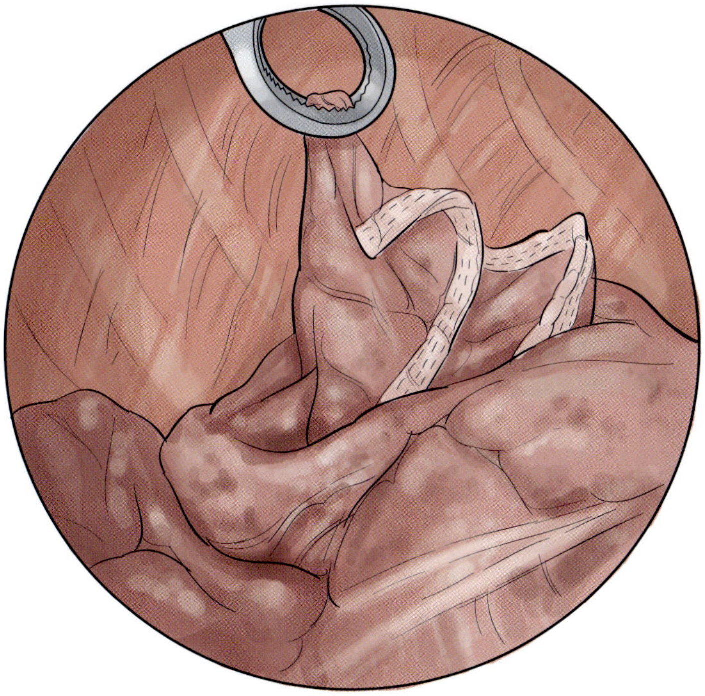

Figure 9-7.

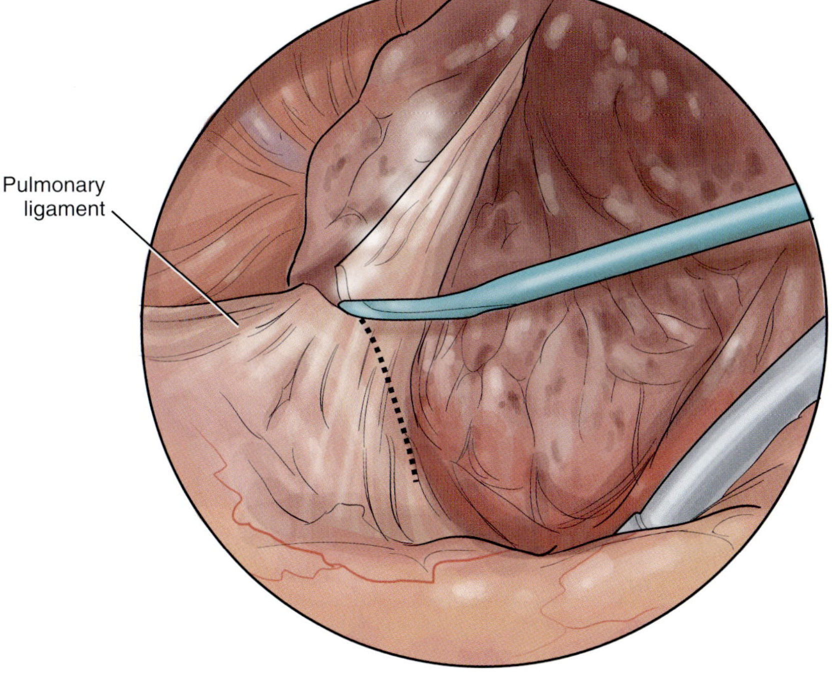

Figure 9-8.

III. ALTERNATIVE TECHNICAL APPROACHES (PRO/CON) AND PEARLS

VATS Anterior Approach

For Bilateral LVRS

- Patient is in the supine position with both arms elevated above the head, with the elbows bent at 90 degrees and the arms supported.
- An inflatable bag placed under each scapula, together with tilting of the operating table away from the surgeon, allows improved access.
- Incisions are made at the fifth intercostal space in the submammary position, in the sixth intercostal space in the anterior axillary line, and in the third intercostal space in the midaxillary line.
- The advantage of this approach is that the patient does not have to be turned during the procedure, and the surgeon simply goes to the opposite side of the patient after finishing the first side.
- The access to posterior and lower zones is less satisfactory compared to the lateral VATS approach as described earlier.

Median Sternotomy Approach

- For patients requiring bilateral LVRS, median sternotomy provides access to both chest cavities using a single incision, which is usually well-tolerated.
- The NETT investigators showed that morbidity and mortality after LVRS was comparable using VATS or the sternotomy approach, as were the functional results. However, the VATS group allowed earlier recovery at a lower cost compared to median sternotomy.

Bronchoscopic Lung Volume Reduction

- A specially designed one-way valve allows air to be vented from an isolated lung segment during normal expiration and prevents air from refilling the lung during expiration.
- The placement of these valves in the segmental bronchi could functionally isolate the airway that supplies the most hyperinflated parts of the emphysematous lungs, favoring deflation and even atelectasis, and thus mimicking LVRS in its contribution to alleviate symptoms.
- The Emphasys (Redwood City, Calif.) endobronchial valve (EBV) is an endobronchial prosthesis designed to both control and redirect airflow. It is a one-way, polymer, duckbill valve that is mounted inside a stainless steel cylinder that is attached to a nickel-titanium (Nitinol) self-expanding retainer. It prevents air from entering the target lung but allows air and mucus to exit (Fig. 9-9).
- Clinical studies have shown that EBV placement is a safe procedure, with significant short-term improvements in functional status, quality of life, and relief of dyspnea in selected patients with emphysema.
- A multicenter analysis confirms that improvement in pulmonary function and exercise tolerance can be achieved in emphysematous patients using EBVs.
- The endobronchial Valve for Emphysema palliatioN Trial (VENT) is a phase III multicenter, prospective, randomized trial, which is currently under way to further evaluate this treatment modality.

Technique of EBV Insertion

- Preoperative CT chest and ventilation/perfusion scans are used to identify bronchial segments for EBV insertion.
- Under total intravenous anesthesia with propofol (Diprivan), the patient is kept in assisted spontaneous ventilation throughout the procedure and placed supine with the head slightly extended.
- A ventilating rigid bronchoscope with a Hopkins telescope (Efer-Dumon Bronchoscope; Efer, La Ciotat, France) is introduced through the mouth into the airway and is then connected to a camera system with the tip of the bronchoscope positioned at the target lobar orifice (Fig. 9-10).
- A flexible delivery catheter is used to place the EBV valve into the targeted bronchial lumen. The delivery catheter is designed to be inserted through a 2.8-mm diameter working channel of a flexible bronchoscope. The flexible bronchoscope carrying the loaded delivery catheter is inserted down the channel of the rigid bronchoscope. The loaded catheter is advanced to the target location and the valve is deployed by actuating a deployment handle, which retracts the distal housing and releases the EBV (Figs. 9-11 and 9-12). The entire procedure is visually monitored by the video bronchoscope. Depending on the exact morbid anatomy, one or more valves are placed in the endobronchial tree.

IV. SPECIAL POSTOPERATIVE CARE

- Thorough bronchial toileting is performed via flexible bronchoscope through the endotracheal tube before extubation.
- Every effort should be made to extubate the patient early to minimize the pressure on the staple lines from positive pressure ventilation.
- Excellent postoperative pain control is vital, and this can be achieved with intercostal infiltration with bupivacaine followed by patient-controlled analgesia with morphine. Others have recommended epidural analgesia with good effect.

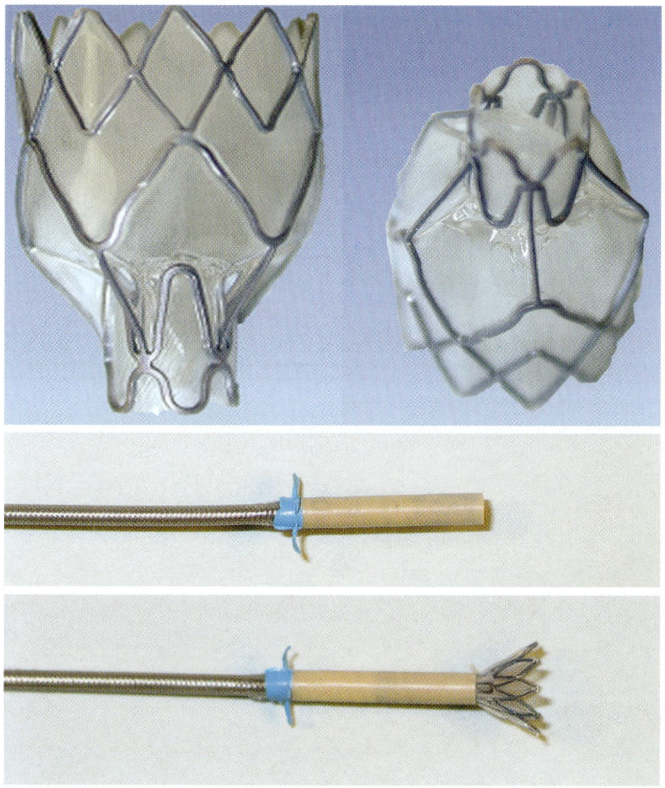

Figure 9-9.

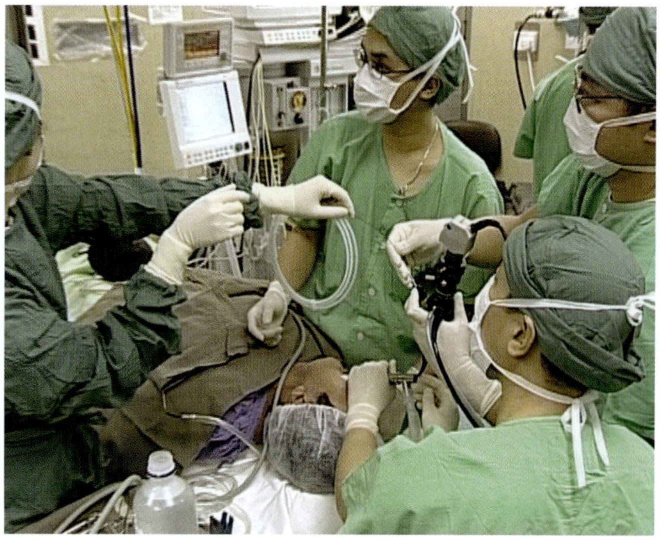

Figure 9-10.

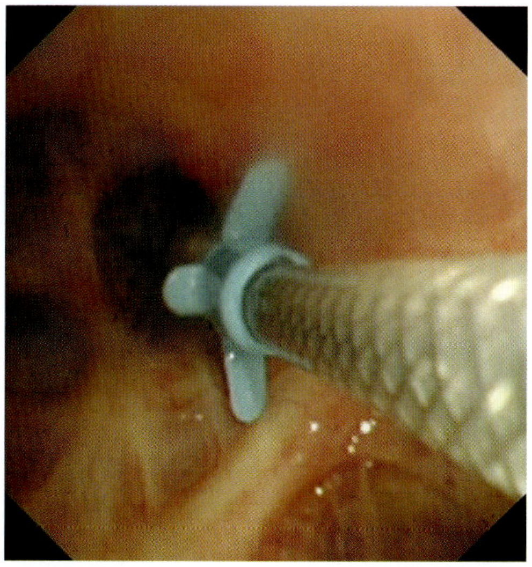

Figure 9-11.

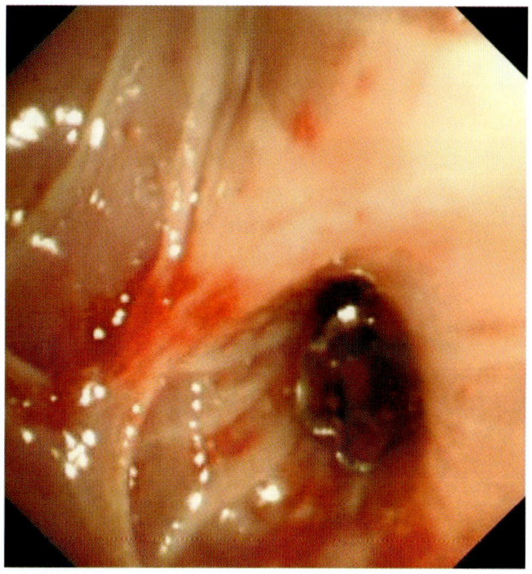

Figure 9-12.

- Our routine is to connect the chest drains to an underwater seal without suction. Suction may promote further air leaks and may damage the already fragile emphysematous lung.
- Chest physiotherapy and incentive spirometry is started on day 1, and early mobilization is encouraged. For patients unable to expectorate effectively, nasopharyngeal suctioning may be needed. Have a low threshold to perform bedside flexible bronchoscopy for patients who have sputum retention despite the foregoing measures.
- The patient is actively monitored for signs of chest infection, and antibiotics are started when indicated.
- For patients who have air leak beyond 1 week, the chest drain is connected to a one-way Heimlich valve bag device to allow discharge, to be reviewed in clinic at regular intervals.

SUGGESTED READINGS

National Emphysema Treatment Trial Research Group: Safety and efficacy of median sternotomy versus video-assisted thoracic surgery for lung volume reduction surgery, *J Thorac Cardiovasc Surg* 127:1350–1360, 2004.

Wan IYP, Toma TP, Geddes DM, et al: Bronchoscopic lung volume reduction for end-stage emphysema: report on the first 98 patients, *Chest* 129:518–526, 2006.

Yim APC, Hwong TMT, Lee TW, et al: Early results of endoscopic lung volume reduction for emphysema, *J Thorac Cardiovasc Surg* 127:1564–1573, 2004.

CHAPTER 10

Chest Wall Resection/ Reconstruction

Antonio Briccoli, MD

I. SPECIAL PREOPERATIVE PREPARATION

- Thoracic wall resections are indicated almost exclusively in neoplastic diseases: in bone and soft tissue tumors, in local recurrences from breast cancer, in radio-induced necroses and infiltrative carcinomas of the lung; less frequent indications include osteomyelitis, specifically of the sternum.
- Preoperative planning must consider the need of oncologically adequate surgery, which requires wide resections that seldom allow for specific functional needs. The thoracic cage has an explicit role in the ventilatory dynamic, behaving like a real bellows: expanding in inspiration, it increases lung capacity and favors assumption of oxygen; contracting during expiration, it allows expulsion of carbon dioxide gas. To maintain this role, reconstructions of the thoracic cage must always allow flexibility. On the other hand, to avoid a harmful flail chest, it must not be excessively elastic, creating a paradoxical dynamic of the reconstructed area.
- Mandatory in preoperative staging is a precise knowledge of tumor extension that determines the correct area of resection.
- Preoperative imaging must give information on both tumor nature and its local extension. Computed tomography (CT) with contrast dye and magnetic resonance imaging (MRI) with gadolinium are useful, but not absolute for a differential diagnosis between benign and malignant lesions.
- To diagnose the nature it is always useful to program a preoperative needle biopsy, preferably CT- or ultrasound-guided. In doubtful diagnoses, the biopsy may be repeated. In case of contradiction between the histologic diagnosis and imaging, an incisional biopsy could be indicated.
- CT and MRI with contrast dye and multiplane reconstruction, particularly for tumors of the superior thoracic wall, allow a definition of tumor extension and its relationship with the underlying vascular structures (Fig. 10-1).
- Besides CT and MRI, ultrasound can be useful in preoperative staging of superficial extension of tumor mass, with the advantage of identifying, especially in recurrences, micronodules that are undetectable by CT and MRI because of their small size.
- Resections of the thoracic cage are divided into anterior (with or without sternum involvement), lateral, and posterior. Anterior and lateral resections, to avoid a harmful flail chest, require specific reconstructive techniques, often unnecessary in posterior resections.

II. OPERATIVE TECHNIQUE

Position

- Position on the operation table varies according to the resection site:
  1. Supine position for anterior resections
  2. Lateral decubitus for lateral resections
  3. Lateral decubitus for posterior resections distant from the spine
  4. Prone position for resections close or extending to the spine

Incision

- The incision can be:
  1. Anterolateral or posterolateral in rib or rib and sternum resections, with the possibility of lateral or craniocaudal extension. This is necessary when a sternum resection or when a muscular rotation flap are also needed.
  2. Presternal median anterior in sternum resections.
- When previous transcutaneous or incisional biopsies have been performed, the area crossed by the trocar or the biopsy scar must be removed with a skin island incision (Fig. 10-2).
- Incision is performed along the rib above or below the previously defined tumor extension. The extension, parallel to the rib margin, is initially limited but sufficient to allow intrapleural finger palpation of the deep tumor mass. It will be laterally widened depending on intraoperative assessment.

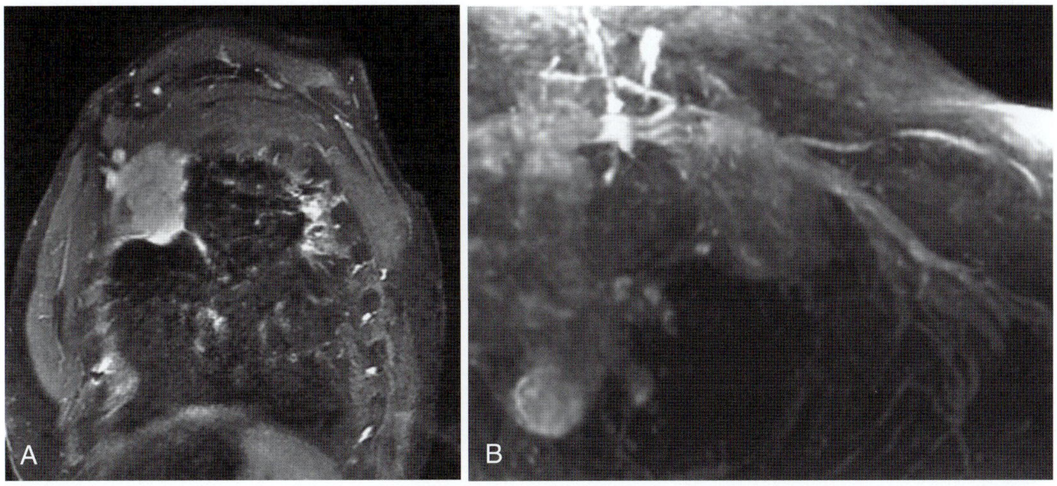

Figure 10-1. **A,** Soft tissue sarcoma of the anterior thoracic wall extending to the costoclavicular area. **B,** Magnetic resonance imaging scan with gadolinium shows the relationship with left subclavian vein.

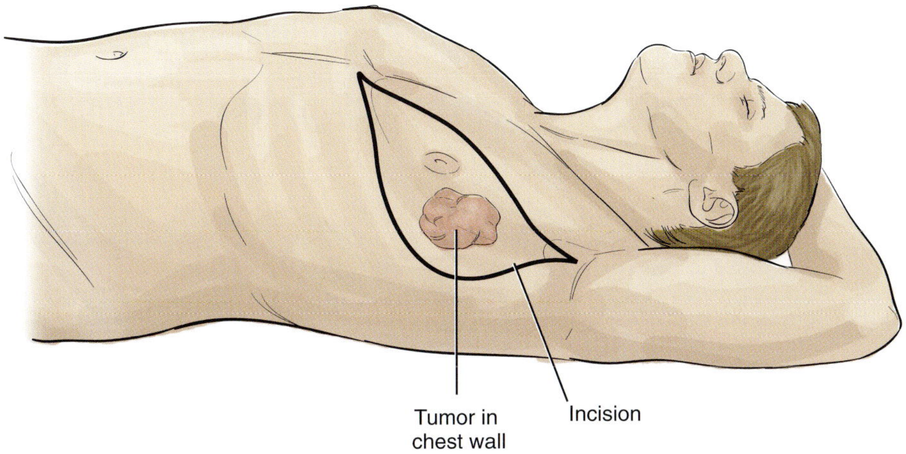

Figure 10-2.

Main Dissection

- Once the resection area is defined, the thoracic wall muscular structures that cover the tumor are dissected with a lateral extension of at least 4 cm from the tumor to avoid local recurrence, including possible previously detected micronodules in case of local recurrence (Fig. 10-3).
- The trocar biopsy pathway or the surgical scar must be included, en bloc with a cutaneous island, in the resection area.
- Possible preservation of superficial muscular structures must be reserved to small bone sarcomas.
- Excluding resections of benign tumors, it is appropriate to perform thoracic wall resections en bloc with cutaneous island, muscles, ribs and sternum, and parietal pleura (Fig. 10-4).
- To define resection margins when tumor extension invades the pleural cavity, it is best to limit the dissection of intercostal muscles and parietal pleura to a healthy area and explore the endopleural tumor margins by finger palpation.

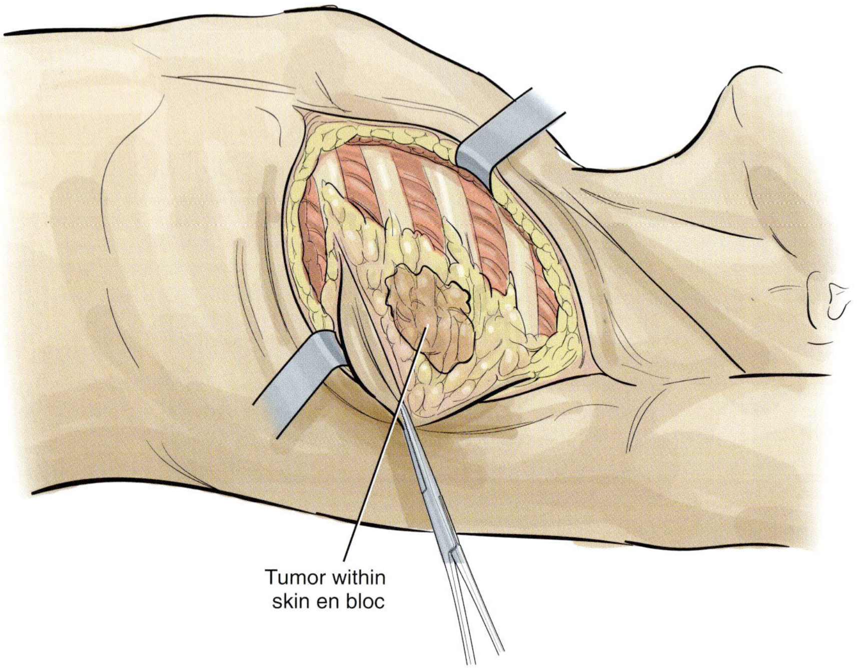

Figure 10-3.

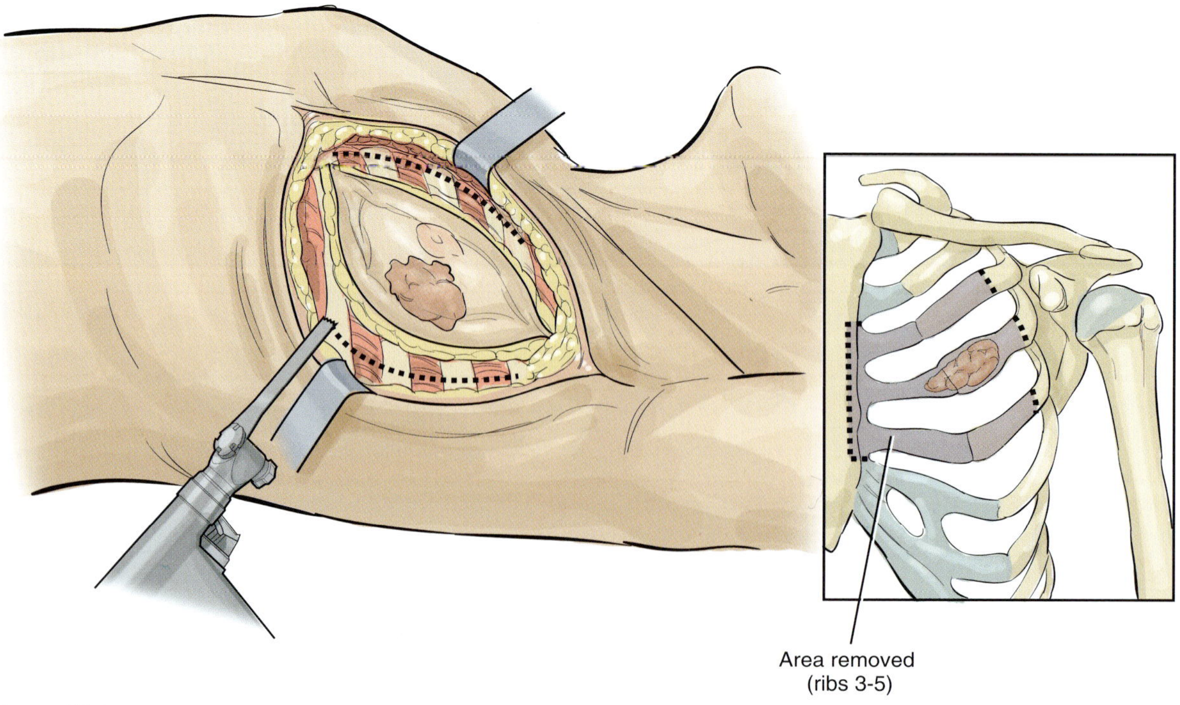

Figure 10-4.

- When the thoracic wall tumor is strictly adherent to the lung, en bloc resection of the tumor and the adjacent lung must be done by wedge resection. The healthy margin of the lung is sutured mechanically or with resorbable thread.
- Resection can be:
  1. *Rib(s)*. In this case, the procedure is a segmental rib resection, made on two spots on the same arc, of one or more ribs; an en bloc resection including the overlying soft tissues is performed, after incision of the periosteum, at a previously established safety distance, including intercostal muscles and underlying parietal pleura. The intercostal corresponding pedicle must be identified, ligated, and dissected beforehand (Fig. 10-5).
  2. *Rib(s) with associated sternum resection*. Here, the rib resection procedure is similar to the preceding, differing in sternum resection. The latter, partial and longitudinal, requires identification, ligature, and dissection of the homolateral internal mammary vascular pedicle before bone resection.
  3. *Sternal*. Partial, subtotal, or total sternum resection may require preliminary disarticulation or resection of the proximal clavicle. In all cases, after monolateral or bilateral ligature and section of the internal mammary vascular pedicles as first-time surgery, the rib-sternum cartilages are dissected. With finger dissection from the suprasternal notch or the xiphoid, the deep plane is isolated from the anterior mediastinum and the sternum sectioned transversely. By proximal and/or lateral traction, the sternum resection is completed en bloc.
- When tumor involves the diaphragm, it is best to remove it en bloc after performing a limited dissection in healthy area, and explore by finger palpation tumor extension below the diaphragm. Diaphragm dissection requires careful hemostasis of the phrenic artery branches, preferably by suture rather than simply by electrocoagulation.
- If resection needs to be extended to the spine, dissection of the paraspinal long muscles is associated with posterior rib resection, disinsertion of the caput costae from the transverse process, or alternatively a resection of the transverse process or marginal osteotomy of vertebral body. Special attention must be given to level D11-L2, avoiding electrocoagulation of the vascular pedicle that branches off from the intercostal artery to supply the spinal cord.
- When postoperative radiotherapy is scheduled, it may be useful to identify soft tissue resection margins with radiopaque clips.

Closure

- Reconstruction of the thoracic wall after simple rib resection does not require particular techniques, except for the need to stabilize the resection stumps to the over- and underlying rib structures.
- Reconstruction of the thoracic wall after extended resections or after sternectomy requires, on the other hand, a choice of suitable materials and procedures to respect the peculiar ventilatory function.

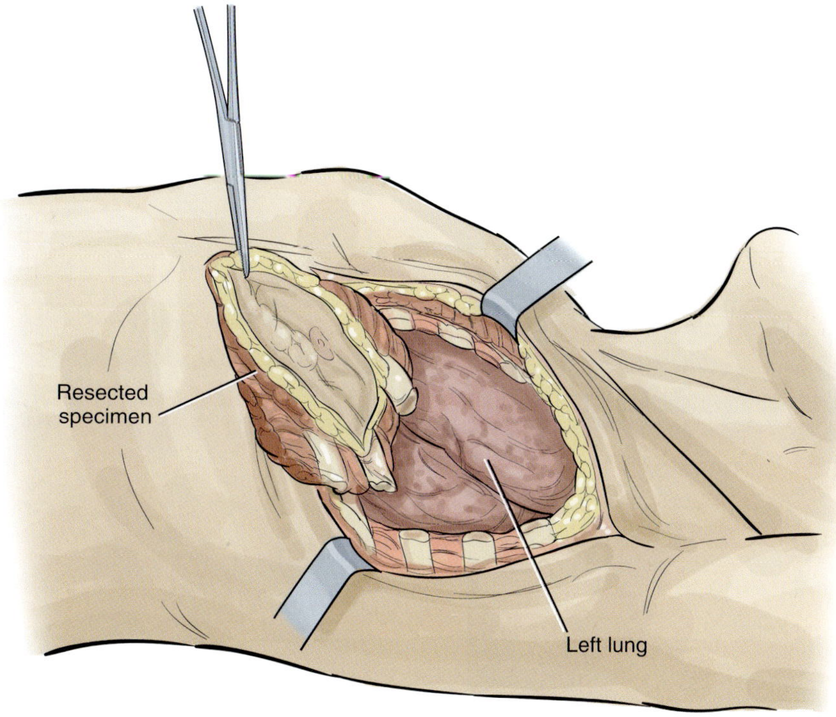

Figure 10-5.

Materials must have enough elasticity to allow expansion and retraction of the thoracic cage. Surgical techniques must prevent excessive elasticity, which causes harmful flail chest, but also avoid inextensible rigid reconstructions.

- Materials generally used are biologic (muscle, fascia lata, bone grafts, dura mater, pericardium, omentum), heteroplastic, and synthetic (sheets and meshes, solid and firm prosthetics, composite, plates and struts) (Fig. 10-6). Personally we prefer fascia lata, autologous or from the bank, which besides having the specific elasticity required, also offers the advantage of fast and easy tissue integration, impermeability, and scarce reactivity that does not causes adherence to the underlying lung parenchyma. It does not require previous treatment with gamma rays, it adapts well to growth in childhood reconstructions, it easily faces to areas requiring reconstruction, and it has a very low risk of infection.
- The use of a more superficial rigid support, anchored to the spared structures of the thoracic cage, where the fascia lata is fixed, avoids all paradoxical movements of the fascia and harmonizes ventilatory dynamics in inspiration and expiration. We use titanium plates, moldable to adapt to the morphology of the area to reconstruct, anchored by nonresorbable sutures to the healthy ribs. In reconstructions of the superior third of the hemithorax, the plate is positioned as the removed rib (Fig. 10-7). In reconstructions of the inferior two thirds of the hemithorax, the plate is positioned longitudinally, bridging the healthy ribs (Fig. 10-8). This is to respect the specific dynamics of the thoracic cage, which in the inferior two thirds must ensure wider expansion. For tumors of the lower thoracic wall, extending to the abdominal wall where the last ribs are removed, the plate is positioned

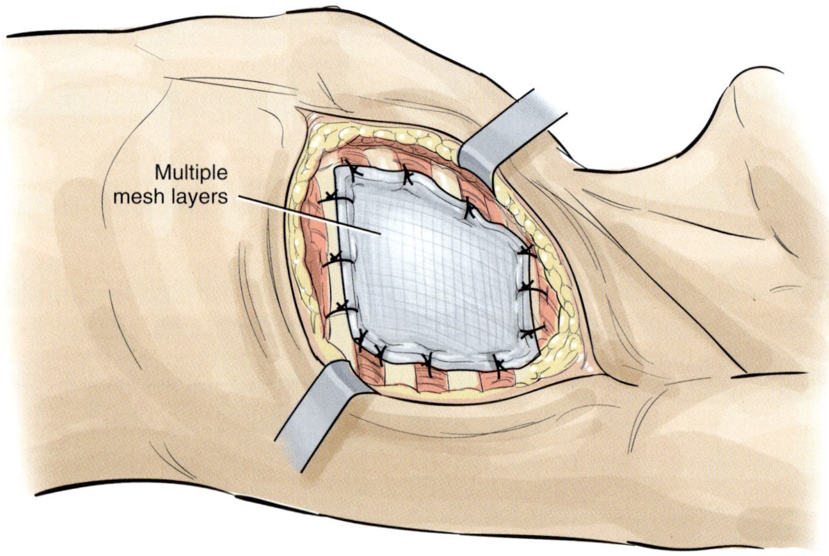

Figure 10-6.

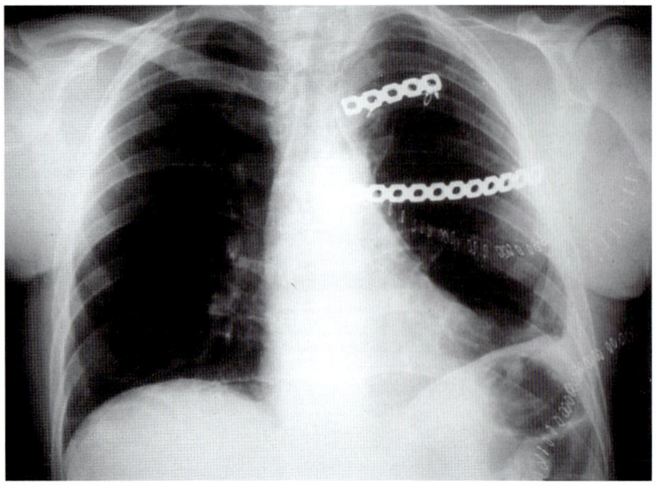

Figure 10-7.

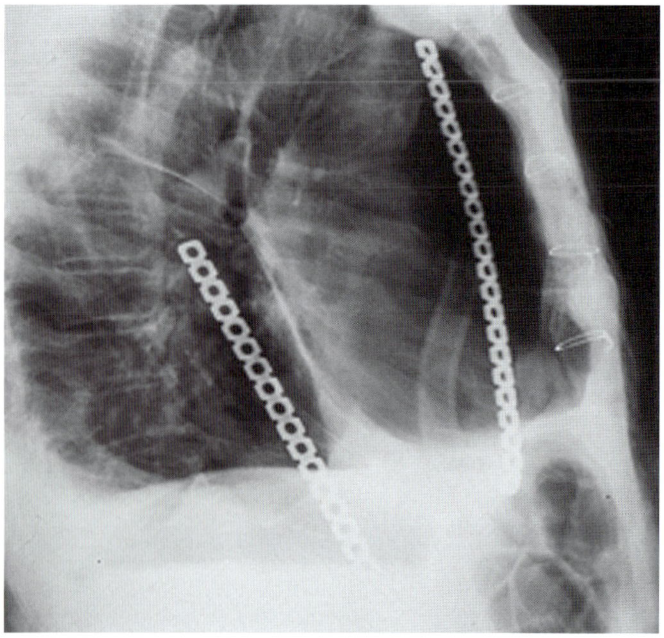

Figure 10-8.

transversely by suturing the rib insertions of the homolateral hemidiaphragm to the anterior face (Fig. 10-9). When performing sternal reconstructions, we use two plates positioned like St. Andrew's cross inserted on the two sides of the hemithorax (Fig. 10-10).

- Plates are stabilized to the skeletal structures with nonresorbable thread.
- When the hemidiaphragm is removed, its reconstruction, if not possible by direct suture of dissected margins, may be performed by a patch of fascia lata (Fig. 10-11).
- Reconstruction is completed by direct suture of residual muscular structures and overlying skin (Fig. 10-12) or with a muscular or myocutaneous rotation flap.

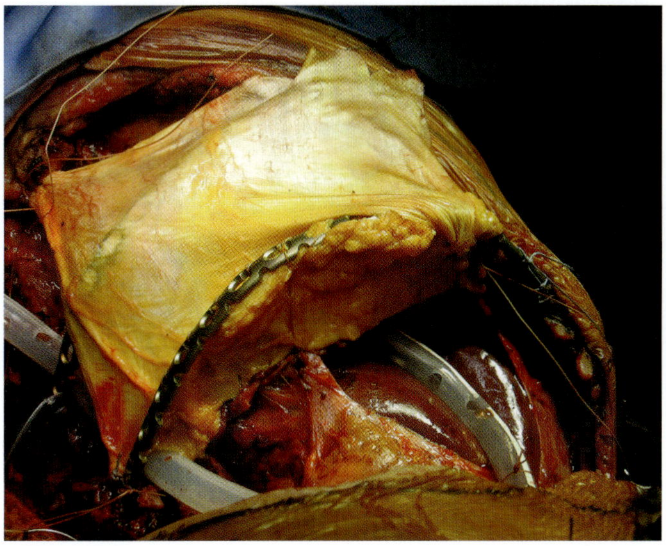

Figure 10-9.

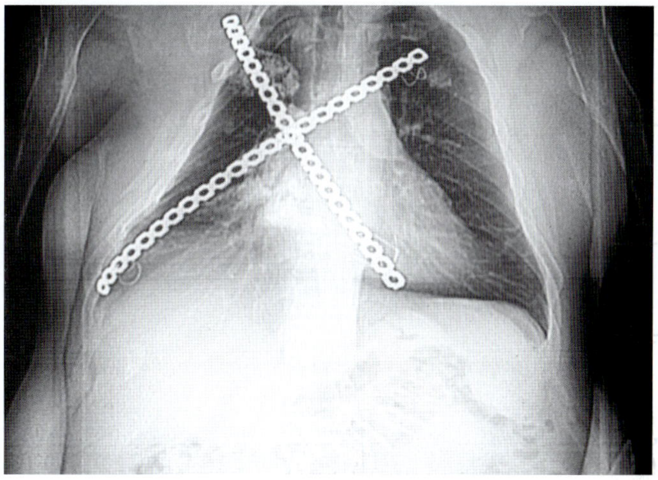

Figure 10-10.

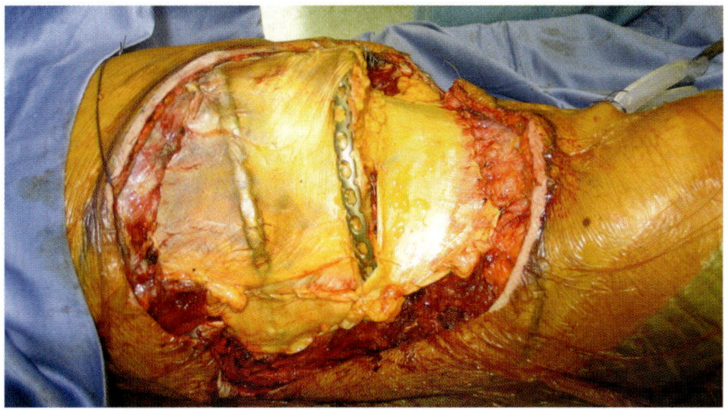

Figure 10-11.

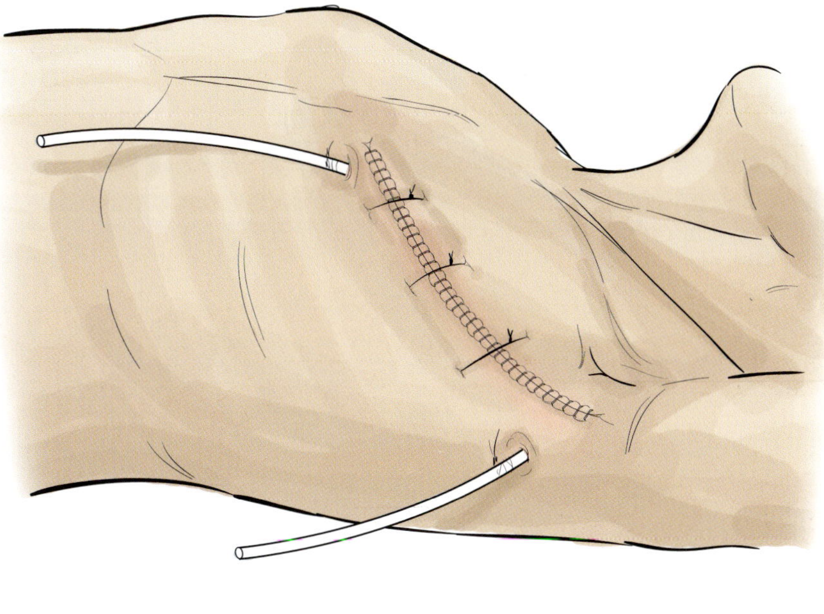

Figure 10-12.

III. ALTERNATIVE TECHNICAL APPROACHES (PRO/CON) AND PEARLS

- Bone graft reconstruction has the disadvantages of difficult fixation of bone stumps, mobility in the respiration phases, preliminary sterilization (if taken from cadaver), and risk of infection. The use of autologous bone graft, even if pedicled, after total sternum resection, has the same disadvantages, but lower risk of infection.
- Reconstructive techniques with synthetic mesh or "sandwich" materials have the advantage of being available at a low cost. The disadvantages are high tissue reactivity, reduced expansion, limited adaptability to growth in childhood, and risk of infection.
- The use of rigid sternum structures, although modeled, has the advantage of good cosmetic results, but these structures have disadvantages similar to those of synthetic materials.
- Anchorage of rigid structures can be done by metal threads. We prefer nonresorbable sutures that are more elastic and do not require crossing the bone, as opposed to metal threads.

IV. SPECIAL POSTOPERATIVE CARE

- Postoperative analgesia is essential to ensure patient collaboration. Epidural analgesia satisfies this need.
- The use of mechanical ventilatory devices such as continuous positive air pressure (CPAP) is also helpful in cases of wall resections associated with lung resection for oncologic needs.
- An orthopneic posture, rehabilitation therapy, and early standing with weight bearing are useful and recommended.

SUGGESTED READINGS

Briccoli A, Galletti S, Salone M, et al: Ultrasonography is superior to computer tomography and magnetic resonance imaging in determining superficial resection margins of malignant chest wall tumors, *J Ultrasound Med* 26:157–162, 2007.

Pearson FG, Hiebert CA, Deslauriers J, et al: *Thoracic surgery*, New York, 1995, Churchill Livingstone.

Skoracki RJ, Chang DW: Reconstruction of the chest wall and thorax, *J Surg Oncol* 94:455–465, 2006.

SECTION III

Esophagus

CHAPTER 11

Radical Esophagectomy with Two- or Three-Field Lymphadenectomy

Toni Lerut, MD, PhD, and Herbert Decaluwe, MD

I. SPECIAL PREOPERATIVE PREPARATION

Understanding Anatomy

- The thoracic esophagus is divided into three parts: upper, middle and lower esophagus. The upper esophagus is the segment between the level of the jugular notch and the carina. The segment of esophagus between the carina and the gastroesophageal junction (GEJ) is divided into two equal parts, the proximal of which is the middle, thoracic esophagus. The lower esophagus comprises the lower thoracic esophagus and the hiatal and abdominal segment of the esophagus. The definition of the esophagogastric esophagus of the cardia is imprecise. True tumors of the cardia are arising from the cardiac epithelium or short segments containing intestinal metaplasia of the GEJ (type II according to Siewert).
- Lymphatic spread is predominantly in the oral direction for tumors located above the carina and in the aboral direction in tumors below the carina and tumors of the cardia. However, cancers of the esophagus and GEJ are notorious for their chaotic lymphatic spread due to bypassing intramural lymphatic channels. As a result, even in carcinoma of the GEJ, cervical lymph node involvement can be seen in up to 15% of cases, and in contrast, upper-third cancers may show lymph node involvement along the lesser curvature and celiac axis in as many as 25% of cases.
- These reflections on anatomy and lymphatic spread are important in relation to the access route at the time of surgery. Cancers of the thoracic esophagus are preferentially approached through a transthoracic route. Supracarinal tumors are best approached from the right side. Infracarinal tumors can be approached either from the right or from the left side, whereas tumors of the GEJ can be approached either from the left side or through a supraumbilical laparotomy and transhiatal dissection and mobilization.

Diagnosis and Staging: Medical Operability

- The cardinal symptom bringing the patient to the doctor is dysphagia. Dysphagia in the majority of cases is reflecting an obstructive tumor and therefore usually an advanced-stage cancer. Diagnosis is confirmed through biopsy at the occasion of a diagnostic esophagoscopy.
- Staging aims at excluding/detecting local invasion into surrounding structures, lymph node metastasis, and organ metastasis resulting in stage grouping according to the Union for International Cancer Control (UICC)/TNM classification.
- Key investigations in this respect are high-resolution computed tomography (CT) scan, echoendoscopy with or without fine-needle aspiration of suspicious lymph nodes at a distance from the primary tumor, positron emission tomography (PET) scan, or integrated PET/CT scan (Figs. 11-1 and 11-2). Careful interpretation of the imaging results is mandatory because of the approximately 25% risk of either under- or overstaging. The latter potentially denies a patient the chance for a treatment with curative option.

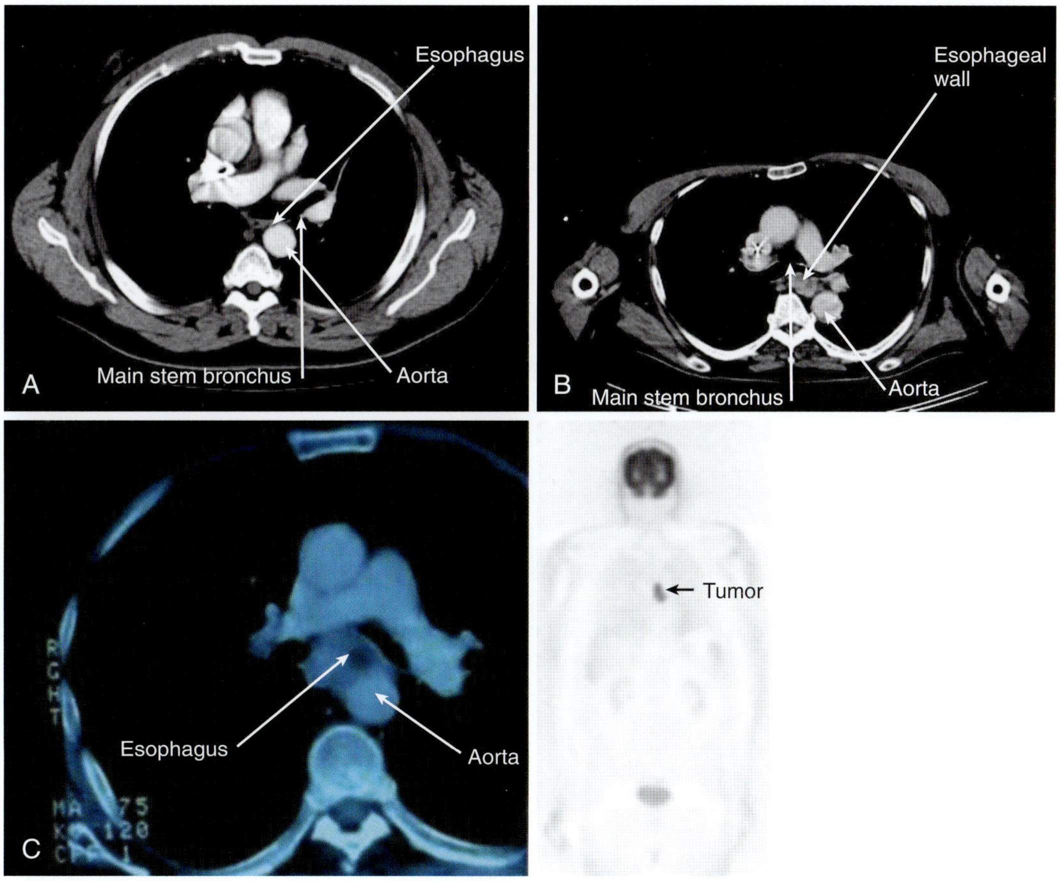

Figure 11-1. **A,** CT scan showing normal topographic configuration of esophagus at level of middle esophagus. **B,** CT scan of a clinical T4 tumor. The esophageal wall is clearly thickened, and there is no fat plane between tumor and posterior wall of main stem bronchus, whereas a clear fat plane is visible as a black line separating esophagus and descending aorta. **C,** CT scan of a clinical T4 tumor: no fat plane between thickened esophagus and bronchi as well as between tumor and aorta and corresponding PET image of the tumor. *CT*, Computed tomography; *PET*, positron emission tomography.

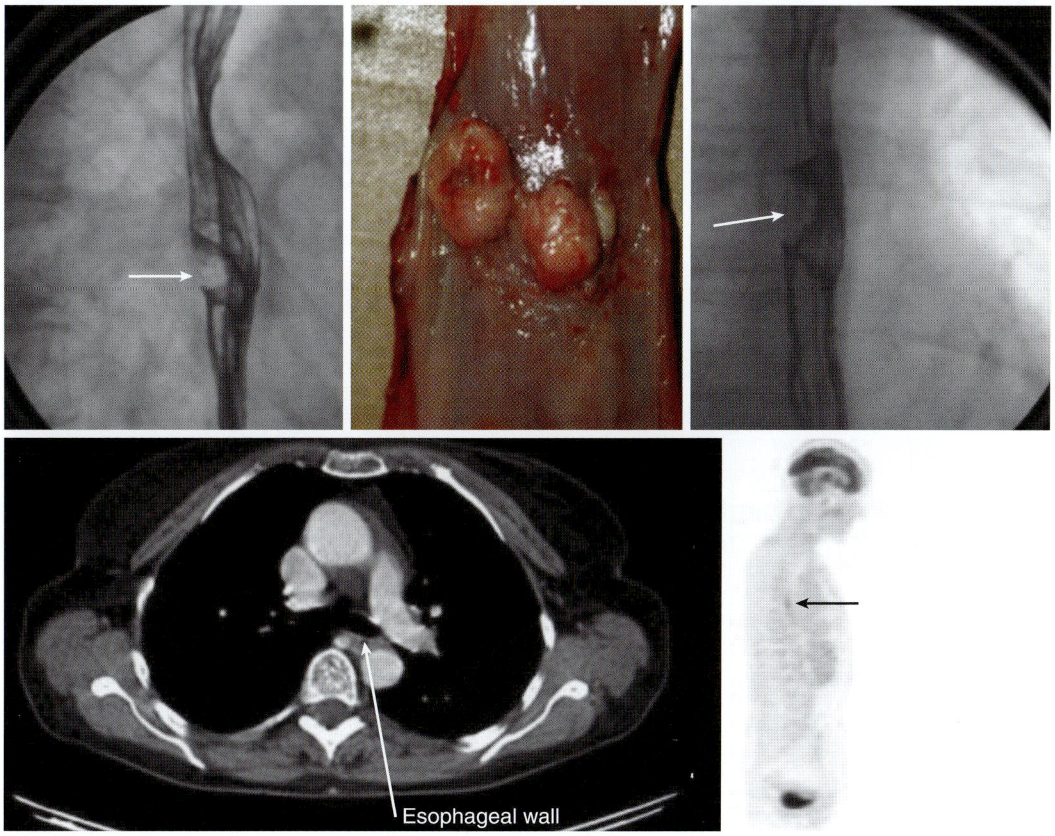

Figure 11-2. Patient with a T2 tumor on echoendoscopy. Barium swallow shows a polypoid like mass (*arrow*). On CT scan the esophageal wall is slightly thickened. PET scan shows an uptake in the midesophagus (*black arrow*). *CT*, Computed tomography; *PET*, positron emission tomography.

- In the absence of organ or distant lymph node metastasis or local invasion, patients are candidates for surgery. In locally advanced tumors, that is, suspicion for incomplete resection of the tumor and/or multiple regional lymph node involvement, induction chemotherapy with or without radiotherapy will precede surgery. Patients with tumors not invading surrounding structure and with no or limited peritumoral node involvement are candidates for primary surgery.
- Given the magnitude of the surgery, medical operability has to be assessed carefully. This includes spirometry including DLCO (diffusion capacity) and cardiac evaluation by electrocardiography and by either stress echocardiography or cycloergometry. The carotid arteries are assessed by Doppler ultrasound.
- Age is not a contraindication for surgery in the absence of significant comorbidity. Tobacco and alcohol abuse is frequently associated with esophageal cancer. Preoperative chest physiotherapy and cessation of smoking and drinking are mandatory. Nutritional condition may require hyperalimentation or gastrostomy tube feeding to convert a physiologically inoperable patient to one able to tolerate the operation. In any case, all existing comorbidities need to be assessed carefully.

Preparation

- It is customary to introduce an epidural catheter before starting anesthesia. This allows analgesia on a permanent basis over 4 to 5 days, allowing patients to cough up their expectorations more comfortably without pain.
- A double-lumen orotracheal tube is preferable, allowing the ipsilateral lung to collapse during the thoracic dissection. Central venous and peripheral arterial lines are part of the routine. It is of paramount importance to restrict intravenous fluid administration to avoid third-space fluid shift into pulmonary tissues manipulated during surgery and subsequent increased risk of pulmonary infection.
- The anesthesiologist should monitor fluid administration on blood pressure rather than on urinary output.

II. OPERATIVE TECHNIQUE: RIGHT-SIDED APPROACH

Position

- Supracarinal tumors are best approached from the right side. The patient is typically positioned in left lateral decubitus position.

Incision

- The chest is entered through the fifth intercostal space (Fig. 11-3), and a rib spreader is introduced.

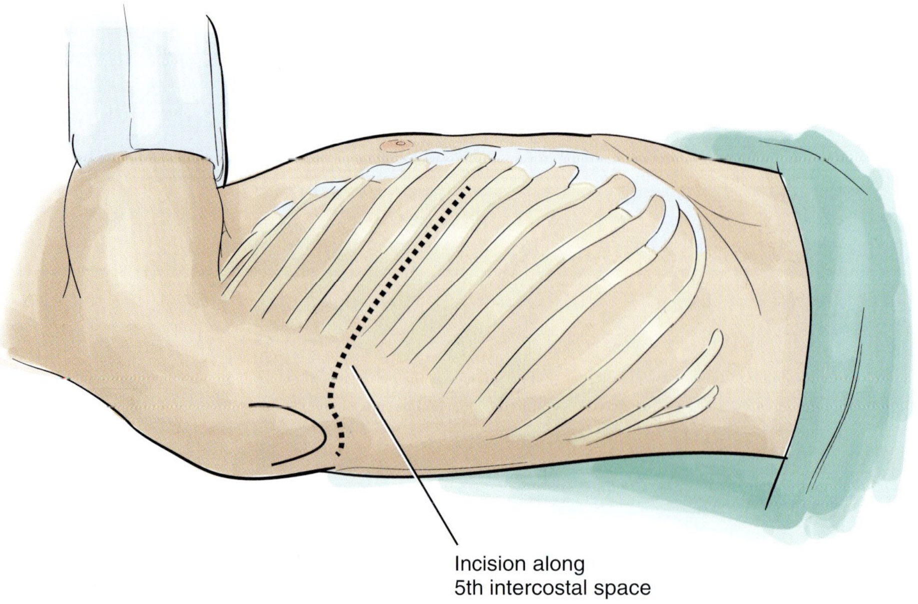

Figure 11-3.

Main Dissection

- After incising the overlying mediastinal pleura along the descending aorta, the azygos vein overlying the esophagus is mobilized, clamped, transected, and ligated.
- The basic principle of the operation consists in a wide peritumoral en bloc resection. This includes all adjacent periesophageal fat, the azygos vein, the thoracic duct, and the surrounding lymph nodes in the posterior mediastinum and subcarinal region. The dissection is commenced by ligating all the branches of the azygos vein and the arterial branches for the esophagus coming from the descending aorta. The thoracic duct is also identified and removed en bloc (Fig. 11-4). The dissection is continued posteriorly behind the esophagus, working toward the anterior side. A dissection plane is then made between the esophagus and pericardium, moving progressively in the cranial direction up to the carinal region, taking the subcarinal lymph nodes en bloc (Fig. 11-5). Both vagal nerves are to be divided,

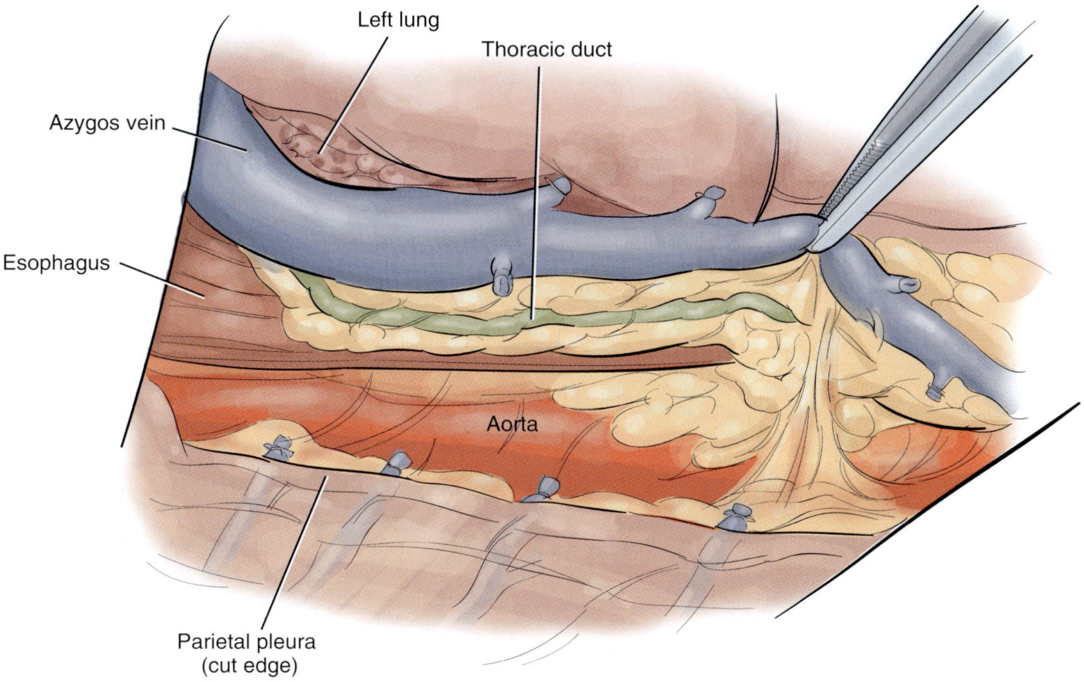

Figure 11-4.

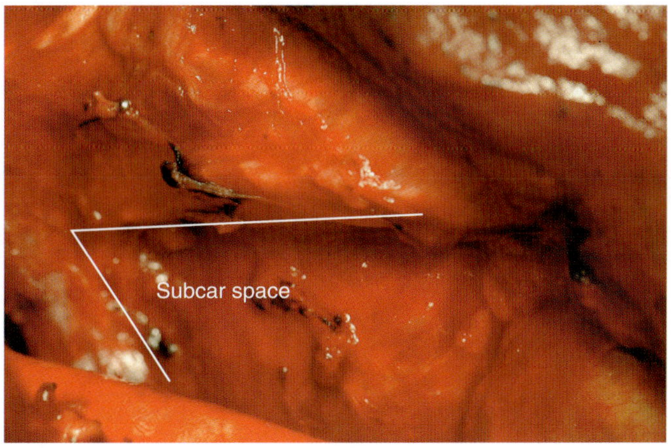

Figure 11-5.

and the dissection is continued up to the apex of the chest. The lymph node dissection in the aorto-pulmonary window and along the recurrent nerves is done separately, and great care is taken not to damage these nerves (Fig. 11-6). The brachiocephalic trunk nodes are the highest nodes removed.

- Downward, the dissection ends at the level of the esophageal hiatus. Incising the phrenoesophageal ligament and underlying peritoneum may facilitate the dissection from below the diaphragm during the abdominal part of the intervention. After closing the chest, the patient is turned to the supine position and prepared for a laparotomy and cervicotomy.
- Laparotomy can be done through a midline vertical supraumbilical incision or through a horizontal incision (Fig. 11-7, *inset*).

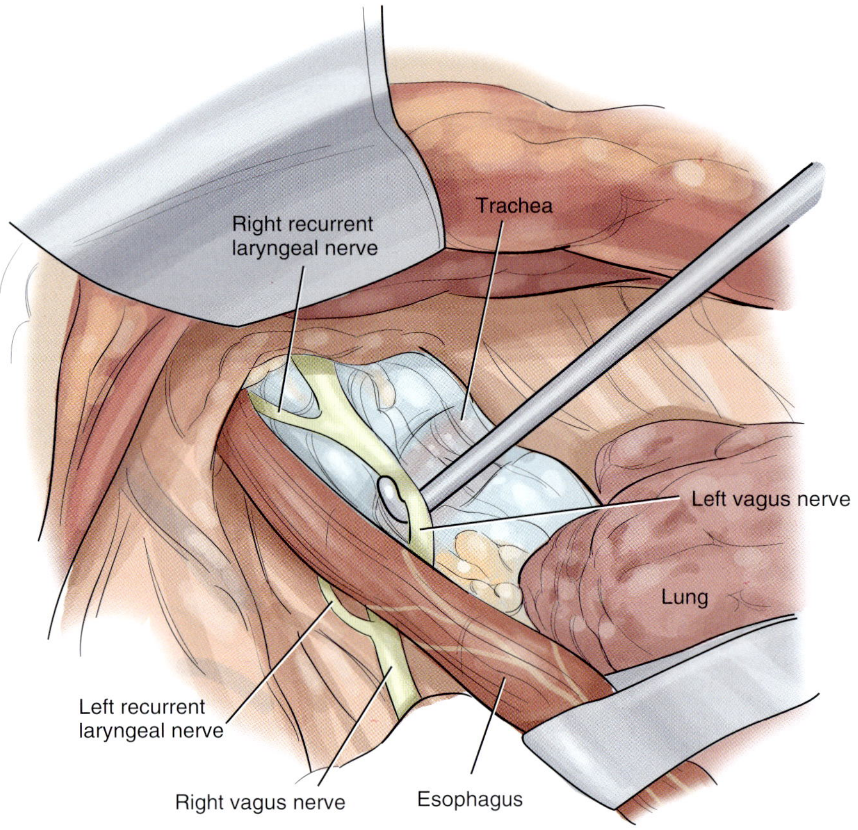

Figure 11-6.

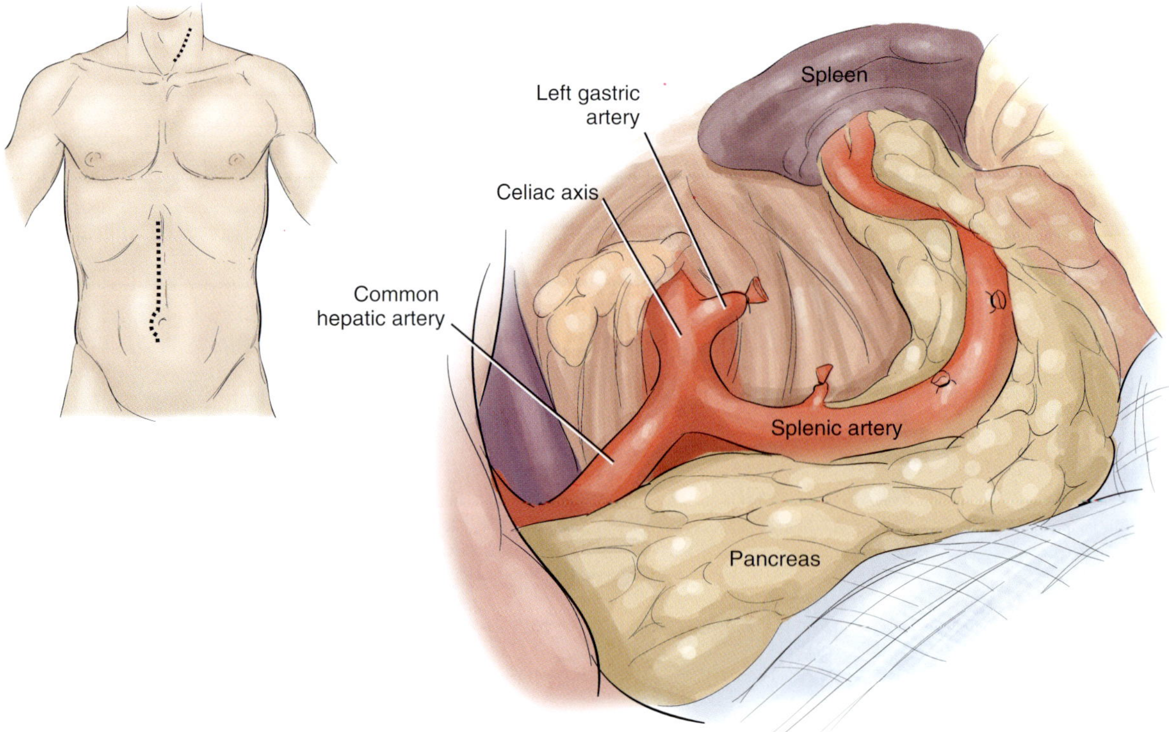

Figure 11-7.

- The left liver lobe is detached from the diaphragm and reclined to the right. Mobilization of stomach starts by dividing the omental branches of the right and left gastroepiploic artery, the short gastric vessels are divided between ligatures or clips, and the mobilization of the fundus is completed by dividing the gastrophrenic attachments up to the left part of the hiatus. The lesser omentum and the vagal branches to the liver are incised and ligated, and the already commenced mobilization of the cardia in the hiatus is completed. Now the lymphadenectomy of the upper abdominal compartment is started by transecting and ligating the left gastric artery and vein and concomitant lymph nodes close to their offspring from the celiac axis. Lymph nodes along the celiac axis, the common hepatic artery, the portal vein, the splenic artery, and the hilum of the spleen are removed separately to obtain a complete level II lymphadenectomy (see Fig. 11-7).
- The stomach is now tubulized, resecting the lesser curvature by using a linear stapler apparatus. The lesser curvature is resected downward to approximately 3 cm above the pylorus. Usually the stapler line is oversewn by a continuous suture (Fig. 11-8). If insufficient length is suspected, a Kocher maneuver is performed to mobilize the duodenum and the head of the pancreas.
- In the case of a two-field lymphadenectomy, a left cervicotomy is made (Fig. 11-9). The sternocleidomastoid muscle and the carotid vessels are retracted laterally. After the inferior thyroid artery is divided,

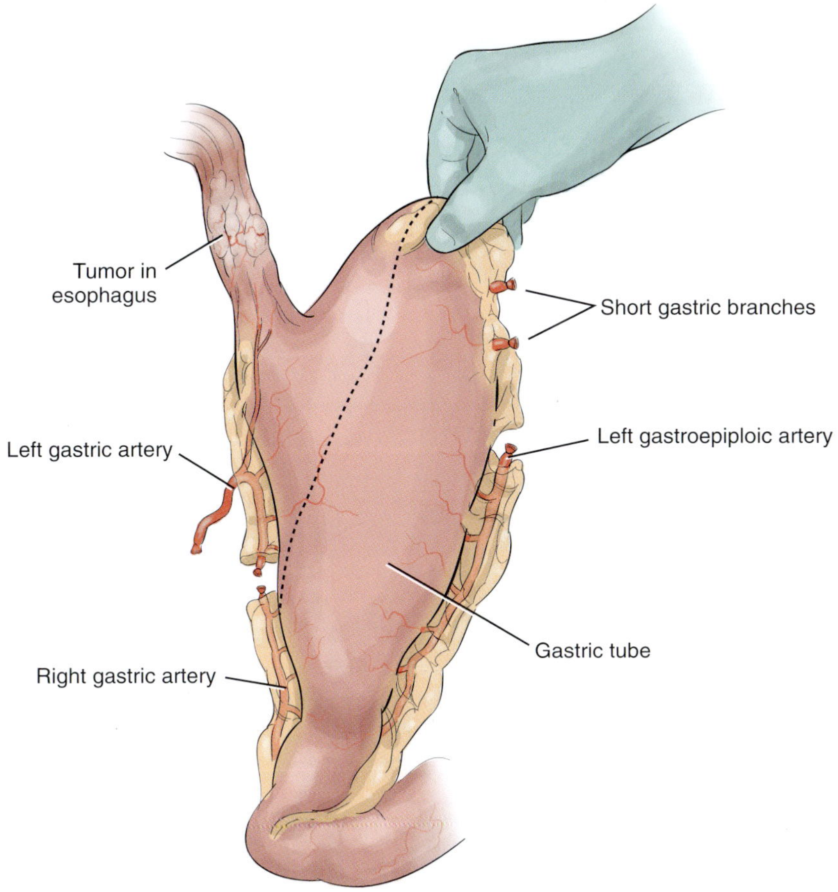

Figure 11-8.

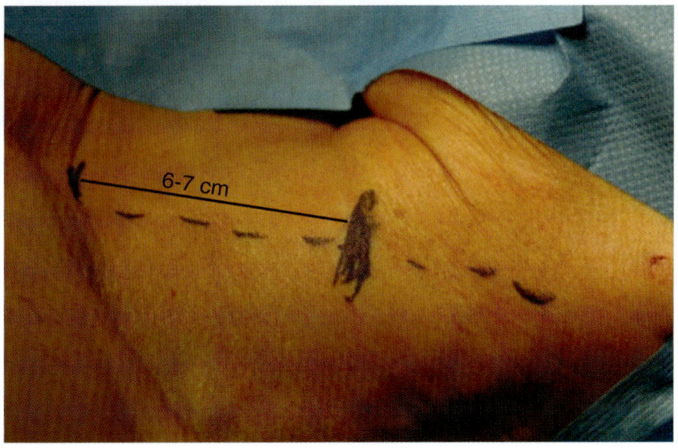

Figure 11-9.

the cervical esophagus becomes readily visible, and usually little dissection is required to complete the esophageal mobilization in the neck.

- The top of the gastric tube, which is temporarily attached to the distal end of the separated lesser curve and the esophagus, is pulled out through the cervical incision until the gastric tube comes into the operative field. After transecting the esophagus, an end-to-side anastomosis is fashioned, usually on the anterior side of the gastric tube. The anastomosis usually is performed in two layers with a continuous running suture: absorbable for the inner layer, nonabsorbable for the outer layer (Fig. 11-10, and see Fig. 11-13).
- When performing a three-field lymphadenectomy (Fig. 11-11), a U-shaped incision is made in the neck 1 cm above the suprasternal notch. The incision is extended upward and laterally along the anterior border of the sternocleidomastoid muscle. The platysma muscle, the omohyoideus and lower third of the strap muscles are then divided. The deep internal cervical nodes (Fig. 11-11, area *A*) medial to the carotid sheet, also known as the recurrent laryngeal chain, are dissected out. Early identification and isolation of recurrent laryngeal nerves is imperative. On the right side, this nerve is somewhat more lateral to the trachea as compared with the left one. Then the deep external (Fig. 11-11, area *B*)

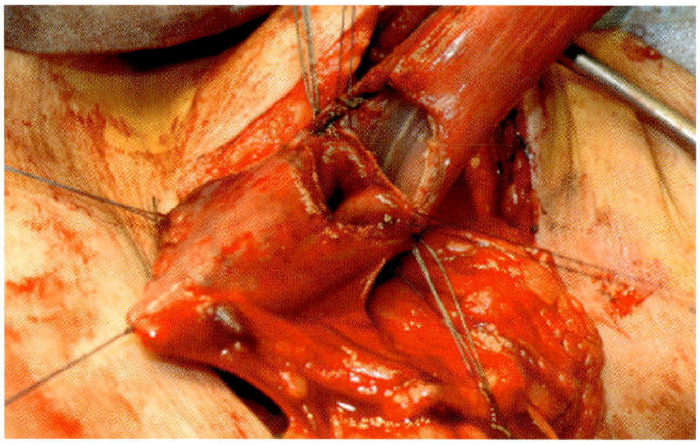

Figure 11-10.

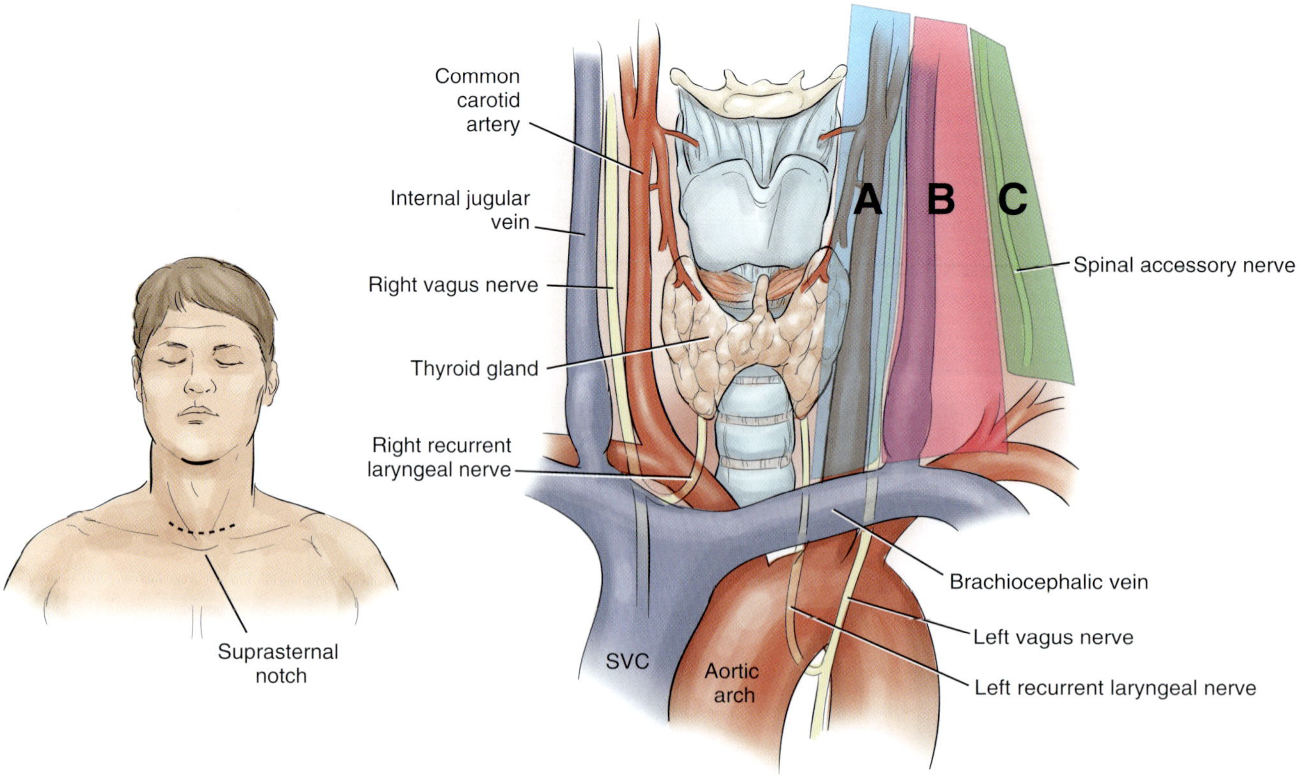

Figure 11-11.

and deep lateral nodes (Fig. 11-11, area *C*) (spinal accessory lymphatic chain) are removed. These nodes are situated lateral to the internal jejunal vein. Vagus and phrenic nerves, as well as the accessory nerves, are to be individually and carefully identified.

Closure

- The laparotomy is closed by approximating the linea alba with continuous 1-0 monofilament suture. The skin is closed with staples. The cervical incision closure involves meticulous approximation of the platysma, and then the skin is closed with staples or subcuticular 4-0 absorbable suture.

III. OPERATIVE TECHNIQUE: LEFT-SIDED APPROACH

- The left thoracic approach is considered by many authors to be the standard approach for carcinoma of the lower esophagus and cardia.

Position

- The patient is placed in the supine position with the left side raised with a wedge to allow full thoracic extension of the thoracoabdominal incision.

Incision

- In this operation, the chest is entered through the sixth intercostal space. After dividing the costal margin, the diaphragm is incised at its periphery using an inverted T-shaped incision; the short limb of the T incises the abdominal wall for a few centimeters. This approach permits optimal direct vision of both the abdomen and chest cavity through a single incision, enabling an optimal radical procedure to be achieved.

Main Dissection

- The entire thoracic esophagus can be dissected through the left-sided approach. The dissection of the esophagus from beneath the aortic arch requires ligation and transection of the bronchial arteries just below the arch. The mobilization is continued by blunt finger dissection behind the aortic arch up into the apex of the chest. The mediastinal pleura above the aortic arch is opened. Lymphadenectomy in both the abdomen and posterior mediastinum is performed as described earlier. After resection of the esophagus, the gastric tube is brought upward through the hiatus and behind the aortic arch. The gastric tube is temporarily fixed to the esophageal stump in the apex of the chest.

Closure

- The incision is then closed, and the patient is turned to the supine position. Through a left cervicotomy, the esophageal stump with the attached gastric tube is exteriorized into the operative field, and a cervical esophagogastrostomy is undertaken.

IV. ALTERNATIVE TECHNICAL APPROACHES (PRO/CON) AND PEARLS

- Using the right-sided approach with the anastomosis performed via a cervical incision as described is called the McKeown procedure (or the so-called three-hole dissection). An alternative technique consists in performing the anastomosis in the top of the chest and is called the Ivor-Lewis procedure (or the so-called two-hole dissection), avoiding a separate incision in the neck.

- The esophagogastrostomy can be performed manually (Fig. 11-12) or by using stapler devices. One can use the circular stapler device or, in particular when performing the anastomosis in the neck, a linear stapler to obtain a so-called semimechanical anastomosis creating a V-shaped enlargement (Fig. 11-13).

Transhiatal Esophagectomy

- This method may be appropriate for tumors originating from the cardia and GEJ.
- The operation is started with a median laparotomy; the incision extends from the xiphoid process to just below the umbilicus. After mobilizing the left liver lobe, the esophageal hiatus can be inspected for invasion of adjacent organs. Subsequently, the stomach is mobilized. The esophagus is freed in the hiatus, and, if necessary, a surrounding cuff of diaphragm can be included in the resection specimen. Next, the central tendon of the left hemidiaphragm is incised, thus opening the lower mediastinum. The periesophageal fatty tissues of the left and right parietal pleura and pericardium are included in the surgical specimen. This procedure can be extended at least as far as the inferior pulmonary veins. The more proximal, and so far unmobilized, part of the (normal) esophagus is bluntly mobilized or stripped, using a vein stripper from the neck. After completion of the intraabdominal dissection, a neoesophagus is created from the stomach. During this procedure, lymph nodes along the right and left gastric artery as well as the common hepatic artery down to the portal vein and along the splenic

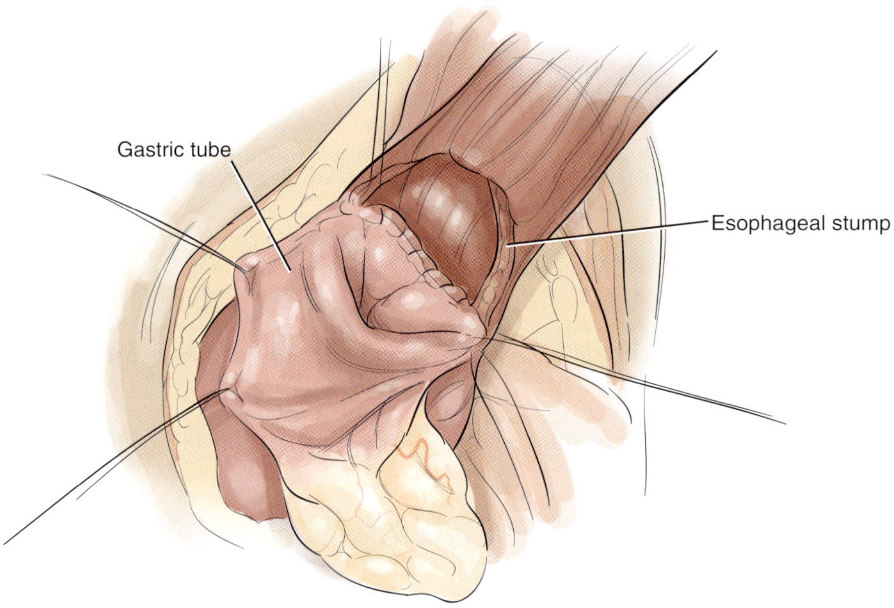

Figure 11-12.

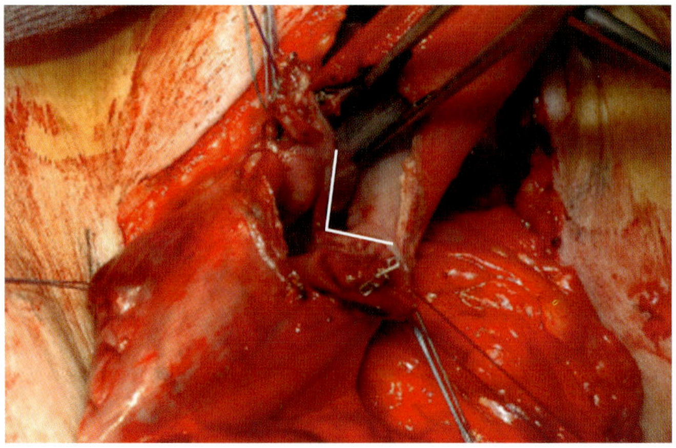

Figure 11-13. Semimechanical anastomosis: the white V-line indicates the staple line resulting in V-shaped widening of the anastomosis.

artery are removed. The gastric tube is pulled/pushed, via the prevertebral route, to the neck where an esophagogastrostomy is created.

Alternatives for Early Carcinoma

- In early carcinoma, in particular T1a in long-segment Barrett, less invasive approaches can be used, because in T1a the likelihood of lymph node involvement is minimal and thus an extensive lymphadenectomy is not necessary. If the Barrett segment is less than 5 cm, a so-called Merendino operation can be used. This operation is done through an upper midline laparotomy and consists in a partial esophagectomy of the lower esophagus and an interposition with a jejunal loop. Both vagal nerves are left intact.
- Another alternative, more suitable in case of early cancer in a long-segment Barrett, is the total thoracoscopic and laparoscopic esophagectomy and reconstruction with the gastric tube. Some authors, however, prefer the transhiatal vagus-sparing esophagectomy followed by a long-segment colon interposition brought up through the posterior mediastinal route. These so-called minimally invasive operations supposedly result in quicker recovery.

V. SPECIAL POSTOPERATIVE CARE

- As in most major thoracic interventions, early extubation is considered beneficial because it allows the patient to resume a normal coughing mechanism, which is responsible for maintaining an unobstructed airway. Combining efficient coughing and chest physiotherapy is of paramount importance in the prevention of pulmonary infection. Equally important is a careful monitoring of the intravenous fluid administration, which should be restricted to avoid transudation of fluid into the lung tissue during surgery with the resulting increased risk for pulmonary infection. Finally, effective analgesia, in particular epidural analgesia, is a key element in helping patients to produce vigorous coughing and clearance of secretions. In case of abundant secretions, liberal use of bronchoscopic aspiration or the use of minitracheostomy may help the patient to overcome reintubation and artificial respiration.
- A nasogastric tube is left in situ until transit is restored. Oral feeding can usually be resumed at day 4 or 5, unless suspicion of anastomotic leak. Signs indicating such event are increasing inflammatory parameters, cervical wound infection, or abcedation followed by salivary drainage. Treatment in the vast majority of cases is conservative until drying up of the salivary fistula. Only in the very rare case of gastric tube necrosis confirmed by endoscopy does reintervention become necessary, that is, taking down the gastric tube and constructing a temporary esophagostomy and feeding jejunostomy. Continuity will be restored after 4 to 6 months, usually by means of a colon interposition.

SUGGESTED READINGS

Altroki N, Skinner D: Should en bloc esophagectomy be the standard of care for esophageal carcinoma? *Ann Surg* 234:581–587, 2001.

Lerut T, Flamen P, Ectors N, et al: Histopathologic validation of lymph node staging with FDG-PET scan in cancer of the esophagus and gastroesophageal junction: a prospective study based on primary surgery with extensive lymphadenectomy, *Ann Surg* 232:743–752, 2000.

Lerut T, Nafteux P, Moons J, et al: Three-field lymphadenectomy for carcinoma of the esophagus and gastroesophageal junction in 174 R0 resections: impact on staging, disease-free survival, and outcome; a plea for adaptation of TNM classification in upper-half esophageal carcinoma, *Ann Surg* 240:962–972; discussion 972–974, 2004.

CHAPTER 12

Transhiatal Esophagectomy via Laparoscopy and Transmediastinal Endodissection

Alberto Peracchia, MD, FACS, and Riccardo Rosati, MD, FACS

I. SPECIAL PREOPERATIVE PREPARATION

Indications

- This operation currently has limited indications, as a thoracoscopic mobilization of the esophagus in prone position has been shown to be safer than the laparoscopic transhiatal approach.
- Surgical planning: to perform a total esophagectomy with laparoscopic gastric tubulization and laparoscopic lymphadenectomy, transhiatal dissection, and cervical esophagogastroplasty via left cervicotomy (see Fig. 12-1).
- Indications to this procedure are:
  - ▲ Multifocal high-grade dysplasia (HGD/T1 carcinoma) on Barrett's esophagus
  - ▲ Resectable carcinoma of the thoracic esophagus stage cT1 or downstaged after neoadjuvant chemoradiation
- For clinical staging and assessment, see Table 12.1.

II. OPERATIVE TECHNIQUE

Position

- General anesthesia is induced with either single- or double-lumen orotracheal intubation.
- Central venous line and arterial monitoring are placed.
- A nasogastric tube is in place to obtain appropriate suction of the gastric content.
- A Foley catheter is placed.
- The patient is placed on the operating table in the lithotomy position with a 20-degree/30-degree reverse Trendelenburg and the surgeon standing between the legs in the standard position for supramesocolic surgery. The first assistant is at the surgeon's right, and the second assistant stays at surgeon's left side. The camera is held by both assistants according to the different phases of the procedure. A roll is placed below the shoulders; the head is hyperextended and turned toward the right. A single skin surgical field is prepared.

Trocar Placement

- Pneumoperitoneum is established with open laparoscopy placing a Hasson trocar in the umbilicus. CO_2 pressure of 12 mm Hg is maintained throughout the procedure. A 30-degree scope is recommended in this case. Four other operating ports are used to access the operative field: the operative trocars (in the surgeon's right and left hands) are 12 mm in diameter and are placed in the left and right hypochondrium, respectively, at the midclavicular line. The first assistant trocar is placed on the transverse umbilical line at its joint with the anterior axillary line. The second assistant trocar is placed below the xiphoid process, slightly at its left (Fig. 12-1).

Main Dissection

- A Kocher maneuver is made, tractioning the duodenum medially and using both sharp and blunt dissection until the retroduodenal vena cava is widely exposed. After this maneuver, if planned, an extramucosal pyloromyotomy (Fig. 12-2, *A*) and pyloroplasty (Fig. 12-2, *B*) are made at this time.

TABLE 12-1 Clinical Staging and Assessment

- Clinical staging of disease:
  - ▲ Endoscopy with biopsy
  - ▲ Endoscopic ultrasound
  - ▲ Abdominal and chest computed tomography scan
  - ▲ In selected cases: neck ultrasound, fluorodeoxyglucose positron emission tomography or computed tomography–positron emission tomography scan, bronchoscopy
- Patient conditions assessment:
  - ▲ Cardiac function
  - ▲ Respiratory function
  - ▲ Liver function
  - ▲ Nutritional status
- Respiratory physiotherapy
- Preparation of the large bowel as for a colonoscopy

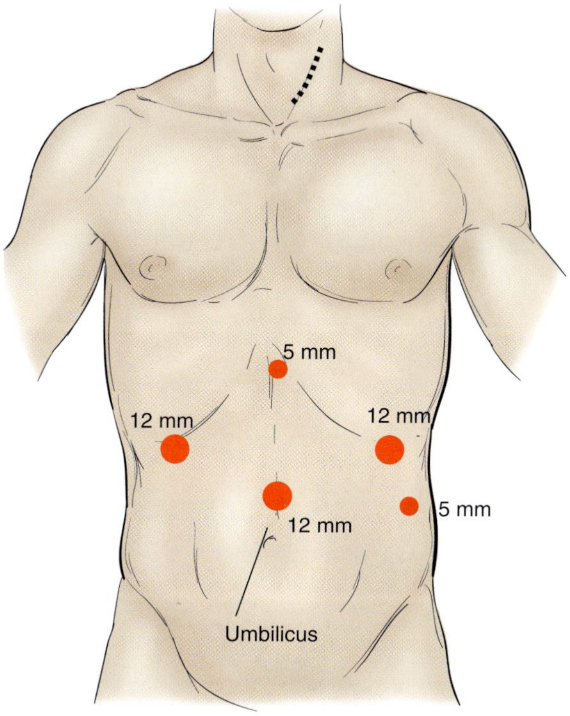

Figure 12-1.

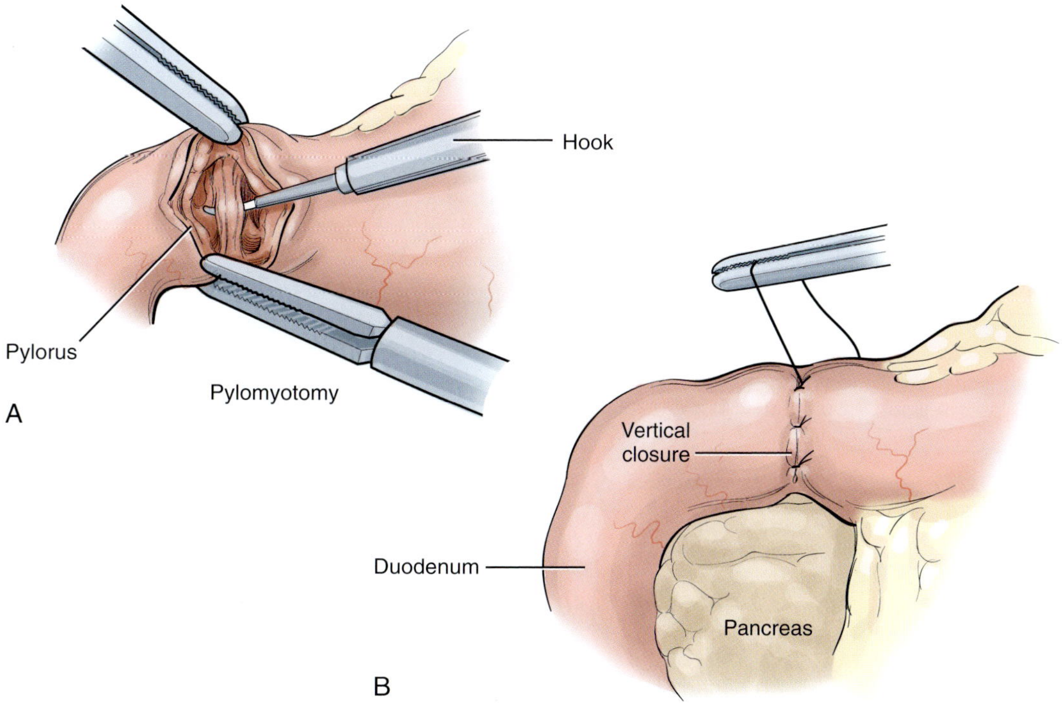

Figure 12-2.

- Gastric mobilization is then started: the stomach is lifted upward and the gastrocolic ligament divided at a safe distance from the right gastroepiploic vascular arcade. Section of the gastrocolic ligament (Fig. 12-3) is made, preferably with the Atlas LigaSure (Valleylab, Boulder, Colo.) or with the Ultracision (Ethicon, Somerville, NJ). The gastrocolic ligament is completely divided from the origin of the right gastroepiploic to the short gastric vessels, allowing the full mobilization of the greater curvature of the stomach. The lesser omentum is also divided just below the margin of the left lobe of the liver (Fig. 12-4). The phrenoesophageal membrane is then divided from right to left, dissecting from above the left diaphragmatic crus. Tractioning the stomach to the left, the peritoneum over the right

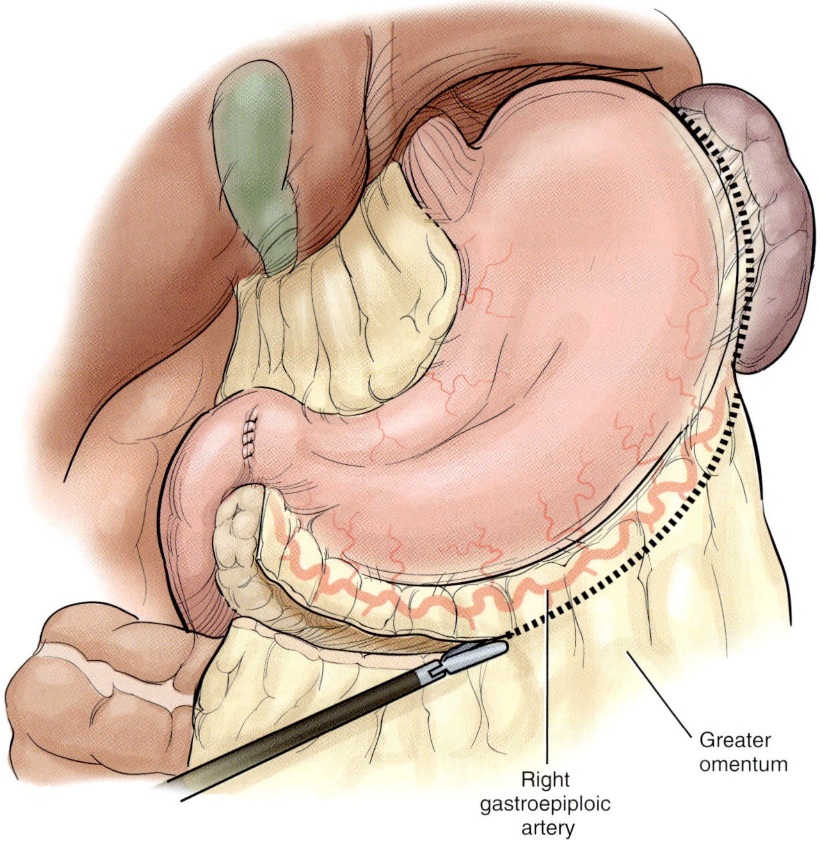

Figure 12-3.

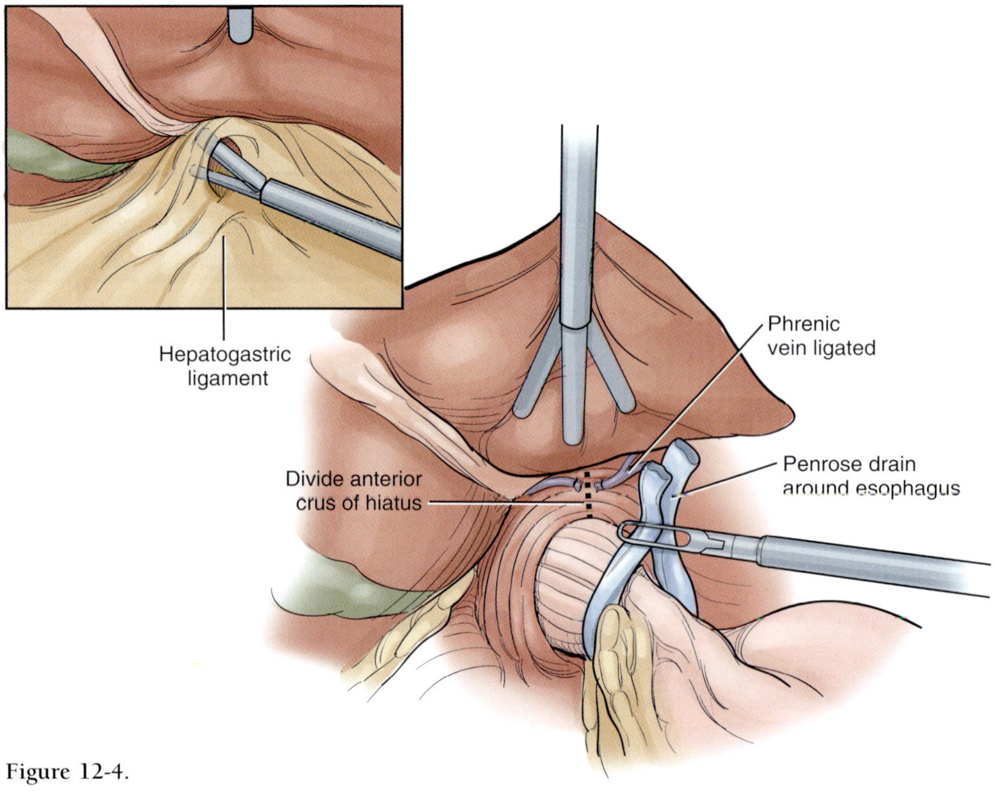

Figure 12-4.

diaphragmatic crus (Fig. 12-5) is then divided, allowing complete encirclement of the abdominal esophagus, which is taped for traction (see Fig. 12-4).

- Dissection on the lesser omentum is extended to the medial border of the common hepatic artery, allowing removal of all the nodes of the hepatogastric area. The stomach is then lifted again to expose the left gastric vascular pedicle and the celiac axis. Incision of the retroperitoneum is made on the pancreatic margin along the hepatic artery. Dissection is made on the arterial wall, excising en bloc all the lymphatic tissue lying on the vessel. Dissection is extended medially at the origin of the left gastric artery and vein (Fig. 12-6), which are clipped and divided.

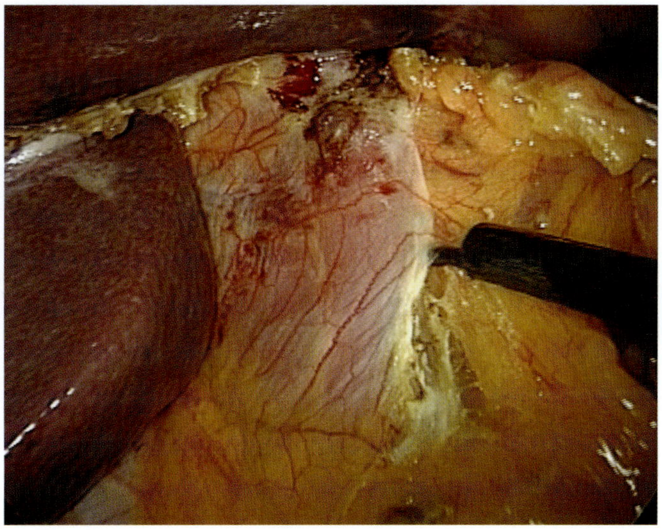

Figure 12-5.

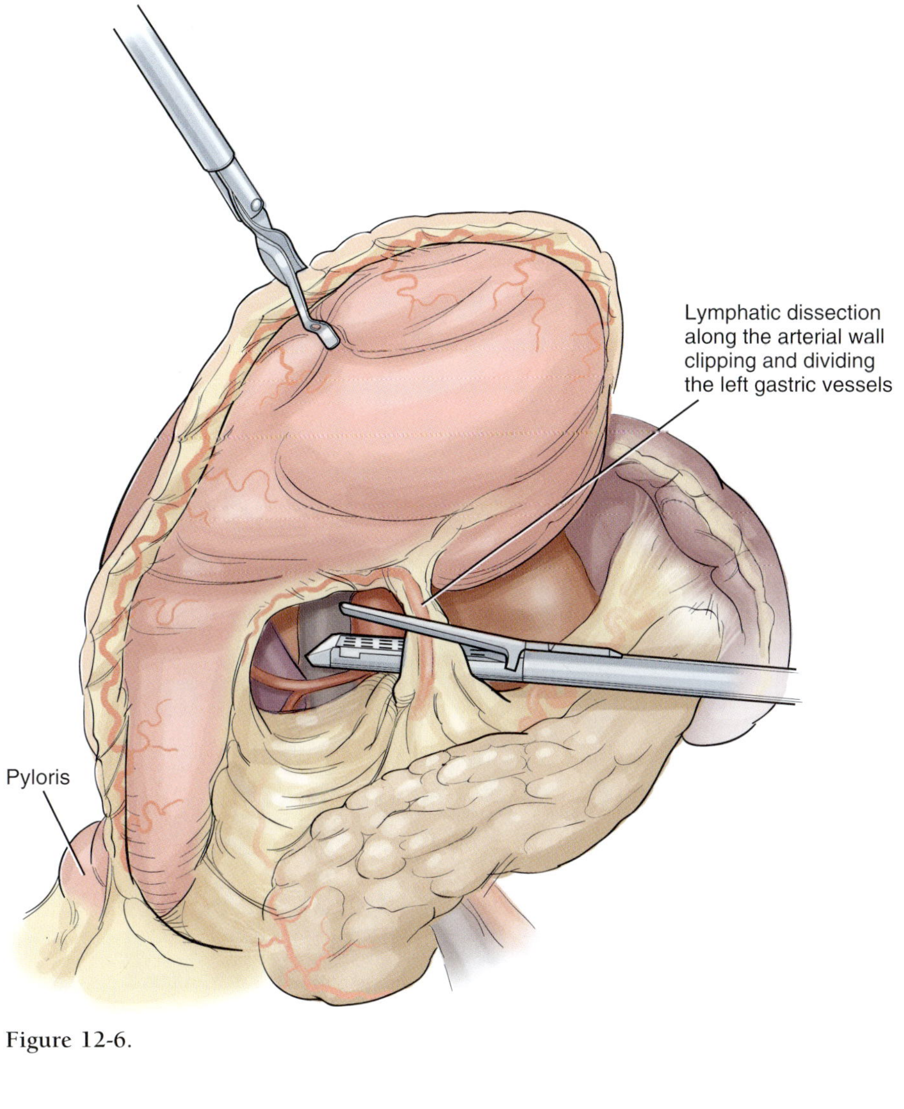

Figure 12-6.

- Dissection is then pushed to the left on the splenic artery, leaving all the lymphatic tissue en bloc with the gastric specimen. According to the surgeon preference, the stomach is then prepared for mediastinal and cervical transposition either as a whole organ or as a gastric tube. In the former case, dissection of the lesser omentum is made on the gastric wall, starting from the level of the pyloric artery, then reaching the cardia. Gastric division is then made with a linear stapler a few centimeters below the cardia to the apex of the gastric fundus. In the latter case, multiple applications of the linear stapler are placed (Fig. 12-7) starting just distally to the angulus, parallel to the greater curvature, reaching the apex of the gastric fundus. In both cases, the gastric staple line might be buttressed with a running, absorbable suture (Fig. 12-8).

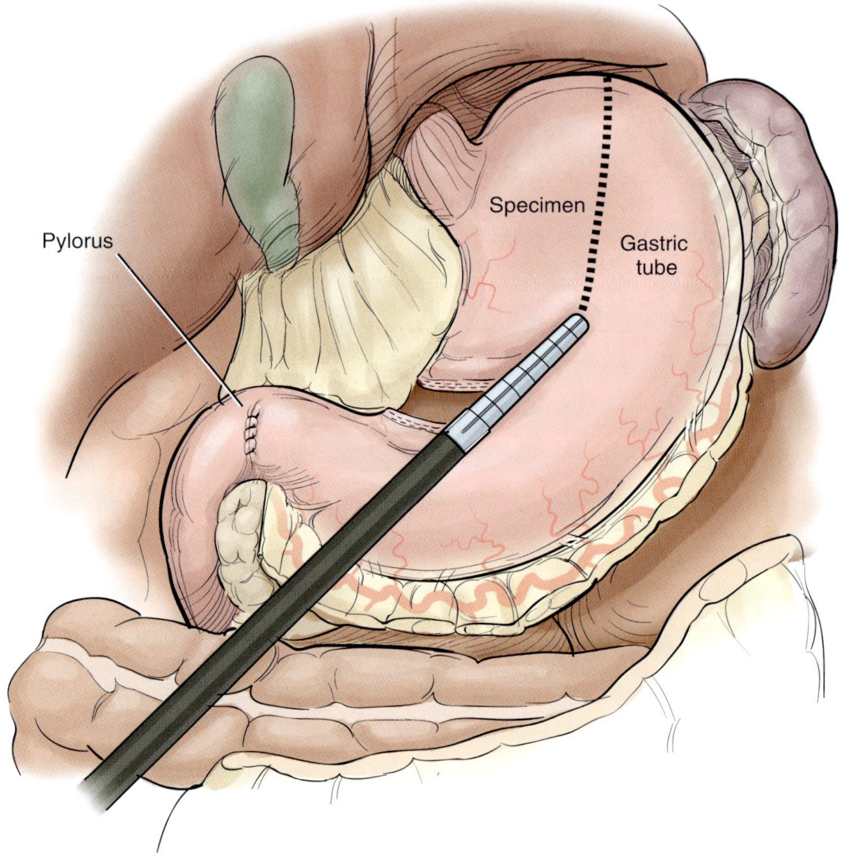

Figure 12-7.

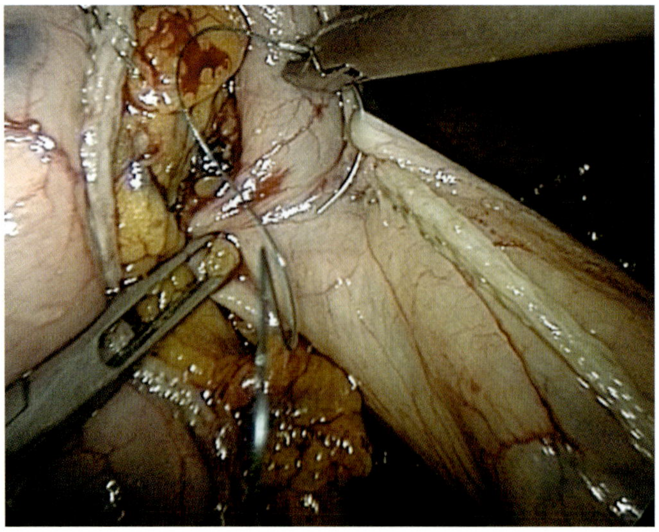

Figure 12-8.

Transmediastinal Dissection

- The mediastinum is entered, staying close to the inner muscular border of the diaphragmatic crura. The plans of dissection are as follows: inferiorly, the anterior wall of the aorta; superiorly, the pericardium; laterally, both the pleura. Dissection is made bluntly and sharply. The use of the Atlas LigaSure (Fig. 12-9) eases this technique: because of its smooth tip, the instrument can be advanced bluntly with no risk of tearing main vascular structures; it can then be activated to cut the minimal vascular pedicles of the esophagus with no bleeding.
- Dissection is moved up in the mediastinum until the tracheal bifurcation is reached.

Cervical Dissection

- A longitudinal incision is made along the border of the sternocleidomastoid muscle from the sternal notch to midway in the mastoid process. Section of the omohyoid muscle and the inferior thyroid artery is made. The thyroid is elevated and a space is created until the prevertebral fascia is reached. The cervical esophagus, which is closely adherent to the inferior face of the thyroid and to the trachea,

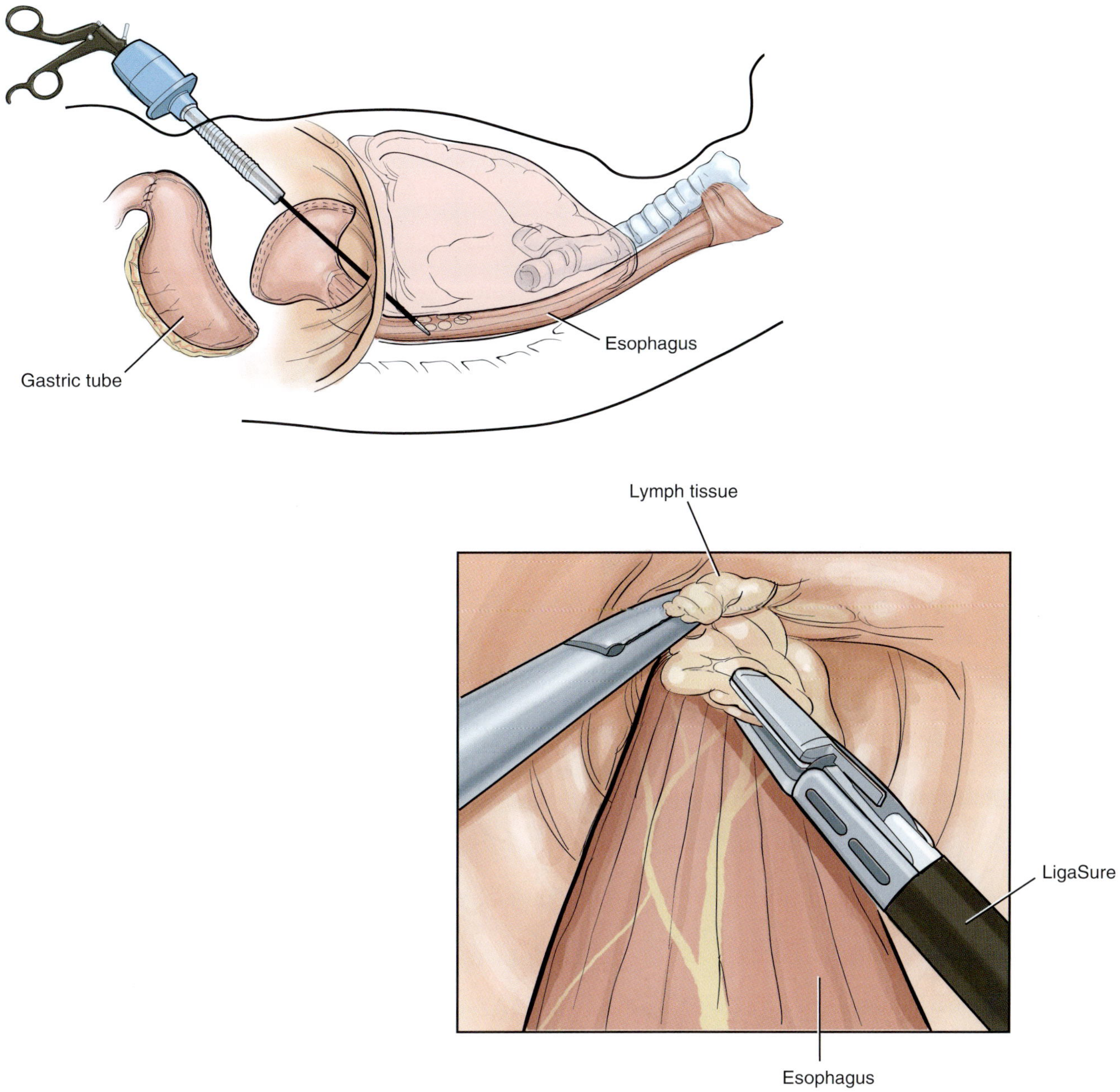

Figure 12-9.

is dissected, encircled (paying attention to the left recurrent laryngeal nerve), and taped for traction. The nasogastric tube is retracted, and the esophagus is cut (Fig. 12-10).

Mediastinal Dissection

- Endomediastinal dissection in the upper mediastinum can be made bluntly as a finger dissection staying adherent to the esophagus. An operative mediastinoscope can also be used for a more precise dissection and hemostasis: either the Buess mediastinoscope (Richard Wolf GMBH, Knittlingen, Germany) or a standard angled operative laparoscope with an applied ogival atraumatic tip (Fig. 12-11). Dissection of the upper mediastinum is pushed downward to reach the tracheal bifurcation.
- A combined dissection is now made by the transhiatal laparoscopic side and by the transmediastinal cervical side until the esophagus is fully mobilized (Fig. 12-12).
- The specimen may then be retrieved from the cervical incision.

Gastric Tube Transposition

- With the help of a tube inserted within the mediastinum from the peritoneal cavity and retrieved from the cervicotomy (Mousseau-Barbin, Porgès, Le Plessis Robinson, France), the stomach is transposed through the mediastinum and reaches the left cervical field. The apex of the gastric tube is sutured to the conic part of the tube, which is gently pulled up from the cervical field. The conical shape of the tube allows a smooth transposition of the stomach, preventing tearing of its vascular pedicle. Once the stomach has reached the neck, a suture is placed that fixes it at the prevertebral fascia and acts as a stay suture.

Anastomosis

- Esophagogastric anastomosis at the neck is performed in a semimechanical fashion according to the technique of Orringer. The apex of the transposed gastric fundus is solidarized with two stay sutures to the posterior esophageal wall, 3 to 4 cm cranially to the stump. A small opening is made on the anterior gastric wall at the level of the esophageal stump, and an EndoGIA II 30 3.5 (United States Surgical, Norwalk, Conn.) is introduced, closed, and fired: this is the mechanical part of the anastomosis, which connects the posterior esophageal wall to the anterior gastric wall (Fig. 12-13).

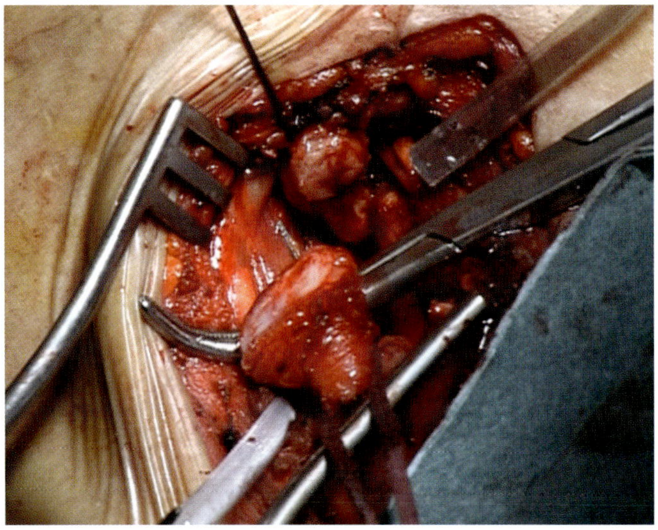

Figure 12-10.

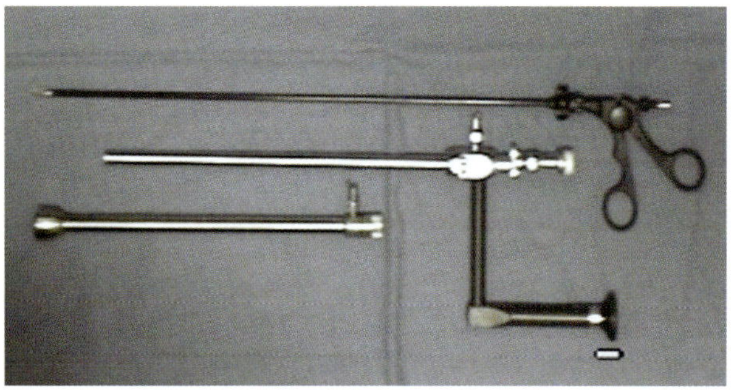

Figure 12-11.

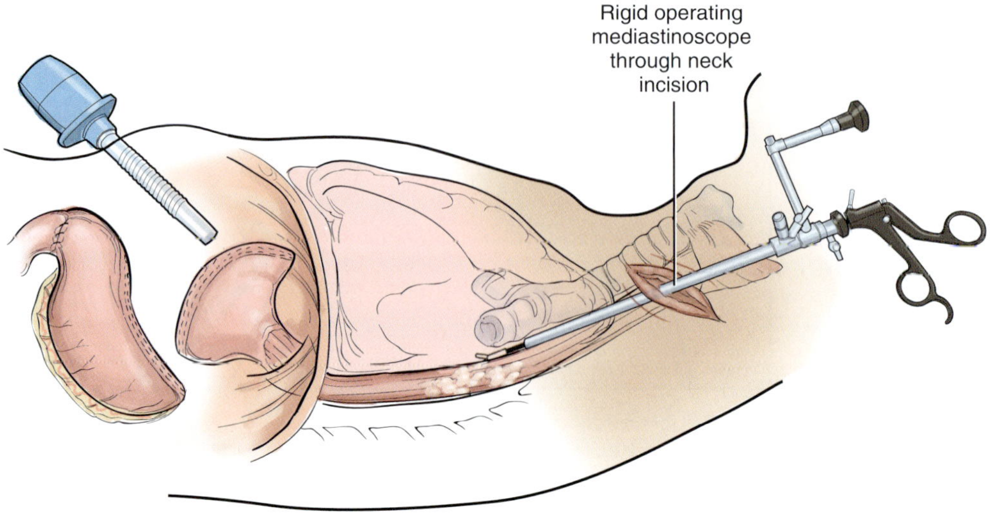

Figure 12-12.

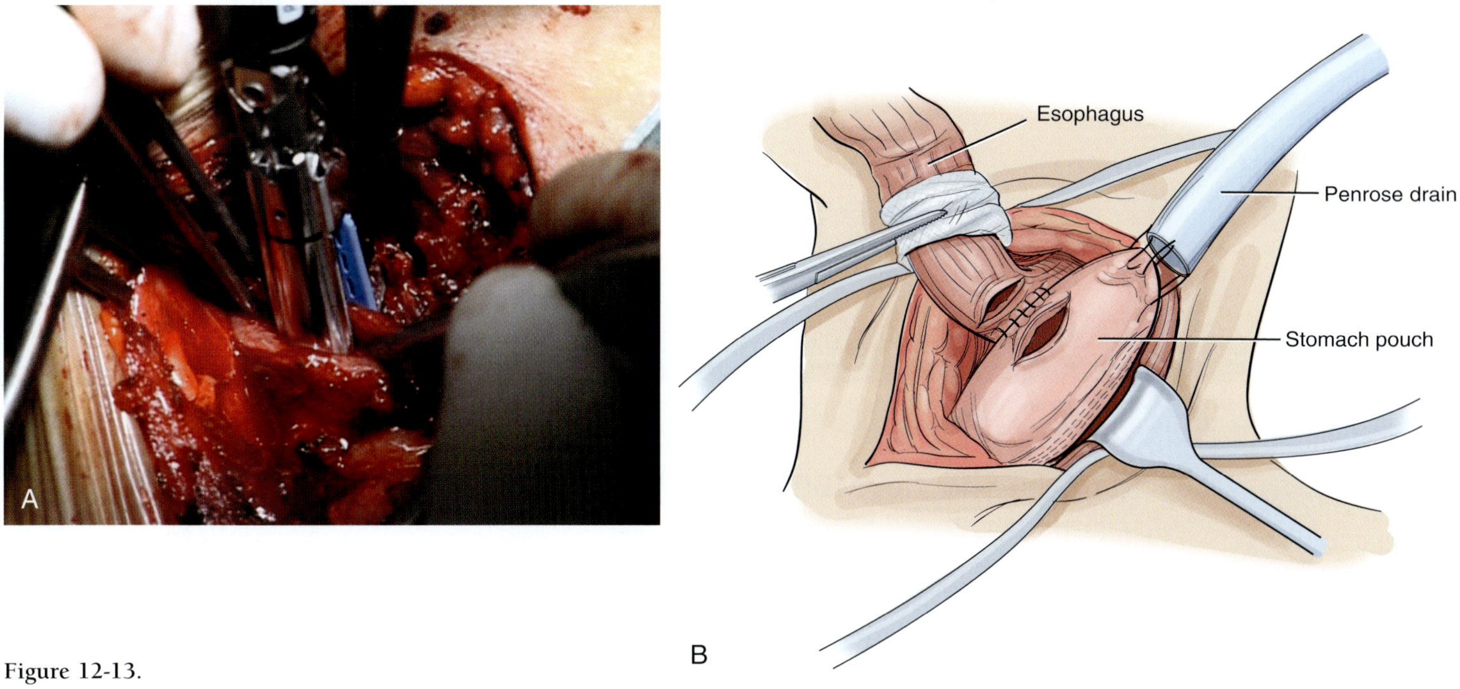

Figure 12-13.

- The anterior part of the anastomosis is generally made manually with absorbable synthetic monofilament in either a single or a double layer, with running or interrupted sutures.
- Once the anastomosis is completed, the nasogastric tube is passed to decompress the transposed stomach.

Closure

- A Penrose drain, which will stay in place for 24 hours, is placed near the anastomosis, and the left cervicotomy is closed.
- In the abdomen, a final inspection is made, and the prepyloric region of the stomach is sutured to both the diaphragmatic crura to prevent migration of the bowel in the mediastinum.

III. ALTERNATIVE TECHNICAL APPROACHES (PRO/CON) AND PEARLS

- Nonsurgical options for HGD on Barrett's esophagus consist of endoscopic mucosal resection (EMR). In experienced hands and selected cases, this might be curative with lesser complications and better quality of life as compared to surgery. Radiofrequency ablation (BarrX) is useful to treat the remaining Barrett's epithelium after EMR.
- However, a large number of patients with a preoperative diagnosis of HGD are in effect understaged, because full histology often reveals invasive adenocarcinoma that carries the risk of nodal metastasis. The need for at least a better staging, if not also for a better prognosis, suggest the performance of esophagectomy and some extent of lymphadenectomy in high-volume centers. In these patients a hybrid approach, with laparoscopic gastric mobilization, tubulization, and abdominal lymphadenectomy combined with an open chest esophagectomy and mediastinal lymphadenectomy, carries the best clinical short- and long-term results.
- In high-risk patients, another nonsurgical option may consist of photodynamic therapy.

IV. SPECIAL POSTOPERATIVE CARE

- Total parenteral nutrition is administered to patients. Oral supplements or immunonutrition is started, if possible, in the early postoperative course (day 3).
- Patients are generally discharged day 7-10, and controlled at office; subsequent controls are scheduled according to the follow-up protocol for cancer of the esophagogastric junction.

SUGGESTED READINGS

Cameron, S: Transhiatal blunt esophagectomy with esophagogastrostomy. In Cameron JL, Sandone C, editors: *Atlas of gastrointestinal surgery*, vol 1, ed 2, Opa-Locka, Fla., 2007, PMPH-USA.

Godiris-Petit G, Munoz-Bongrand N, Honigman I, et al: Minimally invasive esophagectomy: prospective evaluation of laparoscopic gastric mobilization, *Ann Chirurg* 131:189–193, 2006.

Kent MS, Schuchert M, Fernando H, Luketich JD: Minimally invasive esophagectomy: state of the art, *Dis Esophagus* 19:137–145, 2006.

CHAPTER 13

Laparothoracoscopic Esophagectomy

Manisha Shende, MBBS, MS, FACS, and James D. Luketich, MD, FACS

I. SPECIAL PREOPERATIVE PREPARATION

- Patients are carefully evaluated with a complete history and physical examination and are assessed in a preoperative anesthesia unit.
- A thorough staging workup is done. This includes computed tomography of the chest, abdomen, and pelvis; an endoscopic ultrasound; and a positron emission tomography scan.
- Cardiopulmonary evaluation with pulmonary function testing, echocardiogram, and a stress test are done. Smoking cessation is encouraged. Appropriate consultations are obtained as indicated.
- Anticoagulants and antiplatelet medications are discontinued.
- All patients undergo a mechanical prep of the colon a day before surgery.

Anesthesia and Positioning

- All patients receive prophylactic antibiotics before induction, and antiembolism pneumatic stockings are also placed at that time.
- Large-bore intravenous access, arterial line, and Foley catheter are placed. A double-lumen endotracheal tube is placed.
- An upper endoscopy and fiberoptic bronchoscopy is performed. The upper endoscopy confirms the location and extent of tumor or Barrett epithelium and assesses the suitability of the stomach as a conduit and confirms the distal and proximal extent of tumor involvement.

II. OPERATIVE TECHNIQUE: LAPAROSCOPIC PHASE

- The laparoscopic portion is performed first using an Ivor Lewis esophagectomy.

Position

- The patient is placed supine on the operating table on a bean bag. The bean bag is used later on for positioning for the thoracoscopic portion of the operation.
- A footboard is placed.
- Arms are placed on padded arm boards and are extended at the sides.

Incision

- The standard port placement is shown in Figure 13-1; however, this may need to be modified in patients with previous abdominal incisions. A standard Hasson technique is used for abdominal access. A blunt 11-mm port is placed in the right epigastrium through the rectus sheath at a point two thirds of the way down between the xiphoid and the umbilicus.
- Pneumoperitoneum is established to a pressure of 15 mm Hg. The left lobe of the liver is retracted to expose the esophageal hiatus using a Diamond-Flex retractor and held in place with a self-retaining system (Mediplex).
- A thorough laparoscopic staging is performed, and any suspicious lesions are biopsied.

- The dissection starts by dividing the gastrohepatic ligament and exposing the right crus. The upper portion of the left crus is exposed with dissection on the upper phrenogastric attachments. Care is taken during these initial steps to avoid division of the phrenoesophageal ligament and entry into the chest, which leads to loss of intraabdominal pressure and tension pneumothorax.

Main Dissection

- The short gastrics are divided, starting at about the middle of the greater curvature, and the lesser sac is entered. The plane is continued cephalad, freeing up the retrogastric attachments. The plane along the greater curvature is now developed distally, taking care to ensure that the gastroepiploic arcade is not injured (Fig. 13-2). Connecting blood vessels to the omentum are also divided.

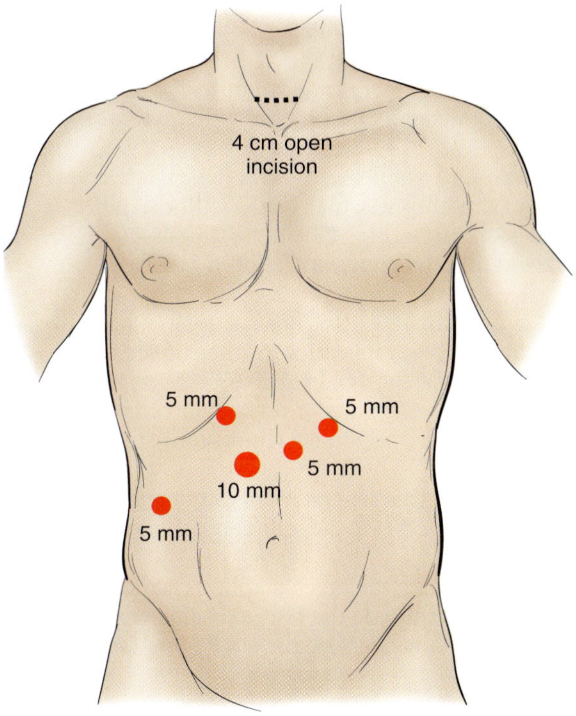

Figure 13-1.

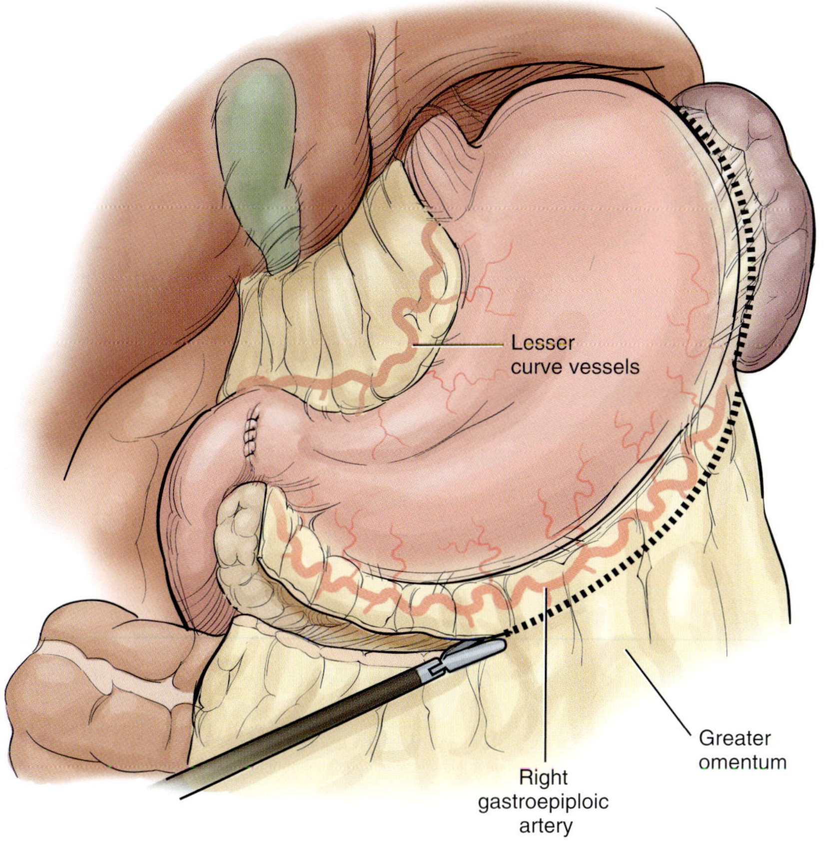

Figure 13-2.

- A Kocher maneuver is performed. Gentle lifting of the pylorus should allow an easy tension-free reach to the right crus.
- At this point, the left gastric pedicle will be easily visible. The lymph nodes and fatty tissue of the celiac axis are swept upward and the left gastric pedicle is divided using an endoscopic vascular stapler (Endo-GIA II, US Surgical, Norwalk, Conn.). Before division of these vessels, a careful assessment of nodal involvement in this area is made. Extensive lymph node involvement in this area may lead to consideration of stopping the procedure.
- Dissection along the left and right crura into the chest cavity is performed. The extent of this depends on the mobility of the tumor and visualization. Ideally, the surgeon carries the laparoscopic dissection plane along the aorta, the left and right pleura, and the pericardium a minimum of 10 cm. The further the extent of this dissection plane, the easier the video-assisted thoracoscopic dissection becomes.
- A pyloroplasty is then performed in a Heineke-Mikulicz fashion (Fig. 13-3). An Endo Stitch (Covidien, Mansfield, Mass.) suture is placed superiorly and inferiorly on the pylorus to provide retraction. Ultrasonic shears are used to incise the pylorus, and the opening is closed transversely using 2-0 interrupted endosutures.
- A Kocher maneuver is performed and the retrogastric and duodenal attachments are carefully dissected to achieve adequate mobilization of the gastric tube. Adequate mobilization should allow the pylorus to easily reach the right crus.
- The gastric tube construction is now initiated by firing the Endo-GIA stapler across the lesser curve vessels and fat at an angle toward the incisura. We generally start with a vascular load, with a staple height of 2.5 mm to minimize small vessel oozing along the lesser curve (Fig. 13-4).
- The angle of the first few staple firings will determine the gastric tube diameter and should be placed accordingly.
- It is preferable to create a relatively narrow gastric tube that is approximately 4 to 5 cm wide. In addition, apply slight caudal and simultaneous cephalad traction during the application of the stapler to keep the gastric tube on slight stretch. This will afford better length of the final tube. An additional 10-mm port placed in the right lower quadrant facilitates placement of a grasper on the antrum to apply countertraction during gastric tube construction. This port site also facilitates jejunostomy tube placement.
- Subsequent firings of the stapler should be maintained in a line parallel to the greater curvature arcade to create a consistent tube width and avoid spiraling (barber-pole effect) of the tubularized gastric conduit.
- The staple load used along the thick, muscular gastric antrum may require the green stapling cartridge (4.8 mm height). As the stapling continues toward the fundus, we generally use the blue loads (3.5 mm height). The staple line is inspected for hemostasis. We generally do not oversew the staple line (see Fig. 13-4).
- An endosuture is used to attach the resected specimen to the gastric tube (Fig. 13-5). This suture should be placed from the tip of the fundic portion of the tube to the lesser curve part of the resected specimen.

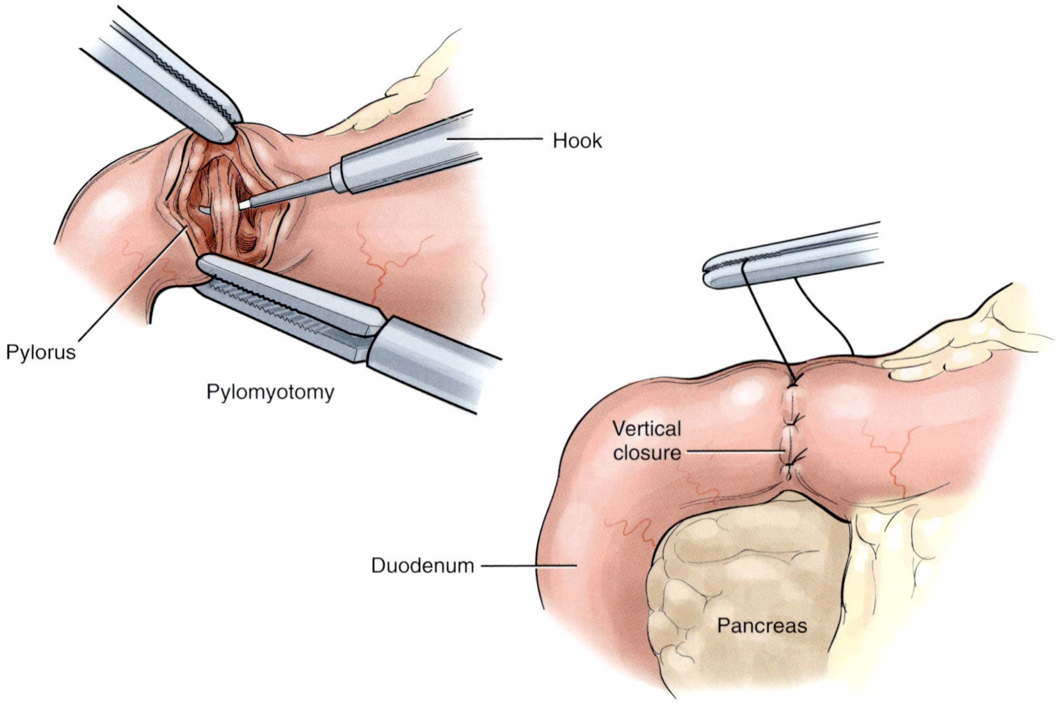

Figure 13-3.

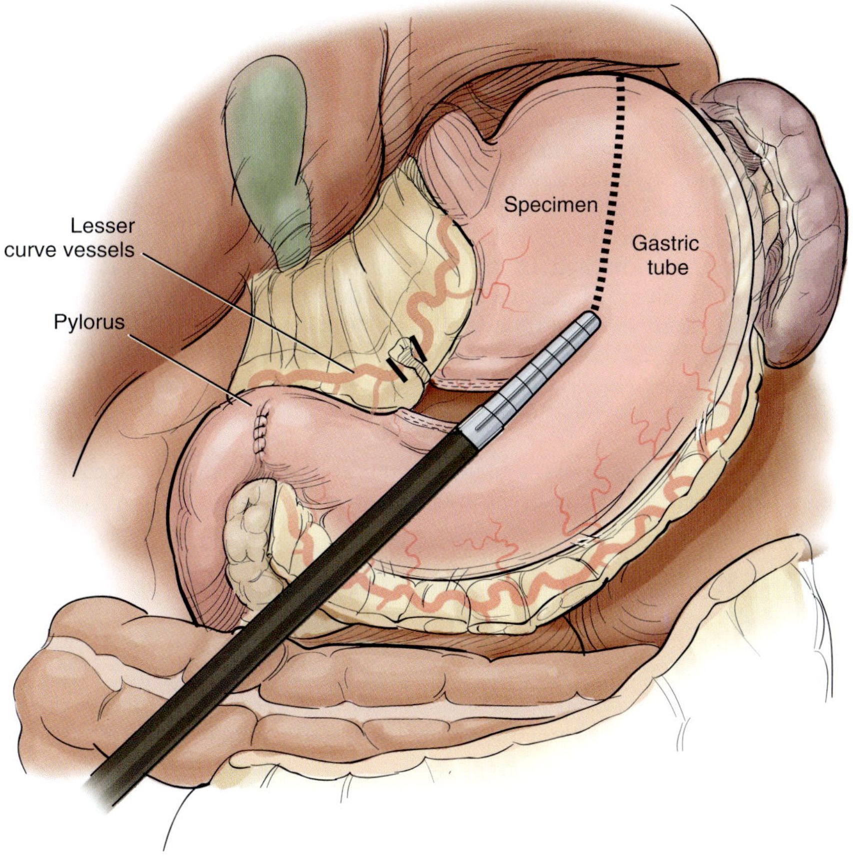

Figure 13-4.

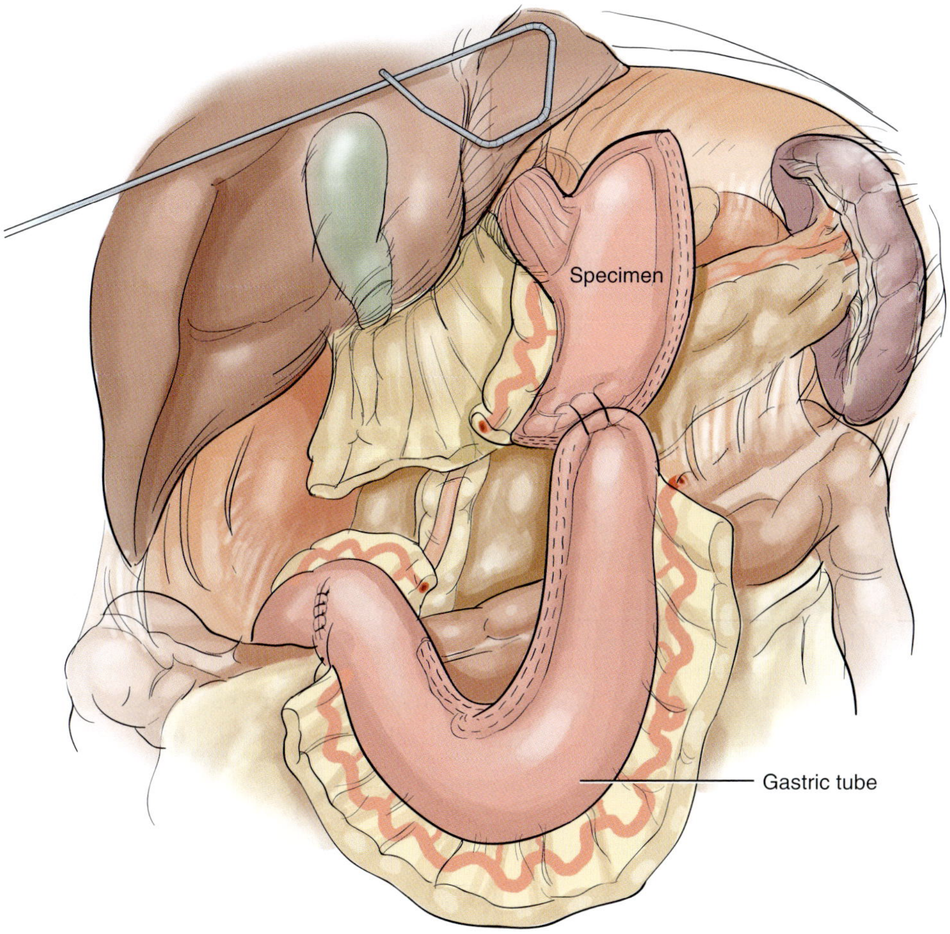

Figure 13-5.

Feeding Jejunostomy

- The transverse colon is retracted cephalad using a grasper applied to the adjacent fatty epiploicae, and the ligament of Treitz is identified.
- Approximately 40 cm from the ligament of Treitz, a loop of jejunum is attached to the anterior abdominal wall in the left lower quadrant using an Endo Stitch.
- A 5-Fr needle catheter feeding jejunostomy tube (Compat Biosystems, Minneapolis) is inserted into the jejunum percutaneously using a Seldinger technique.
- The jejunum is further tacked to the anterior abdominal wall using three additional endosutures as well as a single suture approximately 3 cm distal to the entrance site to prevent torsion. The feeding catheter is secured on the skin, and 10 mL of air is injected rapidly into the small bowel to test for patency and confirm intraluminal placement. If any doubts exist as to true luminal placement, an on-the-table Gastrografin study of the J-tube should be performed.

Closure

- We typically only close the fascia of the main cutdown blunt port site in the right rectus muscle. The other incisions are closed only with a subcuticular stitch for the skin.

III. OPERATIVE TECHNIQUE: THORACOSCOPIC PHASE

Position

- The patient is positioned on a bean bag in a left lateral decubitus position with the right side up. An axillary roll is used and the left arm is positioned on an arm board. The right arm is suspended and the table is flexed.
- Once endotracheal tube positioning has been confirmed, the right lung is deflated.
- The operating table is flexed and placed in slight reverse Trendelenburg position to expand the intercostal spaces and depress the diaphragm (Fig. 13-6).

Incision

- The camera port (10 mm) is placed at the eighth to ninth intercostal space anteriorly.
- A 10-mm port is placed at the eighth or ninth intercostal space 2 cm posterior to the posterior axillary line, for the ultrasonic coagulating shears (US Surgical). Care is taken to avoid placing this port lower, which would make access to the upper chest difficult.
- Two additional ports are placed: one 5-mm port is placed posterior to the tip of the scapula, and one 10-mm port is placed at the fourth intercostal space at the anterior axillary line for lung retraction and countertraction during the esophageal dissection.
- To optimize visualization at the diaphragmatic hiatus, a single retracting Endo Stitch is placed in the central tendon of the diaphragm and brought out of the inferior, anterior chest wall through a 1-mm skin incision. This suture allows downward traction on the diaphragm and excellent exposure of the distal esophagus, thus eliminating the need for an additional retractor.
- After a thorough inspection of the chest, the inferior pulmonary ligament is divided to the level of the inferior pulmonary vein.

Main Dissection

- The mediastinal pleura overlying the esophagus is widely divided from the diaphragm up to the level of the azygos vein, staying close to the pericardium and hilar structures. Great care is used in dissecting near the membranous trachea and bronchi to avoid injury. The azygos vein is then divided using the Endo-GIA vascular stapler (Endo-GIA II, US Surgical).
- The esophagus is then retracted medially, and the parietal pleural is divided just anterior and medial to the line of the azygos vein and thoracic duct. Tributaries from the thoracic duct and azygos are carefully clipped to minimize the potential for chylous leak. Aortoesophageal attachments are also isolated, clipped, and divided.
- Circumferential mobilization of the esophagus is performed up to the level of several centimeters above the azygos vein, including all surrounding lymph nodes, periesophageal tissues, and fat. The precise proximal extent of this dissection may depend on tumor extension and/or gastric conduit length (Fig. 13-7).
- We keep the dissection plane close to the esophagus at the superior extent of the dissection, to avoid injury to either the airway or the recurrent laryngeal nerves. We specifically divide the vagus trunks at the level of the azygos vein to prevent any possible traction injury to the recurrent laryngeal nerves.

Anastomosis

- The posterior ninth interspace port is enlarged to 4 cm, and a wound protector is placed.
- A 28-mm end-to-end anastomosis (EEA) anvil is introduced and placed in the proximal esophageal lumen. It is secured with a purse-string suture using the Endo Stitch device. If a 28-mm EEA will not fit, one can consider gentle dilation of the esophagus with a 30-mL Foley balloon, or downsizing to a 25-mm EEA. We have found the 28-mm EEA superior in terms of esophageal and gastric ring integrity and also lower anastomotic stricture rates.
- The gastric conduit tip is opened, and the stapler is introduced. The point of the EEA exits out of the greater curve 4 to 6 cm distal to the tip, avoiding close proximity to the lesser curve staple line. One may choose to slide the EEA device into the tube further and trim off excess or any potential ischemic gastric conduit tip.

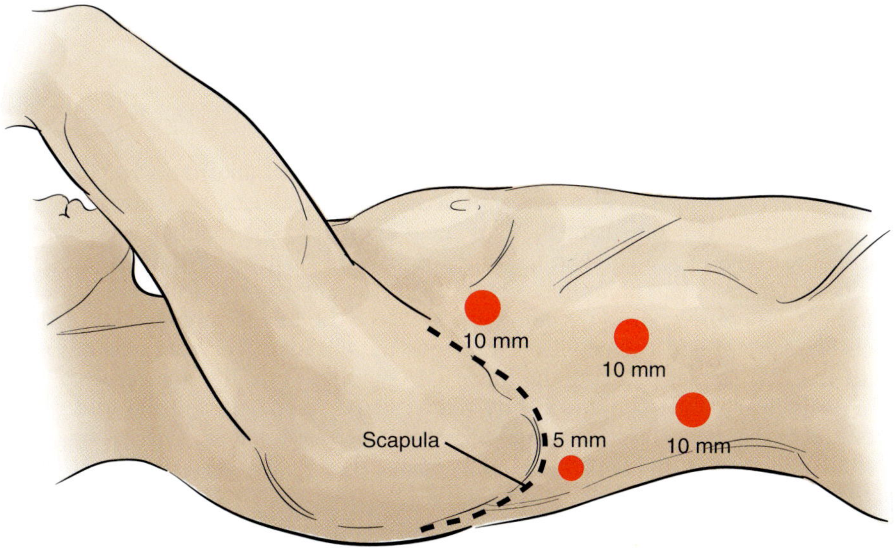

Figure 13-6.

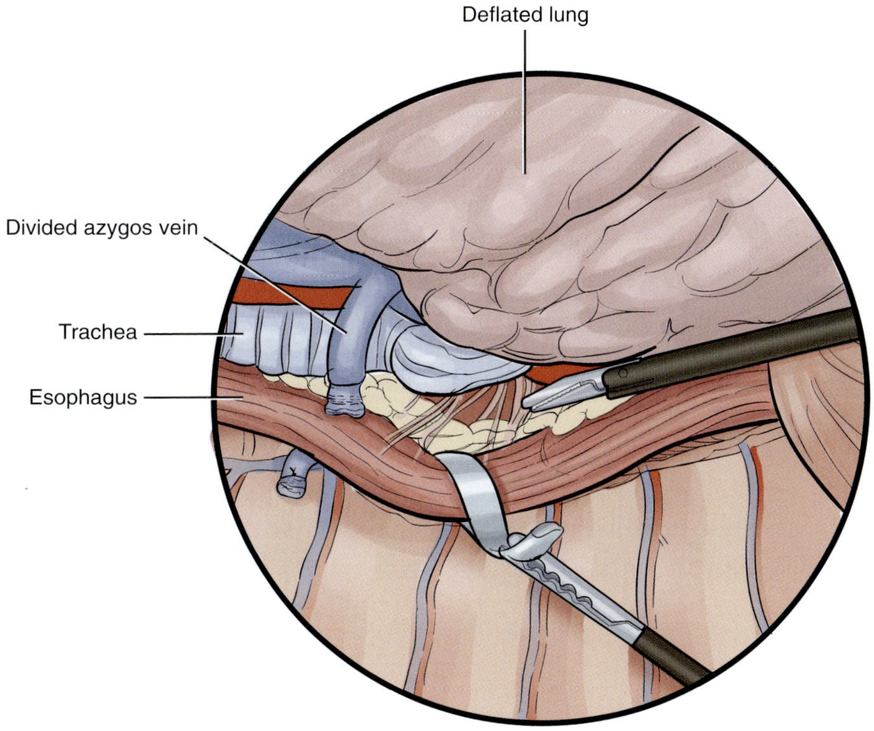

Figure 13-7.

- The EEA device is docked with the anvil and fired.
- The distal gastric tube is amputated with a linear stapling instrument.
- A nasogastric tube is inserted across the anastomosis under direct visualization with the tip positioned in the gastric tube above the pyloroplasty.
- As a final step, any redundant intrathoracic gastric tube is gently tucked back into the abdomen through the diaphragmatic hiatus to facilitate a nice straight gastric tube. The gastric tube is sutured to the crus to avoid delayed hiatal hernia.
- A 28-Fr thoracostomy tube is introduced via the camera access site, and a 10-mm Jackson-Pratt drain is placed in proximity to the anastomosis and brought out through the diaphragm stay suture site. The intercostal nerves (T4-T9) are injected under direct vision with 1 to 2 mL of 0.5% bupivacaine with epinephrine using a thoracoscopic needle.

Closure

- The trocar sites are closed with absorbable suture.
- Toilet bronchoscopy is performed, and the patient is generally extubated in the operating room and placed in the intensive care unit overnight for observation.

IV. ALTERNATIVE TECHNICAL APPROACHES (PRO/CON) AND PEARLS

- Thoracoscopic and laparoscopic esophagectomy with a cervical anastomosis can be performed as a three-stage operation. Initially, the patient is placed in left lateral decubitus position and thoracoscopic esophageal mobilization is done using the Ivor Lewis approach. The esophagus is completely mobilized up to the thoracic inlet. Care is taken to leave the parietal pleura above the azygos vein intact. This limits mediastinal contamination in the event of a cervical anastomotic leak. The patient is then placed supine, and the abdominal portion is commenced. Once the gastric mobilization is done, the cervical collar incision is made and the cervical esophagus mobilized. A cervical anastomosis is performed, either with the EEA stapler or using the linear GIA stapler. Once the anastomosis is completed, the surgeon returns to the abdomen and gently reduces any excess gastric tube into the abdomen. The gastric conduit is then tacked to the hiatus to prevent herniation (Fig. 13-8).

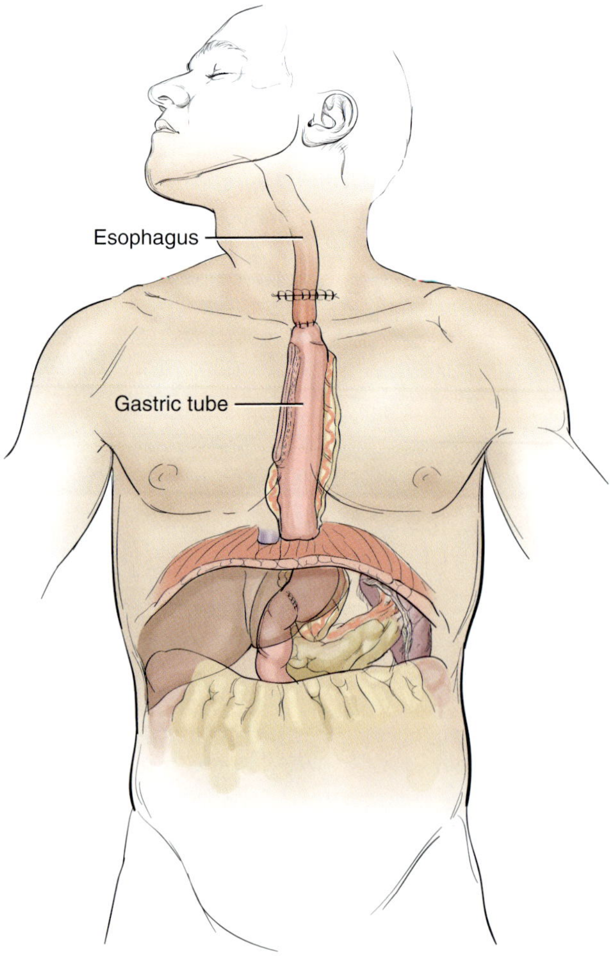

Figure 13-8.

V. SPECIAL POSTOPERATIVE CARE

- Toilet bronchoscopy is done in the operating room before extubation.
- We monitor the patient in an intensive care unit overnight. A Gastrografin swallow is obtained on the third or fourth postoperative day. If no leak is seen, then we start the patient on clear liquids orally, limiting the volume to 1 to 2 ounces per hour. By the time the patient goes home, usually postoperative day 5, he or she is taking full liquids and very soft foods, such as pudding and mashed potatoes. The Jackson-Pratt drain is gently “cracked,” that is, pulled back slightly the day of discharge. The patient is seen in the outpatient clinic at 2 weeks, at which time the drain is removed. The jejunostomy tube is also removed if the patient is taking an adequate oral intake.

SUGGESTED READINGS

Bizekis C, Kent MS, Luketich JD, et al: Initial experience with minimally invasive Ivor Lewis esophagectomy, *Ann Thorac Surg* 82:402–406, 2006.

Kent MS, Schuchert M, Fernando H, Luketich JD: Minimally invasive esophagectomy: state of the art, *Dis Esophagus* 19:137–145, 2006.

Luketich JD, Alvelo-Rivera M, Buenaventura PO, et al: Minimally invasive esophagectomy: outcomes in 222 patients, *Ann Surg* 238:486–494, 2003.

CHAPTER 14

Esophagectomy by Thoracoscopy in Prone Position Followed by Laparoscopy and Cervicotomy

Guy Bernard Cadière, MD, PhD, and Giovanni Dapri, MD, FACS, FASMBS

I. SPECIAL PREOPERATIVE PREPARATION

- In the preoperative workup for esophageal cancer, the patient is submitted to a barium swallow (Fig. 14-1), to gastroscopy with biopsy of the lesion, to a transoral endoscopic ultrasound (Fig. 14-2), to a thoracoabdominal computed tomography (CT) scan, and a positron emission tomography (PET) scan. The patient benefits from neoadjuvant therapy considering the stage of the tumor, as established by the completion of these exams. Other routine preoperative exams, such as chest radiograph, electrocardiogram, biochemical examinations, and anesthesiologist visit, are carried out before surgery.
- The patient is never submitted to an intestinal washout before the operation.
- Perioperative antibiotics (cephalosporin second class) may be continued in the postoperative period, depending on the surgeon's decision. A central venous catheter is positioned in the right subclavicular vein or in the right femoral vein. A double-lumen endotracheal tube is inserted during general anesthesia in supine position.

II. OPERATIVE TECHNIQUE: THORACOSCOPY IN PRONE POSITION

- Minimally invasive esophagectomy includes three steps: (1) thoracoscopy in prone position for the mobilization of the thoracic esophagus and mediastinal lymphadenectomy; (2) laparoscopy in supine position for celiac trunk lymphadenectomy and creation of the gastric tube; and (3) left cervicotomy for esophagogastric anastomosis.
- Full advantage is obtained by the gravity during thoracoscopy in prone position. The lung, which is partially deflated, always remains out of harm's way. This avoids the need for a fourth trocar.
- The esophagus and aortopulmonary lymph nodes are reached under excellent and accurate visualization, and bleeding does not obscure the operative field because blood flows back into the chest cavity.

Position

- The patient is placed in prone position after induction of general anesthesia and insertion of a double-lumen endotracheal tube in supine position. The right arm is placed in front of and beside the head to obtain an open angle between the scapula and spine. The surgeon stands to the patient's right, the camera operator to the surgeon's left, and the scrub nurse to the surgeon's right (Fig. 14-3, *A*).

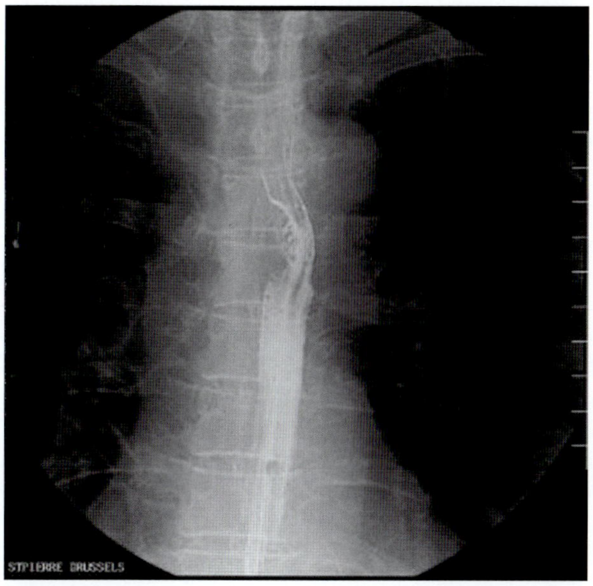

Figure 14-1. Preoperative barium swallow (malignant tumor of the midesophagus).

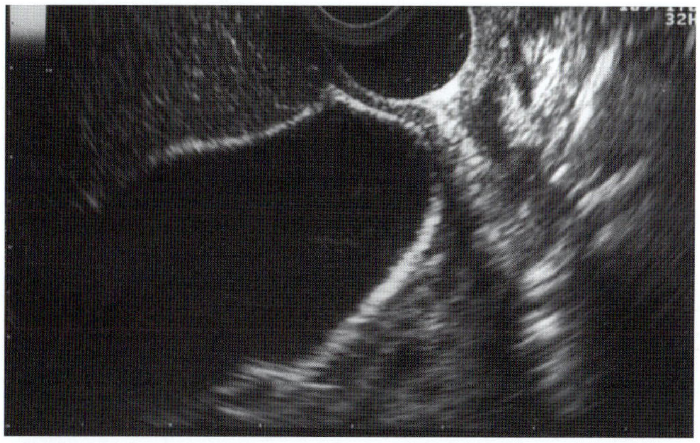

Figure 14-2. Preoperative transoral endoscopic ultrasound (benign tumor of the midesophagus).

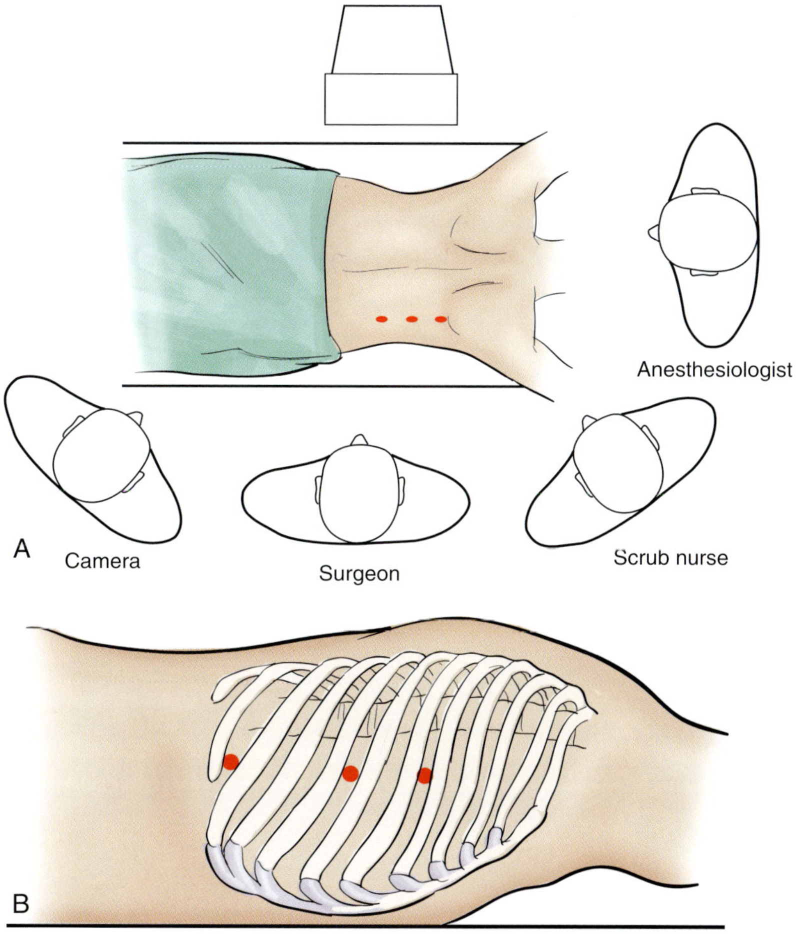

Figure 14-3.

Trocar Placement

- Three trocars are needed for this step: a 10-mm trocar for the 30-degree angled scope is placed in the seventh intercostal space, a 5-mm trocar for the grasping forceps is placed in the tenth intercostal space, and a 5-mm trocar for the coagulating hook is placed in the fifth intercostal space (see Fig. 14-3, *B*). A transitory pneumothorax with CO_2 (6 to 8 mm Hg) is created to achieve a good exposure.
- The lung is then left partially deflated.

Main Dissection

Mobilization of the Intrathoracic Esophagus and Mediastinal Lymphadenectomy

- Thanks to gravity, the cardiopulmonary window drops back and the space of esophageal dissection is directly opened. The mediastinal pleura overlying the esophagus is incised, and the esophagus is circumferentially mobilized along the trachea (Fig. 14-4, *A* and *B*) and the descending aorta (Fig. 14-5), reaching the right crus. All fatty tissue, including lymph nodes, is separated from the pericardium and descending aorta.
- The arch of the azygos vein is isolated, ligated by 2-0 silk stitches and clipped (Fig. 14-6). The para-esophageal, paratracheal, subcarinal, bilateral tracheobronchial, and right peripulmonary artery and

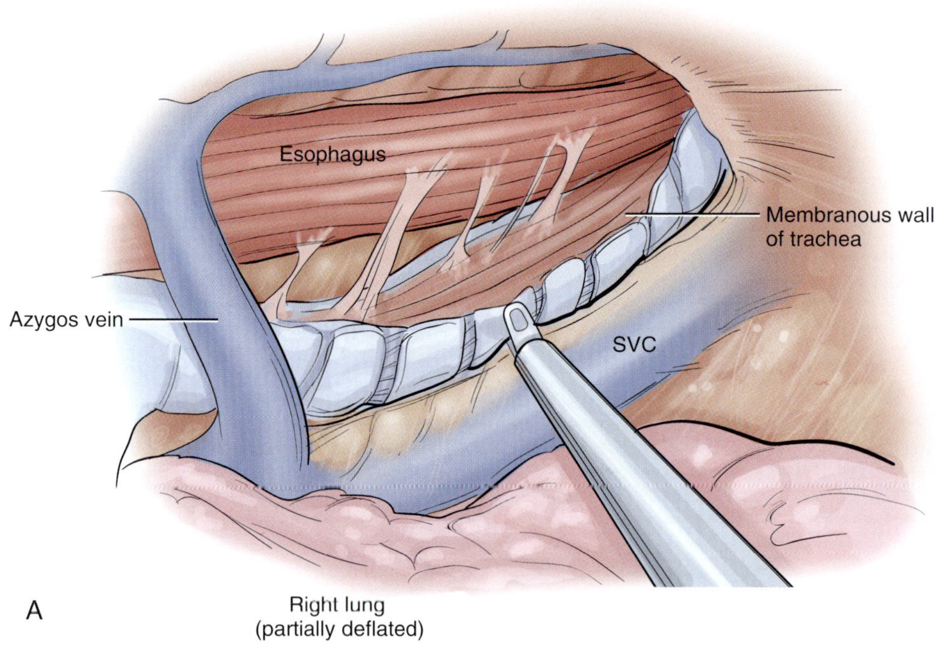

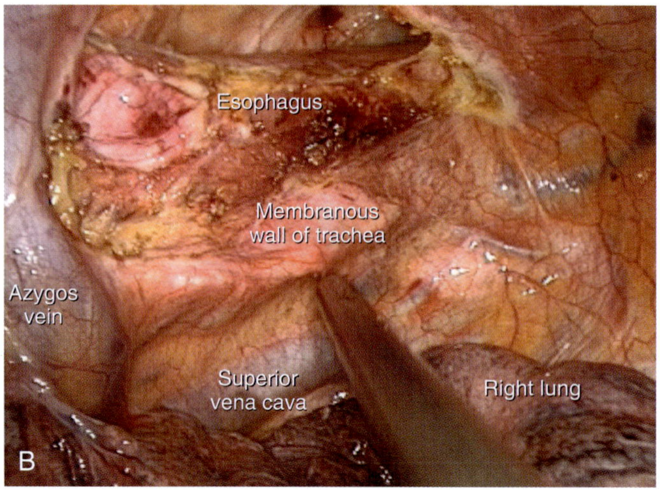

Figure 14-4. *SVC*, Superior vena cava.

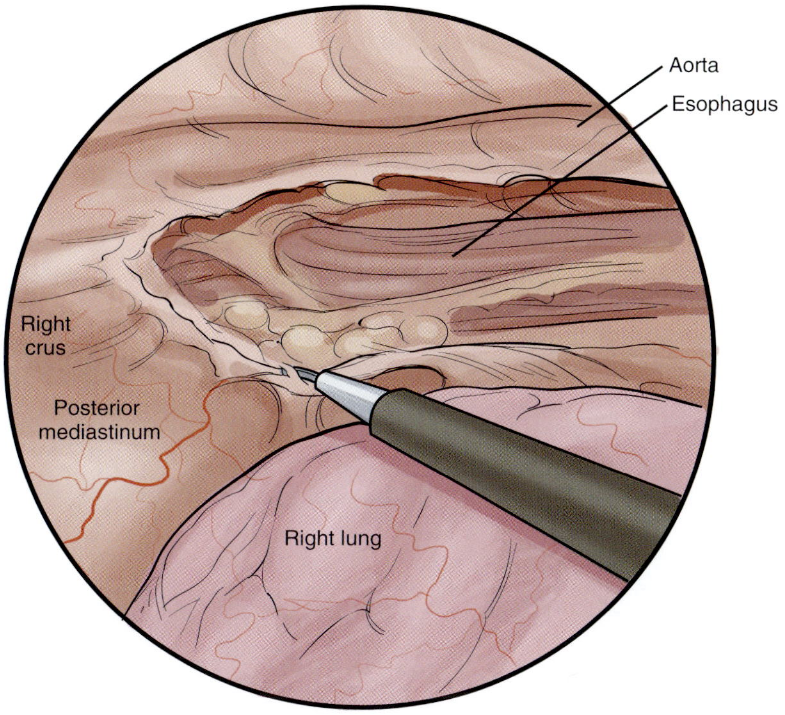

Figure 14-5.

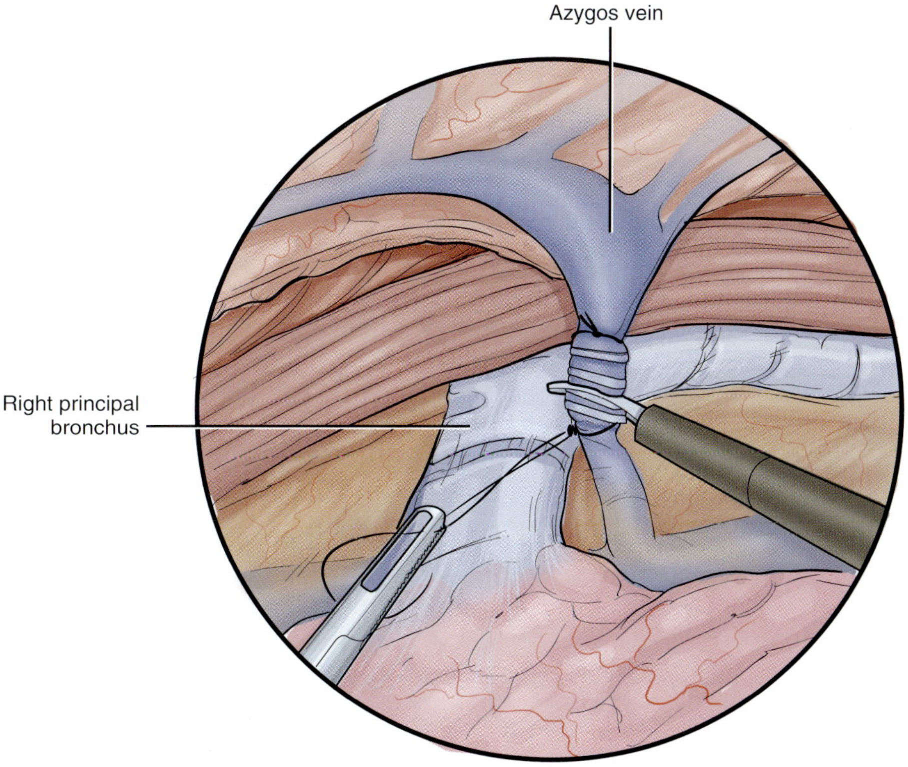

Figure 14-6.

vein lymph nodes are dissected so as to remain en bloc with the surgical specimen (Fig. 14-7). A 28-Fr chest tube is inserted in the eleventh intercostal space on the anterior axillary line at the end of this step.

III. OPERATIVE TECHNIQUE: LAPAROSCOPY IN SUPINE POSITION

Position

- The patient is now placed in supine position with legs separated. The surgeon stands between the patient's legs, the camera operator to the patient's right, the other assistant to the patient's left, and the scrub nurse beside the patient's left leg (Fig. 14-8). The patient is draped so as to allow trocar placement in the abdomen as well as an incision along the left sternocleidomastoid muscle in the neck.

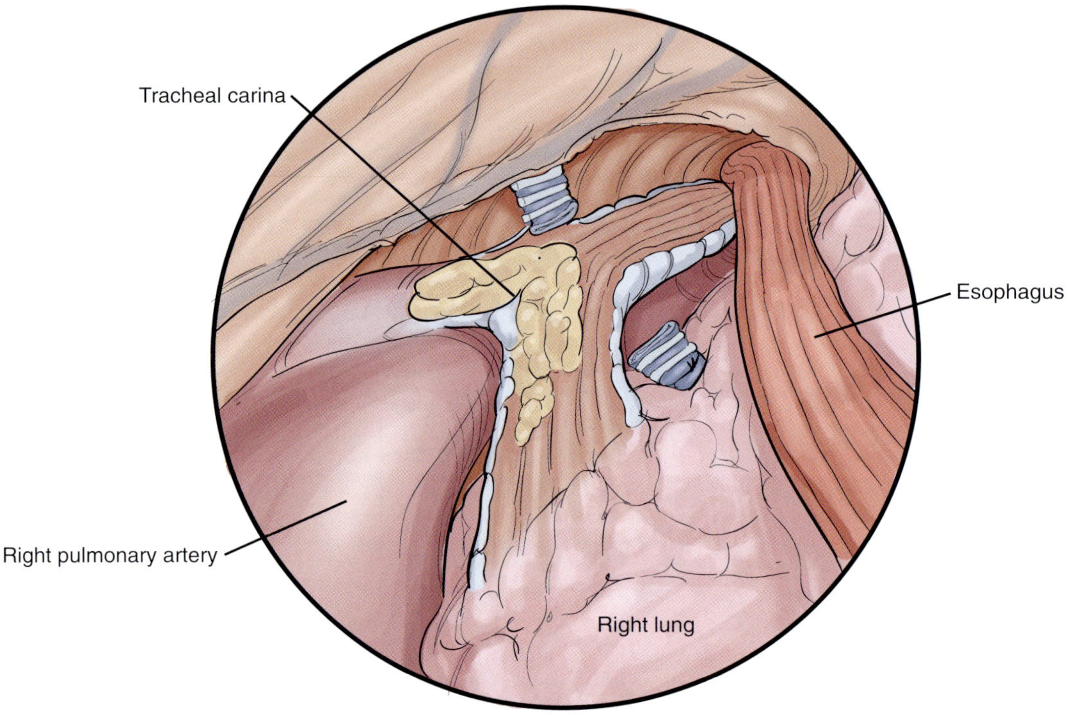

Figure 14-7.

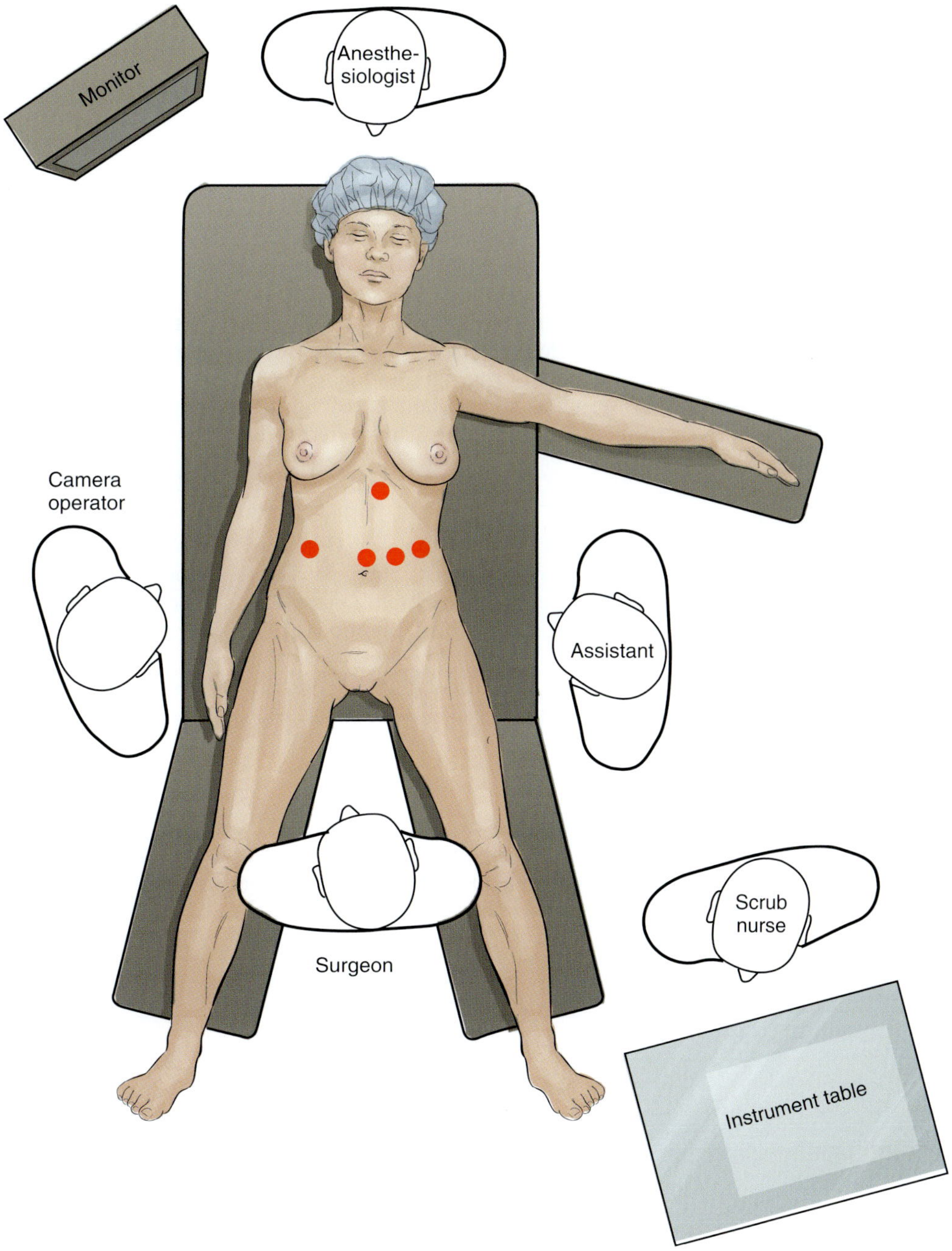
Monitor
Anesthe-
siologist
Camera
operator
Assistant
Surgeon
Scrub
nurse
Instrument table

Figure 14-8.

Trocar Placement

- Five trocars are used for this step: a 10-mm trocar 2 cm above the umbilicus, a 5-mm trocar on the midclavicular line under the left costal margin, a 12-mm trocar halfway between the first two trocars, a 12-mm trocar on the right midclavicular line under the right costal margin, and a 5-mm trocar under the xiphoid access (Fig. 14-9).

Main Dissection

Mobilization of the Esophagogastric Junction

- The dissection of the lesser omentum starts to the left of the right gastric artery and follows the latter toward the hepatic hilus, moving to the left side of the liver until it reaches the right crus (Fig. 14-10). Then the dissections of the anterior sheet of the right and left phrenogastric ligaments is carried out. During the dissection of the right crus, it is important to reach a good opening of the hiatus and to remain at a distance from the tumor. The right crus is dissected to the edge of the aorta.

Mobilization of the Greater Curvature

- The dissection of the gastrocolic ligament, and thus opening of the lesser sac, is carried out just lateral to the gastroepiploic artery and vein (see Fig. 14-10). The lesser sac is opened in the direction of the spleen. Care is always taken not to damage the gastroepiploic vessels. The dissection of the gastrosplenic ligament, reaching the previous dissection of the left phrenogastric ligament, ends this phase of the procedure.
- Subsequently, dissection of the lesser sac is continued in the direction of the gastroduodenal artery.
- The greater omentum is separated from the mesocolon as far as the colic angle. A Kocher maneuver is performed.

Lymphadenectomy of the Celiac Trunk and Ligation of the Left Gastric Vessels

- Visualization of the superior limit of the pancreatic head-body, celiac trunk, and hepatic pedicle is enhanced by the use of a 30-degree angled scope and by pulling the gastric antrum up to the patient's left. The peritoneal sheet that joins the head-body of the pancreas is dissected by the coagulating hook

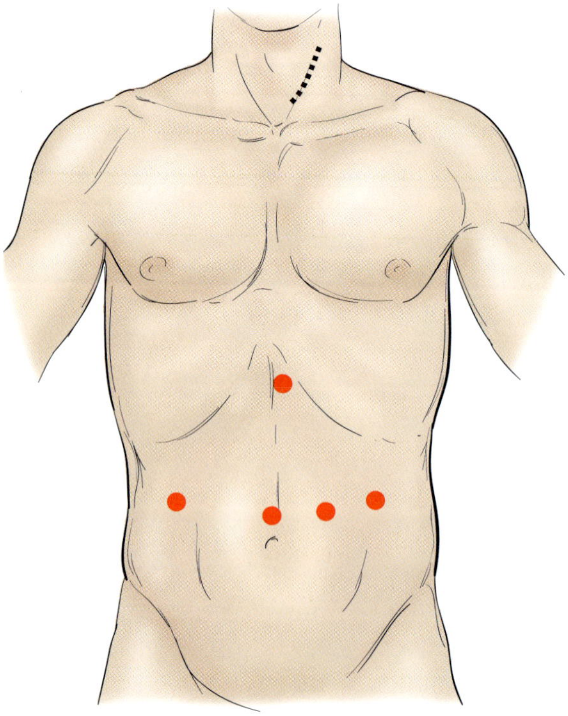

Figure 14-9.

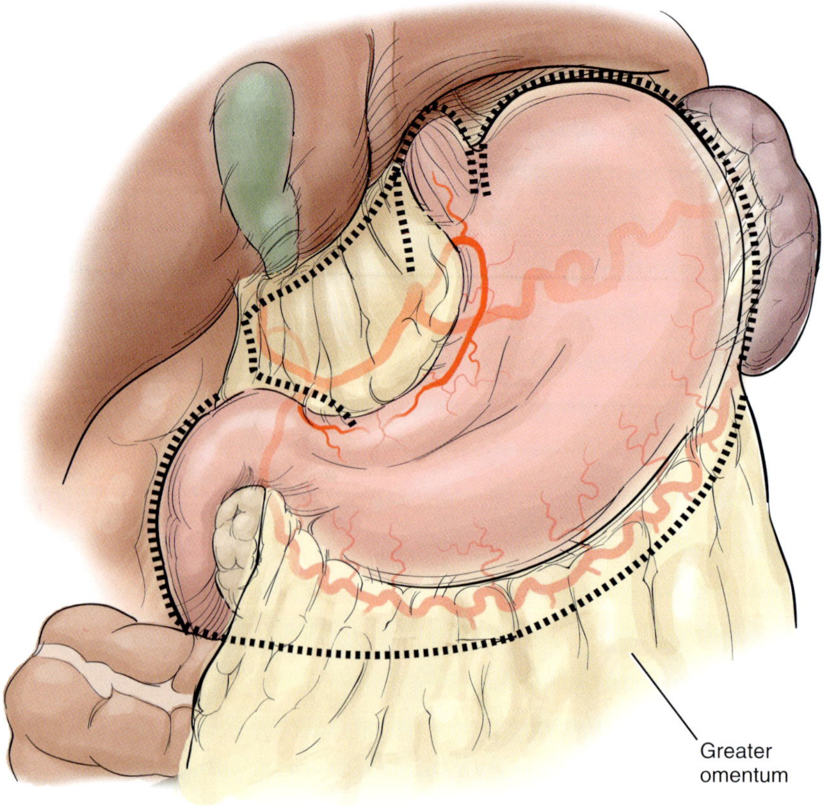

Figure 14-10.

(Fig. 14-11). All lymphoglandular tissue from this point toward the patient's right is sampled, while preserving the right gastric artery and the hepatic pedicle. Skeletonization of the portal vein and hepatic pedicle is performed by the coagulating hook. The assistant pulls the perivascular fatty and lymphoglandular tissue to the patient's left. A careful dissection of the common hepatic artery going upstream reaches the celiac trunk. The left gastric vessels are dissected off, isolated, and divided between clips (Fig. 14-12). Dissection of the lymphoglandular tissue is completed along the abdominal aorta until both crura are reached. A complete mobilization of the stomach has now been performed.

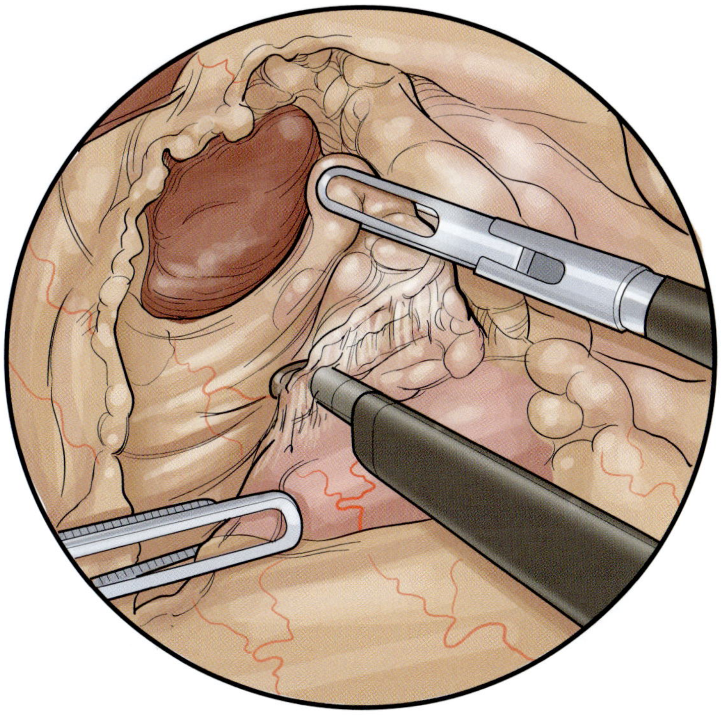

Figure 14-11.

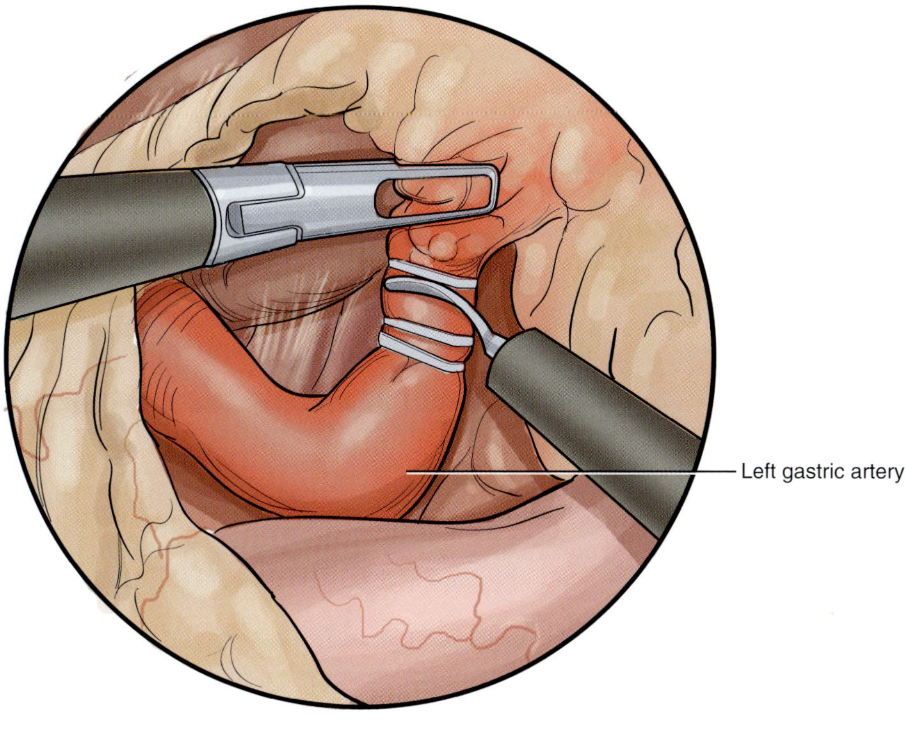

Figure 14-12.

Gastric Tube

- The tubulization is outlined by superficial scoring of the stomach. Tubulization is performed by several applications of a linear stapler blue load. The initial firing of the stapler begins at the level of the crow's foot, perpendicular to the lesser curvature. Other firings are placed parallel to the greater curvature. The section is kept incomplete and ends approximately 4 cm distal to the summit of the fundus (Fig. 14-13). The staple line is reinforced by separate 2-0 silk stitches.

IV. OPERATIVE TECHNIQUE: LEFT CERVICOTOMY

Position

- The patient remains in gynecologic position, and the pneumoperitoneum is deflated. The patient's head is hyperextended and turned toward the right side. The team passes around the neck.

Incision

- An incision is performed lateral to the left sternocleidomastoid muscle.

Main Dissection

Specimen Retrieval and Esophagogastric Anastomosis

- The omohyoid muscle is identified and sectioned. The cleavage planes are easily found because they have already been opened by the pneumothorax created during thoracoscopy. The esophagus is mobilized at its left posterior side until the surgeon can insert a finger in the posterior upper mediastinum, reaching the cervicomediastinal space. The anterior face of the esophagus is separated by the tracheal membrane, until the previous intrathoracic dissection is reached. Lifting of the esophagus containing the tumoral mass (protected by a plastic bag) is achieved under laparoscopic control. A totally mechanical side-to-side esophagogastric anastomosis is performed using three blue loads of the same stapler used for the laparoscopic gastric tube. The first firing is performed by inserting the linear stapler in the upper esophagus and in the gastric tube. The other two firings close the edges of the first one and permit isolation of the surgical specimen from the upper esophagus and from the gastric tube (Fig. 14-14).

Closure

- The procedure ends with the placement of a drain in the neck and in the abdominal hiatus.

V. ALTERNATIVE TECHNICAL APPROACHES (PRO/CON) AND PEARLS

- Esophagectomy is a considerable surgical undertaking because of the need for both abdominal and thoracic approaches. Over the past decade, minimally invasive thoracic and laparoscopic approaches have emerged as effective alternatives to open techniques without compromising pathologic and oncologic outcomes.
- Several minimally invasive approaches have been described for esophagectomy: thoracoscopic in prone position, thoracolaparoscopic, thoracoscopic-assisted, videomediastinoscopic, endoscopic Ivor Lewis, laparoscopic transhiatal, laparoscopic esophagogastrectomy, and laparoscopic-assisted transhiatal. The choice among these approaches is, to a degree, one of personal preference.
- In our department, we routinely perform esophagectomy using three techniques: right thoracoscopy in prone position followed by laparoscopy and left cervicotomy, transhiatal laparoscopy, and thoracolaparoscopic Ivor Lewis (with manual intrathoracic anastomosis). The transhiatal laparoscopic approach appears less invasive than a thoracoscopy in lateral or prone position, but there are some technical disadvantages of the laparoscopic approach, such as the difficulty in mobilizing the middle third of the esophagus because of the limited working space in the mediastinum, the short length of laparoscopic instruments, the difficulty in performing a mediastinal nodal dissection, the exposure of the operative field, and ergonomics.
- To diminish the extent of the upper esophageal blunt dissection and the risk of bleeding and perforation, the thoracoscopic approach is considered by many to be a superior alternative. Thoracoscopic dissection and esophageal mobilization is based on the principle that gravity will enable the cardiopulmonary bloc to fall anteriorly, opening the dissection of the esophagus from the spine. Because the surgeon is positioned in front of the esophagus, the ergonomics of the procedure are maintained

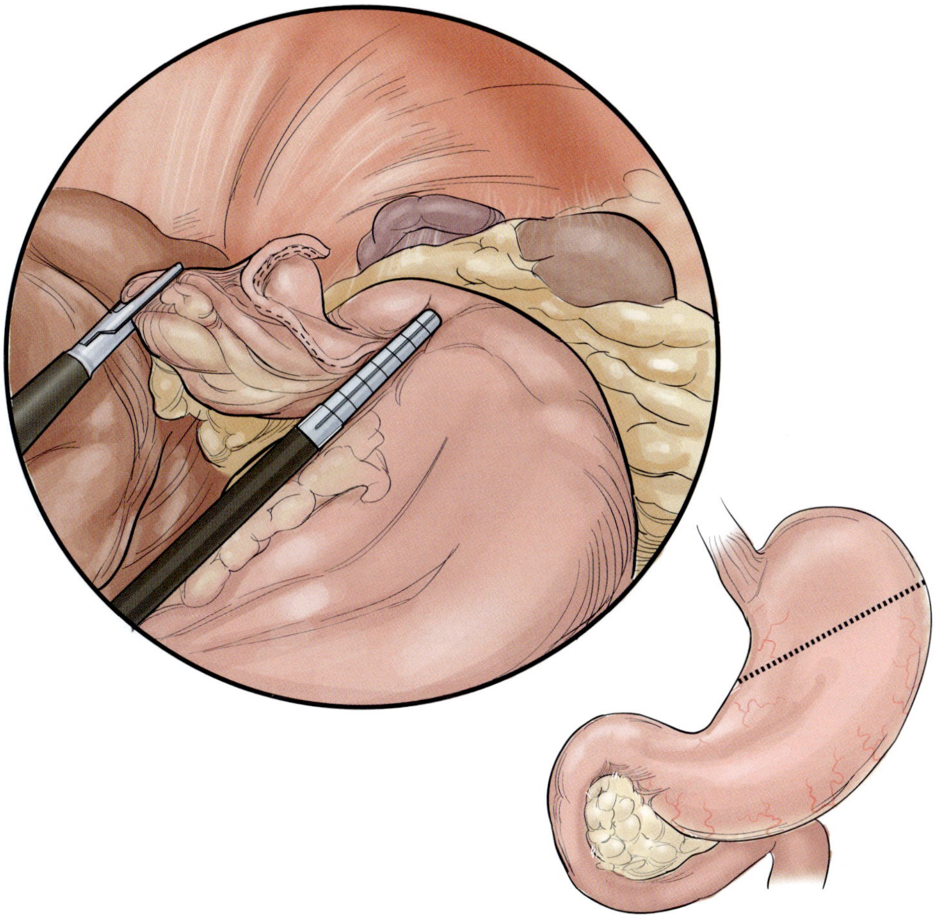

Figure 14-13.

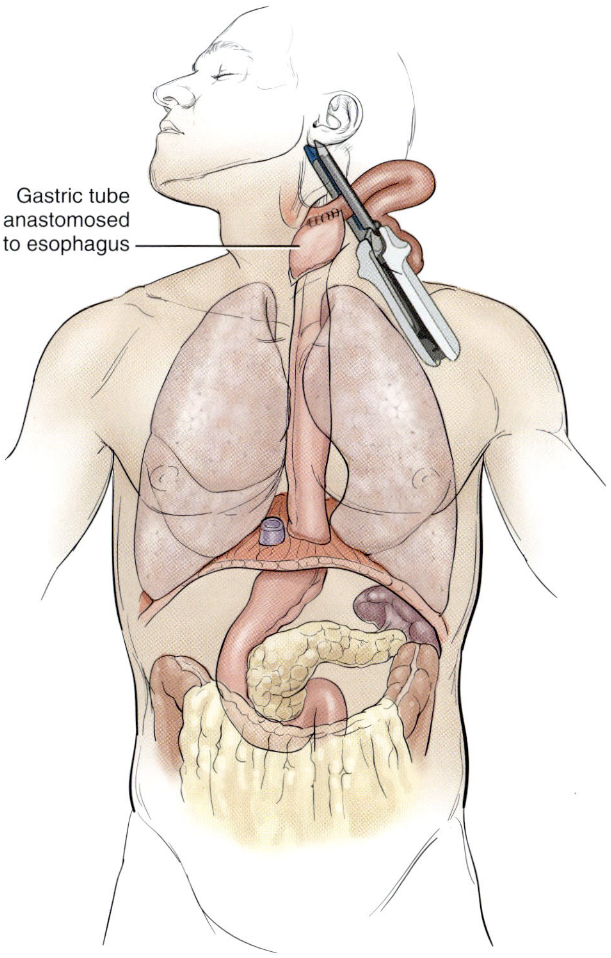

Figure 14-14.

satisfactorily, and the procedure is performed using only three trocars without the need of a fourth trocar for lung retraction. Moreover, even though a double-lumen tube is inserted, the procedure is performed with the lung partially deflated. Exposure is further facilitated by the use of carbon dioxide pneumothorax; in addition to maintaining an adequate operative field, its continuous insufflation aids in the extraction of the smoke created during dissection.

VI. SPECIAL POSTOPERATIVE CARE

- After the operation, the patient is monitored in the intensive care unit for at least the next 48 hours. The nasogastric tube is maintained in place until postoperative day 5. Prevention of deep venous thrombosis is started in the evening of the operation and stopped at complete mobilization of the patient.
- On postoperative day 5, a gastrografin swallow is realized, and if negative, a liquid diet is started. On postoperative day 6 or 7, the drains in the hiatus and in the neck are taken out, respectively.
- If there are no complications, the discharge of the patient can be allowed on postoperative day 10. After the discharge, the patient is followed by the oncologist, nutritionist, and gastroenterologist. Usually a semiliquid diet is started 1 month after surgery. If necessary, adjuvant therapy also is started after 1 month.

SUGGESTED READINGS

Cadiere GB, Dapri G, Himpens J, Fodderie L, Rajan A: Ivor Lewis esophagectomy with manual esogastric anastomosis by thoracoscopy in prone position and laparoscopy, *Surg Endosc* 24:1482–1485, 2010.

Luketich JD, Alvelo-Tivera M, Buenaventura PO, et al: Minimally invasive esophagectomy: outcomes in 222 patients, *Ann Surg* 238:486–494, 2003.

Palanivelu C, Prakash A, Senthilkumar R, et al: Minimally invasive esophagectomy: thoracoscopic mobilization of the esophagus and mediastinal lymphadenectomy in prone position—experience of 130 patients, *J Am Coll Surg* 203:7–16, 2006.

CHAPTER 15

Esophageal Reconstruction with Colonic Interposition

Zeno I. Popovici, MD, PhD

I. SPECIAL PREOPERATIVE PREPARATION

- Pretreatment radiologic imaging of the esophagus provides valuable information that aids in diagnosis and defines the focal extent of the stricture of the esophagus or the pharynx, as well as the etiology (benign or malignant). The current imaging modalities of choice are a barium swallow for benign esophageal stenosis, or contrast-enhanced computed tomography for a malignant tumor of the pharynx and lymph node involvement.
- Cinefluorography through the colon transplant, prolonged fluoroscopy with the image intensifier, and intraluminal pressure studies have not been able to demonstrate peristalsis in either direction. Whether in antiperistaltic or isoperistaltic orientation, when the colon is used as an esophageal substitute, it functions as a passive conduit. There is no progressive peristalsis in the colon, and the peristaltic direction is of no consequence; it functions by gravity.
- There is increasing evidence that the colon, when used as an esophageal substitute, does have a mass contraction of peristaltic action. The combination of gastric peristalsis and the gravity drainage from the interposition produces a yo-yoing of ingested food that may contribute to malabsorption as well as dysphagia.
- Computed tomography of the cervical area should be considered for patients with tumors of the pharynx larger than 3 cm with lymph node involvement. Magnetic resonance imaging is the preferred modality for malignant tumors of the pharynx, as it can provide multiplanar images with better spatial orientation. It also has the advantages that concurrent magnetic resonance angiography can be obtained, allowing delineation of relationships of the tumor to adjacent vascular structure. Dynamic postcontrast images may also facilitate differentiation of the tumor.
- Esophagogastroscopy, esophageal fiberscopy, indirect laryngoscopy, and biopsy are required to establish a definitive histologic diagnosis.
- Colonoscopy is performed in all patients who are considered for colon interposition to evaluate the state of the mucosa, to exclude intrinsic colon disease such as inflammatory bowel disease, malignancy, megadolichocolon, extensive diverticular disease, or multiple colonic polyps. Barium enema is an optional study but may be very useful to detect a previous colic disease (diverticulosis, polyposis, etc.).
- Preoperative selective superior or inferior mesenteric angiography is a necessity in patients older than 50 years to assess the arterial and venous anatomy of the colon and the continuity of the marginal artery of Dwight (particularly of the middle colic Riolan arch), and for arteriosclerosis, which are crucial factors in successful colic interposition.
- The colic veins are orphan ("pauvres parents"). It is our impression that the veins are of even more importance than the arteries. They are more friable, and the least tension may interrupt their continuity, rendering the transplant useless. We believe that the veins are usually the limiting factor in determining the length of viable transplant.
- The antiperistaltic left colic replacement is the most reliable and is advisable particularly for young surgeons with little experience. The left colic pedicle offers the best vascular material for colic interposition. The Y arterial left angle provides the best material for reconstruction.
- Paired relevant radiographic images of angiograms from different perspectives (surgical normal anatomy and pathologic process) made on cadaver specimens will allow the reader to understand

the value of these imaging studies in preparation for the advanced operative procedure. Normal (standard) vascularization represents the ideal type for colonic interposition: a simple pattern with few, strong, long, rectilinear, late-branching colic vessels and a continuous Riolan arch. In contrast with the former, an extremely unfavorable pattern is that of an elderly patient with advanced arteriosclerosis (Figs. 15-1, *A* and *B*, and 15-2, *A* and *B*). Notice the irregularity of the sinuous, tortuous, coiled arteries. The right colic artery (*R*) arising from a common stem with the midcolic artery (M_1), which breaks in a plexus of small vessels, is inadequate for maintaining the viability of the transplant. Likewise, a thin marginal artery and/or failure of the Riolan arch because of the presence of an accessory middle colic artery (M_2) is a contraindication for any kind of colonic plasty. These "anticipatory variants" may provide a practical guide for the operative surgeon dealing with esophageal reconstruction with colon. The veins are even more important that the arteries (Figs. 15-3, *A* and *B*; 15-4, *A*,

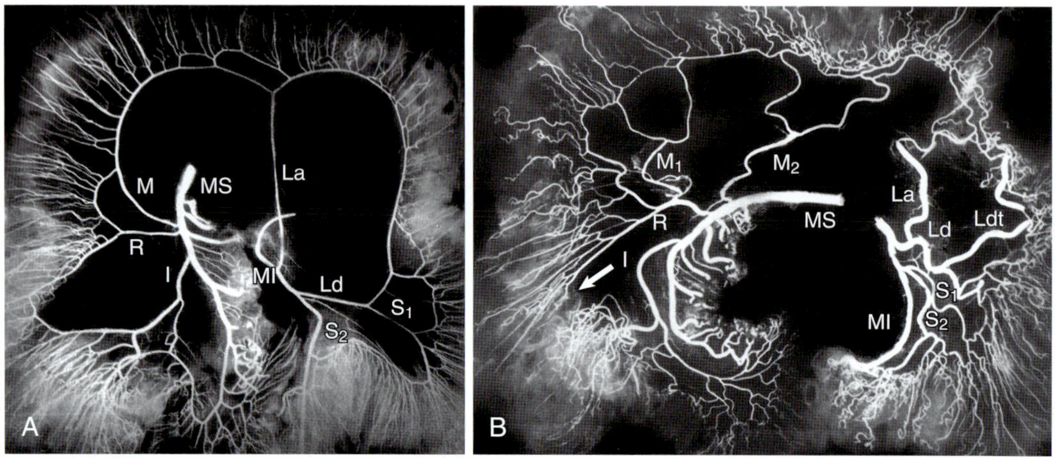

Figure 15-1. **A,** Normal vascularization, illustrating the ideal type for colonic interposition. One can see a variant with separate origin of ascending and descending branches of the left colic artery (*La*, *Ld*). Only two vessels are to be ligated (*M* and *R*). **B,** A contrasting image of arteriosclerosis. Moreover, there is an interruption of the right marginal artery (*arrow*) between the ileocolic (*I*) and right colic artery (*R*), the "critical point" described by Franz, Gosset, and Charrier. M_1, Middle colic artery; M_2, accessory middle colic artery; *MI,* inferior mesenteric artery; *MS,* superior mesenteric artery; S_1 and S_2, sigmoid branches.

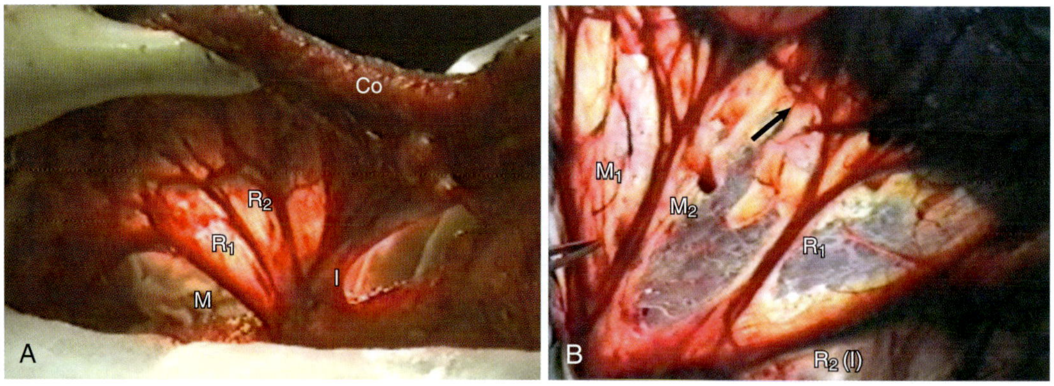

Figure 15-2. **Intraoperative transillumination of the right colon mesentery vessels.** **A,** Early branching type of right colic arteries arising from superior mesenteric artery, at the hepatic flexure realizing a composite (complex) "bouquet" pattern, which is unfavorable for left isoperistaltic colonic interposition. *I,* Ileocolic artery; *M,* middle colic artery; R_1, first right colic artery; R_2, second right colic artery.. One can see skeletonization of the right colic mesentery on both sides to point out the vascular bunch, which will become the pedicle of a left antiperistaltic colonic conduit—Vulliet-Orsoni's procedure (*Co*). See Figure 15-4, *C* [continuation]. **B,** Closer view of early dichotomic bifurcation of *M* and *R*, realizing four right colic arteries: M_1, M_2, R_1, and R_2 (*I*). The last right colic artery is as a matter of fact (actually) the ileocolic artery (*I*). This is a matter of the anatomist's interpretation. Blood supply is unfavorable because of the discontinuity of the marginal artery (*arrow*).

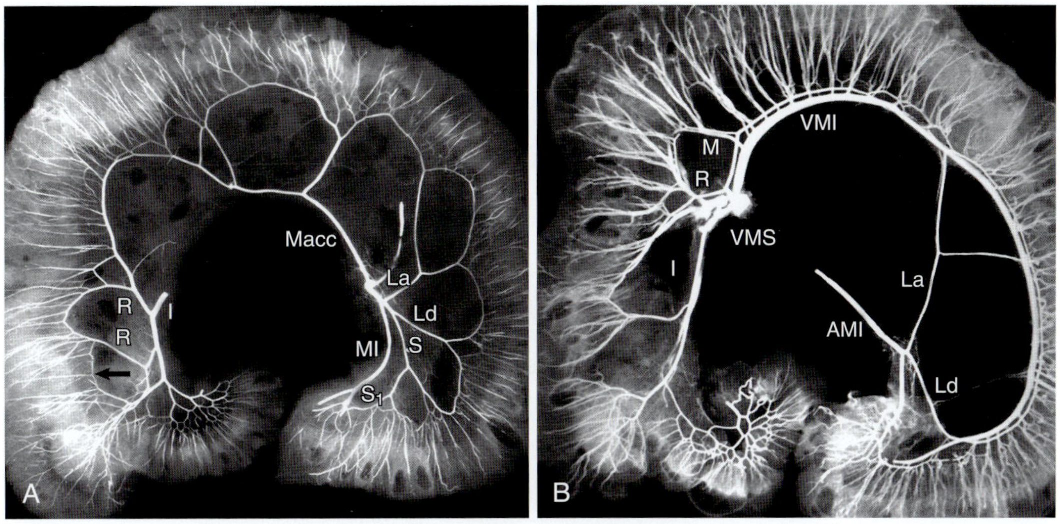

Figure 15-3. **A,** A long accessory midcolic artery (*Macc*) arising from the inferior mesenteric artery (*MI*) and reaching the marginal artery in close proximity with the hepatic flexure. Typical left-predominant pattern. **B,** Failure of inferior mesenteric vein (*VMI*), which was replaced by a large marginal vein directly collecting terminal veins as it courses along the left transverse colon, before entering into the base of the superior mesenteric vein. This pattern was found intraoperatively in three patients.

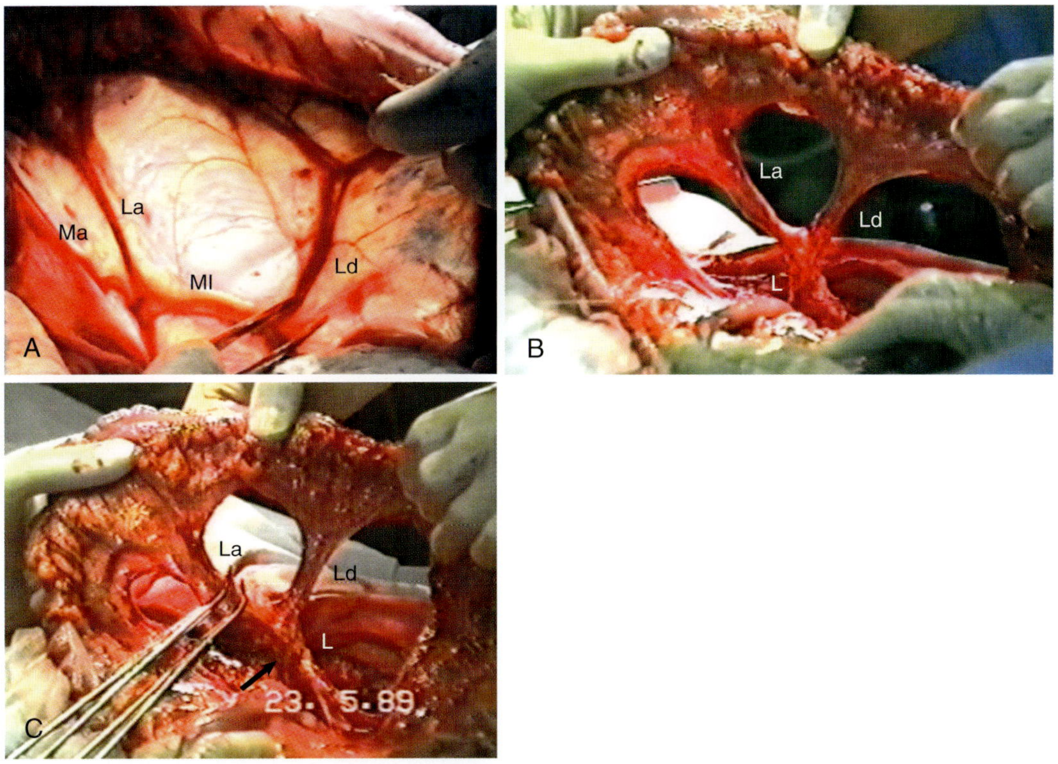

Figure 15-4. **Left colic vessels.** **A,** Very simple left vascular pattern with long nonramified vessels, continuous marginal artery, close to the colon. This is an ideal type for colic interposition. One can see the vascular arch of Treitz, half-arterial and half-venous. *MI,* Inferior mesenteric artery and vein. *La,* Ascending and *Ld,* descending branch of the left colic artery, apparently with separate origin from inferior mesentery artery. The tip of the pickup points to the left colic artery (*L*). *Ma,* Accessory middle colic artery. **B,** The same case after skeletonization and separation of the long left ascending branch (*La*) from the inferior mesenteric vein. One can see the large common trunk of the left colic artery and vein (*L*). Very favorable pattern for esophagocoloplasty. In the left isoperistaltic colon arrangement (procedure of Kelling-Belsey), it is advisable to preserve both branches and the distal segment of left marginal artery as an extended pedicle to improve the blood supply of the graft. **C,** It may also be used in the antiperistaltic orientation (procedure of Vulliet-Orsoni) pedicled on right colic arteries, but this requires dividing both branches. One can see the two long Kelly-Martin Overholt clamps placed on the left ascending artery before division. Compare with Figure 15-2, *A.* We advocate section of the trunk of the left colic artery close to its origin from the inferior mesenteric artery (*arrow*). This will provide a large additional secondary marginal artery for reinforcement of graft circulation ("supercharge").

B, and *C*; 15-5; and 15-6) and are usually the limiting factor in determining the length of viable transplant. The "critical points" of the marginal artery should be carefully checked by painstaking search.

- Intraoperatively, in the classic approach the adequacy of the marginal artery is determined by direct inspection of the colic arteries with the help of transillumination. It was found to be of considerable help to transilluminate the mesentery so as to localize the vessels to be ligated (see Fig. 15-5). A deep second marginal artery may be injured if one is not cognizant of this possibility.
- Pulsed Doppler flowmetry may assist in predicting graft viability.
- *Radionuclide esophageal scintigraphy:* There is a wide range of diagnostic tools to evaluate esophageal dysfunction. However, most of these procedures are invasive and uncomfortable for the patient, limiting reexaminations. The necessity of following up esophageal dysfunction in chronic diseases such as mixed connective tissue diseases may be the indication for performing a radionuclide esophageal scintigraphic study using a semisolid meal with ^{99m}Tc. Their clinical features include characteristics of

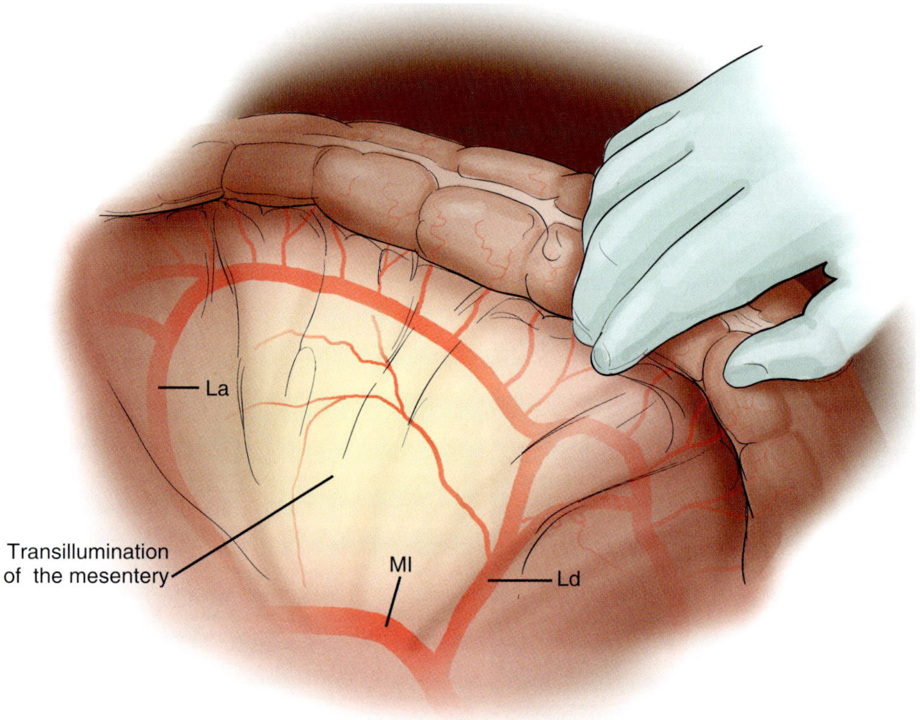

Figure 15-5. *La,* Ascending branch of the left colic artery; *Ld,* descending branch of the left colic artery; *MI,* Inferior mesenteric artery and vein.

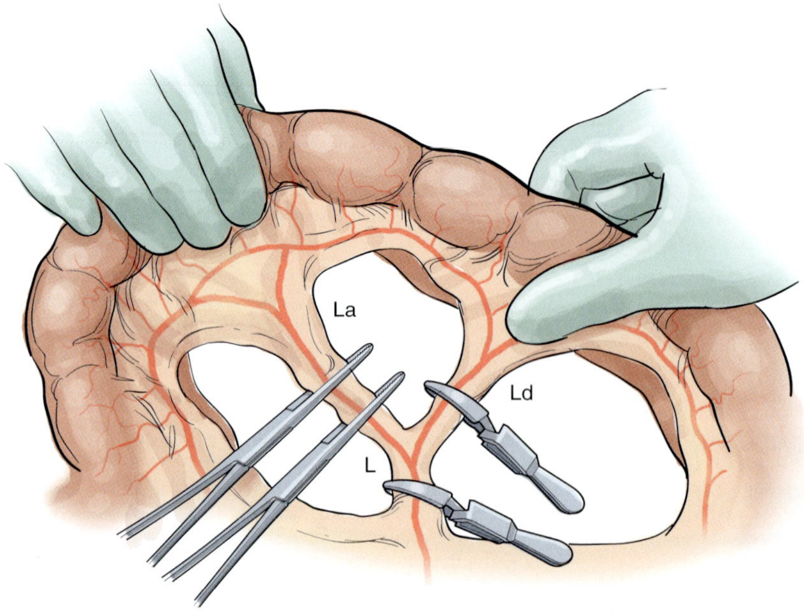

Figure 15-6. *L,* Left colic artery; *La,* ascending and *Ld,* descending branch of the left colic artery.

systemic lupus erythematosus, systemic sclerosis, dermatopolymyositis, Sjögren syndrome, and rheumatoid arthritis. Gastroesophageal reflux has been implicated in the pathogenesis of peptic esophageal strictures. The role of acid and pepsin in the development of laryngeal and pharyngeal injury and carcinoma has been demonstrated. Recent research has shown that in acidic refluxate, pepsin and conjugated bile acids are the most injurious agents affecting laryngeal tissue (laryngopharyngeal reflux). Radionuclide imaging may also be useful to determine delayed postoperative complications after colonic interposition (chronic ischemia of the colonic graft, stenosis of esophagocolic or cologastric anastomosis, gastrocolic reflux, aspiration, and pneumonia).
- *Preoperative colic preparation:* The patient is placed on a high-protein, low-residue diet for 7 to 14 days before the operation. At the beginning, the colon is prepared for 2 to 4 days with neomycin (1 g, 4 times daily), Fleet phosphosoda (½ oz, twice daily), and cleansing enemas using the technique of whole gut lavage. We use 3 to 4 L of Fortrans (Macrogol 4000) peroral solution on the evening before the operation, which ensures the fast evacuation of the entire colon. If dysphagia is total, the solution may be introduced through gastrostomy. Occasionally, total parenteral nutrition may be useful.

Indications

- When the stomach is not available, after esophagogastrectomy, when using the substernal route, when the esophageal replacement must last for a decade or more, when a vagus-sparing esophageal resection can be performed, and in children.
- The colon yielded the best end results as an esophageal substitute.
- *Absolute contraindications:* Intrinsic colon disease such as inflammatory bowel disease, polyposis, diverticulosis, malignancy, inadequate blood supply, and megadolichocolon.
- Colonic interposition has been widely popularized, particularly in the United States, where some have advocated its use as the first choice in esophageal reconstruction. Indications for colonic interposition are given in Box 15-1.

II. OPERATIVE TECHNIQUE

- The classic left isoperistaltic colon replacement is described here.

Position

- The patient is placed in the supine position with the head is turned toward the right side. The patient's neck is extended by inflating a pillow beneath the shoulders. The operative field includes the neck, the anterior chest, and the abdomen from the level of the mandibles to the pubis. The rest of the body is draped.
- The operation is performed by two teams (for the cervical and abdominal stage), reducing the operating time.

Incision

- The peritoneal cavity is entered by the first team through an upper midline abdominal incision from the xiphoid process to well below the umbilicus, visualizing the colon and determining that the left colic artery is large enough, with the marginal vessels, to carry blood supply to the right colon.
- A collar incision or 2-inch-long oblique cervical incision paralleling the anterior border of the sternocleidomastoid muscle (SCM) is made. Inferiorly, this incision extends no further than the suprasternal notch. Alternative incisions may be required in particular instances. An equilateral "collar incision" is

BOX 15-1. Indications for Colonic Interposition

- When the stomach is not available
- When the esophageal replacement must last for a decade or more
- When a vagus-sparing esophageal resection can be performed
- Chemical stenoses
- Chronic gastroesophageal reflux disease (Belsey)
- Barrett esophagus with high-grade dysplasia (DeMeester)
- Achalasia, for a failed or repeat esophagomyotomy
- Congenital esophageal atresia ("Waterston criteria": 6-month-old child, weighing 20 pounds; utilization of the distal esophagus if possible so as to preserve cardioesophageal sphincter)
- Bleeding esophageal varices in portal hypertension after esophagogastrectomy (Montenegro)
- Bypass of tumoral esophagus (palliation)
- Others: cicatricial pemphigoid, diphtheritic croup, Behçet disease

preferred for cosmetic purposes in young females, made in the line of a natural crease approximately 2 cm above the clavicle.

Main Dissection

Abdominal Stage

- The lateral avascular peritoneal attachments of the ascending colon and cecum are severed, and the entire right colon is reflected medially. The left colon is mobilized by coloepiploic dissection and liberation of the splenic flexure, followed by descent of the hepatic flexure of the colon and retroperitoneal dissection in the avascular space of Toldt.
- Once the colon is completely mobilized, the main colic arteries, satellite veins, and marginal artery of Drummond (particularly the arch of Riolan-Haller of transverse colon) are identified by transillumination of the mesocolon (*diaphanoscopy*) (Figs. 15-7, *A* and *B*, and 15-8, *A* and *B*). The middle and right colic artery are identified with their veins and dissected from the mesentery (skeletonization).
- Arterial atraumatic bulldog clamps of Carrel are placed across these vessels to their origin. When placing the arterial clamps across the vessels, the vein should be included in the clamp. This allows observation of the adequacy of the left colic artery to supply the transverse and right colon until the cecum through the marginal artery of Drummond. The colic arterial pulsations should stay under direct vision until the end of the operation.
- The middle and accessory middle colic artery are divided (Fig. 15-9). The various colon grafts are shown in Figure 15-10.

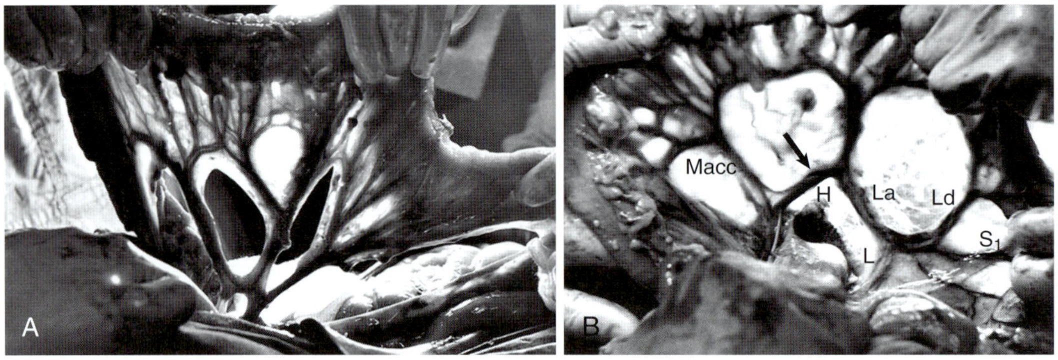

Figure 15-7. **A,** Operative transillumination of the colon mesentery and skeletonization of major vessels, showing early branching midcolic artery and vein. Dissection of the origin of their trunks and preparation for division close to the superior mesenteric vessels. **B,** The accessory midcolic artery originating from the inferior mesenteric artery may dip down toward the roots of the mesentery, giving rise to a complete secondary marginal artery, called by Huard "central intermesenteric anastomosis" (*H*). It was found in our study in 3.2% of patients. In this situation, if the primary marginal artery is weak any colic reconstruction is formally forbidden. *L,* Left colic artery; *La,* ascending left colic artery; *Ld,* descending left colic artery; *Macc,* accessory middle colic artery; S_1, first sigmoid artery.

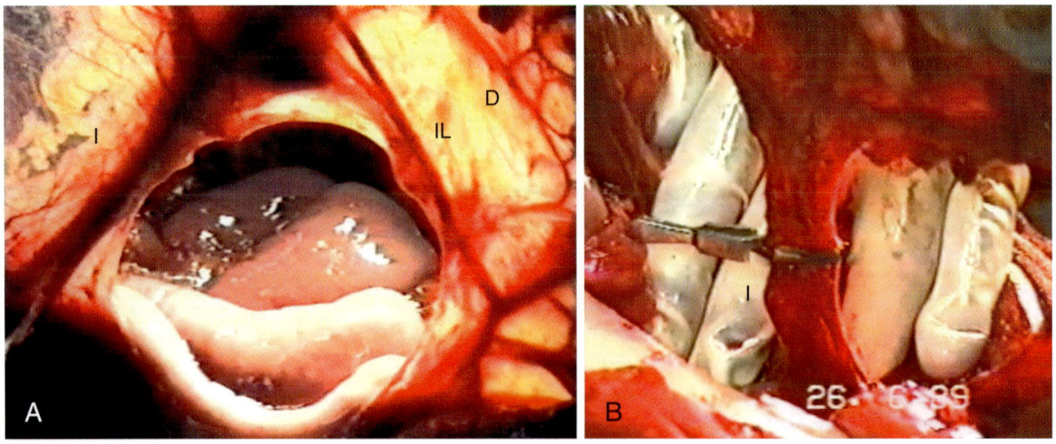

Figure 15-8. **A,** At *left*, the ileocolic artery and vein (*I*), the largest colic vessels (4 mm). Fenestration of the mesentery started at the left side. At *right*, the terminal ileal vessels (*IL*) and ileal marginal artery of Dwight (*D*) with tertiary arches are visible. Through the fenestrated colic mesentery, the small bowel loops are now visible. **B,** Completed free dissection of the ileocolic pedicle (*I*). A bulldog clamp of Carrel is placed across these vessels to their origin. The vein is included in the clamp. This allows observation of the adequacy of the left colic artery to supply the transverse and right colon to the cecum through the marginal artery of Drummond. Division of this ileocolic pedicle is mandatory if the terminal ileum is to be used in continuity with the right colon (procedure of Lafargue) and/or if the ileocecal valve is to be preserved (Dor).

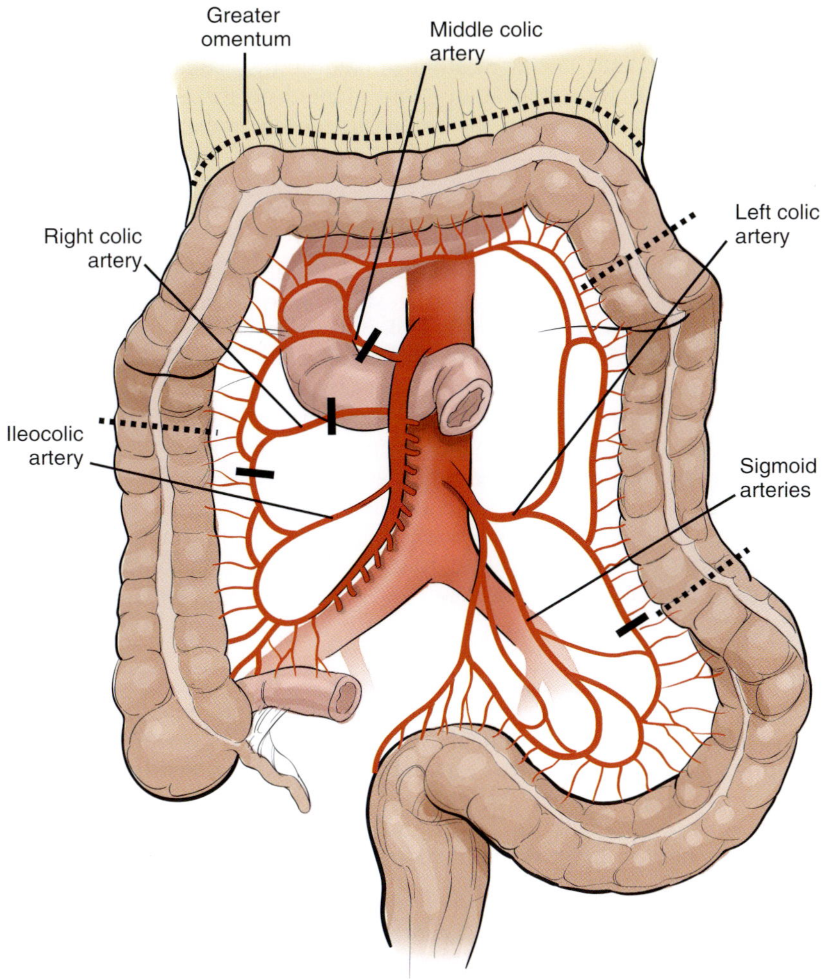

Figure 15-9.

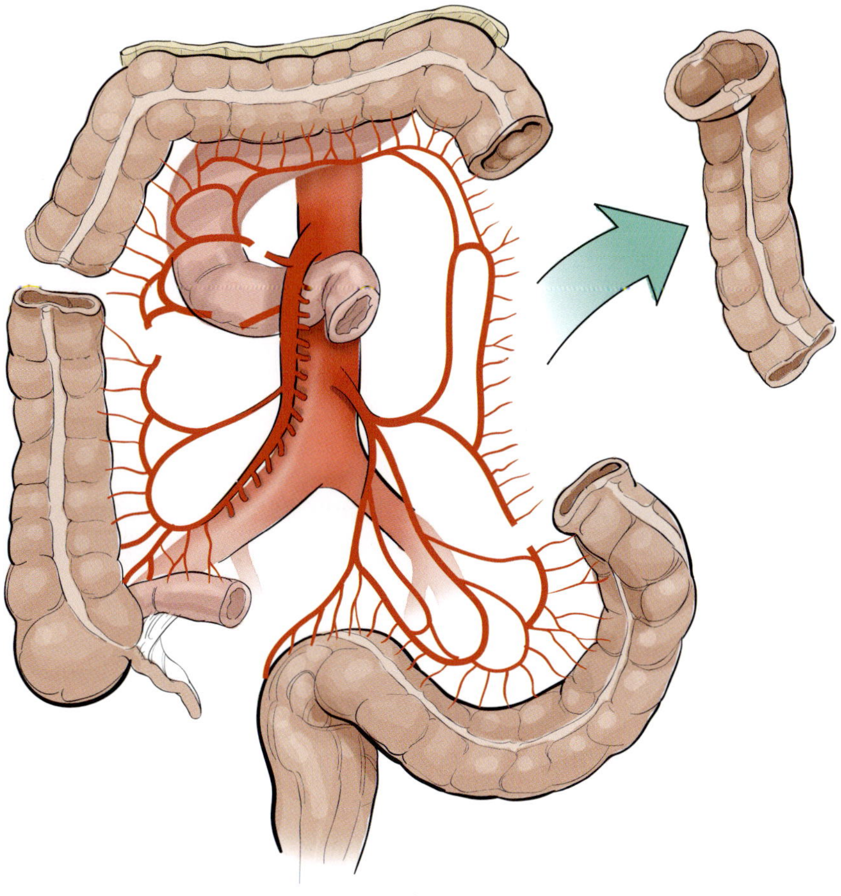

Figure 15-10.

- The length of the colon graft is measured by tethering the colon as much as possible in a cephalad direction on the natural pedicle made by the ascending branch of the left colic artery (first marking stitch). The distance from this point to the angle of the jaw or mastoid (if colon transplantation into the pharynx is planned) is measured liberally with an umbilical tape and marked on the ascending colon with a second marking stitch. One should not measure the colon surface but rather use the marginal artery.

Cervical Stage

- As this latter procedure is being completed, the second team has been preparing the neck by freeing the esophagus at the cervical level and opening the thoracic inlet. Lateral extensions of the deep cervical fascia must be cut to widen the thoracic inlet enough to move the colon to this level.
- The SCM and carotid artery are retracted laterally and the larynx and trachea medially. Posteriorly, the esophagus is resting on the vertebral column and the longus colli muscle. The anterior attachment to the trachea is variable, firm or lax, described by *tracheoesophageal muscle*. Anteriorly it is delimited by the pretracheal fascia, and posteriorly by the prevertebral fascia. The recurrent laryngeal nerve is identified in the sulcus between the esophagus and trachea, close to the esophagus, because of deviation of the esophagus to the left side. The inferior thyroid artery may be divided and ligated, but this is not always necessary in a low cervical dissection (preservation is advocated for providing an improved blood supply of the cervical esophagus, pharynx, trachea, and parathyroid glands). A deep bed of colic transplant is created below the SCM to prevent a late cervical hernia.

Substernal Route

- Following the enlargement of the upper thoracic inlet, the lower end of the mediastinum, anterior to the diaphragm, is opened and the dissection is carried down from above and up from below, with the fingers of both hands of the surgeon approaching each other. An extrapleural tunnel is created in the anterior mediastinum just posterior to the periosteum of the sternum, starting from the sternal notch (space of Burns) and from the xiphoid process to the manubrium by blunt dissection from below and above (Figs. 15-11 and 15-12). The permanent contact with the posterior aspect of sternum is essential.

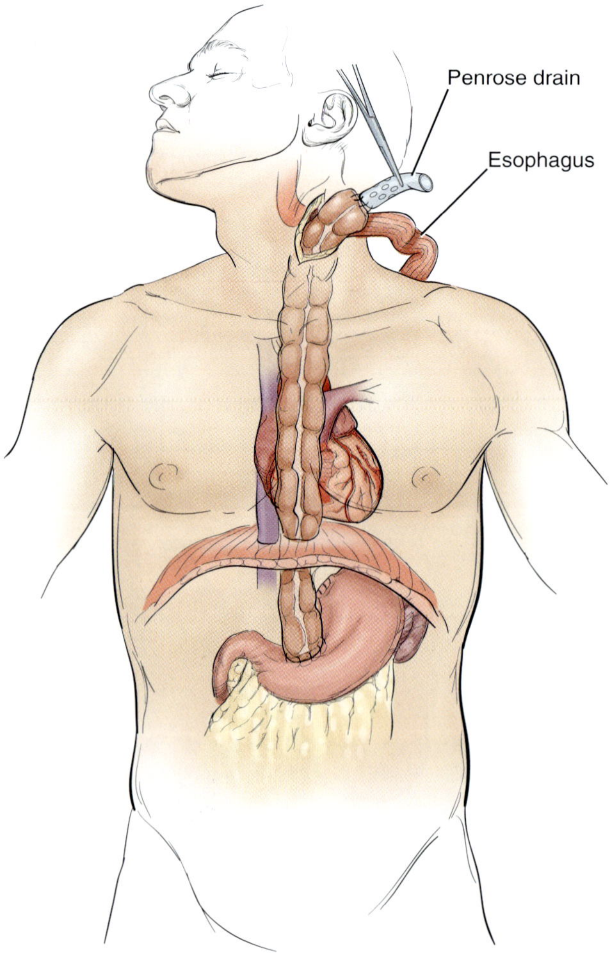

Figure 15-11.

- The proximal end of the graft is sutured inside the funnel of an inverted Mousseau-Barbin tube (Porges Catheter Corp., New York), and a plastic moistened bowel bag is wrapped around the graft and funnel to allow atraumatic passage of the colon through a substernal tunnel. The proximal end of the colon is passed into the neck through this tunnel using a long clamp inserted from above and down to the abdomen. The colon is transplanted behind the stomach and retrosternally into the neck. There must be no torsion or tension on the vascular pedicle. The graft should be fairly vertical to prevent redundancy. The straighter the colon, the better its postoperative function. A straight-line fall works best.
- The left half of the manubrium, the medial end of the first rib, and the sternal head of the left clavicle are occasionally resected to enlarge the thoracic inlet.

Anastomoses

- There are three anastomoses to be carried out. The proximal end of the colon is anastomosed end-to-end to the esophagus in the neck with 4-0 steel filament interrupted sutures (see Fig. 15-12; Fig. 15-13). End-to-end esophagocolostomy is performed in a single-layer fashion using permanent 4-0 steel or monofilament interrupted sutures (see Figs. 15-11 and 15-12). If cervical esophagus is not available, the upper anastomosis should be performed with the pharynx, hypopharynx, or oropharynx. Occasionally, a total pharyngoplasty is mandatory (called *pharyngoplastia vera,* or genuine). Double drainage of the pharynx is an antireflux procedure with particular indications.

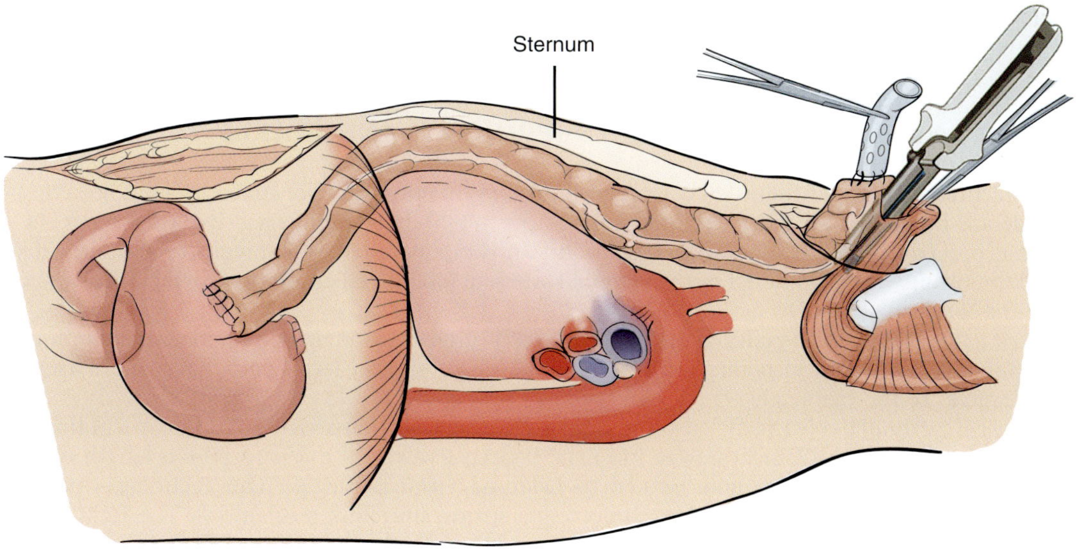

Figure 15-12.

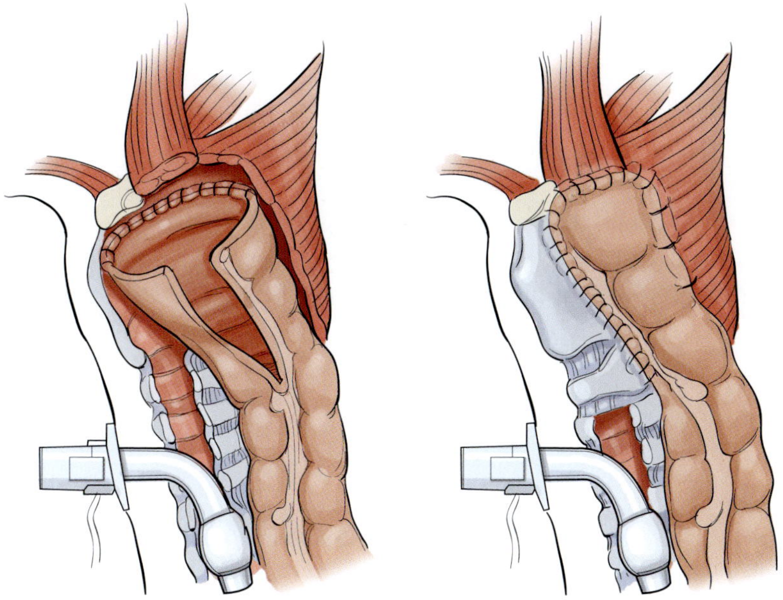

Figure 15-13.

- The distal colonic end is anastomosed terminolateral to the posterior aspect of the stomach in the proximity of the cardia (Fig. 15-14). An end-to-end cologastric anastomosis is placed preferably on the posterior aspect of the vertical segment of the stomach in the proximity of the cardia. Pyloromyotomy, "inkwell" anastomosis, or Nissen valvoplasty (fundoplication) may be optionally added to prevent gastroesophageal reflux. Likewise, a feeding tube gastrostomy may be associated.
- If stomach is not available, the distal end of the colonic graft may be anastomosed with the duodenum or jejunum (Roux-en-Y fashion).
- Bowel continuity is reestablished by an end-to-end colocolic anastomosis in a single layer with interrupted sutures. The defect in the mesentery is closed. If right colon is used, an end-to-end invaginating ileocolostomy is advisable.

Mechanical Autosuture

- The cologastric anastomosis may be carried out using a T-60 stapler to form a triangular orifice (see Fig. 15-12).

Closure

- The abdomen is closed in one layer with continuous 1-0 nonabsorbable monofilament suture and the skin approximated with staples. Drains are placed in the subhepatic area and Douglas cul-de-sac.
- A closed suction drain is placed in the neck and secured with 3-0 nylon. The platysma is approximated with interrupted 3-0 absorbable suture. The skin is closed with a subcuticular closure using 3-0 absorbable suture.

III. ALTERNATIVE TECHNICAL APPROACHES (PRO/CON) AND PEARLS

- The technique of isoperistaltic left colon interposition is the procedure of choice and has been described in detail, because it provides the most satisfactory method for esophageal bypass among the three classic procedures. The technique is isoperistaltic and employs an intestinal segment of middle diameter and uniformity that is bordered by the marginal artery of Riolan-Haller. Alternative technical approaches are the following:
  - ▲ *Left antiperistaltic colon* pedicled on the middle colic artery. Advantages: marginal artery with uniform caliber without critical points; very close to the descending colon, which has a more appropriate diameter to the esophagus.
  - ▲ *Right isoperistaltic colon* pedicled on middle-colic artery with association and/or in continuity with the terminal ileum (2 inches away from the ileocecal valve). If a 15- to 20-cm length of ileum is preserved, the procedure is attributed to Lafargue, from Bordeaux. This technique includes the preservation of the ileocecal valve, conferring a strong antireflux mechanism. The right colon may be prepared as well in antiperistaltic orientation based on the ileocolic artery, but this interposition is rarely used.
  - ▲ *Ileocecoplasty with long ileal loop* (50 cm) pedicled on the ileocolic or midcolic artery. The cecum may be excluded and the distal ileal end anastomosed directly with the stomach, realizing a *total*

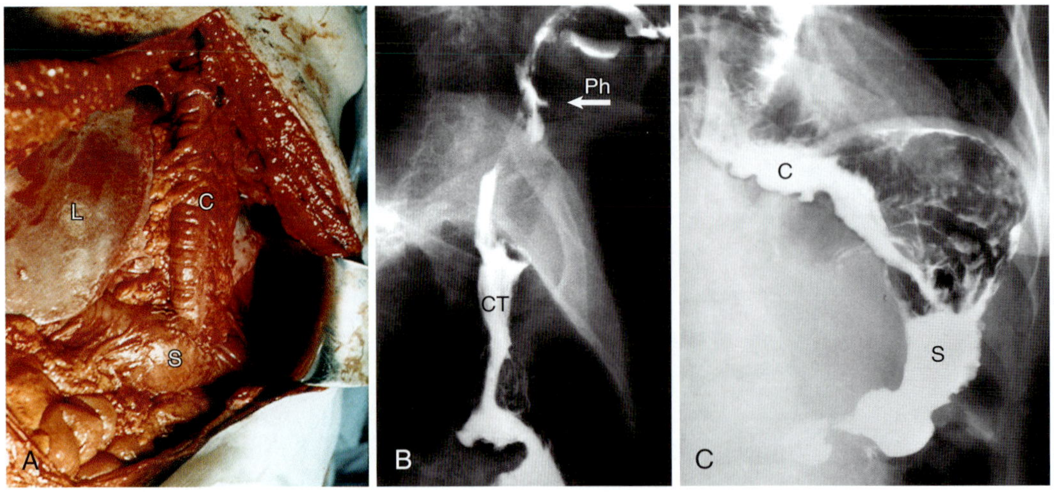

Figure 15-14. **A**, Color operative view of the cologastrostomy (*C*) and the fairly straight abdominal vertical transplant without redundancy passing behind the stomach (*S*) and before the left hepatic lobe (*L*) toward the substernal space. **B**, Radiographic study. **C**, High posterior juxtacardial cologastrostomy.

ileoesophageal interposition. Invaginating ileogastrostomy is preferred. Box resection may be necessary to avoid redundancy and kinking of the interposed ileal loop and to straighten the segment. It was integrated here because the blood supply is provided by the colic vessels and may be useful in repeat esophagoplasty.

▲ *Superlong colic graft* is an original procedure concerning the length of the graft, used particularly in the strictures of the oropharynx, pedicled on the left colic artery, incorporating the splenic flexure, the transverse and ascending colon, and the terminal ileum. This procedure combines the advantages of both isoperistaltic techniques, both the left and the right colic transplants. Therefore we have termed it the *Kelling-Roith procedure*.

▲ *Continuous colic loop* is a simple and safe original procedure, which does not involve a septic stage caused by colic transection and lessens the risk of necrosis of the graft in elderly or poor-risk patients with precarious blood supply. The distal colonic conduit is anastomosed distally side-to-side to the stomach and is associated with a constrictive ligation of the colon, immediately below the anastomosis.

- *Route of the colon* may be substernal (standard), antethoracic, or posterior mediastinal (after transhiatal esophagectomy). Colon interposition in the bed of the esophagus is associated with the least number of functional problems. Rarely, a transplanted colon can be placed in the left pleural cavity, lying behind the lung root. This site allows preservation of the cardioesophageal sphincter (important in children).
- The substernal route is the most common. A left-neck anastomosis is technically easier to perform because the esophagus presents more to the left at this level and the risk of recurrent laryngeal nerve injury may be less than if the reconstruction was performed in the right neck. Some authors advocate splitting the sternum to create a larger space for the conduit and to avoid kinking of the pedicle as it enters the neck. These authors encountered problems with immediate graft ischemia in those patients in whom they attempted a tunneled substernal approach. As a result of this experience, they have abandoned this method for complex reconstructions. By performing a formal sternotomy, they have found that a larger space can be developed, aided by mobilization of the brachiocephalic (innominate) vein.
- A retrosternal route for esophageal reconstruction is created easily with the tips of the fingers of the surgeon's open hand. It is important to ensure an adequate passageway through the thoracic inlet. One way to do this is for the surgeon to pass at least three fingers through this space from below.
- Resection of the clavicular head and a portion of the manubrium sometimes is necessary to provide sufficient space at the thoracic inlet for passage of a reconstructive organ through a substernal route.
- *Hemimanubriectomy* describes the boundaries of the resection of half of the manubrium, the medial end of the first rib, and the sternal head of the left clavicle to increase the size of the thoracic inlet when the substernal route is used to bring a large colon and/or cecum into the neck.
- *Total manubriectomy* is used in mediastinal tracheostomy and cervical exenteration in total circumferential pharyngolaryngectomy for carcinoma ("surgery of salvation") or stomal recurrences after laryngectomy and/or supraaortic or cervicothoracic esophageal carcinoma (Nissen). The inferior section passes through sternomanubrial junction (Louis angle). A pectoralis major myocutaneous island flap is required to cover the space and prevent rupture of the innominate artery. It is preferable to carry out only cervical rather than total esophagectomy ("pull-through"), which determines tracheal devascularization and anonymous artery rupture.
- The straighter the colon, the better its postoperative function. One disadvantage of the colon is a tendency to dilate and elongate with time (secondary megadolichocolon) resulting in dysphagia. To avoid this complication, the surgeon must not be timid in resecting a redundant lower segment so that the shortest possible tube is interposed. A narrower space will keep the colon straight in the midline. The shorter straight route facilitates food passage by gravity.
- A two-stage operation is preferred in children and in colonic pharyngeal reconstruction.
- Resection of the esophagus is advocated only in malignancy because the operative risk would be unduly increased by the resection, and the incidence of development of carcinoma in the remainder esophagus after colic bypass is less than 2%. If the esophagus is left in place, complications due to secretions or infection may occur: chronic mediastinal abscess, traction type hiatal hernia, and/or carcinoma in the remainder esophagus.
- Continuity is reestablished in the cervical region in all cases because intrathoracic anastomosis stricture will almost invariably occur.
- Partial colic plasties (small graft/long pedicle, "like a bean on a stalk") are uncommonly used for replacement of the cervical esophagus due to the frequent injury of the marginal artery. In contrast, they are employed more frequently for bleeding esophageal varices and in resection for peptic esophageal stricture after partial esophagogastrectomy.
- *Repeat esophagoplasty* may be a formidable procedure with high morbidity and mortality. Composite grafts (named by us "kaleidoscopic plasty") are any grafts that use tissue from more than one source (visceral or cutaneous), pedicled or free revascularized. The incidence of malignant transformation in these multivisceral plasties is higher in these cases, and prompt resection of the graft is required.
- It is important to have a flexible approach with regard to the surgical techniques employed. This is a complex group of patients, and more than one technique is necessary for their optimal management.

The majority of authors have performed a single procedure of colonic interposition all their lives, using the left or the right colon. Our philosophy is not to use a single procedure, and this is the dominant attitude currently. The choice of procedure should be determined by the pattern of blood supply.

- One should start with the mobilization of the right colon, and if available, an ileocecal transplant with a long ileum (50 cm), vascularized by the ileocolic artery, should be performed. This procedure requires transection of the distal segment of superior mesenteric artery above its bifurcation. If this arrangement is not feasible, the ileocolic artery may be divided, blood supply being provided by the right and/or midcolic artery, and the right colon may be used for interposition. Likewise, further on, one could gently slide toward left in a clockwise direction, reaching the left colic flexure and performing a transverse colic transplant, in either the iso- or the antiperistaltic direction. Finally, if all previous setups were not feasible, the last resort remains the entire descending colon in antiperistaltic orientation, pedicled on the left colic artery. If the transplant is too short, the upper segment of the rectum may be incorporated in continuity with the sigmoid. This mobile policy or "balanced operation" is opposed to the classic rigid approach relying on a single type of colic interposition.
- Free colic grafts are still uncommon in limited fibrous strictures of the cervical esophagus and pharynx or after pharyngolaryngectomy for carcinoma. Free ileocolon transfer after hypopharyngolaryngo-esophagectomy has been used for speech rehabilitation. The ileocecal valve works to prevent aspiration and also as the vibration source when speaking, so that tracheostomy is unnecessary. Recently an impact on outcome was made through additional microvascular anastomosis—"supercharge"—on colon interposition for esophageal replacement. A particular indication remains when marginal viability of the graft is suspected intraoperatively.
- Colon interposition, like other complex procedures, has a definite and considerable learning curve until its intricate details are mastered. Graft necrosis occurs in approximately 5% to 10% of patients and can be a life-threatening event. The procedure is technically demanding and requires a great deal of experience, particularly when assessing the adequacy of the blood supply to the graft.

IV. SPECIAL POSTOPERATIVE CARE

- Fluid is administered liberally because of the propensity to third spacing after a procedure of this magnitude (colloid solutions, lactated Ringer's solution). Hypovolemia and hypotension must be avoided to prevent splanchnic vasoconstriction, which can result in ischemic injury to the colon graft.
- The patient should remain intubated during the initial recovery.
- The nasogastric tube should be kept on suction postoperatively, until gastrointestinal function returns.
- Gastrostomy feedings should be supplemented.
- Graft ischemia should be detected before the development of septic complications (base deficit and/or increased lactate level, "cervical open-window" method, or pulsed Doppler flowmetry).
- Low-dose dopamine, 3 mcg/min, should be given to reduce splanchnic vasoconstriction.
- The specific intraoperative complications that may be encountered are acute ischemia of the colonic graft, venous infarction, twisting or rupture of the colic pedicle, hemo- or pneumothorax, cardiac arrest during substernal passing of the graft, mediastinal hematoma, and contamination of the peritoneal cavity or mediastinum.
- The specific immediate postoperative complications that may be encountered are necrosis of the transplant, peritonitis, cervical anastomosis leak, cologastrostomy or colocolostomy fistula, cervicomediastinitis, hemoperitoneum, cervical hematoma, upper gastrointestinal hemorrhage, perforation of colonic diverticulum, gaseous gangrene of portal system with jejunal and hepatic necrosis, and early intestinal obstruction. Ischemia and necrosis are frequently catastrophic, unless patients are managed appropriately in the acute stages. Conduit necrosis requires the patient to be aggressively resuscitated and immediately returned to the operating room for defunctioning with a cervical esophagostomy, resection of the necrotic conduit, and insertion of a feeding jejunostomy. These procedures can be life saving. Further reconstruction in reversing the esophageal discontinuity is challenging, and the commonly used conduits are either a colonic interposition or a jejunal transfer. The risk of complications and the length of stay in the hospital and intensive care unit are higher in patients having reconstruction with jejunum. Given this, the colon is our first choice in esophageal replacement. Other advantages of using the colon include its relatively straight mesentery, and increased length that can be mobilized on its pedicle. The jejunal mesentery is more irregular, having a tendency to "accordion." The maximum length of jejunum that can survive on a single pedicle is 30 cm; anything longer than this (which is frequently needed to reach the cervical anastomosis or the pharynx) must be supercharged with a microvascular anastomosis in the neck.
- The specific delayed complications that may be encountered with colic interposition are subacute or chronic ischemia of the colic graft, stenosis of esophagocolic and/or cologastric anastomosis, delayed intestinal obstruction (adhesions, intussusception, compression, or twisting/torsion around the colic vascular pedicle), upward herniation and kinking of a redundant transplant, upper thoracic inlet syndrome, native esophageal repermeation, spontaneous perforation of the distal esophagus, development of cysts in the cicatrized remnants of the thoracic esophagus, chronic mediastinal abscess with

bronchoesophageal fistula, corrosive carcinoma of the esophagus, peptic gastrocolic anastomotic ulcer, recurrent ulceration and colopericardial fistula, gastrocolic reflux disease, chronic aspiration and pneumonia, active antiperistaltic (reverse) activity, secondary megadolichocolon, cervical hernia, dumping syndrome, retardation of growth, poor gastric emptying, sensation of frustration in the chest while eating, late infarction of remaining colon, and malignant transformation of the colonic graft.

SUGGESTED READINGS

DeMeester SR: Colon interposition following esophagectomy, *Dis Esophagus* 14:169–172, 2001.

Popovici Z: A new philosophy in esophageal reconstruction with colon: a thirty-year experience, *Dis Esophagus* 16:323–327, 2003. (A personal series of 347 operated cases with 4.6% mortality.)

Renzulli P, Joeris A, Strobel O, et al: Colon interposition for esophageal replacement: a single-center experience, *Langenbecks Arch Surg* 389:128–133, 2004.

CHAPTER 16

Operative Approach to Zenker Diverticulum

Richard L. Scher, MD, FACS

I. SPECIAL PREOPERATIVE PREPARATION

- Zenker diverticulum (ZD) is the most common type of esophageal diverticulum.
- ZD is a pulsion diverticulum with herniation of pharyngeal mucosa proximal to the upper esophageal sphincter between the cricopharyngeal and inferior constrictor muscles.
- ZD most commonly presents in the elderly during the seventh and eighth decades of life.
- Etiology is unknown, but probably related to some factor(s) associated with upper esophageal sphincter dysfunction.
- Common presenting symptoms include dysphagia, food regurgitation, coughing, mucus in throat, weight loss, aspiration.
- Diagnosis made definitively with contrast radiography of the pharynx and esophagus (barium swallow) (Fig. 16-1).
- ZD may also be identified by upper aerodigestive tract endoscopy.
- Differential diagnosis includes cricopharyngeal achalasia, esophageal dysmotility/achalasia, gastroesophageal reflux, esophageal web/stricture, thoracic or epiphrenic esophageal diverticula.

II. OPERATIVE TECHNIQUE: EXTERNAL APPROACHES

- There are a variety of external approaches, most including performance of cricopharyngeal myotomy.

Position

- The patient is positioned supine, with the head in slight extension using a shoulder roll placed transversely under the scapulae to aid in exposure of the pharyngoesophageal region (Fig. 16-2).
- The entire neck from the lower border of the mandible to below the clavicle is prepped and draped.

Incision

- Generally all external procedures use a transcervical approach to the ZD using a left lateral neck incision, unless the diverticulum is found on the right side by preoperative barium esophagram.
- Before incision, cervical esophagoscopy is performed to identify the diverticulum and pack it with gauze to help in identification during surgical exposure.
- An esophageal dilator is inserted into the esophagus during endoscopy to assist in cricopharyngeal myotomy and minimize the risk of esophageal stenosis if excision of the diverticulum is performed.
- The incision can be placed along the anterior border of the sternocleidomastoid muscle, but a curvilinear transverse incision placed at the level of the cricoid cartilage provides excellent exposure and improved postoperative cosmesis (see Fig. 16-2).

Main Dissection

- Subplatysmal skin flaps are raised superiorly to the level of the upper edge of the thyroid cartilage and inferiorly to the clavicle.
- Fascial attachments along the anterior border of the sternocleidomastoid muscle are then incised and the muscle retracted laterally.
- The sternohyoid and sternothyroid strap muscles are identified and retracted anteromedially. The omohyoid muscle can either be retracted, or divided if additional exposure is required, with reapproximation during wound closure.

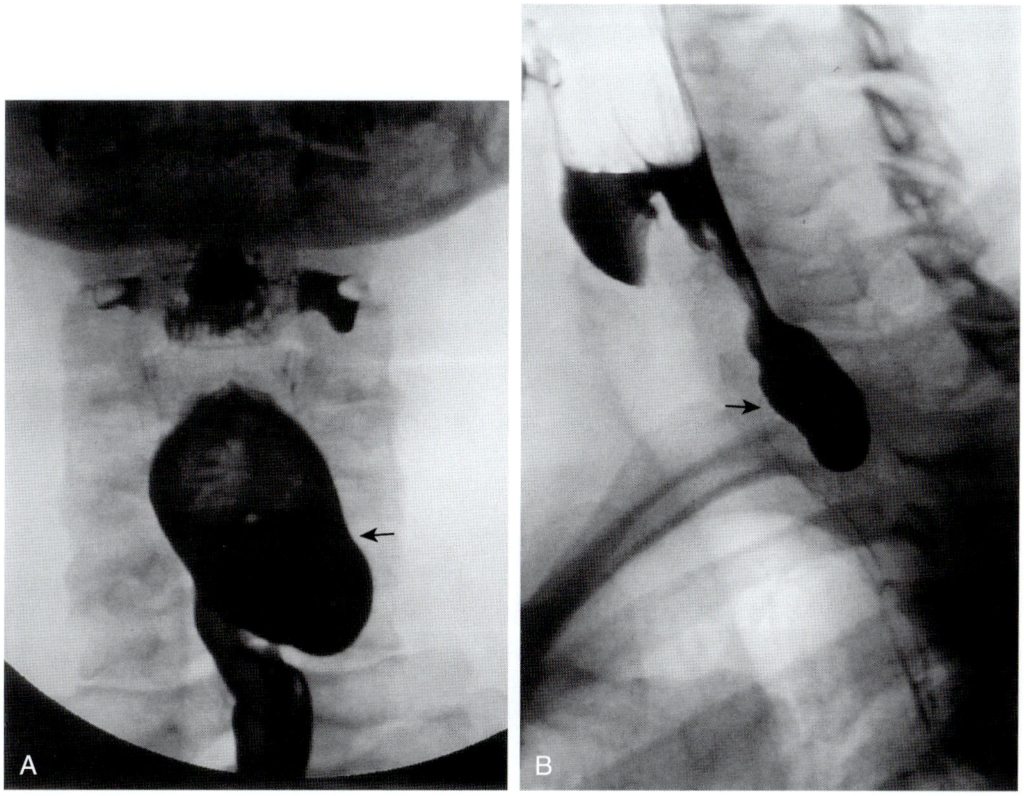

Figure 16-1. Barium swallow study demonstrating Zenker diverticulum (*arrows*). Anterior (**A**) and lateral (**B**) views. *(From Scher RL: Zenker's diverticulum. In Cummings CW, Flint PW, Haughey BH, et al, editors:* Otolaryngology: head and neck surgery, *ed 5, Philadelphia, 2010, Mosby, p 989, Fig. 74-5.)*

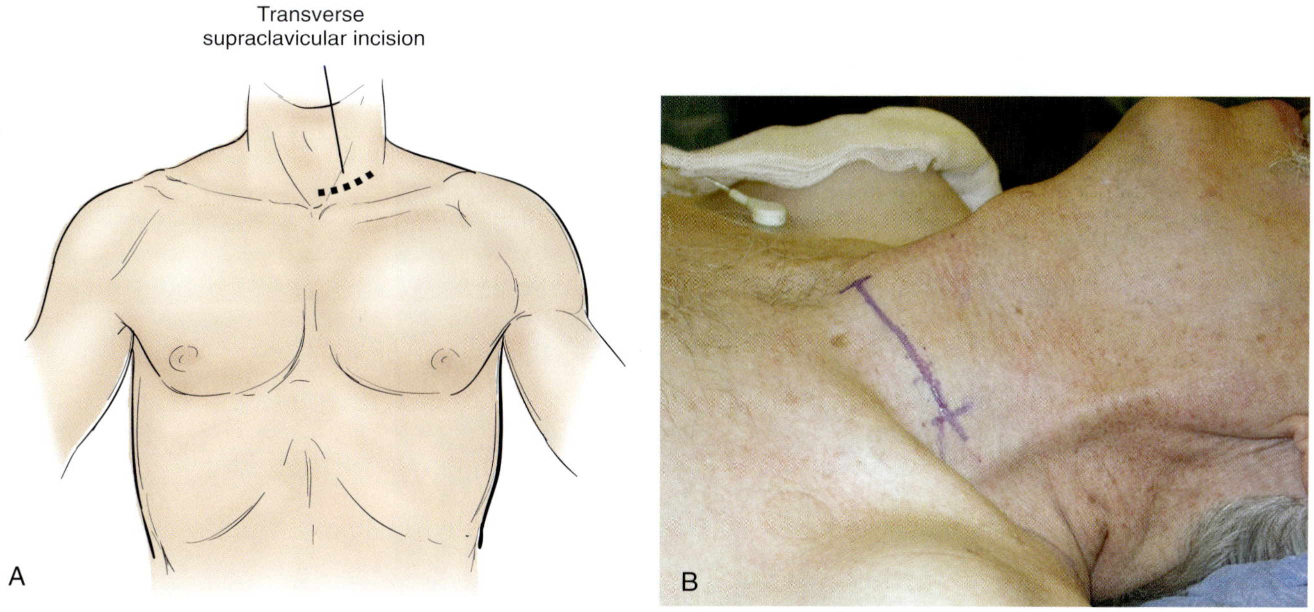

Figure 16-2.

- Blunt dissection is used to expose the posterior aspect of the inferior pharynx, larynx, and cervical esophagus, with palpation to confirm the position of the cricoid cartilage.
- The thyroid gland is retracted anteriorly, with identification and preservation of the recurrent laryngeal nerve. The middle thyroid vein is ligated and divided, allowing lateral retraction of the carotid artery and internal jugular vein.
- The diverticulum is identified inferior and posterior to the muscular attachment of the inferior constrictor muscle to the cricoid cartilage (Fig. 16-3).
- The fascial attachments around the diverticulum are sharply and bluntly dissected to allow the diverticulum to be freed and mobilized from the surrounding tissues down to its base attachment to the hypopharynx.
- A cricopharyngeal myotomy is performed (Fig. 16-4).
- The diverticulum is then excised using a stapling technique.
- Small diverticula less than 2 cm long may be treated by cricopharyngeal myotomy.

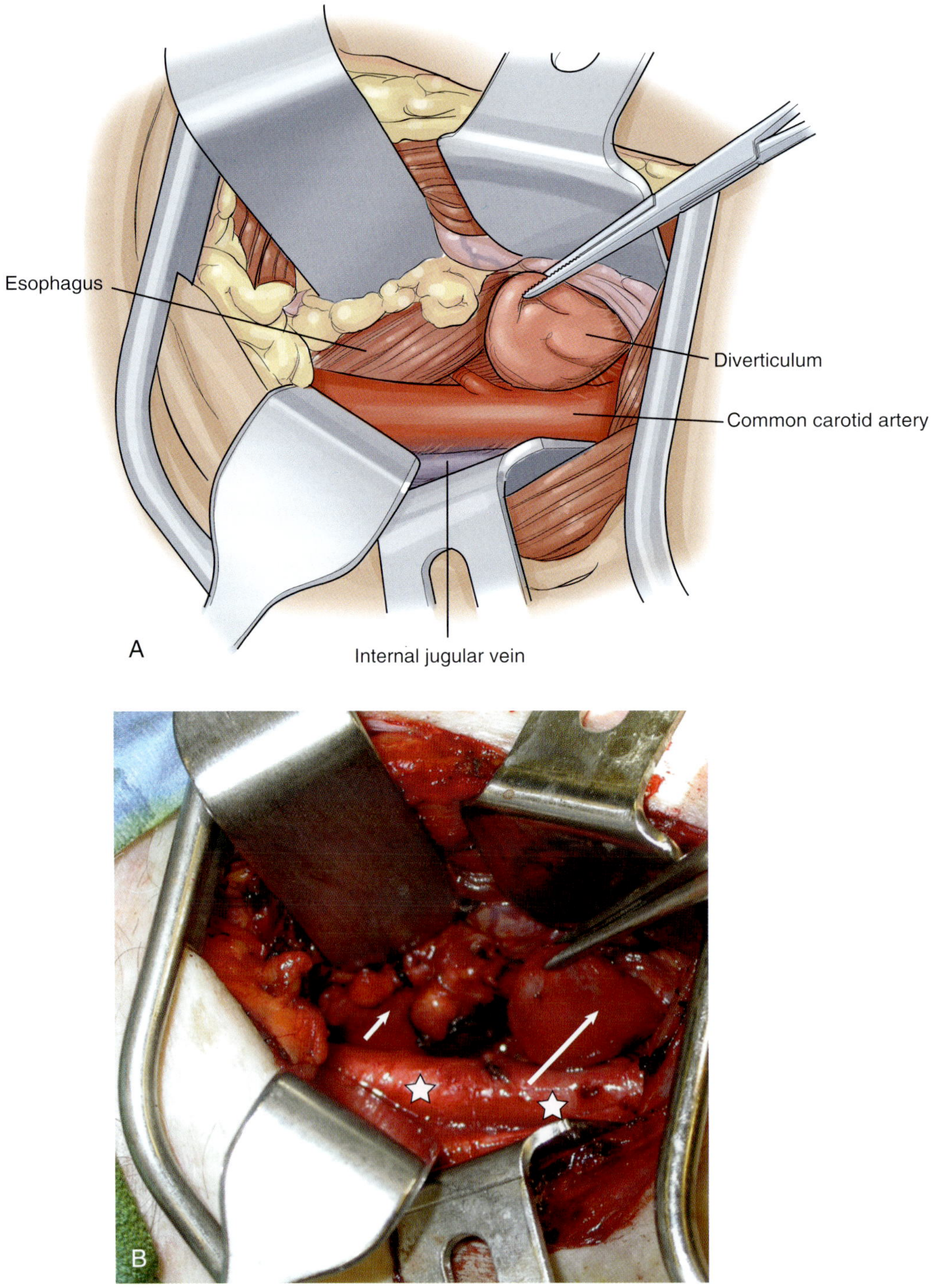

Figure 16-3. Exposure of the diverticulum (*long arrow*) and the esophagus (*short arrow*) is accomplished after retraction of the strap muscles of the neck, the internal jugular vein, and common carotid artery (*stars*).

Closure

- A suction drain is placed in the wound and the incision closed.
- A nasogastric tube may be placed for possible postoperative feeding, but most patients are observed overnight with nothing by mouth and then started on a clear liquid diet on the first day after surgery if no signs of complication exist.
- Diet is then advanced to full liquids and soft foods.
- Perioperative antibiotics are used and continued for 24 hours.

III. OPERATIVE TECHNIQUE: ENDOSCOPIC APPROACH

- Endoscopic techniques involve visualization of the ZD using a modified laryngoscope with division of the common wall between the diverticulum and esophagus using electrocautery, carbon dioxide laser, or staples.
- Endoscopic staple diverticulostomy has proven to be the treatment of choice for patients with ZD.

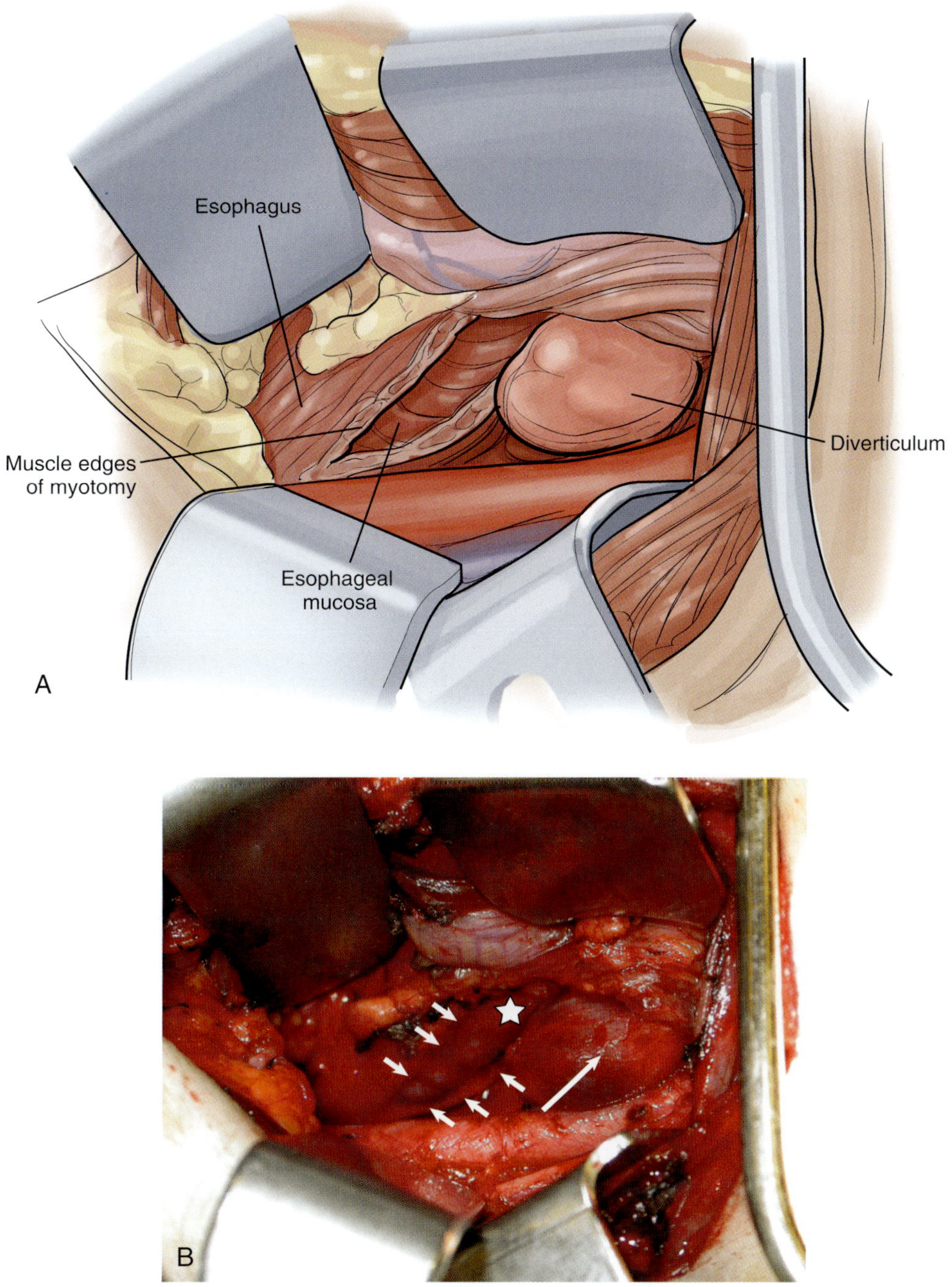

Figure 16-4. The diverticulum (*long arrow*) is mobilized from surrounding fascia before excision, and a cricopharyngeal myotomy is performed. The muscle edges of the myotomy (*short arrows*) and the esophageal mucosa (*star*) are visible after the myotomy.

Position

- The procedure is performed with the patient under general anesthesia with an endotracheal tube and positioned supine with the head in slight extension.

Incision

- A dental guard is used to protect the teeth, when present, and the Weerda bivalved laryngoscope (Karl Storz, Culver City, Calif.) is introduced into the oral cavity and positioned posterior to the larynx to expose the common wall between the esophagus and diverticulum (Fig. 16-5).
- A magnified view of the operative field and all manipulations is achieved by using a rigid 0-degree telescope connected to a video camera.

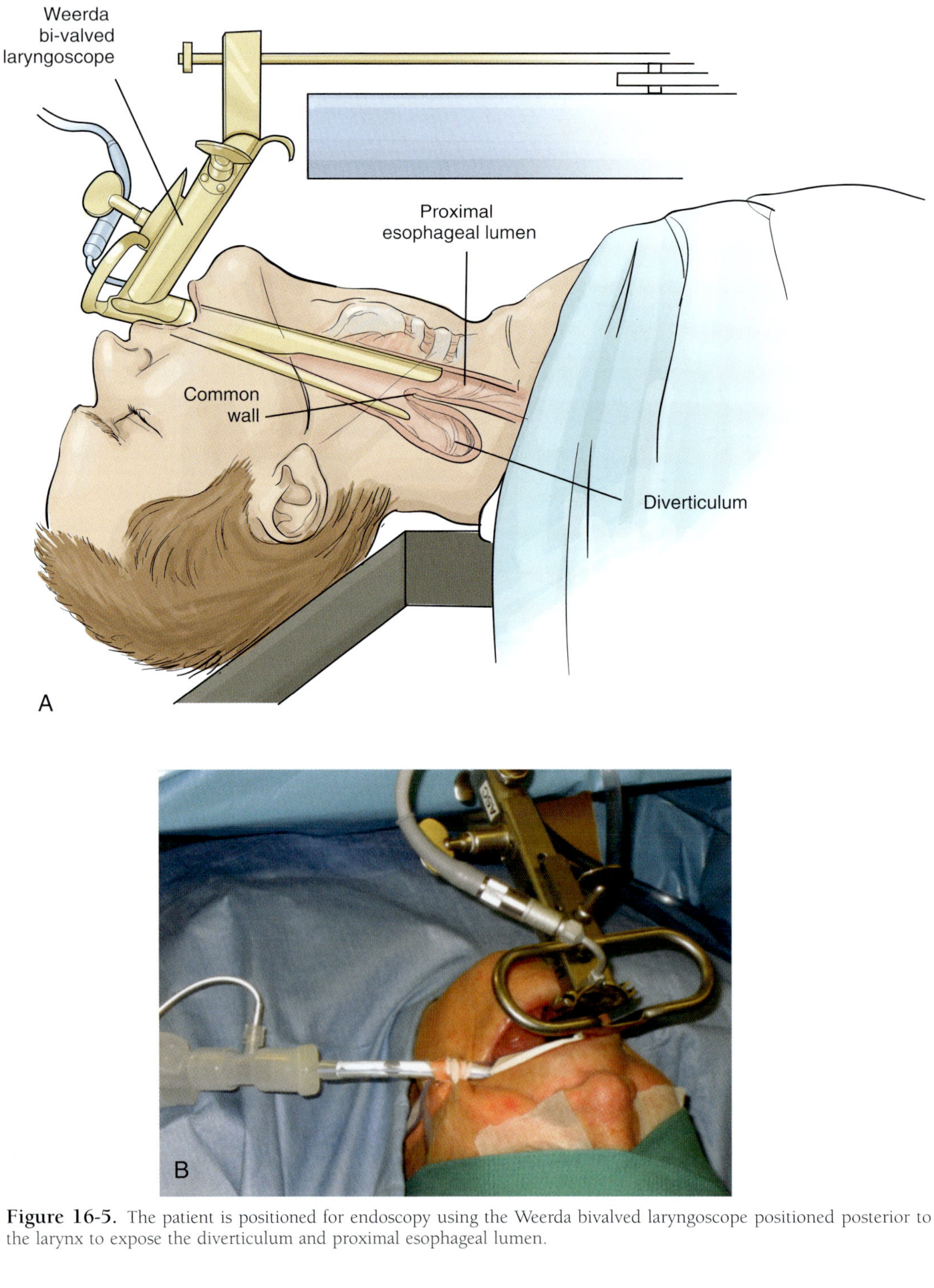

Figure 16-5. The patient is positioned for endoscopy using the Weerda bivalved laryngoscope positioned posterior to the larynx to expose the diverticulum and proximal esophageal lumen.

Main Dissection

- Retraction sutures are placed through the lateral edges of the common wall using the Endostitch Autosuture device (United States Surgical Corp., Norwalk, Conn.). The sutures allow tension to be placed on the common wall to help with positioning of the stapler blades for small diverticula (<2 cm) and for assistance in countertraction when reinserting the stapler blades for a second or third cut in large diverticula (>3.5 cm).
- The diverticulum's common wall is divided using the disposable Endo-GIA 30 stapler (US Surgical Corp.). The stapler blade containing the staple cartridge is placed into the esophageal lumen, and the opposite blade is placed in the diverticulum (Fig. 16-6).

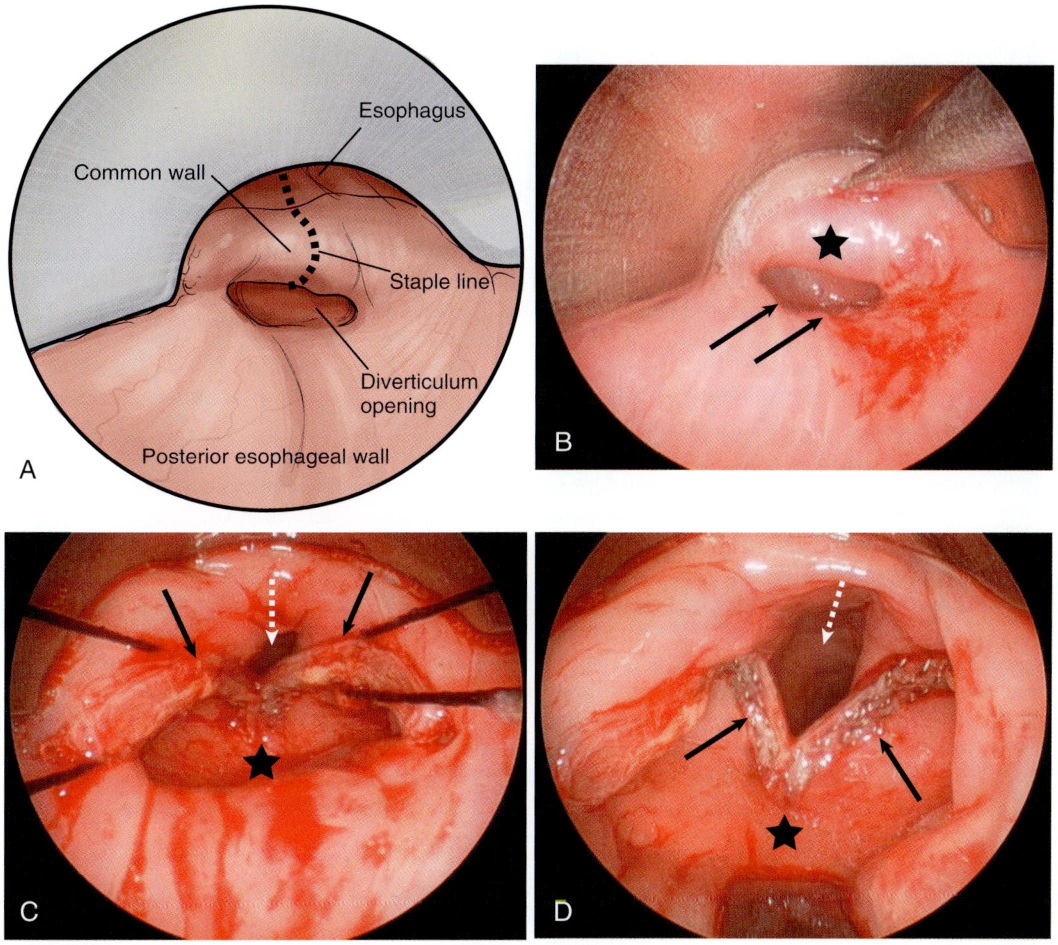

Figure 16-6. **A**, Endoscopic view of the diverticulum during endoscopic staple diverticulostomy. **B**, The diverticulum (*arrows*) is seen posterior to the common wall (*star*) with the esophagus. **C**, The Endo-GIA 30 stapler has been used to create a diverticulostomy (*arrows*) between the diverticulum (*star*) and esophagus (*dashed arrow*). Retraction sutures are placed before endoscopic stapling. **D**, Completion of the procedure with a wide-open diverticulostomy (*arrows*) between the diverticulum (*star*) and esophagus (*dashed arrow*). Staples are seen along each side of the diverticulostomy extending distal to the division of the common wall.

- The stapler blades are closed around the common wall with their position confirmed visually with the telescope. The stapler is activated allowing simultaneous cutting and stapling of the common wall.
- Multiple applications may be necessary for large diverticula (Fig. 16-7).

Closure

- The retraction sutures are then removed after the esophagodiverticulostomy is completed (see Fig. 16-7; see also Fig. 16-6).
- The telescope is used to examine the esophagus, diverticulum, and incised common wall for any evidence of perforation or foreign debris such as loose staples, which are removed.
- Patients are observed postoperatively for 2 to 3 hours to assess for complications.
- Clear liquids are started on the day of surgery, if there is no evidence of complication, and continued until the first postoperative morning, when regular diet is resumed as tolerated.
- Most patients are discharged home the day of surgery, unless hospitalization is required for care of coexistent illness or surgical complication.
- Antibiotics are not routinely administered perioperatively.
- Postoperative esophageal radiography is not performed except to assess for possible complications, or for long-term assessment of recurrence of symptoms after initial successful resolution of dysphagia.

IV. ALTERNATIVE TECHNICAL APPROACHES (PRO/CON) AND PEARLS

- Endoscopic treatment using the carbon dioxide laser to divide the common wall has been extensively reported. Although good success at symptom relief can be achieved, the risk of morbidity, especially infection, is higher than with the endoscopic stapling technique.
- There are limitations to the stapling technique, though few in number. Exposure of the diverticulum may be difficult or impossible because of patient anatomy such as kyphosis, large cervical osteophytes, or small oropharyngeal opening. In these cases, endoscopic treatment should be attempted, but if unsuccessful, an external approach will be necessary if indicated.
- In patients with a small ZD (<2 cm), an insufficient endoscopic cricopharyngeal myotomy may be performed, although placement of retraction sutures improves the ability to expose and adequately divide the common wall. Even with these sutures, adequate retraction of the common wall may not be possible in patients with recurrent small ZD after prior external approaches secondary to extraluminal fibrosis.
- The endoscopic approach may be used for recurrence of the diverticulum after either prior endoscopic or external treatment approaches, with excellent symptom relief and low morbidity.
- Larger diverticula are readily managed using the endoscopic staple technique, and large diverticulum size is not a contraindication to use of this approach.
- Some have proposed that by removing the distal part of the Endo-GIA 30 stapler anvil, a more complete division of the common wall to the bottom of the diverticulum can be accomplished. This introduces avoidable risks to the procedure by potentially affecting the integrity of the staple closure. We have found such a modification unnecessary and advise against altering the stapler in this way.

V. SPECIAL POSTOPERATIVE CARE

- The major intraoperative complication of surgery to treat ZD includes iatrogenic perforation of the pharynx or esophagus. If recognized, these should be repaired immediately. Endoscopic repair during endoscopic treatment is possible using endosuturing techniques. Antibiotics should be given in this situation, and the patient should be monitored appropriately.
- Delayed perforation is very uncommon with the endoscopic staple approach. Signs of perforation that should be monitored postoperatively include tachycardia, subcutaneous emphysema, back or chest pain, and fever. Suspicion of perforation should lead to evaluation by barium esophagram along with immediate administration of antibiotics and avoidance of oral intake.
- Recurrent laryngeal nerve injury is a recognized complication of external approaches. If seen with the endoscopic approach, it is likely to be related to endotracheal tube or laryngoscope pressure and is almost sure to be transient.
- Recurrence of ZD after both external and endoscopic approaches is possible. Revision surgery should be performed endoscopically in these cases if possible.
- If no signs of immediate complication exist, and endoscopic treatment was technically appropriate, patients are observed in the postoperative care unit for 2 to 3 hours. Clear liquid diet is started and continued for 24 hours. Patients are then allowed to advance their diet and activity as tolerated with no restrictions.

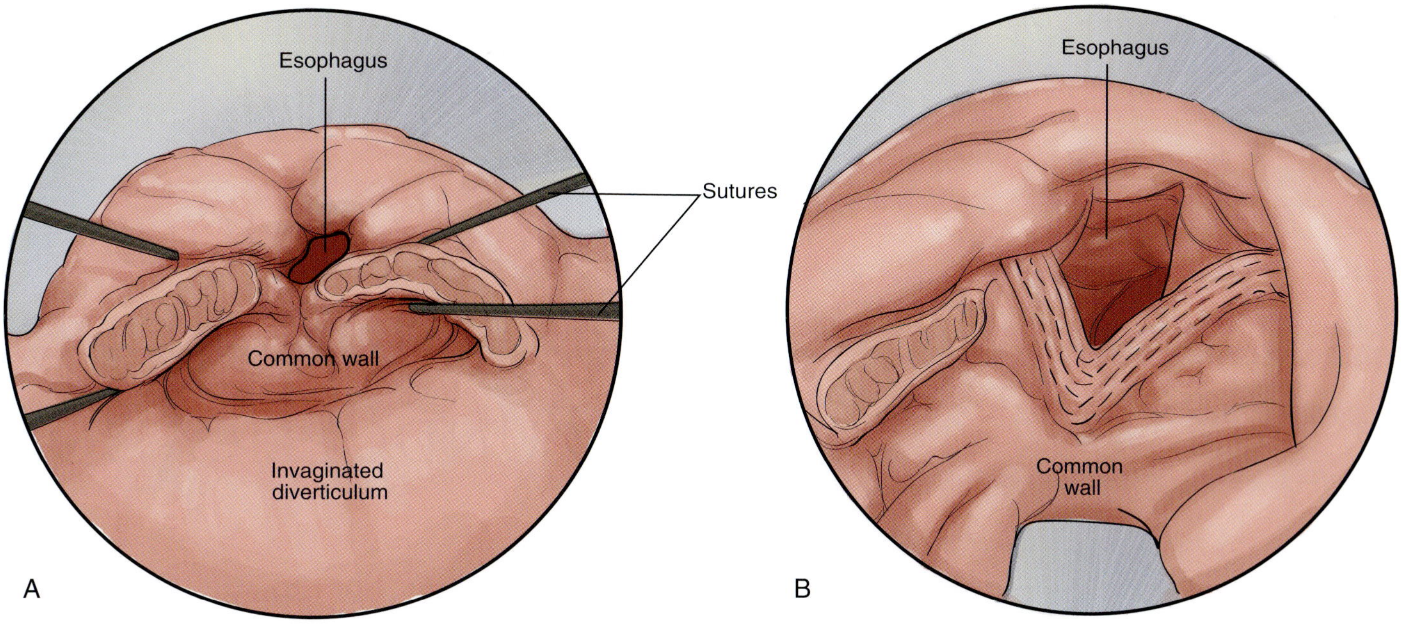

Figure 16-7.

SUGGESTED READINGS

Chang CY, Payyapilli RJ, Scher RL: Endoscopic staple diverticulostomy for Zenker's diverticulum: review of literature and experience in 159 consecutive cases, *Laryngoscope* 113:957–965, 2003.

Chang CY, Scher RL: Zenker's diverticulum. In Cummings CW, editor: *Otolaryngology: head and neck surgery*, ed 4, Philadelphia, 2005, Mosby, p 1878.

Scher RL: Endoscopic staple diverticulostomy for recurrent Zenker's diverticulum, *Laryngoscope* 113:63–67, 2003.

CHAPTER 17

Transthoracic Fundoplication: Belsey Fundoplication

Arjun Pennathur, MD, FACS, and James D. Luketich, MD, FACS

I. SPECIAL PREOPERATIVE PREPARATION

- The Belsey transthoracic fundoplication is a particularly useful approach in patients who need fundoplication but have a "hostile" abdomen due to multiple previous surgeries. It is also of use in patients who have had multiple previous transabdominal antireflux procedures. In addition, it is a useful approach when a partial fundoplication is planned after a transthoracic myotomy for a motility disorder such as achalasia, diffuse esophageal spasm, or pulsion diverticula.
- The workup for the patient who requires a redo antireflux procedure, in particular, should be thorough and comprehensive. The patient's original indication and history along with the operative report should be thoroughly reviewed. Specific notes should be made about the definition of the gastroesophageal junction, dissection of the fat pad, preservation of the vagus, closure of the crura, size of the bougie, and technical details of construction of the fundoplication itself.
- Complete workup includes esophagogastroduodenoscopy, barium swallow, manometry, and pH monitoring. In patients requiring redo surgery, a gastric emptying study is also typically obtained.

II. OPERATIVE TECHNIQUE

Position

- The patient is intubated with a double-lumen endotracheal tube in the operating room. The position of the tube is verified by bronchoscopy. In addition to adequate venous access and a Foley catheter, an arterial line is also placed. An epidural catheter is placed to optimize postoperative pain control.
- An on-table esophagogastroduodenoscopy is then performed by the surgeon. Specific note is made of hiatal hernia, Barrett esophagus, and any other complications of reflux disease.
- The patient is placed in a right lateral decubitus position. The pressure points are padded, and sequential compression devices are placed on the lower extremities.
- The table is flexed above the hip, and the patient is further secured to the table with a belt.

Incision

- A posterolateral thoracotomy is then performed, and the chest is entered through the seventh or eighth intercostal space (Fig. 17-1).
- The incision is made directly over the rib space. A 1-cm segment of the eighth or ninth rib is excised posteriorly.
- After placement of the retractor, the ribs are separated to the minimal extent possible. A 5-cm opening is generally sufficient.

Main Dissection

Exposure and Mobilization

- The collapsed left lung is retracted superiorly, and the inferior pulmonary ligament is divided (Fig. 17-2).
- The esophagus is dissected between the hiatus and the inferior pulmonary vein by freeing up the mediastinal attachments. It is important to mobilize the esophagus along with the vagus nerve. Care should be taken not to injure the vagus. In addition, avoid entry into the contralateral pleural space.

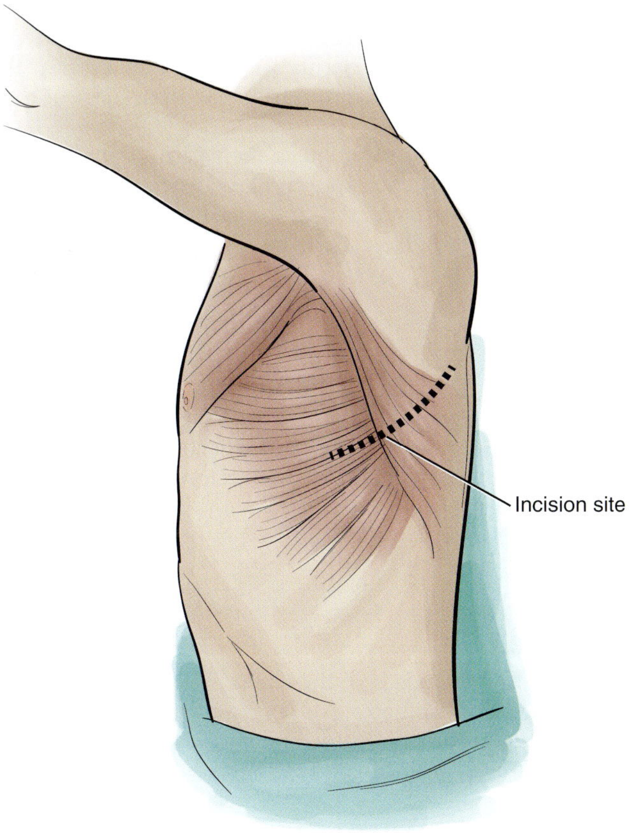

Figure 17-1.

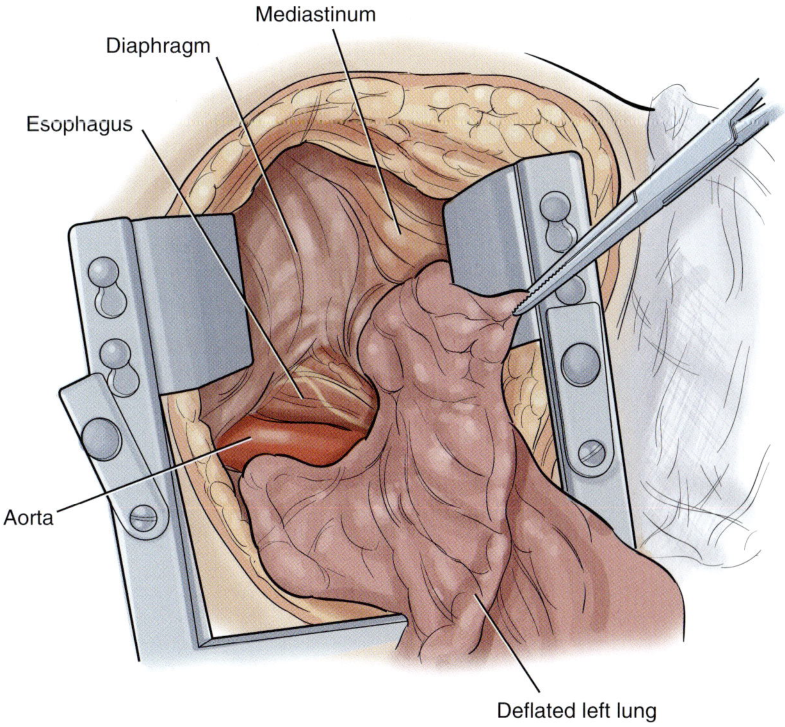

Figure 17-2.

A Penrose drain is placed after circumferential mobilization, and this is used for traction as the esophagus is mobilized (Fig. 17-3).

- The esophagus is released from the diaphragmatic hiatus to the inferior pulmonary vein. When a shortened esophagus is suspected, the esophagus should be mobilized to the aortic arch. In some instances, a gastroplasty may be added when there is persistent esophageal shortening despite complete mobilization of the esophagus. The following description applies when no esophageal shortening is present.

Mobilization of the Gastroesophageal Junction

- When there is no hiatal hernia, the rim of the hiatus is grasped with an Allis clamp, and the phreno-esophageal membrane is divided. The peritoneal cavity is then entered through the hiatus (see Fig. 17-3). When a hiatal hernia is present, the hernia sac can be entered near the hiatus. It is again important to be careful to preserve the vagus nerve during the dissection of the sac. In moderate to large hernia, the sac is excised.
- Divide the retroperitoneal attachments to mobilize the gastroesophageal junction (GEJ).
- An inconstant artery ("Belsey artery") communicating between the left gastric and the inferior phrenic artery should be divided. This is encountered in the posteromedial dissection, and it is important to control these vessels before division.
- Expose the crural decussation.

Mobilization of the Stomach

- Excise the GEJ fat pad to define the GEJ.
- Divide the upper short gastrics to mobilize the fundus. The gastric fundus should be adequately mobilized to prevent tension after completion of the fundoplication (Fig. 17-3). It is also important to make an assessment of esophageal length and whether a tension-free fundoplication can be performed. As mentioned earlier, if there is concern for esophageal shortening, complete mobilization of the esophagus should be performed; a gastroplasty should be performed if there is persistent shortening after complete mobilization.

Approximation of the Crura

- It is important to clearly define the edges of the crura.
- The crural sutures are placed but not tied.
- Place no. 0 silk or similar nonabsorbable sutures, 1 cm apart.
- A spoon-shaped retractor is used, with care taken not to injure the intraabdominal structures such as the spleen, liver, and bowel.
- Usually three to four sutures are needed. Do not tie the sutures.

Fundoplication

- The stomach is mobilized posteriorly into the chest.
- A 54-Fr bougie is then placed in the esophagus across the GEJ.
- A 240- to 270-degree wrap is then performed as follows. The first row of mattress sutures is performed with 2-0 silk on an atraumatic needle. Three mattress sutures are placed, about 1 cm apart. The first row of sutures is placed about 1 cm cephalad to the GEJ in the esophagus and 1 cm distal to the GEJ in the stomach, care being taken to preserve the vagus nerves (Fig. 17-4). The most posterior stitch is anterior to the left vagus nerve and medial stitch is placed adjacent to the right vagus nerve. Each suture should capture approximately 0.5 cm of tissue between its entry and exit points. It is critical to incorporate the submucosa of the esophagus and stomach. It is important to not make the sutures too tight, and this should be done by vision more than by feel.

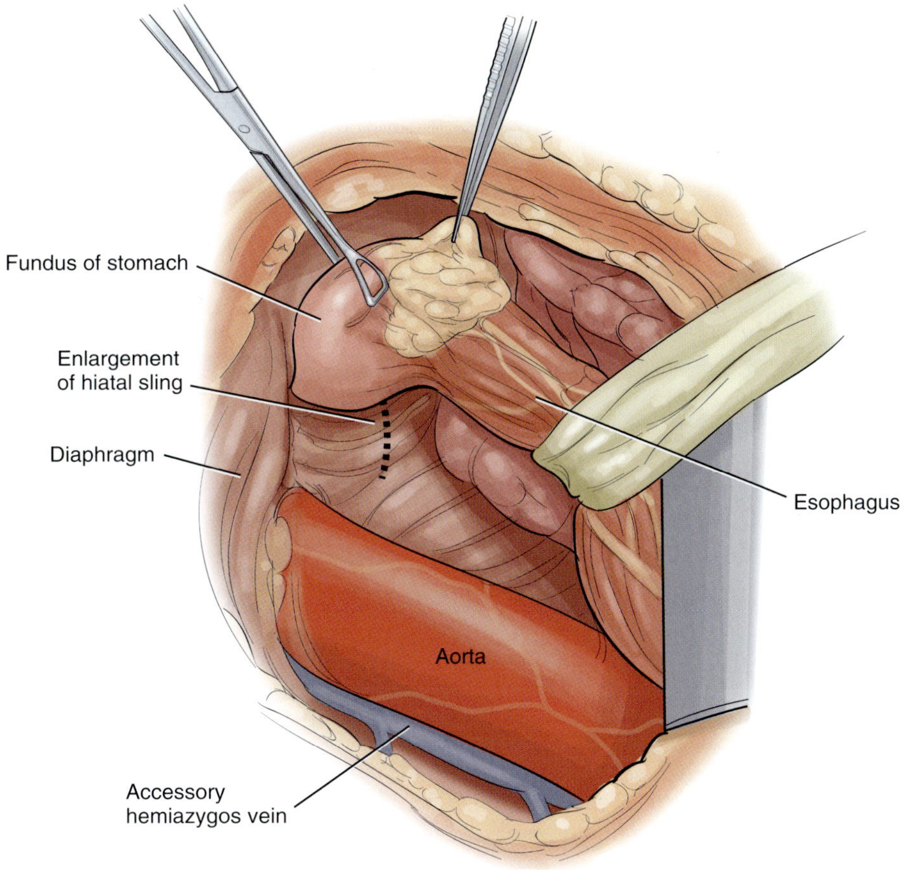

Figure 17-3.

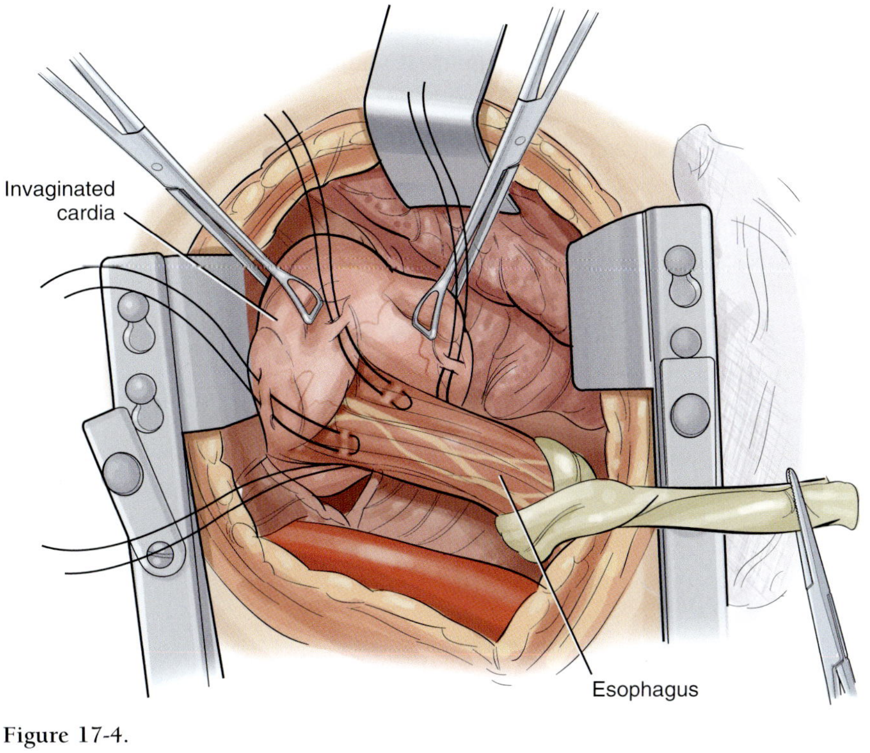

Figure 17-4.

- The second row of mattress sutures is then placed, incorporating the esophagus, stomach, and diaphragm. These sutures are placed about 1 to 1.5 cm proximal and distal to the first row in the esophagus and the stomach. Each suture should capture approximately 0.5 cm of tissue between its entry and exit points. (Fig. 17-5). A modified teaspoon is then placed through the hiatus to protect the abdominal viscera, and the suture is passed through the diaphragm. Three sutures are placed but not tied.
- The partial wrap is then reduced into the abdomen. Once reduced into the abdomen, the sutures are pulled up tight and are then tied (Fig. 17-6).
- The bougie is removed. The crural sutures are then tied, starting at the most posterior suture. Care must to be taken to not make this too tight. After crural sutures are tied, the index finger up to the distal interphalangeal joint should be able to slide easily along the posteromedial aspect of the crus.

Closure

- A nasogastric tube is then placed and guided into the stomach by the surgeon.
- A 28-Fr thoracostomy tube is then placed to drain the pleural space.
- The incision is then approximated in layers.

III. ALTERNATIVE TECHNICAL APPROACHES (PRO/CON) AND PEARLS

- It is important to recognize esophageal shortening when it is present. If there is concern about esophageal shortening, full mobilization of the esophagus up to the aortic arch is performed. If esophageal shortening is present after complete mobilization, a gastroplasty (Pearson) should be added to the repair.
- Identify and preserve both vagi.
- The bougie should be passed by the surgeon.
- Similarly, the nasogastric tube should be passed with the surgeon's hands guiding the tube.

IV. SPECIAL POSTOPERATIVE CARE

- Keep the patient from retching or vomiting in the postoperative period. Antiemetics should be given prophylactically.
- The nasogastric tube should be functional to avoid postoperative gastric distention. The patency and function of the nasogastric tube should be ensured by the staff taking care of the patient.
- When gastrointestinal function has resumed, and the nasogastric tube drainage is low, the nasogastric tube is removed and the patient is started on clear liquids.
- Patients are typically discharged on a soft diet.
- Stool softeners are prescribed while the patient is on pain medications.
- Patients are specifically instructed not to strain or to lift weights greater than 10 lb for a minimum of 2 months.

SUGGESTED READINGS

Champion JK: Thoracoscopic Belsey fundoplication with 5-year outcomes, *Surg Endosc* 17:1212–1215, 2003. Review.

Migliore M, Arcerito M, Vagliasindi A, et al: The place of Belsey Mark IV fundoplication in the era of laparoscopic surgery, *Eur J Cardiothorac Surg* 24:625–630, 2003.

Nguyen NT, Schauer PR, Hutson W, et al: Preliminary results of thoracoscopic Belsey Mark IV antireflux procedure, *Surg Laparosc Endosc* 8:185–188, 1998.

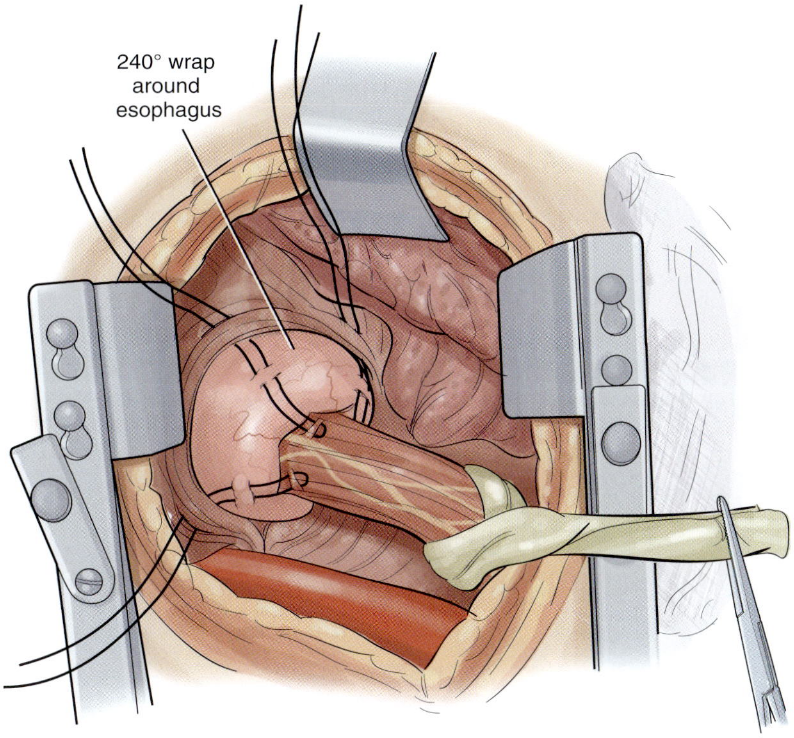

Figure 17-5.

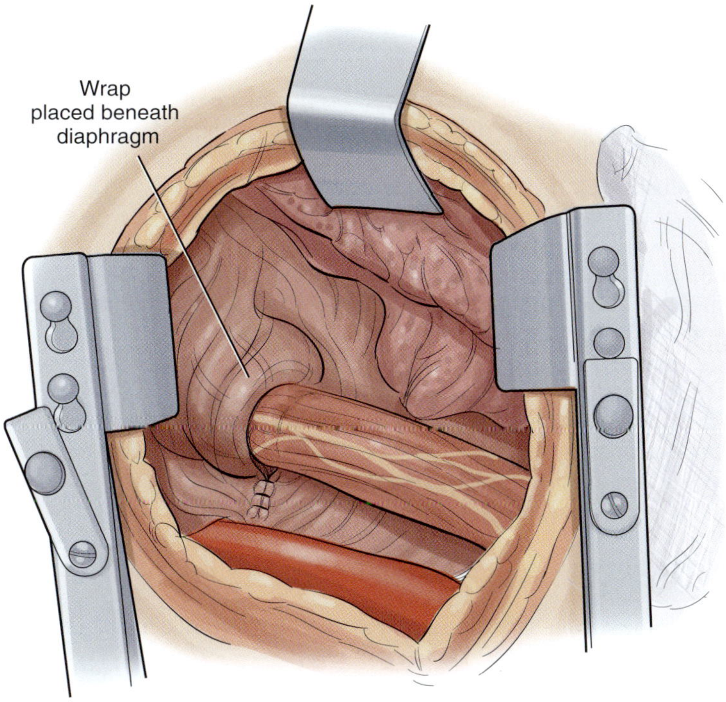

Figure 17-6.

CHAPTER 18

Laparoscopic Approach for Achalasia and Epiphrenic Diverticulum

Alberto Peracchia, MD, FACS, and Riccardo Rosati, MD, FACS

I. SPECIAL PREOPERATIVE PREPARATION

Achalasia

- Surgical planning: to perform a laparoscopic esophagocardiomyotomy with an anterior (Dor) antireflux wrap.
- Barium swallow provides important information on the shape of the esophagus and the possible presence of a sigmoid appearance of the distal part of the viscus (Fig. 18-1). It also determines the diameter of the esophageal lumen and allows the Eckart classification of the disease. Normally the gastric air located in the fundus is not visible in achalasic patients.
- Endoscopy rules out any synchronous malignancy and determines the degree of mucosal damage due to esophagitis caused by food stagnation.
- Stationary manometry is diagnostic. It shows 100% of synchronous waves in the esophageal body and generally a hypertonic lower esophageal sphincter that does not relax on swallowing (Fig. 18-2). Residual pressure is normally high, greater than 4 mm Hg.
- Twenty-four-hour pH or impedance monitoring is an interesting baseline test to be compared with long-term objective postsurgical evaluation. Very often the results of this test are positive because the lack of peristalsis: even a single reflux gives a high percentage of time with pH less than 4 because there is no clearing capacity of the esophagus itself. Impedance evaluation can discriminate acid, nonacid (saliva that goes up and down many times before reaching the stomach), and gaseous reflux.

Epiphrenic Diverticulum

- Surgical planning: to perform a laparoscopic transhiatal diverticulectomy combined with esophagocardiomyotomy and partial (Dor/Toupet) antireflux wrap.
- Barium swallow shows the true dimension of the diverticular pouch, the side on which it protrudes, the status of the esophageal body above the diverticulum (very often there are multiple diverticula), the distance of the pouch from the cardia, and any presence of an associated hiatal hernia (Fig. 18-3).
- Endoscopy rules out malignancy within the mucosa of the diverticular pouch. It gives the exact length of the diverticular neck and the distance of its lower margin from the cardia.
- Stationary manometry is rarely diagnostic of the motor disorder underlying the diverticulum formation. However, it may detect an associated abnormality such as an achalasic sphincter or aspecific motor abnormalities. Even if normal, a motor disorder is usually suspected. A longer manometric monitoring (e.g., 24-hr manometry) is investigational and has no clinical role.
- Twenty-four-hour pH or impedance monitoring should always be performed if the patient complains of reflux symptoms or if a hiatal hernia is associated. It also gives the baseline test to be compared with long-term objective postsurgical evaluation.

Barium Swallow and Manometry

- Figure 18-1 is a preoperative upper gastrointestinal examination of a grade II achalasia: the tightness of the distal esophagus and the height of the barium column above the cardia are well visible
- Figure 18-3 is an upper gastrointestinal examination of a right-sided epiphrenic diverticulum situated 8 cm above the cardia and with a diverticular neck of 4 cm.
- Figure 18-2 illustrates the manometric pattern of an achalasia: the simultaneous waves are clearly visible with the concurrent lack of opening of the lower esophageal sphincter.

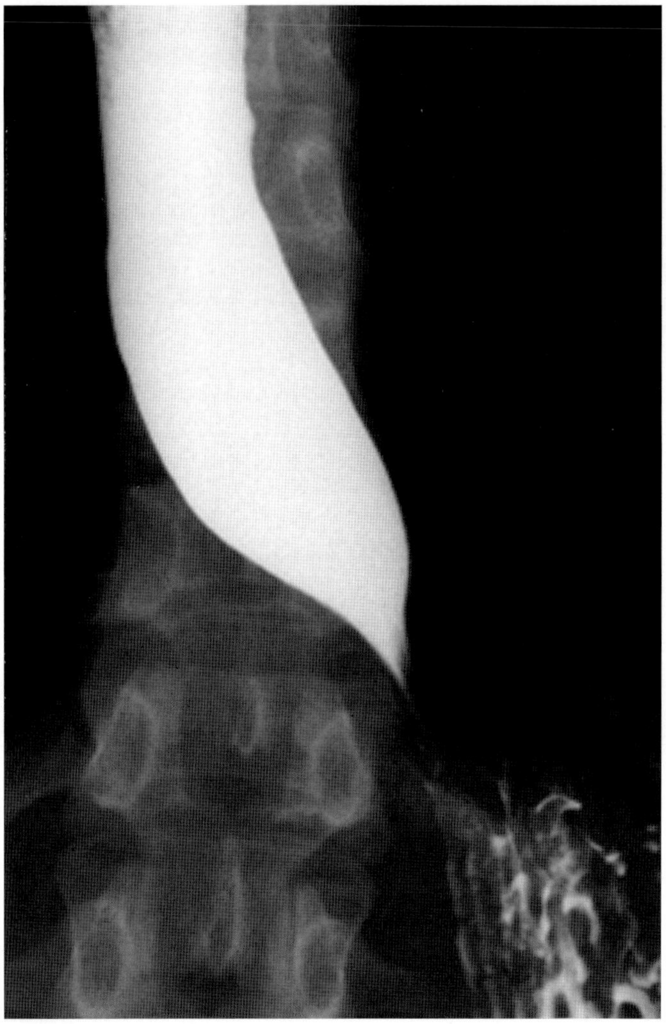

Figure 18-1.

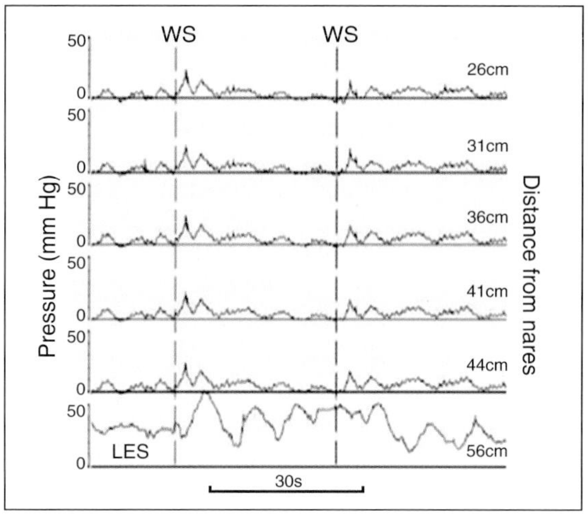

Figure 18-2.

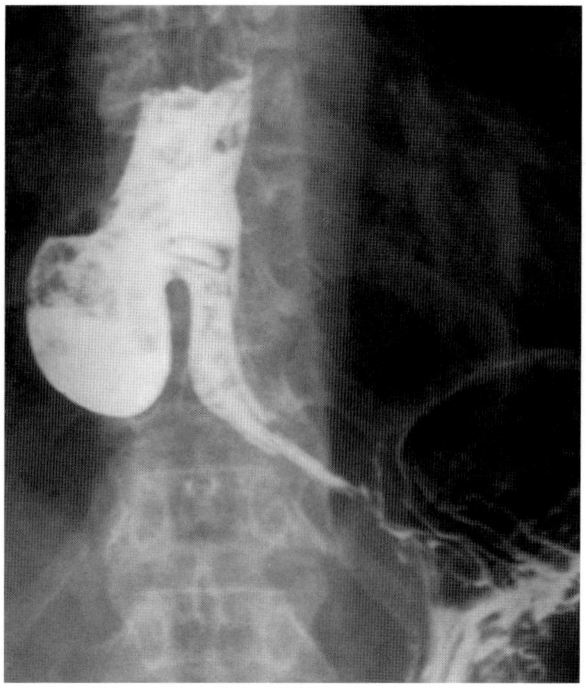

Figure 18-3.

II. OPERATIVE TECHNIQUE

Position

- The patient is placed on the operating table in the lithotomy position with a 20- to 30-degree reverse Trendelenburg and the surgeon standing between the legs in the standard position for surgery of the hiatal region. The first assistant, at the surgeon's right, holds the camera and a retracting grasper placed below the gastroesophageal junction. The second assistant may also stay on the surgeon's right, holding the liver retractor placed from the subxiphoidal port. Flexible endoscopic equipment is placed near the patient's head (the procedure is performed through laparoscopy under simultaneous endoscopic control).
- A nasogastric tube is in place to obtain appropriate suction of the gastric contents.

Trocar Placement

- Pneumoperitoneum is established, and five operating ports are used to access the operative field (Fig. 18-4). A 30-degree scope is recommended in this case. The camera port is placed at the left of the midline at the lower third of the xiphoumbilical line: the greater the patient's body mass index, the more the port is moved cranially. The operative trocars (surgeon's right and left hands) are placed some centimeters cranially to the camera port near the costal margin of the left and right hypochondrium, respectively. The first assistant trocar is placed on the transverse umbilical line at its joint with the anterior axillary line. The second assistant trocar is placed below the xiphoid process, slightly at its left. Port placement is the same for both achalasia and diverticulum.

Main Dissection

Achalasia

- Once the peritoneal cavity is entered, a 5-mm retractor is placed to elevate the left lobe of the liver, and the instrument inserted through the left lateral trocar gently grasps the stomach, giving appropriate traction inferiorly and laterally. Using the coagulating hook, the gastrophrenic ligament is incised and the cardial fat pad is removed with bipolar forceps. The phrenoesophageal membrane is slightly incised just between the diaphragmatic crura to free only the anterior aspect of the esophageal wall (Fig. 18-5).
- Myotomy is started, with the hook making a small vertical incision of the muscular wall just until the submucosal layer is reached. Intraoperative simultaneous endoscopy is performed. The endoscope is

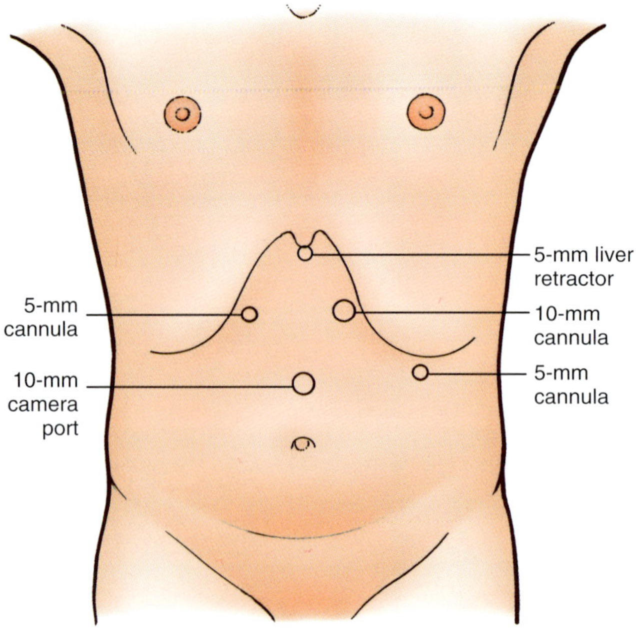

Figure 18-4.

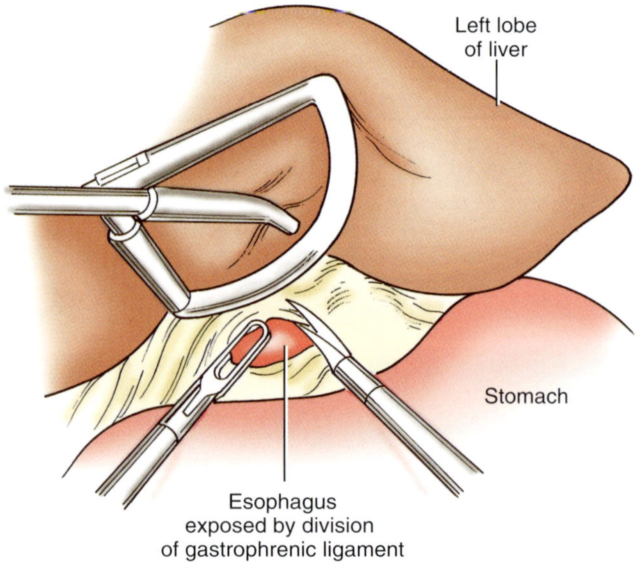

Figure 18-5.

advanced in the esophagus, and transillumination ensures that the correct plan has been prepared by the surgeon. Once the proper plan has been identified, the myotomy scissor (Peracchia-Rosati myotomy scissors; Microfrance, Saint Aubin Le Monial, France) is inserted through the operative port (Fig. 18-6). The scissors are gently pushed upward, realizing a dissection of both the muscular layers along the submucosal plan because of their blunt and fully insulated tip (Fig. 18-7). Once the muscle is dissected from the submucosa, it is then cut, with liberal use of monopolar cautery. No risk of injury to the underlying mucosa occurs because of the particular shape and material of the scissors tip.

- The use of cautery allows sharp and clean myotomy edges along all the myotomy length. Once the esophageal myotomy is judged sufficient in length (approximately 6 to 8 cm), the surgeon addresses the cardial part of the myotomy. This is made with the myotomy hook and is extended for almost 2 cm on the oblique fibers of the cardia. In this area, a very fragile mucosa is usually encountered, especially in patients with previous endoscopic treatments (i.e., pneumatic dilations or botulinum toxin injections), and the risk of inadvertent mucosal tear is particularly high. If tears occur, mucosal sutures with 5-0 absorbable interrupted stitches are placed.
- Once the myotomy is completed, the endoscope is advanced into the stomach. This ensures mucosal integrity and completeness of myotomy. It is then retracted and a nasogastric tube is gently placed into the stomach, as it will stay in place for 24 hours postoperatively.

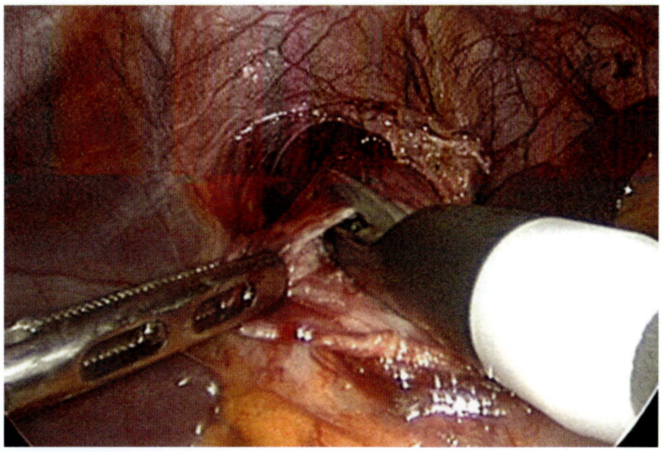

Figure 18-6.

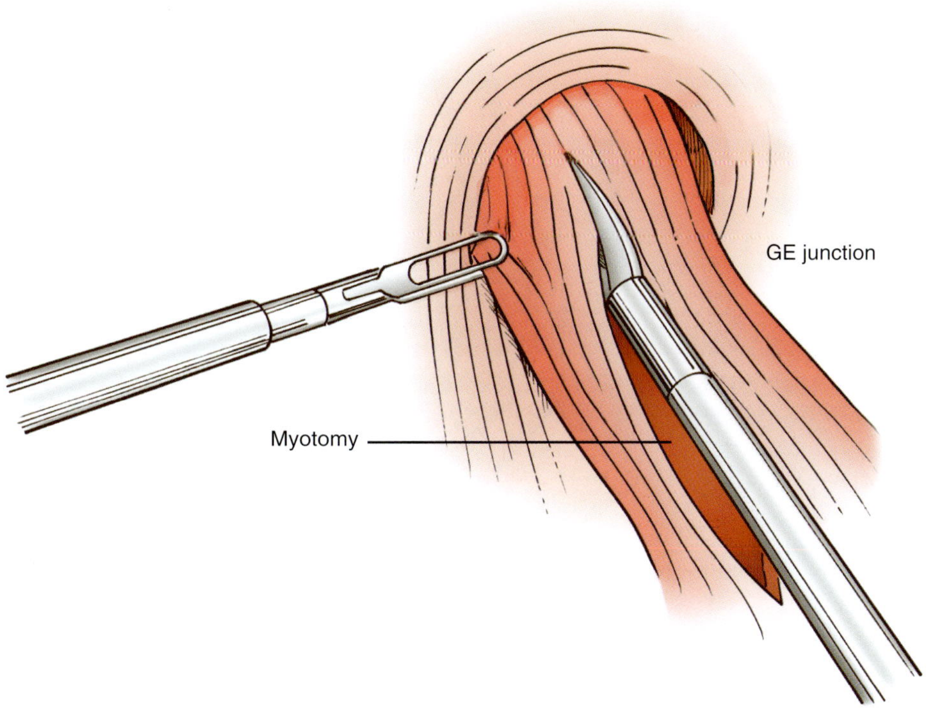

Figure 18-7.

- The antireflux wrap is then constructed. Because achalasia is a primary motor disorder, we believe that a total fundoplication increases the esophageal outflow pressure too much. We believe that a careful technique with minimal esophageal dissection, such as the technique we describe here, is crucial to minimize the risk of postoperative reflux. A partial anterior antireflux wrap according to the Dor technique is good enough to prevent reflux. The anterior fundic wall is sutured first to the left and then to the right muscular edges of the myotomy with three to five interrupted sutures for each side. The cranial sutures of both sides also include the upper part of the crura to keep the myotomy edges in an open position and to prevent their approximation by scarring. A 3-0 braided suture is used with intracorporeal knotting technique. The anterior fundus covers the myotomy area as a patch, thus protecting it from possible postoperative leaks due to undetected thermal injuries or iatrogenic tears.
- Irrigation of the operative field and placement of a soft rubber Penrose drain complete the procedure.

Epiphrenic Diverticulum

- Once the peritoneal cavity is entered, a 5-mm retractor is placed to elevate the left lobe of the liver, and the instrument inserted through the left lateral trocar gently grasps the stomach, giving appropriate traction inferiorly and laterally. After incision of the phrenoesophageal membrane, dissection is begun on the right crus. It is then moved along the esophageal ring to the upper part of the left crus. The right crus is then dissected downward and the esophagus is completely encircled with a soft Penrose drain used for traction. Mediastinal dissection is then started sharply, using both scissors and hook, and bluntly with smooth instruments and swabs staying close to the esophageal surface until the diverticular pouch is reached. A flexible endoscope is advanced into the esophageal lumen at the level of the diverticular neck. Inflation, deflation, and transillumination of the diverticular pouch are of the utmost importance to ease safe dissection. The pouch must be thoroughly dissected until the diverticular neck is completely dissected from all adherent tissue. Special attention should be paid to the upper corner of the neck that shall be free from adherences. Care should be taken to avoid injury to the pleural sacs.
- An Endo Universal Roticulator stapler (United States Surgical Corporation, Norwalk, Conn.) with a parenchymal cartridge is introduced through the operative trocar placed in the left upper quadrant and is advanced to the level of the diverticular neck. The stapler jaws are thus parallel to the longitudinal axis of the esophagus, and the suture will not result in any blind pouch (Fig. 18-8). The endoscope in the stomach also acts to correctly calibrate the esophageal lumen in order not to narrow it too much. Further stapler application might be necessary to completely cut and suture the diverticular

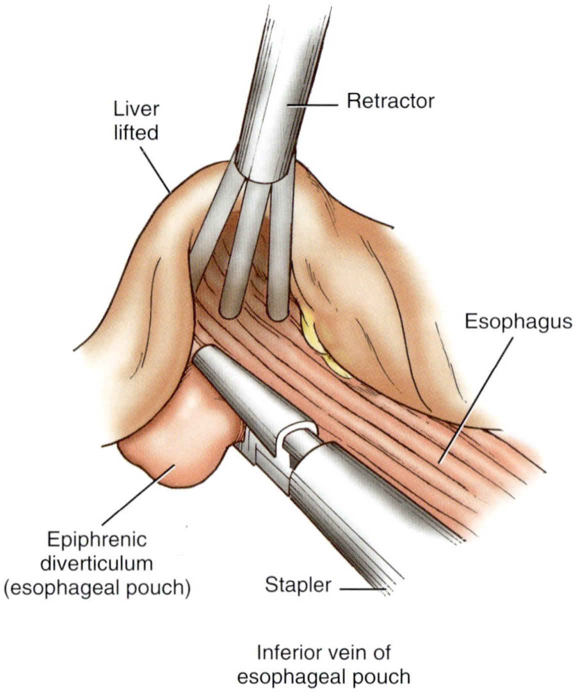

Figure 18-8.

neck, depending on its length. The pouch is removed and extracted in a specimen bag. Two or three interrupted nonabsorbable sutures might be placed to buttress the muscular layer over the suture.

- A myotomy is performed on the esophageal wall opposite to the diverticular neck. Longitudinal and circular muscular fibers are divided and the submucosal plane carefully dissected as for achalasia, with both the myotomy scissors and the hook. The myotomy is extended cranially, above the upper limit of the diverticular neck, and distally for almost 1.5 cm onto the cardia (Fig. 18-9, *A*). Endoscopic inspection of the suture line and myotomy is performed to ensure absence of inadvertent injuries.
- A posterior closure of the hiatus is then accomplished with two or three interrupted sutures. The partial fundoplication is then constructed. The anterior wrap (Dor) is performed with the anterior fundic wall sutured to the muscular edges of the myotomy (see Fig. 18-9, *B* and *C*). The cranial sutures attach the fundus also to the superior part of the crura (see Fig. 18-9, *D*). If the posterior wrap (Toupet) is chosen because of concurrent hiatal hernia or symptoms of gastroesophageal reflux disease, the gastric fundus is placed behind the esophagus without sectioning the short gastric vessels. The fundus is sutured to the right crus and to both the right and left sides of the esophagus. A rubber drain is positioned near the stapled suture of the diverticular neck. A nasogastric tube is left in place.
- Irrigation of the operative field and placement of a soft rubber Penrose drain complete the procedure.

Closure

- Both for achalasia and for epiphrenic diverticulum, trocars are extracted under direct vision. Normally, 5-mm port sites are not closed, whereas 5- to 12-mm sites are closed either by direct external suture from outside or by a full-thickness suture with the aid of a "suture passer" placed before trocar extraction.

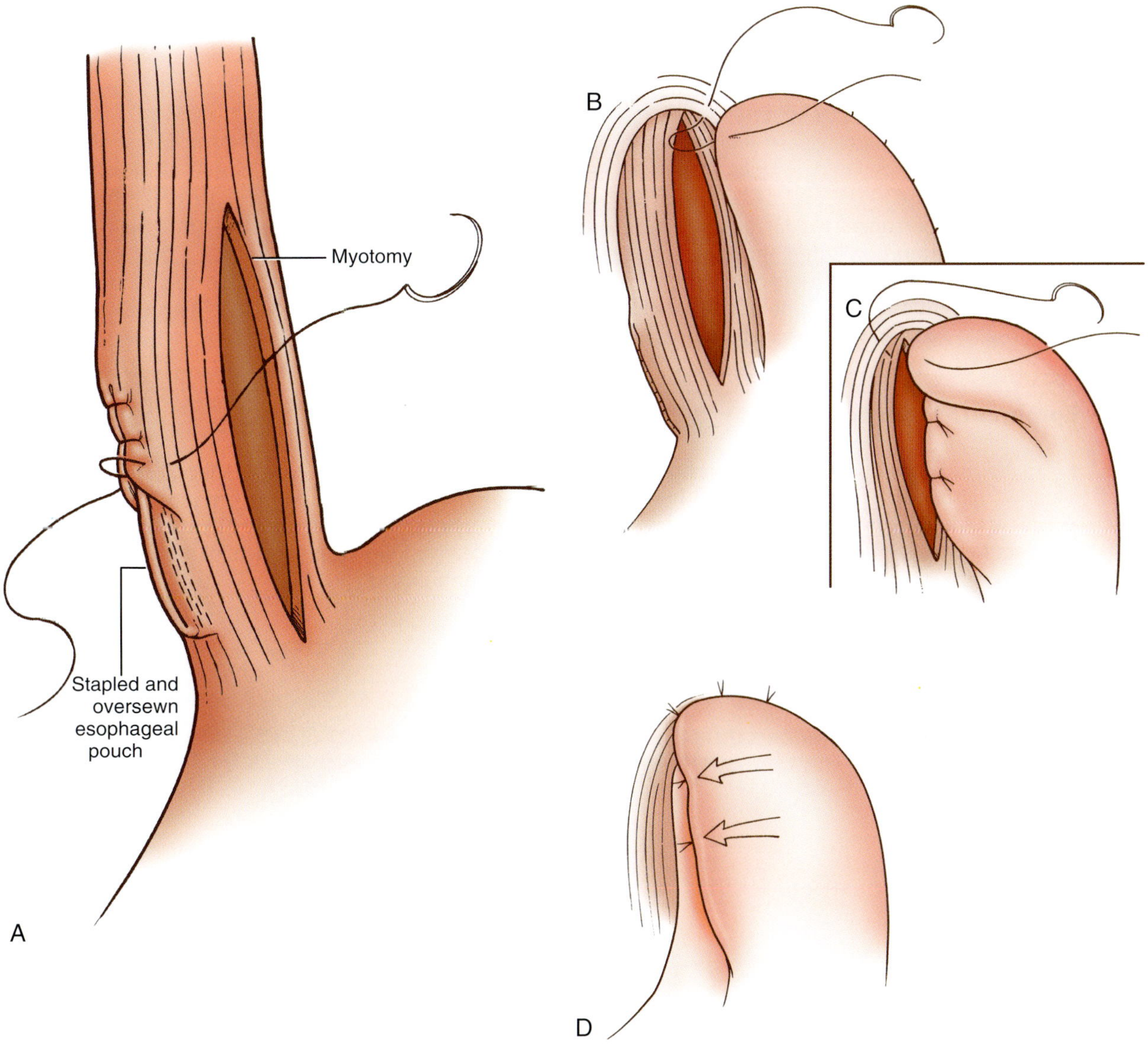

Figure 18-9.

III. ALTERNATIVE TECHNICAL APPROACHES (PRO/CON) AND PEARLS

Achalasia

- Nonsurgical options consist of endoscopic treatment: botulinum toxin injections and pneumatic dilatation of the cardia have been employed. As for endoscopic injections, all the prospective studies have shown that the clinical result is good in a large group of patients, but it is temporary: a loss of effectiveness is recorded with repeated injections. Pneumatic dilatation has a good effect, even if it is repeated twice or more. It carries a higher risk of perforation or long-term reflux as compared to surgical myotomy.
- Surgical options, with both open and minimally invasive access, might record abdominal or thoracic (left thoracotomy or thoracoscopy) approaches. The abdominal approach is recognized as superior because it allows an easier myotomy on the gastric site and an easier antireflux procedure.
- The discussion still exists on which antireflux wrap should be preferred: as stated earlier, with our technique of minimal dissection, we believe that the partial anterior wrap according to Dor is good enough to guarantee for reflux protection. Because the cardiomyotomy procedure is performed to relieve dysphagia, it does not seem appropriate to perform a wrap that carries a high incidence of postoperative dysphagia just to prevent a possible long-term complication.

Epiphrenic Diverticulum

- Nonsurgical options consist of watchful waiting for asymptomatic patients, because the natural history of the disease does not show any disease-related complications for these patients.
- Open surgery is classically performed: diverticulectomy, myotomy, and Belsey Mark IV partial fundoplication through the left chest.
- Thoracoscopic diverticulectomy has been described in the past but has been abandoned because of suboptimal clinical results.

IV. SPECIAL POSTOPERATIVE CARE

Achalasia

- On the first postoperative day, a Gastrografin swallow is obtained. This allows nasogastric tube removal and resumption of a liquid and then soft diet (from day 2) .
- Patients are generally discharged on day 3, with follow-ups at 7 and 30 days. No medications are prescribed unless the patient is symptomatic. At 1 year, objective follow-up consists of barium swallow, endoscopy, stationary manometry, and 24-hr impedance monitoring.

Epiphrenic Diverticulum

- On the third postoperative day, a Gastrografin swallow is obtained to check for esophageal suture. This allows nasogastric tube removal and resumption of a liquid and then soft diet (from day 4) .
- Patients are generally discharged on day 5, with follow-ups at 7 and 30 days. No medications are prescribed unless the patient is symptomatic. At 1 year, objective follow-up consists of barium swallow, endoscopy, stationary manometry, and 24-hr impedance monitoring.

SUGGESTED READINGS

Rosati R, Fumagalli U, Bona S, et al: Diverticulectomy, myotomy and fundoplication through laparoscopy: a new option to treat epiphrenic esophageal diverticula? *Ann Surg* 227:174–178, 1998.

Rosati R, Fumagalli U, Bona S, et al: Laparoscopic treatment of epiphrenic diverticula, *J Laparosc Surg Adv Surg Tech* 11:371–375, 2001.

Rosati R, Fumagalli U, Bonavina L, et al: Laparoscopic approach to esophageal achalasia, *Am J Surg* 169:424–427, 1995.

SECTION IV

Stomach/Small Intestine

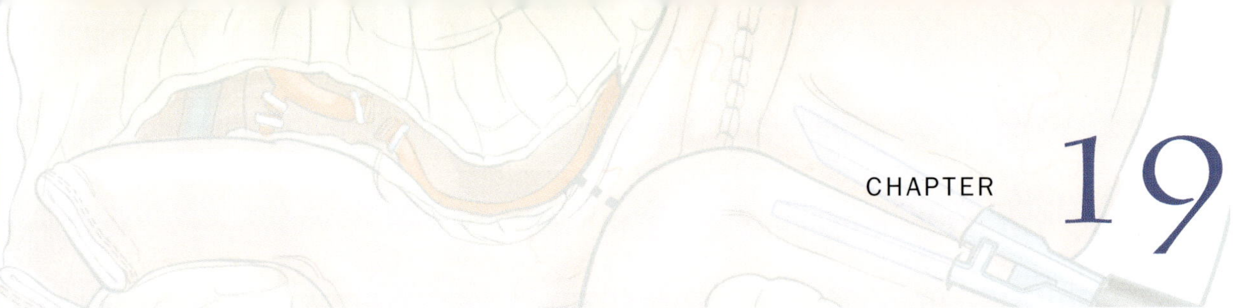

CHAPTER 19

Total Gastrectomy with D2 Lymph Node Dissection

Mitsuru Sasako, MD, PhD, and Takeo Fukagawa, MD, PhD

I. SPECIAL PREOPERATIVE PREPARATION

- Upper gastrointestinal endoscopy is mandatory to confirm histologic diagnosis and decide the tumor depth and surface spread in the stomach, including proximal and distal tumor margins. Endoscopic ultrasonography is sometimes used to diagnose the tumor depth in the wall and also is useful to detect submucosal or deeper infiltration without superficial mucosal change, especially in cases of diffuse cancer such as linitis plastica.
- Upper gastrointestinal barium meal study is still often used in Japan for better understanding the tumor location and unclear proximal invasion of cancer, which could be shown by rigidity of the stomach wall in x-ray studies.
- Thin-sliced enhanced computed tomography (CT) scan is mandatory for staging advanced gastric cancer. Regarding the primary tumor, this examination is not so useful but sometimes helps to detect wall thickening and esophageal invasion. Using contrast medium for vascular structure is very useful to diagnose hepatic lesions and lymph node metastasis. Any lymph nodes enhanced and larger than 10 mm are likely to be metastatic. Highly enhanced small spots in the omentum correspond to peritoneal metastasis. Ascites detected by CT scan suggests existence of peritoneal metastasis when the amount is moderate or more.
- Staging laparoscopy is the only way to detect small peritoneal metastasis less than 3 to 4 mm in size. Inferior surface of the bilateral diaphragm, both lateral gutters, the inner peritoneum of the anterior abdominal wall, and the pelvic area including the pouch of Douglas should be observed carefully. To completely rule out peritoneal metastasis requires the observation of the entire mesentery of both small and large intestine, which is sometimes technically difficult and requires patience on the part of the examiner. Washing cytology is recommended for detecting invisible metastasis.
- Although the indication of splenectomy remains controversial, splenectomy is often avoided when the tumor is not located near the greater curvature. Not only CT scan but also barium meal study are often helpful for this purpose.
- It is important that the surgeon understand the various assignments of the lymph node stations in the upper abdomen.

II. OPERATIVE TECHNIQUE

Position

- The supine position is usual. If the tumor is invading the esophagus more than 3 cm, sometimes right semilateral position is used for left thoracoabdominal oblique incision. In this position, intraabdominal procedures are usually done in supine position, and intrathoracic procedures are carried out by turning the patient nearly to the right lateral position by tilting the table.

Incision

- For slim or medium-sized patients, upper median incision is commonly used. For obese or deep-bodied patients, roof-type or Mercedes-type incisions are preferred (Fig. 19-1). The difference between these two is an additional short median incision at the top. In any case, good retractors to pull up the costal margins are essential for good access to the esophagogastric junction.

Main Dissection

- Staging is confirmed by observing the tumor surface (T factor) and the entire surface of the visceral and parietal peritoneum to exclude peritoneal seeding. The liver surface should carefully be observed and palpated to detect small metastatic nodules located on the liver surface, which sometimes cannot be detected by CT scan. Additional detection of metastatic nodes by observation or palpation is not easy, because most large nodal metastases can be diagnosed preoperatively, and about 40% of metastatic nodes are 5 mm or less in size. Only nodal metastases that involve the surfaces of nodes or the surrounding tissue can be recognized as metastatic regardless of their size.
- If there is no factor hampering curative resection, surgeons must decide whether a total gastrectomy is mandatory. It is desirable to gain sufficient information about proximal extension by several examination modalities. Principally, a surgical margin of at least 2 cm and 5 cm is needed for expanding and infiltrating type tumors, respectively. Palpation during surgery allows detection of unexpected wall thickness, which should be regarded as a part of discrete invasion.
- A D2 total gastrectomy includes complete omentectomy and lymph node dissection of the first- and second-tier nodes. Inclusion of complete bursectomy and splenectomy is controversial, but they are not indicated at least for T1 tumors. These two procedures are regarded as standard in many Japanese cancer hospitals, whereas spleen preservation is recommended in most Western specialist centers. Recently the Maruyama index has been used to evaluate the quantitative risk of residual nodal diseases. According to this program, many patients with T3/T4 tumors of the greater curvature should have a Maruyama index greater than 5, if splenectomy is not carried out. To evaluate the clinical value of splenectomy for advanced gastric cancer that does not involve the greater curvature, the Japan Clinical Oncology Group is carrying out a large multicenter randomized controlled trial. The results of this study will be available in 2 years.
- Operation is started by omentectomy with or without bursectomy. In any case, right to the middle colic vessels, the omental bursa is closed and should be opened along this line to gain access the proper layer for lymph node dissection of the infrapyloric area. Thus the right one third of the anterior sheet of the transverse mesocolon should be resected together with the omentum (Fig. 19-2).

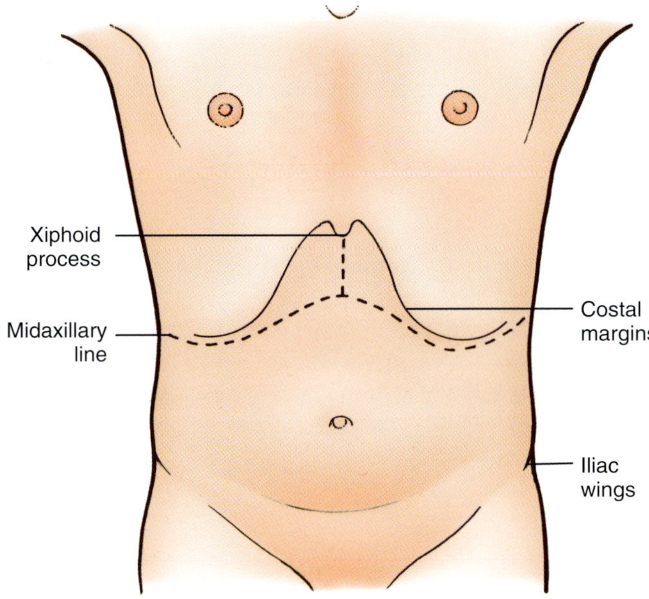

Figure 19-1.

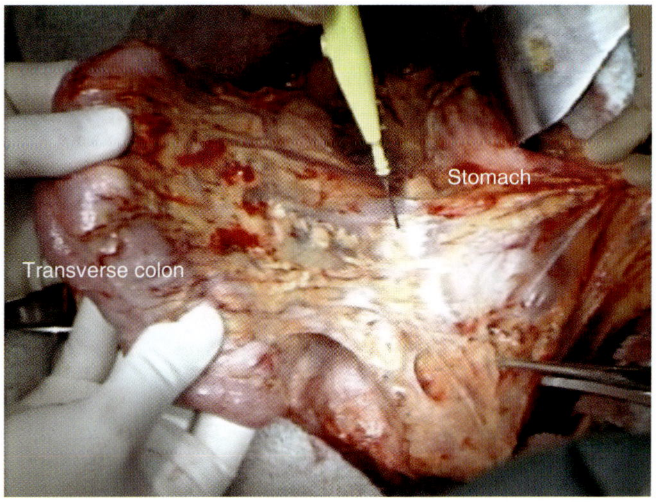

Figure 19-2.

- The right gastroepiploic vein is located at the same level as the posterior surface of the pancreas, which is deeper than the level of the origin of the right gastroepiploic artery (RGEA), arising from the gastroduodenal artery (GDA) on the anterior surface of the pancreas. Ligate and dissect this vein first and then change the layer from behind the pancreas to the surface of the pancreas (Fig. 19-3, *A* and *B*). A few vessels coming from the inferior border of the pancreas to the anterior sheet of the mesocolon should be ligated and divided. The pancreatic capsule at the neck should be dissected toward the duodenum to access the GDA. By following the GDA caudally, the origin of the RGEA is found easily. After division of this artery, the inferior pyloric artery, another branch from the GDA or RGEA, should also be ligated and divided. Before coming up to the lesser curvature, it is recommended to dissect the GDA to the bifurcation of the common hepatic artery.
- The serosa of the hepatoduodenal ligament should be incised to separate the right one third untouched and the left two thirds for nodal dissection (Fig. 19-4). The supraduodenal arteries, which come from the GDA in most cases, should first be ligated and divided on the superior border of the duodenum. This makes a wide window cranial to the duodenum, and the GDA is directly observed (Fig. 19-5). Small branches, often accompanied by nerve fibers, should be ligated along the GDA. Following the GDA cephalad, the origin of the proper hepatic artery (PHA) or the left hepatic artery is easily found. In the majority of cases, the right gastric artery branches off from the PHA, but occasionally from the GDA or from the left hepatic artery. In the last variation, the origin of the left hepatic artery might be mistaken for the right gastric artery. After division of the right gastric artery, the duodenum is transected and closed by a liner stapler.
- The stomach can now be pulled up for good access to the superior border of the pancreas. In the left lateral part of the hepatoduodenal ligament, lymph nodes left to the portal vein are dissected in connection with common hepatic artery (CHA) nodes (Fig. 19-6). In cases where there are no macroscopic metastatic nodes, autonomic nerve fibers surrounding the CHA, splenic artery, left gastric artery (LGA), and celiac artery should be preserved to minimize the functional disturbance to the pancreas, the biliary tract, and the intestines. Especially, the large fiber of the celiac ganglion and its branches can be preserved (Fig. 19-7). When T1 tumors are treated, the celiac branch of the posterior vagal nerve is often preserved, considering the relative low incidence of nodal metastasis in this area.
- The location of the left gastric vein varies. The most common site is to the right of the celiac and behind the CHA, which flow into either the splenic or portal vein (Fig. 19-8). In other cases, it crosses

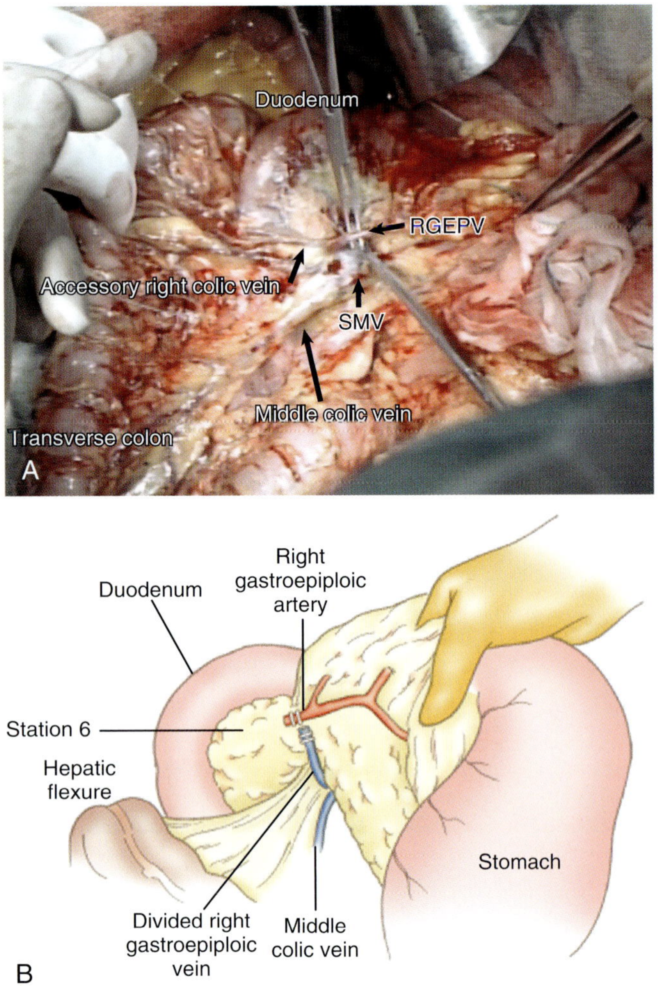

Figure 19-3. *RGEPV*, Right gastroepiploic vein; *SMV*, superior mesenteric vein.

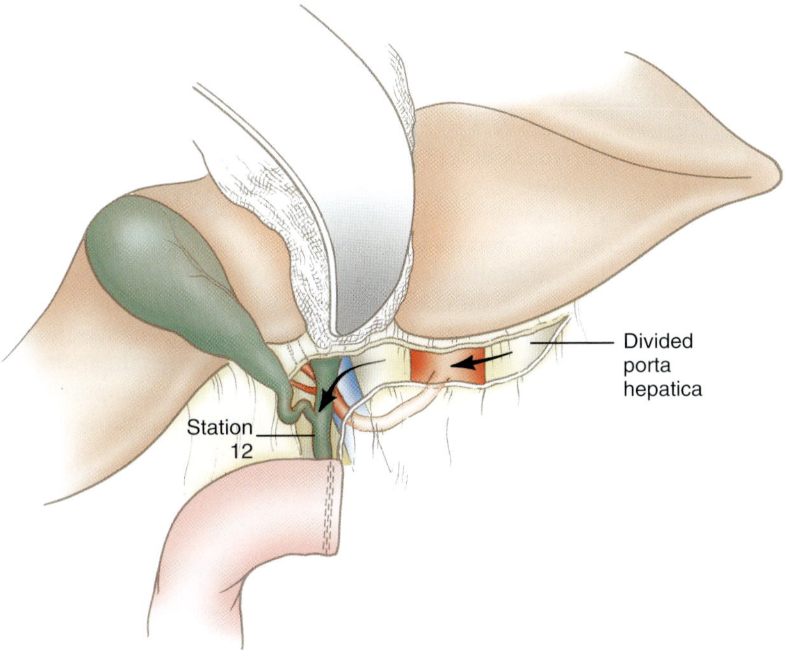

Figure 19-4.

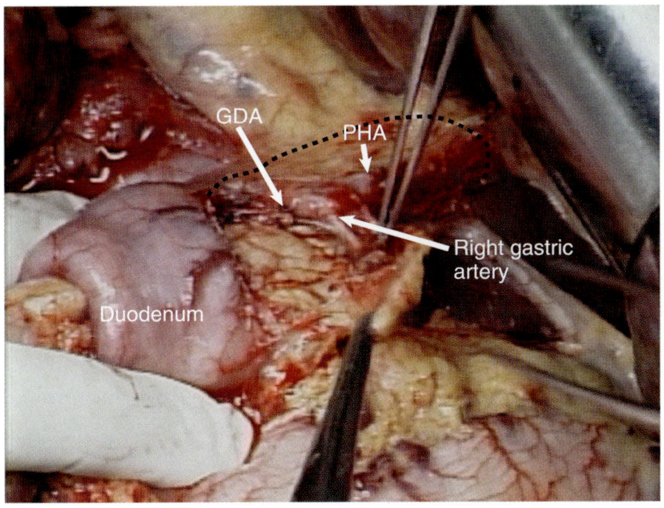

Figure 19-5. *GDA*, Gastroduodenal artery; *PHA*, proper hepatic artery.

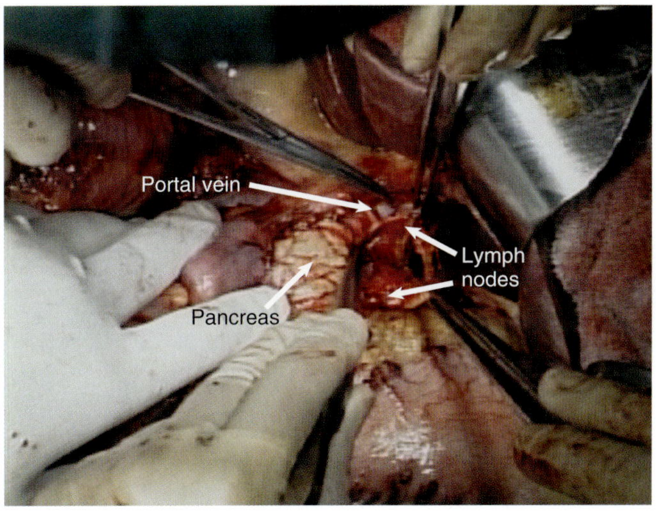

Figure 19-6.

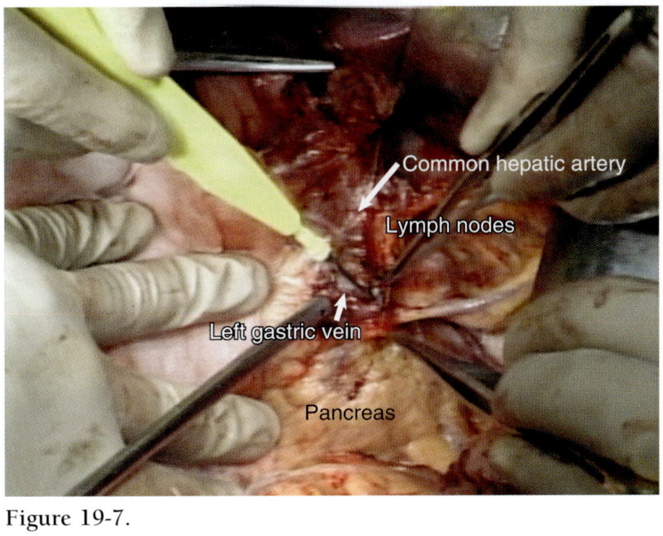

Figure 19-7.

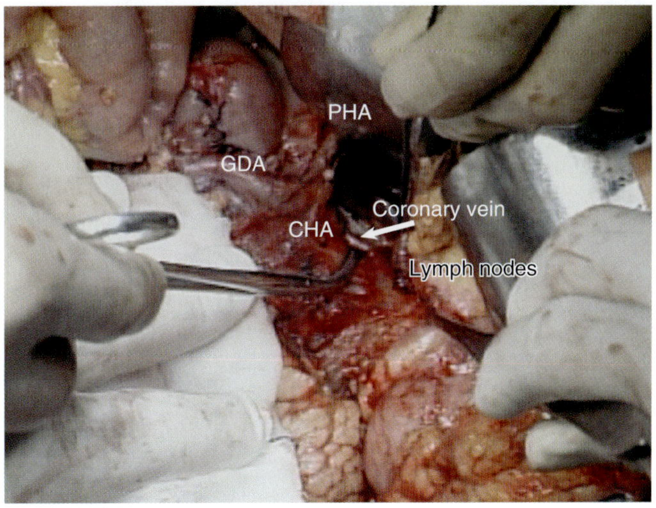

Figure 19-8. *CHA*, Common hepatic artery; *GDA*, gastroduodenal artery; *PHA*, proper hepatic artery.

above the CHA or splenic artery and flows into the splenic vein. The posterior border of the lymph node dissection is the fascia of the crura. After ligation and division of the LGA (Fig. 19-9), dissection on the surface of the right crus should be continued to the left side on the left crus and then on the Gerota fascia. Keeping this layer as the posterior border is essential to carry out the complete nodal dissection along the splenic artery and vein. Returning to the pancreatic surface, dissection of splenic artery should be continued up to about two thirds of the whole length of the splenic artery (Fig. 19-10).

- If the spleen is preserved without mobilizing the organ, dissection of the splenic hilar nodes cannot be complete. For advanced tumors involving the stomach wall near the greater curvature, complete dissection including splenectomy may have benefits that outweigh its disadvantages. Dissection of splenic artery nodes is still possible all along the splenic vessels to the splenic hilum, even preserving the spleen (Fig. 19-11). In this procedure, the posterior gastric artery and vein are encountered in the middle of the splenic vessels in most cases (Fig. 19-12). In some patients, the posterior gastric artery comes from the upper polar artery near the spleen. For such patients, the major branch coming cephalad from the splenic artery should carefully be followed to exclude the possibility of being the upper polar artery. Lymph nodes exist on the anterior side of the artery and on the posterior side of the vessels. During dissection, several vessels between the splenic artery trunk and the pancreatic parenchyma should carefully be preserved. The left gastroepiploic vessels can found near the inferior pole of the spleen at the tip of the pancreatic tail (Fig. 19-13). They are usually the last branches of the splenic vessels. When the splenic artery has already been dissected to the pancreatic tail, the origin of the left gastroepiploic vessels and the short gastric vessels can also be found. They should be ligated and divided as close as possible to their origin.
- In the case of pancreas-preserving total gastrectomy with splenectomy (the Maruyama method), the pancreatic body and tail should be extensively mobilized from the inferior to the superior border of the pancreas on the layer of the fusion fascia and more laterally on the Gerota fascia (Fig. 19-14). The lateral retroperitoneum should be divided at the end of this process from the inferior to the superior pole of the spleen. Dissection of the splenic artery nodes should be carried out in the same way as in the spleen preservation technique until near the splenic hilum. The splenic artery should be preserved at least until the origin of the great pancreatic artery, and if possible, to the origin of the pancreatic tail artery, whereas the splenic vein should be preserved as long as possible to the distal tip of the pancreatic tail to avoid congestion of the tail (Fig. 19-15). When the primary tumor or the metastatic nodes adhere to or invade the pancreas, the organ distal to the involved part should be resected together with the spleen.
- Continuing the incision of the lateral retroperitoneum of the spleen toward the left side of the esophageal hiatus, the cardioesophageal branch from the inferior phrenic vessels should be ligated and divided. The lymph nodes along this branch are regarded as perigastric nodes, often metastatic from the tumor of the cardia.
- The esophagus is dissected from the inner membrane covering the inner surface of the crura of the hiatus. Then the anterior and posterior vagal trunk should be divided at appropriate positions according to the resection line based on the proximal invasion of the tumor. The esophagus is resected and the whole stomach is taken out with or without the spleen (and pancreatic tail for T4).

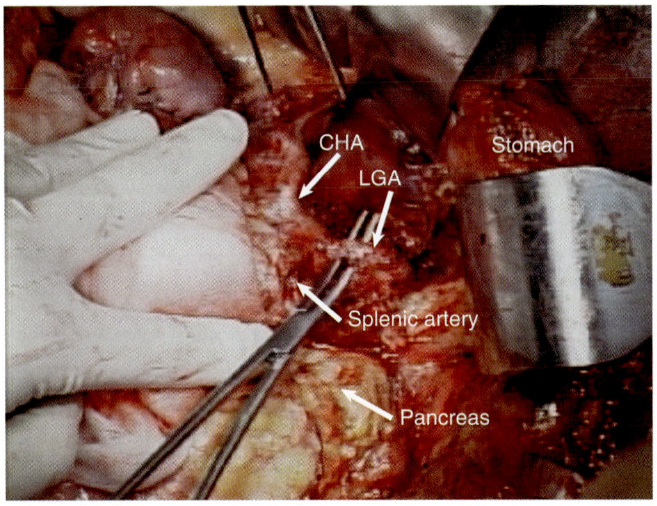

Figure 19-9. *CHA*, Common hepatic artery; *LGA*, left gastric artery.

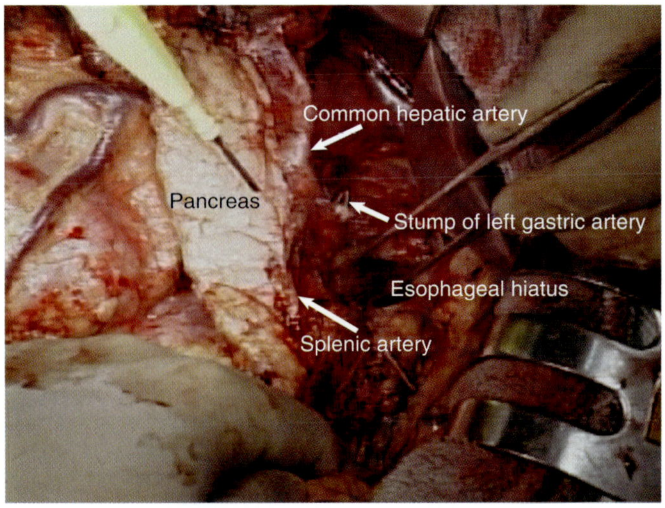

Figure 19-10.

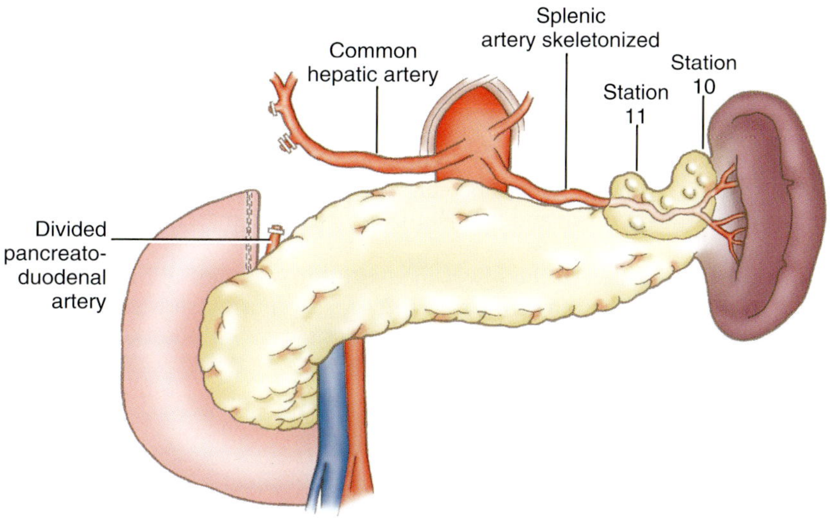

Figure 19-11.

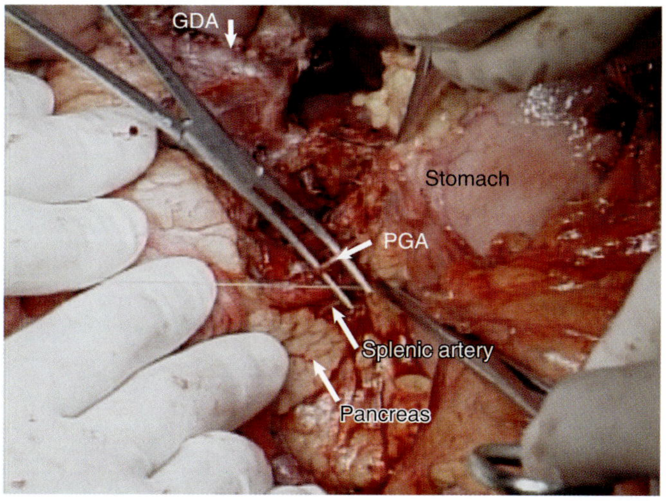

Figure 19-12. *GDA*, Gastroduodenal artery; *PGA*, Posterior gastric artery.

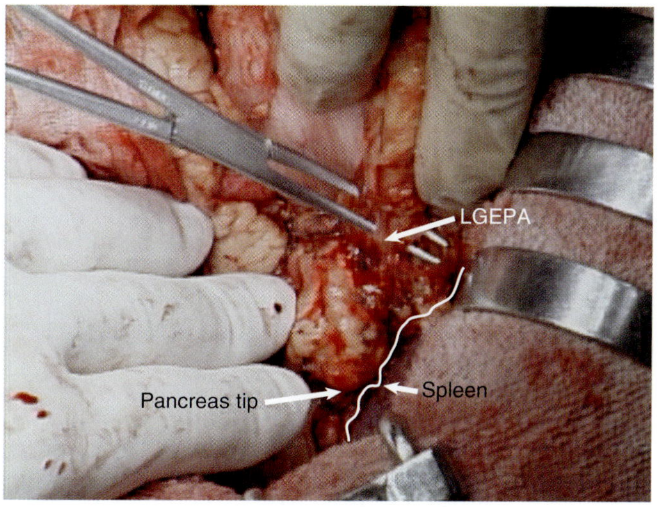

Figure 19-13. *LGEPA*, Left gastroepiploic artery.

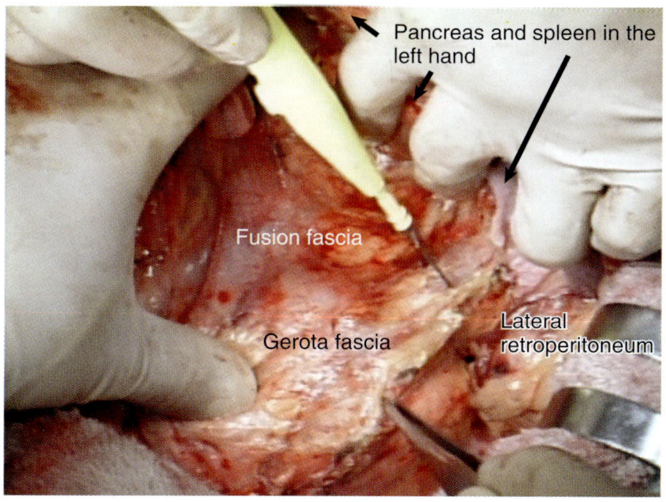

Figure 19-14.

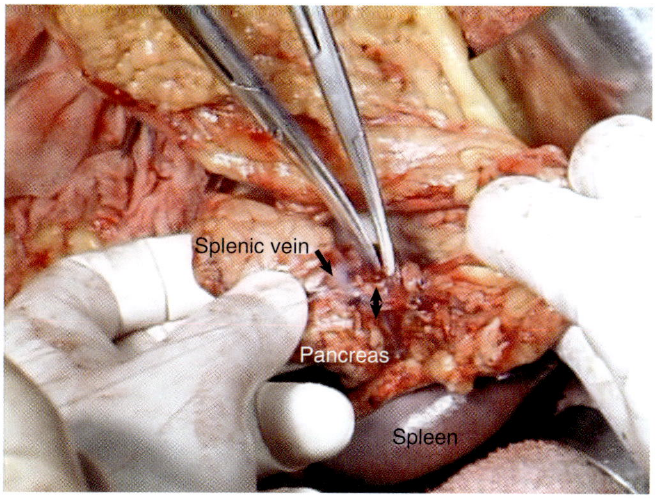

Figure 19-15.

Reconstruction

- The most commonly used reconstruction is still the simple Roux-en-Y method. Principles of safe esophagojejuno anastomosis (EJA) are as follows:
  - ▲ Use a circular stapler.
  - ▲ Make an end-to-side EJA.
  - ▲ Make the jejunal stump as small as 3 to 4 cm.
  - ▲ Bring up the jejunum through the mesocolon (retrocolic).
  - ▲ Make the jejunum straight down and fix it at the orifice of the mesenteric hole at about 10 cm below the EJA.
- In the case of high EJA, located in the lower mediastinum, division of one jejunal artery and vein is recommended to minimize the tension at the EJA. Anastomosis using jejunum is more affected by tension than by blood supply, unlike colonic anastomosis.

Closure

- The midline incision is closed with continuous 1-0 monofilament suture. For a subcostal incision, the muscles of the anterior abdominal wall are closed in layers with 1-0 monofilament suture. Skin is closed with staples,

III. ALTERNATIVE TECHNICAL APPROACHES (PRO/CON) AND PEARLS

- Until recently, there has been a hot discussion between the East and the West regarding optimal lymph node dissection. However, evidence has finally led to the global acceptance of D2 dissection among surgical oncologists.
- In the Dutch and Medical Research Council D1 and D2 trials, splenectomy and distal pancreatectomy was the most often requested procedure in a D2 total gastrectomy in the protocols. Retrospective analyses of these studies proved that the high postoperative mortality and morbidity could be attributed to the combined resection of these organs. Therefore, in the West, if patients need to be treated by total gastrectomy, doing the procedure without distal pancreatectomy or splenectomy is recommended. This suggestion can be applied only when the tumor has no possibility of indiscrete invasion to the gastrosplenic ligament. Even in such cases, it is recommended to ligate and cut the short gastric vessels at their origins. Lymph nodes along the splenic vessels should be dissected at least proximal to the origin of the posterior splenic vessels.
- For T1 tumors that have little possibility of nodal metastasis to the splenic hilum nodes, splenectomy should be avoided.

IV. SPECIAL POSTOPERATIVE CARE

Fluid Balance after Extended Lymphadenectomy

- After D2 total gastrectomy, a large amount of lymphatic fluid flows into the free space, causing remarkable intravascular hypovolemia for a couple of days after surgery. Sufficient fluid should thus be given intravenously for this period, with careful observation of the turning point when fluid starts to flow back suddenly into the vascular space. If this change of fluid balance is overlooked and too much fluid is given, overhydration may result in pulmonary complications.

Most Common Surgical Complications

- The most frequent and serious complication is pancreatic juice leakage, which is usually followed by intraabdominal abscess. The incidence of this complication depends on the method of dissection; 30% to 40% after pancreaticosplenectomy, 15% to 20% after pancreas-preserving total gastrectomy with splenectomy, and 3% to 5% after total gastrectomy preserving both spleen and pancreas. Anastomotic leakage occurs in 2% to 5% of patients with ordinary total gastrectomy and 5% to 8% of patients with mediastinal anastomosis. Duodenal stump leakage may also occasionally be fatal, but incidence is less than 1%.

Treatment of Intraabdominal Infectious Complication

- Intraabdominal abscess should be treated by drainage and irrigation if needed. If the infection is well localized and controlled by drainage, continuous irrigation is not mandatory but often shortens the time healing. Leakage followed by panperitonitis should be treated as in emergency cases of panperitonitis. A large subphrenic abscess with pancreatic leak or necrosis or with anastomotic leakage should be treated with extensive continuous irrigation.

SUGGESTED READINGS

Hundahl SA, Macdonald JS, Benedetti J, et al: Surgical treatment variation in a prospective, randomized trial of chemoradiotherapy in gastric cancer: the effect of undertreatment, *Ann Surg Oncol* 9:278–286, 2002.

National Comprehensive Cancer Network: NCCN clinical practice guidelines in oncology, *Gastric cancer*, version 2.2011. Available at http://www.nccn.org.

Okines A, Verheij M, Allum W, et al: Gastric cancer: ESMO Clinical Practice Guidelines for diagnosis, treatment and follow-up, *Ann Oncol* 21:v50–54, 2010.

Sasako M, Kurokawa Y: Challenges in performing surgical randomized controlled trials in Japan, *Surgery* 145:598–602, 2009.

Sasako M, Sakuramoto S, Katai H, et al: Five-year outcomes of a randomized phase III trial comparing adjuvant chemotherapy with S-1 versus surgery alone in stage II or III gastric cancer, *J Clin Oncol* 29: 387–4393, 2011.

Songun I, Putter H, Kranenbarg EM, et al: Surgical treatment of gastric cancer: 15-year follow-up results of the randomized nationwide Dutch D1D2 trial, *Lancet Oncol* 11:439–449, 2010.

CHAPTER 20

Laparoscopy-Assisted Distal Gastrectomy with Lymphadenectomy

Seigo Kitano, MD, PhD, FACS, and Norio Shiraishi, MD, PhD

I. SPECIAL PREOPERATIVE PREPARATION

Indications

- The indications for laparoscopy-assisted distal gastrectomy (LADG) are early gastric cancer (EGC) with risk of lymph node metastasis located in the distal two thirds of the stomach, an area that is not indicated for endoscopic treatment, and advanced gastric cancer (AGC) without serosal exposure (T2N0, T2N1).
- The Japanese Gastric Cancer Association guidelines define EGC with risk of lymph node metastasis as follows:
  1. Well-differentiated mucosal cancer of more than 2.0 cm in diameter
  2. Well-differentiated mucosal cancer with ulceration
  3. Poorly differentiated mucosal cancer
  4. Submucosal cancer
- Because the effect of CO_2 pneumoperitoneum and laparoscopic procedures on dissemination of cancer cells from the serosal surface of the stomach is not clear, the indications for treatment of AGC by LADG are limited.

Preoperative Evaluation

- Histologic type, size, and depth of wall invasion of the cancer are evaluated by endoscopic examination (Fig. 20-1, *A* and *B*) and barium meal study.
- Preoperative cancer staging (Table 20-1) is determined on the basis of abdominal ultrasonography and computed tomography imaging examinations.
- These examinations provide valuable information on lymph node metastasis (Fig. 20-2), hematogenous metastasis such as liver and lung metastasis, and peritoneal dissemination.
- Three types of laparoscopic lymph node dissections are performed in LADG: perigastric lymph node dissection (D1+α) only, additional lymph node dissection along the common hepatic artery (D1+β), and extended lymph node dissection (D2).
- The benefit to survival following D2 lymph node dissection is still controversial. In Japan, to completely control the local cancer, the type of lymph node dissection to be performed is determined on the basis of preoperative clinical cancer staging.
- D1+β lymph node dissection is the most commonly performed type during LADG. LADG with D2 lymph node dissection is performed only by surgeons with advanced skills and only in a limited number of departments.
- General preoperative evaluation of the patient is carried out as it is for open gastrectomy.
- LADG should be performed carefully in obese patients (BMI>30) because of the high rate of operative complications.

II. OPERATIVE TECHNIQUE

- Herein the techniques of LADG with D1+β lymph node dissection are introduced.

Position

- The patient is placed supine in the 20-degree reverse Trendelenburg position with the legs spread (Fig. 20-3).
- The surgeon stands between the patient's abducted legs. The laparoscopist is at the patient's right side, and the technical assistant is at the patient's left side.
- The laparoscopic monitor is positioned at the left side of the patient's head.

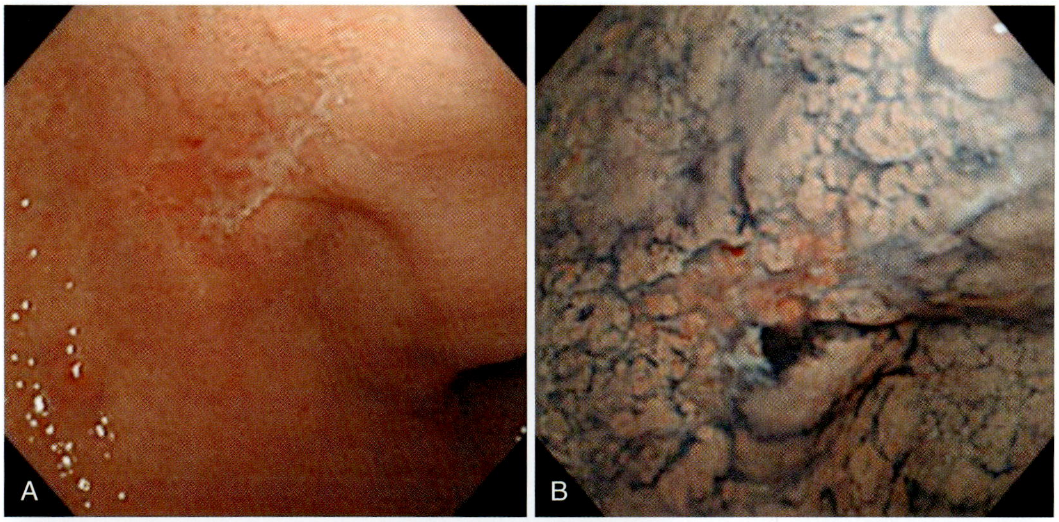

Figure 20-1. Endoscopic examination of histologic type, size, and depth of wall invasion of the cancer.

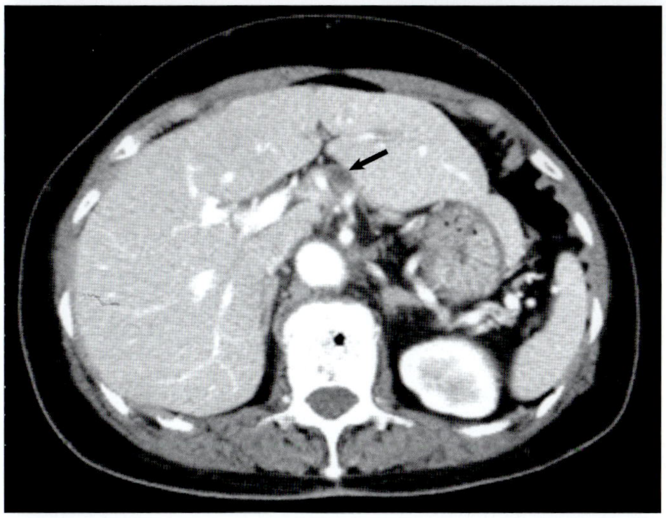

Figure 20-2. Computed tomography (CT) imaging examination for lymph node metastasis, hematogenous metastasis, and peritoneal dissemination.

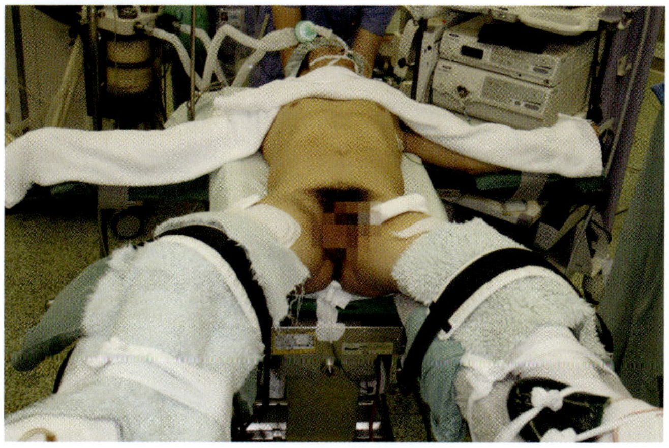

Figure 20-3.

TABLE 20-1 Gastric Cancer Staging

	N0	N1	N2	N3	P0H1 N2~
T1 (M · SM)	Ia	Ib	II	IIIa	IVa
T2 (MP · SS)	Ib	II	IIIa	IIIb	
T3 (SE)	II	IIIa	IIIb	IVa	
T4 (SI)	IIIa	IIIb	IVa	IVb	
P0H1 T3~	IVa				

From Japanese Gastric Cancer Association: Japanese classification of gastric carcinoma, ed 2, *Gastric Cancer* 1:10–24, 1998.
H, Hematogenous metastasis; *N0-N3,* lymph node metastasis; *P,* peritoneal dissemination; *T1-4,* cancer depth.

Trocar Placement

- A Hasson-type trocar is inserted in the subumbilical position using open techniques (Fig. 20-4).
- After a CO_2 pneumoperitoneum of 10 mm Hg is created and the laparoscope is inserted into the abdominal cavity, the liver, peritoneal surfaces, and stomach are carefully observed.
- Thereafter, four trocars are inserted into the upper abdomen (Fig. 20-5, *A* and *B*).

Main Dissection

Laparoscopic Procedures

The Greater Curvature Area

- The greater omentum and gastrocolic ligamentum are stretched by lifting the stomach with assistant's grasping forceps, and they are opened using laparoscopic coagulation shears (LCS) (Fig. 20-6). The greater omentum and gastrocolic ligamentum are then divided about 3 to 5 cm from the gastroepiploic arcade toward the spleen (Fig. 20-7).
- Dissection of the gastrosplenic ligamentum at the lower end of the spleen enables exposure of the left gastroepiploic vessels (Fig. 20-8). After clipping, these vessels are cut with the LCS.
- The no. 4sb lymph nodes are dissected, and then the greater omentum and gastrocolic ligamentum are dissected distally toward the infrapyloric area.

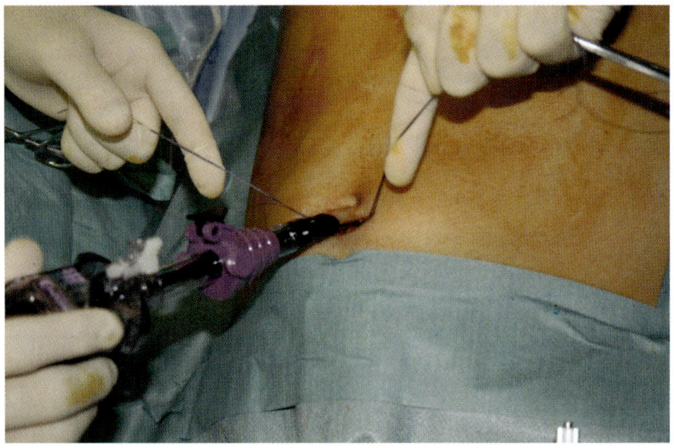

Figure 20-4.

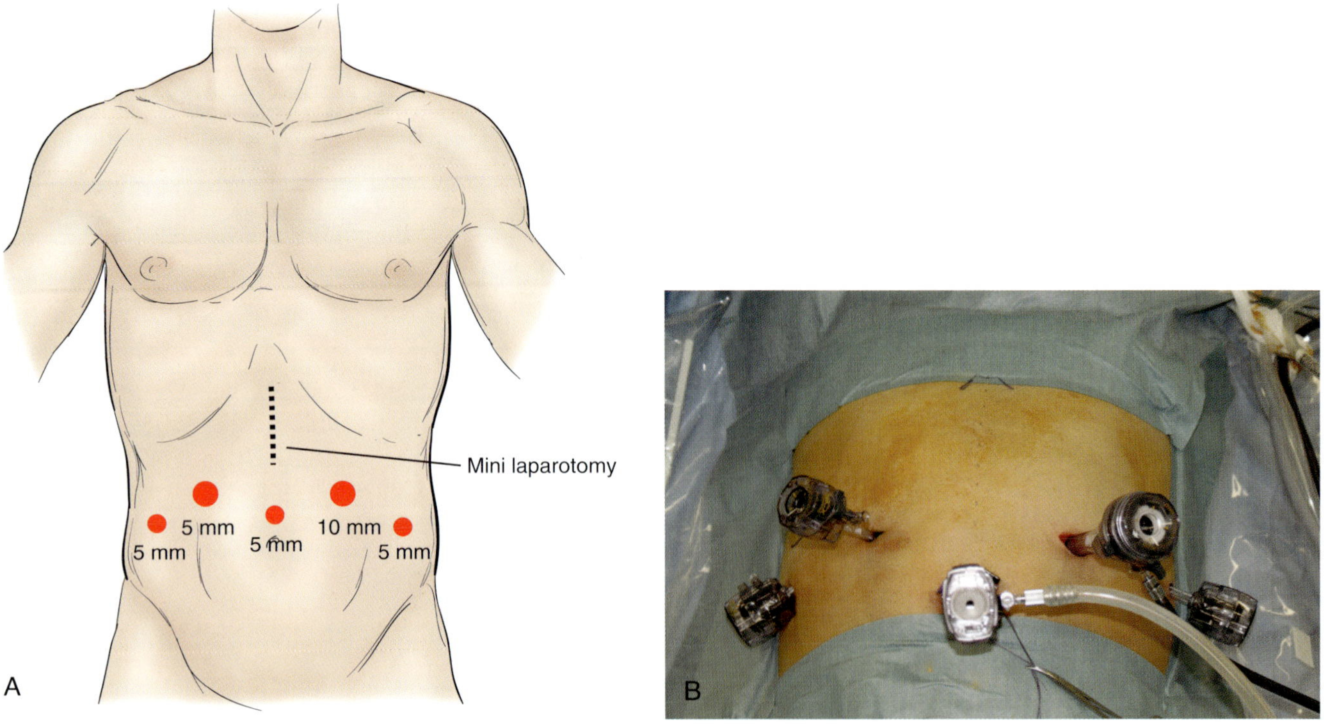

Figure 20-5.

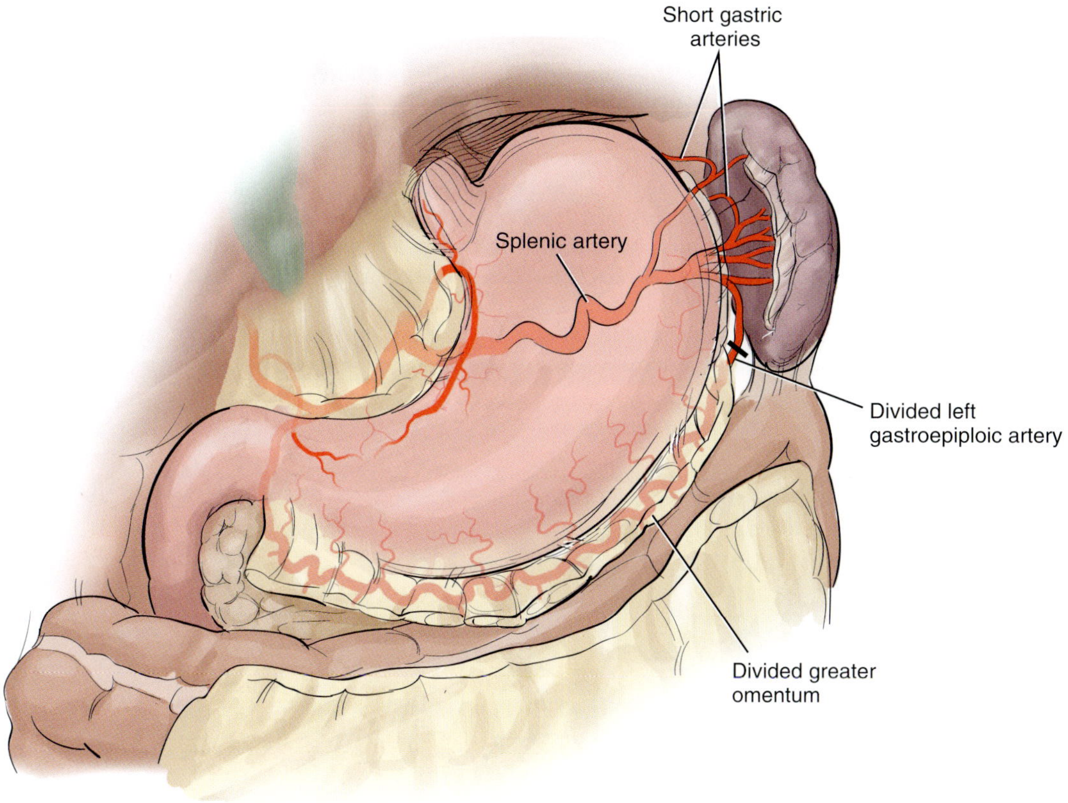

Figure 20-6.

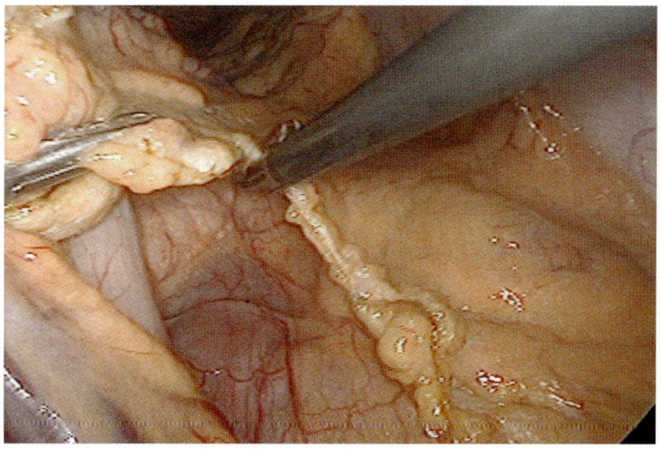

Figure 20-7.

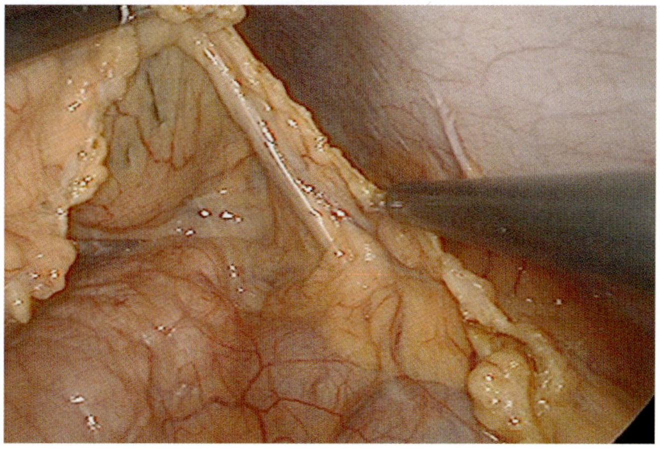

Figure 20-8.

- After dissecting the greater omentum and gastrocolic ligamentum in the infrapyloric area layer by layer, the inferior plate of the pancreatic head is exposed to identify the root of the gastroepiploic vein. This vein is clipped and divided (infrapyloric lymph node [no. 6] dissection) (Fig. 20-9).
- The gastroduodenal artery is located on the anterior surface of the pancreas, and the root of the right gastric artery can then be easily identified. The right gastric artery is clipped and divided, and then the branches of the infraduodenal artery are divided with the LCS.

The Lesser Curvature Area

- After the liver is lifted using a snake-type retractor, the lesser omentum is opened and divided toward the esophagocardial junction (Fig. 20-10). The lesser omentum is then divided toward the hepatoduodenal ligamentum.
- The right gastric artery is lifted with the assistant's grasping forceps, and a hole is made in the upper area above the bulbus of the duodenum.

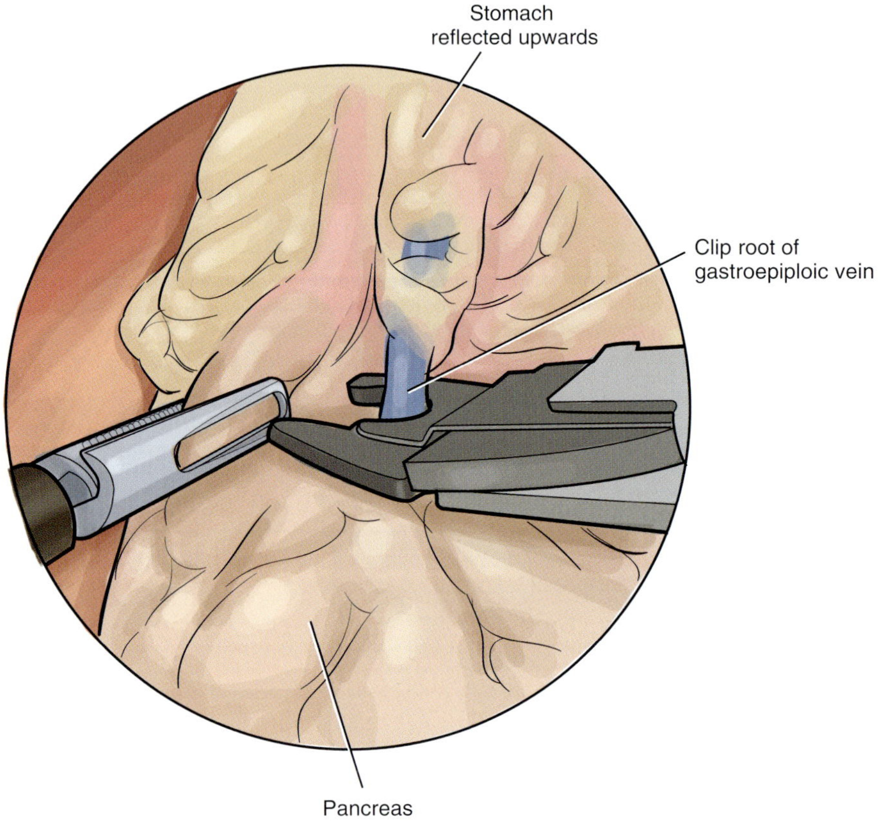

Figure 20-9.

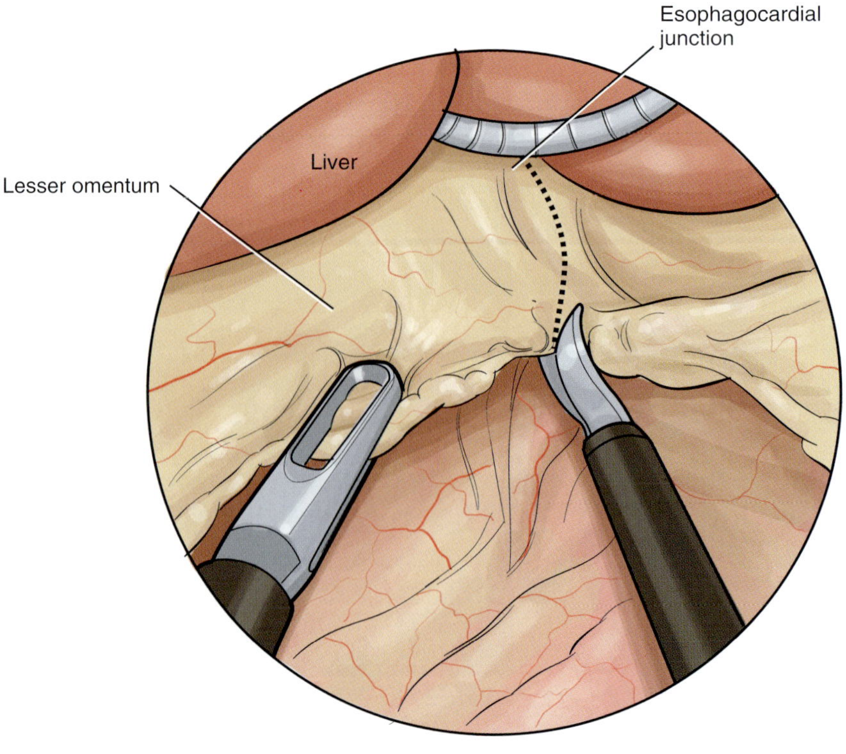

Figure 20-10.

- After transection of the duodenum with a laparoscopic linear cutter, lifting the stump of the stomach enables the root of the right gastric artery to be identified. The right gastric artery is divided, allowing the dissection of the suprapyloric lymph nodes (no. 5) (Fig. 20-11).
- The gastropancreatic ligament is stretched to identify the root of the left gastric artery, and the peritoneum on the right crux of the diaphragm is opened.
- The lymph nodes along the left gastric artery and the celiac artery are dissected, and the left gastric artery is clipped and divided (see Fig. 20-11).
- The peritoneum along the upper side of the pancreas is opened from the hepatoduodenal ligamentum to the root of the left gastric artery, and the left gastric vein is then easily exposed. After clipping and dividing the left gastric vein, the lymph nodes along the common hepatic artery are dissected (Fig. 20-12).

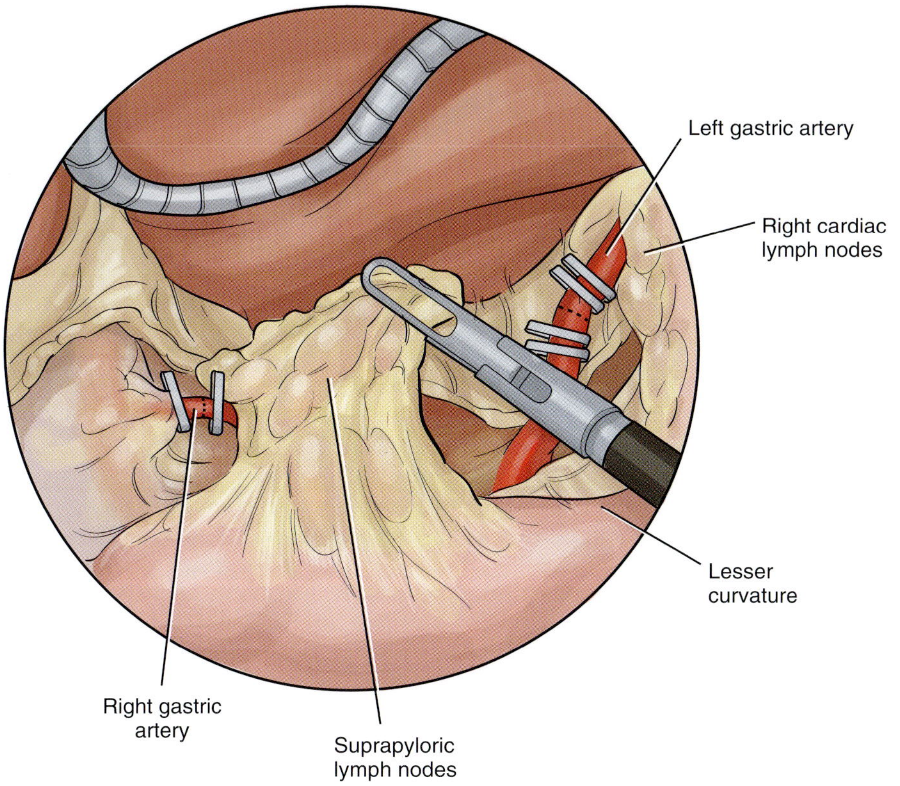

Figure 20-11.

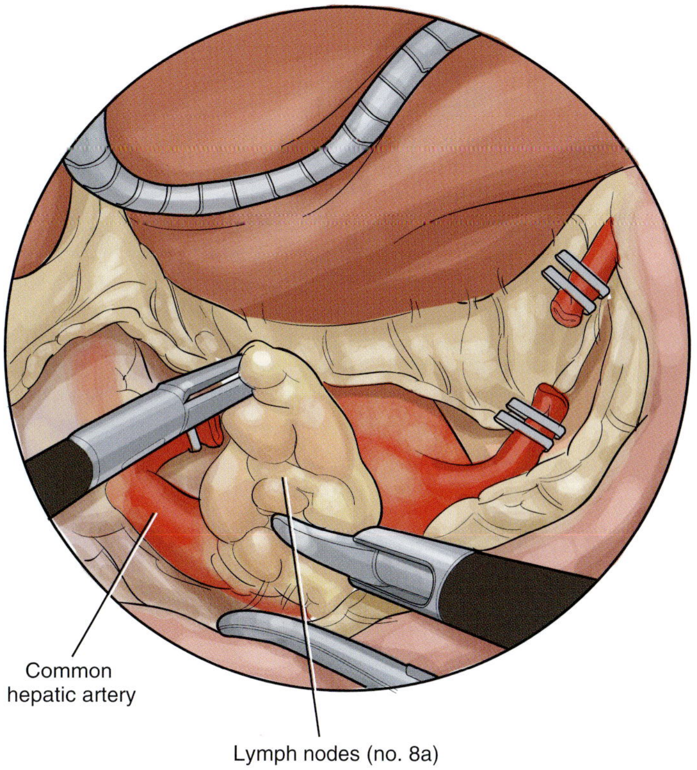

Figure 20-12.

- The right cardiac and superior lymph nodes along the lesser curvature (nos. 1 and 3) are dissected. During dissection of these lymph nodes, the vagal nerves are divided.

Procedures Performed through Mini Laparotomy

- After mobilization of the distal stomach with laparoscopic techniques, a 5-cm mini laparotomy is performed in the upper abdomen 2 cm lateral to the left of midline. The laparotomy wound is protected and opened with a wound-sealing device.
- The distal stomach is exteriorized through the mini laparotomy, and distal gastrectomy is carried out using open techniques (Fig. 20-13).
- Reconstruction after gastrectomy is performed by the Roux-en-Y method.
- After the pneumoperitoneum is recreated, the ligament of Treitz is located. The jejunum is marked at a point 30 cm distal to the ligament of Treitz and pulled out through the mini laparotomy.
- Gastrojejunostomy and jejunojejunostomy are performed through the mini laparotomy with a functional end-to-end anastomotic method using a linear cutter. These methods of reconstruction used in LADG are the same as those used in open gastrectomy.

Closure

- After the anastomosis is carried out, the pneumoperitoneum is recreated. Hemostasis and lavage of the abdominal cavity are performed, and then a closed drain is placed.
- The mini laparotomy and trocar wounds are closed (Fig. 20-14).

III. ALTERNATIVE TECHNICAL APPROACHES (PRO/CON) AND PEARLS

- With the development of laparoscopic shears, division of vessels can be carried out safely. Combined use of ultrasonic coagulation shears and the vessel sealing system are especially helpful in LADG.
- During dissection of organs with the ultrasonic coagulation shears, mist can disturb the laparoscopic operative field. Thus, use of ultrasonic coagulation shears with an auto-exhaust system is recommended.
- To improve patient postoperative quality of life, laparoscopic pylorus-preserving gastrectomy and laparoscopic vagus-nerve–preserving gastrectomy have been developed.
- Proximal gastrectomy and total gastrectomy have also been attempted laparoscopically for the treatment of proximal EGC and AGC.

IV. SPECIAL POSTOPERATIVE CARE

- LADG is less invasive than open distal gastrectomy (ODG) and offers several advantages over ODG, including earlier patient recovery, earlier recovery of intestinal movement, less pain, and a shorter hospital stay.
- The ninth national survey conducted by the JSES showed the incidences of intraoperative and postoperative complications associated with LADG to be 1.3% and 8.2%, respectively. The incidence appears to be similar to that with ODG.
- Laparoscopic surgeons have developed advanced techniques as their learning curves have improved, resulting in a decrease in the incidence of operative complications.
- The most common intraoperative complications of LADG are bleeding and injury to other organs. The most common bleeding sites are located in the upper area of the stomach. Injuries to the spleen and pancreas occur during dissection of the left and right gastroepiploic vessels.
- Common postoperative complications include wound infection, pancreatic injury, and anastomotic problems such as stenosis and leakage.
- There are few reports on the long-term outcome after LADG. Although patient long-term quality of life after LADG is the same as that after ODG, the incidence of adhesive ileus is lower with LADG than with ODG.

SUGGESTED READINGS

Hoshino S, Arimoto Y, Ohtani H, et al: Meta-analysis of short-term outcomes after laparoscopy-assisted distal gastrectomy, *World J Gastroenterol* 12:7676–7683, 2006.

Kitano S, Iso Y, Moriyama M, et al: Laparoscopy-assisted Billroth I gastrectomy, *Surg Laparosc Endosc* 4:146–148, 1994.

Kitano S, Shiraishi N, Uyama I, et al: A multicenter study on oncologic outcome of laparoscopic gastrectomy for early cancer in Japan, *Ann Surg* 245:68–72, 2007.

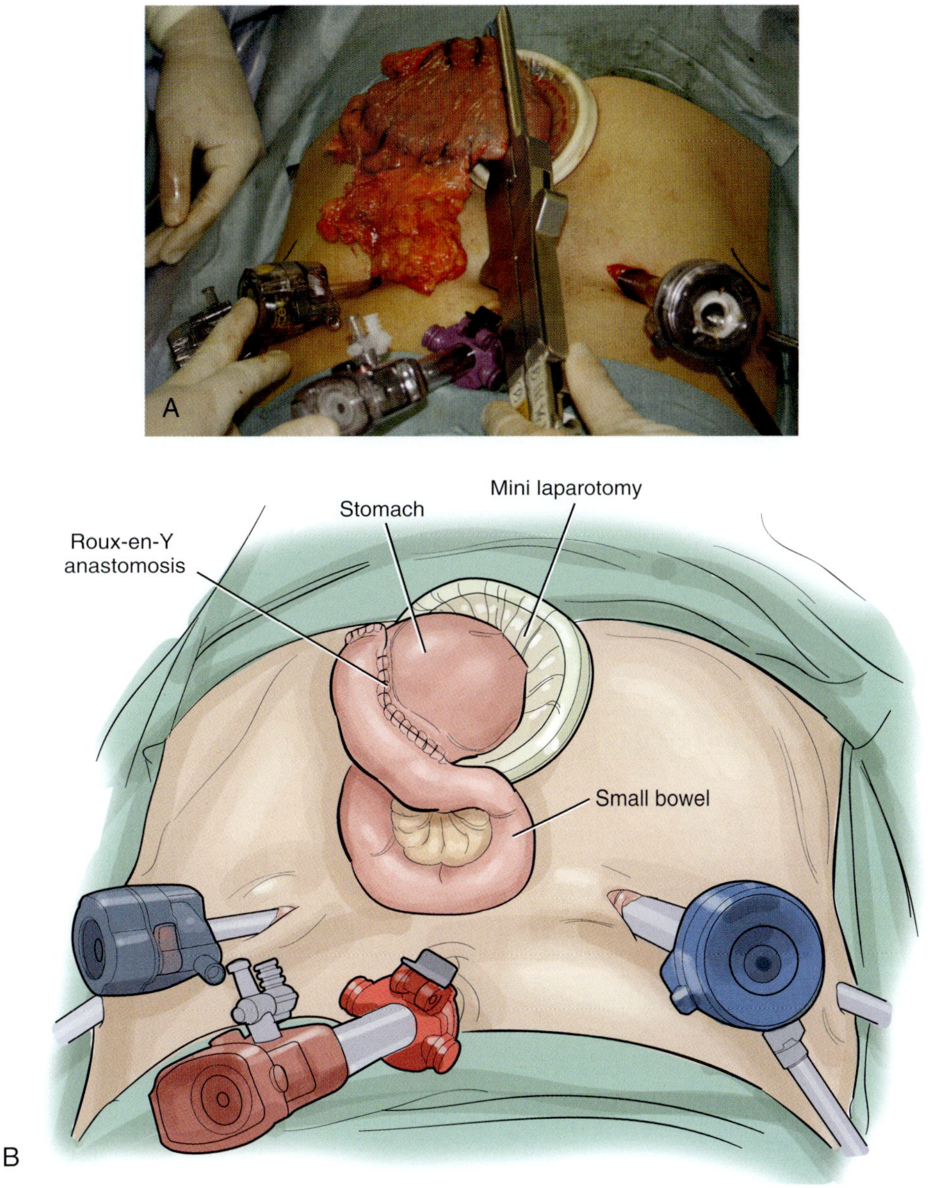

Figure 20-13.

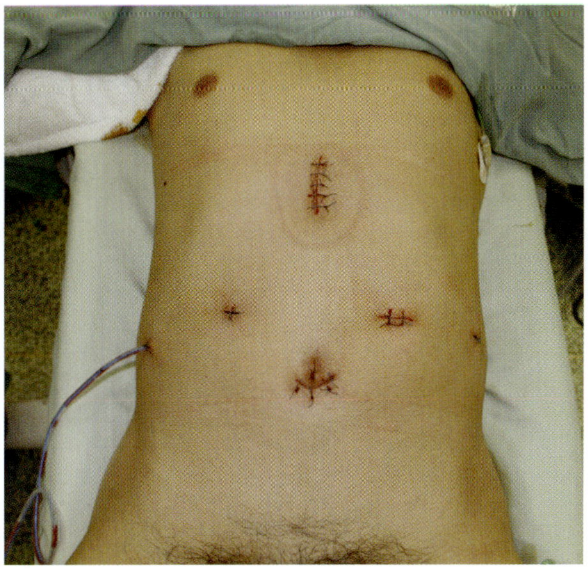

Figure 20-14.

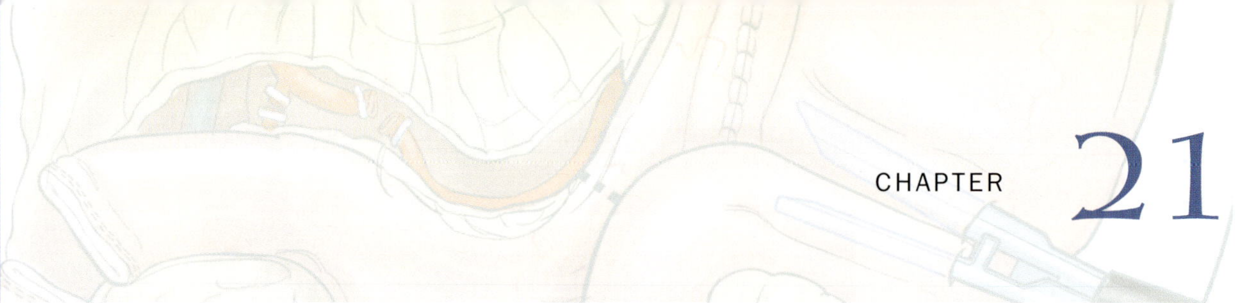

CHAPTER 21

Laparoscopic Vagotomy and Seromyotomy with Antrectomy

Namir Katkhouda, MD, FACS

I. SPECIAL PREOPERATIVE PREPARATION

- Eradication of *Helicobacter pylori* is very effective in treating patients with peptic ulcer disease. Despite medical control, complications can arise such as obstruction or intractability. Acid suppression surgery is reserved for this population. Acute complications such as perforation or hemorrhage are managed emergently, usually without an acid-suppressive procedure.
- Endoscopic examination of the upper intestinal tract is necessary to diagnose and follow peptic ulcer disease. Biopsy of the ulcer should be taken to examine for malignancy and for presence of *Helicobacter pylori*.

II. OPERATIVE TECHNIQUE

Position

- A low lithotomy position is used, with the surgeon standing in the middle and assistants on the sides of the patient.

Incision

- See Figure 21-1.
- The first trocar for a 30-degree scope and high-definition camera (Karl-Storz) is inserted above the umbilicus.
- A 5-mm subxiphoid trocar is placed for liver retraction.
- Additional 5-mm trocars are inserted in the midclavicular line two finger breadths beneath the left and right subcostal margin.
- The last trocar, a 10- to 12-mm operating port, is inserted 6 cm to the left of the umbilicus.

Main Dissection

- The operation begins by dissecting the avascular portion of the lesser omentum to enter the lesser sac. The right crus is identified, and the esophagus is dissected away from it.
- The right posterior vagus nerve is identified as a thick white filament that can be easily freed from the esophageal wall. The nerve is excised between two clips and passed off for pathologic examination.
- A trucal vagotomy is performed but another alternative is one described by Taylor known as the anterior seromyotomy. Anterior lesser curvature seromyotomy begins at the cardiac incision and is extended in a curved fashion 1.5 cm away from the lesser curvature (see Fig. 21-1). Seromyotomy should be extended to 6 cm from the pylorus. Seromyotomy is performed using the hook with electrocautery or harmonic shears. Mucosa should be checked for perforation using methylene blue dye.

- For obstructive ulcer disease, antrectomy and Billroth II gastrojejunostomy is then performed with a primary hand-sewn anastomosis. It is also possible to perform the anastomosis using staplers.
- For the antrectomy and Billroth II gastrojejunostomy, the following steps are followed:
  1. Mobilization of the greater curvature to the level of the desired antrectomy, outside the gastroepiploic arcade using the harmonic shears (Fig. 21-2).

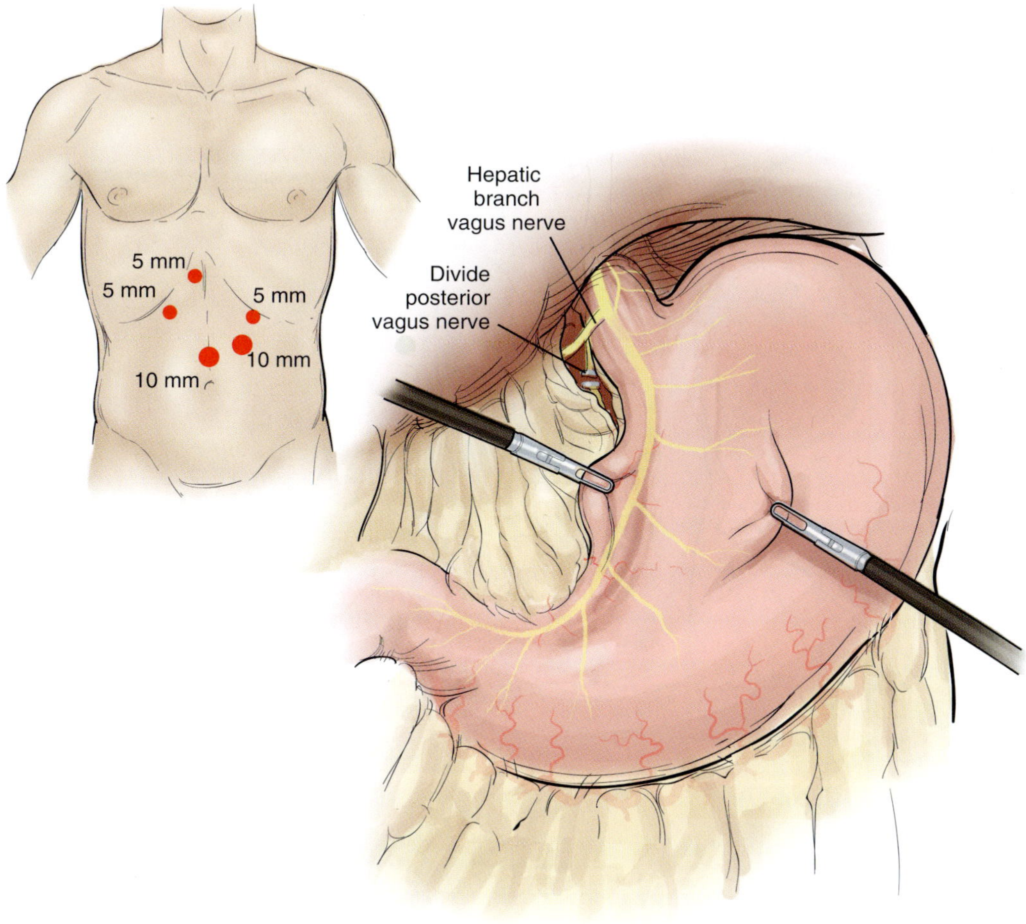

Figure 21-1.

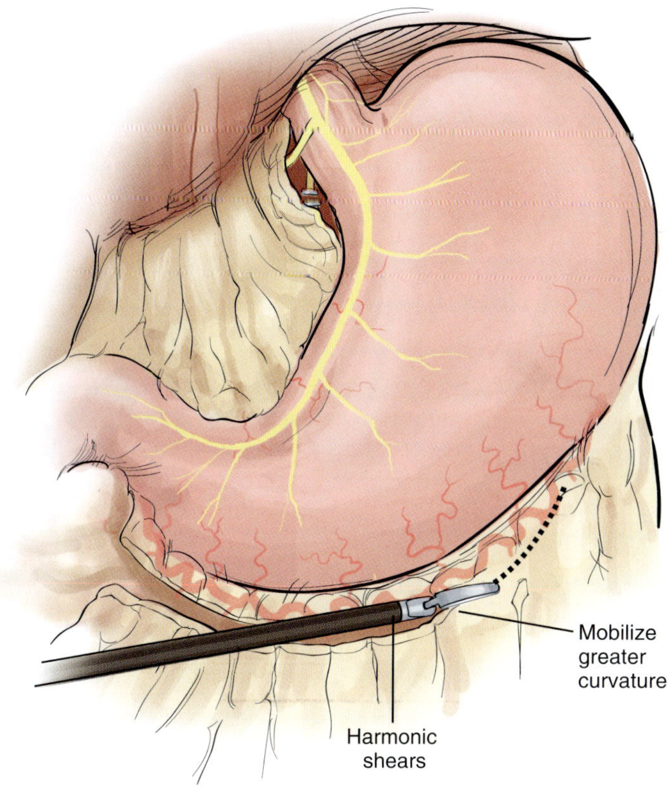

Figure 21-2.

2. Mobilization of the lesser curvature with the ligation of the right gastric artery (Fig. 21-3).
3. Division of the duodenum distal to the ulcer inflammation and proximal to the hepatic portal using a linear stapler (Fig. 21-4). At this point two options for reconstruction are possible: extracorporeal anastomosis by delivering the specimen through an extended 10-mm incision (Fig. 21-5), and intracorporeal anastomosis (Fig. 21-6).

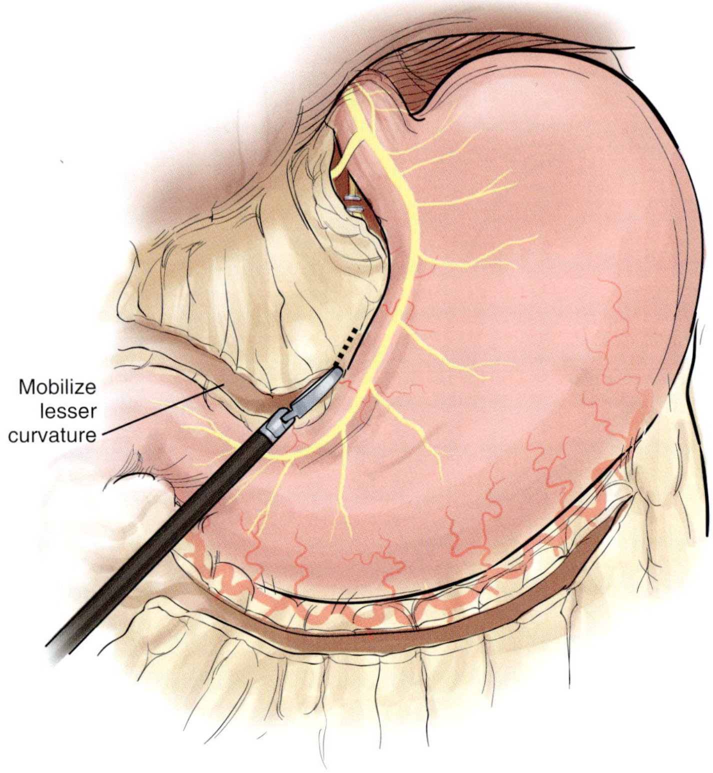

Figure 21-3.

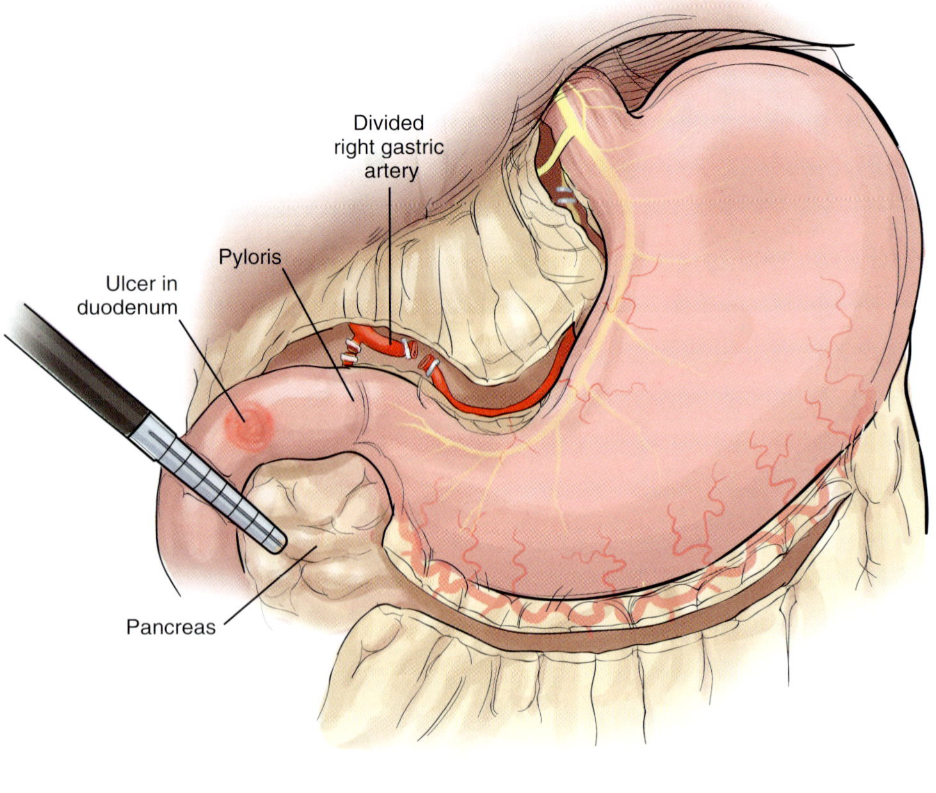

Figure 21-4.

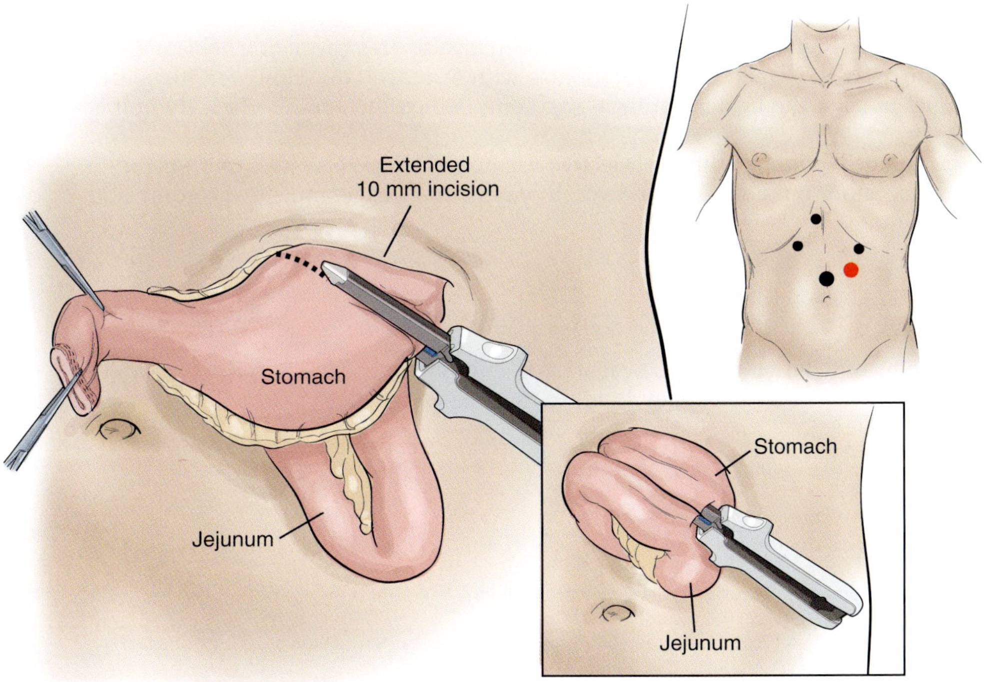

Figure 21-5.

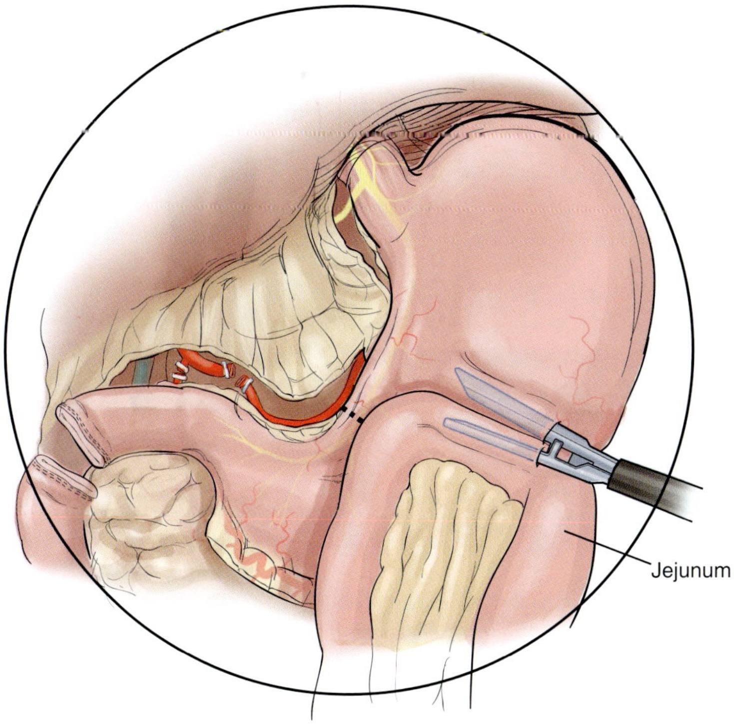

Figure 21-6.

Closure

- Use of the Optiview trocar (Ethicon Endo-Surgery, Cincinnati) alleviates the need to close the port incisions. The only part that needs closure is the incision used for extracorporeal anastomosis and/or the delivery of the specimen.

III. ALTERNATIVE TECHNICAL APPROACHES (PRO/CON) AND PEARLS

- Bilateral truncal vagotomy with drainage procedure is an alternative to this procedure. It is a faster operation and does not carry a risk of mucosal perforation as with seromyotomy. However, it exposes the patient to the complications of the bilateral truncal vagotomy, which include diarrhea, dumping, and gastroparesis.
- The other alternative technique would be a highly selective vagotomy. This is also an easier operation and has the benefit of being more physiologic. However, there is a risk of incomplete vagotomy and therefore higher recurrence rate.

IV. SPECIAL POSTOPERATIVE CARE

- Known risks of seromyotomy and antrectomy are bezoars and dumping.
- Endoscopic surveillance is warranted to detect any long-term malignant changes.

SUGGESTED READINGS

Katkhouda N, Mouiel J: A new technique of surgical treatment of chronic duodenal ulcer without laparotomy by videocoelioscopy, *Am J Surg* 161:361–364, 1991.

Shapiro S, Gordon L, Dayhkovsky L, et al: Development of laparoscopic anterior seromyotomy and right posterior truncal vagotomy for ulcer prophylaxis, *J Laparoendosc Surg* 1:277–286, 1991.

Zanchi P, Schlumph R, Aras N, et al: Laparoscopic anterior extended seromyotomy with posterior truncal vagotomy: an experimental study, *Surg Laparosc Endosc* 7:42–46, 1997.

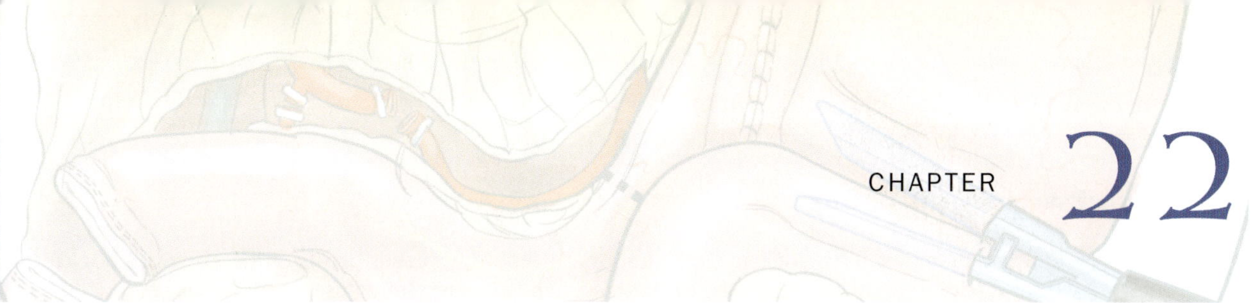

CHAPTER 22

Laparoscopic Roux-en-Y Gastric Bypass Surgery

Mohamed Ali, MD, and Henry Buchwald, MD, PhD

I. SPECIAL PREOPERATIVE PREPARATION

Physiologic Testing

Cardiac Evaluation

- Consider in patients with metabolic syndrome, high body mass index (greater than 50 kg/m^2), symptoms of cardiovascular disease, age greater than 50 years, and immobility.

Pulmonary Evaluation

- Patients should be screened for obstructive sleep apnea (OSA) syndrome by symptom inventory and confirmed by sleep study, if OSA is severe.
- Patients with OSA should receive constant positive airway pressure therapy and use it in the perioperative period.
- Arterial blood gas evaluation on room air should be considered in patients with severe OSA to obtain a preoperative baseline and to evaluate for obesity-hypoventilation syndrome.
- Patients with significant severe obesity-hypoventilation syndrome (hypoxia and hypercarbia) should be evaluated for pulmonary hypertension and right heart failure by echocardiography and/or right heart catheterization.
- Asthma is common in morbid obesity, and severe asthma may be considered for pulmonary function testing.

Gastrointestinal Evaluation

- Esophagogastroduodenoscopy should be considered in all patients with history of significant gastroesophageal reflux, chronic nonsteroidal antiinflammatory drug use, or peptic ulcer disease.
- Gastric emptying should be evaluated in patients with history of delayed gastric emptying or symptoms (e.g., bloating).
- All patients should be screened by history and symptoms for irritable bowel syndrome, as symptoms can worsen following surgery and can counteract certain bariatric procedures.

Cancer Surveillance

- Breast cancer, colon cancer, prostate cancer, and endometrial cancer can occur more frequently in obese patients.
- Screening for these malignancies (or record of it) should be a part of the preoperative evaluation.

Coagulation Evaluation

- Obese individuals are at higher risk for venous thromboembolic events (VTE) (i.e., deep vein thrombosis, pulmonary embolism).
- History of VTE should be elicited and carefully evaluated.
- A preoperative vena cava filter can be considered in high-risk patients.

Psychological Testing

- All patients considered for bariatric surgery are generally prescribed to undergo psychological evaluation to identify psychopathology, eating disorders, coping strategies, or addictive personality traits.

Nutritional Preparation

- Education in proper nutrition (e.g., caloric intake, reading food labels) should be completed before surgery.
- Patients should be educated regarding the nutritional deficiencies that can follow gastric bypass.
  - Micronutrients such as calcium (due to bypass of duodenum and change in enterohepatic circulation), iron (bypass of the duodenum), vitamin B_{12} (decreased intrinsic factor), other B vitamins, vitamin D, and vitamin C need to be supplemented after surgery.
  - Patients should be evaluated for deficiency before surgery and appropriately supplemented.
  - Patients should be educated about the signs and symptoms of these deficiencies.
- Patients should be educated about post–gastric bypass nutrition.
  - Restriction of oral intake predisposes patients to malnutrition, protein deficiency, and dehydration.
  - The early caloric goal is 600 to 800 kcal/day.
  - Long-term, patients should consume 1000 to 1200 kcal/day.
  - Patients should understand calorie counting, protein calculations, and the importance of hydration.

II. OPERATIVE TECHNIQUE

Position

- The patient should be secured to the operating table to accommodate for position changes, especially reverse Trendelenburg (Fig. 22-1).
- Upper extremities, lower extremities, and back should be carefully positioned and padded to prevent nerve injury and crush muscle injury.

Trocar Placement

- Five to six ports are typically used for laparoscopic Roux-en-Y gastric bypass surgery (LRYGB). The surgeon is positioned on the patient's right (see Fig. 22-1).

Main Dissection

Creation of Alimentary (Roux) Limb

- The transverse mesocolon is identified and opened anteriorly and to the left of the ligament of Treitz (Fig. 22-2).

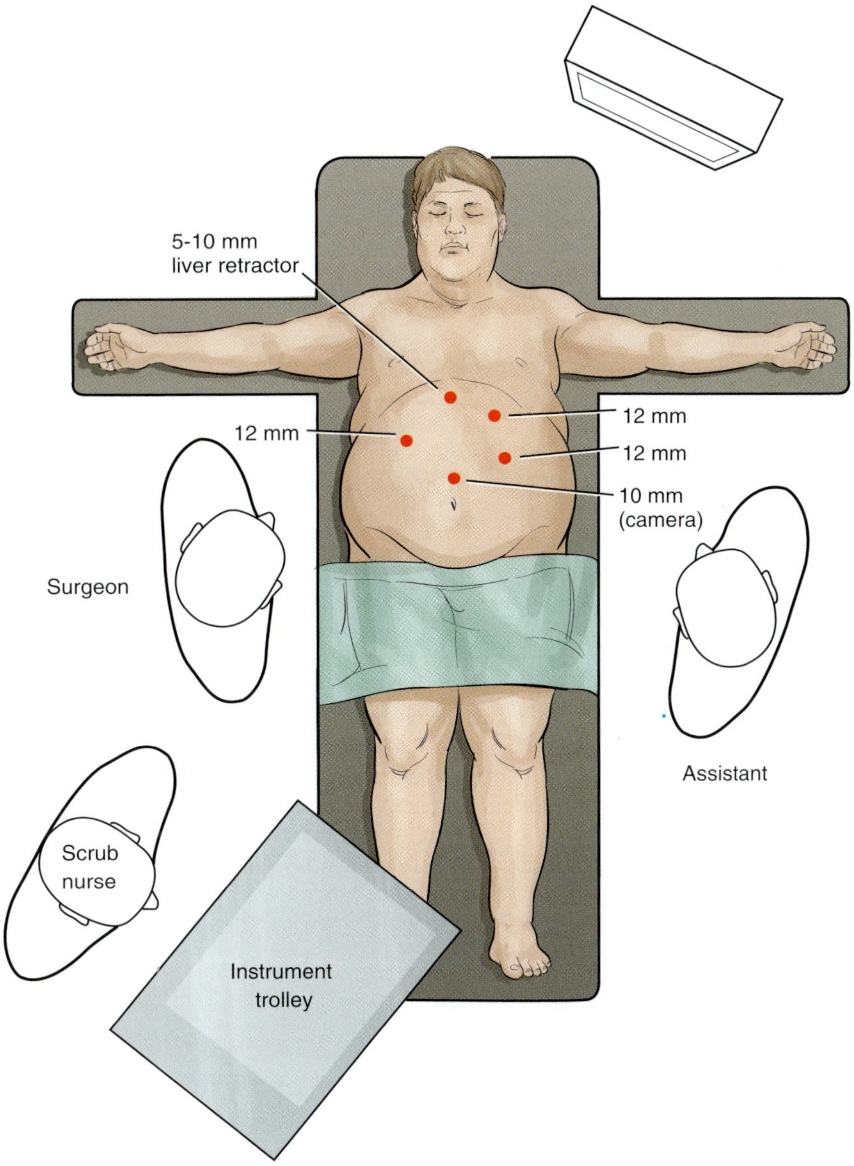

Figure 22-1.

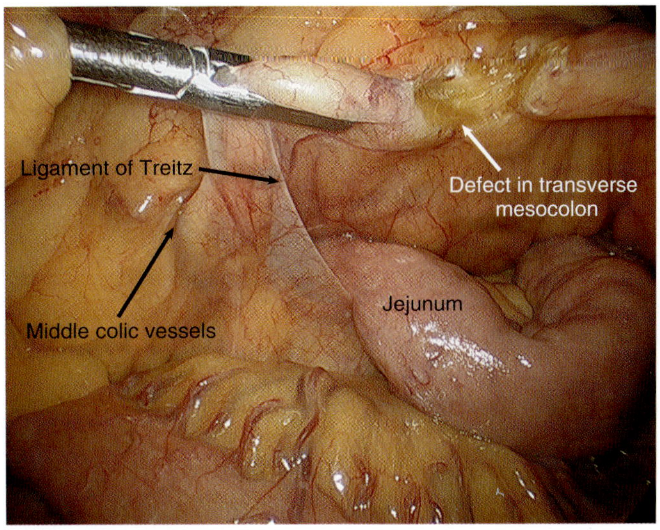

Figure 22-2.

- The proximal jejunum is measured 40 cm from the ligament of Treitz and divided to create the biliopancreatic limb (Fig. 22-3).
- The distal jejunum is measured 75 cm or 100 cm and anastomosed side-to-side with the biliopancreatic limb (jejunojejunostomy), using the linear stapler and oversewing the anastomosis (Fig. 22-4, *A* and *B*).
- The alimentary limb is placed into the mesocolic defect for retrocolic, retrogastric tunneling to the upper abdomen (Fig. 22-5).

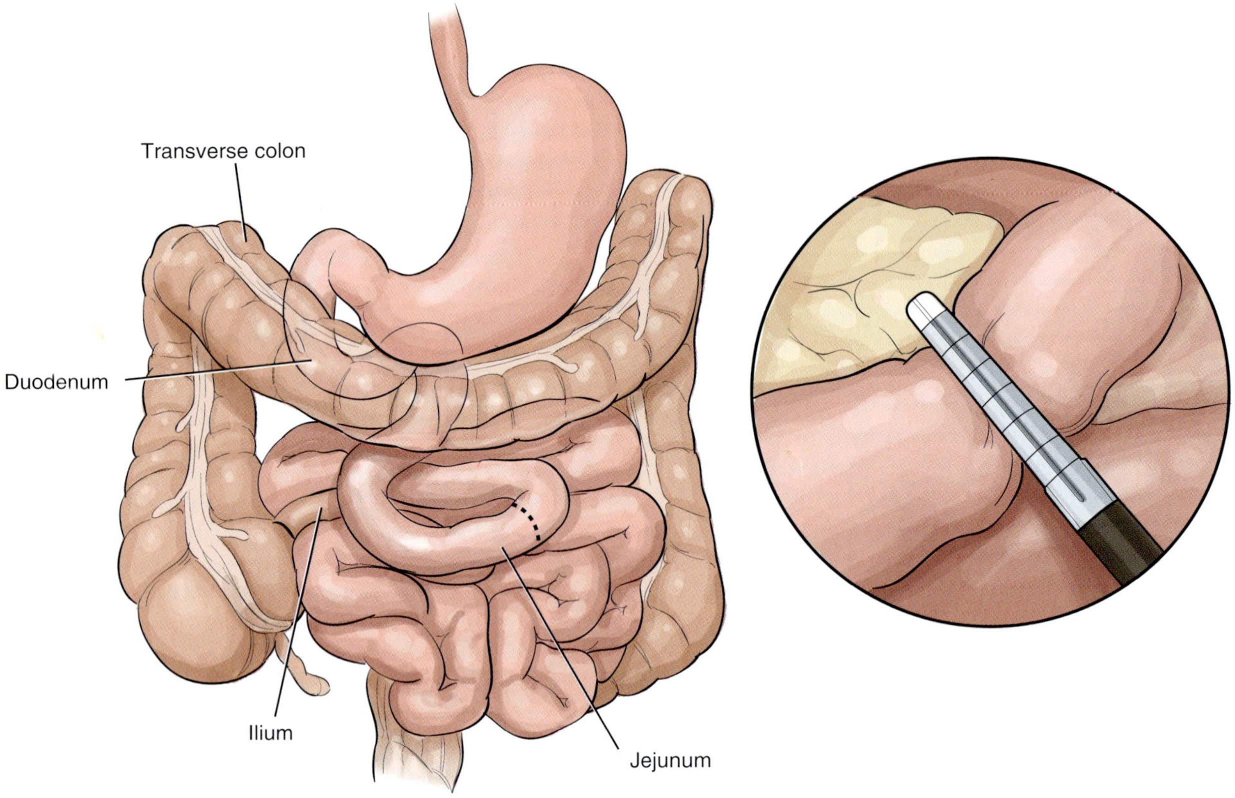

Figure 22-3.

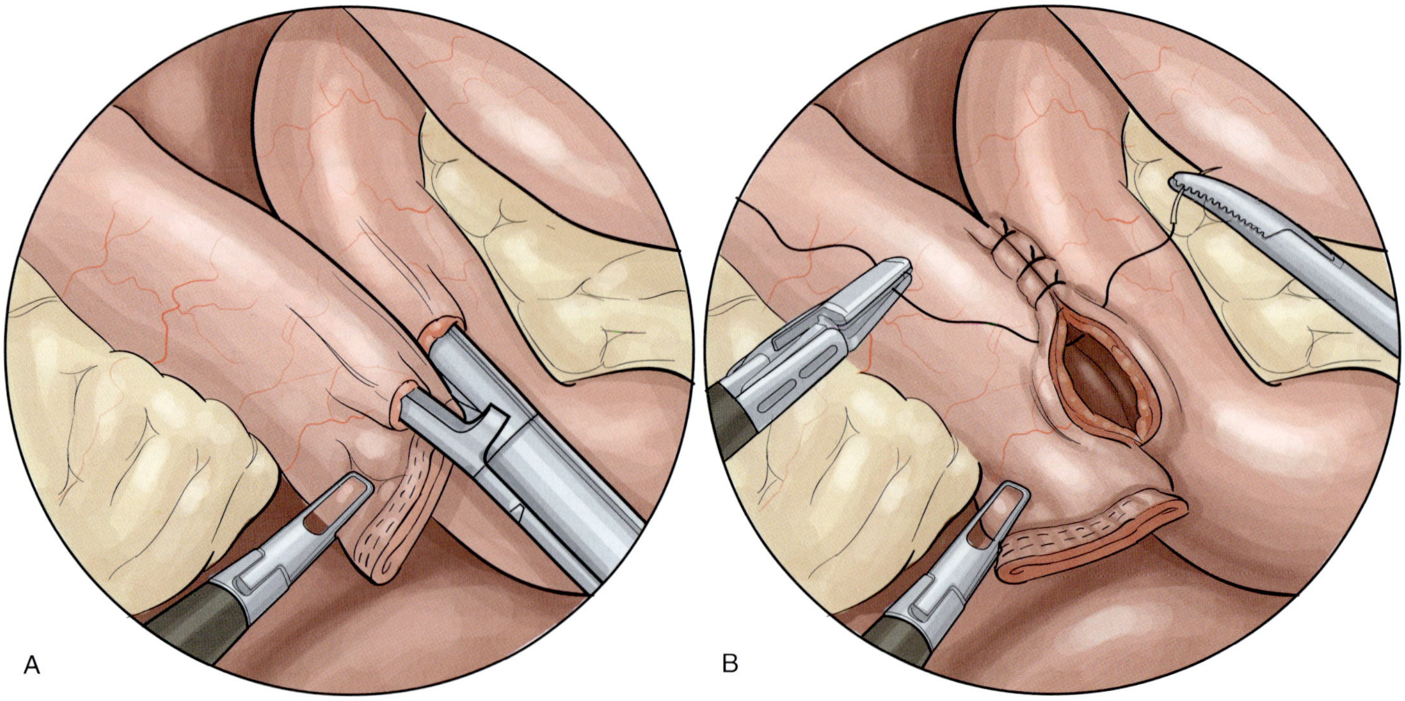

Figure 22-4.

Creation of Gastric Pouch

- Gastric pouch volume should be 30 mL or less and based on the lesser curvature (all of the distensible fundus should be excluded).
- The left lobe of the liver is retracted, and the gastrohepatic ligament is divided below the first set of feeding vessels (Fig. 22-6).
- The lesser curvature of the stomach is divided (pars flaccida technique) near the angularis.
- Successive stapler firings with the linear stapler divide the gastric pouch from the remnant stomach (care should be taken to ensure complete division) (Fig. 22-7).
- The posterior aspect of the gastric pouch is freed from overlying tissue in preparation for anastomosis of the alimentary limb to the posterior aspect of the pouch.

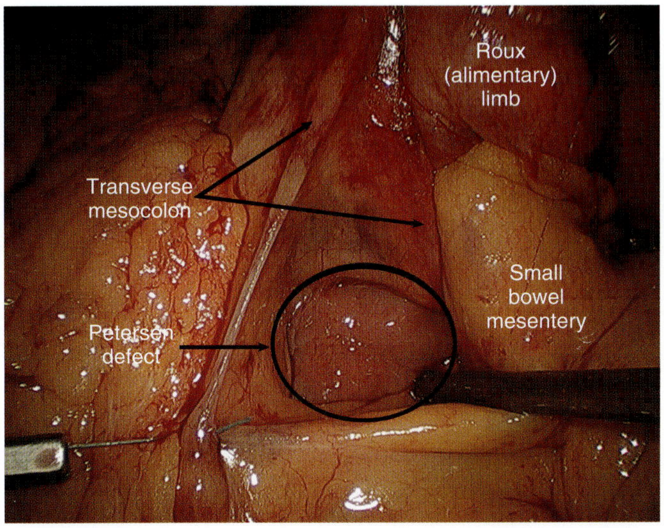

Figure 22-5.

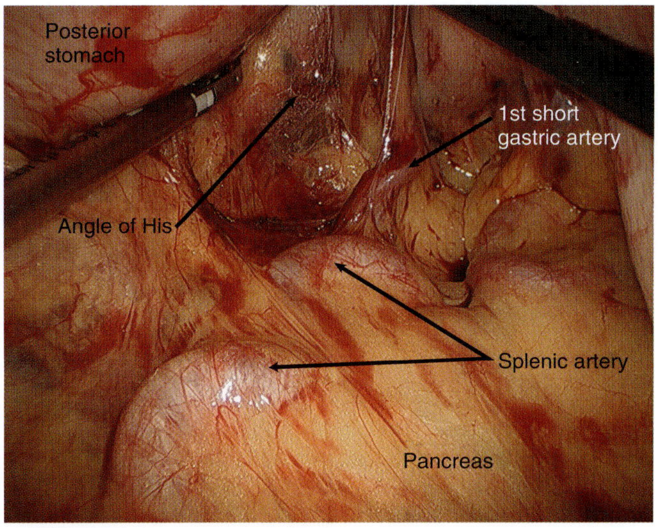

Figure 22-6.

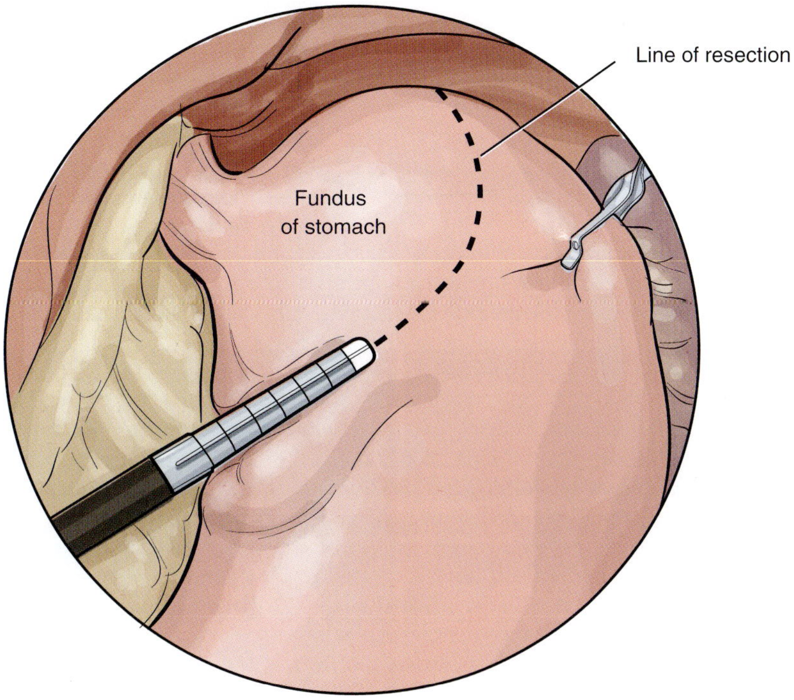

Figure 22-7.

Creation of Gastrojejunostomy

- The alimentary limb is delivered into the upper abdomen and oriented to ensure that it is not rotated (Fig. 22-8).
- The posterior outer layer of the gastrojejunostomy (GJ) is performed with a running suture.
- The posterior inner layer is created with a linear surgical stapler.
- The anterior inner and anterior outer anastomotic layers are performed with running suture (Fig. 22-9, *A* and *B*).
- A bowel clamp is placed on the alimentary limb, and air is insufflated through an endoscope inside the lumen of the gastric pouch while the anastomosis is externally submerged in saline.
- Any area with bubbles is reinforced to create an airtight anastomosis.
- Figure 22-10 shows the completed surgery.

Closure

- A closed suction drain may or may not be left posterior to the GJ for the early postoperative period.

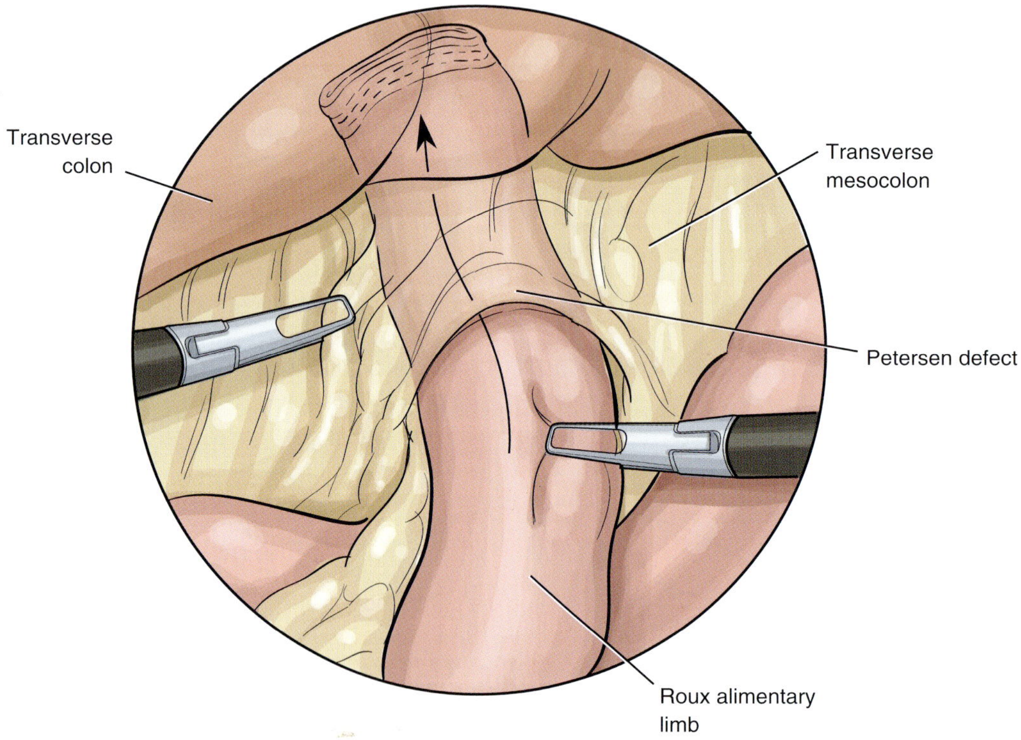

Figure 22-8.

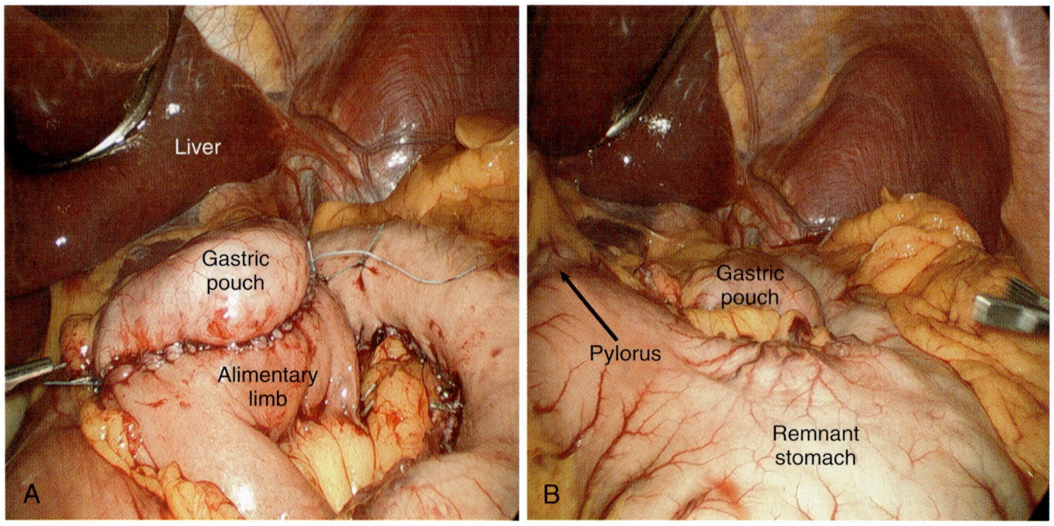

Figure 22-9.

III. ALTERNATIVE TECHNICAL APPROACHES (PRO/CON) AND PEARLS

Route of Alimentary Limb

- The alimentary limb can be routed in the antecolic, antegastric position. This avoids creation of a window in the transverse mesocolon. Most surgeons using this approach do not close any defects. This technique may require division of the greater omentum to reduce tension. Internal hernia can still develop.
- The alimentary limb can be routed in the retrocolic, retrogastric position. This is the shortest route to the upper abdomen (less tension on the anastomosis), and it requires closure of mesenteric defects to prevent internal hernia (Fig. 22-11). This route is potentially more difficult to access during a revision operation.

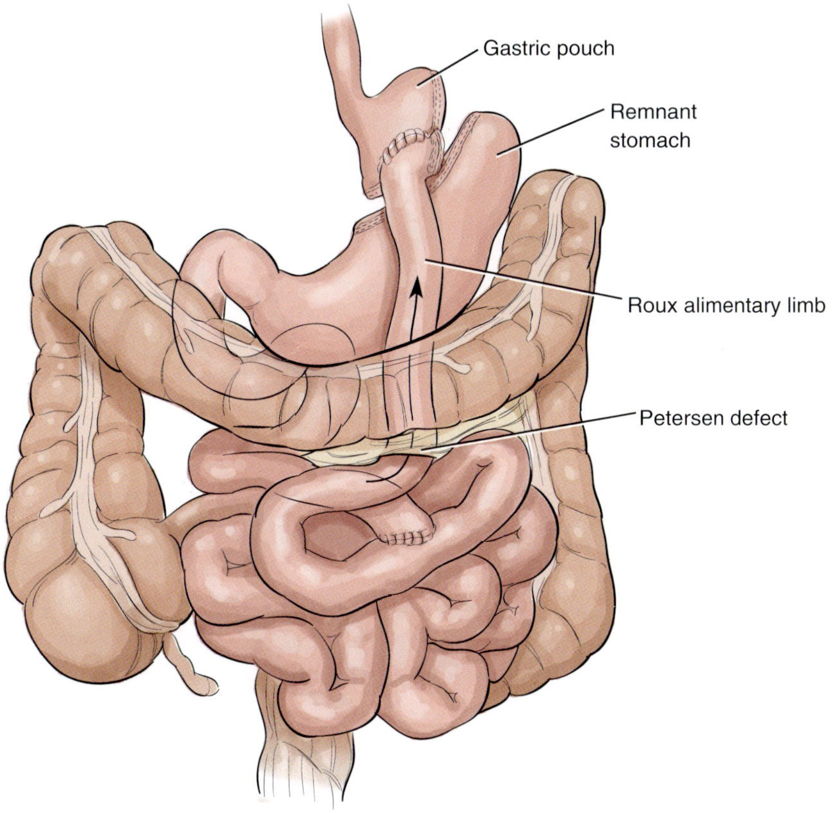

Figure 22-10.

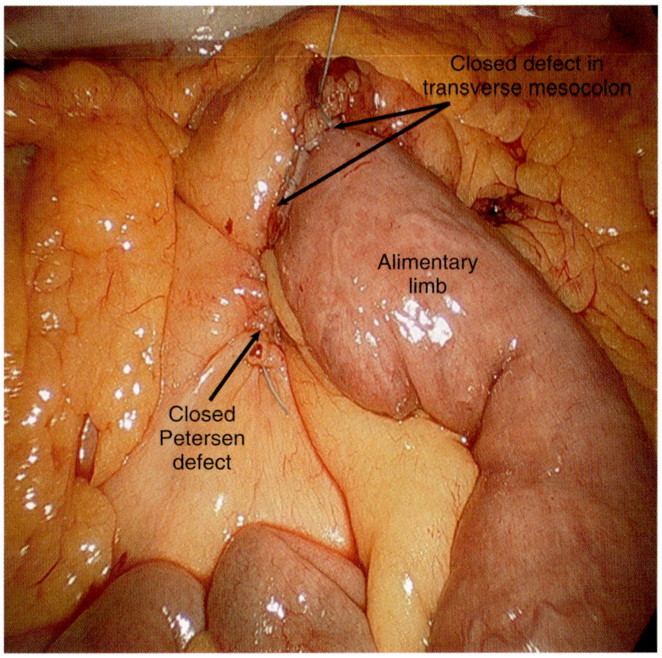

Figure 22-11.

TABLE 22-1 GJ Construction

HAND-SEWN	LINEAR-STAPLED	CIRCULAR-STAPLED
Low leak rate	Low leak rate	Low leak rate
Low stricture rate	Low stricture rate (similar to hand-sewn)	Higher stricture rate than hand-sewn and linear-stapled
Fewer marginal ulcers	More marginal ulcers than hand-sewn, but same as circular	More marginal ulcers than hand-sewn but same as linear
Technically more demanding and requires more time	Usually reinforced with an outer sutured layer	Technically easier to perform
Usually performed in two layers		

Gastrojejunostomy Construction

- For a comparison of different methods of GJ construction, see Table 22-1.

Mesenteric Defects

- Mesenteric defects occur from dividing and rerouting the small bowel and opening the mesocolon. Bowel can herniate into these defects, leading to incarceration, strangulation, and ischemia. Mesenteric defects should be closed during gastric bypass.

IV. SPECIAL POSTOPERATIVE CARE

- Long-term postoperative care is critical for the gastric bypass patient. Bariatric programs should aim to follow patients for a minimum of 5 years after surgery, and preferably for a lifetime.

Weight Loss

- Following LRYGB, patients can expect to lose about two thirds or more of excess body weight (starting weight – ideal body weight) in the first year.
- Weight loss is more pronounced early in the postoperative course, and the rate of weight loss begins to decrease after the first 6 months.
- Patients who exercise regularly have better weight loss and experience less pronounced plateaus in weight loss.
- Most patients regain about 15% of weight between 18 and 24 months after surgery.
- Maintenance of 50% or greater of excess body weight loss is considered surgical success.

Nutrition

- Early after surgery, the patient should focus on protein (60 to 80 g/day) and hydration (1.5 to 2 L fluid/day) and avoid carbohydrates. Multivitamins should be taken daily.
- Later, the patient should focus on portion control with variety of intake, avoiding simple sugars. Micronutrient supplementation (vitamin B_{12}, calcium, iron, thiamine, folic acid, multivitamins) is important. Changes in body composition will occur to increase muscle mass as adipose tissue decreases.

Changes in Medical Comorbidities

- Surveillance for improvement of medical problems is crucial, particularly in light of changing requirement for medications.
- Some comorbidities (e.g., diabetes mellitus, hypertension, dyslipidemia, reflux) respond quickly (days to weeks) and independently of weight loss.
- Other comorbidities (e.g., sleep apnea, degenerative joint disease, urinary stress incontinence) respond as a function of weight loss and change later.

Complications

- Gastrointestinal leak is the most common cause of mortality after LRYGB and can occur for any area of division and anastomosis of the gastrointestinal tract (pouch, GJ, remnant stomach, jejunojejunostomy). Diagnosis is by physical examination and a clinical course indicating sepsis. Contrast swallow evaluation can be used as an adjunct to diagnosis.
- VTE is more common among obese patients. Pulmonary embolism is the second most common cause of death after LRYGB. VTE prophylaxis is a critical component of bariatric patient care and should include chemoprophylaxis unless contraindicated.
- GJ complications can include marginal ulcer and GJ stricture, which occur in 2% to 20% of patients. Marginal ulcer occurs most commonly within the first 6 months after surgery and can usually be treated medically; surgery is reserved for refractory or complicated (hemorrhage, perforation) cases. GJ stricture often responds to endoscopic balloon dilatation and rarely requires further surgery.

SUGGESTED READINGS

Buchwald H: *Buchwald's atlas of metabolic and bariatric surgical techniques and procedures*, Philadelphia, 2011, Saunders.

Buchwald H, Avidor Y, Braunwald E, et al: Bariatric surgery: a systematic review and meta-analysis, *JAMA* 292:1724–1737, 2004.

Pories WJ, Swanson MS, MacDonald KG, et al: Who would have thought it? An operation proves to be the most effective therapy for adult-onset diabetes mellitus, *Ann Surg* 222:339–352, 1995.

CHAPTER 23

Laparoscopic Adjustable Gastric Banding

Guy Bernard Cadière, MD, PhD, and Giovanni Dapri, MD, FACS, FASMBS

I. SPECIAL PREOPERATIVE PREPARATION

- The patient is evaluated by the psychologist, nutritionist, and endocrinologist. If the patient is a candidate for obesity surgery, he or she will be submitted to other exams: gastroscopy, blood tests (general and specific tests), abdominal ultrasound, chest radiograph, electrocardiogram, and anesthesiologist consultation. In case of suspicion of sleep apnea, the patient will be examined through polysomnography, and in case of suspicion of arthrosis, the patient will be studied by specific radiographs. Finally, the patient will be evaluated by the surgeon, and the bariatric procedure (e.g., gastric banding, gastric bypass, sleeve gastrectomy, duodenal switch, biliopancreatic diversion) will be chosen considering the results of each consultation and exam.

II. OPERATIVE TECHNIQUE

Position

- The patient is positioned supine with the legs apart, and carefully strapped to the operating table. The arms are placed in abduction. Shoulder supports are placed as well, and extreme care is taken to pad the pressure points and articulations with foam cushions (Fig. 23-1).
- The surgeon stands between the patient's legs, the camera operator to the patient's right, the assistant to the patient's left, and the nurse between the assistant and the surgeon (see Fig. 23-1).

Incision

- Abdominal insufflation up to 16 mm Hg is obtained by the insertion of a Veress needle at the left upper quadrant. Abdominal trocars are placed as follows:
  - ▲ A 10-mm trocar for the optical system (30-degree angled scope) just to the left of the midline, 20 cm distal to the xiphoid
  - ▲ A 10- to 15-mm trocar on the left anterior axillary line 5 mm distal to the costal margin
  - ▲ A 5-mm trocar in the left upper quadrant on the midclavicular line and between the first and second trocar
  - ▲ A 5-mm trocar in the right upper quadrant on the right midclavicular line
  - ▲ A 5- or 10-mm trocar just distal and to the left of the xiphoid (see Fig. 23-1)

Main Dissection

Dissection of the Phrenogastric Ligament and the Retrogastric Area

- The grasper in the most lateral left trocar pulls the gastric fundus caudally to put the phrenogastric ligament under tension. A small window is created in this ligament using the coagulating hook. Location of this window is usually halfway between the upper pole of the spleen and the esophagus, just to the left side of the left crus (Fig. 23-2).
- The hepatogastric ligament is opened widely. The base of the right crus covered by the peritoneal sheet (posterior layer of the hepatogastric ligament) is identified and the peritoneal sheet is incised (Fig. 23-3).

Retrogastric Tunnel

- A grasper introduced in the right upper quadrant is advanced from the right crus to the left, staying close to the hiatus under direct vision. The instrument is pushed until its tip becomes visible in the dissection area of the phrenogastric ligament (Fig. 23-4).

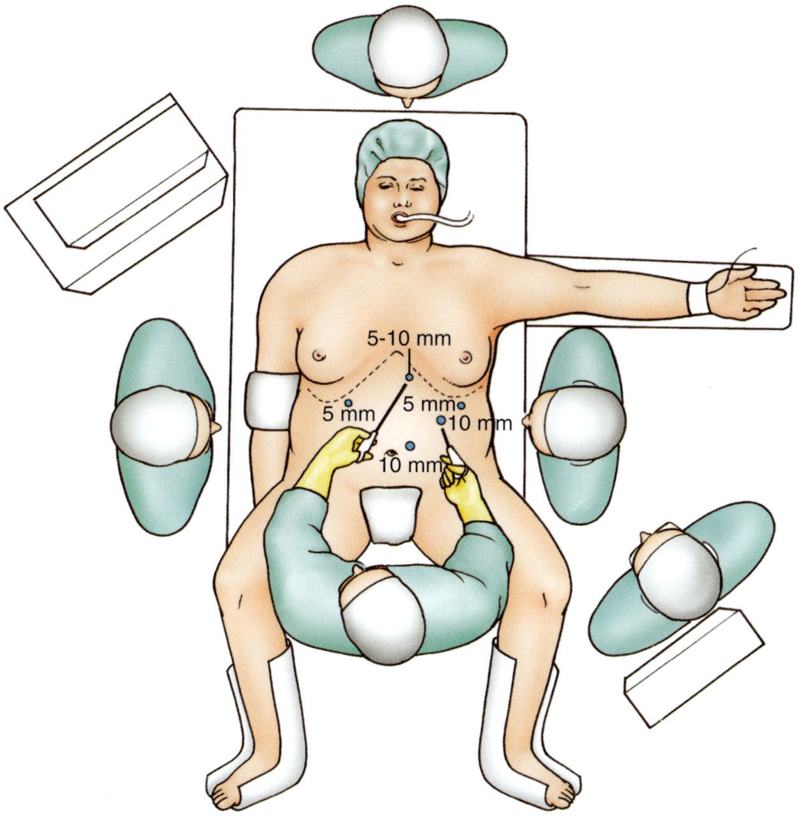

Figure 23-1.

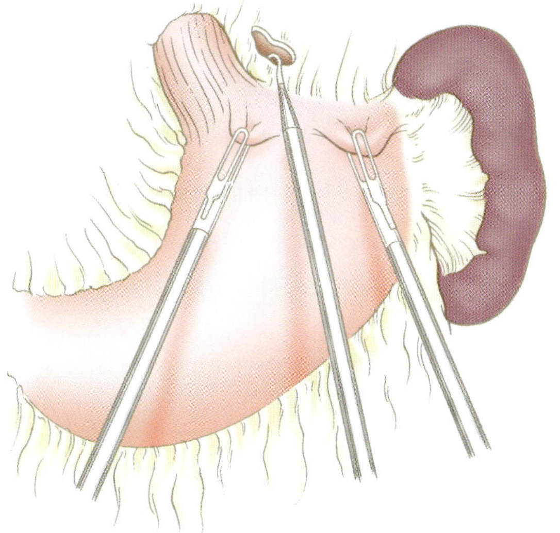

Figure 23-2.

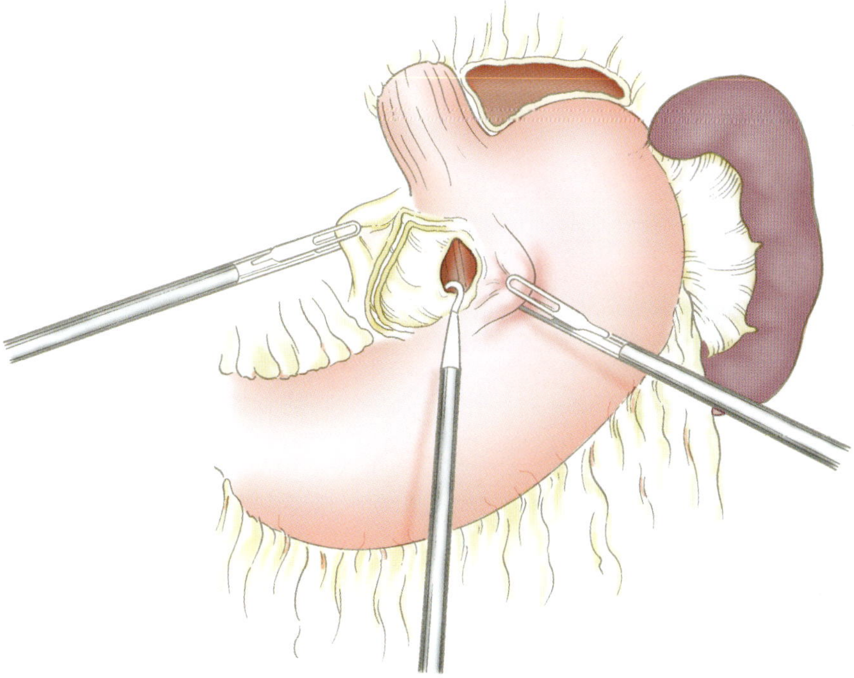

Figure 23-3.

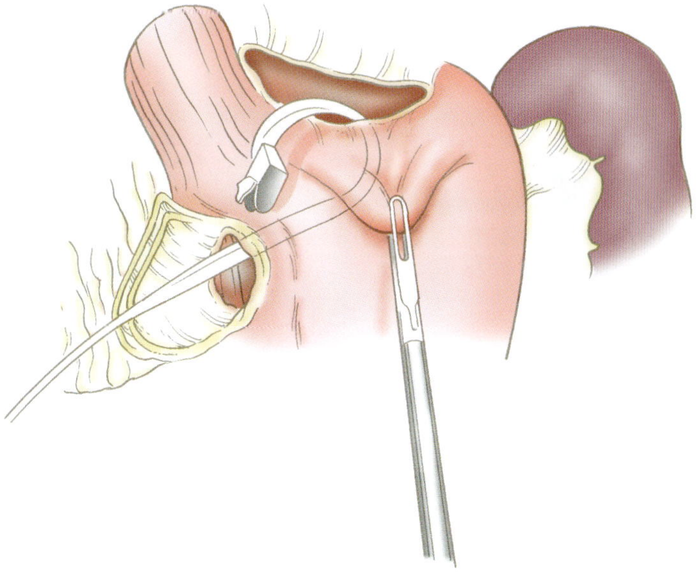

Figure 23-4.

Introduction and Placement of the Adjustable Gastric Banding

- The most lateral 10-mm trocar is replaced by a 12-15 mm trocar. A silicone band with its tubing is introduced intraperitoneally. The band is grasped by the grasping forceps and looped around the stomach at the level of dissection (Fig. 23-4). The tip of the tubing is introduced in the locking area of the band.
- The anesthesiologist introduces a balloon-tipped orogastric tube inside the stomach, and 25 mL of air is insufflated in the balloon. The tube is pulled back until it sits snugly below the esophageal junction. The band is tightened around the stomach and locked (Fig. 23-5, *A*). Four to five stitches (2-0 silk) are placed between the serosa of the stomach just above and below the band to avoid slipping (see Fig. 23-5, *B*).

Closure

- The 12-15 mm port is removed, and the nonkinking tube is cut to an appropriate length and connected to the injection port.
- The port is buried, convex side up, and stitched to the parietal fascia overlying the costal margin to the left. The band is deflated (Fig. 23-6).
- The ports are removed, and the skin is closed with absorbable sutures.

III. ALTERNATIVE TECHNICAL APPROACHES (PRO/CON) AND PEARLS

- A traditional classification of the different procedures for the treatment of morbid obesity is based on their mode of action. Three groups can be identified:
  - ▲ Restrictive procedures
  - ▲ Mixed restrictive and malabsorptive procedures
  - ▲ Malabsorptive procedures
- Adjustable gastric banding is one of the restrictive procedures besides sleeve gastrectomy and vertical banded gastroplasty. The most common restrictive and malabsorptive procedure is Roux-en-Y gastric bypass. Malabsorptive procedures are biliopancreatic diversion and duodenal switch.
- The principle of adjustable gastric banding is to reduce the stomach's volume by dividing it into two parts. The first compartment has a volume of 25 mL, the equivalent of 2 tablespoons. The second compartment is the rest of the stomach. As soon as one ingests two spoonfuls, the first compartment is filled and one experiences a feeling of fullness. Because it takes a long time for the first compartment to empty because of the narrow outlet, more food can only be ingested after substantial time has elapsed. One must therefore eat at a much slower pace. Because of that slower pace, the satiety center has the time to be stimulated. As the hunger sensation is no longer present, overall food intake is reduced.
- The advantages of adjustable gastric banding regarding other bariatric procedures are reversibility, absence of mortality, low morbidity, and low learning curve. The major advantage of this procedure is the possibility to adjust the size of the outlet (stoma) without anesthesia, as the stoma size can be

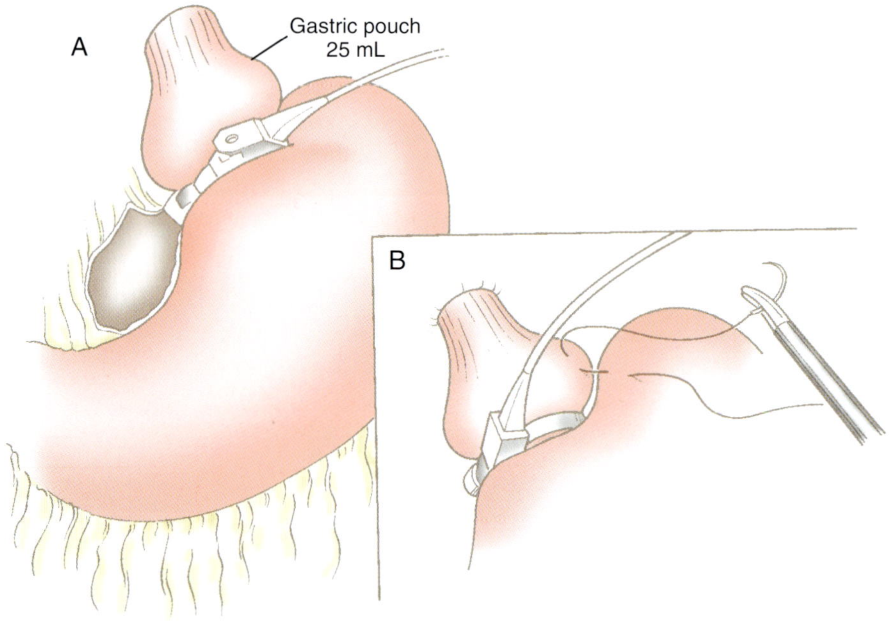

Figure 23-5.

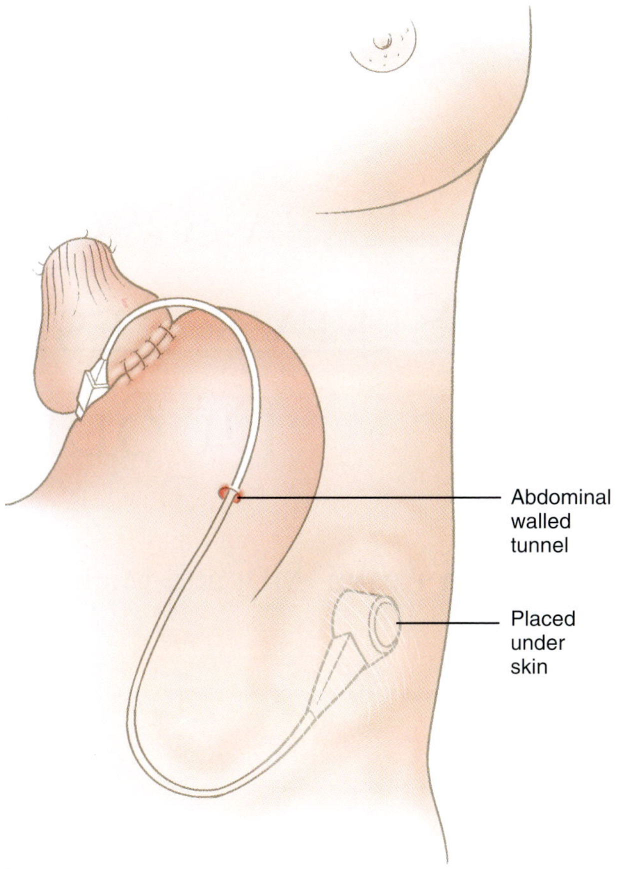

Figure 23-6.

readily adjusted by injecting or withdrawing saline via the percutaneous access port, thereby inflating or deflating the inflatable portion of the silicone band. The adjustments should be based on objective criteria, including documented dietary inquiry, postoperative weight loss curves, and radiologic studies. In case of inefficacy or complications such as gastric pouch dilation and gastric erosion, removal of the band is possible, and removal with conversion into another procedure is a valuable option.

IV. SPECIAL POSTOPERATIVE CARE

- On postoperative day 1, a gastrografin swallow is performed, and if there is a adequate passage and the test confirms the band is in the correct position, the patient is authorized to leave the hospital on a liquid diet.
- The adjustment is performed by the radiologist 1 month later. Stoma size will be established depending on complications (reflux, food intolerance), the weight loss curve, and results of the radiograph.

SUGGESTED READINGS

Ponce J, Paynter S, Fromm R: Laparoscopic adjustable gastric banding: 1014 consecutive cases, *J Am Coll Surg* 201:529–535, 2005.

Steffen R, Biertho L, Ricklin T, et al: Laparoscopic Swedish adjustable gastric banding: a five year prospective study, *Obes Surg* 13:404–411, 2003.

Suter M, Calmes JM, Paroz A, Giusti V: A 10-year experience with laparoscopic gastric banding for morbid obesity: high long-term complication and failure rates, *Obes Surg* 16:829–835, 2006.

CHAPTER 24

Laparoscopic Gastric Sleeve Resection with Duodenal Switch

Manish Parikh, MD, and Michel Gagner, MD, FRCSC, FACS

I. SPECIAL PREOPERATIVE PREPARATION

- Esophagogastroduodenoscopy to exclude gastric or duodenal pathology, including *Helicobacter pylori* infection. If *H. pylori* is present, patients are treated before surgery.
- Upper gastrointestinal series if the patient has had a prior bariatric procedure.
- Medical clearance.
- Psychiatric evaluation and instruction by registered dietitian or nutritionist.
- Screening colonoscopy if over age 50.
- Evaluation for obstructive sleep apnea (if applicable).
- Clear liquid diet the day before surgery.

II. OPERATIVE TECHNIQUE

Position

- An Alphastar table (Maquet, Rastatt, Germany) with foot-plate attachments is used.
- A French, split-leg position is used, with the legs abducted, but not flexed, and properly secured.
- The surgeon stands between the patient's legs, the first assistant (liver retractor and camera holder) stands on the patient's right, and the second assistant stands on the patent's left.

Incision (Trocar Placement)

- There are seven trocars in total (Fig. 24-1):
  - ▲ A 10-mm trocar at the umbilicus (we prefer the open technique to enter the peritoneal cavity); diagnostic laparoscopy is then performed with the 10-mm, 30-degree laparoscope.
  - ▲ Three 10-12 mm trocars—one in the left epigastric paramedian position for optics and one in the right subcostal position in the midclavicular line (liver retraction) and one in the subxiphoid position
  - ▲ Two 10-15 mm trocars—one in the left midclavicular line, four finger breadths inferior to the costal margin and one in the right midclavicular line, just superior to the umbilicus.
  - ▲ A 5-mm port in the left anterior axillary line lateral to the trocar.
- A second insufflator is attached to optimize pneumoperitoneum (15 mm Hg carbon dioxide)

Main Dissection

- We prefer to start with the sleeve gastrectomy rather than the distal ileoileostomy because occasionally patients cannot tolerate pneumoperitoneum and may require a shortened procedure. In these cases, performing a sleeve gastrectomy alone permits an effective and abbreviated procedure without compromising the patient. Several months later (after significant weight loss has taken place), the patient may return for completion duodenal switch.

Sleeve Gastrectomy

- The patient is placed in steep reverse Trendelenburg position, and the table is tilted right side down to optimize visualization of the gastroesophageal junction.
- The laparoscope is placed through the 10-mm left epigastric paramedian trocar. If the stomach is distended, the anesthesiologist should place an orogastric tube to decompress the stomach; this tube must be removed as soon as the stomach is decompressed to avoid any problems during subsequent stapling.
- A 10-mm liver retractor (fan-type retractor) is placed through the right subcostal port to retract the liver anteriorly and to expose the entire stomach and gastroesophageal junction. The surgeon's working ports are the subxiphoid trocar and the left subcostal trocar. The second assistant retracts the omentum laterally with a bowel grasper through the 5-mm left lateral trocar.
- Dissection begins along the distal greater curvature by dividing the branches of the gastroepiploic artery near the gastric wall with the ultrasonic scalpel. The greater curvature is devascularized in this manner

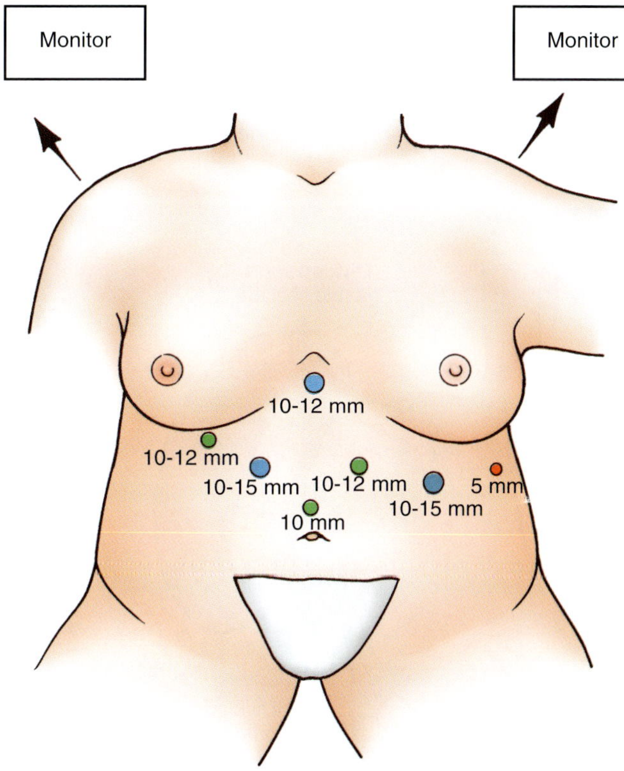

Figure 24-1.

proximally to the level of the left crus (including division of the short gastric vessels, Fig. 24-2, *A*). The second assistant's grasper is frequently repositioned superiorly to maximize retraction. Exposure while dividing the short gastric vessels and dissecting near the left crus is often difficult. Helpful maneuvers include the following:

- ▲ Place the second assistant's grasper on the lateral fold of the omentum (in the midgastrosplenic ligament) and retract this laterally toward the spleen
- ▲ Temporarily increase the pneumoperitoneum to 20 mm Hg
- ▲ Place the patient in maximal reverse Trendelenburg position
- ▲ Tilt the patient more toward the right side
- ▲ Ask the anesthesiologist to give an additional dose of paralytics
- ▲ Position the second assistant on the posterior fundus and retract this toward the patient's right side

- Occasionally an additional 5-mm trocar is required to retract the perigastric fat and adequately expose the gastroesophageal junction.
- All posterior attachments to the pancreas must be freed, taking care not to injure the splenic artery. Placing the second assistant's graspers on the posterior fundus and retracting this toward the patient's right shoulder exposes these attachments. It is important to divide these attachments before stapling, because these attachments can tear and create significant bleeding. However, one must not be too aggressive near the lesser curvature, because the blood supply to the sleeve will come from the lesser curvature vasculature only.
- Now the left crus can be visualized by lifting the stomach anteriorly. The left crus and the gastroesophageal junction must be completely exposed. The ligament attaching the stomach and diaphragm must be divided. The anterior perigastric fat just to the left of the gastroesophageal junction must be cleared to minimize tissue thickness during subsequent stapling. However, avoid dissecting to the right of the gastroesophageal junction because of risk of injury to the vagus nerve. If the patient has a significant hiatal hernia, this should be reduced, because failure to recognize or repair a herniated fundus may lead to weight loss failure and reflux after sleeve gastrectomy.
- Next, the remainder of the greater curvature is liberated distally to 2 cm beyond the pylorus. The second assistant retracts the greater curvature anteriorly toward the patient's right shoulder. The surgeon's left hand grasps the fat of the gastrocolic ligament (via the right midclavicular trocar) and retracts it caudad. The surgeon's right hand manipulates the ultrasonic scalpel. The remainder of the gastrocolic ligament between the antrum and gastroepiploic arcade is divided with the ultrasonic scalpel.

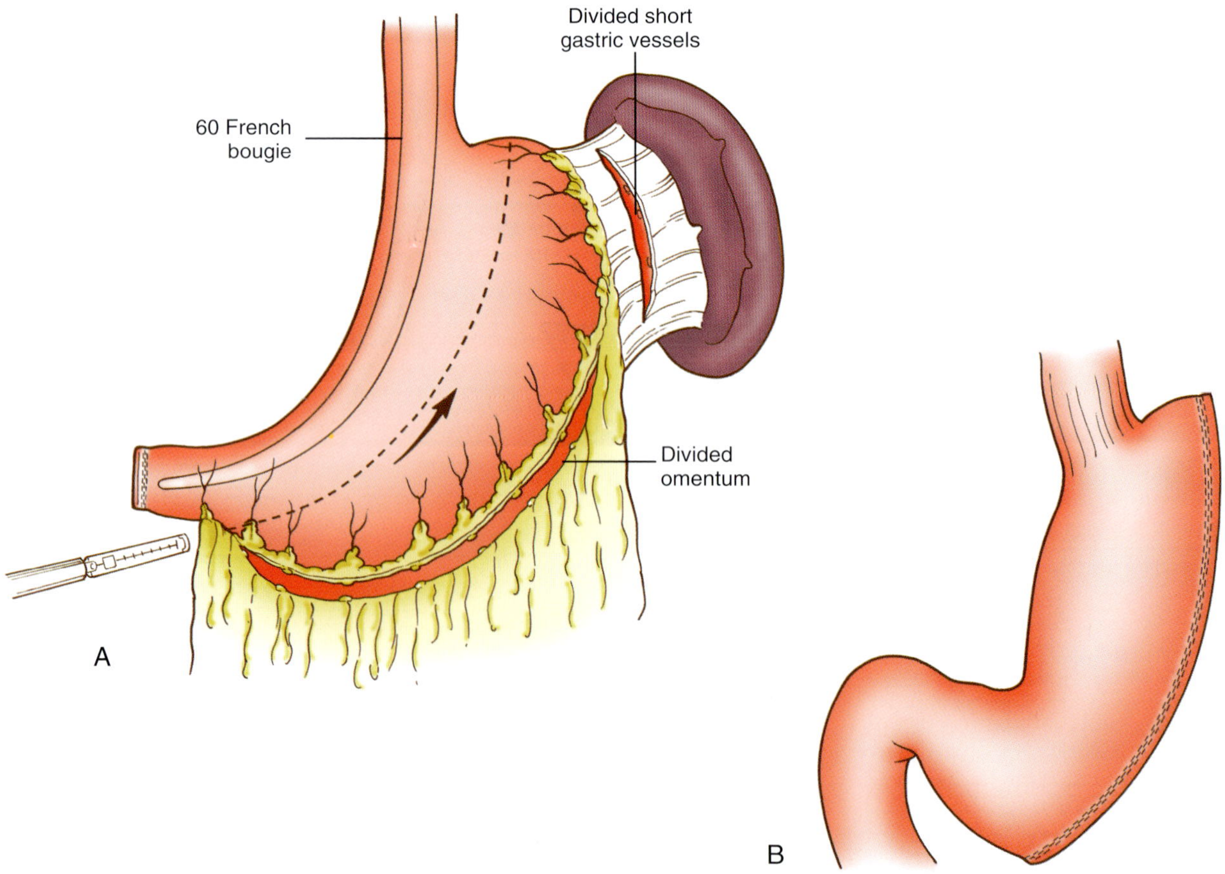

Figure 24-2.

- Instrument palpation is used to confirm the anatomic position of the pylorus. Approximately 6 to 8 cm proximal to the pylorus (at the level of the "crow's foot," just distal to the incisura), the sleeve gastrectomy is begun along the greater curvature (Fig. 24-2). Initiating the sleeve less than 6 cm proximal to the pylorus may compromise the antrum and could lead to gastric emptying problems.
- The surgeon's left hand holds the 4.8-mm linear stapler (60-mm length) through the right midclavicular trocar. The second assistant retracts the body of the stomach toward the patient's left side. The stapler should be positioned such that at least 2 cm of anterior stomach serosa is visible between the stapler and lesser curvature.
- The first two firings of the stapler are performed, aiming approximately 2 cm away from the lesser curvature. These firings should be done slowly, because the stomach is thickest in this area. Additional sutures are required if the tissue is too thick for the stapler. We routinely use buttress material (Bioabsorbable Seamguard; Gore, Flagstaff, Ariz.) similar to the Maxon suture (United States Surgical, Norwalk, Conn.), which is sandwiched between, over, and below the anterior and posterior gastric wall. This bioabsorbable material reduces staple-line hemorrhage and possibly the leakage rate.
- The anesthesiologist inserts a 60-Fr orogastric bougie. Under laparoscopic vision, the bougie is aligned medially along the lesser curvature into the duodenum. Two bowel graspers can be used to help direct the bougie posteriorly into the sleeve toward the pylorus. Inserting the bougie after the first two stapler firings helps align the bougie along the lesser curvature (see Fig. 24-2, *A*). For all duodenal switch cases, we currently use the 60-Fr bougie to ensure enough volume of the stomach to permit adequate protein intake. (For primary sleeve gastrectomy, we use a 40 Fr bougie).
- The remainder of the sleeve gastrectomy is completed by sequential firings of the 4.8-mm linear stapler along the bougie toward the angle of His (see Fig. 24-2, *B*). Although we have used the 3.5-mm linear stapler in the past, we believe that it is safest to use the 4.8-mm linear stapler for the entire sleeve gastrectomy because of the thick stomach in these morbidly obese patients. The differences in hemostasis between the two staplers are no longer seen with the routine use of the buttressing Seamguard material. The surgeon's right hand holds the stapler via the left midclavicular trocar and aims toward the left crus; the surgeon's left hand (via the subxiphoid trocar) grasps the anterior wall of the stomach and retracts this toward the patient's right side. The second assistant holds the posterior wall of the stomach and retracts this toward the patient's left side. A total of five to six staple firings are typically required to complete the sleeve. The anesthesiologist must pay careful attention that the bougie does not retract during stapling to prevent the tip of the bougie from being incorporated into the staple line.
- Next, the anesthesiologist removes the bougie. Figure-eight 3-0 Maxon (monofilament absorbable) sutures are placed at the apex of the sleeve gastrectomy (the area most prone to developing leaks), at the intersections of the staple lines (also prone to suboptimal healing), and at the most distal end of the staple line (the thickest part of stomach). The second assistant can retract the stomach toward the patient's right side to help expose the apex of the sleeve.
- If there is any doubt about the integrity of the staple line, a methylene blue test should be performed before proceeding to the next stage. The anesthesiologist inserts an 18-Fr orogastric tube. The surgeon clamps near the pylorus, and the anesthesiologist injects methylene blue mixed with saline through the tube. Approximately 120 mL is required to distend the sleeve. Another option is to insert a gastroscope and check for leak (and intraluminal bleeding) via air insufflation; this latter option is used less often because of the tendency of air to pass through the pylorus and distend the small bowel.
- The right midclavicular trocar site is enlarged, the abdominal wall is dilated with an atraumatic clamp (the circular stapler will be introduced through this site later), a large impermeable bag is introduced, and the specimen is extracted. Grasping the end of the sleeve and pulling it out progressively may make extraction easier and require less abdominal wall dilation.

Duodenal Transection and Preparation for Duodenoileostomy

- The pylorus and first portion of duodenum are palpated. Any remaining branches between the gastroepiploic arcade and the antrum/pylorus are divided with the ultrasonic scalpel, proceeding toward the inferior aspect of the first portion of the duodenum. Typically, the dissection extends to just beyond the vascular complex inferior to the pylorus. It is important to avoid hemostatic clips in this area (especially on the duodenal side) to prevent having clips interfere with the staple line. Any duodenal adhesions from prior cholecystectomy must be divided at this time.
- The retroduodenal and supraduodenal tissue are dissected free with the ultrasonic scalpel. The second assistant retracts the stomach laterally and anteriorly so the surgeon can see both the greater curvature and the posterior stomach for the retroduodenal dissection. The gastroduodenal artery, which lies posteriorly between the first and second portion of duodenum, marks the distal aspect of dissection.
- Using a 10-mm right-angle dissector, a 1-cm window (enough to accommodate a linear stapler) is made posterior and superior to the duodenum, medial to the common bile duct. Ideally, the supraduodenal window is between the serosa of the duodenum and the pyloric branches of the right gastric artery, thus maximizing blood supply to the subsequent anastomosis.
- The duodenum is transected with a 3.5-mm Endo GIA linear stapler (60-mm length; Tyco Healthcare) buttressed with Bioabsorbable Seamguard, leaving a 2- to 5-cm duodenal cuff (typically via the left

midclavicular trocar; Fig. 24-3). Sometimes, the right midclavicular trocar provides a better angle for transection. The second assistant retracts the antrum toward the patient's left side to facilitate this. The Seamguard buttressing material obviates the need to oversew the duodenal stump.

- If the surgeon is faced with a scenario where he or she is unable to complete the supraduodenal window, an alternate method is to transect the inferior two thirds of the duodenum with the linear stapler, complete the supraduodenal window, and then transect the remaining duodenum with another firing of the stapler.
- We prefer to use a circular stapler for the duodenoileostomy, specifically the CEEA 21 (Tyco Healthcare). The CEEA 25 is too large for the ileum and frequently tears the ileum during insertion. The 21 anvil is delivered transabdominally through the right midclavicular trocar site (Fig. 24-4). The 21 anvil is problematic to deliver through the proximal duodenal stump using the modified nasogastric tube-anvil apparatus commonly used for gastric bypass because it does not flex and traverses the pylorus only with some difficulty.
- The ultrasonic scalpel is used to remove 1 to 2 cm of the proximal duodenal staple line, and the base of the 21 anvil is placed into the duodenal lumen. Once the anvil is in place, it is secured with a 3-0 Prolene purse-string suture.
- Next the surgeon must assess the ability of the ileum to be brought toward the duodenum antecolic and in a tension-free manner. Particularly in patients with bulky omentum, one must divide the omentum along its right lateral third to facilitate subsequent passage of the ileum toward the duodenum. It is important that the right side of the omentum (and not the left side as commonly done in gastric bypass) is divided, because an oblique line runs from the ileocecal valve toward the pylorus.

Small Bowel Measurement

- The surgeon and first assistant move to the patient's left side. The patient is placed in the Trendelenburg position and then tilted left side down to aid in exposure of the ileocecal region.
- With the laparoscope in the left epigastric paramedian port and the surgeon's working hands in the subxiphoid and umbilical ports, the distal small intestine is measured from the ileocecal valve using a 50-cm umbilical tape. Flat 5-mm forceps (Dorsey, Karl Storz; Tuttlingen, Germany) are used to avoid serosal tears during measurements. Any adhesions that prevent proper measurement of the small intestine (e.g., prior lower abdominal or pelvic surgery) must be divided. The umbilical tape should

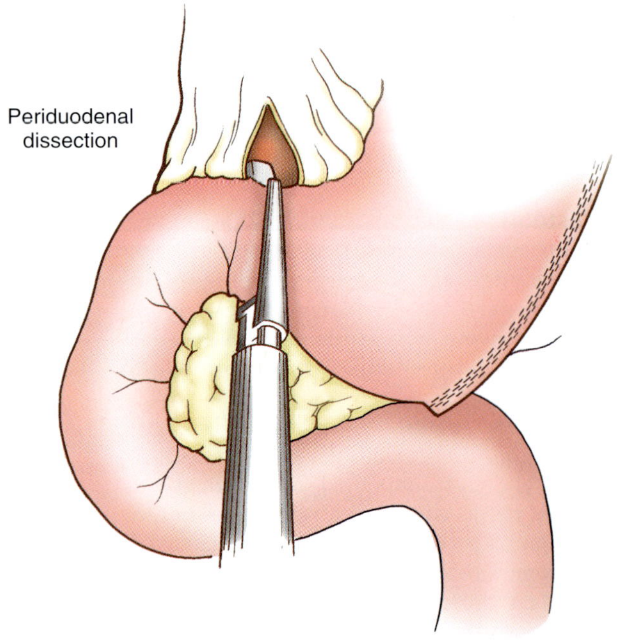

Figure 24-3.

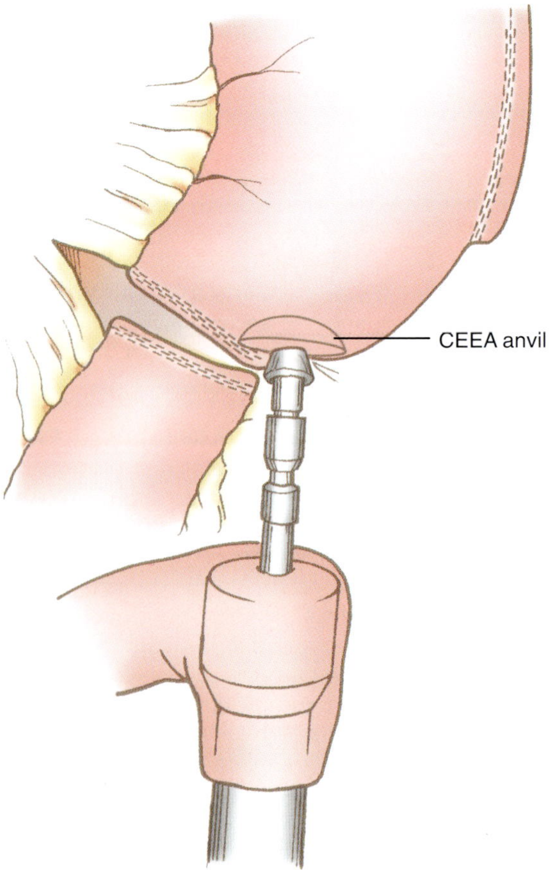

Figure 24-4.

be kept on the antimesenteric side during measurements. We prefer umbilical tape for these measurements because it is a more reliable method of measuring small intestine versus estimating distances with a bowel grasper.

- At 100 cm proximal to the ileocecal valve, clips are placed on the ileal mesentery (to mark the site of anastomosis of the future common channel). Another 150 cm is measured proximally from this point (future alimentary limb). Here, a window is made in the ileal mesentery with a 10-mm right-angle clamp. It is best to not dissect directly on the bowel wall, because the mesentery advances over the intestinal wall in the morbidly obese. Instead, make the window in the mesentery approximately 1 cm away from the bowel wall.
- The ileum is transected with a 2.5-mm linear stapler (45-mm length is adequate) buttressed with Bioabsorbable Seamguard (via the left midclavicular trocar). The ultrasonic scalpel is used to divide another 1 to 2 cm of mesentery between the two ends of bowel. Dividing more than 1 to 2 cm of mesentery is unnecessary and places the subsequent anastomosis at risk of becoming ischemic.
- The grasper remains on the distal bowel (with the umbilical tape) to maintain proper orientation. The staple line and buttress material are completely excised from the distal ileum to permit entry of the 21-mm circular stapler. The umbilical tape is then removed. Care is taken to ensure that there is no twisting of the mesentery or misidentification of bowel limbs by running the bowel again from the ileocecal valve proximally to the transected (and opened) ileum.

Duodenoileal Anastomosis

- A suture is attached to the spike of the CEEA 21 for easy retrieval. The CEEA 21 is secured to a plastic camera drape (for wound protection) with a Steri-Strip and is introduced via the right midclavicular trocar site.
- Three graspers are used to triangulate the opened end of the ileum: two are placed at the 2 o'clock and 10 o'clock positions, and a third grasper is placed at the 6 o'clock position adjacent to the mesentery.
- The stapler is gently maneuvered into the distal ileal enterotomy and advanced cephalad in a clockwise manner toward the duodenal cuff containing the anvil. The first two graspers are removed. The grasper at 6:00 remains in place to prevent the stapler from coming out of the bowel. It is critical that the ileum be brought toward the duodenum (and not vice versa) under minimal or no tension. The omentum needs to be divided to facilitate this, as described earlier.
- The first assistant moves between the patient's legs, and the surgeon remains on the patient's left (second assistant remains on the patient's right to retracting the liver anteriorly).
- The white plastic perforator is advanced through the antimesenteric wall of the ileum approximately 6 to 7 cm distal to the opened ileum. The spike is removed by grasping the suture attached to the spike. The anvil (in the duodenum) is then united with the stapler. It is important that there be no tissue between the ileum and duodenum and no pinching of the bowel wall (which can create an obstruction later).
- The stapler is fired, and an end-to-side anastomosis is created. The CEEA 21 is not a flipped-top; therefore two to three rotations of the stapler are required in conjunction with countertraction on the antrum to pull the CEEA through the anastomosis.
- Next, the Steri-Strip holding the wound protector is removed, and the CEEA is removed from the trocar site while advancing the wound protector over the tip of the stapler to prevent the stapler from contacting the wound.
- The surgeon returns to stand between the patient's legs, and the first assistant returns to the patient's right side. The right midclavicular trocar is reinserted.
- The open ileal limb is inspected for bleeding. Any oozing emanating from the enterotomy may indicate bleeding from the duodenoileostomy and must be further evaluated. If there is no bleeding from the open limb, a 2.5-mm linear stapler (45-mm length) buttressed with Bioabsorbable Seamguard (via the subxiphoid or the left midclavicular trocar) is used to transect the blind limb. The tips of the stapler must be in the ileal mesentery to ensure that the opened ileum has been completely closed (otherwise a leak can occur into the mesentery). The specimen is extracted from the right midclavicular trocar site.
- The duodenoileostomy staple line (including the upper and lower corners) is reinforced with a running 3-0 Maxon suture. We prefer monofilament absorbable sutures because permanent sutures (e.g., silk sutures) have been associated with marginal ulcers and strictures. One helpful maneuver to provide adequate exposure of the superior corner (where leaks are most prone to occur) is to place the second assistant's graspers on the antrum and retract this toward the patient's left lower quadrant to pull the anastomosis toward the midline. To facilitate exposure of the posterior aspect of the staple line, the second assistant should grasp the posterior antrum and gently retract this toward the patient's right shoulder.
- Next, the anesthesiologist inserts an 18-Fr orogastric tube just proximal to the anastomosis and then instills approximately 120 mL methylene blue mixed with saline with a Tumi syringe. Simultaneously, the surgeon clamps the ileum distal to the duodenoileostomy. The area around the anastomosis is irrigated with saline to help identify any methylene blue. Once the test has been completed and no leak has been identified, the gastric sleeve is completely aspirated and the orogastric tube is removed.

Distal Ileoileostomy

- The surgeon and first assistant return to the patient's left side, and the laparoscope is placed through the left epigastric paramedian trocar. The table is tilted left side down, and the patient is placed in slight Trendelenburg position.
- The surgeon uses 5-mm bowel graspers in the subxiphoid and umbilical port to run the alimentary limb from the duodenoileostomy distally to the level of the previously placed clips on the ileal mesentery (at 100 cm proximal to the ileocecal valve).
- We prefer the "M" triple-staple technique, which is a completely stapled anastomosis that provides a large patent anastomosis while avoiding the risk of narrowing the bowel lumen during closure of the enterotomy (Fig. 24-5). The clips on the ileal mesentery are removed.
- An enterotomy is made with the ultrasonic scalpel on the antimesenteric side of the marked ileum. Another enterotomy is made approximately 1 to 2 cm away from the stapled end of the proximal ileum. The stapled proximal ileum (biliopancreatic limb) should be on the patient's left, and the alimentary limb should be on the patient's right side. Again, one must take care that there has been no twisting of the mesentery and that both staples are fired on the antimesenteric border to avoid ischemia.
- The 2.5-mm linear stapler (60-mm length) is introduced through the subxiphoid trocar, aiming toward the pelvis. It is best to insert the larger jaw of the stapler into the proximal ileum (larger diameter) and the smaller jaw into the distal ileum (narrower). A standard side-to-side anastomosis is created between the biliopancreatic limb and the last 100 cm of distal ileum.
- Through the same enterotomy, the linear stapler (2.5 mm, 60-mm length) is then fired between the alimentary limb and the common channel. A third firing of the 2.5-mm linear stapler (via the left midclavicular Versaport) closes the enterotomy transversely. The specimen is removed without contaminating the wound. An alternate option for enterotomy closure is to carefully close the enterotomy with a running 2-0 silk suture, in one or two layers.

Closure of Mesenteric Defects

- We recommend complete closure of all mesenteric defects to avoid internal hernias and their associated complications. With the same position (surgeon and first assistant on the patient's left side), the ileoileostomy mesenteric defect is closed with a running 2-0 silk suture (24-cm length). We prefer to incorporate the serosa of the ileum in the last stitch of this closure.
- The surgeon then returns to a position between the patient's legs to close the Petersen defect. The patient is placed in slight reverse Trendelenburg position. Sometimes it is necessary to insert an additional 5-mm trocar in the left lower quadrant to optimize suturing angles.
- The omentum is retracted superiorly to the transverse colon. The first assistant grasps the epiploic appendage of the transverse colon and retracts this cephalad. Now this space between the transverse colon mesentery and the ileal mesentery should be completely exposed, and this defect is closed with a running 2-0 silk suture.
- We prefer to close this from the patient's left side because there is a wider space on the left and because closure from the left side permits visualization of the ligament of Treitz and helps the surgeon avoid catching proximal jejunum in the closure. The final stitch should approximate the transverse colon serosa to the ileum serosa, because mesenteric fat closure alone may eventually (with significant weight loss) enlarge and lead to an internal hernia. It is imperative to completely close these defects, especially at the root of the mesentery, because a small defect may be more susceptible to incarceration than the initially large patent defect.

Closure

- The sleeve gastrectomy staple line, duodenoileostomy, and ileoileostomy are all inspected for any evidence of bleeding or leakage. The final anatomic configuration is shown in Figure 24-6. The biliopancreatic limb must be coming from the patient's left side, and the alimentary limb and common channel must be on the patient's right side.
- We do not routinely place any drains or a nasogastric tube.
- All fascial defects larger than 5 mm are closed with a suture-passing device (Karl Storz) with 0-Vicryl sutures. The umbilical site is usually closed under direct vision with a no. 1 Prolene suture. Skin incisions are closed with subcuticular absorbable monofilament sutures.

III. ALTERNATIVE TECHNICAL APPROACHES (PRO/CON) AND PEARLS

- Although we prefer to use the circular stapler (CEEA 21) for construction of the duodenoileostomy, there are several alternatives:
  - ▲ Linear stapler (side-to-side anastomosis, 3.5-mm blue cartridge): Place one jaw of the linear stapler in the ileum, bring it up to the duodenum and place the second jaw into the duodenotomy, and

then fire the stapler. The enterotomy may be closed with a running suture. The downside of this approach is that a large enterotomy inevitably results, which needs to be closed primarily.
  - ▲ Hand-sewn technique—two layers, end-to-end or end-to-side: This has a difficult learning curve and is associated with the longest operative time.
  - ▲ Hand-assisted—through a small midline incision: This may be useful for surgeons early in their learning curve. However, this approach may provide fewer benefits (e.g., wound complications, analgesic requirements, postoperative recovery) compared to the completely laparoscopic approach.
- Originally, most surgeons avoided the circular stapler because of the difficulty experienced placing the anvil into position, especially when trying to pass the anvil through the pylorus (using the modified nasogastric-tube apparatus). We have adapted our technique to position the anvil via duodenotomy (followed by Prolene purse-string suture to secure the anvil in place), and this has significantly reduced our operative time.
- Alternate techniques for the ileoileostomy include hand-sewn (associated with longer operating times) and the double-stapled technique (biliopancreatic limb to common channel and closure of enterotomy). Our concern with the latter technique is that this may narrow the common channel during closure of the enterotomy, particularly because of the smaller-diameter ileum.
- The most critical factor that results in a leak at the duodenoileostomy is exaggerated tension at the anastomosis. Maneuvers to eliminate tension at the anastomosis include:
  - ▲ Division of the omentum needs along its right lateral aspect
  - ▲ Mobilization of the right colon
  - ▲ Division of blood vessels superior to the pylorus—one must be cautious, because this may compromise the blood supply to the anastomosis.
- We have not found retrocolic duodenoileostomy to be necessary. The foregoing maneuvers should ensure a tension-free anastomosis; moreover, we generally avoid retrocolic construction because of its association with increased incidence of internal hernias.
- The surgeon should always consider the two-stage approach in the high-risk superobese or in the patient who cannot tolerate prolonged pneumoperitoneum, who has extensive intraabdominal adhesions, or who lacks adequate working space despite higher pneumoperitoneum pressures. A two-stage approach (laparoscopic sleeve gastrectomy followed by completion duodenal switch 6 to 12 months later) has the advantages of technical facility, shorter operative times, and interval weight loss between stages, which in turn results in decreased morbidity in this high-risk group.

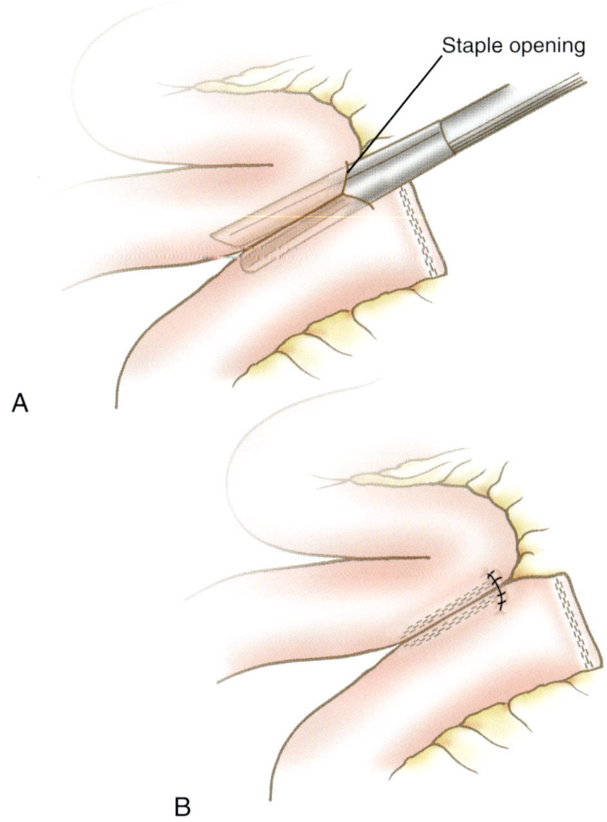

Figure 24-5.

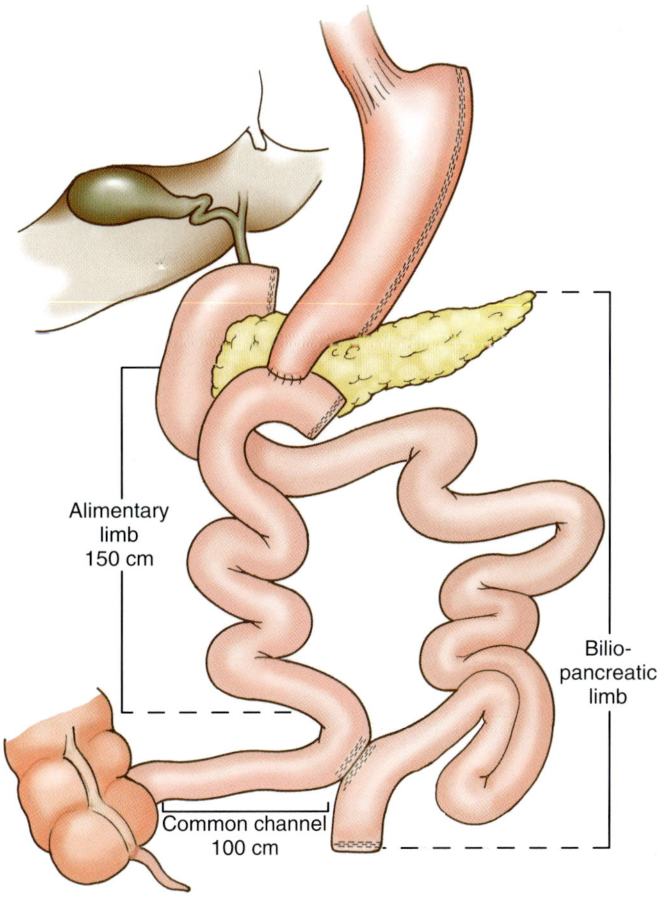

Figure 24-6.

- It is advisable to keep the total operative time to less than 4 hours to avoid the attendant risks (pulmonary, thromboembolic, and rhabdomyolysis) of prolonged general anesthesia, especially in the high-risk bariatric patient.

IV. SPECIAL POSTOPERATIVE CARE

- Patients are closely monitored for at least 6 hours.
- Patients are placed on continuous positive airway pressure if sleep apnea is present or suspected.
- Maintenance intravenous fluids are continued to ensure urine output of at least 0.5 to 1 mL/kg/hr.
- Early ambulation is critical—the majority of our patients ambulate the very evening of surgery.
- We use postoperative upper gastrointestinal contrast studies selectively:
  - In cases of any intraoperative technical difficulties (such as positive methylene blue test requiring additional sutures)
  - For patients who manifest signs and symptoms concerning for leak (e.g., fever greater than 38.5° C, tachycardia, tachypnea, somnolence, and failure to thrive)
- Patients usually require an intravenous patient-controlled analgesic pump for the first 2 days.
- Patients receive clear liquids on the first postoperative day. If they do well, their Foley catheters are removed and they are weaned off the intravenous fluids.
- Patients are advanced to a pureed diet the next day.
- Our nutritionist sees all patients postoperatively, and their dietary recommendations are reviewed.
- Patients are usually discharged home by the third postoperative day on a pureed diet and oral analgesics.
- Patients are seen 4 weeks after discharge. They receive follow-up nutritional counseling for a protein-enriched diet and are given twice-daily multivitamins, oral calcium supplements, iron, and fat-soluble vitamins.
- Patients with intact gallbladders are prescribed ursodiol 300 mg twice daily for 6 months for gallstone prophylaxis.
- At 3 months postoperatively, a thorough nutritional evaluation is performed, including serum levels of iron, ferritin, B_{12}, folate, albumin, parathyroid hormone, calcium, phosphorus, alkaline phosphatase, zinc, selenium, lipids, vitamins A and D, total protein, and hematology panels.

Intraoperative/Immediate/Late Complications

- The most dreaded complication is leakage either along the gastric staple line, the duodenoileostomy or the ileoileostomy. As with all bariatric procedures, the surgeon should reexplore if the patient manifests any signs of an anastomotic leak (e.g., tachycardia, fever, severe abdominal pain, or mental status changes). We currently routinely use a staple-line buttressing material (Bioabsorbable Seamguard) that has been shown to be safe and effective in reducing staple-line hemorrhage and leakage along the sleeve gastrectomy staple line. Routine intraoperative testing of the duodenoileostomy (with methylene blue) is also important to detect leakage that can be repaired at the time of the operation. Maneuvers to ensure a tension-free duodenoileostomy were described earlier.
- Although nutritional side effects exist with this procedure, they are significantly less compared to the biliopancreatic diversion alone. It is important that the common channel be at least 100 cm, because the incidence of significant nutritional side effects is much greater with a shorter common channel. For this reason, we routinely use umbilical tape to ensure accurate measurements of the common channel.
- All mesenteric defects must be completely closed to avoid internal hernias and their associated complications. We prefer to incorporate a superficial bite in the bowel serosa during the final closure stitch, because mesenteric closure alone may eventually (with loss of mesenteric fat) enlarge and lead to an internal hernia. One must completely close these defects, especially at the root of the mesentery, because a small defect may be even more susceptible to incarceration than the initially large patent defect.

SUGGESTED READINGS

Bellanger DE, Greenway FL: Laparoscopic sleeve gastrectomy, 529 cases without a leak: short-term results and technical considerations, *Obes Surg* 21:146–150, 2011.

Moy J, Pomp A, Dakin G, et al: Laparoscopic sleeve gastrectomy for morbid obesity, *Am J Surg* 196:e56–e59, 2008.

Søvik TT, Taha O, Aasheim ET, et al: Randomized clinical trial of laparoscopic gastric bypass versus laparoscopic duodenal switch for superobesity, *Br J Surg* 97:160–166, 2010.

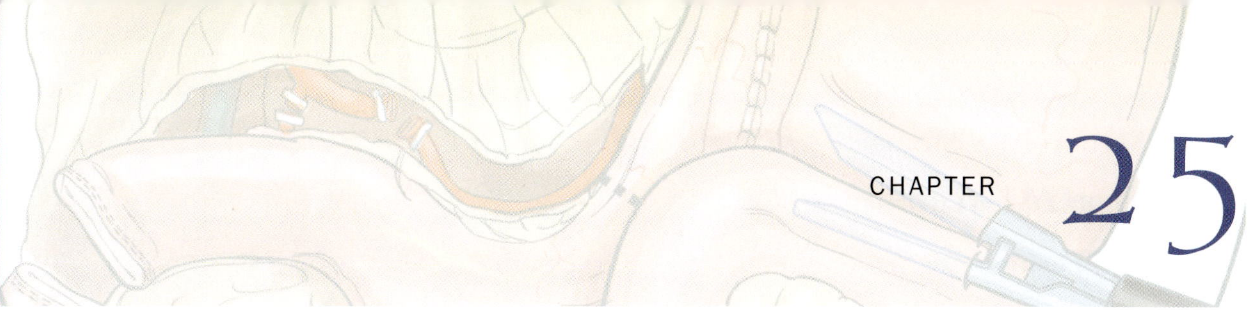

CHAPTER 25

Laparoscopic Nissen Fundoplication

Manish Parikh, MD, and Michel Gagner, MD, FRCSC, FACS

I. SPECIAL PREOPERATIVE PREPARATION

- Evaluation begins with a meticulous history and physical. A thorough inquiry into all medications taken, including nonprescription medications (nonsteroidal antiinflammatory drugs, iron, vitamins, etc.) is warranted. A patient history reporting the cessation of gastroesophageal reflux symptoms with acid suppression and conversely the return of symptoms with cessation of therapy confirms the clinical diagnosis of gastroesophageal reflux disease (GERD). Physical exam should focus on possible systemic causes of esophageal symptoms, such as scleroderma, collagen vascular diseases, and diabetic neuropathy.
- Barium esophagram is typically the first study obtained in patients with clinical GERD. This exam provides detailed anatomic evaluation and some functional assessment of esophageal peristalsis. It can also identify esophageal stricture, shortening, large hiatal hernias, and other factors that may affect the complexity of surgical repair.
- Routine esophagogastroduodenoscopy (EGD) is the primary tool to evaluate the esophageal and gastric mucosa for esophagitis and Barrett esophagus (and possible malignancy). It is important to ascertain the presence or absence of Barrett esophagus (by biopsy) before surgical treatment is undertaken. If Barrett esophagus with high-grade dysplasia is found, esophagectomy is indicated because up to 50% of these patients have underlying adenocarcinoma. EGD also helps delineate the anatomy in terms of esophageal length and size of hiatal hernia.
- Esophageal manometry provides an objective assessment of esophageal pressures, peristalsis of the esophageal body and coordination of muscular activity. It identifies the length, location, and pressure of the lower esophageal sphincter (LES). A motility abnormality seen on manometry warrants a partial fundoplication instead of a 360-degree wrap. Findings consistent with reflux include:
  - ▲ LES pressure less than 6 mm Hg (normal is 15 mm Hg)
  - ▲ LES overall length less than 2 cm
  - ▲ Intraabdominal length less than 1 cm
- 24-hour pH monitoring is still considered the gold standard to diagnose reflux disease, especially in those patients with atypical presentations of GERD. It is also useful to establish a record of the patient's pretreatment condition and compare this several months postoperatively to document control of acid reflux. The patient must be off H_2 blockers for at least 3 days and proton-pump inhibitors for at least 14 days before testing. Generally, this test is considered positive if the patient has more than 1.5 hours of pH less than 4 during the daytime, or any nocturnal evidence of pH less than 4.
- Gastric emptying studies (scintigraphy) are occasionally warranted in patients with significant nausea and vomiting, belching, early satiety, or those with severe insulin-dependent diabetes.
- The ideal GERD patient who presents for laparoscopic fundoplication is one whose preoperative workup reveals a small hiatal hernia (less than 5 cm), no GERD-related complications (stricture, Barrett esophagus), and a normal esophageal body and hypotensive LES on manometry.

II. OPERATIVE TECHNIQUE

Position

- See Figure 25-1.
- An Alphastar table (Maquet; Rastatt, Germany) with foot-plate attachments is used.
- A French, split-leg position is used, with the legs abducted, but not flexed, and properly secured.
- The surgeon stands between the patient's legs, the camera operator stands on the patient's right, and the second assistant stands on the patent's left.

Incision (Trocar Placement)

- A total of five trocars are used (Fig. 25-1):
  - ▲ A 10-mm trocar at the umbilicus (we prefer the open technique to enter the peritoneal cavity); diagnostic laparoscopy is then performed with the 10-mm, 30-degree laparoscope
  - ▲ A 10-mm port in the right subcostal position in the midclavicular line (liver retraction)
  - ▲ Two 5-mm ports: subxiphoid position (surgeon's left hand) and left anterior axillary line (second assistant)
- Occasionally, if the patient is obese, an additional 10-mm trocar can be placed in the left epigastric paramedian position for better optics.
- A second insufflator is attached to optimize pneumoperitoneum (15 mm Hg carbon dioxide). An orogastric tube is temporarily placed by the anesthesiologist to decompress the stomach.

Main Dissection

Hiatal Dissection and Mobilization of the Fundus

- The patient is placed in steep reverse Trendelenburg position to permit gravity to retract the abdominal contents inferiorly and expose the hiatus.
- The left lateral segment of the liver is retracted anteriorly and superiorly with a handheld liver retractor.

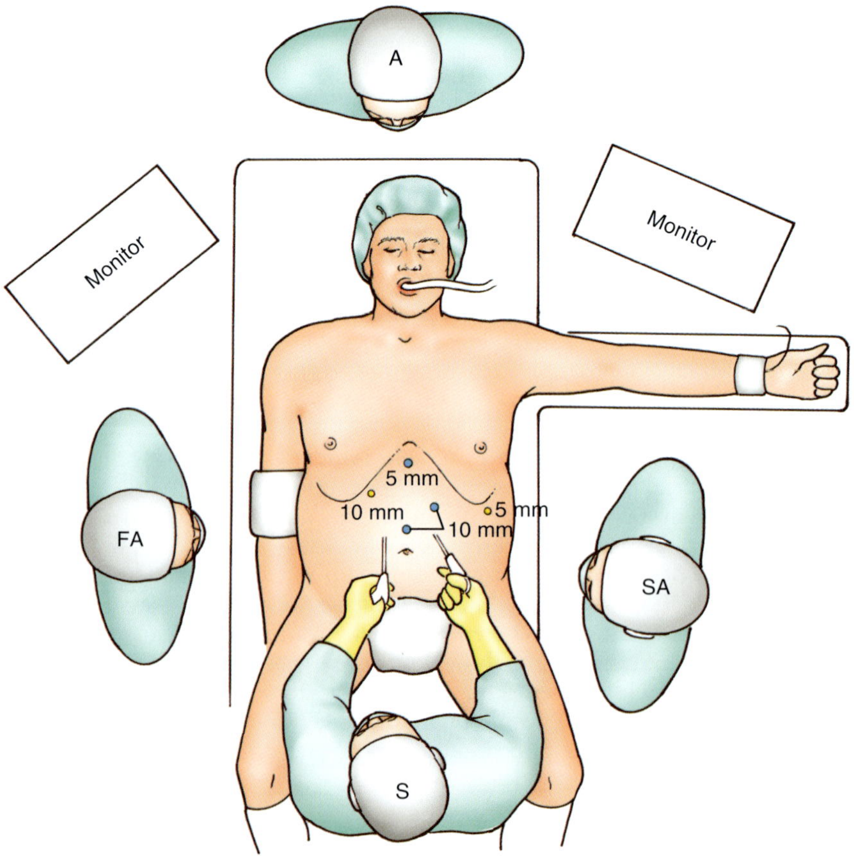

Figure 25-1. *A,* Anesthesiologist; *FA,* first assistant; *S,* surgeon; *SA,* second assistant.

- The second assistant's grasper is placed on the gastric cardia, and this is retracted inferiorly and to the left to place the gastrohepatic omentum on stretch. The transparent lesser omentum is incised just superior to the hepatic branch of the vagus nerve to expose (from right to left) the caudate lobe, right crus, esophageal hiatus, and, if present, hiatal hernia (Fig. 25-2, *A*). An aberrant left hepatic artery, which can be present in up to 20% of patients, should be preserved.
- The peritoneum over the right crus is incised with the hook electrocautery or ultrasonic scalpel. Mobilization of the medial edge of the crus is then carried out superiorly to the apex of the hiatus and inferiorly to the confluence of the right and left crura. A plane must be established between the right crus and the esophagus, taking care to preserve the vagus nerves with the esophagus. The surgeon's left instrument pushes the right crus laterally, and the right instrument gently sweeps the esophagus and periesophageal tissue to the left to bluntly mobilize the distal esophagus. The right (posterior) vagus should be identified and swept with the esophagus to the left.
- Inferiorly, the confluence of the right and left crura is exposed, allowing the early development of a posterior window behind the esophagus and stomach through which the fundoplication will subsequently be passed (see Fig. 25-2, *B*).

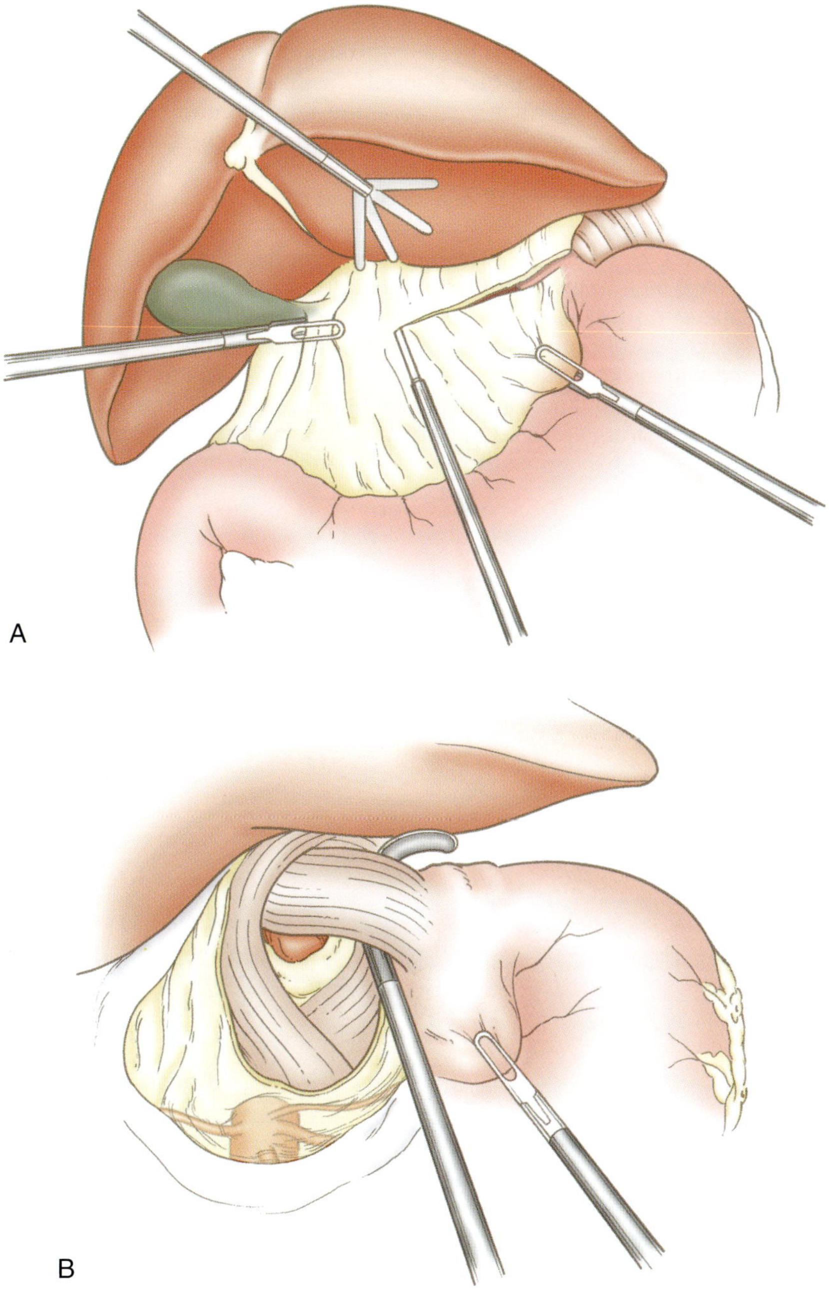

Figure 25-2.

- Dissection continues superiorly to the level of the anterior crural confluence. The phrenoesophageal ligament is divided. If a hiatal hernia is present, this must be reduced. The second assistant retracts the stomach to the right and inferiorly to better expose the left crus (posteromedial aspect). The left (anterior) vagus should be identified, because it often is intimately associated with the left crus and can be injured during this time. Exposure of the inferior aspect of the left crus is difficult because the left crus curves behind the esophagus. Complete exposure of the left crus is often facilitated by first mobilizing the gastric fundus.
- An area along the proximal greater curvature is chosen for entry into the lesser sac, usually 10 to 15 cm inferior to the angle of His. The branches of the gastroepiploic artery near the gastric wall are divided with the ultrasonic scalpel. The short gastric vessels are dissected and divided with the ultrasonic scalpel until the left crus is exposed. The second assistant's grasper is frequently repositioned superiorly to maximize retraction. Division of the most superior short gastric vessel exposes the peritoneum over the left crus. Division of this peritoneum causes the spleen to fall away from the operative field and now allows mobilization of the inferior aspect of the left crus.
- The posterior window behind the distal esophagus and proximal stomach is completed by dividing all attachments between the esophagus and the inferior crural confluence. With the stomach retracted toward the left and inferiorly, place a 7-inch-long, ¼-inch wide Penrose drain through the posterior window (Fig. 25-3). Both ends of the Penrose are grasped, and a clip is applied. The second assistant then holds the Penrose drain to provide better esophageal retraction while the posterior window is widened.
- The esophagus is mobilized to increase the intraabdominal esophageal length by dividing its attachments in the posterior mediastinum as cranially as possible. Use the Penrose drain to optimize exposure posteriorly and laterally. The esophagus is freed in this manner from the pleura, aorta, and lateral crural attachments. Dissecting laterally in the hiatus should be avoided because of the risk of breaching the pleura. If the pleural space is inadvertently entered, the surgeon must communicate with the anesthesiologist to monitor airway pressures and ventilation. Generally, chest tubes are not necessary.

Crural Approximation

- There should be at least 2 to 3 cm of intraabdominal esophagus present once traction is released. If not, further esophageal mobilization within the mediastinum or an esophageal lengthening procedure (e.g., Collis gastroplasty) is necessary.
- Gentle traction on the Penrose drain anteriorly and to the left exposes the hiatus. A posterior crural repair is performed with several interrupted figure-of-eight 2-0 Ticron sutures (Sherwood-Davis and Geck, St. Louis). Intracorporeal knots are preferred because they minimize crural tension and traction and prevent splitting or tearing of the crura during approximation. The crura are reapproximated until a 5-mm instrument fits snugly between the last crural stitch and the esophagus (see Fig. 25-3). Failure to adequately close the hiatus may result in transthoracic migration of the fundoplication.

Creation of the Floppy Fundoplication

- The mobilized gastric fundus is placed near the left crus.
- With the second assistant retracting the Penrose anteriorly, an atraumatic grasper is passed through the posterior window. The fundus is gently grasped and delivered through the window and placed to the right of the esophagus (Fig. 25-4). Any bluish discoloration of the fundus indicates that the

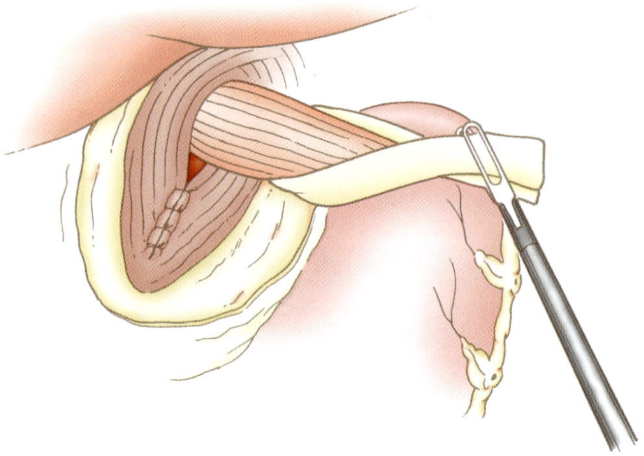

Figure 25-3.

retroesophageal space is too narrow and further dissection is needed. Both the anterior and posterior fundus should be manipulated to ensure that it envelops the esophagus without twisting ("the shoe-shine maneuver"; see Fig. 25-4). The wrapped fundus is then released. If it retracts, more fundic attachments need to be divided to eliminate this tension. Insufficient mobilization of the fundus will lead to a tight or twisted fundoplication. The Penrose drain is removed.

- The esophagogastric fat pad on the anterior esophageal wall is removed to allow a clear area for placement of the fundoplication. The anterior vagus nerve should be avoided (the cleared area should be to the right of the midline).
- The first suture is the lowest suture, ensuring that the fundoplication is constructed on the distal esophagus and not the cardia of the stomach. We prefer Ticron sutures because we have experienced dissolution of silk sutures. A 2-0 Ticron seromuscular suture is placed through the fundus to the left of the esophagus. This stitch is then positioned 5 to 10 mm above the esophagogastric junction, passing through the anterior wall of the esophagus. Although ideally the bite must pass through the inner circular layer of muscle, it is important that the suture not breach the lumen. Finally, this suture passes through the fundus to the right of the esophagus, and then the knot is tied with minimal traction on the esophagus or stomach (Fig. 25-5). An identical suture is placed 8 to 10 mm superior to this suture. A third and final suture is placed 8 to 10 mm superior to the second suture. Ideally all bites try to incorporate the esophagus, although sometimes this is not possible depending on the path of the

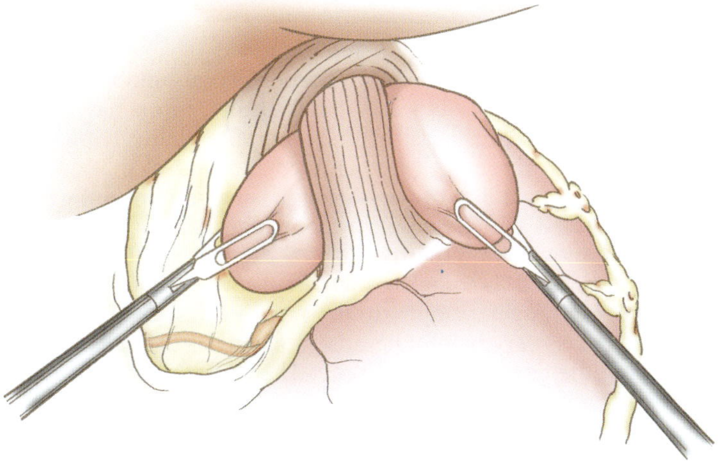

Figure 25-4.

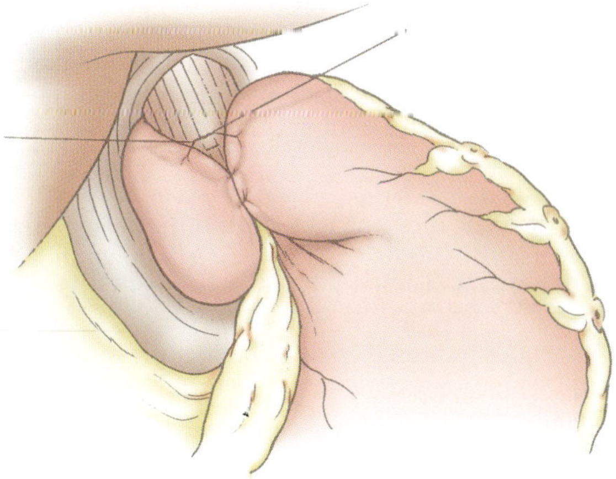

Figure 25-5.

anterior vagus nerve. Inspection of the fundoplication should confirm that it is loose, approximately 2 cm in length, and rests in the abdomen without any tension (see Fig. 25-5).

Closure

- The right subcostal trocar site is closed with a 0-vicryl figure-of-eight suture via the suture-passing device (Karl Storz, Tuttlingen, Germany). The umbilical port is closed under direct vision with a no. 1 Prolene suture. Skin incisions are closed with subcuticular absorbable monofilament sutures.

III. ALTERNATIVE TECHNICAL APPROACHES (PRO/CON) AND PEARLS

- Some surgeons prefer to not routinely divide the short gastric vessels (Nissen-Rosetti modification). With this modification, the gastric fundus is not completely mobilized. Thus the fundoplication is constructed with the anterior gastric wall only (and not the anterior and posterior walls as with conventional Nissen fundoplication). Advantages include shorter operative time and potentially decreased bleeding. Disadvantages include possibly increased rotational tension and less experience with division of short gastric vessels if not done routinely. Also, most surgeons believe that the rate of persistent dysphagia is less with routine division of the short gastric vessels. Especially for the short "floppy" fundoplication, we advocate routine division of the short gastric vessels, full mobilization of the posterior aspect of the fundus, and division of posterior adhesions to the left crus and pancreas. Division of these attachments decreases the rotational stress or tension of the fundoplication and long-term failure rate.
- In patients with inadequate esophageal motility (amplitude less than 45 mm Hg), a partial fundoplication (270-degree Toupet) is indicated. This is a posterior partial fundoplication, 3 to 4 cm long, constructed via six interrupted sutures. The first 2-0 Ticron suture approximates the right lateral esophageal wall 3 to 4 cm superior to the esophagogastric junction to the fundus lying to the right of the esophagus. This suture is also passed through the superomedial aspect of the right crus before it is tied. A second suture is placed 1 to 2 cm inferiorly between the lateral esophageal wall and the gastric fundus. The final third suture is placed 1 to 2 cm below the second suture (5 mm superior to the esophagogastric junction), again approximating the right lateral esophageal wall and fundus. On the left side, three identical sutures are placed to complete the partial fundoplication.
- The periesophageal dissection is where injury to the vagus nerves commonly occurs. Placing a Penrose drain around the esophagus is very helpful because it facilitates dissection of the posterior esophagus and allows direct view of the retroesophageal space. The fat pad at the gastroesophageal junction is a good retractor. Another useful tool is intraoperative endoscopy. The light from the endoscope can maintain identification of the esophagus at all times during a difficult hiatal dissection. Intraoperative endoscopy also allows assessment of the esophagus and stomach to exclude perforation or to evaluate the fundoplication.
- An alternate sequence of dissection, especially useful for the surgeon early in his or her learning curve, is to take down the short gastric vessels first and proceed superiorly along the fundus to the left crus. This way, one is less likely to dissect into the esophagus.
- Pledgets are sometimes required for a more secure crural closure, especially if the tissue is very attenuated. Some surgeons advocate mesh reinforcement, particularly for a large hiatal defect. Long-term data, especially regarding the risk of erosion, are still pending. Transdiaphragmatic herniation of the fundoplication usually occurs posteriorly, where there are few adhesions anchoring the fundoplication to the crura. For this reason, some surgeons place a suture between the fundoplication and the crura. The key technical points to minimize this complication are:
  - ▲ Extensive esophageal mobilization.
  - ▲ Secure diaphragmatic closure.
  - ▲ Esophageal lengthening (if 3 cm of esophagus does not remain intraabdominal in a tension-free manner). Most can be managed with extensive transmediastinal mobilization of the esophagus (to the level of the aortic arch). The remainder requires a formal lengthening procedure (such as a Collis gastroplasty).
  - ▲ Avoidance of events leading to increased intraabdominal pressure (retching, coughing, straining to lift/urinate/defecate, etc.). Thus, it is important to treat nausea aggressively and to use Foley catheters and stool softeners liberally.

IV. SPECIAL POSTOPERATIVE CARE

- Patients are closely monitored for at least 4 hours. Nasogastric tubes are not necessary for most uncomplicated operations. Patients usually require an intravenous patient-controlled analgesic pump for the first 24 hours. Standing intravenous antiemetics (metoclopramide 10 mg three times daily; ondansetron) are used to prevent dry heaving or retching, which may disrupt the fundoplication. It is important to do everything possible to avoid dry heaving or vomiting, because failures are correlated with early postoperative vomiting and other diaphragmatic stressors (dry heaving or retching).

- It is not uncommon for a patient to exhibit cervical and mediastinal emphysema. Usually observation alone is adequate. For the patient with a pneumothorax, observation is adequate; chest tubes are rarely required.
- Patients receive clear liquids on the first postoperative day. If they tolerate clear liquids and their pain is well controlled with crushed or liquid pain medications, they can be discharged home on a pureed diet for the following 2 weeks. The patient receives dietary instructions, including eating multiple small meals; chewing thoroughly; and avoiding high-fat foods, excessive caffeine, alcohol, and carbonated beverages.
- Upper gastrointestinal contrast studies are used selectively—for patients who have severe abdominal pain or who vomit early.
- For the asymptomatic patient, symptom follow-up evaluation is adequate, and routine physiologic testing is unnecessary. However, routine postoperative pH testing should be performed in patients with continuing or recurrent reflux symptoms and should be considered in patients with Barrett esophagus. Routine endoscopy with biopsy should be performed in patients with known Barrett esophagus as well.

SUGGESTED READINGS

Broeders JA, Rijnhart-de Jong HG, Draaisma WA, et al: Ten-year outcome of laparoscopic and conventional Nissen fundoplication: randomized clinical trial, *Ann Surg* 25:698–706, 2009.

Rice TW, Gagner M: Laparoscopic antireflux surgery, *Semin Thorac Cardiovasc Surg* 9:173–187, 1997. Review.

Stylopoulos N, Rattner DW: The history of hiatal hernia surgery: from Bowditch to laparoscopy, *Ann Surg* 241:185–193, 2005. Review.

CHAPTER 26

Laparoscopic Paraesophageal Hernia Repair

Helen J. Sohn, MD, and Namir Katkhouda, MD, FACS

I. SPECIAL PREOPERATIVE PREPARATION

- Contrast swallow study is used to diagnose a patient with suspicion of paraesophageal hernia. In addition to providing the diagnosis, it provides important anatomical information needed for surgical consideration such as the size of the herniation, location of the gastroesophageal junction, and esophageal motility and length (Fig. 26-1).
- Upper endoscopy is necessary to evaluate intraluminal pathology. Esophageal mucosa should be examined for columnarization of the epithelium, ulcerations, or strictures from repeated episodes of acid reflux. Stomach can exhibit signs of chronic pressure at the level of the hiatus such as ulcerations, erosions, and ischemia.
- Esophageal manometry and pH analyses are used in evaluating patients with reflux symptoms. Herniation of the stomach and/or gastroesophageal junction can make placement of the catheter difficult, and it should be placed under endoscopic guidance.
- Cardiopulmonary status of the patient should be carefully examined. Patients with paraesophageal hernia are often elderly and tend to be high-risk operative candidates. Asymptomatic or minimally symptomatic patients with poor cardiopulmonary status should be managed expectantly. On the other hand, compromised pulmonary status due to repeated aspiration episodes should prompt surgical repair of the paraesophageal hernia.

II. OPERATIVE TECHNIQUE

Position

- Low lithotomy position allows the operating surgeon to stand between the legs.
- The patient should be in steep reverse Trendelenburg position to aid in the exposure of the hiatus and mediastinum. It is prudent to securely fasten the patient to prevent slipping during positioning.

Incision

- See Figure 26-2.
- Standard five-port laparoscopic Nissen fundoplication incisions include following:
  - ▲ A 10- to 12-mm midline camera port is placed one third of the way between the umbilicus and xiphoid process. The next four ports are placed after adequate insufflation of the abdominal cavity.
  - ▲ Right and left subcostal operating ports are placed in the midclavicular line. The left-sided port should be 10 mm to accommodate suture passage.
  - ▲ A left lateral 5-mm port is placed for the retracting assistant.
  - ▲ A subxiphoid liver retractor port is placed. A Nathanson liver retractor is inserted in place of a 5-mm trocar and attached to a self retainer after proper positioning.

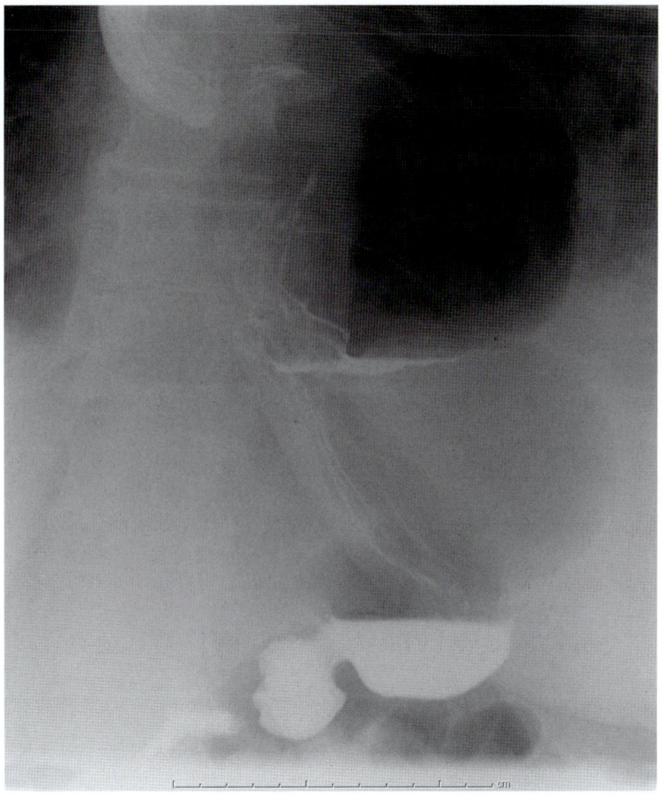

Figure 26-1.

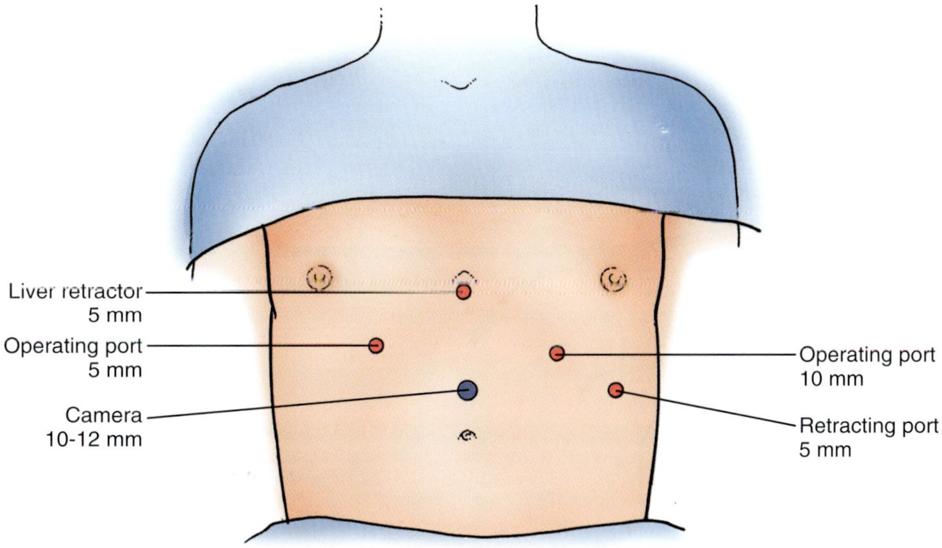

Figure 26-2.

Main Dissection

- Reduction of the hernia sac is the first of four main aspects of the procedure. The hernia sac is located anterior to the passage of the esophagus through the hiatus. After reduction of the herniated stomach (Fig. 26-3), the sac is incised along the medial border of the right crus and is bluntly reflected off of its mediastinal attachments. The incision on the hernia sac is carried out anteriorly and toward the left crus, which is followed until the hernia sac is attached only at the gastroesophageal junction. Note that the stomach may not stay reduced until the sac is completely reduced.
- Mediastinal dissection is important in mobilizing the esophagus to gain the maximum length to ensure that the gastroesophageal junction remains intraabdominal. Penrose placed around the distal esophagus can aid in retraction without undue trauma (Fig. 26-4). Care should be exercised to avoid injury to the vagus nerves and the pleura as well as the esophagus.
- The hernia sac can then be excised after being fully reduced from the mediastinum to help better identify gastroesophageal junction and to minimize hernia recurrence. Again, care should be exercised to avoid injuring the vagus nerve.
- Approximation of the crural defect is the next step. Heavy nonabsorbable suture such as 1-0 Ethibond should be used to approximate the left and right crus posteriorly, starting at the desiccation. It is very important to obtain enough width of the muscle and the overlying fascia without strangulating the muscle or putting undue tension on the repair itself (see Fig. 26-4, *A* and *B*).

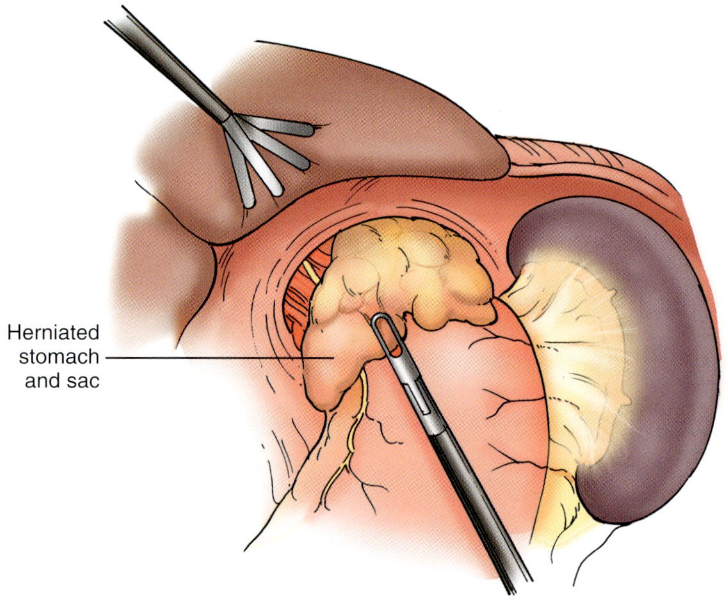

Figure 26-3.

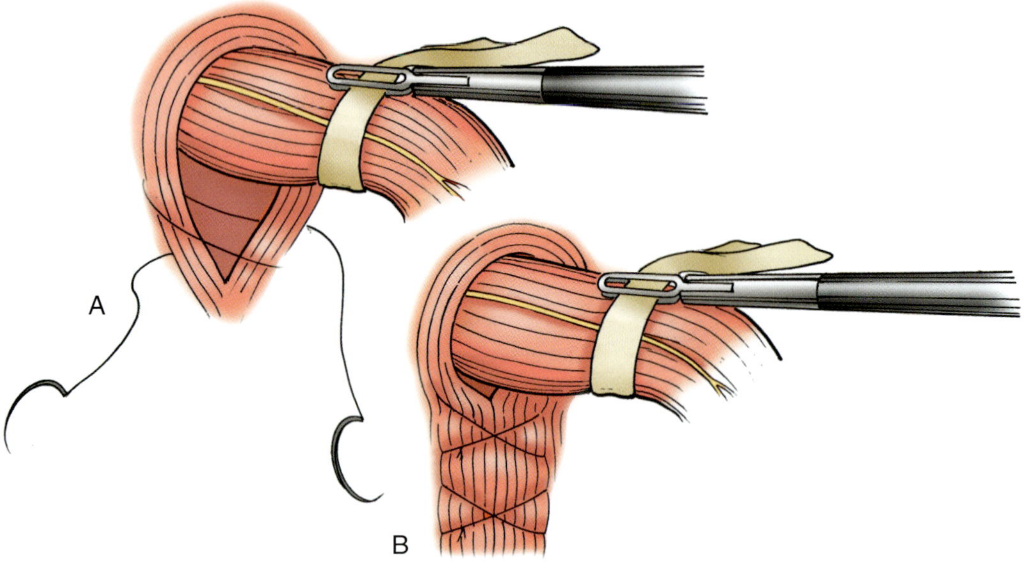

Figure 26-4.

- The procedure should be concluded with a full or partial fundoplication. The posterior fundus is freed and passed behind the isolated intraabdominal esophagus; if necessary, some of the short gastric vessels are divided (Fig. 26-5). This is done not only to prevent a high rate of symptomatic postoperative reflux but also to anchor the gastroesophageal junction below the diaphragm. The full wrap should be done floppy over a 60-Fr bougie to avoid postoperative dysphagia (Fig. 26-6). Preoperative esophageal manometry is useful in determining whether a partial or a full fundoplication may be tolerated.

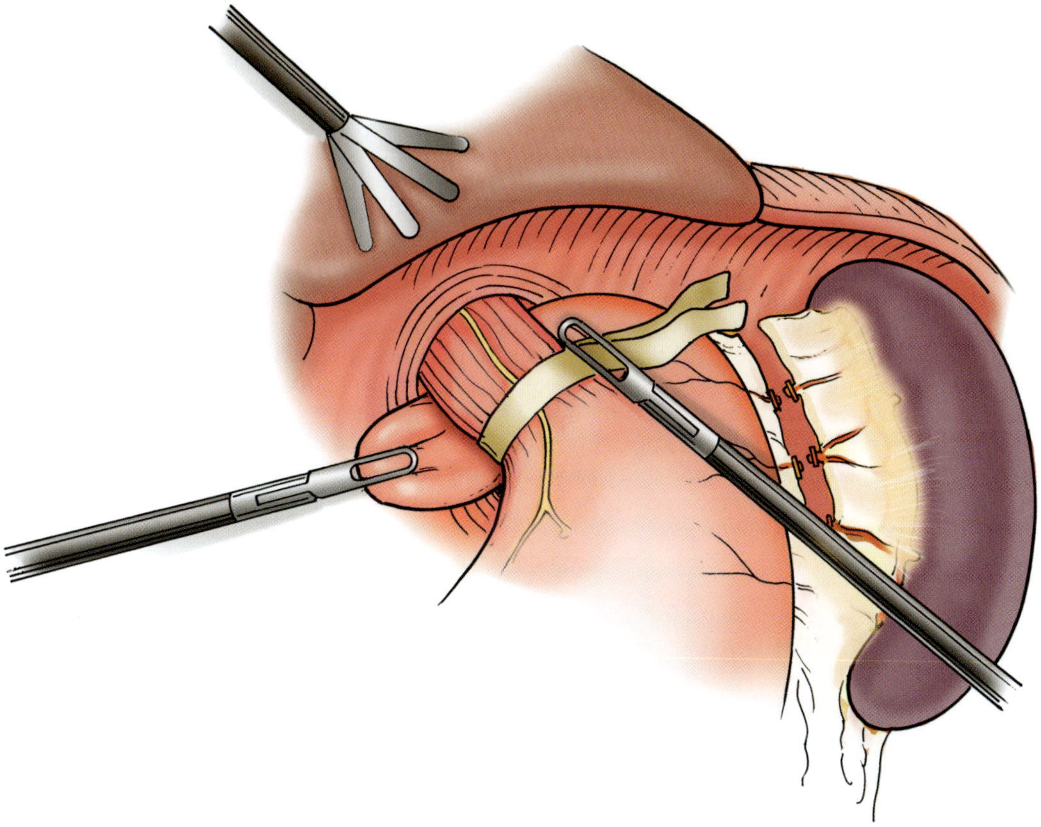

Figure 26-5.

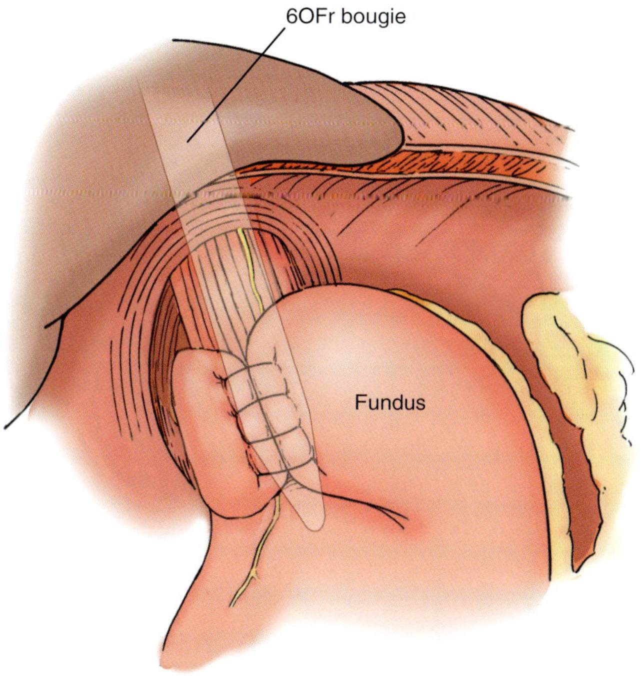

Figure 26-6.

Closure

- Port sites larger than 10 mm should be closed at the fascial level. All other sites are closed at the skin level.

III. ALTERNATIVE TECHNICAL APPROACHES (PROS/CONS) AND PEARLS

- The open versus laparoscopic approaches have been compared. The laparoscopic approach has been found to have less morbidity and mortality and a shorter hospital stay, as well as shorter time to recovery. A transthoracic approach should be considered when esophageal shortening is suspected to gain access to the level of the aortic arch for complete esophageal mobilization.
- Synthetic or biologic mesh has been used to obtain tension-free crural closure, and recent reports state reduced recurrence rates with the use of mesh. But fear of esophageal erosion and stricture have steered most surgeons away from using any type of mesh at the hiatus. With low recurrence rates achieved by obtaining the maximal esophageal length via extensive mediastinal dissection and anchoring achieved by a wrap, mesh onlay should be reserved for massive hiatal defects or extremely poor underlying tissue.
- Gastropexy and gastrostomy have been used to anchor the stomach intraabdominally so as to minimize recurrence. Gastrostomy may be useful in patients who need supplemental nutritional support postoperatively. Fundoplication achieves a similar anchoring effect with an added antireflux benefit.
- Full versus partial fundoplication is another heated controversy in paraesophageal hernia repair. The full wrap can produce greater dysphagia, especially in patients with poor esophageal motility that is difficult to determine preoperatively because of the obstructive nature of the hernia. The partial wrap has not been proved to be as good as the full wrap in preventing long-term reflux. The partial wrap should be considered only in patients with poor esophageal motility.
- The need for an esophageal lengthening procedure cannot be accurately determined preoperatively. It should be contemplated intraoperatively only after maximum esophageal length has been obtained via appropriate mediastinal dissection. Collis-Nissen gastroplasty can then be done laparoscopically by performing a stapled wedge fundectomy and creating the wrap over the staple line.

IV. SPECIAL POSTOPERATIVE CARE

- A routine intraabdominal or nasogastric drain is not used.
- A contrast swallow study should be done on postoperative day 1.
- Port-site hernia should be suspected in any patient with bowel obstruction after a laparoscopic procedure.
- Postoperative dysphagia or heartburn symptoms can occur from edema around the gastroesophageal junction. Symptoms that do not resolve with time should prompt further investigation.

SUGGESTED READINGS

Lal DR, Pellegrini CA, Oelschlager BK: Laparoscopic repair of paraesophageal hernia, *Surg Clin North Am* 85:105–118, 2005.
Rosen MJ, Ponsky JL: Laparoscopic paraesophageal hernia repair, *Oper Tech Gen Surg* 8:127–135, 2006.
Stylopoulos N, Rattner DW: The history of hiatal hernia surgery from Bowditch to laparoscopy, *Ann Surg* 241:185–193, 2005.

SECTION V

Pancreas

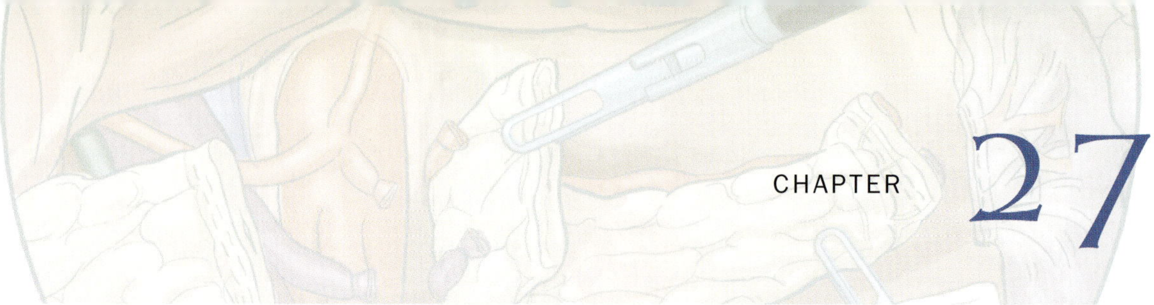

CHAPTER 27

Pancreaticoduodenectomy with or without Distal Gastrectomy and Radical Lymphadenectomy

Ernest L. Rosato, MD, and Charles J. Yeo, MD

I. SPECIAL PREOPERATIVE PREPARATION

- Preoperative preparation begins at the time of initial office evaluation. All patients are educated regarding a critical pathway (Fig. 27-1) designed to improve patient safety and reduce perioperative morbidity, mortality, and length of stay. The operative procedure is reviewed in detail. The postoperative care plan is outlined for the patient. We target an intended discharge date of postoperative day 6 or 7 following the Whipple resection.
- Three-dimensional computed tomography (CT) has evolved as the predominant modality for diagnosis and preoperative staging of periampullary malignancies before Whipple resection (Fig. 27-2). It generates detailed, volume-rendered CT data that are processed and displayed in three dimensions. This allows for enhanced assessment of vascular invasion of both the arterial and venous system by periampullary malignancies (Figs. 27-3 and 27-4). It also detects mesenteric venous thromboses, arterial anatomic variations, and arterial stenoses that may influence operative planning. Last, it can detect metastatic solid organ and peritoneal implants of 1 cm or greater diameter.
- Magnetic resonance imaging (MRI) is an effective tool for diagnosing and staging periampullary malignancies, which we use selectively. It is particularly useful in patients who have intravenous contrast allergy or chronic renal insufficiency and in whom the use of standard CT scan vascular contrast could be problematic. MRI may be more sensitive in the diagnosis of liver metastases. T1-weighted images of the pancreas can detect and better characterize equivocal pancreatic lesions when CT scan has been unable to definitely diagnose a parenchymal abnormality.
- Endoscopic ultrasound uses an ultrasound probe, endoscopically directed through the sweep of the duodenum and proximal antrum. This allows for direct ultrasound imaging of the periampullary region through the wall of the antrum and the first, second, and third portions of the duodenum. It offers

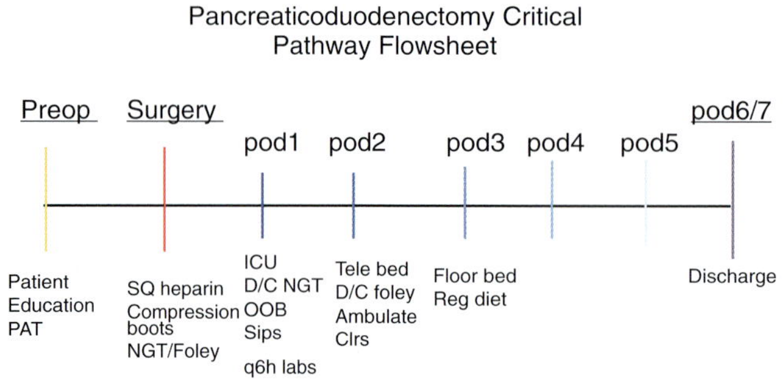

Figure 27-1. *pod,* Postoperative day.

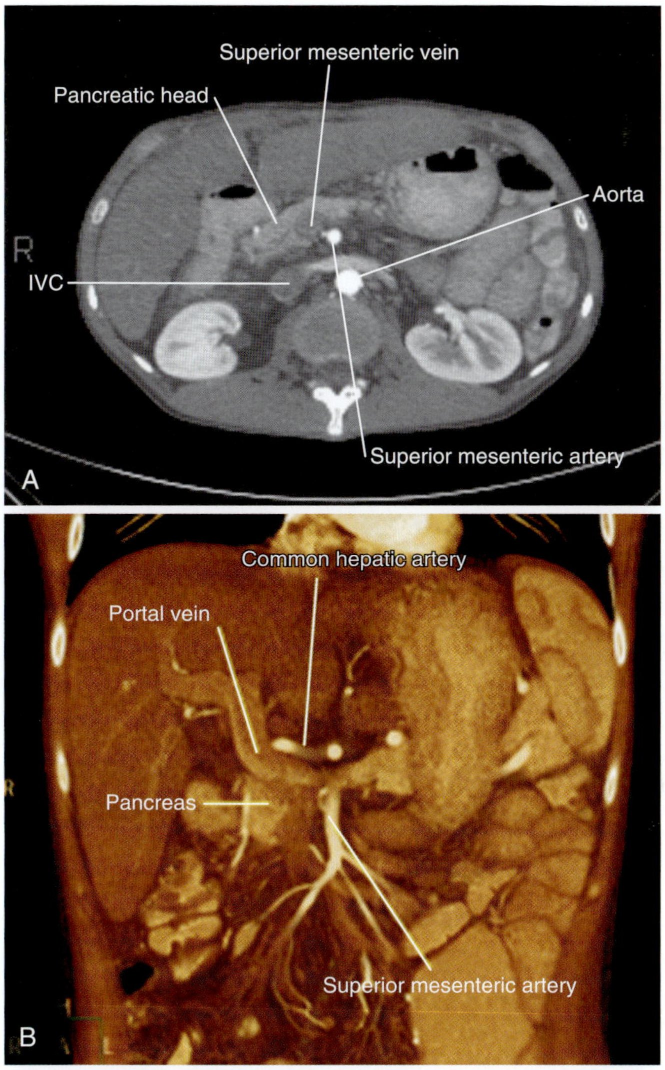

Figure 27-2. **A**, Axial CT image illustrating the normal anatomy of the pancreas and surrounding mesenteric vasculature. **B**, Normal coronal view of the pancreas and surrounding vascular structures. *IVC,* Inferior vena cava.

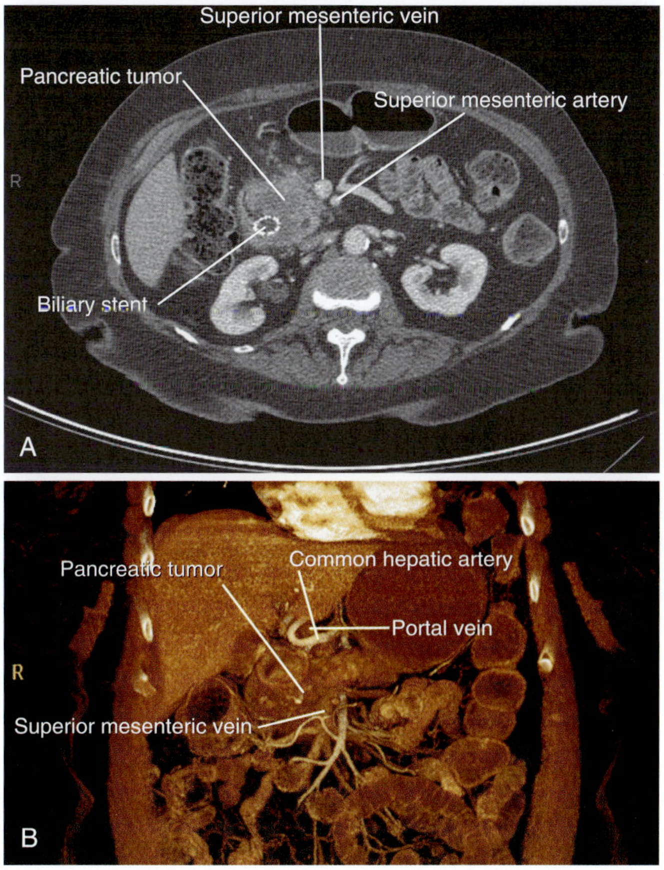

Figure 27-3. Axial image of a resectable pancreatic carcinoma (**A**) and a coronal view of the same pancreatic head neoplasm (**B**). Note the clean plane between the tumor and the mesenteric vein and artery as well as the absence of metastatic spread.

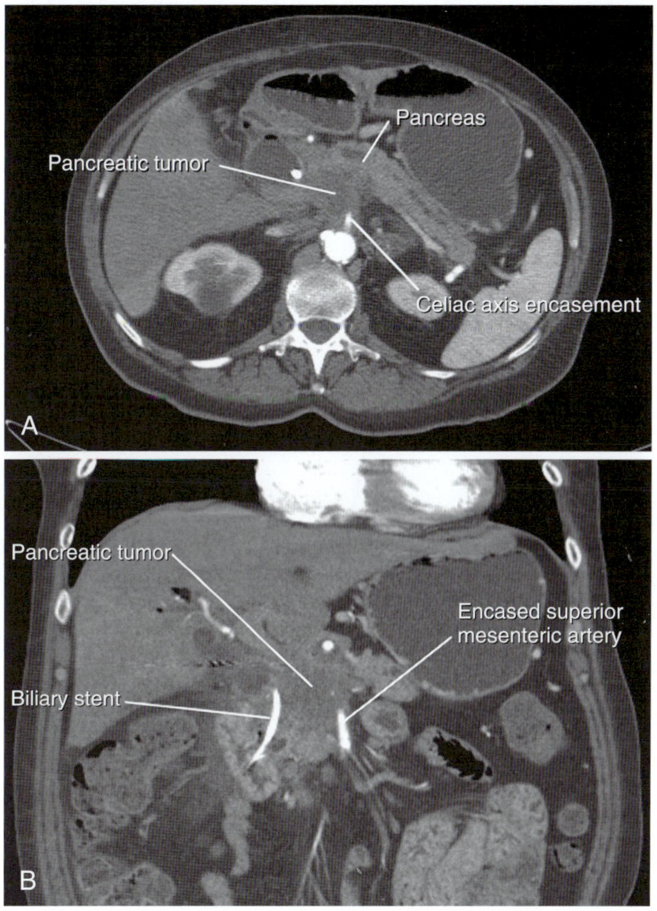

Figure 27-4. **A**, Axial image of a locally advanced unresectable pancreatic head carcinoma. The celiac axis is encased. **B**, The coronal view shows the superior mesenteric artery encased by tumor.

greater sensitivity than CT scan or MRI for detecting small periampullary neoplasms. Lesions as small as 5 mm can be reliably detected with this technology. Endoscopic ultrasound enables local examination of the vascular structures and surrounding lymph nodes and, when combined with ultrasound-guided fine-needle aspiration (FNA), can provide tissue sampling of the primary tumor and surrounding lymph nodes. This technique is very user dependent and requires skilled application and interpretation of the ultrasound images for reliable results. Additionally, in most cases, positive or negative results from the FNA do not alter the decision to offer resection.

- Positron emission tomography scan uses a radiolabeled glucose molecule ([18F] fluorodeoxyglucose) that is preferentially metabolized by the rapidly dividing tumor cells. This gives an image of functional tumor burden. It can be fused with CT scan images to give coarse anatomic and functional tumor staging details. It is not currently the standard of care for staging periampullary malignancies.
- Preoperative tissue diagnosis by FNA is neither required nor pursued in those patients who are considered candidates for pancreatic resection.

II. OPERATIVE TECHNIQUE

- The following text outlines the standard steps performed during pancreaticoduodenectomy at our institution. It is important to remember that the order of the steps can be changed as needed to facilitate safe exposure and removal of pancreatic head, neck, and uncinate neoplasms.

Position

- The patient is placed in the supine position. Pneumatic compression boots and subcutaneous heparin are administered before the induction of anesthesia. Prophylactic intravenous antibiotics are administered within 1 hour of the incision. The abdomen is clipped (hair removal) and prepped from nipples to pubis. If there is concern for vascular resection during the procedure, the left neck and bilateral upper legs and groin are shaved and prepped so as to facilitate access to the internal jugular vein and saphenous vein, respectively.

Incision

- A standard midline incision (Fig. 27-5) is used to gain access to the abdomen. This typically extends from the xiphoid to the lower abdomen and allows for complete examination of the peritoneal cavity and exposure of the root of the mesentery if vascular reconstruction is necessary.
- Alternatively, an extended right subcostal incision can be used. This may facilitate exposure of the right upper quadrant and pancreatic head regions in patients who have a short trunk or are morbidly obese. We use this incision infrequently because of its discomfort and the need to divide muscle, nerves, and blood vessels.

Main Dissection

- A complete abdominal exploration is performed to rule out peritoneal and solid organ metastases. The liver surfaces should be palpated anteriorly and posteriorly. The small and large bowel are examined

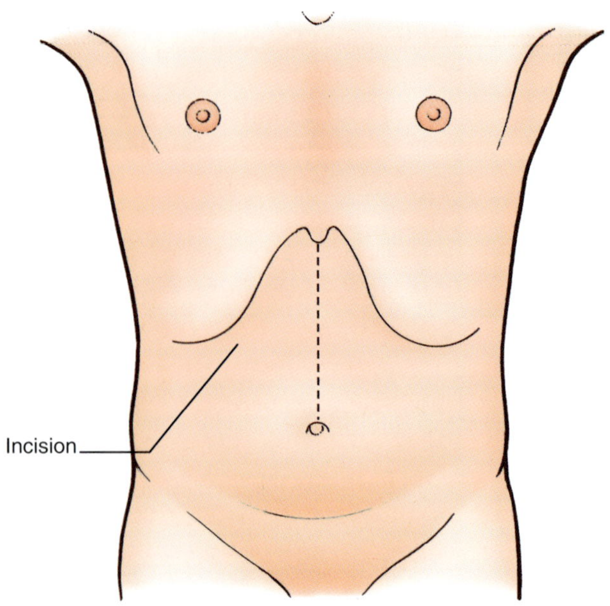

Figure 27-5.

in sequence from the ligament of Treitz to the rectum. The mesentery and peritoneal surfaces are examined for nodal enlargement and peritoneal implants. The periumbilical and round ligament surfaces should be palpated for tumor implants. Last, the root of the mesentery should be evaluated for any suspicious lymphadenopathy in the area of the proximal jejunum. Suspicious lesions outside of the resection zone should be sampled for frozen-section examination to rule out distant spread.

- The celiac axis and gastrocolic ligament are examined to rule out metastatic adenopathy. The periportal and hilar lymph nodes are examined.
- An extensive Kocher maneuver is performed by lifting the duodenum from the retroperitoneum and elevating the head of the pancreas with its neoplastic process from the underlying vena cava. The uncinate process is elevated out of the retroperitoneum, and the superior mesenteric artery is palpated and confirmed to be free of tumor involvement (Fig. 27-6). Of note, careful review of the CT images usually defines the extent of vascular involvement better than direct palpation at this point in the procedure.
- The porta hepatis is assessed by first taking the gallbladder down from fundus to infundibulum with ligation of the cystic artery and cystic duct. This exposes the lateral border of the common bile duct. The common hepatic artery and gastroduodenal artery junction are identified, as is the proper hepatic artery. Either the common bile duct or the common hepatic duct is cleared of overlying tissue, carefully encircled with a vessel loop, elevated, and divided (Fig. 27-7). This exposes the anterior surface of the portal vein, which can be traced down to the neck of the pancreatic gland. Palpation posterior and lateral to the common bile duct will identify a replaced right hepatic artery—an important variant to recognize before division of the bile duct. A temporary occlusion of the gastroduodenal artery is performed to ensure that good flow remains in the common hepatic and particularly the proper hepatic arteries, signifying a widely patent celiac axis. A bulldog clamp is applied to the proximal hepatic duct to control bile outflow. Early division of the common hepatic duct facilitates dissection of the anterior and lateral wall of the portal vein and untethers the head of the pancreas to allow for safe caudal dissection in the retropancreatic tunnel.
- The anterior and lateral aspects of the portal vein are dissected under direct vision from the overlying pancreatic neck and head region containing the neoplasm (see Fig. 27-6). Alternatively, the lesser sac can be opened and the mesenteric vein identified by tracing the duodenum around to its third portion where the lateral wall of the vein is identified as it issues from under the neck of the pancreas and over the third portion of the duodenum. The superior mesenteric vein also can be identified by tracing the right gastroepiploic vein and the middle colic vein down to the anterior surface of the retroperitoneum, where they form a common trunk that enters the superior mesenteric vein just inferior to the neck of the pancreatic gland. The superior mesenteric vein can be carefully cleared of its overlying peritoneal covering. Under direct vision, dissection is continued cephalad along the surface of the mesenteric vein and under the neck of the pancreas to allow for safe separation of the overlying pancreas and tumor-bearing head.

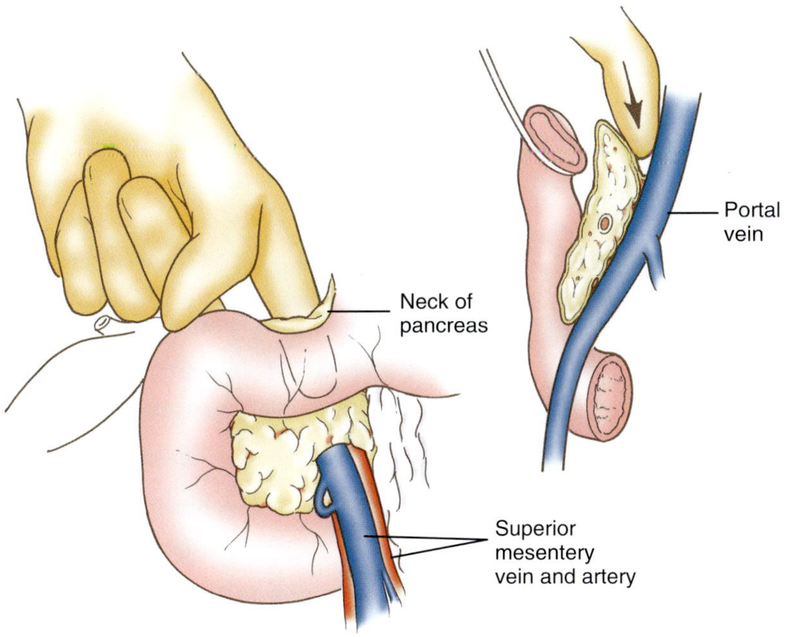

Figure 27-6.

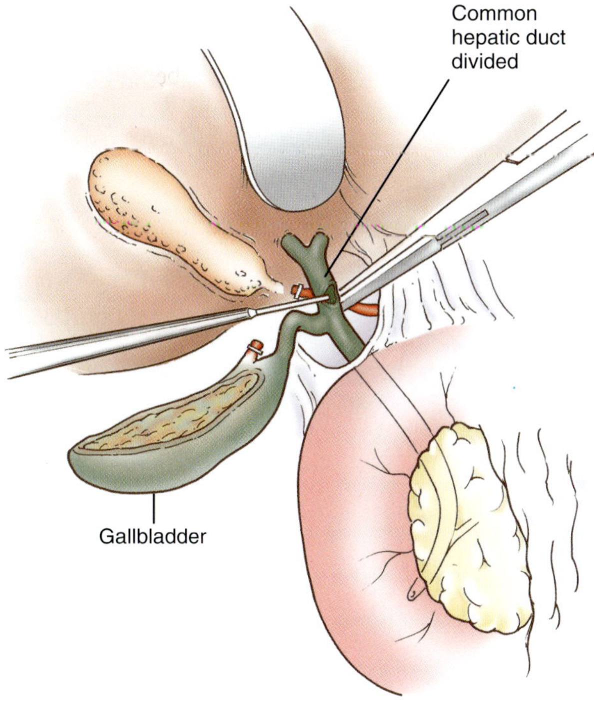

Figure 27-7.

- Once resectability is confirmed, the gastroduodenal artery is divided between 0-silk ties complimented by 2-0 silk suture ligatures (Fig. 27-8, *A*). If pylorus preservation is planned, the gastrohepatic ligament is divided with electrocautery. Vascular and lymphatic bundles are secured between 2-0 silk ties and divided sharply. Dissection is continued along the superior aspect of duodenum, approximately 2 to 3 cm distal to the pylorus. This dissection is repeated along the greater curvature. The duodenum is divided roughly 3 cm distal to the pylorus using a gastrointestinal stapling device.
- Next, the neck of the pancreas is divided with the electrocautery over a gloved finger or Penrose drain to protect the underlying portal–superior mesenteric vein confluence (see Fig. 27-8, *A*). The pancreatic duct is visualized during its dissection and identified for the upcoming anastomosis. Vascular pedicles along the cephalad and caudad portions of the pancreas may be oversewn with 3-0 silk suture ligatures if cautery is not effective at controlling bleeding.
- The neck, head, and uncinate are now carefully separated from the branches of the portal and superior mesenteric veins. This is performed with gentle dissection and careful ligation of these fine venous tributaries that drain from the pancreas into the portal and superior mesenteric veins. Great care is taken to prevent injury to the superior mesenteric vein, as control of bleeding can be difficult.
- The uncinate is dissected under the portal–superior mesenteric vein confluence, and the lateral wall of the superior mesenteric artery is palpated. The uncinate tissue and adjoining lymphatics are taken with the specimen by serial clamping and skeletonization of the lateral wall of the superior mesenteric artery until the specimen can be freed (see Fig. 27-8, *B*). This allows for complete removal of the retroperitoneal uncinate process and all draining lymphatics in the region. We believe it is imperative to skeletonize the lateral aspect of the superior mesenteric artery to avoid leaving retained pancreatic tissue on the artery.
- At this point, the proximal jejunum is divided at the ligament of Treitz. The mesentery of the duodenum is carefully divided between 2-0 silk ties, and mobilization is carried out in a left-to-right fashion under the mesenteric vessels. The third and fourth portions of the duodenum are delivered into the right upper quadrant, behind the superior mesenteric artery and vein.
- The specimen, which has been marked to identify the cut surface of the bile duct, the pancreatic neck, and uncinate margin as well as the proximal and distal duodenal margin, is sent for frozen section. Surgical margin status and tumor pathology are determined before reconstruction.
- If radical dissection is desired, the distal 20% to 30% of the stomach is divided with a gastrointestinal stapling device, and the nodal tissues of the gastrohepatic ligament, antrum, and greater curvature are carefully dissected and taken with the specimen en bloc. The distal gastrectomy includes lymph node stations 5 and 6 (superior and inferior pyloric nodes) and some nodes from stations 3 and 4 (gastric greater and lesser curve nodes). The retroperitoneal lymph node dissection extends from the right renal hilum to the left lateral border of the aorta in the horizontal axis and from the portal vein to below the third portion of the duodenum in the vertical axis. The retroperitoneal lymph node tissues contain nodes harvested from stations 16a2 and 16b1 (aortocaval nodes from celiac to inferior mesenteric artery) and also include sampling of celiac nodal station 9 (Fig. 27-9).
- The ligament of Treitz mesenteric defect is closed with an interrupted or running 2-0 or 3-0 silk suture to prevent internal herniation.
- A retrocolic window to the right of the mesenteric vessels is created that allows delivery of the proximal jejunal limb into the right upper quadrant.
- The pancreaticojejunostomy can be performed in many ways. We prefer either a duct-to-mucosa or invagination technique. In the duct-to-mucosa anastomosis, the outer layer is performed with 3-0 silk suture between serosa of bowel and capsule of the pancreatic remnant. An inner layer of 4-0 absorbable monofilament sutures is placed between pancreatic duct and bowel mucosa over a no. 5 or no. 8 French stent which can be removed following completion of the anastomoses (Fig. 27-10, *A* and *B*).

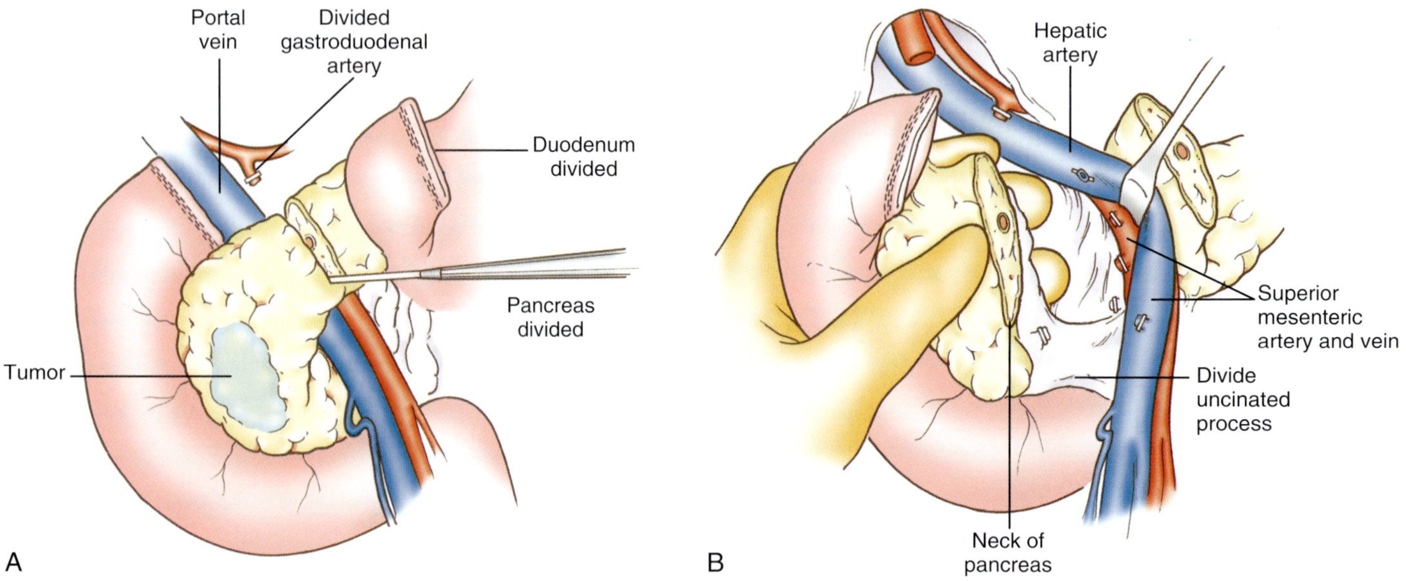

Figure 27-8.

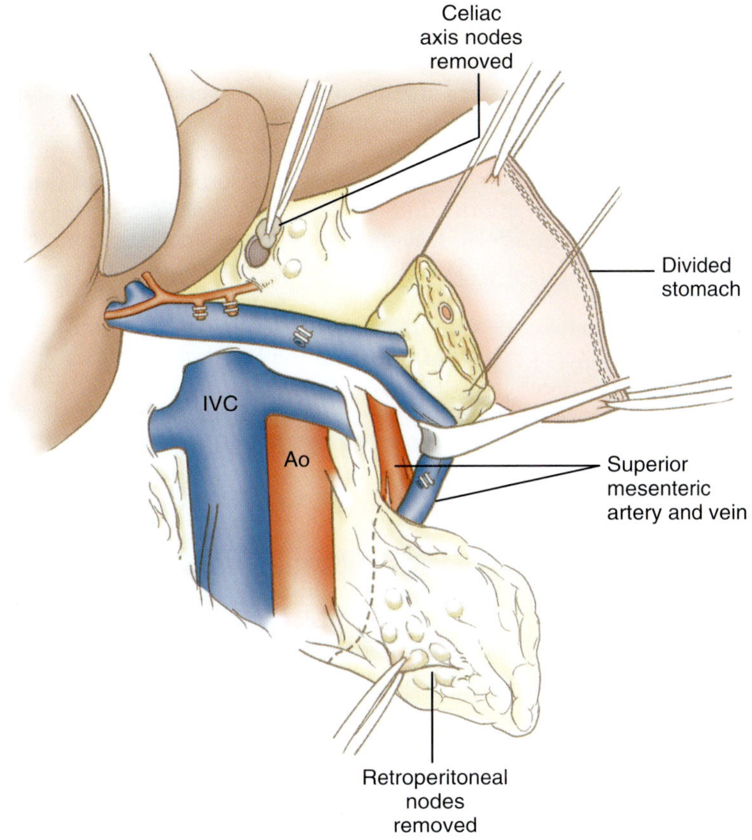

Figure 27-9. *Ao,* Aorta; *IVC,* inferior vena cava.

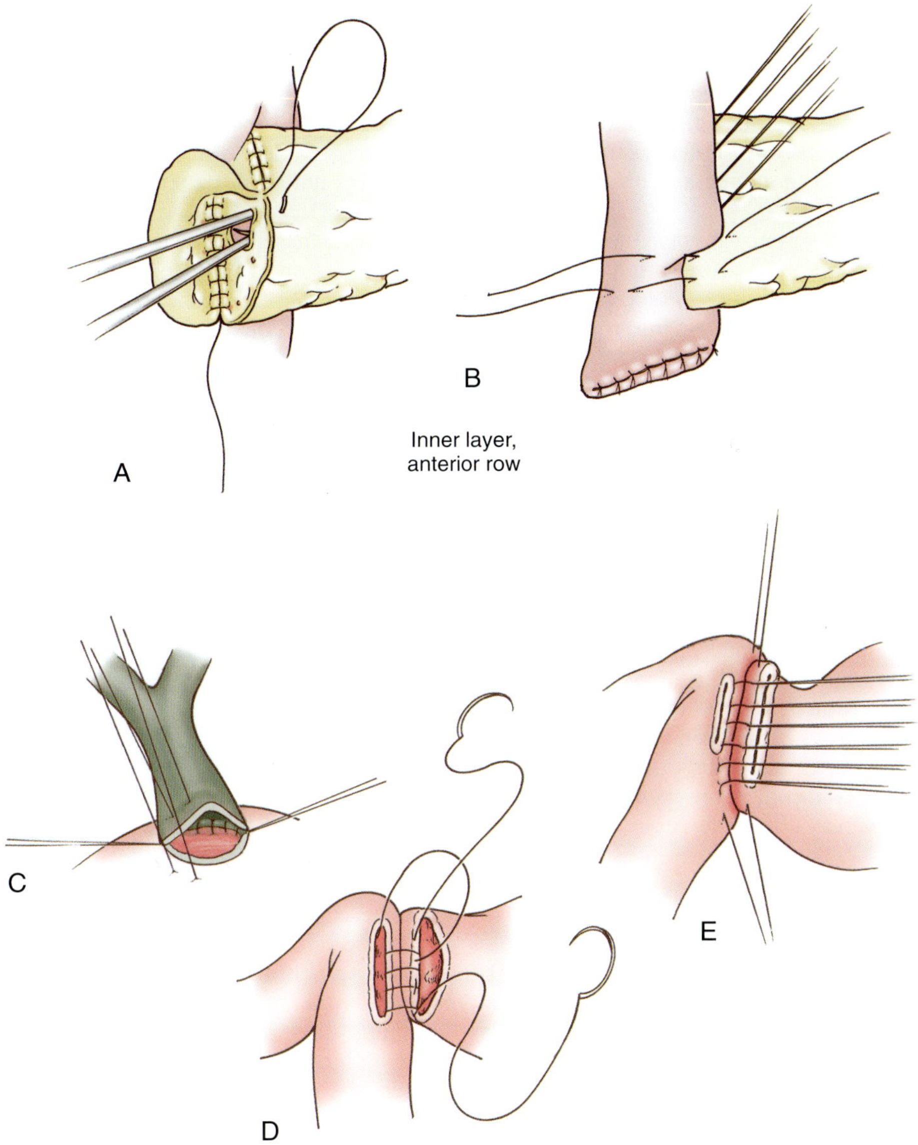

Figure 27-10.

Alternatively, a "dunking" or invagination anastomosis can be performed with an outer layer of serosa to pancreatic capsule sutures of 3-0 silk and an inner layer of running 3-0 Vicryl suture.

- A standard hepaticojejunostomy is performed between the common hepatic duct and side jejunum in a single layer using interrupted 5-0 or 4-0 monofilament absorbable suture (see Fig. 27-10, *C*).
- The duodenojejunostomy can be performed in two layers using an outer layer of 3-0 silk and an inner layer of 3-0 Vicryl suture (see Fig. 27-10, *D* and *E*). If a classic pancreaticoduodenectomy is performed (to include a distal gastrectomy), a standard stapled or hand-sewn two-layer gastrojejunal anastomosis is performed.
- Feeding tubes are not routinely used. We typically place two $\frac{3}{16}$-inch round Jackson-Pratt drains. The right drain resides near the hepaticojejunostomy, and the left drain is placed cephalad to the pancreaticojejunostomy. These are brought out through stab incisions in the lateral abdominal wall. Irrigation with saline allows for clearance of any blood clots and operative debris.

Closure

- The wound is closed in a single layer with a running no. 2 nylon suture or no. 1 absorbable monofilament suture and either skin staples or subcuticular suture, depending on the degree of soilage. Retention sutures are placed in patients who are at high risk for wound dehiscence. Dressings are applied, and the patient is returned to the intensive care unit (ICU), where standard postoperative orders (i.e., monitor blood pressure, hemoglobin, urine output, electrolytes, lactate level, and liver function) are followed.

III. ALTERNATIVE TECHNICAL APPROACHES (PRO/CON) AND PEARLS

- The use of the harmonic shears and bipolar cautery can facilitate dissection of the perigastric and duodenal tissues and minimize blood loss. These must be used with caution, because lateral thermal energy spread can injure tissues in close proximity. They can also be used to mobilize the third and fourth portions of the duodenum.
- The neck of the pancreas, when soft, can be easily divided with a gastrointestinal anastomosis stapling device to help minimize leak at the cut surface of the pancreas. The pancreatic duct is carefully exposed by removing those staples that have secured it. Again, a duct-to-mucosa reconstruction can be performed over a 5- or 8-Fr stent using 4-0 monofilament absorbable suture and an outer layer of either 3-0 silk or 3-0 monofilament absorbable suture, or an invagination pancreaticojejunostomy can be performed.
- In the event of vascular involvement of the portal or superior mesenteric vein, control can be achieved proximally on the superior mesenteric vein by careful dissection around the vein with caution taken to avoid injury to any posterior venous branches. Usually the vein is most easily dissected close to the neck of the gland as it enters into the lateral attachment of the uncinate process. This can be controlled with a vessel loop or vascular clamp. Proximally, the portal vein is easily dissected and encircled for control. The neck of the gland can be dissected off of the underlying superior mesenteric artery in a plane that is lateral to the bulk of the tumor burden. Once the splenic vein and superior mesenteric artery have been identified, dissection can then occur in a left-to-right direction. This also allows for encirclement of the splenic vein, which completes vascular control in this area. Dissection can then be safely carried out with both inflow and outflow control maintained; if the tumor is found to be inseparable or if an inadvertent tear is encountered during mobilization of the tumor, blood loss is minimized. If 30% or less of the mesenteric or portal vein is resected, this can be patched with a saphenous vein patch (Fig. 27-11, *A* and *B*). Alternatively, reconstruction can be carried out by direct vein mobilization and reanastomosis for short-segment vein resection or using interposition grafts of internal jugular or the left renal vein, which provide for an adequate size match (see Fig. 27-11, *C*).
- In those tumors anterior to the portal–superior mesenteric vein confluence, where it may be unsafe to dissect the tumor from the underlying venous structures, dissection from the left, as noted previously, as well as from the right, can facilitate safe tumor resection. In this "artery-first" technique, the uncinate process can be carefully dissected from the lateral wall of the superior mesenteric artery between suture ligatures or using one of the thermal dissection devices. This allows for mobilization of the right portion of the pancreas off of the superior mesenteric artery such that the lateral wall of the portal vein is exposed, facilitating removal of the tumor that may be invading the anterior portion of the portal–superior mesenteric vein confluence.
- Positive margins at the hepatic duct and pancreatic neck can and should be resected. This may require resection of the hepatic duct up to the level of the hepatic hilum and/or completion pancreatectomy to achieve negative margin status. Positive margins at the level of the uncinate cannot be cleared with additional surgery, because we routinely skeletonize the portal and superior mesenteric veins and the lateral aspect of the superior mesenteric artery. Titanium clips should remain along the margins of resection, especially if there is suspicion of close or microscopic positive margin status at the time of resection, to assist with planning of postoperative external beam radiation therapy.

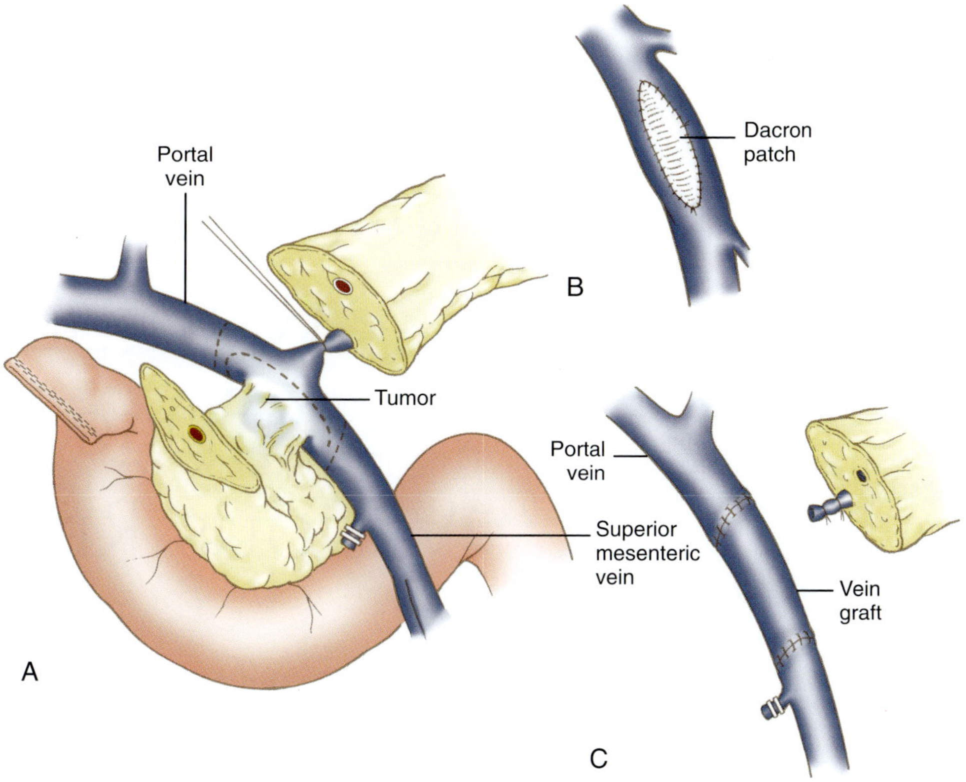

Figure 27-11.

- Clips should be left to mark the superior, inferior, medial, and lateral extent of retroperitoneal lymphadenectomy during radical pancreaticoduodenectomy.

IV. SPECIAL POSTOPERATIVE CARE

- Postoperatively, patients are placed in an ICU setting to allow careful hemodynamic monitoring and hourly assessment of urinary output. On postoperative day 1, they are transferred to a step-down ICU and ambulated, and nasogastric tubes are removed. Clear liquids are started on postoperative day 2.
- On postoperative day 3 or 4, the least draining Jackson-Pratt is removed, the diet is advanced, and patients are encouraged to ambulate. Between postoperative days 4 and 5, ambulation is increased and the remaining Jackson-Pratt drain removed. Discharge is targeted for postoperative day 6 or 7, assuming no complications. Patients with malignant pathology are seen by our oncology consultants while hospitalized to allow introduction of the topic of postoperative adjuvant therapy.
- Deviations from the postoperative critical pathway are handled through standard sets of interventions to minimize morbidity and speed discharge.
- Patients are seen in follow-up between 2 and 4 weeks postoperatively for review of their pathology and adjuvant therapy planning.

SUGGESTED READINGS

Kennedy EP, Rosato EL, Sauter PK, et al: Initiation of a critical pathway for pancreaticoduodenal at an academic institution—the first step in multidisciplinary team building, *J Am Coll Surg* 204:917–924, 2007.

Riall TS, Cameron JL, Yeo CJ, et al: Pancreaticoduodenectomy with or without distal gastrectomy and extended retroperitoneal lymphadenectomy for periampullary adenocarcinoma: update on 5-year survival, *J Gastrointest Surg* 9:1191–1206, 2005.

Yeo CJ, Cameron JL, Lilliemoe KD, et al: Pancreaticoduodenectomy with or without distal gastrectomy and extended retroperitoneal lymphadenectomy for periampullary adenocarcinoma. Part II: Randomized controlled trial evaluating survival, morbidity and mortality, *Ann Surg* 236:355–368, 2002.

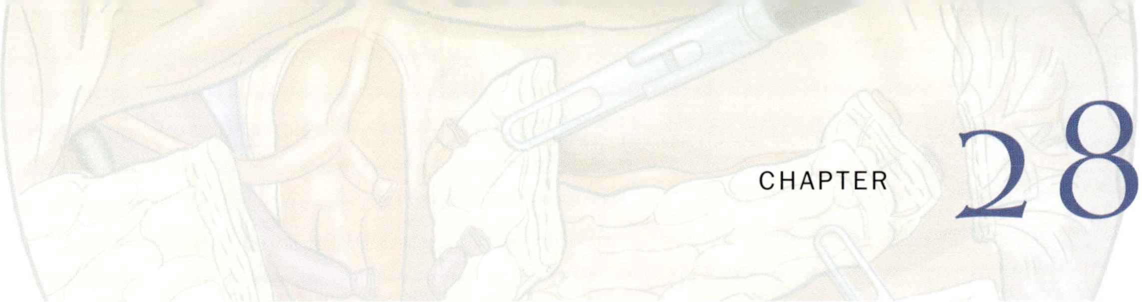

CHAPTER 28

Pancreaticoduodenectomy with Superior Mesentericoportal Venous Resection

N.J. Lygidakis, MD, PhD, FRCST(H), FJSS(H), and Sandesh Kumar Sharma, MS

I. SPECIAL PREOPERATIVE PREPARATION

- A thorough preoperative workup includes routine laboratory evaluation, liver function test, coagulation profile, tumor marker study, upper gastrointestinal study to see secondary varices, and Doppler ultrasound of the mesentericoportal axis to look for portomesenteric invasion of the tumor. Detailed radiologic evaluation with contrast-enhanced computed tomography (CECT) and magnetic resonance imaging (MRI) with angiographic sequences are of paramount importance before undertaking pancreaticoduodenectomy with portomesenteric reconstruction in cases of pancreatic malignancy with vascular invasion.
- Doppler ultrasound is useful to see any obvious liver secondary metastases or cholangitic abscesses. Doppler also aids in assessment of the grade of portal hypertension. However, because of the anatomic location of the pancreas, other modalities such as triple-phase CECT and MRI angiography have become modalities of choice depending on the availability of local expertise.
- Endoscopic sonography has reemerged as a competitive or slightly better modality for the detailed evaluation of mesentericoportal invasion as compared to CECT. Endoscopic sonography also provides the option of tissue sampling. However, it is a highly operator-dependent technique.
- CECT with triple-phase and vascular reconstruction images (Fig. 28-1) is the most widely used modality for the complete evaluation of the pancreatic tumor, revealing its extent and the grade of vascular invasion of the mesentericoportal axis. It is considered the gold standard and is the most widely used modality for preoperative evaluation of pancreatic tumors.
- MRI with angiographic sequences (Fig. 28-2) is gradually replacing computed tomography (CT) in many centers as it can provide multiplanar images with excellent angiographic details. It also provides detailed ductal anatomy and an excellent road map of biliary pancreatic anatomy, and has fewer biliary stent artifacts as compared with CT.
- Laparoscopic ultrasound has not contributed much in avoiding or providing additional detail. It is also highly operator-dependent and requires a high level of expertise.
- Intraoperative ultrasound can be an adjunct to such advanced cases, as it can be a useful tool to evaluate the quality of the vascular reconstruction.

II. OPERATIVE TECHNIQUE

Position

- The patient is positioned supine with the head elevated about 15 degrees and a bolster under the subcostal margin. This helps to make the pancreas more prominent and is particularly helpful for the obese patient.

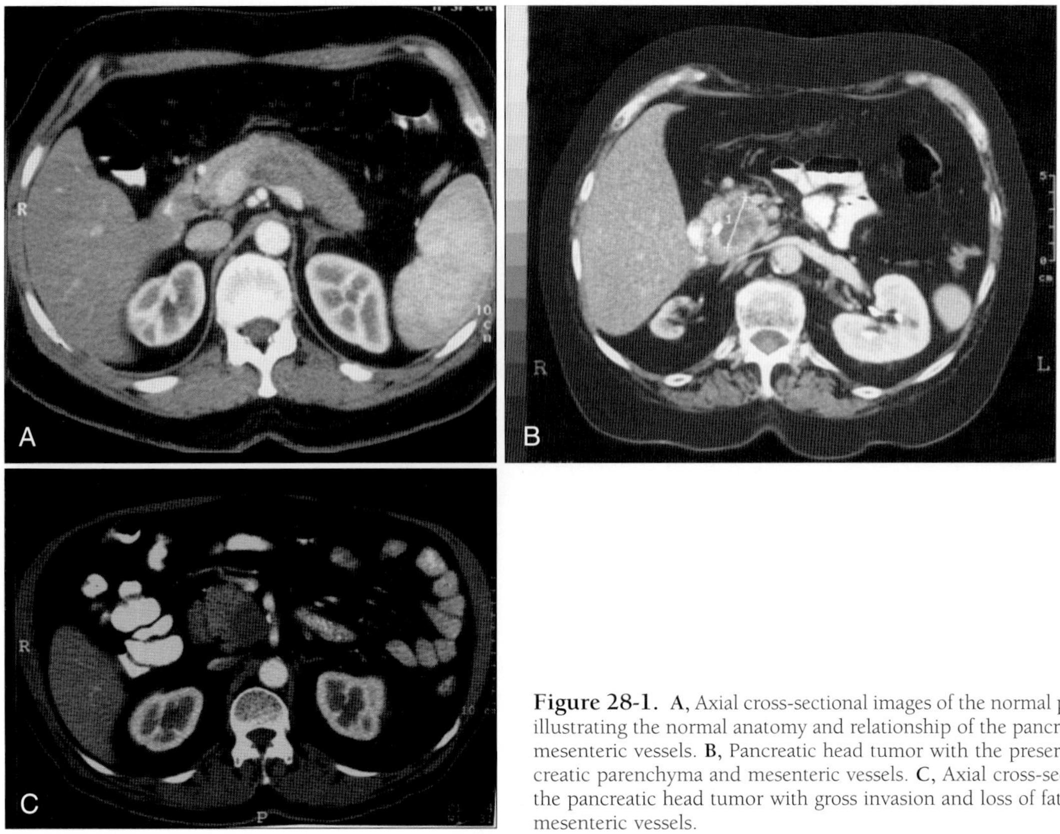

Figure 28-1. **A**, Axial cross-sectional images of the normal pancreas at the level of mesenteric vessels illustrating the normal anatomy and relationship of the pancreatic head and uncinate process with the mesenteric vessels. **B**, Pancreatic head tumor with the preservation of the fat plane between the pancreatic parenchyma and mesenteric vessels. **C**, Axial cross-sectional computed tomography images of the pancreatic head tumor with gross invasion and loss of fat plane between the parenchyma and the mesenteric vessels.

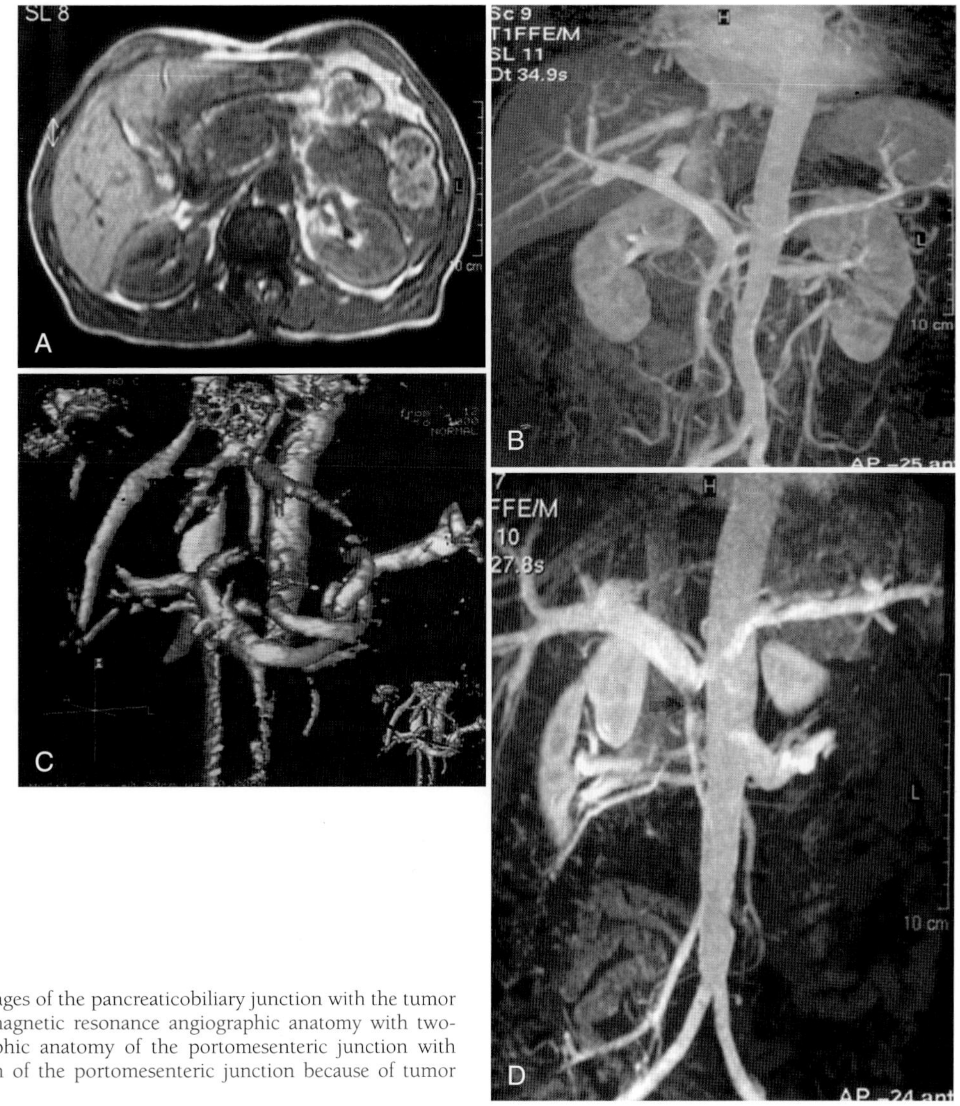

Figure 28-2. **A**, Axial T2 magnetic resonance images of the pancreaticobiliary junction with the tumor in the head region. **B**, Normal portomesenteric magnetic resonance angiographic anatomy with two-dimensional reconstruction. **C**, Normal angiographic anatomy of the portomesenteric junction with three-dimensional reconstruction. **D**, Compression of the portomesenteric junction because of tumor (*arrow*).

Incision

- A bilateral subcostal incision with both costal margins retracted by self-retaining retractors gives good exposure to the operative field. The liver is further retracted by a self-retaining blade, allowing good exposure of hepaticoduodenal structures.
- Careful surveillance and detailed exploration is performed of the whole abdomen, including the undersurface of both domes of the diaphragm, peritoneum, base of the mesentery, and pelvis for any peritoneal seeding or metastatic deposit.
- Careful mobilization of the transverse colon from its hepatic attachment is done (Cattel maneuver), as this provides good exposure to the operating field and avoids any inadvertent injury to the colon (Fig. 28-3).
- Next step is the liberal kocherization from the first part of the duodenum up to the fourth part (to the ligament of Treitz). Posteriorly, the inferior vena cava and aorta should be visible. This helps in radical clearance of the lymphatics and also marks the limit of posterior dissection.
- Once properly kocherized, the pancreas can be held and lifted up and to the right with the surgeon's left finger posteriorly and thumb anteriorly, after opening the gastrocolic omentum. Thorough assessment of further operability and vascular invasion should be assessed by intraoperative ultrasound with a Doppler probe to determine the vascular involvement and plan accordingly.
- The gallbladder is dissected from the liver bed, and the cholecystectomy is performed in standard fashion. The fascial covering over the hepatoduodenal ligament is dissected, and a sling is passed around the common bile duct and retracted to the right. This exposes the portal vein posteriorly and allows lymphatic clearance. A vascular sling is also passed around the portal vein to help in achieving cephalic control during the anticipated portal venous reconstruction.
- The common bile duct can be divided at his stage above the junction of the cystic duct. The lower cut end is oversewn with suture (Fig. 28-4). The cut upper end of the common bile duct should be temporarily closed with vascular forceps to avoid bile spillage over the operating field.
- Dissection of the hepaticoduodenal ligament is further continued. The fascial (adventitial) covering over the hepaticoduodenal ligament is dissected over the first part of duodenum, and the gastroduodenal artery is identified, skeletonized, doubly ligated proximally with Prolene 3-0 suture, and divided. Care must be taken at this stage to avoid damage to the common hepatic artery. It is not always necessary to skeletonize the hepatic artery, as long as lymphatic clearance can be adequately achieved. However, few centers routinely advocate this step to clear the lymphatics around the proper hepatic artery.
- The gastrocolic omentum is divided at this stage. Meticulous separation of the posterior layer of the mesocolon and fourth layer of the omentum is done up to the base of the middle colic vessel, reaching the base of the mesentery where the superior mesenteric vessels can be seen. Superiorly, the stomach can be divided at the level of the antrum using an Endo GIA stapler. This will further provide clear access to the upper border of the pancreatic head (Fig. 28-5).

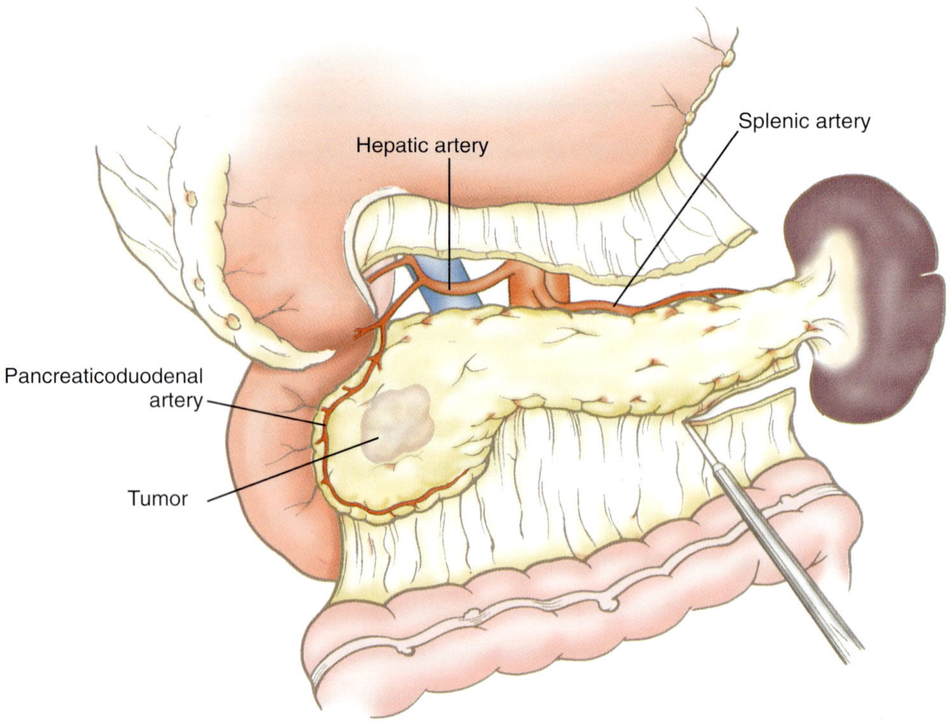

Figure 28-3.

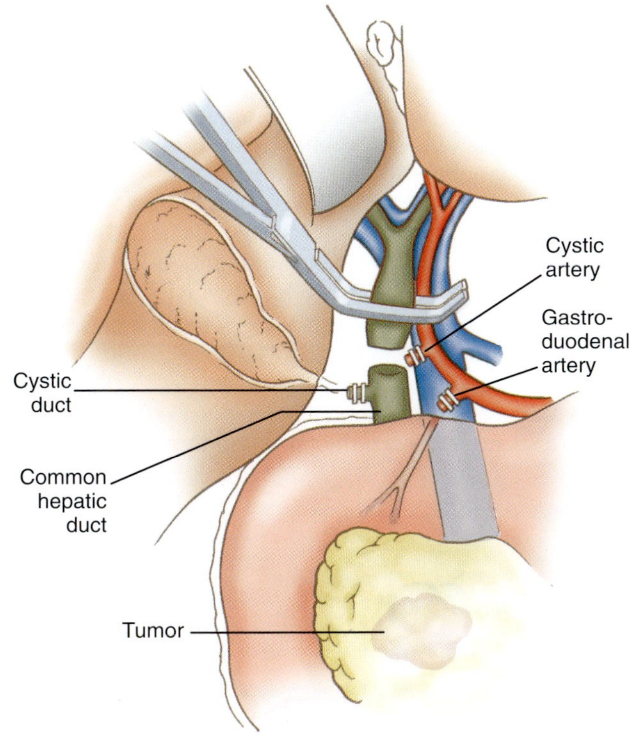

Figure 28-4.

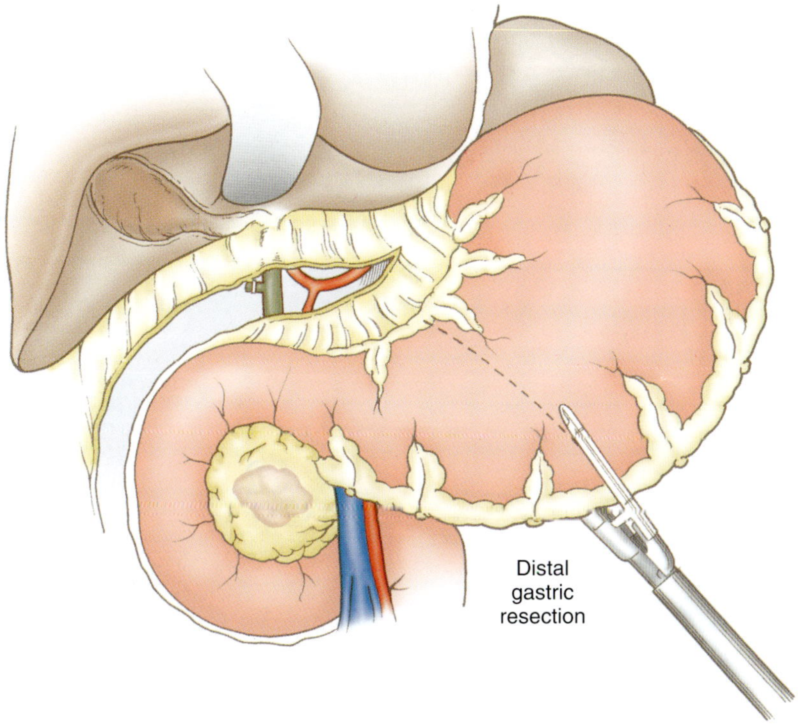

Figure 28-5.

- The next step is to create a tunnel across the pancreatic isthmus between the mesenteric vessels and pancreatic parenchyma. This is the most vital step for further safe pancreatic parenchyma division (Fig. 28-6). If there is any vascular infiltration by tumor, normally a tunnel cannot be created. At this point, preparation for the vascular reconstruction should be done by taking control of the portal vein proximally and the superior mesenteric vein inferiorly. It is also important to control and ligate the splenic vein to prevent back bleeding. The splenic vein can be safely ligated in the majority of cases, as the short gastric vein takes care of venous drainage of the spleen. However, the spleen should be observed for any congestion, and if splenic congestion is seen, splenectomy should be performed before venous reconstruction.
- I prefer to divide the first part of the jejunum and bring the cut end underneath the mesenteric vessels to the right of the patient. This helps create better orientation for the future vascular reconstruction. However, this step makes pancreaticoduodenectomy irreversible.

Main Dissection

- Once vascular control is achieved, four traction sutures using Vicryl 2-0 are applied at the superior and inferior border of the pancreas between the proposed line of division. These sutures help in lifting

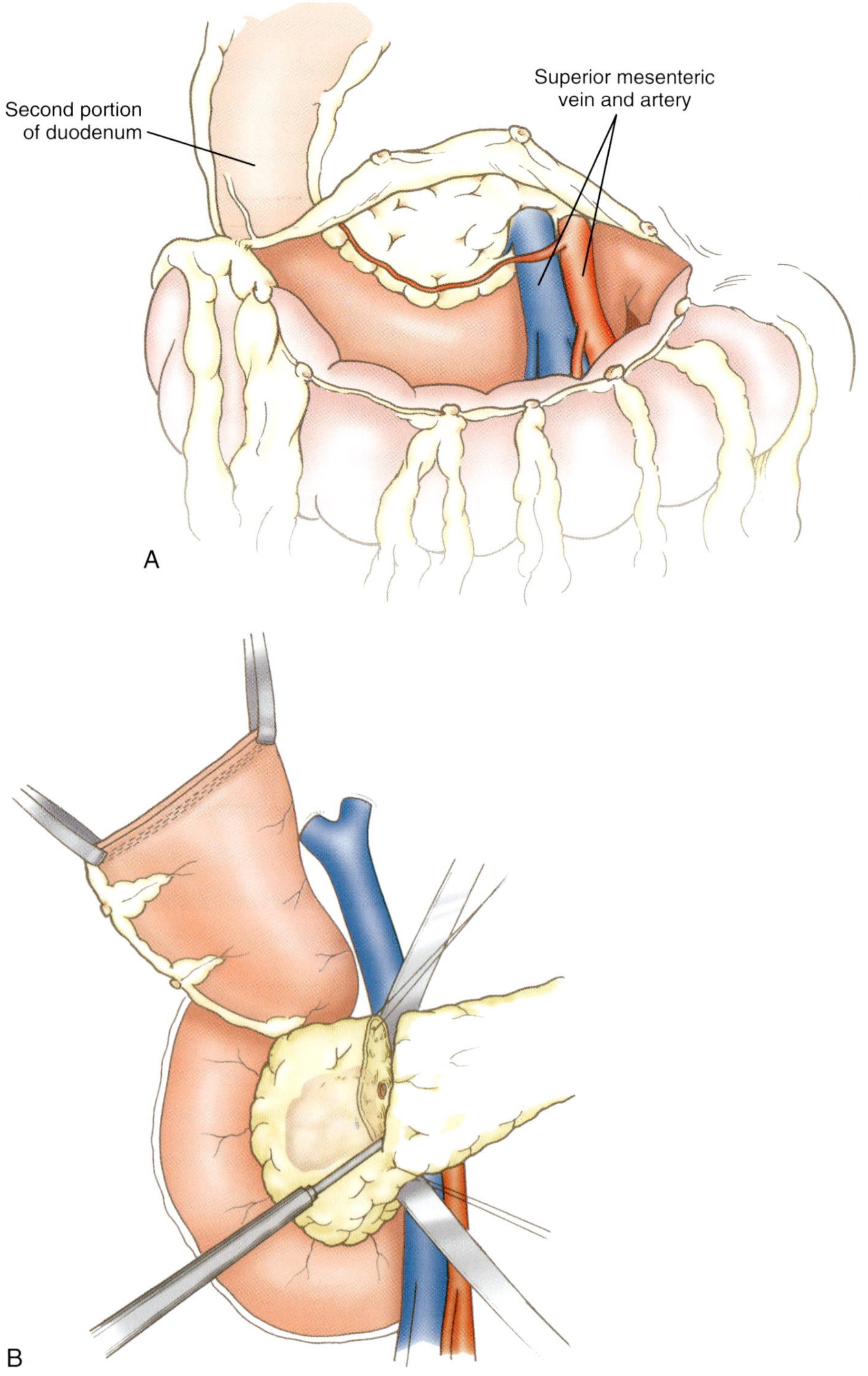

Figure 28-6.

and retracting the pancreas and also provide hemostasis. Pancreatic parenchymal transaction can be started using diathermy or a scalpel knife (I prefer to use diathermy for the soft pancreas and a scalpel knife for the firm pancreas). Once more than half of the pancreas is transected and the portal vein starts appearing, further transection should be done after controlling the portal flow by tightening the vascular loop (Fig. 28-7). A vascular Satinsky clamp is applied to the splenic vein if it is visible in field. Further parenchymal transection proceeds, and pancreaticoduodenectomy is completed by carefully dissecting the pancreaticoduodenal specimen with the tumor mass from the retroperitoneal adventitia. All smaller veins draining directly from the pancreas to the portal vein are carefully clipped or suture ligated at this point. Lateral retraction of the superior mesenteric artery using a vascular sling further aids in lymphatic clearance around the superior mesenteric artery. In cases of partial infiltration of the portal vein, a vascular clamp is applied sideways to the portal vein and the tumor is excised, taking the lateral cuff of the portal vein. After completing the parenchymal transection, the portal vein can be repaired using fine Prolene (5-0 monofilament nonabsorbable) suture. A segmental loss of portal vein that cannot be brought together in an end-to-end fashion needs portal vein substitution using either a venous graft (from the great saphenous vein) or a Gore-Tex graft (6-mm diameter) (Fig. 28-8).

- I prefer to use a Gore-Tex graft of 6-mm size because it is less prone to kinking and is available in various sizes and lengths.
- The graft is sutured to the divided proximal and distal end of the portal vein using 5-0 Prolene by standard vascular suturing technique (Fig. 28-9). Once the portal substitution is complete, the vascular clamp and vascular sling of the cephalic end are released first, and then the caudal clamp and sling are

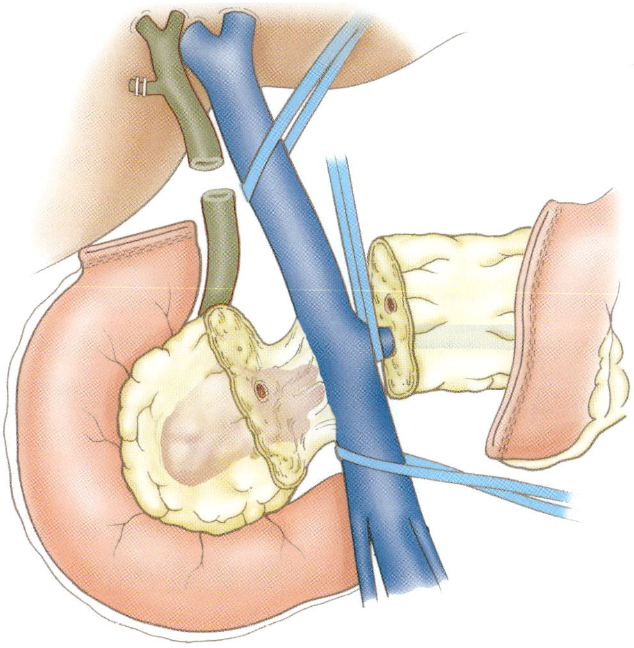

Figure 28-7.

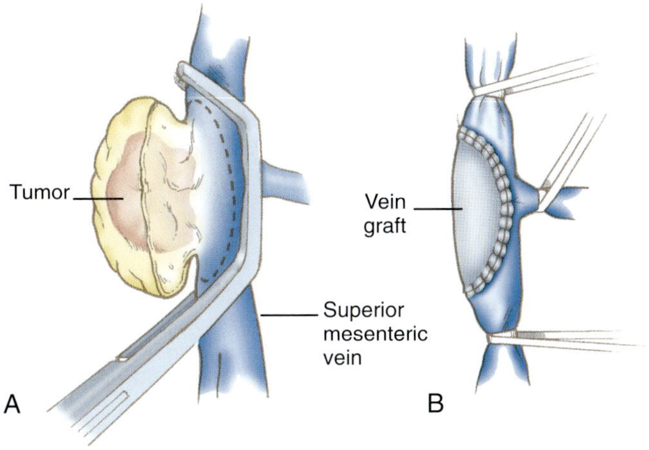

Figure 28-8.

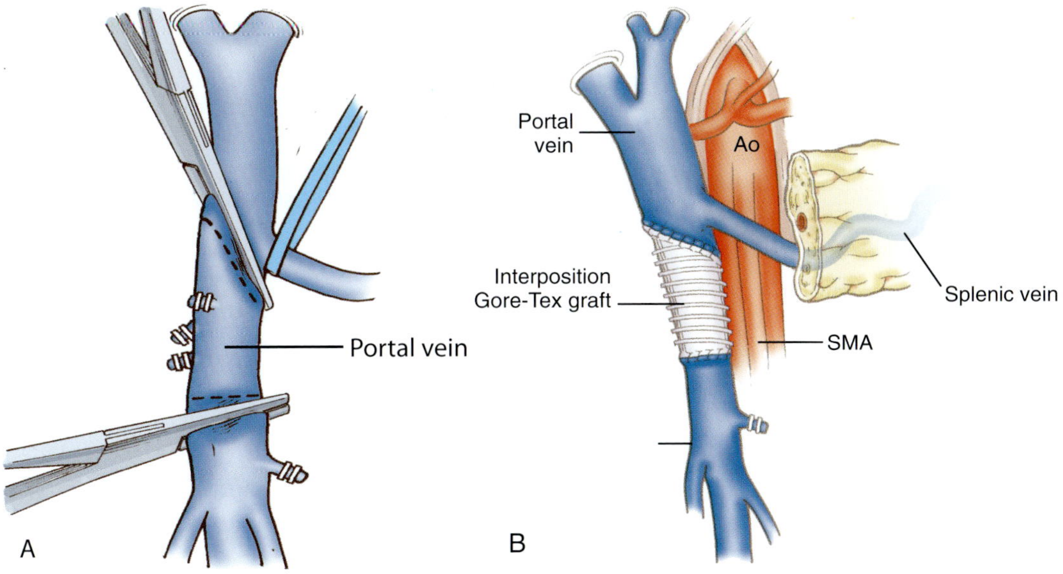

Figure 28-9. *Ao,* Aorta; *SMA,* superior mesenteric artery; *SMV,* superior mesenteric vein.

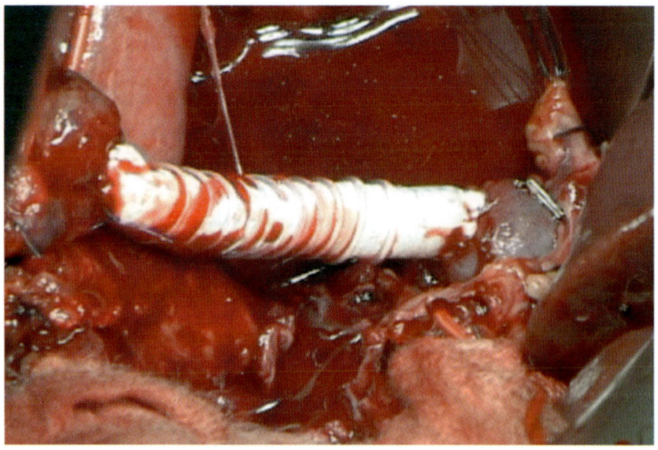

Figure 28-10.

released later (Fig. 28-10). Flow across the graft can be ascertained by intraoperative Doppler study or using the finger to feel the distensibility of the graft. At this point, I prefer to give an intravenous (IV) bolus of unfractionated heparin, 5000 international units, to prevent acute graft venous thrombosis.
- After completing the vascular reconstruction, the specimen should be sent for frozen section, and the cut margins should be analyzed to confirm R0 resection. If cut margins are positive, a further total pancreatectomy is completed.
- Further gastrointestinal continuity is established by doing an end-to-side duct-to-mucosal pancreaticojejunostomy and hepaticojejunostomy using a separate jejunal loop for pancreaticobiliary reconstruction and gastrojejunal anastomosis (double-loop reconstruction).

Closure

- After gastrointestinal continuity is established, two Penrose drains are placed in the subhepatic and lesser sac, brought separately away from the main incision to the right and left anterior axillary line, and fixed to skin with 2-0 silk suture.
- After complete hemostasis is achieved, the abdomen is closed using continuous-loop polydioxanone surgical suture.
- Skin approximation is done using interrupted nylon 2-0 suture.

III. ALTERNATIVE TECHNICAL APPROACHES (PRO/CON) AND PEARLS

- In cases of mesentericoportal invasion, alternatively total spleno-pancreaticoduodenectomy is advocated. This helps in avoiding the pancreatic gastrointestinal anastomosis and assures radicality. However, the patient is subjected to crippling diabetes with high susceptibility to opportunistic postsplenectomy sepsis that may be overwhelming.
- Instead of using the Gore-Tex graft, an autologous venous graft from the saphenous vein can be used for portal venous reconstruction.
- Gastrointestinal continuity can be established with a single Roux-en-Y jejunal loop. Alternatively, a pancreaticogastric anastomosis can be performed instead of pancreaticojejunal.

IV. SPECIAL POSTOPERATIVE CARE

- The patient is electively ventilated for the first 24 hours with intensive monitoring performed for the next 48 hours in the intensive care unit.
- Subcutaneous double-dose low–molecular-weight heparin is given to avoid deep vein thrombosis and prevent graft thrombosis.
- Blood sugar is tightly controlled using insulin infusion to maintain the blood sugar level.
- We routinely give octreotide (Sandostatin) 100 mcg three times daily, administered subcutaneously, for the next 5 days to reduce the chance of disruption of the pancreatic anastomosis.
- Early ambulation and chest physiotherapy are highly encouraged.
- A prophylactic wide-spectrum IV antibiotic is given for 5 days.
- Prophylaxis (pneumococcal vaccine) against *Pneumococcus* infection is highly recommended for post-splenectomy status.

SUGGESTED READINGS

Jain S, Sacchi M, Vrachnos P, Lygidakis NJ: Carcinoma of the pancreas with portal vein involvement—our experience with a modified technique of resection, *Hepatogastroenterology* 52:1596–1600, 2005.

Lygidakis NJ, Jain S, Sacchi M, Vrachnos P: Reappraisal of a method of reconstruction after pancreaticoduodenectomy, *Hepatogastroenterology* 52:1077–1082, 2005.

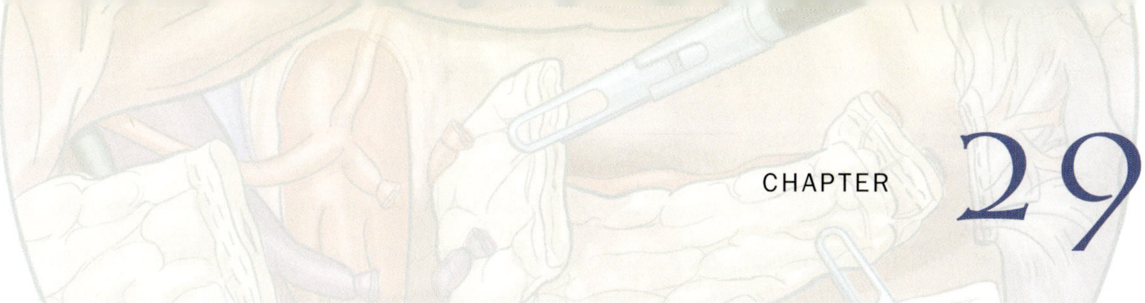

CHAPTER 29

Distal Subtotal Pancreatectomy with and without Spleen Preservation

Laureano Fernández-Cruz, MD, FRCS Ed(Hon), FCRSI(Hon)

I. SPECIAL PREOPERATIVE PREPARATION

Introduction

- Distal pancreatic resection (DPR) has been performed over the years for management of patients diagnosed with inflammatory pancreatic disorders for chronic pancreatitis and for tumors localized in the body and tail of the pancreas. However, the technique is usually not performed in the same manner by all surgeons.
- In general, distal pancreatectomy is performed en bloc along with resection of the spleen. Most of the time, the en bloc pancreatic-spleen resection is performed for technical reasons; it makes the operation short and easy but does not offer any special advantage for the patient. Overwhelming sepsis after distal pancreatectomy and splenectomy has been reported.
- One alternative technique involves preserving both the splenic artery and vein. In another technique of distal pancreatectomy, splenic vessels are ligated both at the level of transection of the pancreas and again at the splenic hilum, leaving the spleen to survive on blood flow through the short gastric vessels. Others have described techniques whereby the pancreas is dissected off the splenic vessels completely. In recent years, the laparoscopic approach has been introduced, with all the advantages of a minimally invasive procedure.

Fundamental Differences between Laparoscopic and Open Approaches

- The primary differences between the two procedures are the method of access (length and number of abdominal incisions), the method of exposure, and the extent of operative trauma.
- Open DPR is commonly performed through an upper abdominal incision, whereas laparoscopic DPR is performed through four or five small abdominal incisions.
- The method of exposure during open distal pancreatectomy involves the use of abdominal wall retractors and mechanical retraction of the abdominal viscera. In contrast, the method of exposure during laparoscopic DPR involves the use of pneumoperitoneum to create a working space and gravidity for displacement of the abdominal viscera.
- By reducing the length of the surgical incision and eliminating the need for mechanical retraction of the abdominal wall and viscera, we believe that the operative trauma after laparoscopic DPR is reduced compared with that of open DPR.

II. OPERATIVE TECHNIQUE: OPEN APPROACH

Position

- The patient is placed in the supine position.

Incision

- A bilateral subcostal, straight transverse incision or midline incision can be used.

Main Dissection

- The planning of the operation can be distal pancreatectomy with en bloc splenectomy or spleen-preserving distal pancreatectomy with or without splenic vessels preservation.

Distal Pancreatectomy with en Bloc Splenectomy

- In division of the gastrocolic omentum, the body-tail of the pancreas is best exposed by displacing the omentum and the colon with its mesocolon inferiorly away from the pancreas. The dissection is continued up to the uppermost short gastric vessels, which are ligated and divided.
- Division of adhesions between the posterior wall of the stomach and pancreas allows the stomach to be retracted superiorly. The celiac axis is visualized at the upper border of the body of the pancreas; the hepatic artery is identified and freed from the superior margin of the pancreas; this artery is then followed to the left until it merges with the splenic artery at its origin from the celiac trunk. The splenic artery is ligated and divided (Fig. 29-1).
- The posterior aspect of the body of the pancreas is mobilized out of the retroperitoneum until the superior mesenteric vein is clearly identified (see Fig. 29-1). A tape is passed around the neck of the pancreas after dissecting the mesenteric-portal vein axis from the neck of the pancreas. The body of the pancreas is further mobilized until the inferior mesenteric vein is identified and divided. The dissection of the inferior border of the pancreas is continued and extended beneath the pancreas, where there is often an avascular plane. At this point the splenic hilum is visualized.
- After dissecting the body-tail of the pancreas, the lienorenal and lienophrenic ligament are divided. The spleen (free from the diaphragm) and tail of the pancreas are dissected from the posterior abdominal wall; the dissection is continued to the neck of the pancreas. With the splenopancreatic block fully mobilized and brought over the right side of the patient, the splenic vein is dissected onto the portal vein and oversewn on the portal vein (Fig. 29-2).
- The left pancreas is now attached to the head of the pancreas by a narrow neck of tissue; we favor transection of the pancreas by means of a 60-mm linear stapling device (see Fig. 29-2). Another option is that transection of the pancreas can be performed by using electrocautery: to prevent pancreatic fistula, a row of Prolene 3-0 sutures is placed in a figure-of-eight fashion over the end of the pancreas; a separated suture is placed in a mattress fashion around the divided pancreatic duct. Further refinement is transection of the pancreas by the ultrasonic dissector: during the transection procedure, even small pancreatic ducts and vessels are adequately exposed, tied proximally, and divided. The pancreatic stump is left open without parenchymal suturing.

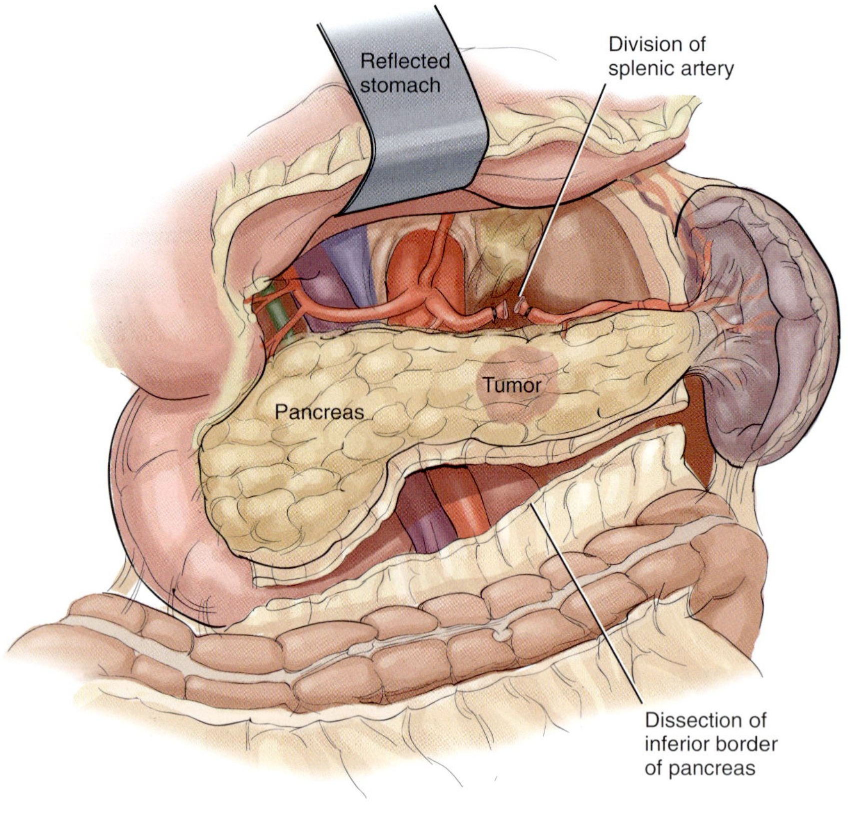

Figure 29-1.

Spleen-Preserving Distal Pancreatectomy

- When performing spleen-preserving distal pancreatectomy, we have two alternatives: spleen salvage with or without splenic vessel preservation.
- In the latter technique, after division of the gastrocolic omentum, the splenic artery is ligated and divided (Fig. 29-3).
- The posterior aspect of the body-tail of the pancreas is mobilized out of the retroperitoneum until the splenic hilum is clearly identified.

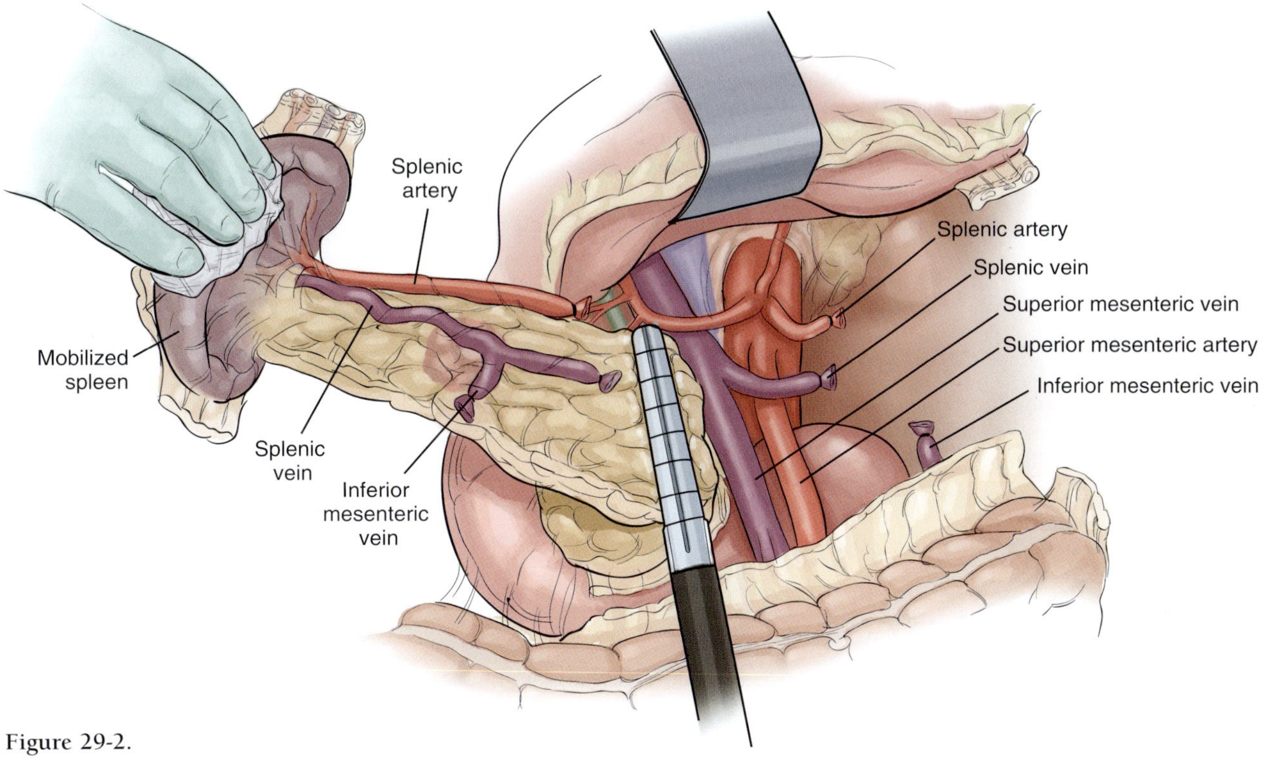

Figure 29-2.

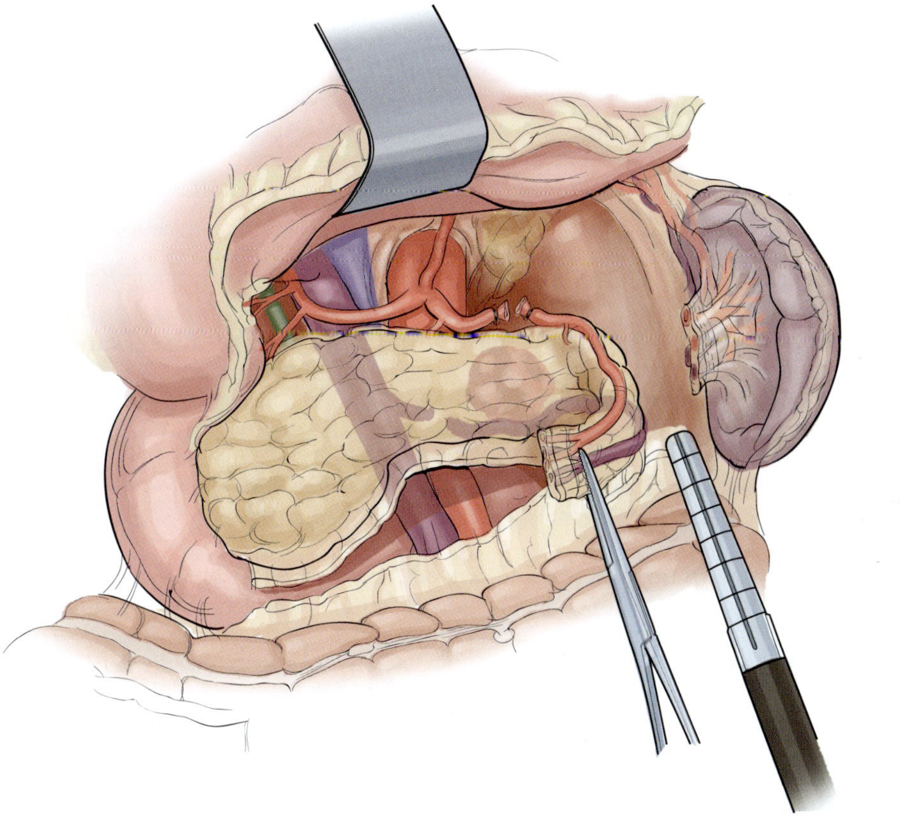

Figure 29-3.

- A 60-mm linear stapler is placed between the distal end of the tail of the pancreas and the splenic hilum (including the entry of the short gastric vessels and the left gastroepiploic vessels). The spleen is kept vascularized solely from these vessels (see Fig. 29-3).
- The body-tail of the pancreas is then brought over the right of the patient. The splenic vein is identified, ligated, and divided at its junction with mesenteric-portal vein axis (see Fig. 29-3).
- Transection of the pancreas is performed as described earlier (see Fig. 29-2).
- In the technique of spleen-preserving distal pancreatectomy with splenic vessel preservation, the dissection of the superior and inferior border of the pancreas is performed as described previously, to identify the splenic artery emerging from the celiac trunk and the splenic vein–superior mesenteric vein junction.
- A tunnel behind the neck of the pancreas is created between the splenic vessels and the posterior wall of the pancreas to allow transection of the neck of the pancreas by using a 30-mm staple device.
- The splenic artery and the splenic vein are carefully dissected from the posterior aspect of the pancreas until the splenic hilum is reached. Much of this can be done bluntly, but there are small vessels between the pancreas and the splenic vessels that need to be identified, then coagulated or ligated and divided.
- A 30-mm linear stapling device will divide the vascular attachments between the tail of the pancreas and the splenic hilum.

Closure

- A midline incision is closed by approximating the linea alba with 1-0 monofilament suture. A bilateral subcostal incision is closed in layers by approximating the anterior abdominal wall muscles with 1-0 monofilament suture.

III. OPERATIVE TECHNIQUE: LAPAROSCOPIC SURGERY

Position

- Using our approach, the patient is placed in the half-lateral position with the left side up. The surgeon and assistant stand on the left side of the patient and the camera person and scrub nurse on the opposite side.

Trocar Placement

- Four 10- to 12-mm trocars are inserted in the abdominal wall 3 to 4 cm above the umbilicus, on the xiphoid area, subcostal on the midaxillary line, and subcostal to the midclavicular line.
- Two monitors are used. CO_2 pneumoperitoneum is used. Abdominal pressure is monitored and maintained at 14 mm Hg. A 308 scope is used. The liver is explored visually and by laparoscopic ultrasonography (7.5-MHz probe, 10-mm diameter; B-K Medical, Gentolfe, Denmark).

Main Dissection

Spleen-Preserving Distal Pancreatectomy with Splenic Vessel Preservation

- The first step is to start sectioning the lienorenal ligament and dissecting the subjacent fascia lateral to the spleen. The splenocolic ligament is divided using a Harmonic scalpel or LigaSure device. The splenic flexure of the colon is mobilized downward. The gastrocolic omentum is widely opened up to the level of the mesenteric vessels, and the body-tail of the pancreas is then visualized. The anterior aspect of the pancreas is exposed by dividing the adhesions between the posterior surface of the stomach and the pancreas. Care must be taken to preserve the short gastric and the left gastroepiploic vessels.
- The inferior border of the pancreas is dissected, and the body and tail of the pancreas are completely detached from the retroperitoneum. This mobilization of the left pancreas allows visualization of the posterior wall of the gland, where the splenic vein is easily identified (Fig. 29-4). The splenic vein is pushed away from the posterior pancreatic wall by gentle blunt dissection. Visual magnification through the laparoscope permits excellent control of the small pancreatic veins, which are coagulated using the LigaSure device or the Harmonic scalpel, or clipped with titanium clips. A tunnel is created between the splenic vein and the pancreas. The splenic artery is identified through this space using blunt careful dissection with a curve dissector.
- The pancreas is then transected with a 60-mm endoscopic linear stapler (Fig. 29-5). Usually two stapler applications are necessary.

- The tail of the pancreas is then grasped and retracted anteriorly with a 5-mm forceps, and traction is applied to expose the small branches of the splenic artery and vein, which are coagulated using the LigaSure device (see Fig. 29-5). The dissection is continued laterally until the splenic hilum is reached. The vascular area connecting the end of the tail of the pancreas and the spleen is transected with a 60-mm endoscopic linear stapler (Endo GIA). Another option is to preserve the spleen, where the

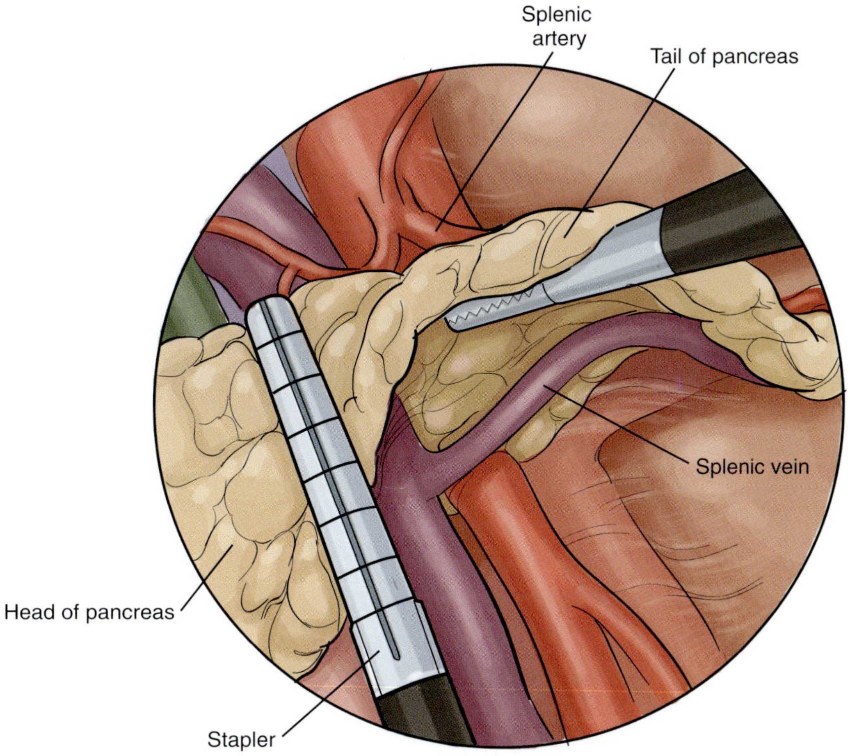

Figure 29-4.

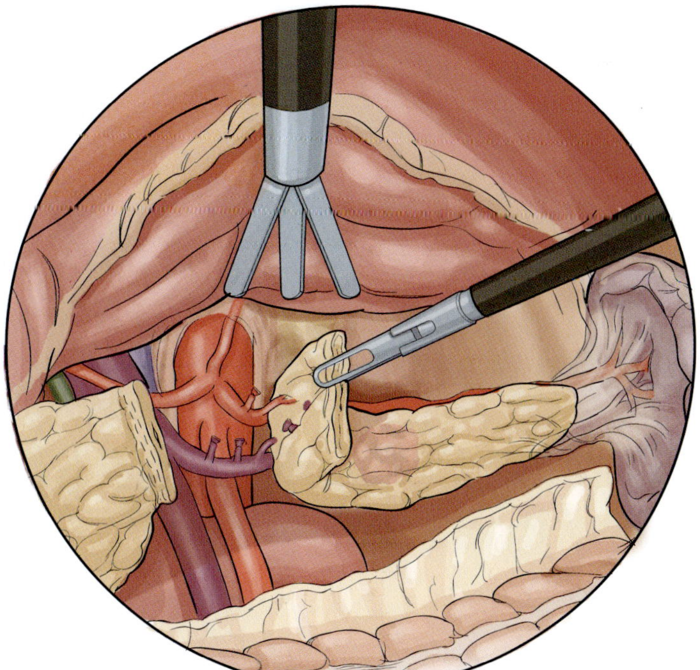

Figure 29-5.

small vessels connecting the tail of the pancreas with the splenic vessel, are exposed and then ligated and coagulated (Fig. 29-6).

Spleen-Preserving Distal Pancreatectomy without Splenic Vessel Preservation

- This technique follows the same surgical steps as described previously, until the plane behind the neck-body of the pancreas and in front of the superior mesenteric and portal veins is reached. At this point, the splenic vein is divided between clips (Fig. 29-7).
- The use of laparoscopic ultrasonography demarcates the line of pancreatic transection 2 cm away from the tumor.
- After pancreatic transection, the splenic artery is divided between clips.

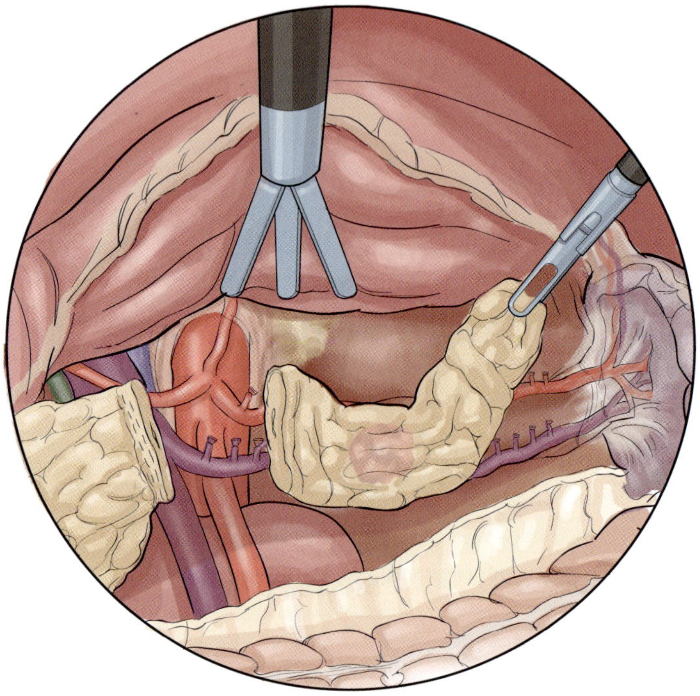

Figure 29-6.

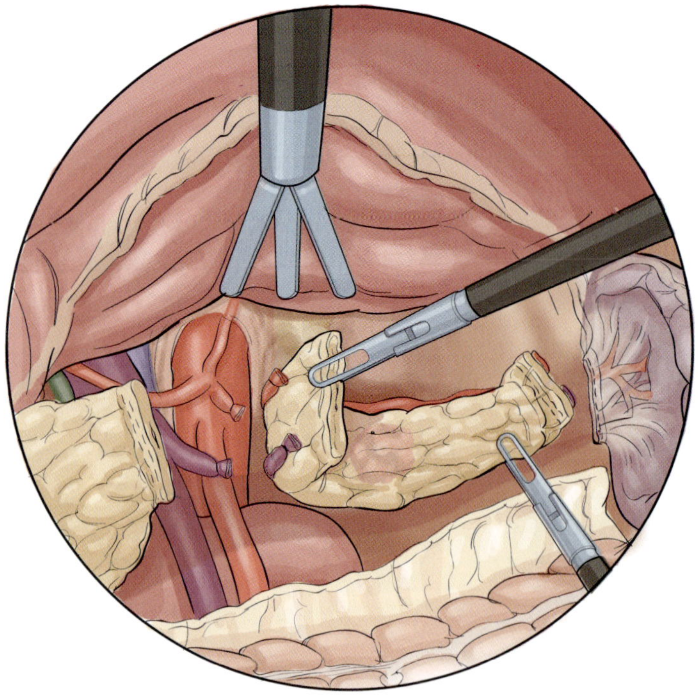

Figure 29-7.

- The left pancreas is then lifted and mobilized posteriorly with the splenic artery and vein. The latter are clipped and divided or transected with the Endo GIA as they emerge from the pancreatic tail to enter the hilum of the spleen.
- The spleen is kept vascularized solely from the short gastric vessels and the left gastroepiploic vessels (see Fig. 29-7).

Closure

- The ports are removed, and the 10-mm fascial defect can be closed using the Endo Stitch technique. Skin is closed with subcuticular 4-0 absorbable suture.

IV. ALTERNATIVE TECHNICAL APPROACHES (PRO/CON) AND PEARLS

Radical Antegrade Modular Pancreatosplenectomy

- This technique is recommended in patients who have adenocarcinoma of the body and tail of the pancreas. In this method, dissection proceeds from right to left in one of two posterior dissection planes to achieve negative posterior resection margins.
- The neck of the pancreas is divided after dissection of the lymph nodes on the left border of the proper hepatic artery, portal vein, and common hepatic artery.
- Performance of the celiac node dissection at this time exposes the origin of the splenic artery, and it is ligated and divided closely at this point.
- The splenic vein is isolated at its junction with the superior mesenteric vein and divided. The plane of the dissection now proceeds vertically in the sagittal plane, dividing fat and fibrotic tissue until the superior mesenteric artery is encountered. The lymph nodes anterior to the aorta (between the celiac artery and the superior mesenteric artery) and those anterior to the left of the superior mesenteric artery are taken with this step.
- When the planned posterior plane is anterior to the adrenal, the dissection on the aorta is carried no farther. If the planned posterior plane of dissection is posterior to the adrenal, the dissection is carried down the left side of the aorta in the sagittal plane onto the diaphragm.

V. SPECIAL POSTOPERATIVE CARE

- One of the most serious complications of DPR is the development of a postoperative pancreatic fistula, which may lead to a subphrenic abscess, sepsis, or lethal arterial bleeding. Factors that have been implicated as potentially important in the development of pancreatic leak include the method of pancreatic stump closure, the underlying disease process (e.g., chronic pancreatitis, benign tumors, malignant tumors, or trauma), and concomitant splenectomy.
- Postoperative pain is an important measure of outcome because it can be measured objectively. The degree of pain after open DPR is associated with the length of surgical incision, the extent of operative dissection, and operative trauma. The results from our own series demonstrated that for patients undergoing laparoscopic DPR, the amount of pain medication was not different from that required by patients undergoing laparoscopic cholecystectomy.
- The reduced incidence of wound infections after laparoscopic DPR is one of the recognized advantages of the laparoscopic approach. Furthermore, another clinical advantage of the laparoscopic DPR is the reduced incidence of a late incisional hernia.

SUGGESTED READINGS

Fernández-Cruz L, Cosa R, Blanco L, et al: Curative laparoscopic ressection for pancreatic neoplasms: a critical analysis from a single institution, *J Gastrointest Surg* 11:1607–1622, 2007.

Marbrut JY, Fernández-Cruz L, Azagra JS, et al: Laparoscopic pancreatic resection: results of a multicenter European study of 127 patients, *Surgery* 137:597–605, 2005.

Strassberg SM, Drebin JA, Linehan D: Radical antegrade modular pancreatosplenectomy, *Surgery* 133:521–527, 2003.

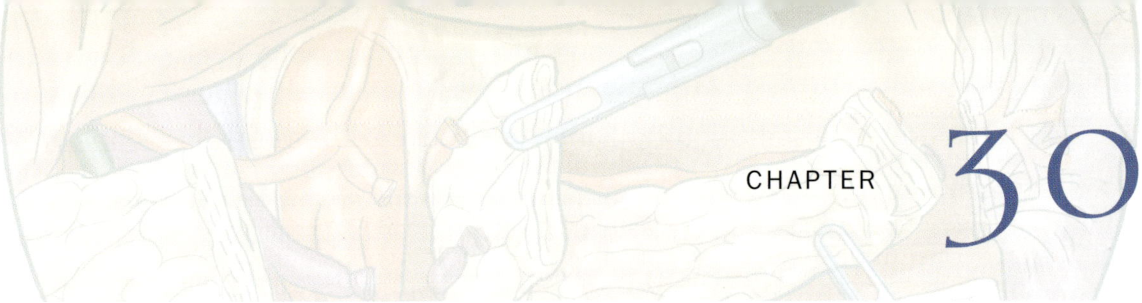

CHAPTER 30

Total Pancreatectomy

A.R. Moossa, MD, FACS, FRCS, and Jacqueline Y. Tracey, MD, FACS

I. SPECIAL PREOPERATIVE PREPARATION

Indications

- Diffuse intraductal papillary mucin-producing neoplasms
- Multicentric tumors
- Rare giant tumors—that is, cystadenomas, cystadenocarcinomas, and sarcomas
- Positive distal margin on frozen section during a Whipple resection
- Chronic pancreatitis with endocrine and exocrine pancreatic insufficiency
- Uncontrolled pancreatic fistula with sepsis or hemorrhage following a Whipple resection

Contraindications

- Distant metastases
- Inability to manage diabetes
- Invasion of portal or superior mesenteric vein or artery

Preoperative Imaging

- A pancreatic protocol abdominal computed tomography is the best test to assess tumor size, extrapancreatic invasion, nodal enlargement, and involvement of major vessels. If the tumor appears resectable on imaging, there is no need to perform a preoperative biopsy.
- Magnetic resonance cholangiopancreatography may become the preferred imaging modality in the future.
- If invasion of major vessels is unclear, an endoscopic ultrasound can be useful.
- Diagnostic endoscopic retrograde cholangiopancreatography and/or percutaneous transhepatic cholangiogram with or without biliary decompression are both avoided. Preoperative biliary manipulation is associated with increased morbidity.

Preoperative Labs

- Laboratory tests include a hemogram, chemistry panel, liver function tests, coagulation panel, and tumor markers (CEA and CA 19-9).

Other

- Mechanical bowel preparation is recommended.
- The patient is immunized against encapsulated organisms, including *Meningococcus, Haemophilus influenzae,* and *Pneumococcus*, several days before the operation. Vitamin K is also given at this time.

Informed Consent

- The surgeon must have a minimum of one comprehensive documented discussion, in simple terms, with the patient and relatives.

Immediate Preoperative Preparation

- Prophylactic antibiotics are given along with vitamin K and a proton pump inhibitor.
- Preoperative and intraoperative communication with the anesthesiologist regarding blood glucose monitoring and blood loss is paramount.

The Operation

- Preexploration laparoscopy is not routinely performed.
- The seven sacred principles of the operation can be summarized as follows: access, exposure, assistance, recognition and mobilization of anatomic structures, adherence to recognized tissue planes, and careful homeostasis.
- The anatomic extent of the operation and reconstruction is shown in Figure 30-1.

II. OPERATIVE TECHNIQUE

Position

- The supine position with a bilateral subcostal incision is preferred.

Incision

- A long vertical midline incision is used if the patient has a long narrow subcostal angle.
- The falciform ligament is preserved for later use.
- The liver and peritoneal cavity are inspected for metastatic disease. The root of the mesentery in the region of the transverse mesocolon and the ligament of Treitz are carefully inspected for puckering or tenting. The presence of portal hypertension in association with these findings implies invasion of the root of the mesentery and occlusion of the superior mesenteric vein, which indicates unresectability. If there is any question of tumor extension, a biopsy is taken for frozen-section histology.

Main Dissection

Posterior Approach (Extensive Kocher Maneuver)

- Mobilize the hepatic flexure of the colon.

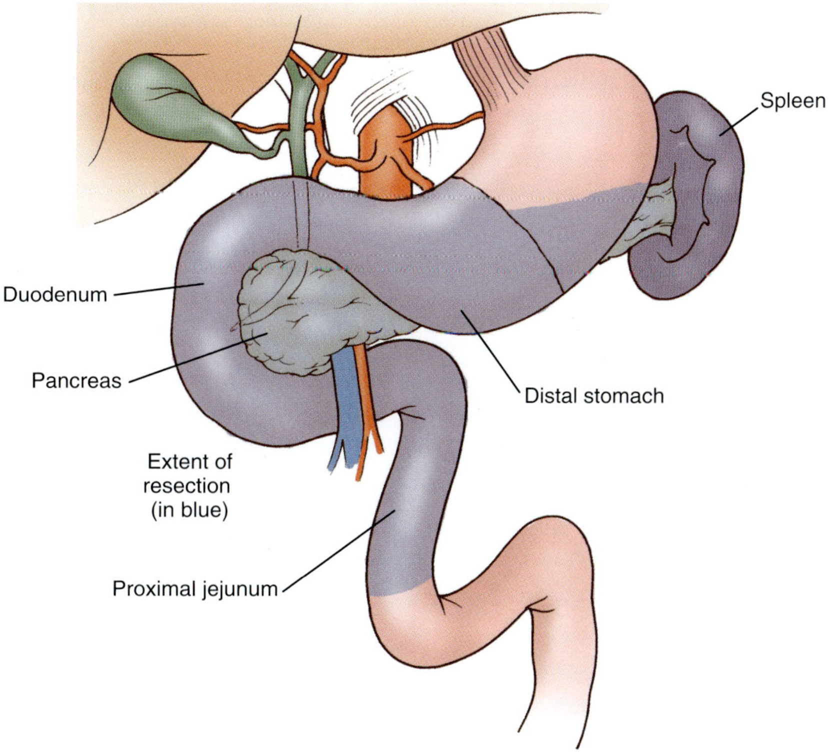

Figure 30-1.

- Incise the peritoneum lateral to the second part of the duodenum, opening the foramen of Winslow superiorly down to the third part of the duodenum where the superior mesenteric vessels cross (Fig. 30-2).
- Expose the right kidney, the right renal vessels, the vena cava, gonadal veins, and the left renal vein.
- Palpate the posterior aspect of the uncinate process to appreciate the tumor and its lateral relationship to the superior mesenteric vessels (Fig. 30-3).
- With posterior palpation, look for a potential anatomic variant, present in about 30% of individuals, the right hepatic artery (replaced right), or common hepatic artery (replaced common) originating from the superior mesenteric artery and coursing upward, behind the uncinate process and common bile duct.

Anterior Approach

- Detach the omentum from the transverse colon along the avascular plane to enter the lesser sac. Elevate the stomach and omentum to expose the pancreas (Fig. 30-4).
- Follow the middle colic vein to its junction with the superior mesenteric vein just below the neck of the pancreas.

Superior Approach

- Transversely incise the peritoneum overlying the portal triad and strip inferiorly all the soft tissue and lymphatics overlying the hepatic artery, the common hepatic duct, and the portal vein.
- Detach the gallbladder fundus first, then ligate and divide the cystic artery as usual.
- Encircle and divide the common hepatic duct. Place stay sutures on the distal bile duct and use it for traction while developing the plane anterior to the portal vein.
- Ligate and divide the gastroduodenal artery as it leaves the hepatic artery.
- If there is no invasion, this plane anterior to the portal vein can be gently opened (Fig. 30-5).

Mobilization and Transection of the Stomach

- Detach the omentum from the greater curve of the stomach; ligate the right gastroepiploic vessels and their gastric branches. Ligate and divide the left gastroepiploic vessel and the lowest short gastric vessels at this point in the procedure or after the spleen has been mobilized (Fig. 30-6).
- Elevate the stomach anteriorly. If "pylorus preservation" is desired, divide the first part of the duodenum.
- Alternatively, if an antrectomy is to be performed, ligate and divide the right gastric at its origin from the hepatic or gastroduodenal artery.
- Ligate and divide the terminal branches of the left gastric artery at the junction of the antrum and body of the stomach (crow's feet).
- Preserve the main trunk of the left gastric artery and its esophageal branches.
- Transect the stomach at the level of the incisura.

Mobilization of the Spleen and Pancreatic Tail

- Retract the dome of the spleen in the direction of the right iliac fossa. Divide the tensed posterior leaf of the lienorenal ligament in front of the left kidney and the splenocolic ligament.
- Mobilize anteriorly the spleen and tail of the pancreas using blunt dissection. The uppermost two or three short gastric vessels can now be easily ligated and divided if they were not previously.

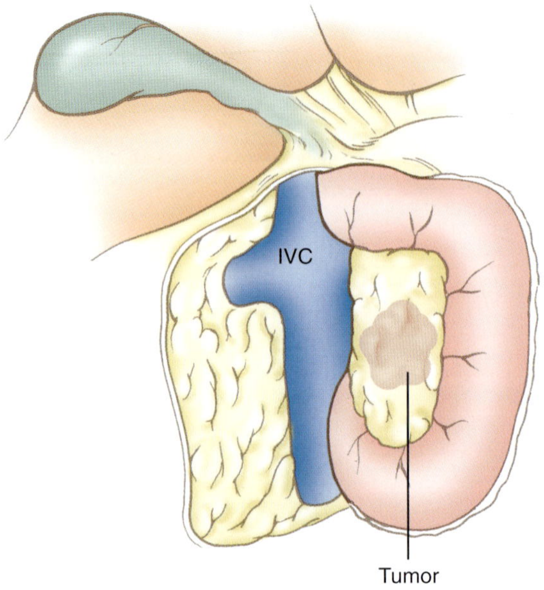

Figure 30-2. *IVC,* Inferior vena cava.

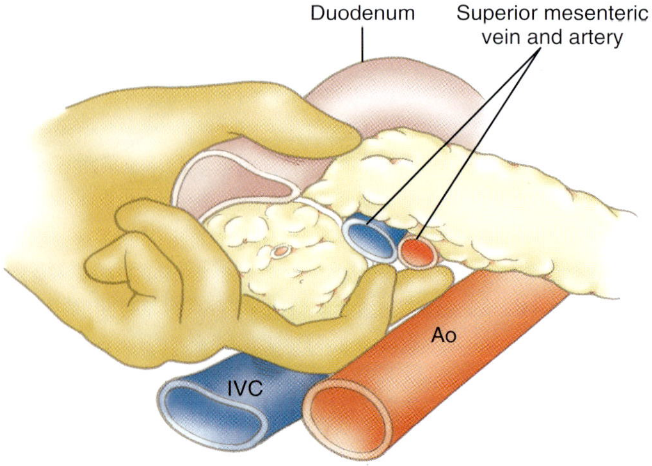

Figure 30-3. *Ao,* Aorta; *IVC,* inferior vena cava.

- The inferior mesenteric vein is dealt with according to the anatomic variation of its termination. If it enters the splenic vein, it is ligated and divided close to the entry. If it enters the superior mesenteric vein, it is not disturbed.
- Doubly ligate and divide the splenic artery at its origin from the celiac axis.
- Doubly ligate and divide the splenic vein close to its junction with the portal vein. This allows the neck of the pancreas to be elevated from the anterior aspect of the portal and superior mesenteric veins. The spleen and the left pancreas are rotated to the right.
- Three areas now attach the specimen: the uncinate process and its fibrofatty adherence to the superior mesenteric vessels, the upper small bowel with its midgut vascular attachments, and the peritoneum around the ligament of Treitz.

Freeing the Uncinate Process

- Retract the uncinate process laterally and the portal vein–superior mesenteric vein axis medially. Small venous branches are ligated and divided.
- At this point, the posterior-lateral segment of the portal vein/superior mesenteric vein axis may be found to be invaded by tumor. If the invasion is minimal, apply a Satinsky clamp and excise the lateral

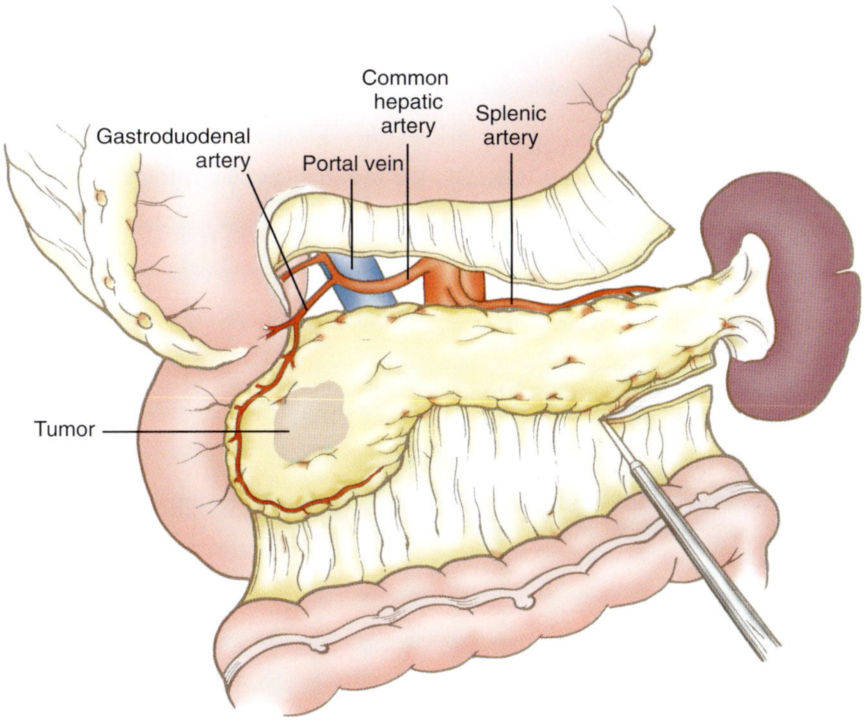

Figure 30-4.

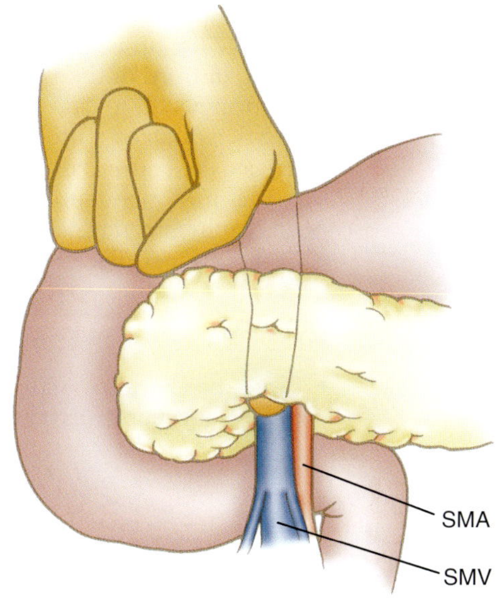

Figure 30-5. *SMA,* Superior mesenteric artery; *SMV,* superior mesenteric vein.

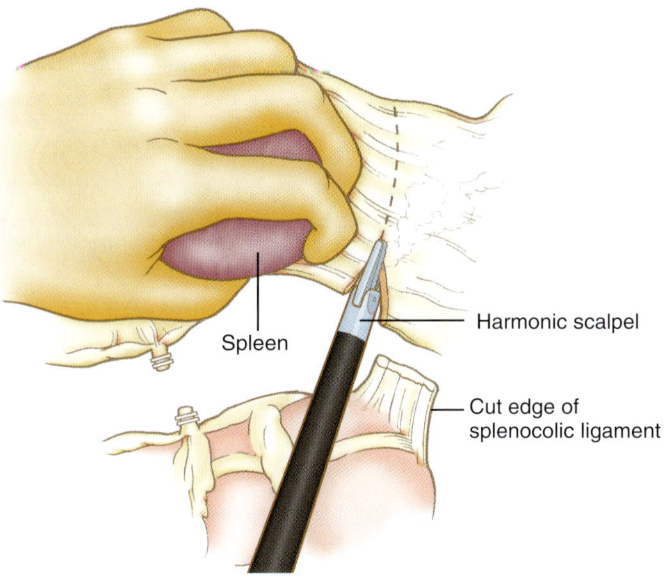

Figure 30-6.

edge of the vein along with the specimen (Fig. 30-7). Alternatively, resect a short segment of the vein with the specimen and perform an end-to-end anastomosis.

- Retract the venous trunk medially using a vein retractor, revealing the posterior bridge of tissue between the superior mesenteric artery and the uncinate process (Fig. 30-8). Before division, it is important to carefully palpate the uncinate process once more, posteriorly, to check for a possible replaced right or common hepatic artery in that location.
- The multiple small arterial branches from the superior mesenteric artery to the uncinate process are not easily seen. Stay on the adventitia of the superior mesenteric artery and sequentially separate the tissue using a right-angle clamp or hemoclips to ligate and divide the fibrofatty tissue.

Division of the Ligament of Treitz and the Proximal Jejunum

- Expose and divide the ligament of Treitz under the transverse mesocolon so that the duodenojejunal junction is free except for its vascular attachments. Free the upper jejunum by ligating and dividing the inferior pancreaticoduodenal vessels and the upper jejunal branches of the superior mesenteric vessels. Herniate the small bowel beneath the root of the mesentery into the right upper quadrant, where it can be divided to free the entire specimen.

Reconstruction

- Oversew the staple line of the upper proximal jejunum and the distal stomach with interrupted seromuscular sutures.
- Create an end-to-side hepaticojejunostomy using a single layer of full-thickness interrupted absorbable sutures, care being taken to achieve mucosa-to-mucosa apposition.
- Use the falciform ligament as a buttressing patch to hold the upper jejunum behind and around the biliary-enteric anastomosis, helping to relieve tension on the anastomosis.
- Arrange the upper jejunum to create a new "C-loop," which is tacked to the residual lateral peritoneal lining in front of the right renal capsule.
- Perform a side-to-side posterior retrocolic gastrojejunostomy. If the anastomosis is stapled, the staple line is reinforced with interrupted seromuscular sutures.
- Irrigate the entire abdomen and check for hemostasis. Place two Jackson-Pratt or similar suction drains to drain the right subhepatic space posterior to the biliary-enteric anastomosis and the left posterior subdiaphragmatic space.
- Ensure proper placement of the nasogastric tube.

Closure

- Close the abdomen with no. 1 Maxon sutures in two layers and approximate the skin with staples. If there is a generous layer of subcutaneous tissue, vertical mattress nylon sutures are used.

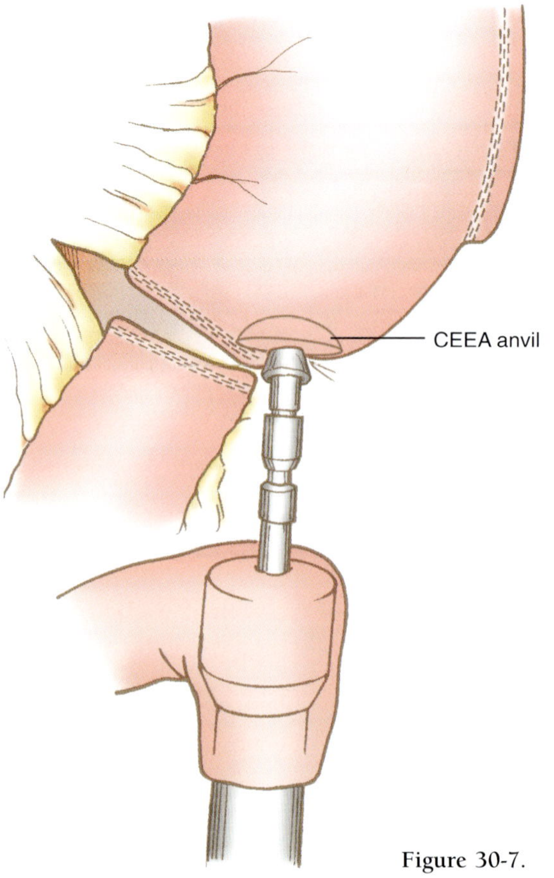

Figure 30-7.

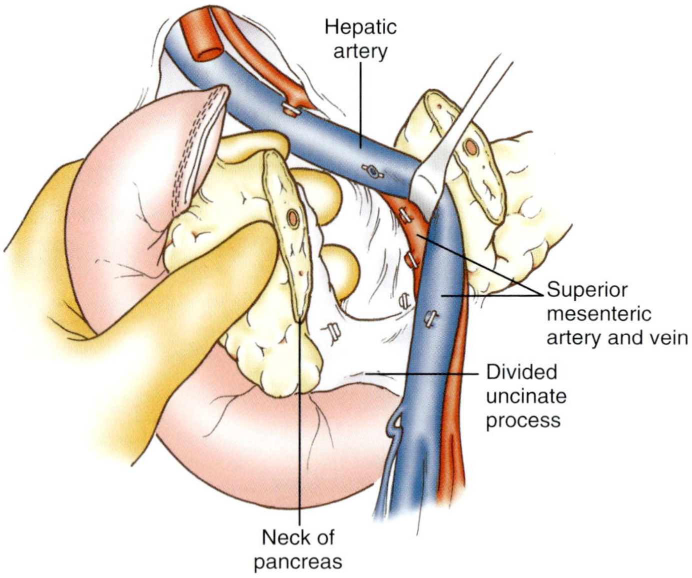

Figure 30-8.

III. ALTERNATIVE TECHNICAL APPROACHES (PRO/CON) AND PEARLS

- Splenic preservation: with benign disease only.
- Pylorus preservation: benign disease. Increased incidence of delayed gastric emptying.

IV. SPECIAL POSTOPERATIVE CARE

- Blood glucose is strictly maintained between 70 and 140 mg/dL.
- The nasogastric suction tube and the Jackson-Pratt drains are removed on the fourth or fifth postoperative day. Antibiotics are used perioperatively only.
- When eating, the patient is instructed to take small, frequent, low-fat, high-carbohydrate and -protein meals together with pancreatic enzyme supplements and a proton pump inhibitor.
- Teaching of blood glucose management and insulin administration is important.

Complications

Intraoperative Complications
- Hemorrhage is the most frequent. A thorough knowledge and appreciation of standard anatomy along with its variants is important. It is further controlled by meticulous dissection and ligation of all vessels along with replacement of blood and clotting factors as deemed appropriate.

Immediate Postoperative Complications
- Hemorrhage is most common.
- Hemobilia may develop.
- Generalized sepsis, mesenteric arterial and venous thrombosis, renal failure, hepatic failure, myocardial infarction, congestive heart failure, cerebrovascular accident, and pulmonary embolism may all occur.

Intermediate Complications
- Delayed gastric emptying occurs in roughly 20% to 30% of patients with pylorus preservation and is usually self-limiting.
- Other nonfatal complications may include urinary tract infection, pneumonitis, small bowel obstruction, wound dehiscence, atrial fibrillation, and, occasionally, bile leaks and bilomas. Intraabdominal abscesses and wound infection may develop, especially if the patient's biliary tree was stented preoperatively. Fecal fistulas and gastrojejunocolic fistulas are exceptionally rare but may occur.
- The incidence of upper gastrointestinal bleeding due to stress ulceration or marginal ulceration has decreased with adequate pharmacologic suppression of gastric acid secretion.

Late Complications
- Recurrent cancer leading to jaundice, cholangitis, gastric outlet obstruction, and small bowel obstruction may occur. On occasion, patients may develop complications due to adhesions. In addition, cholangitis secondary to intestinal biliary reflux and gastroesophageal reflux disease may occur.

Exocrine Insufficiency
- Steatorrhea may lead to dehydration, malabsorption, and weight loss.

Endocrine Insufficiency
- The resulting diabetic state necessitates comprehensive education for the patient and relatives.
- It is important to start teaching the patient to monitor his or her own blood sugar regularly at least two times a day and to self administer insulin to maintain a blood glucose level between 70 and 140 mg/dL.

Short-Term Outcome
- The operative mortality should not exceed 1% to 2% in experienced hands. The overall operative morbidity is around 40%.

Long-Term Outcome
- The long-term mortality is dependent on the type and stage of the pancreatic tumor and its response to postoperative adjuvant therapy.

SUGGESTED READINGS

Casadei R, Monari F, Buscemi S, et al: Total pancreatectomy: indications, operative technique, and results: a single centre experience and review of literature, *Updates Surg* 62:41–46, 2010.

Heidt DG, Burant C, Simeone DM: Total pancreatectomy: indications, operative technique, and postoperative sequelae, *J Gastrointest Surg* 11:209–216, 2007.

Müller MW, Freiss H, Kleeff J, et al: Total pancreatectomy—renaissance of a formerly abandoned surgical procedure? *Ann Surg* 246:966–975, 2007

CHAPTER 31

Central Pancreatectomy

Irinel Popescu, MD

I. SPECIAL PREOPERATIVE PREPARATION

- The preoperative diagnosis is important when planning a central pancreatectomy, because the operation has very specific indications.
- In benign cystic lesions, the operation is recommended most of the time. The arguments in favor of resection are the malignant potential of both mucinous and serous cysts and their dimensions, with frequent involvement of the duct of Wirsung.
- In solid tumors, the main indications are neuroendocrine tumors. In this case, if the tumor is not very large and the duct of Wirsung is not involved, an enucleation can be sufficient. Therefore, a histologic diagnosis and the precise anatomic position and relations of the tumor with the vessels and the duct of Wirsung are mandatory for a final decision.
- For the rare cases of pancreatic metastases (from renal cancer, melanoma, etc.), central resection is preferred to enucleation for oncologic reasons.
- Ultrasonography (US) (including endoscopic US; Fig. 31-1), computed tomography (CT) scan, and magnetic resonance imaging can provide an accurate diagnosis.
- Thus, the location of the tumor (at the left of the gastroduodenal artery), the diameter and the solid or cystic nature are assessed (Figs. 31-2 and 31-3, *A* and *B*).
- The relation with the duct of Wirsung is very important. When the duct is involved, enucleation is not possible and a resection should be performed (Fig. 31-4, *A* and *B*).
- Tumor markers (CA 19-9, CEA) can be useful for differentiating a benign tumor from a malignant one.
- Octreotide scan scintigraphy is used for the diagnosis of endocrine tumors.
- Intra-arterial calcium stimulating test is useful for the diagnosis of insulinoma.
- Glycemia and glucose tolerance test are indicated to evaluate the postoperative diabetes risk.
- Fine-needle biopsy (US- or CT-guided) can help in differentiating mucinous from serous adenoma and in finding malignant cells in solid tumors (Fig. 31-5). All these are important criteria for a final surgical decision.

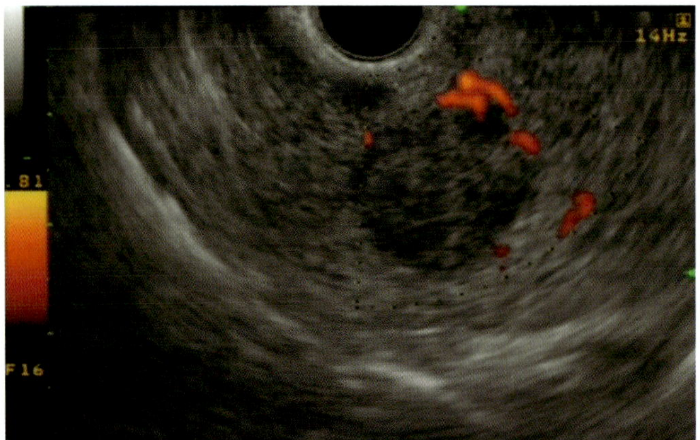

Figure 31-1. Endoscopic ultrasound: a hypoechoic mass inside the pancreatic body.

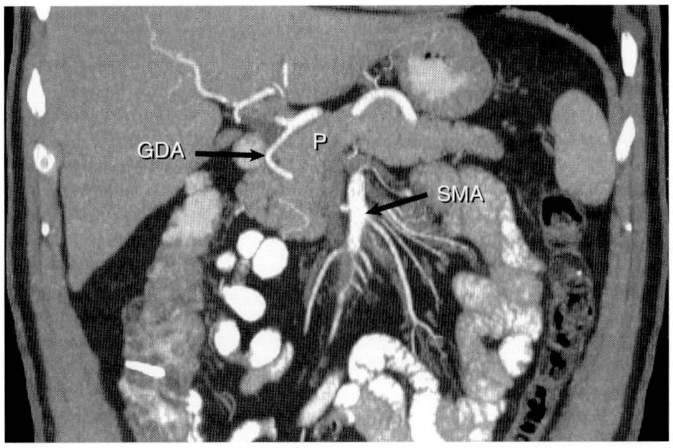

Figure 31-2. Computed tomography angiography reconstruction: normal view of the pancreas and main arterial vessels. *GDA,* Gastroduodenal artery; *P,* pancreas; *SMA,* superior mesenteric artery.

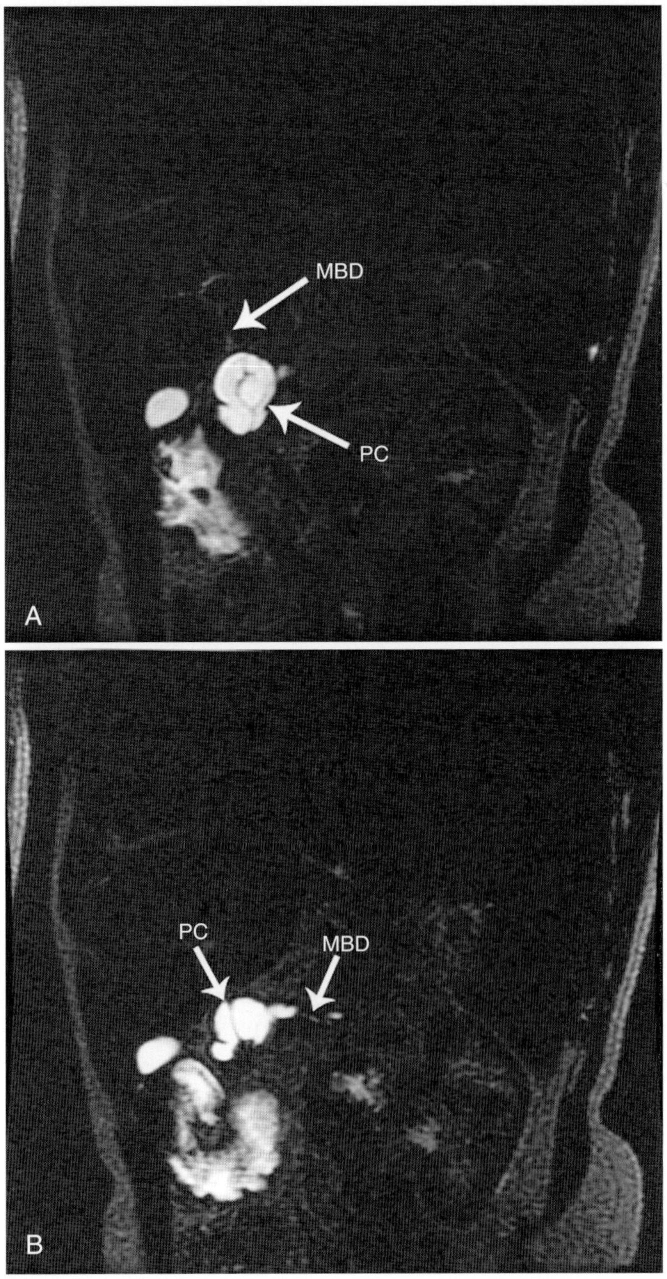

Figure 31-4. Magnetic resonance cholangiopancreatography—thin slice 250 TE (echo time). The cyst (*PC*) presents an irregular form and multiple septa inside. **A,** Main biliary duct (*MBD*) is thin. **B,** Main pancreatic duct (*MPD*) is also thin except a small segment dilated because of tumor compression.

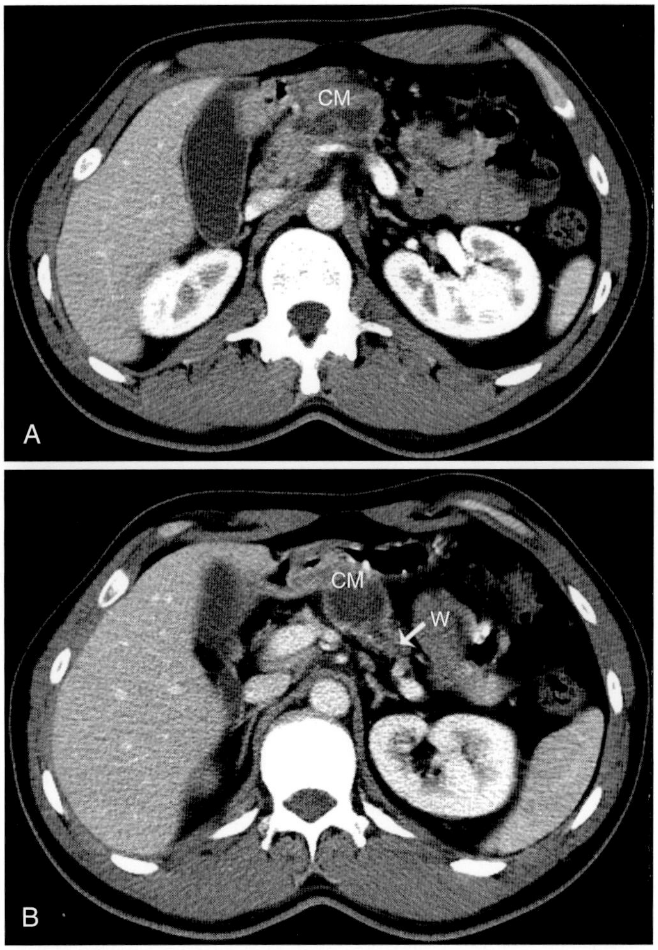

Figure 31-3. Contrast-enhanced computed tomography of a cystic pancreatic tumor. A, Well-circumscribed cystic mass (*CM*) with a thin wall and small enhanced septa in the pancreas body. **B,** The duct of Wirsung (*W*) is dilated at the contact with the cyst.

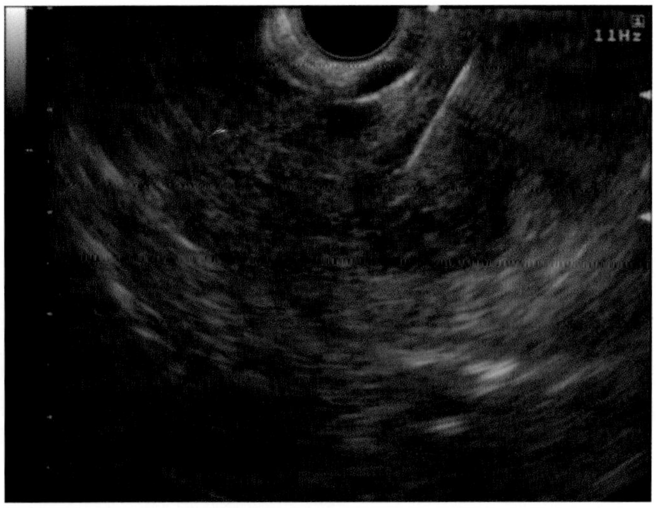

Figure 31-5. Endoscopic ultrasound: the fine needle inside the tumor.

II. OPERATIVE TECHNIQUE

Position

- The patient is in the supine position, with the abdomen prepped and draped from the lower thorax to the suprapubic area.

Incision

- A midline incision is preferred in thin and lanky patients, whereas a transverse incision is performed in obese, thick, or stocky patients.

Main Dissection

- A complete exploration of the abdomen is mandatory because it can reveal other tumor locations, liver metastases, local recurrence, and so forth.
- The lesser sac is entered either through detachment of the greater omentum from the transverse colon or through division and ligation of the vessels of the greater omentum.
- The next step is a complete exploration of the pancreas, including visual inspection, palpation, and intraoperative US.
- The first assessment is to determine whether the lesion is benign (in malignant tumors, except for small metastases, central pancreatectomy is not indicated because of the safety margins required and of the associated lymphadenectomy, both precluding limited resections).
  - It is better to have a preoperative diagnosis of malignancy that can be obtained through a fine-needle biopsy. If this is not done, the intraoperative approach is rather to resect the specimen and ask for a frozen section than to perform an intraoperative fine-needle biopsy.
- A second aspect that must be evaluated from the beginning is the position of the tumor:
  - At the right border, the tumor should be located to the left of the gastroduodenal artery; otherwise, a resection of the pancreatic head is indicated.
  - At the left border, the tumor should leave at least 5 cm of uninvolved pancreas; otherwise, a left pancreatectomy (or splenopancreatectomy) is indicated (in this case the benefit of leaving just a small amount of pancreatic tissue is minimal and does not outweigh the risk of postoperative pancreatic fistula).
  - The degree of involvement of the pancreatic parenchyma: small and superficial tumors can benefit from an enucleation, whereas larger or deeply located tumors will require a central resection.
  - The relation of the tumor with the pancreatic duct and with the splenic and mesenteric vessels (these elements are assessed by intraoperative US): tumors that involve the pancreatic duct must be resected.
- The peritoneum is incised at the upper and lower border of the pancreas (Fig. 31-6).

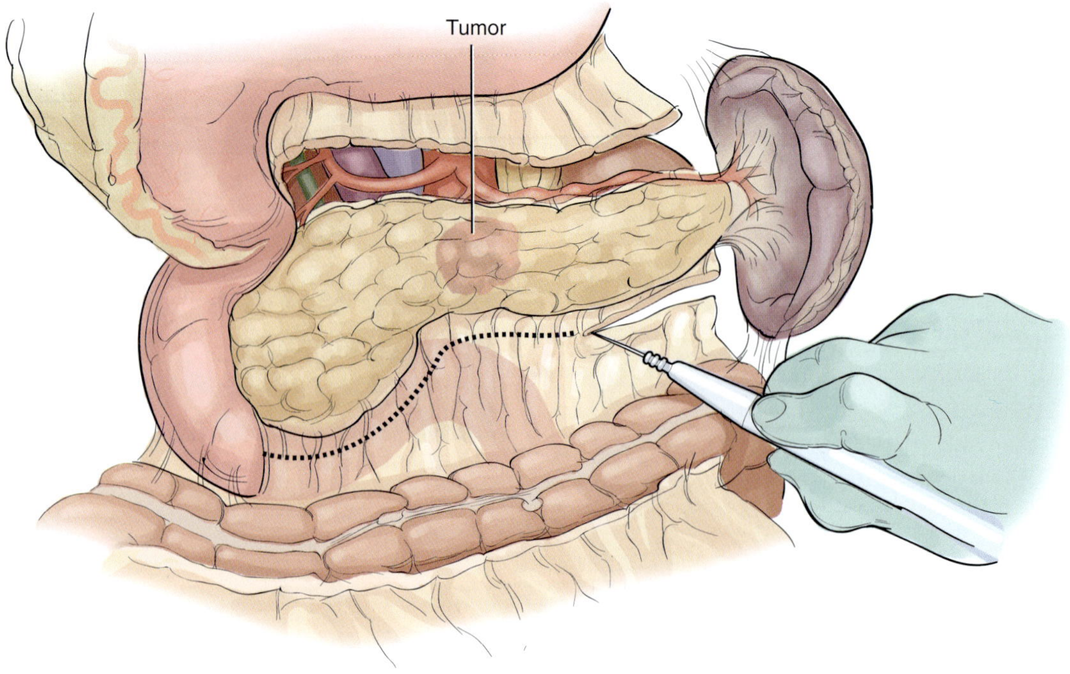

Figure 31-6.

- The most important maneuver is the separation of the portomesenteric axis from the pancreas (Fig. 31-7); this is performed digitally. When the separation is complete, a tape is introduced through the created tunnel, lifting the pancreas. In the area to be resected, the splenic artery is located superiorly and the portal vein inferiorly and posteriorly. Therefore, arterial and venous branches for the pancreas are encountered at these levels. These branches should be ligated and divided until a 1-cm margin is reached on the left side of the tumor. This can be done after the division of the pancreas on the right side of the tumor (which makes the maneuver easier) (Fig. 31-8). On the right side, it is usually

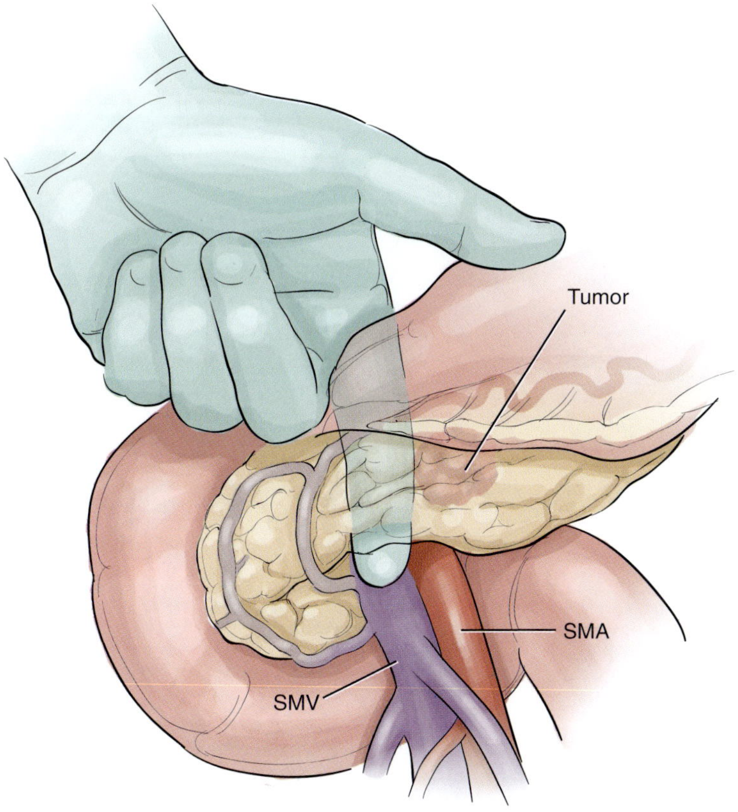

Figure 31-7. *SMA,* Superior mesenteric artery; *SMV,* superior mesenteric vein.

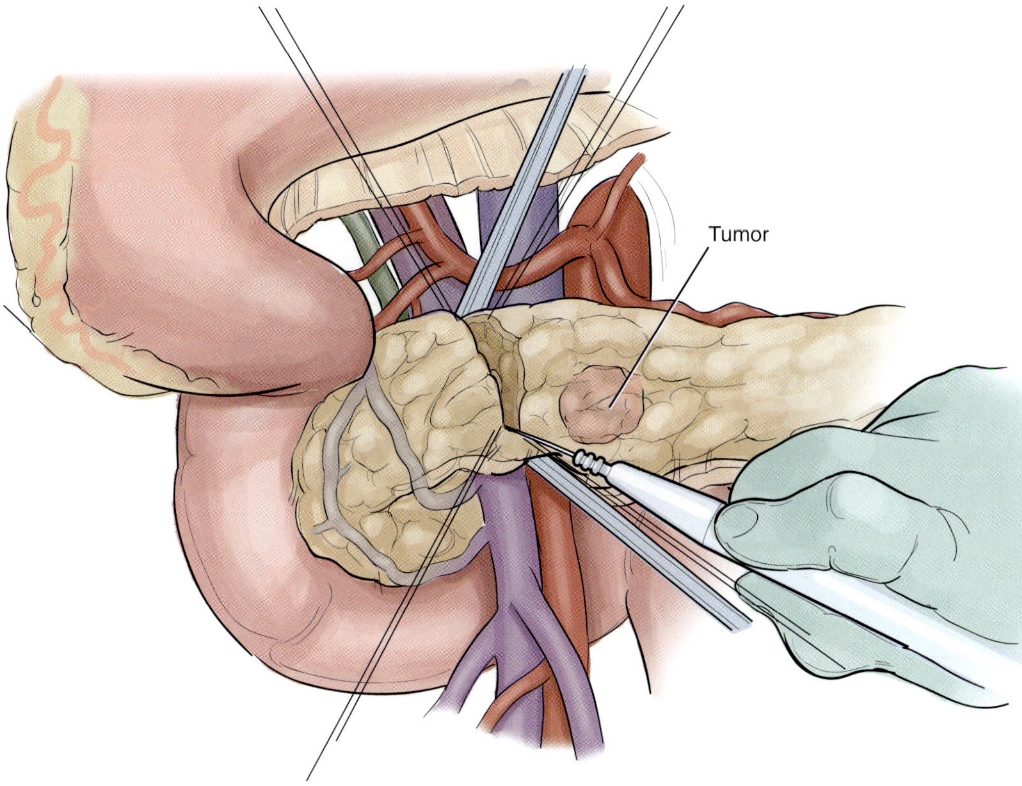

Figure 31-8.

necessary to dissect the hepatic artery for a distance of a few centimeters. Sometimes, a dorsal pancreatic artery can emerge, most often from the splenic artery, very rarely from the hepatic artery. If it is of a significant size, the central pancreatectomy should be converted into a left (distal) pancreatectomy, because of the risk of ischemia of the pancreatic tail. A second tape is introduced behind the pancreas at the level of the division line on the left side.

- The pancreas is transected first on the right side, at the level of the tape that is used to protect the portal vein (Figs. 31-9 and 31-10). The division of the pancreas can be done with the scalpel or by electrocautery. When the scalpel is used, the cut surface has many bleeding points that should be

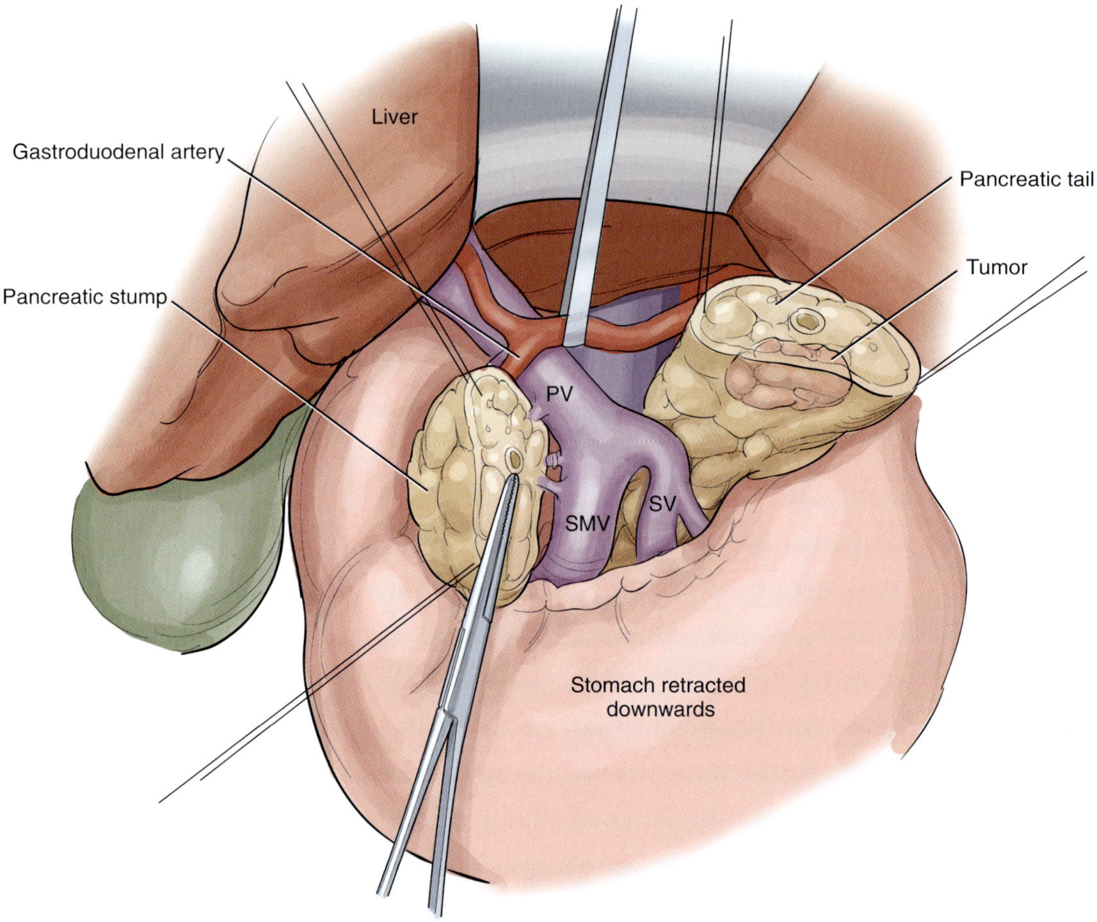

Figure 31-9. *PV,* Portal vein; *SMV,* superior mesenteric vein; *SV,* splenic vein.

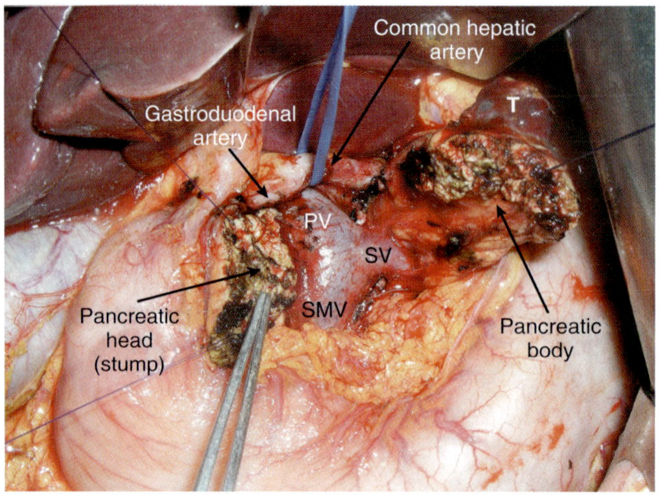

Figure 31-10. Transection of the pancreas at the left of the gastroduodenal artery. *PV,* Portal vein; *SMV,* superior mesenteric vein; *SV,* splenic vein; *T,* tumor.

carefully controlled with stitches or electric coagulation. This is partially avoided when using electrocautery, which is considered, however, more aggressive for the pancreatic tissue and therefore more prone to a risk of fistula. The right pancreatic stump is closed using a separate stitch on the duct of Wirsung (if this can be identified) and separate stitches of 4-0 Prolene between the anterior and the posterior margin (Figs. 31-11 and 31-12).

- The dissection continues to the left. If there are any other branches of the splenic vein or artery still attached to the area to be removed, these are carefully ligated and divided. The pancreas is sectioned at the level of the left tape in the same manner as described earlier.

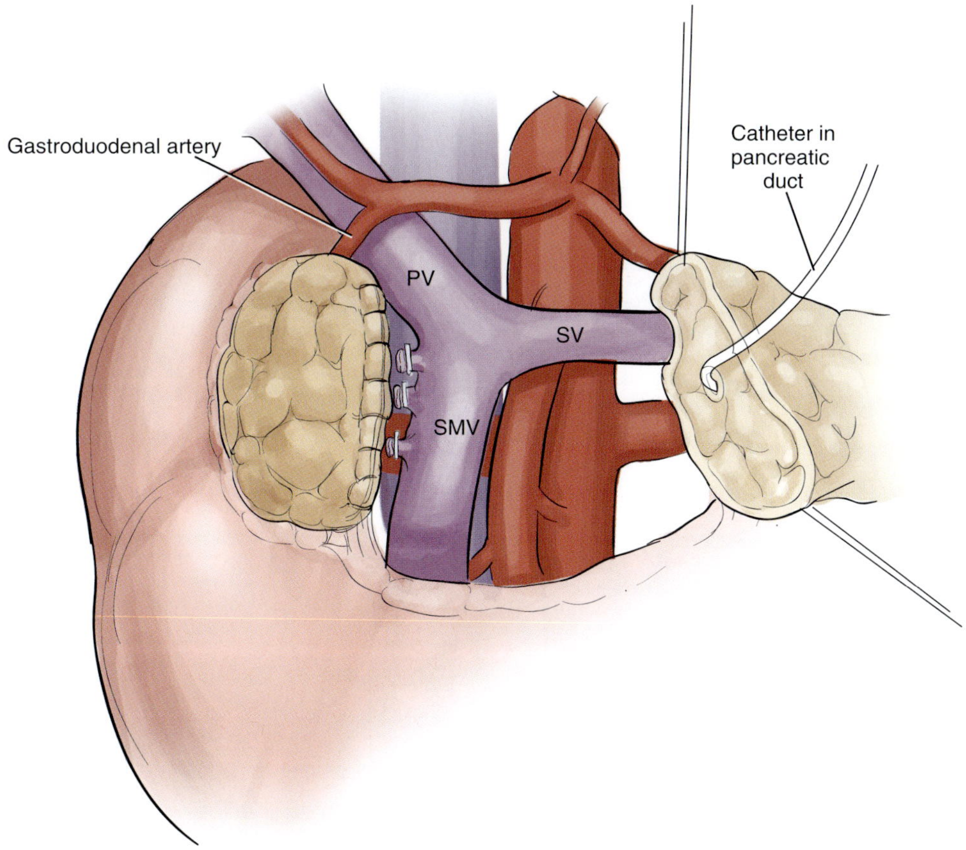

Figure 31-11. *PV,* Portal vein; *SMV,* superior mesenteric vein; *SV,* splenic vein.

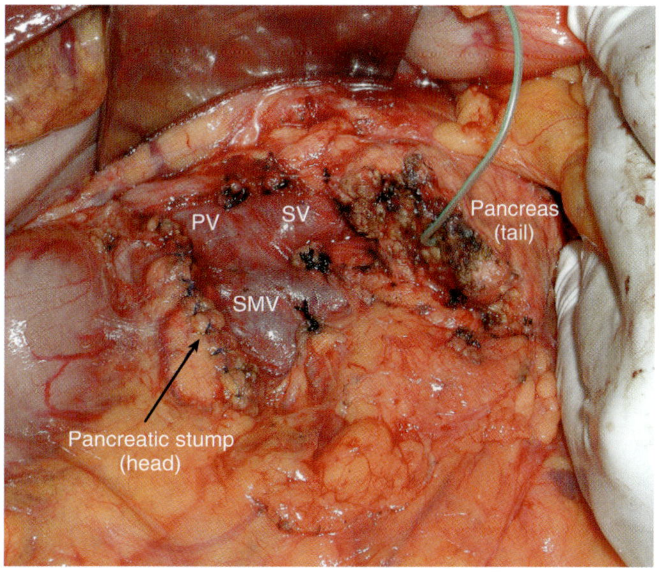

Figure 31-12. Intraoperative view after the removal of the specimen. The duct of Wirsung in the pancreatic tail is stented. *PV,* Portal vein; *SMV,* superior mesenteric vein; *SV,* splenic vein.

- The duct of Wirsung is identified, and a stent is introduced inside and anchored with Prolene (see Figs. 31-11 and 31-12). A Roux-en-Y small bowel loop is made from the proximal jejunum using a linear stapler. The distal end is brought through the transverse mesocolon, and an end-to-side anastomosis with the pancreatic stump is performed (Figs. 31-13 and 31-14). One layer of 5-0 polydioxanone (PDS) interrupted sutures is used. The proximal end of the small bowel is implanted in an end-to-side manner into the distal end, at approximately 50 cm distance from the anastomosis with the pancreas. The enteroenteric anastomosis is performed manually, in two layers of 4-0 running PDS.
- Additional stitches of 4-0 PDS are used to close the mesenteric defect.

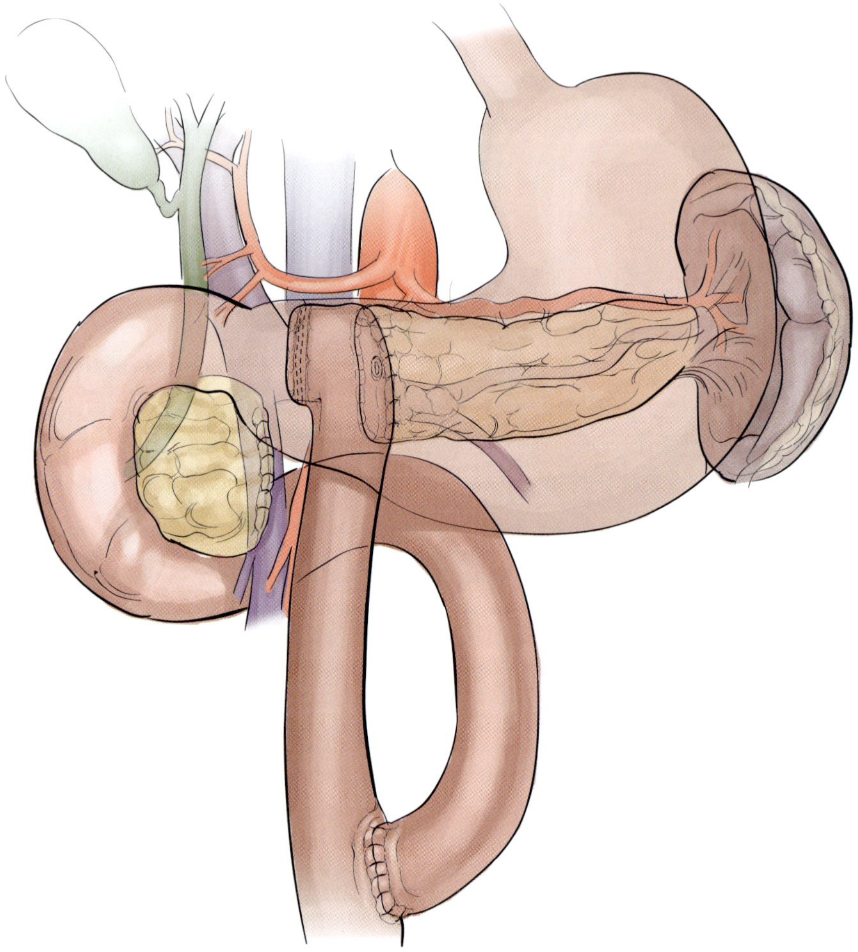

Figure 31-13.

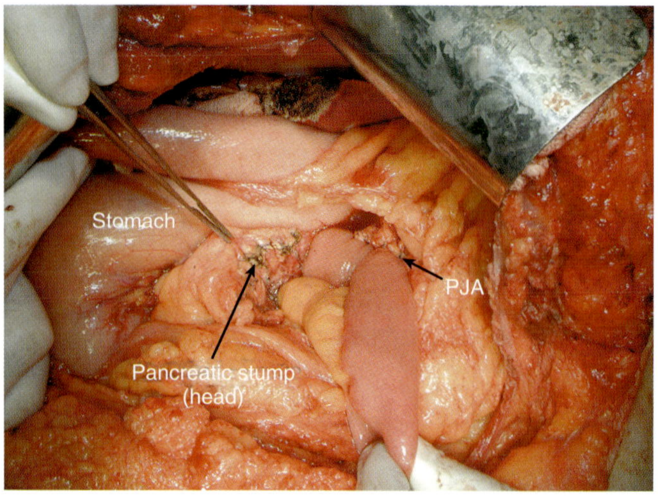

Figure 31-14. The terminolateral pancreaticojejunal anastomosis (*PJA*) with a Roux-en-Y small bowel loop. The stump of the pancreatic head is closed with separate stitches.

Closure

- Drains are placed in the proximity of the pancreatic stump and of the pancreaticojejunal anastomosis.
- The abdomen is closed using a running suture of no. 1 (loop) nonabsorbable monofilament suture.
- The skin is carefully closed with staples.
- Intravenous somatostatin can be started during the operation.

III. ALTERNATIVE TECHNICAL APPROACHES (PROS/CONS) AND PEARLS

- Because pancreatic fistula is the main complication after this operation, various methods have been employed to avoid it.
- If the caliber of the duct of Wirsung is large enough, stenting might not be necessary, and a direct anastomosis of the duct with the small bowel can be performed.
- A second layer of sutures can be added at the two corners of the pancreaticojejunal anastomosis and on the anterior face of the anastomosis.
- The pancreaticogastrostomy is an alternative that avoids the operative steps in the inframesocolic compartment and the preparation of the Roux-en-Y loop. The stomach is incised longitudinally on the posterior face for an appropriate distance, and the pancreatic stump is anastomosed with interrupted stitches of 4-0 PDS to the stomach. A second layer of stitches is recommended. There is no need to stent the pancreatic duct.
- Recently, the central pancreatectomy has been performed laparoscopically. Dissection is similar to the open approach. To cut the pancreas on the right side, a linear stapler can be used. There is no need for additional stitches in this case. Alternatively, the LigaSure (Tyco-Valleylab, Boulder, Colo.) or the Harmonic scalpel (Ethicon Endo-Surgery, Cincinnati) can be used. These can produce a good division of the pancreas and seal the duct of Wirsung at the same time. In both cases, suture of the pancreatic stump is necessary, as in the open technique. On the left side, either LigaSure or Harmonic scalpel is used for cutting the pancreas. The rest of the technique is similar to the open approach but requires appropriate skill with laparoscopic digestive anastomoses.

IV. SPECIAL POSTOPERATIVE CARE

- Somatostatin administration should be continued postoperatively.
- The patient should be closely monitored, because bleeding episodes (from the pancreatic stump, the Roux-en-Y anastomosis, or other sources) may occur and sometimes may require early reoperation.
- The drains must be monitored, and if there is a suspicion of pancreatic fistula, amylase should be determined in the drainage fluid.
- Fistulas from the proximal stump are rare and have a better course, with small output and spontaneous closure.
- Fistulas from the pancreaticoenteric anastomosis are more difficult to treat and take a longer time to close. Complications such as intraabdominal abscesses are more frequent and require either percutaneous drainage or reoperation. Fistulas that do not close spontaneously may also require reoperation and redoing of the pancreaticojejunal anastomosis.
- US monitoring is mandatory. Peripancreatic fluid collections require CT scan and percutaneous drainage.
- Glycemia also should be monitored, because there is a definite risk of diabetes, even after such limited resections.
- Both the exocrine and endocrine function need to be monitored for the long term.

SUGGESTED READINGS

Iacono C, Bortolasi L, Serio G: Indications and technique of central pancreatectomy—early and late results, *Langenbecks Arch Surg* 390:266–271, 2005.

Sauvanet A, Partensky C, Sastre B, et al: Medial pancreatectomy: a multi-institutional retrospective study of 53 patients by the French Pancreas Club, *Surgery* 132:836–843, 2002.

Vibert E, Regimbeau JM, Sauvanet A: Technique de la pancreatectomie mediane, *Ann Chir* 128:268–272, 2003.

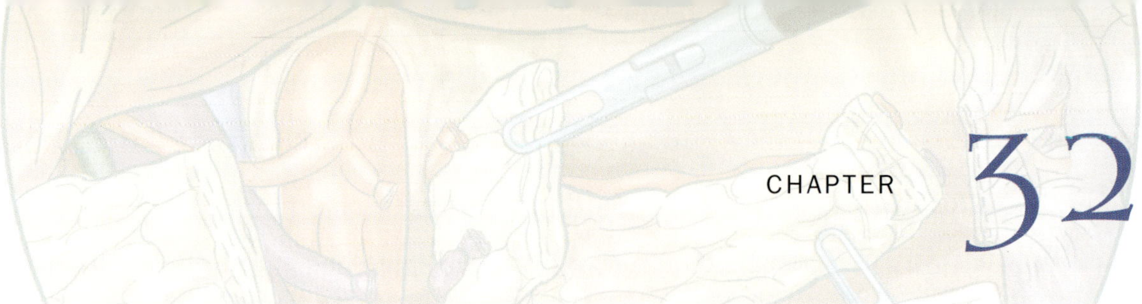

CHAPTER 32

Extended Pancreatectomy with Resection of the Celiac Axis (Appleby Operation)

Irinel Popescu, MD

I. SPECIAL PREOPERATIVE PREPARATION

- The preoperative diagnosis starts with ultrasonography. A description of the tumor (dimensions, local invasion, vascular invasion) is obtained as a preliminary step.
- Computed tomography (CT) scan and magnetic resonance imaging confirm the ultrasonographic findings and provide detailed information about the tumor. Currently, CT angiography has almost completely replaced arteriography. Contrast CT is mandatory for evaluating the limits of the tumor, its structure and its relation with the surrounding tissues (Figs. 32-1 and 32-2).
- Tumoral invasion of the celiac axis or of the common hepatic artery (CHA) is the key element for planning the operative strategy.
- The anatomic basis of the Appleby operation is the restoration of hepatic flow via the gastroduodenal artery (GDA) from the superior mesenteric artery (SMA) in the case of ligation of the celiac trunk or of the CHA (Figs. 32-3 and 32-4).
- A percutaneous or endoscopic biopsy may provide the histologic diagnosis.
- Signs of metastatic disease (liver or lung metastases, peritoneal carcinomatosis, and ascites) are a clear contraindication for resection.
- Elevated markers (CA 19-9, CEA) are usually a bad prognostic sign and can be taken into consideration for a final decision on resection.
- When the disease is confined only to the pancreas, a splenopancreatectomy with celiac axis resection can be performed.

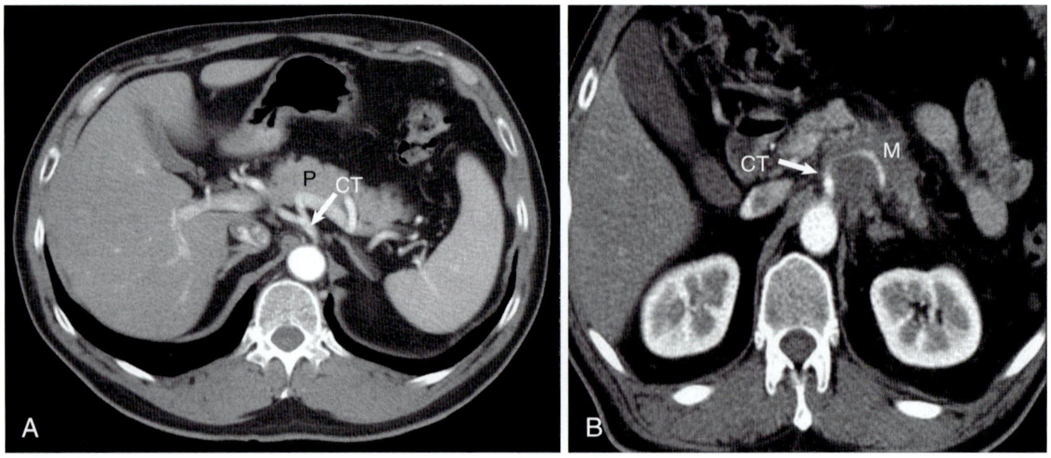

Figure 32-1. **A,** Normal view of the pancreas (*P*) and the origin of celiac trunk (*CT*)—axial plane in spiral computed tomography. **B,** Axial image shows a hypodense mass (*M*) in the pancreas body invading the CT.

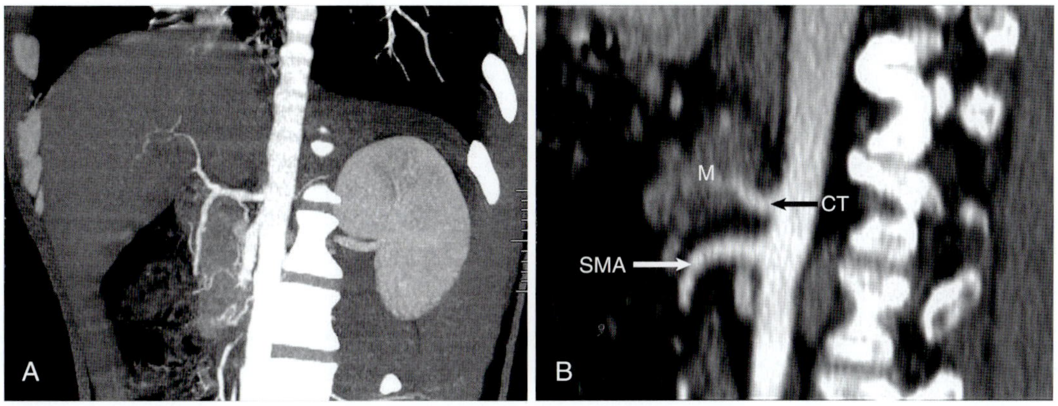

Figure 32-2. **A**, Normal computed tomography angiogram reconstruction. **B**, Computed tomography angiogram (maximum intensity projection) shows irregular encasement at the origin of celiac trunk (*CT*) and a noninvaded superior mesenteric artery (*SMA*).

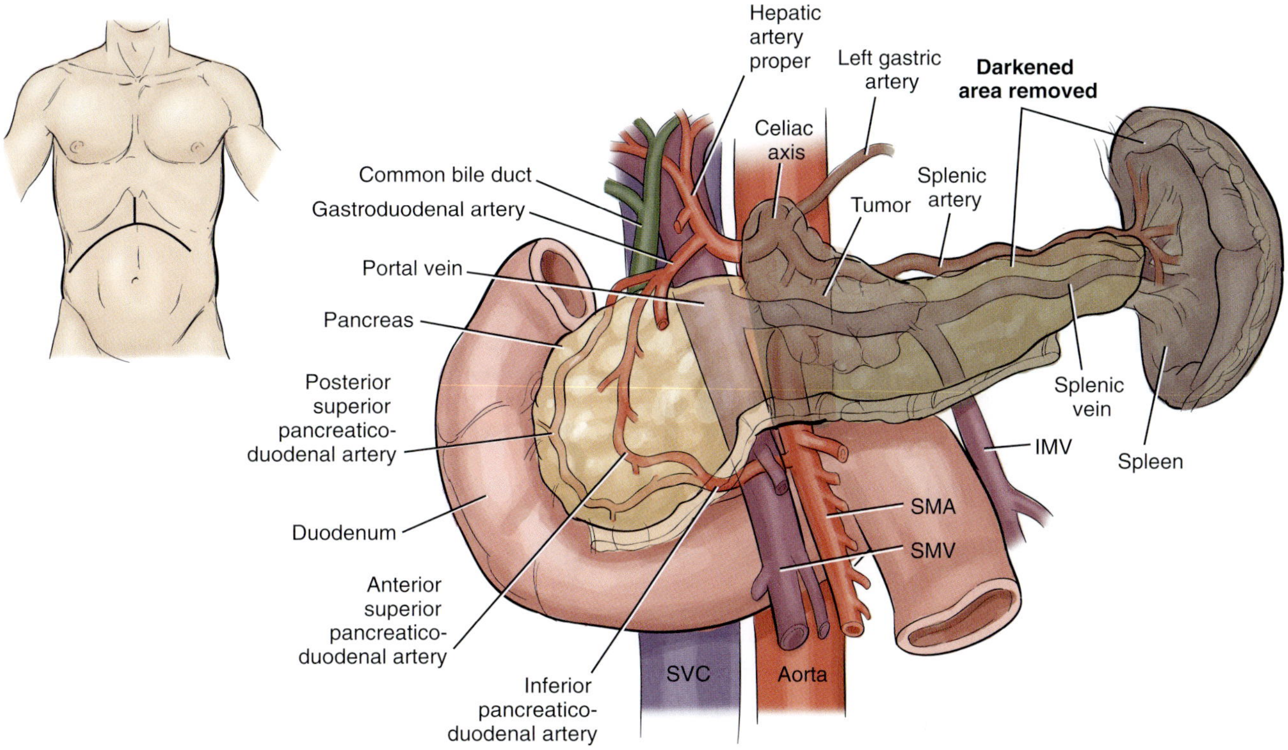

Figure 32-3. *IMV,* Inferior mesenteric vein; *SMA,* superior mesenteric artery; *SMV,* superior mesenteric vein; *SVC,* superior vena cava.

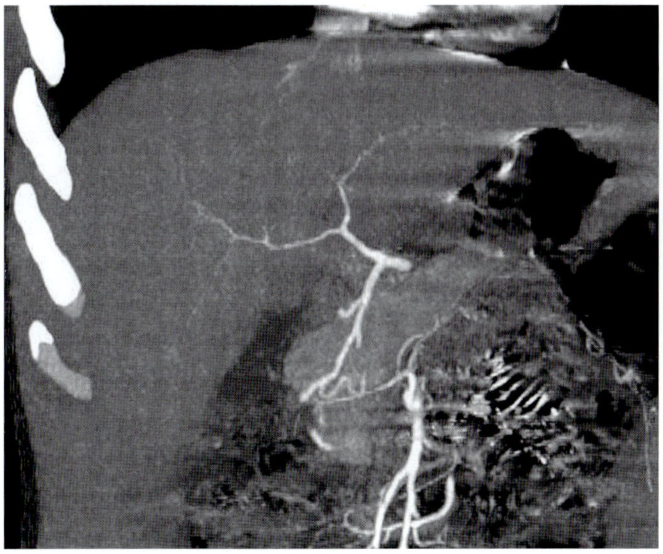

Figure 32-4. Computed tomography angiography reconstruction showing collaterals between gastroduodenal artery and superior mesenteric artery at the level of the pancreatic head, through the pancreaticoduodenal arcades.

- It is important to determine that the SMA is not invaded. Its invasion will be a clear sign of nonresectability for oncologic and technical reasons:
  - ▲ The prognosis is very bad in case of invasion.
  - ▲ The inferior pancreatic arteries, branches of the SMA, are the vessels that reestablish the flow through the GDA, and their resection could completely compromise the arterial circulation of the liver.
- It is also important to assess that the proper hepatic artery and the GDA are not invaded.
- Embolization of the CHA before the operation can aid the development of collateral circulation.

II. OPERATIVE TECHNIQUE

- The aim of the operation is an R0 en bloc resection.

Position

- The patient is in the supine position, with the surgeon on the right side and the first assistant on the left side.

Incision

- A bilateral subcostal incision is preferred, with a xiphoid extension ("Mercedes-Benz") (see Fig. 32-3, *inset*). A long midline incision starting at the xiphoid and ending below the umbilicus could also be adequate, especially in thin patients. The operative field should be optimally exposed. An abdominal retractor with bilateral subcostal retraction is necessary.

Main Dissection

- The exploration of the abdominal cavity includes inspection, palpation, and intraoperative ultrasonography.
- Distant metastases (liver, peritoneum) will be searched for because they contraindicate the resection.
- The local invasion must be evaluated. The invasion of the SMA is a key element that also precludes a resection. The retropancreatic space, just above the left renal vein, is the advisable place to look for it. The Kocher maneuver is necessary. This maneuver is recommended in all cases because it allows a good assessment of the retropancreatic space in the cephalic area (invasion at this level contraindicates the operation).
- Next, the hepatic artery is examined: the GDA must not be invaded and must have a good caliber. The proper hepatic artery must also not be invaded. To be sure there is an adequate flow coming from the GDA, the CHA is clamped; the pulse in the proper hepatic artery is assessed and the flow is measured with a flowmeter or through Doppler ultrasonography (Fig. 32-5). The intrahepatic arterial circulation is assessed with Doppler ultrasound examination after clamping the CHA. The lesser sac is entered through the gastrocolic omentum, ligating and dividing the epiploic vessels, or through coloepiploic detachment. The lesser omentum is divided completely. The hepatic artery is dissected starting from the hepatic pedicle toward the celiac trunk; the GDA is exposed and dissected for a length of 1 to 2 cm. The dissection of the hepatic artery stops at the takeoff of the splenic artery or at the place of tumoral invasion (when this extends to the CHA); 2-0 silk ties are tied on the artery, which is then transected.
- The portal vein is dissected supra- and infrapancreatically. The surgeon's finger is introduced into the plane between the pancreas and the portal vein, creating a tunnel between the two, where a tape is introduced.

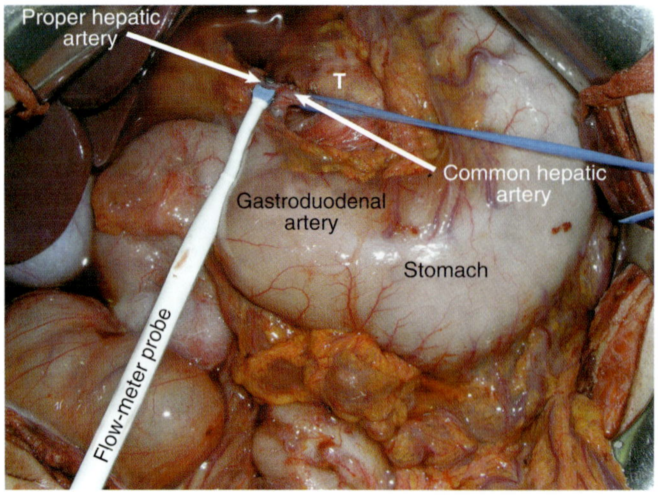

Figure 32-5. Assessment of the hepatic arterial flow after clamping the common hepatic artery. *T*, Tumor.

- The pancreas is divided at this level, above the tape, using either a scalpel (in this case completing the hemostasis with 5-0 Prolene stitches and electrocoagulation) or an electrocautery. The duct of Wirsung is closed separately with a stitch of 5-0 Prolene. The pancreatic stump is oversewn with separate stitches of 4-0 Prolene.
- When the portal vein is exposed with the portosplenic confluence, the splenic vein can be divided between clamps and the two ends can be oversewn with 5-0 Prolene.
- When the stomach is not invaded, it can be preserved, but the right gastric and right gastroepiploic arteries should also be preserved (Fig. 32-6).
- The left gastric artery and vein are ligated and divided above the pancreas and close to the stomach (Fig. 32-7).

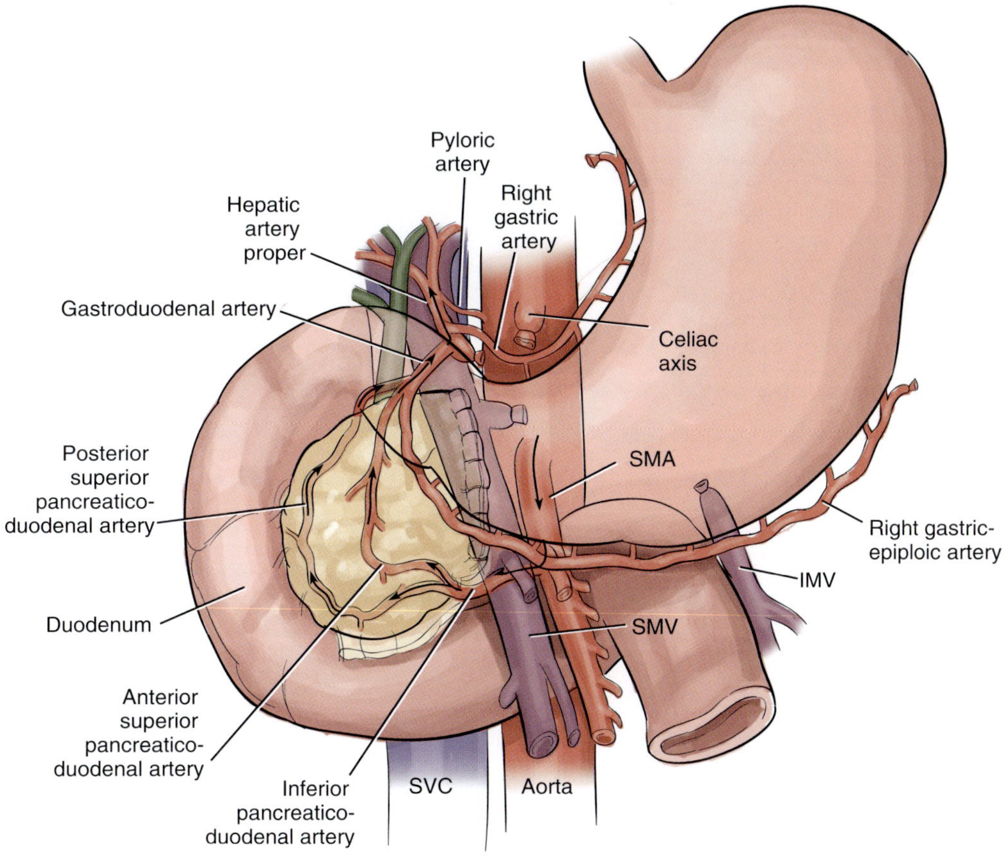

Figure 32-6. *IMV,* Inferior mesenteric vein; *SMA,* superior mesenteric artery; *SMV,* superior mesenteric vein; *SVC,* superior vena cava.

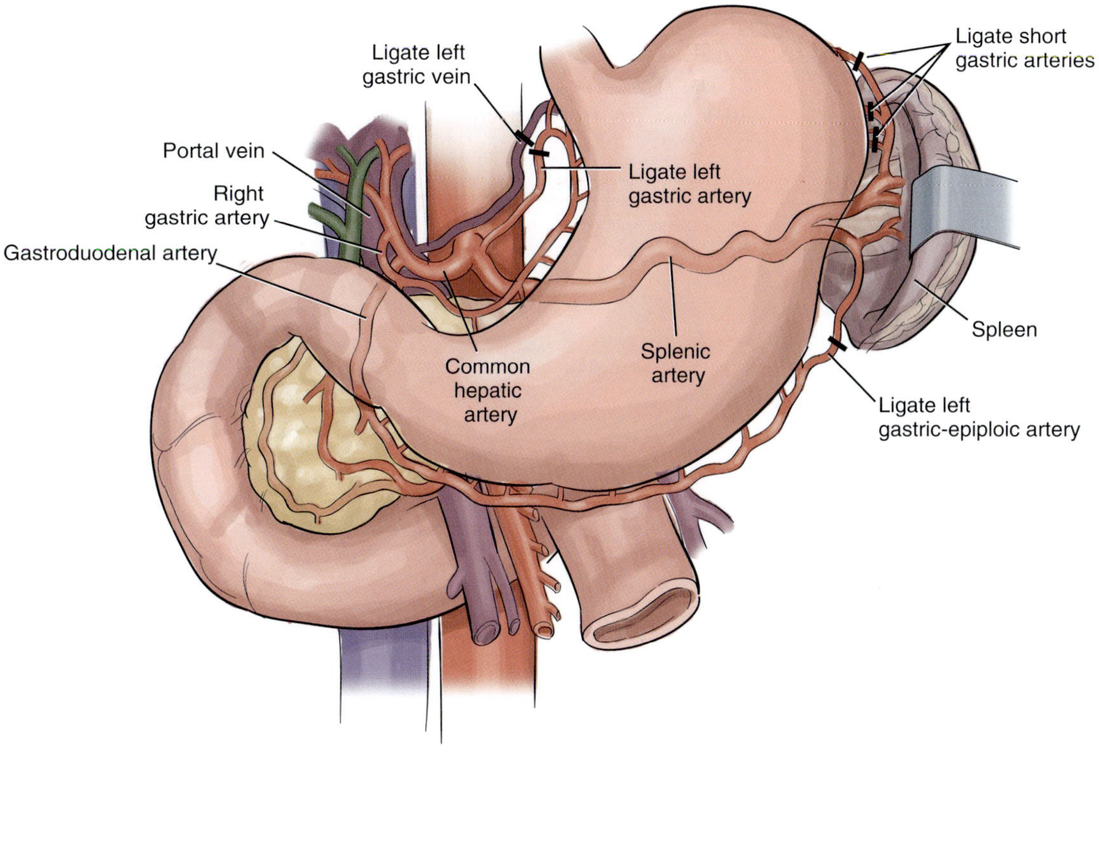

Figure 32-7.

- The left gastroepiploic vessels and the short gastric vessels are divided and ligated (see Fig. 32-7).
- After the incision of the infrapancreatic peritoneum, the inferior mesenteric vein is ligated and divided (Fig. 32-8).
- The splenocolic and splenorenal ligaments are divided (see Fig. 32-8).
- The spleen is mobilized from the lateral and superior attachments toward the right, together with the pancreatic tail and body. At the level of the celiac trunk, a clamp is applied behind the tumor mass and immediately in front of the aorta, and the trunk is ligated and divided (Fig. 32-9). Then, the entire specimen is removed (Fig. 32-10).

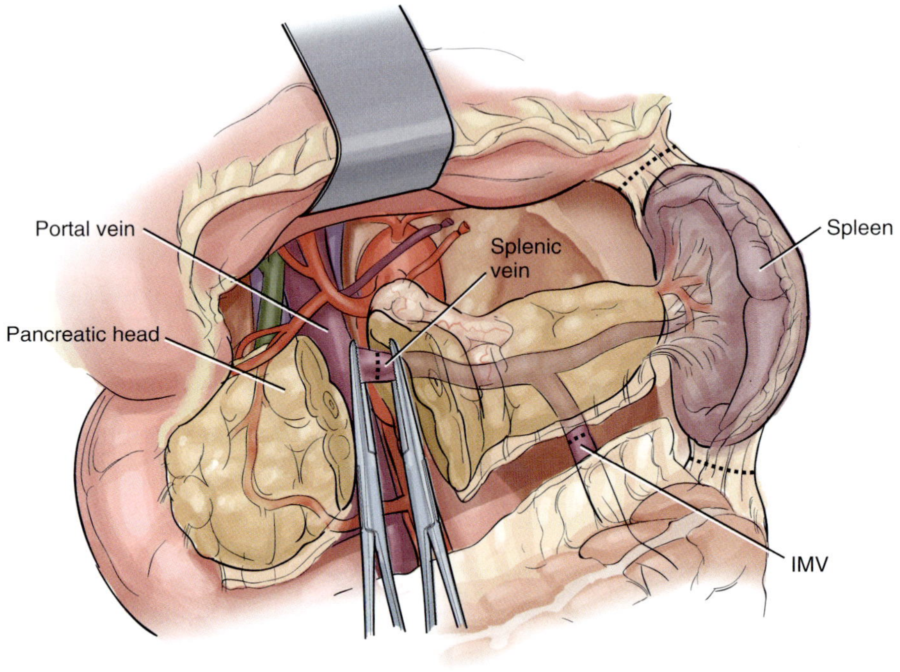

Figure 32-8. *IMV,* Inferior mesenteric vein.

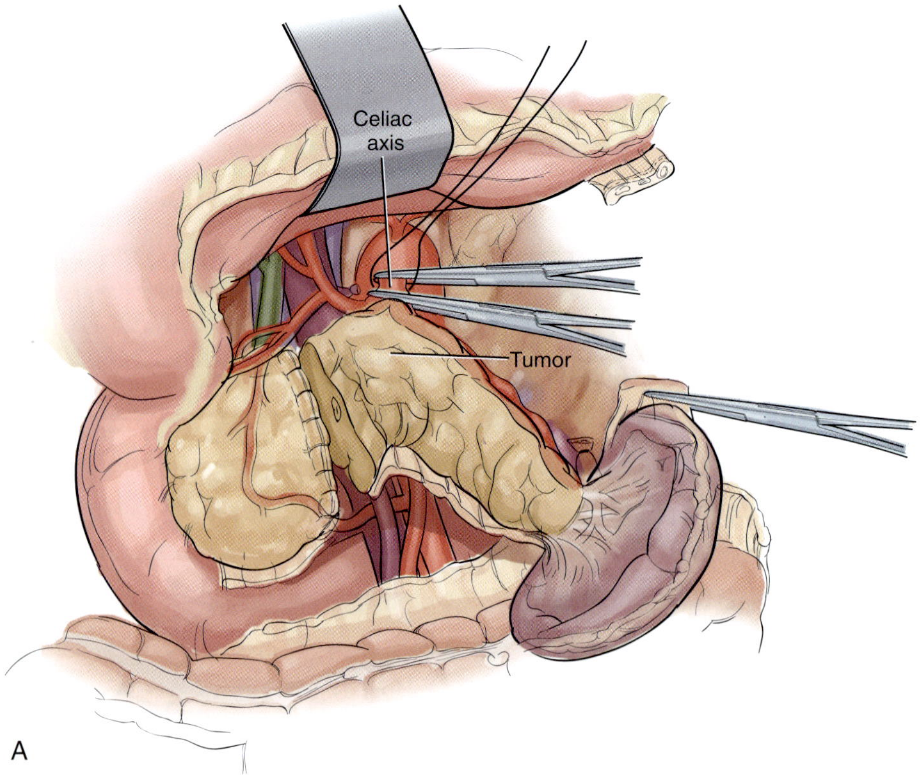

Figure 32-9. Isolation of the celiac axis in a case of Appleby procedure associated with total gastrectomy. *P*, Head of pancreas; *T*, tumor.

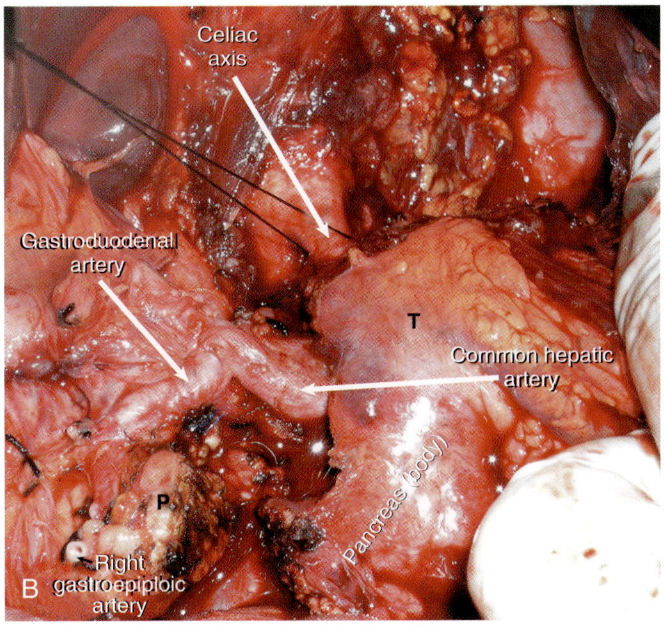

Figure 32-9, cont'd. For legend see opposite page.

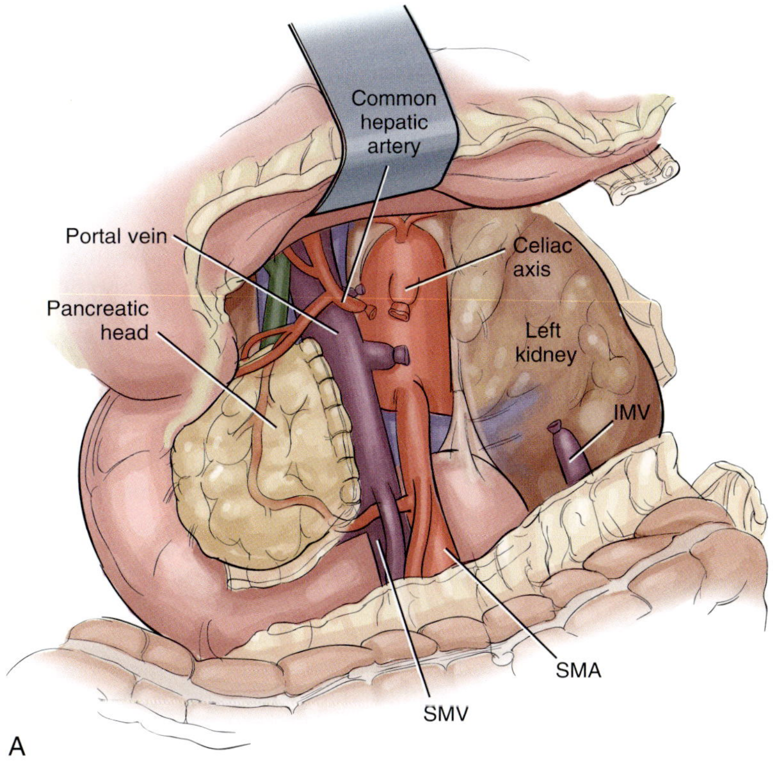

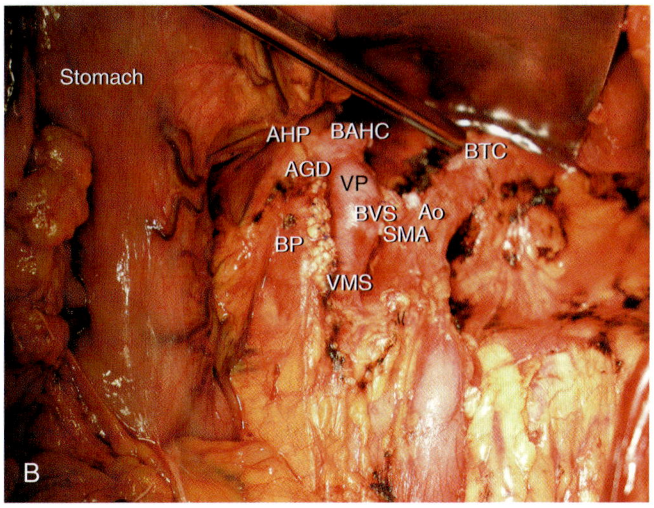

Figure 32-10. Final appearance after Appleby procedure with gastric preservation. *AGD,* Gastroduodenal artery; *AHP,* proper hepatic artery; *Ao,* aorta; *BAHC,* common hepatic artery stump; *BP,* pancreatic stump; *BTC,* celiac trunk stump; *BVS,* splenic vein stump; *IMV,* inferior mesenteric vein; *SMA,* superior mesenteric artery; *SMV,* superior mesenteric vein; *VMS,* superior mesenteric vein; *VP,* portal vein.

- The area is inspected for possible remnant tissue; if any is found, it should be removed. Particular importance is attributed to the lymph nodes; when detected, they should be removed, because lymph node metastases are frequent. This is the case for periaortic lymph nodes and the nodes at the origin of the SMA. If there is any suspicion of residual tissue at the level of the pancreatic stump, a frozen section is performed; if the margin is positive, a total pancreatectomy is necessary.
- The viability of the liver and of the stomach is reevaluated.

Closure

- Careful hemostasis in the splenic fossa and retropancreatic area is performed.
- Drains are placed near the pancreatic stump and in the splenic fossa.
- The abdomen is closed using a running no. 1 suture (loop) of nonabsorbable monofilament.

III. ALTERNATIVE TECHNICAL APPROACHES (PRO/CON) AND PEARLS

- If the stomach is invaded, it must be resected en bloc with the specimen. It is worth noting that the Appleby operation was originally performed for gastric cancer with invasion of the pancreas and of the celiac trunk. In these situations, the greater omentum is also removed. The right gastric artery and the right gastroepiploic artery are ligated and divided, and a linear cutter is applied immediately below the pylorus. The esophagus is also transected. The stomach remains attached to the splenopancreatic bloc; therefore, the left gastroepiploic vessels and the short gastric vessels are kept. Digestive continuity is reestablished through an esophagojejunal anastomosis with a Roux-en-Y loop.
- Invasion of the portal vein does not necessarily preclude the operation, although the prognosis in such cases is poor. Resection of the invaded segment will be followed by reconstruction either through an end-to-end anastomosis or using a venous or a synthetic graft.
- The celiac trunk can be controlled at its origin, by dissecting the supraceliac aorta until the emergence of the trunk is reached. The trunk is then ligated and divided. This maneuver is easier when the stomach is removed.
- If the flow in the proper hepatic artery is insufficient after clamping the CHA, a direct anastomosis between the origin of the celiac trunk and the proper hepatic artery is performed, or a venous graft can be interposed between the celiac stump and the hepatic artery.
- Anatomic variants of the hepatic arteries are possible. A right hepatic branch from the SMA does not change the situation too much, and a good flow in the GDA is necessary. A totally replaced hepatic artery from the SMA makes the situation favorable because, in that case, ligation of the celiac trunk does not affect liver vascularization. A left hepatic branch from the left gastric artery creates a difficult situation, because there is no satisfactory alternative blood supply to the left side of the liver. There is no predictive factor regarding the fate of this territory, which sometimes manages to develop collateral circulation from the surrounding areas (falciform ligament, diaphragm, the contralateral circulation), or necrosis.
- The splenopancreatic bloc can be mobilized and resected from right to left. In this case, the pancreatic body, at the level of the isthmus, where it was divided from the pancreatic head, is mobilized toward the left. The left gastric artery and vein are ligated and divided above the pancreas. The celiac trunk is ligated and divided above and behind the invaded area, in front of the aorta; the inferior mesenteric vein is ligated in the infrapancreatic portion before joining the splenic vein. The posterior mobilization and dissection continues to the left of the aorta, until it reaches the spleen, which is mobilized from its attachments and removed with the entire specimen.
- The Appleby operation can also be performed for recurrences of pancreatic and gastric cancer. In such cases, the principles remain the same, but the local anatomy is strongly modified; therefore the dissection can be more difficult.

IV. SPECIAL POSTOPERATIVE CARE

- Serum glutamic-oxaloacetic transaminase, serum glutamic-pyruvic transaminase, and bilirubin are monitored in the postoperative period in order to assess the hepatic function.
- Doppler ultrasound examination is used to assess the hepatic arterial flow.
- Ultrasonography is also used for detecting any intraabdominal fluid collections.
- The drains in the proximity of the pancreatic stump are monitored to detect a pancreatic fistula. Fistulas of the proximal pancreatic stump usually have a more favorable course and close spontaneously most of the time.
- Glycemia also must be monitored, because such an extensive resection can induce diabetes.
- The most notable immediate effect of the operation can be the relief of pain.
- In the long run, local recurrence rate is low for an R0 resection, and the evolution of the disease is most often characterized by the development of liver metastases.

SUGGESTED READINGS

Gagandeep S, Artinyan A, Jabbour N, et al: Extended pancreatectomy with resection of the celiac axis: the modified Appleby operation, *Am J Surg* 192:330–335, 2006.

Hirai I, Kimura W, Kamiga M, et al: The significance of intraoperative Doppler ultrasonography in evaluating hepatic arterial flow when assessing the indications for the Appleby procedure for pancreatic body cancer, *J Hepatobiliary Pancreat Surg* 12:55–60, 2005.

Yamaguchi K, Nakano K, Kobayashi K, et al: Appleby operation for pancreatic body-tail carcinoma: report of three cases, *Surg Today* 33:873–878, 2003. Review.

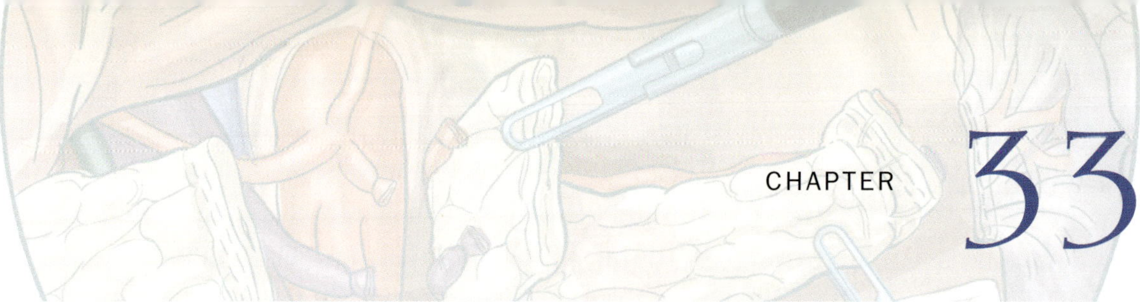

CHAPTER 33

Beger and Frey Procedure for Chronic Pancreatitis

Hans G. Beger, MD, MD(Hon), FACS(Hon), JSS(Hon), and Bertram Poch, MD

I. SPECIAL PREOPERATIVE PREPARATION

Indications for Surgery

- Chronic pancreatitis is a disease of the exocrine pancreatic tissue compartment that in the late course extends to the endocrine tissue. After a preclinical period of 3 to 12 years, a majority of patients develop upper abdominal pain as the first sign of the disease. Continuous alcohol consumption and cigarette smoking enhance the progression of chronic pancreatitis. In the late stage, local complications are caused by the progressing inflammatory process.
- An indication to change from medical to surgical treatment is severe medically intractable upper abdominal pain and development of clinically relevant local complications.
- About 30% to 50% of patients develop an inflammatory mass in the pancreatic head (contrast-enhanced computed tomography [CECT] investigation). A common bile duct stenosis is objectified by endoscopic retrograde cholangiopancreatography in about 30% of patients.
- Severe stenosis of the duodenum has been observed in 7% of patients, causing a gastric outlet syndrome.
- Compression or occlusion of the portal, splenic, and mesenteric vein is observed in about 15% of patients.
- The association of chronic pancreatitis and ductal pancreatic cancer has been found in about 6% of patients.
- Pseudocystic lesions less than 4 to 6 cm in diameter in the pancreatic tissue or outside of the pancreas are present in 15% to 25% of patients.
- A duodenum-preserving pancreatic head resection (Beger procedure) is indicated in advanced chronic pancreatitis with an inflammatory mass in the head of the pancreas, in common bile duct stenosis after failure of biliary stenting, and in cases with severe stenosis of the peripapillary duodenum. The Frey procedure is a combination of coring out the head of the pancreas with main duct drainage. It is indicated in patients who show a dilated pancreatic main duct with absence of side brunch duct stenoses and absence of an inflammatory mass of the head.
- The diagnosis of chronic pancreatitis is based on the pain history and imaging data using CECT: tissue calcifications, intrapancreatic cystic cavities, and enlargement of the pancreas (Fig. 33-1).
- Magnetic resonance cholangiopancreatography/endoscopic retrograde cholangiopancreatography: pancreatic main duct dilatation, common bile duct stenosis, side-branch duct stenosis or dilatations
- Exocrine function is tested by fecal fat content.
- Patients with advanced chronic pancreatitis show exocrine insufficiency with the consequence of increased fat content in stools.
- Endocrine function is objectivized by measuring H5B1A in the blood and by an oral glucose tolerance test.
- About 20% of surgical patients have insulin-dependent diabetes; 15% to 20% exhibit glucose intolerance but do not need medication.
- The preoperative workup includes upper gastrointestinal-tract anomalies, using gastroduodenoscopy and endoscopic sonography. In patients with ascites, the portohepatic vessels must be checked by computed tomography angiography.

II. OPERATIVE TECHNIQUE: BEGER PROCEDURE

Position

- The patient is placed in supine position.

Incision

- To gain access to the upper abdomen, an upper abdominal midline incision between the xiphoid and navel is performed. A paracostal transverse incision is time consuming, requires ligation of vessels, and results in a transection of both sides of the rectus muscle. A midline incision is a quick and bloodless access.

Main Dissection

- After exposition of the upper abdominal cavity and exclusion of cross pathologic changes of the stomach, duodenum, and liver, exposure of the pancreatic head takes place by performing two separate steps:
  - ▲ Transection of the gastrocolic ligament, preserving the gastrocolic vessels.
  - ▲ Transection of the duodenocolic ligament to expose the uncinate process and the postpapillary duodenum.
- After this, a Kocher maneuver is performed to mobilize the pancreatic head dorsally, avoiding any transection of vessels near the hepatoduodenal ligament (see Fig. 33-5).
- To perform a subtotal resection of the pancreatic head, it is beneficial to identify and curb the common bile duct in the hepatoduodenal ligament, the common hepatic artery, and the superior mesenteric vein (below the uncinate process). All three structures are curbed with a vessel loop. The tunneling of the pancreatic neck in front of the portal vein is a decisive step. In more than 90% of patients, it is an easy and bloodless dissection. In patients with inflammatory connections between the dorsal pancreas and the wall of the portal vein, the risk of portal vein leakage is increased. Portal vein bleeding following dorsal pancreatic head dissection will be adequately managed when the portal vein in the hepatoduodenal ligament is identified and curbed by a loop.
- In patients with thrombosis of the portal vein, tunneling of the pancreatic neck from the portal vein should be avoided.
- After completion of transection of the neck, a silk banding with ligation of the pancreatic neck is carried out to compress vessels and the pancreatic duct.

Subtotal Resection of the Head

- Transection of the pancreatic head on the duodenal edge of the portal vein takes place by lifting the loop around the left pancreas. Usually two major vessels are transected: the great pancreatic artery and the transverse artery. To close the vessels, four separate stitches are necessary. The pancreatic main duct is identified, and a cuff of 2 to 5 mm of the duct wall is preserved.

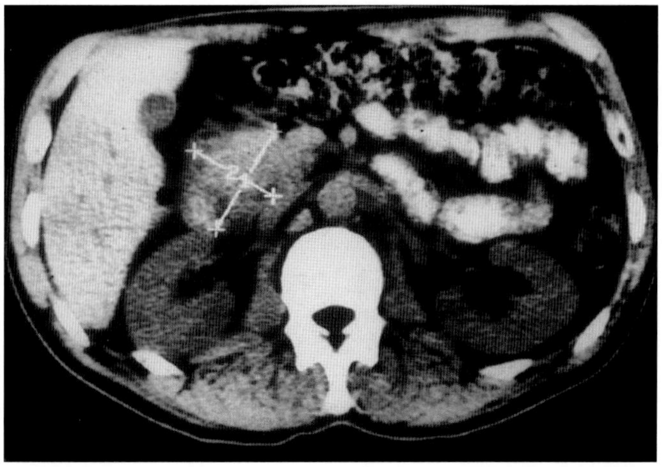

Figure 33-1. Contrast-enhanced computed tomography in chronic pancreatitis shows a head enlargement or an inflammatory mass of the pancreatic head in greater than 50% of patients presenting for surgical treatment.

- After complete transection and finishing blind vessel suturing, rotation of the pancreatic head with the duodenum into a ventral dorsal position at 90 degrees exposes the head for subtotal resection. Some veins carrying blood from the head directly to the portal vein must be ligated (Fig. 33-2).
- The incision line is marked by 3 to 5 sutures on the dorsal and 3 to 5 sutures on the ventral pancreatic head. With the left hand behind the head of the pancreas, a subtotal section of the pancreatic head starts from dorsal, preserving the dorsal pancreatic tissue capsule. Meticulous suturing of small blood vessels on the cut surface is mandatory (Fig. 33-3).
- Excision of the pancreatic head toward the intrapancreatic segment of the common bile duct, starting dorsally, enables the identification of the wall of the intrapancreatic bile duct.
- To avoid injury of the intrapancreatic common bile duct, a small incision in the supraduodenal duct segment in the hepatoduodenal ligament with intraductal placement of an Olivesonde into the papillary segment is helpful.
- The dissection of the pancreatic head tissue from the wall of the common bile duct is performed by blunt dissection. Subtotal resection of the pancreatic head results in a decompression of the common

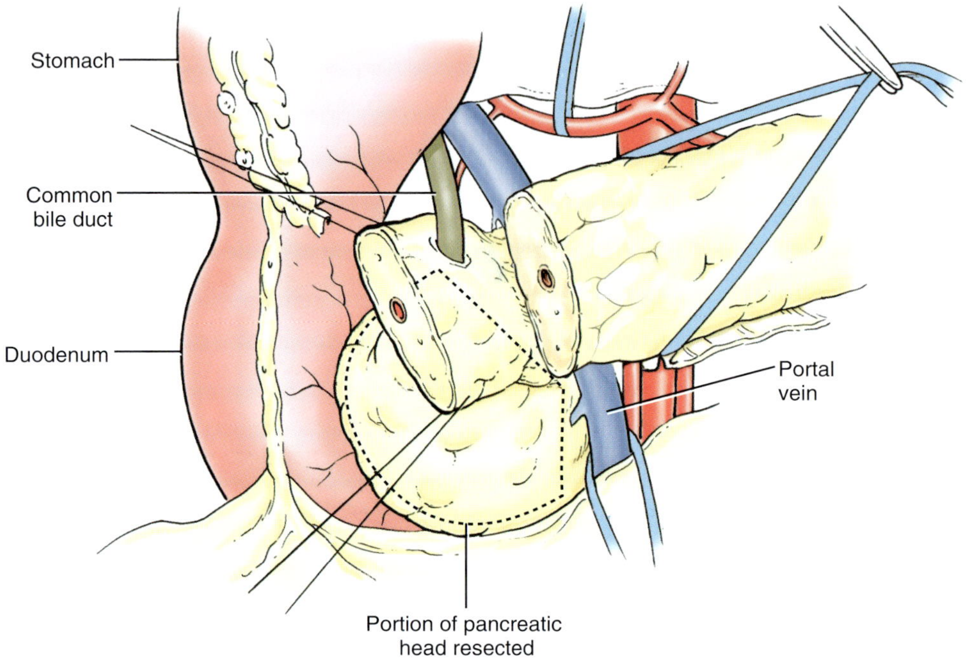

Figure 33-2.

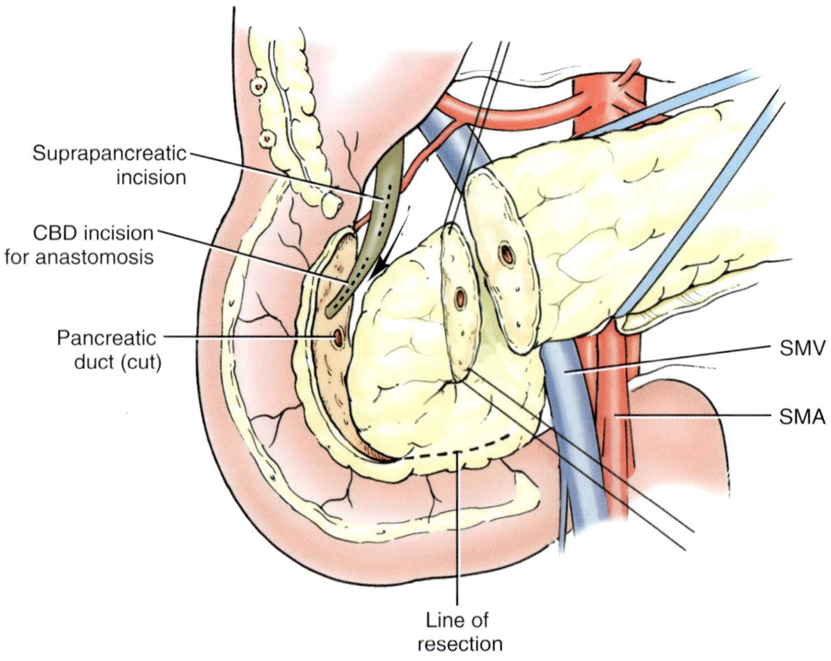

Figure 33-3. *CBD,* Common bile duct; *SMA,* superior mesenteric artery; *SMV,* superior mesenteric vein.

bile duct. In case of a inflammatory process in the duct wall with narrowing of the prepapillary segment of the bile duct, opening of the bile duct is needed (Fig. 33-4, *A*).

- After completion of subtotal pancreatic head resection, a shell-like remnant of the duodenal pancreatic head remains; ventrally a distance of 5 mm to the duodenal wall, preserving the pancreaticoduodenal arcades, and dorsally a 2.5- to 3-cm shell-like remnant is maintained (see Fig. 33-4, *B*; Fig. 33-5). A frozen section from the center of the inflammatory mass and from the cut surface of the left pancreas is recommended. The pancreatic main duct is measured in the lengths up to the tail of the pancreas, and intraductal pancreatic stones are removed.

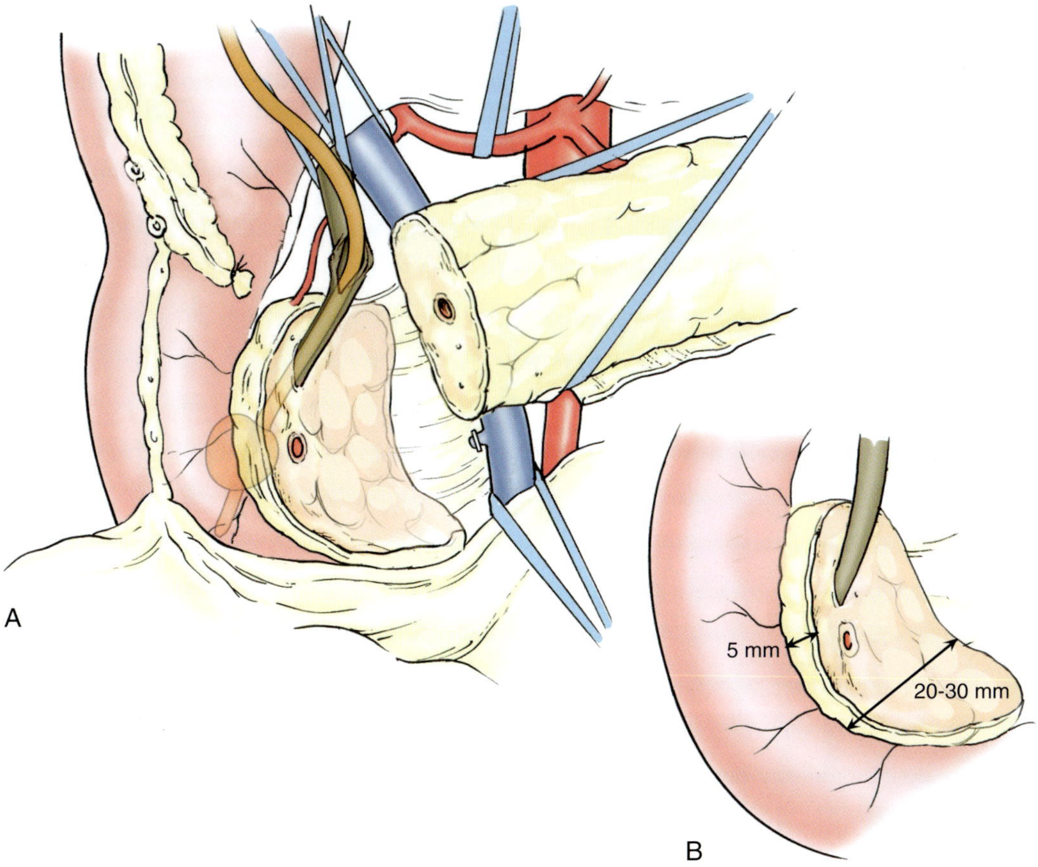

Figure 33-4.

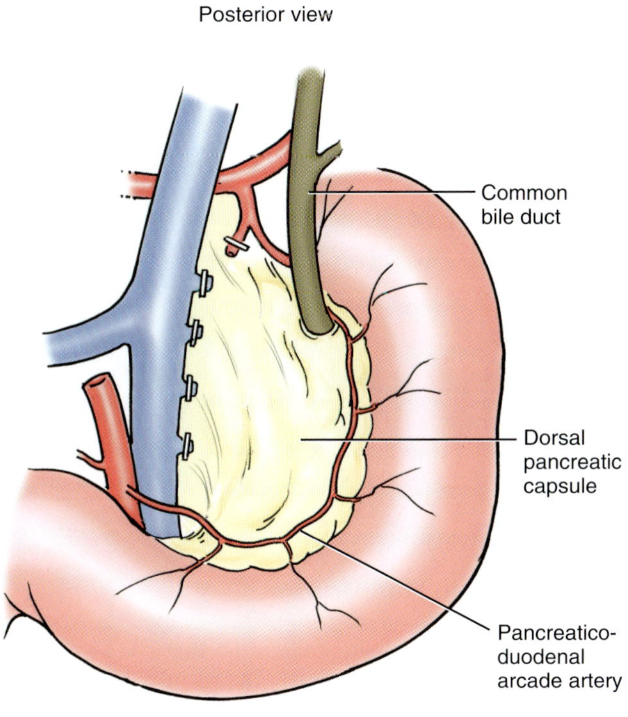

Figure 33-5.

Reconstruction after Subtotal Head Resection

- The aboral jejunal loop is transected about 20 cm distal to the ligament of Treitz using stapler devices. The jejunal loop is transposed through a retrocolic mesenteric cleft, right of the middle colic artery to the level of the pancreatic head.
- The connection between the left pancreas and the excluded jejunal loop is performed as a side-to-end, two-layer anastomosis, with interrupted resorbable, monofilament sutures. The mucosa-to-mucosa anastomosis between the jejunum and the duct wall using 6-0 sutures is a safe but demanding technique. The cut surface of the left pancreas is covered in the outer layer by single-stitch circular sutures between the seromuscularis and the pancreatic tissue, using 4-0 monofilament material.
- A side-to-end anastomosis between the jejunal loop with the shell-like remnant of the head of the pancreas, about 8-cm distal of the left pancreatic anastomosis, follows. The incision of the jejunum is 4- to 5-cm in length. The inner layer of the anastomosis is sutured continuously. The outer layer, between the pancreatic capsule and the seromuscular layer of the jejunum, is performed as an interrupted single-stitch technique. The inner layer is sutured between the pancreatic tissue and the mucosa. The outer layer includes the pancreatic capsule and the seromuscular layer of the jejunum (Fig. 33-6).
- To restore the continuity of the upper gastrointestinal tract, an enteroanastomosis (Roux-en-Y) is carried out 20 cm distal to the pancreatic head below the mesentery of the transverse colon. In the authors' experience, a two-layer continuously sutured anastomosis, using 5-0 for the inner layer and 4-0 for the outer layer, is a safe technique.

III. OPERATIVE TECHNIQUE: FREY PROCEDURE

- In 1986, Charles Frey published a modification of the duodenum-preserving subtotal pancreatic head resection for chronic pancreatitis by coring out parts of the head of the pancreas, in addition to a side-to-side pancreatic duct anastomosis. This technique resembles the Partington-Rochelle procedure with additional excision of the ventral part of the pancreatic head. In the first three cases about 6 g of pancreatic head tissue was reported to be cored out. The Frey-Izbicki technique, which is widely used in the United States, includes an extended coring-out technique of the ventral part of the pancreatic head.
- An excluded jejunal loop is used for reconstruction of the pancreatic duct and the rest of the pancreatic head. The anastomosis is performed as a single-layer, continuous suturing of the jejunum and the pancreatic parenchyma. Extensive coring-out of the ventral pancreatic head tissue may lead to decompression of the narrowed intrapancreatic segment of the common bile duct. To achieve long-term pain control, the major goal of the coring-out technique is to achieve subtotal extirpation of the pancreatic head (Fig. 33-7).
- Partial resection or coring-out of the inflammatory pancreatic head may result in reoccurrence of pain or persistence of narrowing of the intrapancreatic common bile duct.
- In patients with an inflammatory mass in the head of the pancreas, a subtotal resection of the pancreatic head, using the Beger procedure, is the most adequate surgical technique to ensure long-term pain control.
- In patients with chronic pancreatitis and a dilated pancreatic main duct with absence of side-branch duct stenosis, in which an inflammatory mass of the head of the pancreas is not dominant, the Frey procedure is advantageous in regard to permanent pain control, maintenance of endocrine functions, and quality of life.

IV. ALTERNATIVE TECHNICAL APPROACHES (PRO/CON) AND PEARLS

- There are some situations in which modifications of the main approach may be needed.

Biliary Modification

- In patients with a prepapillary common bile duct stenosis that persists after subtotal resection of the pancreatic head because of an inflammatory process in the wall of the bile duct, an additional connection to the jejunum is performed. Depending on the the length of the common bile duct stenosis, an incision of up to 1.0 cm with oval excision of the wall is made. Suturing with a jejunal loop is unnecessary because this biliary connection is included in the jejunal anastomosis with the rest of the pancreatic head.

Pancreatic Main Duct Drainage Modification

- Chronic pancreatitis with a dilated pancreatic main duct that shows multiple stenoses in the left pancreas and absence of side-branch duct obstructions, the main pancreatic duct is longitudinally opened on its ventral surface, extending the incision toward the tail of the pancreas. A side-to-side anastomosis is performed, using the Partington-Rochelle technique for duct-jejunal anastomosis. Continuous suture

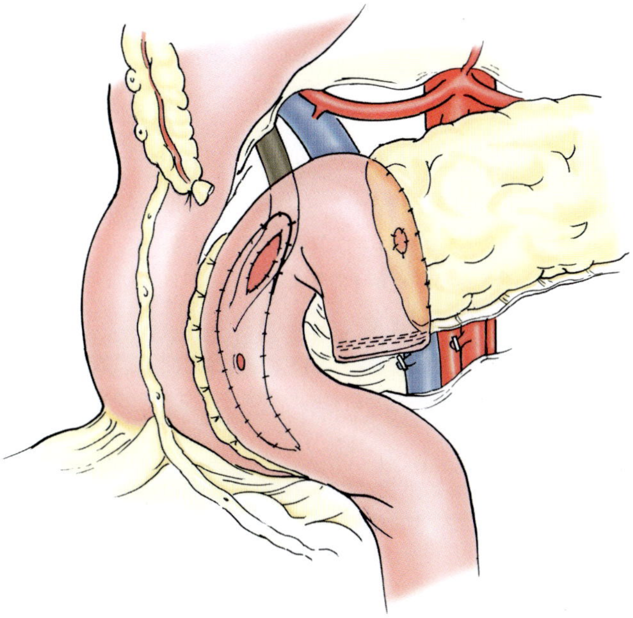

Figure 33-6.

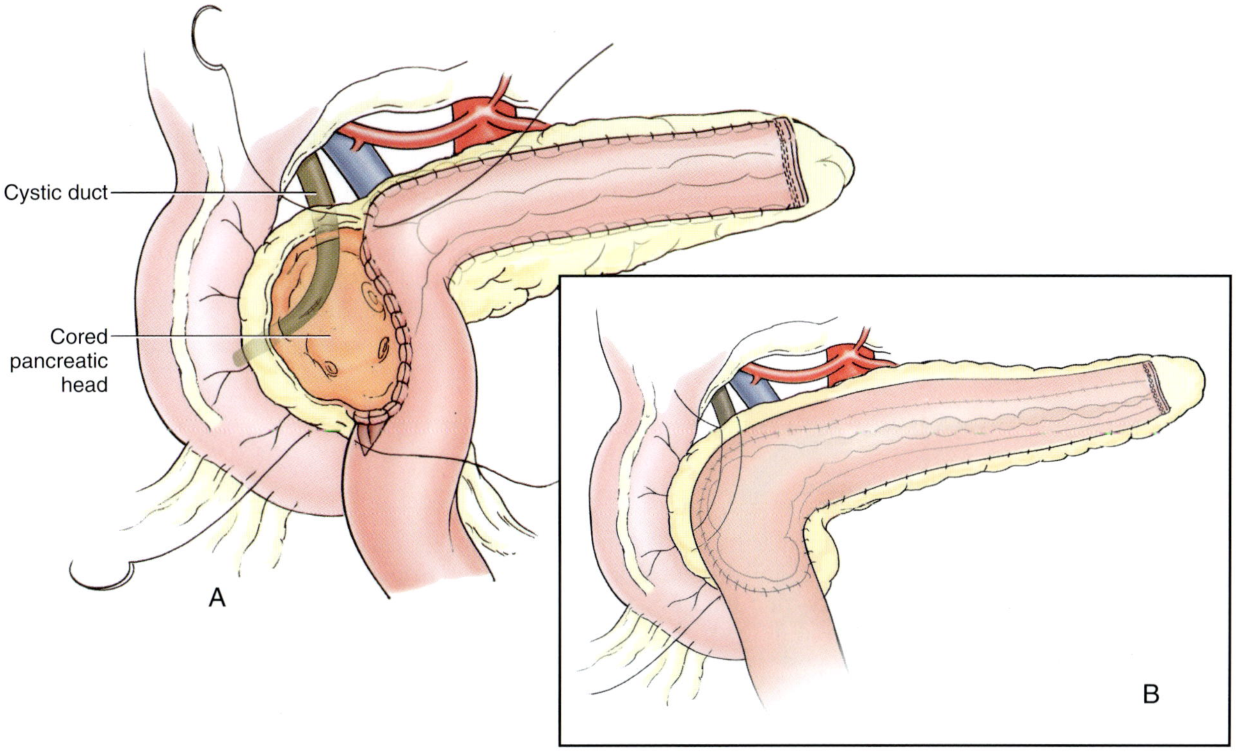

Figure 33-7.

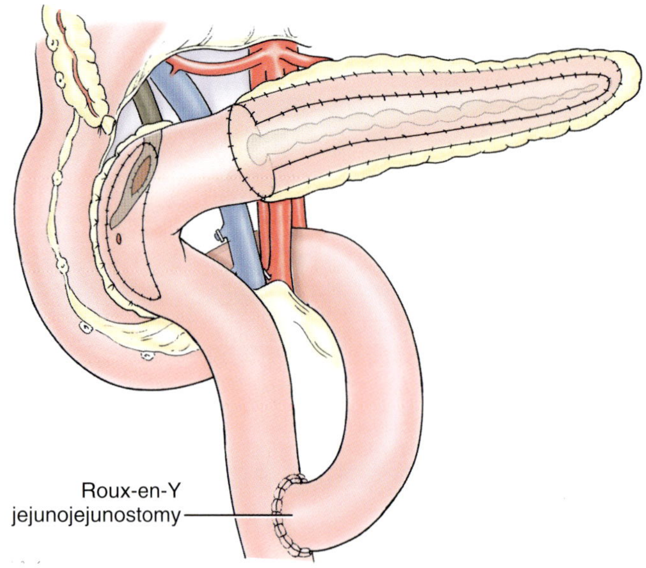

Figure 33-8.

lines, using 4-0 monofilament, resorbable sutures, are carried out, except for the anastomosis between the cut surfaces of the left pancreas (Fig. 33-8).

Total Pancreatic Head Resection

- In chronic pancreatitis, in which the inflammatory process is extended to the pancreatic tissue between common bile duct and duodenal wall, creating a rimmed pancreatitis, total pancreatic head resection is indicated.
- The dissection of the pancreatic head starts from the postpyloric duodenal wall toward the papilla and from the uncinate process toward the papilla.
- Because of the transection of the ventral and posterior inferior vessel arcades, between the superior mesenteric artery and the gastroduodenal artery, the peripapillary segment of the duodenum must be included in the resection to avoid an ischemic lesion. After careful dissection of the pancreatic head up to the prepapillary level, a transection of the duodenal papillary segment is performed, using a stapler twice. Transection of the suprapancreatic common bile duct is the final step of total head extirpation.
- In addition to pancreatic anastomosis of the left pancreas, reconstruction necessitates an end-to-end anastomosis between the proximal and distal duodenum and end-to-side anastomosis between the supraduodenal common bile duct and the duodenum. The biliary anastomosis is performed with a continuous single-layer suturing.

V. SPECIAL POSTOPERATIVE CARE

Early Postoperative Course

- Postoperative local complications after the Beger and Frey procedures are rare. Local bleeding, which appears as intestinal blood loss, and anastomotic leakage, which primarily is objectified by appearance of intestinal contents, amylase-rich fluid evacuation in the drainage fluid, and the development of a pancreatic fistula, are observed in fewer than 5% of patients. Mild laboratory signs of pancreatitis are frequent, lasting only a few postoperative days.
- Systemic complications regarding pulmonary dysfunction are observed in about 10% of patients. The patients do not suffer a delay of gastric emptying, except for those with a segmental resection of the duodenum. Most of the patients are on regular oral nutritional status on the third postoperative day.

SUGGESTED READINGS

Beger HG, Schlosser W, Poch B, Gansauge F: Inflammatory mass in the head of pancreas. In Beger HG, Warshaw AL, Buechler MW, et al, editors: *The pancreas*, London, 1998, Blackwell Science, pp 757–760.

Frey CF, Smith GJ: Description and rationale of a new operation for chronic pancreatitis, *Pancreas* 2:701–707, 1987.

Itzbicki JR, Bloechle C, Broering DC, et al: Extended drainage versus resection in surgery for chronic pancreatitis: a prospective randomized trial comparing the longitudinal pancreatico-jejunostomy combined with local pancreatic head excision with the pylorus-preserving pancreatoduodenectomy, *Ann Surg* 228:771–779, 1998.

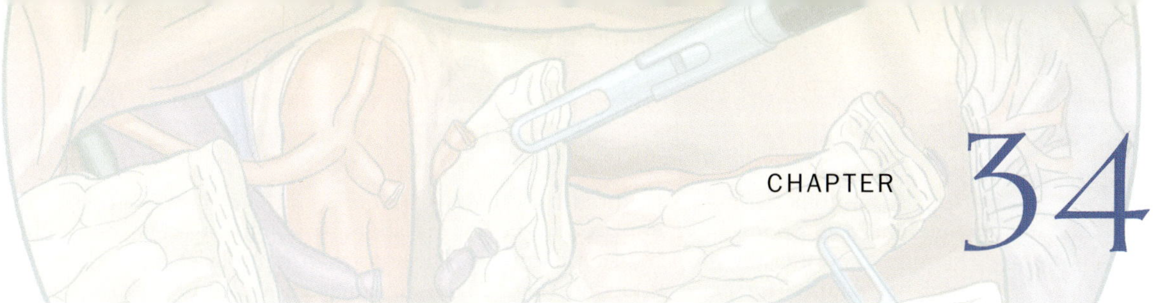

CHAPTER 34

Laparoscopic Pancreatic Pseudocyst Drainage

Adrian E. Park, MD, FRCSC, FACS, FCS (ECSA), and Stephen M. Kavic, MD, FACS

I. SPECIAL PREOPERATIVE PREPARATION

- Pancreatic pseudocysts are defined by consensus as fluid collections that persist for more than 1 month and have a well-defined wall. They may communicate with the pancreatic ductal system.
- Abdominal computerized tomography scanning is considered the single best study for definition of pancreatic pseudocysts.
- Endoscopic ultrasound may help define the extent and precise location of the pseudocyst as well as aid in operative planning.
- Endoscopic retrograde cholangiopancreatography has been used in many centers for diagnosis of ductal communication; however, it is limited by its invasive nature if the question is purely diagnostic.
- Magnetic resonance cholangiopancreatography also defines pancreatic ductal and pseudocyst anatomy. Abnormalities in ductal anatomy occur with some frequency in patients with pseudocysts, with most estimates running at approximately one half of patients.
- Aspiration of the cyst fluid may help differentiate pseudocysts from cystic neoplasms of the pancreas. Pseudocyst fluid is typically high in amylase, low in viscosity, and negative for tumor markers such as CEA, CA-125, and CA 19-9.
- Management options include nonoperative, observational therapy with repeated imaging as follow-up. Patients who are asymptomatic with pseudocysts that are either stable or decreasing in size may avoid the operating room. Approximately one half of patients with pseudocysts may be treated nonoperatively with anticipated resolution of the pseudocyst; the single best predictor of success is pseudocyst diameter.
- Percutaneous drainage is available as a treatment option. Percutaneous drainage is the preferred technique for the management of a pancreatic abscess. In the elective setting, the role of percutaneous drainage has not been precisely defined, as the majority of patients require further therapy. Pseudocyst recurrence rates following percutaneous drainage exceed 50%. Contraindications include pancreatic necrosis, hemorrhage, and multiple small cysts.
- Endoscopic therapies include transmural drainage as well as pancreatic stenting. Excellent initial results have been obtained at some centers; long-term follow-up data regarding recurrence and success are still evolving.

II. OPERATIVE TECHNIQUE

Position

- The patient is placed in either a "low lithotomy" or split-leg position. The surgeon operates standing between the patient's legs. The patient's arms are tucked at each side, allowing more flexibility for port placement and positioning of assistants. On occasion a roll will be placed under the patient's left side to provide elevation of the spleen should posterior hilar access be required during the procedure.

Incision

- Pneumoperitoneum is achieved either by the Hasson technique or Veress needle depending on surgeon experience and practice. All trocars must be introduced under direct visualization. As with all minimally invasive procedures, placement of trocars must first take into account ergonomic and ease-of-access factors followed by aesthetic considerations. To that end the longest (10-mm) incision is made in the superior umbilical rim. This is used for camera placement and later introduction of the endostapler. Five-millimeter ports are then placed in the left midabdomen, high epigastric, and right midabdomen, slightly inferior to the umbilicus. Occasionally a fifth port—5-mm placed in the left lower quadrant—will be required for extra retraction (Fig. 34-1). An angled (30-degree) 5-mm laparoscope is used mainly through the umbilical port. It may then be moved between ports as needed. The midabdominal ports allow passage of the surgeon's left- and right-hand instruments. With more caudally extending pseudocysts, these ports may need to be placed more inferiorly. The epigastric port is used to retract mainly the stomach and gastrocolic omentum.

Main Dissection

- Based on review of computed tomography images of the pseudocyst location with the pancreas and initial laparoscopic survey, a position along the greater curve of the stomach is grasped and entry is made into the lesser sac (Fig. 34-2). When dividing the gastrocolic ligament (with ultrasonic dissection, electrocautery, radiofrequency device, clips, or stapler), care must be taken to ensure adequate access to the inferior and most medial aspect of the pseudocyst (Fig. 34-3). It is not vital that full lateral and superior access be as generously established.

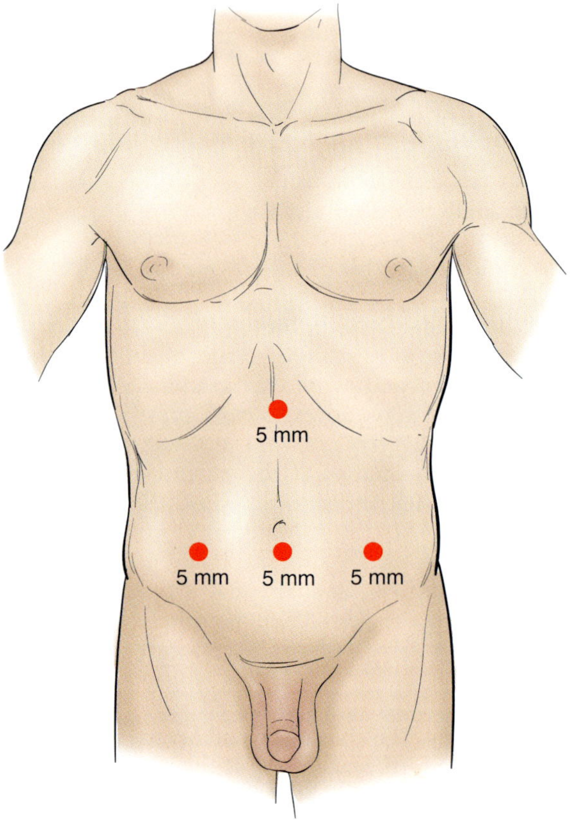

Figure 34-1.

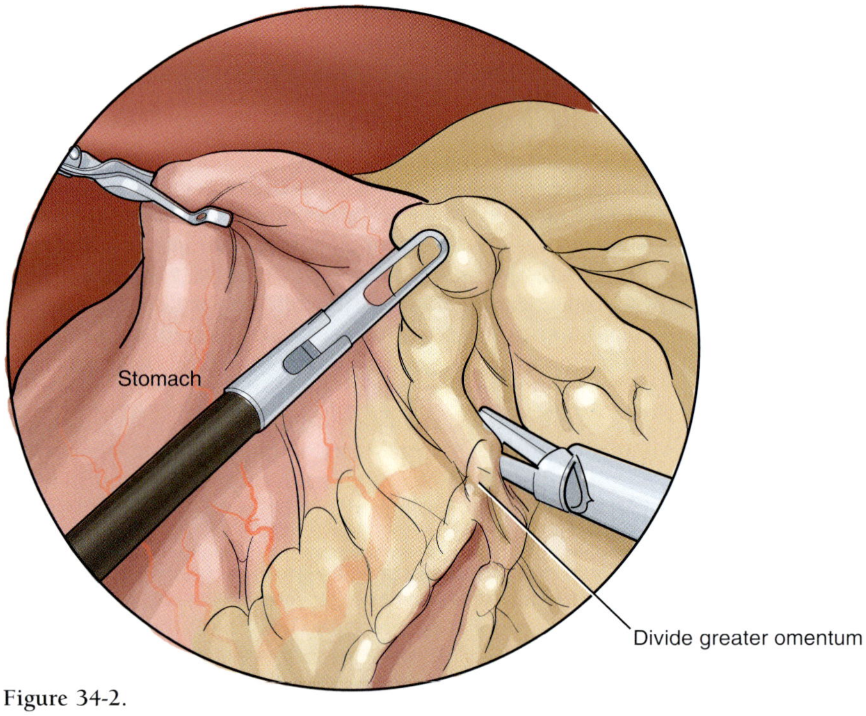

Figure 34-2.

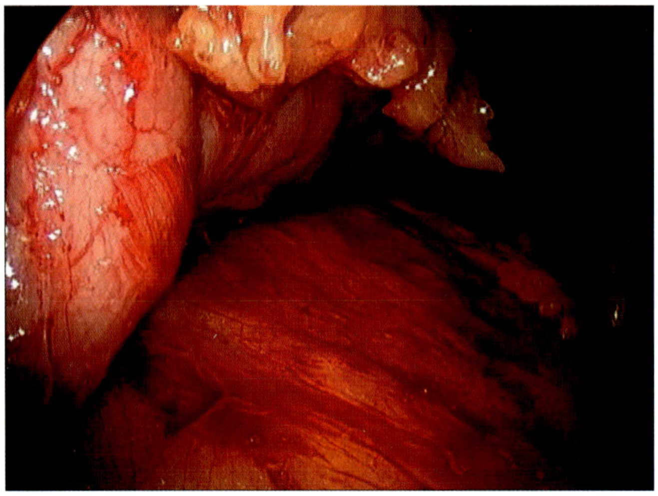
Figure 34-3.

- If there is any doubt about the pseudocyst's location, a laparoscopic ultrasound probe can be used for location purposes. An aspiration needle can also be used (Fig. 34-4).
- A window into the lesser sac is created, extending at least 10 cm along the greater curve of the stomach. Often the lesser sac is significantly obliterated by peripancreatic inflammation and foreshortening and thickening of the transverse colon mesentery. Through this window, the posterior stomach/cyst interface is explored. The ideal location of the cyst gastrostomy will be at that position of adequate stomach/cyst fusion that is most medial and dependent in the cyst. This is often a point more caudal than initially suspected; for this reason, during trocar placement, the left- and right-sided ports may need to migrate well infraumbilical to allow comfortable working angles as the case progresses.
- A cystotomy is made at the selected position (see earlier discussion) using sharp dissection, the ultrasonic dissector, or electrocautery. A gush of cyst fluid usually results. Samples of this fluid as well as a biopsy of the cyst wall via the cystotomy are sent for cytology, biochemical analysis, and histology. Through the enlarged cystotomy, a laparoscopic exploration and evacuation of the pseudocyst is undertaken. Debridement as indicated can also be accomplished (Figs. 34-5 and 34-6).

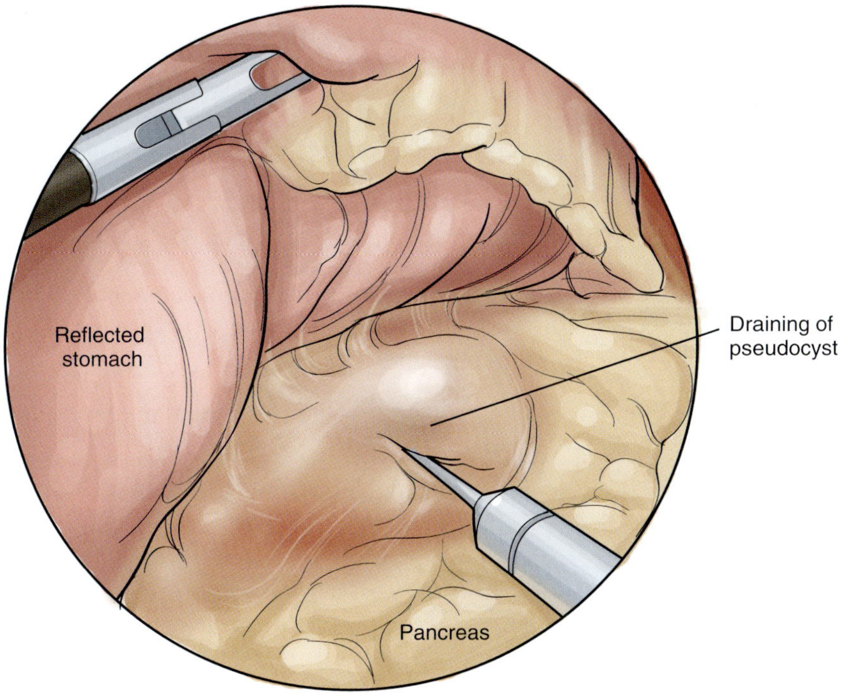

Figure 34-4.

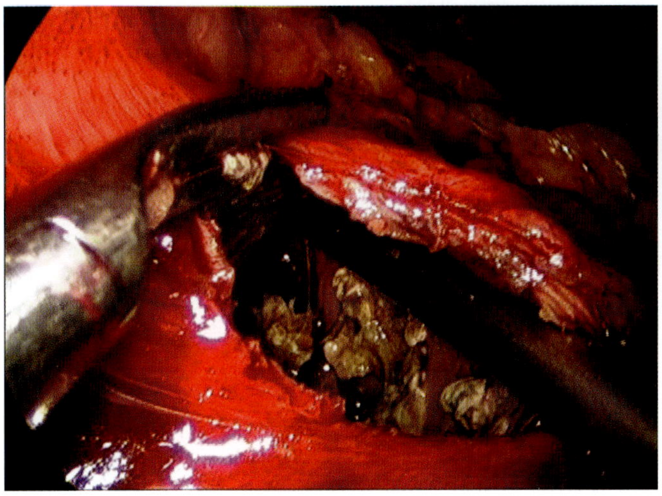

Figure 34-5.

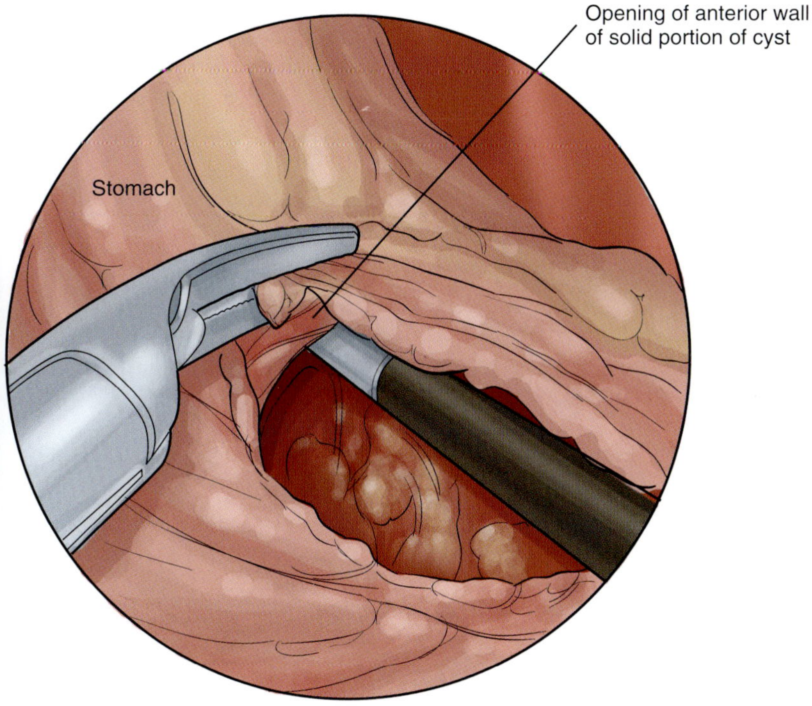

Figure 34-6.

- A gastrotomy just en face to the cystotomy gives access to the stomach. A gastroscope within the stomach allows monitoring of this process as well as subsequent examination of the anastomosis and endoscopic exploration of the pseudocyst.
- An articulating endoscopic stapling device with a 60-mm (blue) cartridge is then introduced with one jaw through the gastrotomy and one through the cystotomy (Fig. 34-7). When the jaws are approximated and the device fired, a stapled, hemostatic cystogastrostomy results. The cystotomy/gastrotomy have been rendered in continuity, and at this stage the single "otomy" must be sutured closed. In securing the corner stitches, both distally and proximally, it is of vital importance to ensure full-thickness bites with no gap between the staple line and stitch. The authors prefer use of interrupted silk sutures to close the "otomy." Thus, the resulting cystogastrostomy is entirely hemostatic and hydrostatic via both staples and sutures (Fig. 34-8).
- The stomach is gently insufflated with the gastroscope, while saline is irrigated along the suture line to identify a possible leak (Fig. 34-9). The gastroscope is advanced through the anastomosis to ensure patency and hemostasis, for example. The stomach is then desufflated and the scope removed.
- A drain drawn through the left-sided 5-mm port side is placed near the cystogastrostomy, within the lesser sac (Fig. 34-10).
- Instrument and trocars are removed following a final laparoscopic survey. Fascia on the supraumbilical port site is closed. All sites are then closed with subcutaneous absorbable sutures.
- If location of the cyst or inadequate fusion of gastric and cyst wall preclude the possibility of cyst gastrostomy function, then a cyst jejunostomy should be considered.
- A 40-cm Roux limb is created in the standard fashion with several applications of the endostapling device. Following completion of the jejunojejunostomy (stapled or sutured), the mesenteric defect is closed. The Roux limb is drawn antecolic.
- The cyst jejunostomy is created in much the same way as the cyst gastrostomy. Access is gained to the lesser sac and cyst via a window in the gastrocolic omentum. The cystotomy is made, and the cyst is evacuated and prepared for anastomosis. An enterotomy is made in the Roux limb approximately 8 cm from the stapled end. One arm of the endostapler is passed through the cystotomy and the other arm through the enterotomy. The arms are approximated and the staples deployed.

Closure

- The larger "otomy" is then closed via interrupted silk sutures, as previously described. A drain is placed in proximity to the anastomosis.

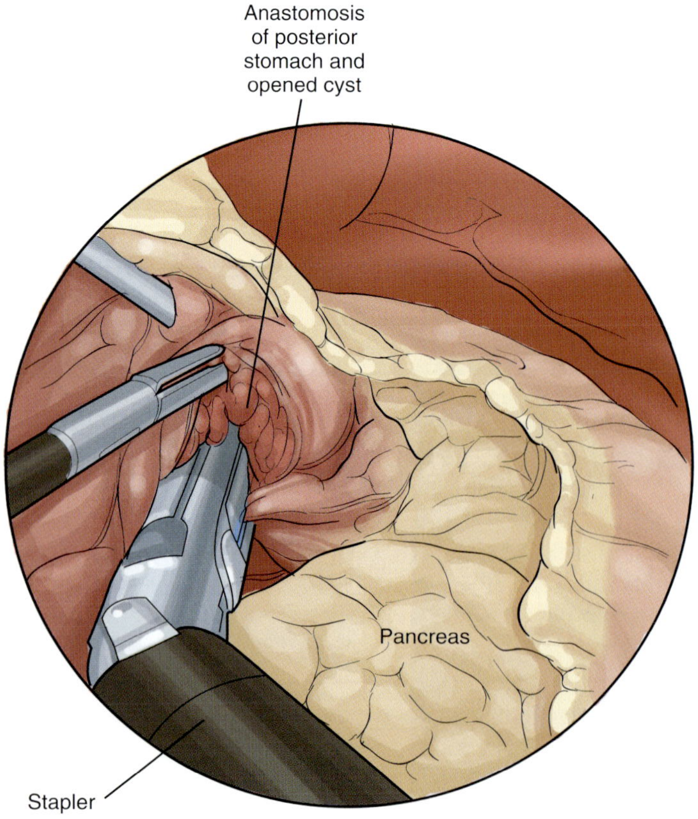

Figure 34-7.

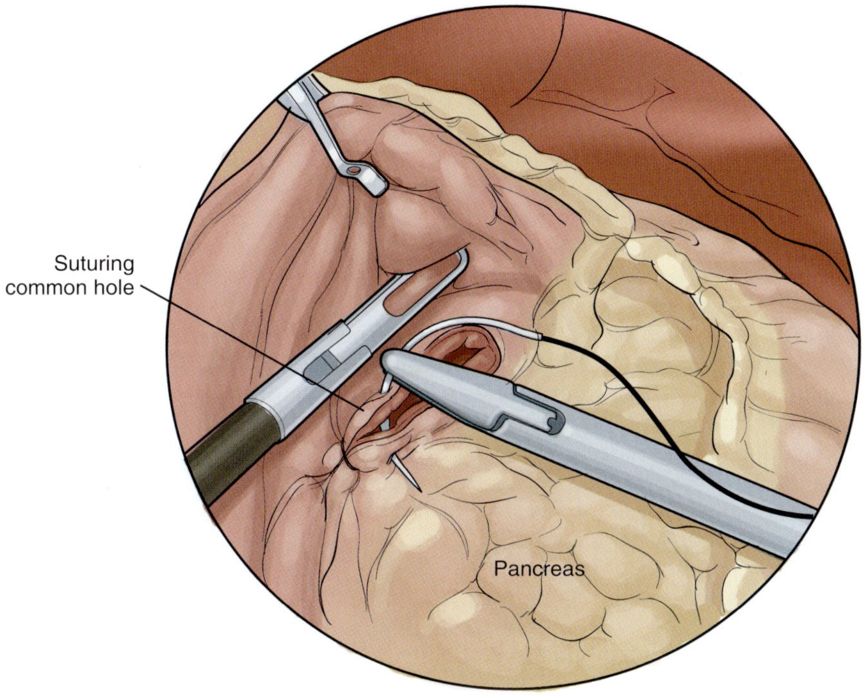

Figure 34-8.

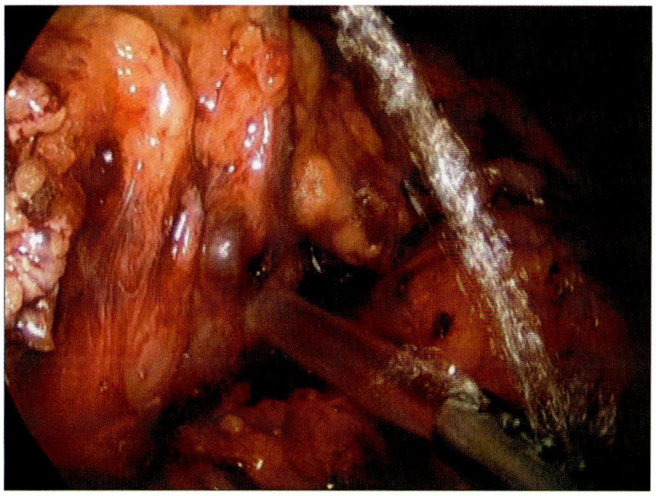

Figure 34-9.

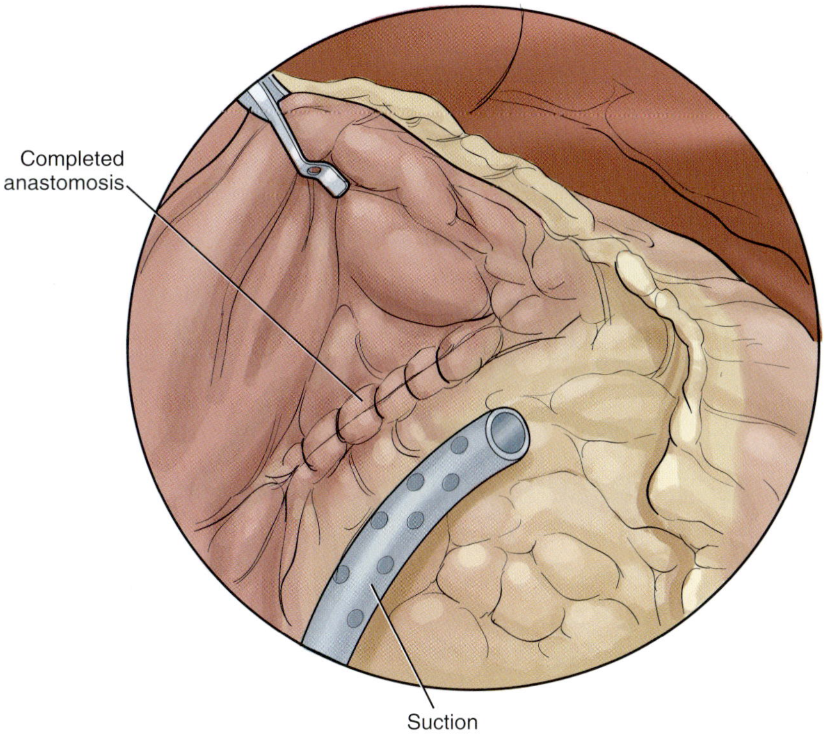

Figure 34-10.

III. ALTERNATIVE TECHNICAL APPROACHES (PRO/CON) AND PEARLS

- A few other techniques of minimally invasive cyst gastrostomy that differ significantly from the lesser sac approach have been described. In the laparoendoscopic or intragastric approach, an endoscope is placed into the stomach, and two 5-mm ports are passed through the anterior abdominal wall and into the stomach. The endoscope provides illumination and visualization, and the cyst gastrotomy is performed by introducing instruments through the intragastric working ports. The cyst gastrotomy is made by means of sharp dissection and electrocautery or ultrasonic dissection. The integrity of the anastomosis is dependent solely on the fusion of the posterior gastric wall and cyst. The authors have performed intragastric suturing for hemostasis when indicated. This is technically very demanding and time-consuming. A third 5-mm transgastric port for a laparoscope provides better visualization, but the working space remains very limited. Once the intragastric work is completed, the trocars are withdrawn from the stomach and the gastrotomies are closed laparoscopically with single silk sutures.
- The advantage of this technique resides largely in the minimal footprint of only two or three 5-mm incisions. The disadvantages include the technical difficulty of performing the procedure, the risk of bleeding from the cyst gastrostomy, the difficulty in securing a sutured hemostatic/hydrostatic anastomosis, and the creation of two or three separate gastrotomies apart from the cyst gastrostomy.
- Another technique involves creating a large anterior gastrotomy by which means the postgastric wall is accessed. The cyst gastrostomy is performed transgastrically (vs. intragastrically) and can be sutured or stapled with greater facility.
- Technique pros: Easier access to postgastric wall; ability to perform stapled or sutured hemostatic anastomosis.
- Technique cons: Creation of two large gastrotomies; risk of spillage of gastric contents while working transgastrically; angles to suture and staple can be difficult.
- By contrast, the pros of the lesser sac approach are many: no anterior gastrotomy(ies), entirely hemostatic/hydrostatic anastomosis, technically easier access for stapling/suturing, and best access to assess cyst/stomach interface and fusion. A con to this approach is that surgeons must be comfortable with laparoscopic suturing.

IV. SPECIAL POSTOPERATIVE CARE

- The principal intraoperative complications include hemorrhage and leak.
- The risk of hemorrhage may be increased for patients in whom the pseudocyst has eroded into a vessel wall and permitted the development of a pseudoaneurysm. The most commonly involved vessel is the splenic artery, although the gastroduodenal and pancreaticoduodenal arteries may be involved.
- Surgeons in the operating room must be aware that patients with pseudocysts may also have a higher incidence of splenic vein thrombosis, which may lead to gastric varices or splenomegaly.
- Meticulous attention to closure of enterotomies minimizes the overall risk of leak. The risk may be increased for patients in whom the pseudocyst wall is not well established.
- Most patients may be rapidly advanced on diet and do not require prolonged antibiotic therapy. The usual precautions with regard to deep venous thrombosis prophylaxis should be employed.

SUGGESTED READINGS

Behrns KE, Ben-David K: Surgical therapy of pancreatic pseudocysts, *J Gastrointest Surg* 12:2231–2239, 2008.

Park A, Heniford T: Therapeutic laparoscopy of the pancreas, *Ann Surg* 236:149–158, 2002.

Park A, Heniford T: Minimally invasive pancreatic pseudocyst surgery. In Targanona EM, Trias M, editors: *Advances in minimally invasive therapy and new technologies in general and digestive surgery*, New York (Barcelona), 2003, Springer, pp 316–320.

SECTION VI

Spleen

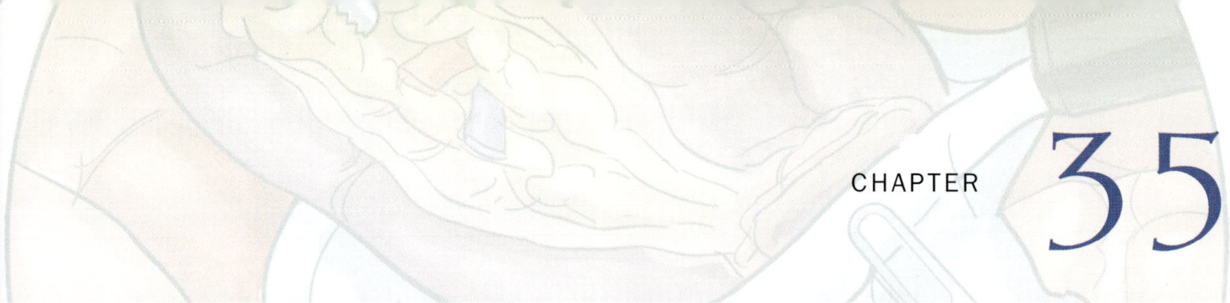

CHAPTER 35

Laparoscopic Splenectomy

Samer S. Deeba, MD, MD(res), MRCS(Eng), and Ara Darzi, PC, KBE, HonFREng, FMedSci

I. SPECIAL PREOPERATIVE PREPARATION

Indications

- Hematologic diseases are the most common indication for laparoscopic splenectomy (LS). The spleen does not reach gigantic sizes in these disorders and thus a laparoscopic approach is deemed the gold standard; typically the spleen cephalocaudal diameter will be less than 20- cm. The disorders best treated with LS are idiopathic thrombocytopenic purpura, thrombotic thrombocytopenic purpura, spherocytosis, sickle cell anemia, idiopathic autoimmune hemolytic anemia, and thalassemia.
- Secondary hypersplenism is also treated by LS. Cirrhosis, cystic fibrosis, and bone marrow proliferative disorders are included in the above.
- Primary hematologic malignancies are also approached by LS such as lymphomas and leukemias (primarily chronic lymphocytic leukemia, myeloid metaplasia, and multiple myelomas).
- Other etiologies such as Felty syndrome, sarcoidosis, Gaucher disease, abscesses, infarcts, cysts, and primary tumors of the spleen are also approached by LS.

Preparation

- Vaccination against pneumococcus should be done at least 1 week in advance of the planned LS. If the vaccine was not given at that time, then it is best given 2 weeks after the operation, and during that period it is recommended that the patient be covered by prophylactic antibiotics. The patient should be free of any infectious process at the time of immunization. Long-term antibiotics have not been proven to be efficacious in avoiding infections, but nonetheless, they are prescribed generously when infection occurs.
- Preoperative imaging is for diagnosis and surgery planning. An ultrasound is best for delineating the three-dimensional size of the spleen. Ultrasound is later complemented with a computed tomography (CT) scan of the abdomen to visualize the enlarged spleen with respect to the organs in its vicinity, such as the stomach, pancreas, and colon. In addition, a CT with arterial contrast can delineate any vascular anomalies in the hilum of the spleen, which the surgeon should be aware of to avoid intraoperative bleeding. A CT scan is also very useful in excluding the presence of accessory spleens that may also be enlarged (Fig. 35-1).
- Complete blood count should be checked a few hours before the planned procedure and platelet units cross-matched and available. The platelet count should be on the order of 100 when a planned LS is under way, and the patient should be transfused if the count is less than that.

II. OPERATIVE TECHNIQUE

Position

- Nasogastric and urinary drainage is routine.
- The patient is positioned in a right lateral semidecubitus position with the lateral axis of the body from shoulder blade to shoulder blade forming an angle of 45 to 60 degrees with the operating table and the patient's left arm fixed over the head in a splint. The table can be turned further to place the patient in a full right lateral decubitus position, if needed for larger spleens. The table is also tilted at the umbilical level, which hyperextends the abdomen, thus providing more working space for the surgeon. It also keeps the intraabdominal organs tucked by gravity in the dependent gutters away from the spleen. In this position the spleen hangs from its dorsolateral fixation and the exposure of its hilum is easier. The weight of the spleen also puts tension on the diaphragmatic attachments and better exposes them for an easier dissection (Fig. 35-2).

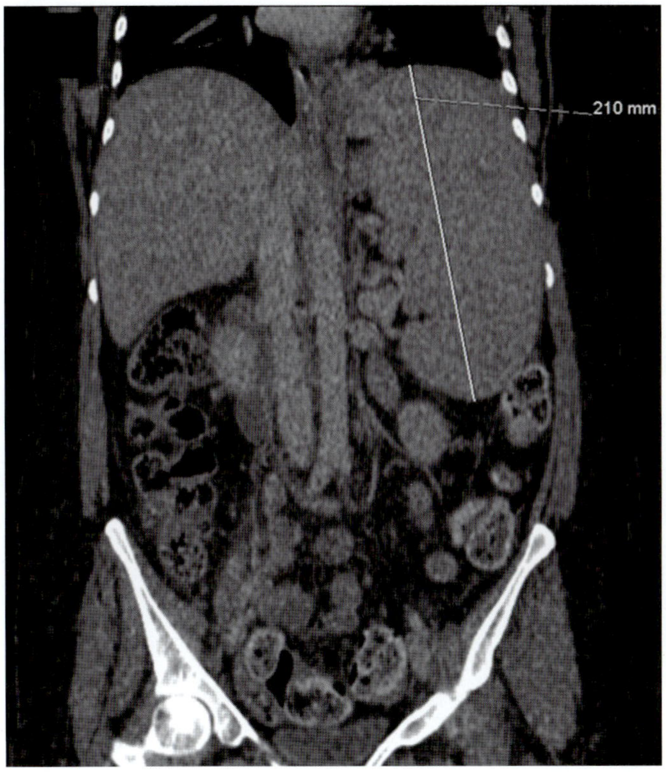

Figure 35-1. Computed tomography scan coronal section showing splenomegaly in a myelofibrosis patient with a cephalocaudal spleen length of 21 cm.

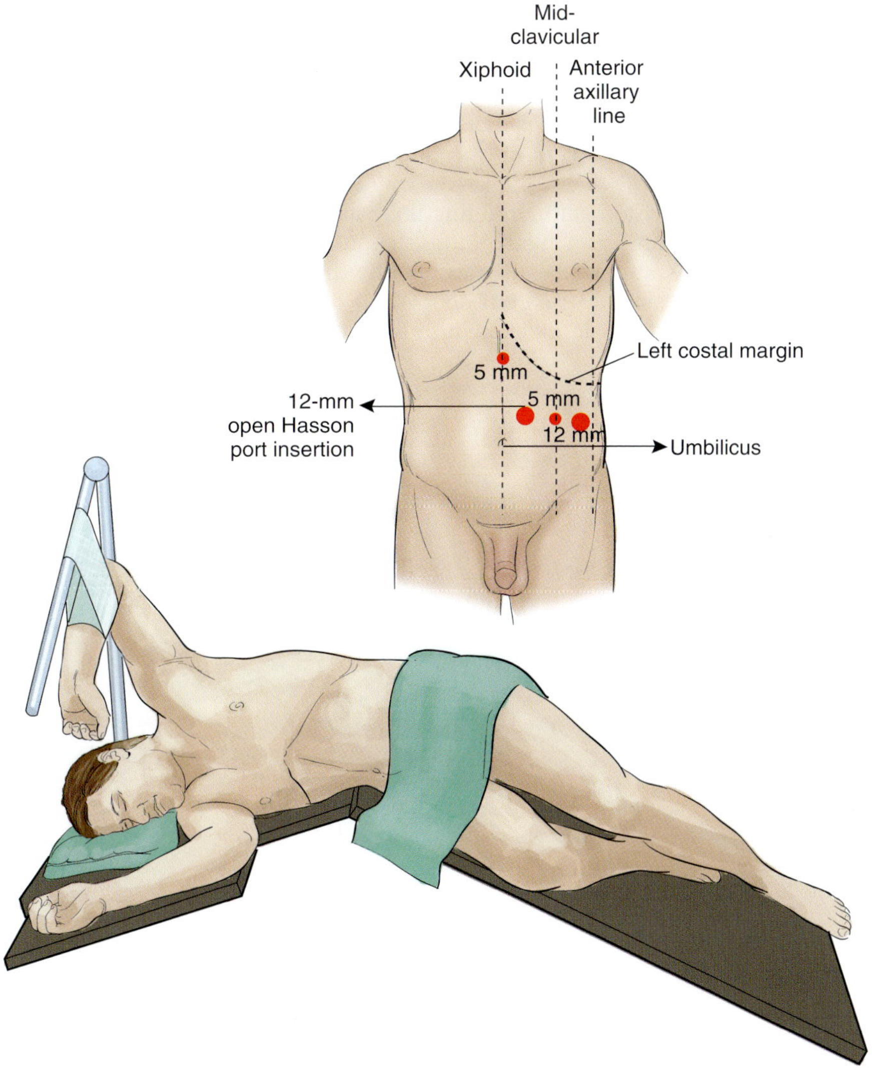

Figure 35-2.

- Nasogastric suctioning is used to deflate the stomach.
- The surgeon and the assistant stand on the abdominal side of the patient with the assistant in the more cephalad position.

Trocar Placement

- First port pneumoperitoneum is achieved by an open cutdown of an 11-mm Hasson port just left and superior to the umbilicus. A 30-degree scope is used because it allows for better visualization of the hilum and areas deep in the abdomen and behind organs.
- A 12-mm port is inserted under vision at the lower left costal margin two finger breadths lower than the margin at the level of the anterior axillary line. This is used for the surgeon's right-hand instrument and the introduction of stapling devices and the LigaSure device (Valleylab, Boulder, Colo.) in the abdomen.
- A 5-mm port is introduced under vision at the level of the left costal margin two finger breadths below the margin at the level of the midclavicular line. This is used for the surgeon's left-hand instrument and for aiding in dissection and traction.
- Another 5-mm port is inserted in the epigastric area three finger breadths below the xiphoid process. This aids in introduction of traction instruments by the assistant (see Fig. 35-2).
- The abdomen is explored, searching for accessory spleens around the splenic hilum; the greater curve of the stomach; and the gastrocolic, gastrosplenic, and splenocolic ligaments. This confirms that there are no accessory spleens, confirming the preoperative CT scans.

Main Dissection

- There are two recommended approaches: the suspended pedicle and the hanging spleen approach.
- In the suspended pedicle approach:
  - ▲ The mobilization of the spleen is carried out as in open approach.
  - ▲ The splenocolic and the splenophrenic ligaments are divided with the LigaSure. Then the gastrosplenic ligament is divided with meticulous dissection of the short gastric arteries (Fig. 35-3), which can be controlled either by the 10-mm endoclipper or by the LigaSure.
  - ▲ The splenic hilum and the vascular pedicle are the only attachments of the spleen remaining. Care must be taken in handling the spleen in traction because it no longer has the support of the abdominal wall, and traction on its parenchyma can cause a tear in the capsule and excessive bleeding, obscuring the surgeon's vision, and rendering the patient unstable. We advise the introduction of a small tonsil swab to be used as a cushion for traction by a metal instrument.
  - ▲ A Maryland dissector is used to dissect and identify the splenic artery and usually two veins (Fig. 35-4, *A* and *B*). Dissection is carried out about 2 to 3 cm away from the hilum before the vessels branch as they near the splenic parenchyma. After their control, the vessels are transected by a

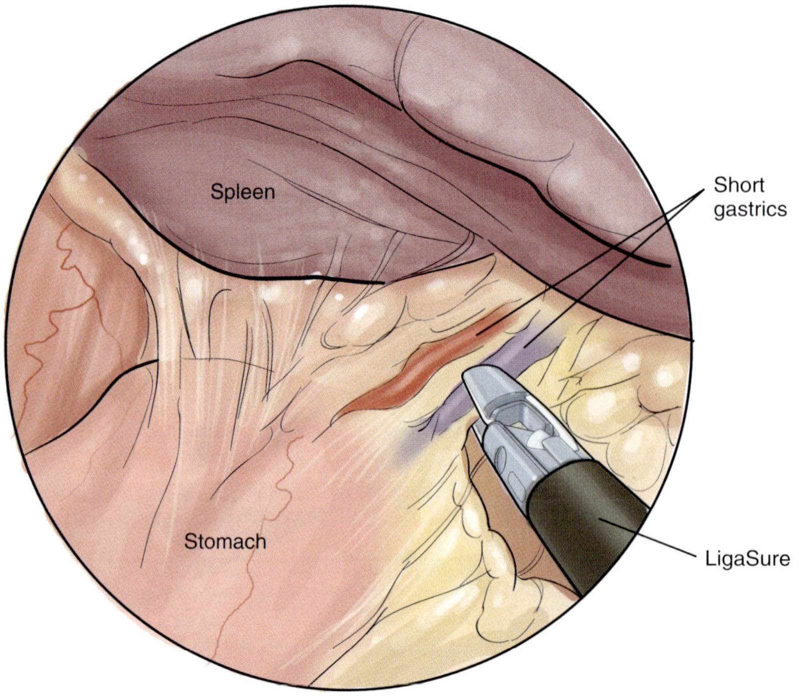

Figure 35-3.

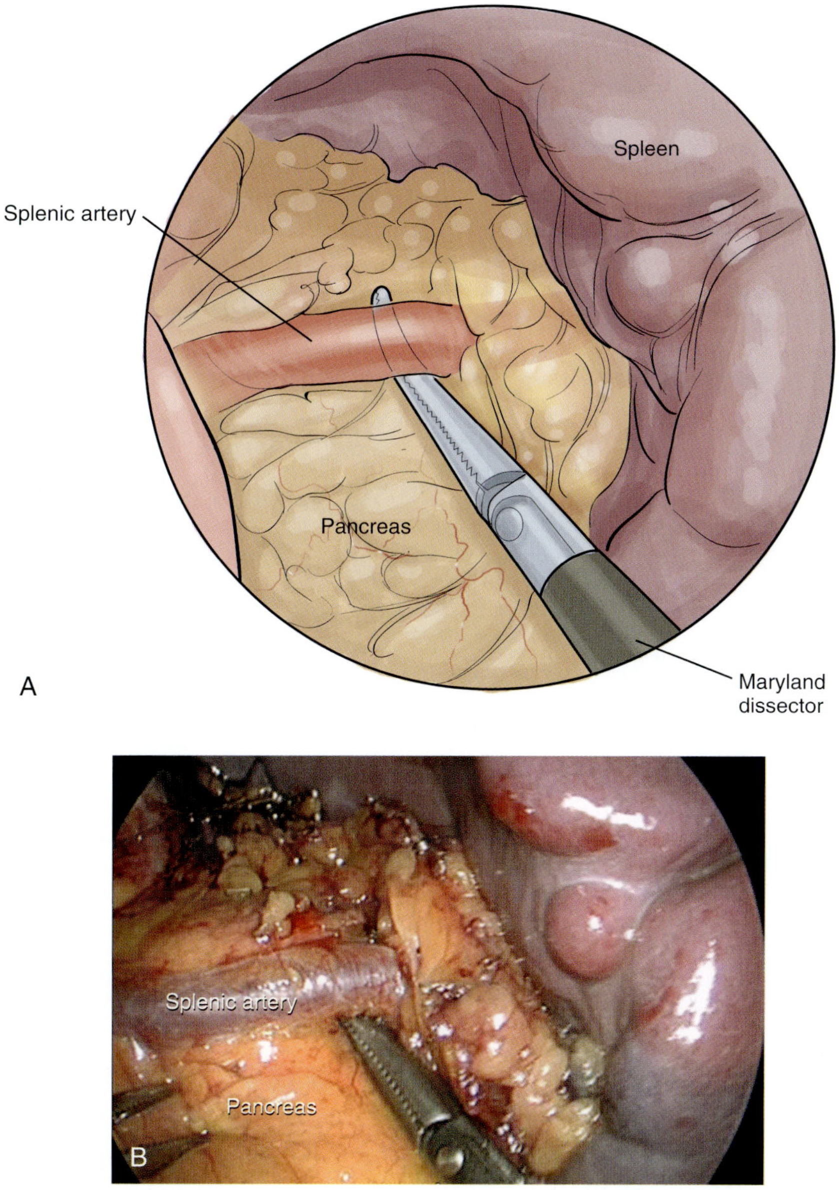
Spleen
Splenic artery
Pancreas
Maryland dissector
A
Splenic artery
Pancreas
B

Figure 35-4.

vascular Endo GIA stapling device (Covidien, Mansfield, Mass.) introduced through the 12-mm trocar. Some surgeons perform an en bloc transection, whereas others transect the vessels in separate stages. There is no difference, and we advocate the one-stage transection because it saves time and cost and is safe. Arteriovenous fistulas from single transections are extremely rare (Figs. 35-5, *A* and *B*; 35-6, *A* and *B*; and 35-7).

- In the hanging spleen approach:
  - ▲ In the hanging spleen approach, the attachments of the spleen are left intact until the hilum is dissected and controlled. We recommend this approach.
  - ▲ After transection of the hilar vessels, the short gastric arteries and the gastrosplenic ligament are divided with the LigaSure.

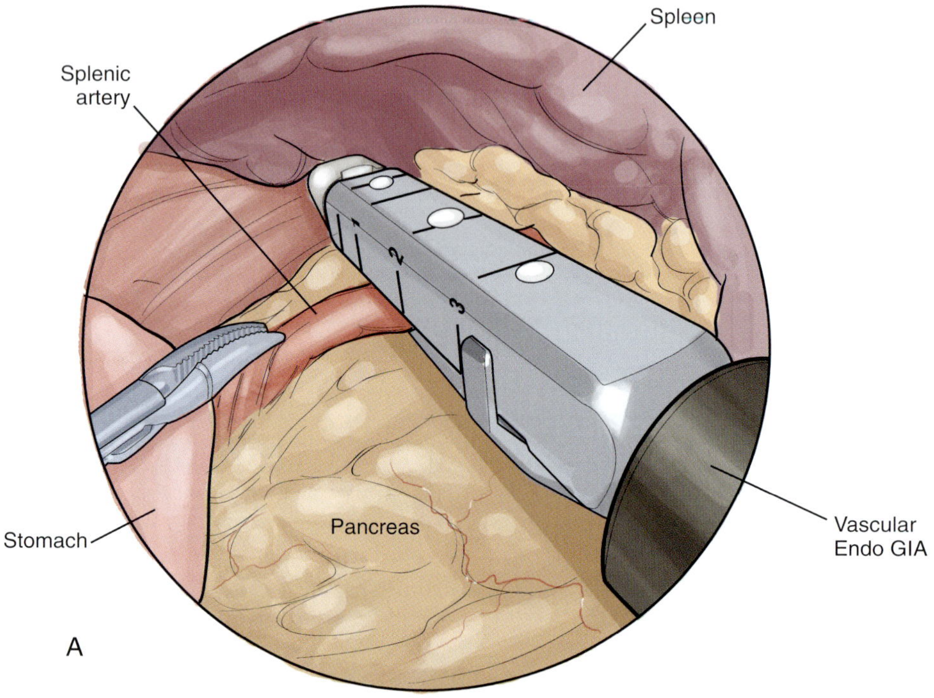

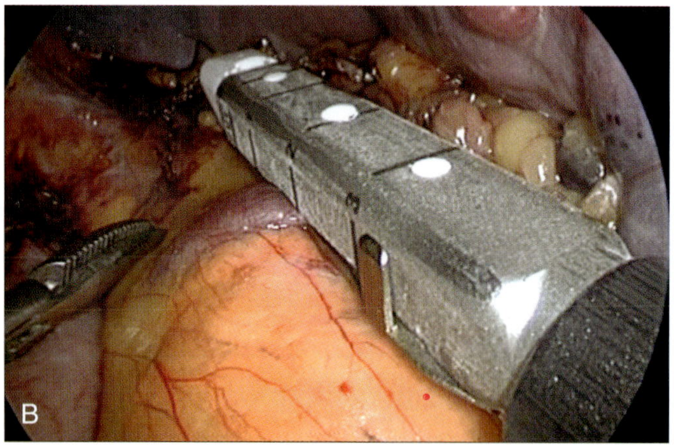

Figure 35-5.

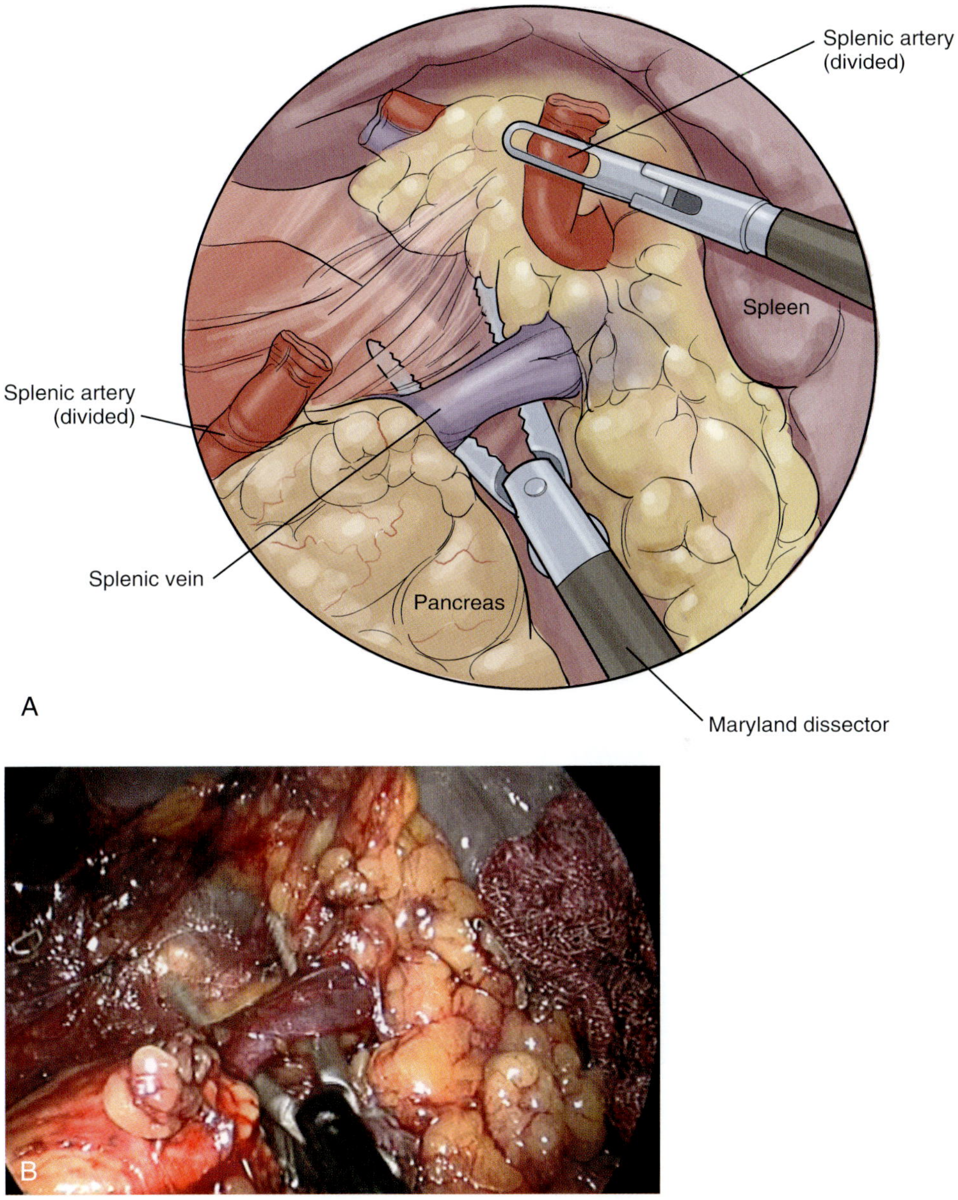

Figure 35-6.

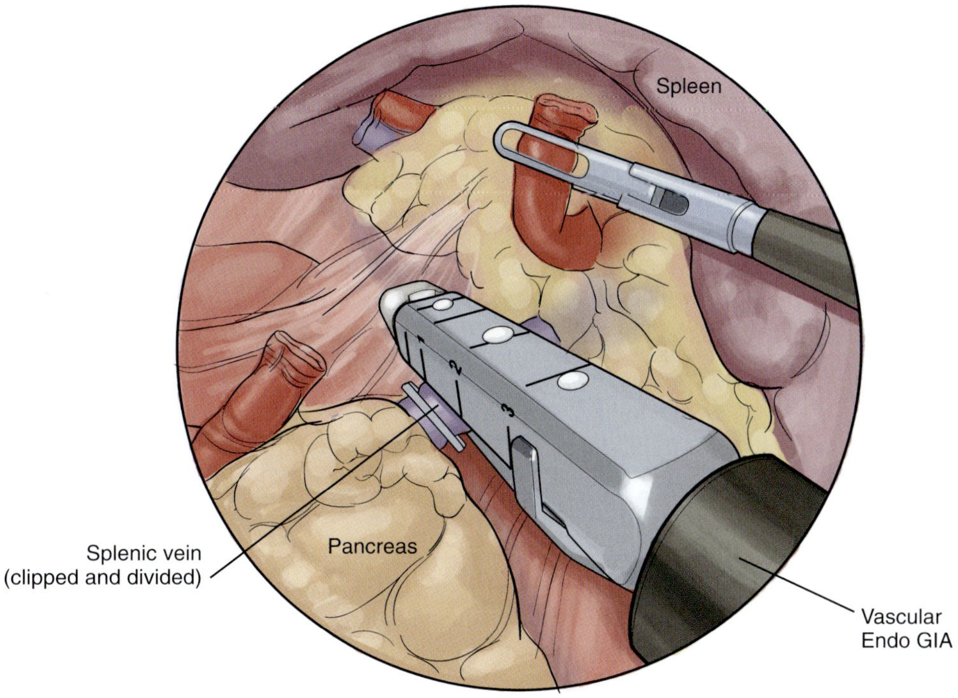

Figure 35-7.

  - ▲ The spleen is now denuded of all its vascular supply. The remaining ligaments are then divided from the abdominal wall to free the spleen (Fig. 35-8).
- In both techniques, when dissecting the hilum, extra care must be taken to avoid the pancreatic tail, which is in contact with the hilum in about 30% of patients and separated from the hilum by about 2 cm in 70% of patients. Meticulous dissection is warranted to free the tail, because pancreatic injuries of the tail can lead to pancreatitis, fistulas, cysts, abscesses, and, most dreaded, pancreatic leaks.
- The free spleen is now put in an endobag ready for delivery (Fig. 35-9).
- A 4-cm incision is made low in the lower left quadrant, and a muscle-splitting technique is used to enter the abdomen. The spleen is then delivered by opening the endobag through that incision, and morcellation of the spleen is performed. Care must be taken not to spill any of the contents in the abdomen, because there is a chance of seeding accessory spleens or even splenosis. If a specimen is needed intact for histologic assessment of a malignancy, the incision is elongated for adequate delivery.
- Hemostasis is checked.
- A drain is left in the splenic fossa for 24 to 48 hours postoperatively, especially if a pancreatic injury is suspected or the hemostasis was less than adequate.

Closure

- The incision in the left lower quadrant is closed using no. 1 loop nylon running sutures for the abdominal fascia and skin clips for the skin. The 12-mm and the umbilical port abdominal fascia are closed using size 1 absorbable suture, and skin clips are used for the skin of all the port sites.

III. ALTERNATIVE TECHNICAL APPROACHES (PRO/CON) AND PEARLS

Hand-Assisted Laparoscopic Splenectomy

- This technique is of benefit when operating on spleens larger than 20 cm.
- A hand port is deployed in the lower left quadrant or in the lower midline at the beginning of the operation, just after pneumoperitoneum is achieved. This assists the surgeon by allowing insertion of the surgeon's left hand to aid in traction, dissection, vascular control of the splenic pedicle, and to feel for accessory spleens.
- Fewer ports are needed.
- The surgeon might feel more secure controlling the pedicle proximally with his fingers while transecting the pedicle with a vascular Endo GIA.
- Traction is also made easier and safer when the surgeon uses his fingers rather than the metal laparoscopic instruments.
- The incision for the hand port is then used for specimen delivery.
- Contrary to that reported in the literature, operative time seems to be shorter and hospital stays and analgesia requirements are not increased.

Partial Splenectomy

- In this technique, a pole of the spleen is resected, leaving the main body of the spleen in place for immunologic purposes, especially in young patients.
- Partial LS is sometimes warranted in painful splenic cysts, benign tumors (such as hamartomas, fibromas, and pulpomas), infarcts, and intrasplenic pancreatic cysts.
- The preoperative care and positioning of the patient as well as the ports in the abdomen are the same as in regular LS.
- Operative procedure:
  - ▲ Mobilization: Only the part of the spleen that needs resection is mobilized. If the lower pole is to be resected, the omental connections and the branches of the gastroepiploic artery that are feeding through the ligament are controlled by LigaSure. The artery feeding the lower pole is then dissected and controlled. If the upper pole is being resected, dissection begins at the upper hilum, and the short gastric vessels are controlled, after which the artery of the upper pole is identified, clipped, and cut.
  - ▲ Parenchyma resection: After vascular control, the area that needs resection usually delineates itself by becoming paler. The transection is done by a vascular Endo GIA through the 12-mm port. The instrument is used to gently grasp the parenchyma and, when locked, is fired. Additional clips or sutures can be used to achieve hemostasis for breakthrough bleeding from the staple line. Tamponade with Surgicel (Johnson & Johnson, Langhorne, Pa.) usually controls the raw edge bleeding. The raw edges can also be sprayed with collagen sealant, readily available in the market.

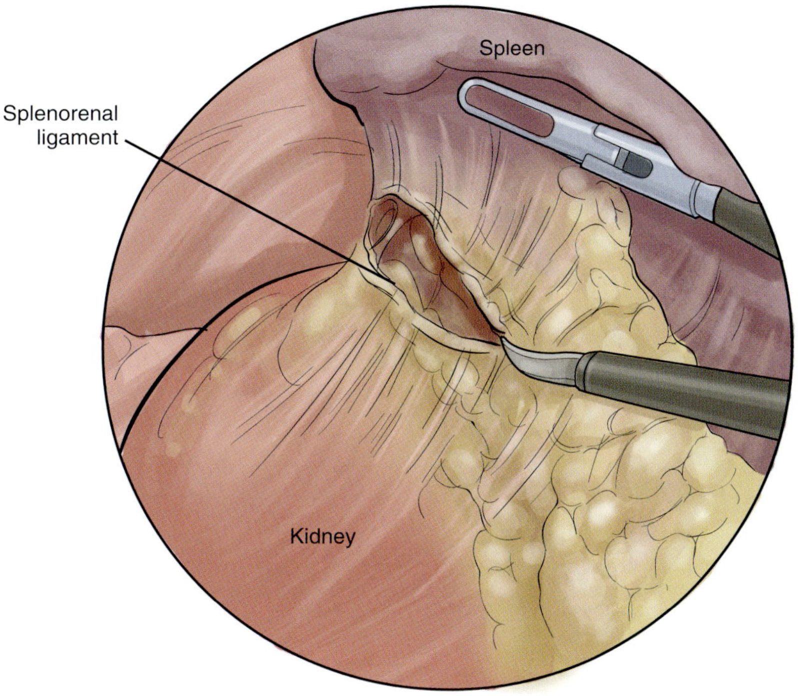

Figure 35-8.

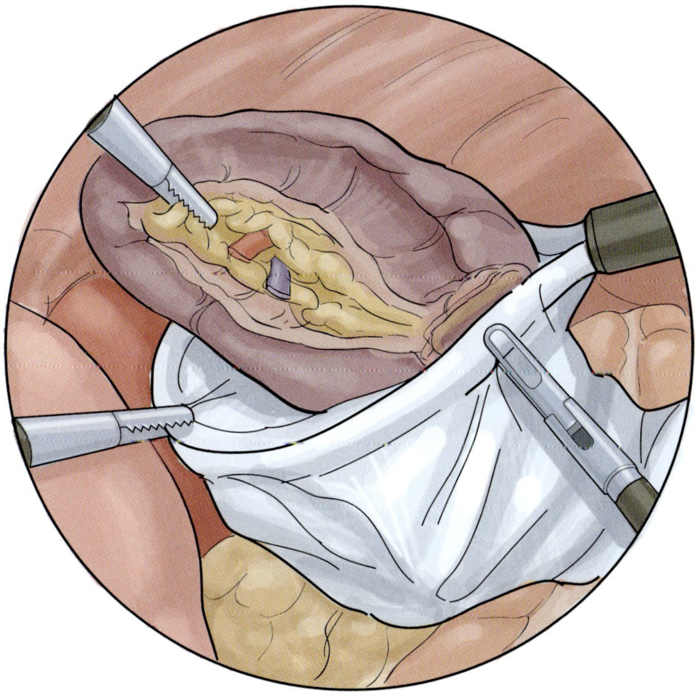

Figure 35-9.

- ▲ The specimen is removed with an endobag through the 12-mm port site. An extension to 2 cm is more than enough for delivery after morcellation of the specimen.
- ▲ Closure is done in a similar manner to LS.

IV. SPECIAL POSTOPERATIVE CARE

- A nasogastric tube is left in place until the patient is awake and nausea subsides.
- Oral fluids are started the night of the operation and advanced to a regular diet as the patient tolerates the next day.
- The abdominal drain is withdrawn after it dries out, usually in the next 24 hours.
- The patient ambulates and the urinary catheter is removed the next day after the operation.
- Thromboprophylaxis is done according to routine.
- The patient can be discharged home on the second day after the operation if the platelet count is normal.

SUGGESTED READINGS

Dexter SP, Martin IG, Alao D, et al: Laparoscopic splenectomy. The suspended pedicle technique, *Surg Endosc* 10:393–396, 1996.

Park A, Targarona EM, Trias M: Laparoscopic surgery of the spleen: state of the art, *Langenbecks Arch Surg* 386:230–239, 2001.

Rosen M, Brody F, Walsh RM, Ponsky J: Hand-assisted laparoscopic splenectomy vs. conventional laparoscopic splenectomy in cases of splenomegaly, *Arch Surg* 137:1348–1352, 2002.

SECTION VII

Hepatobiliary

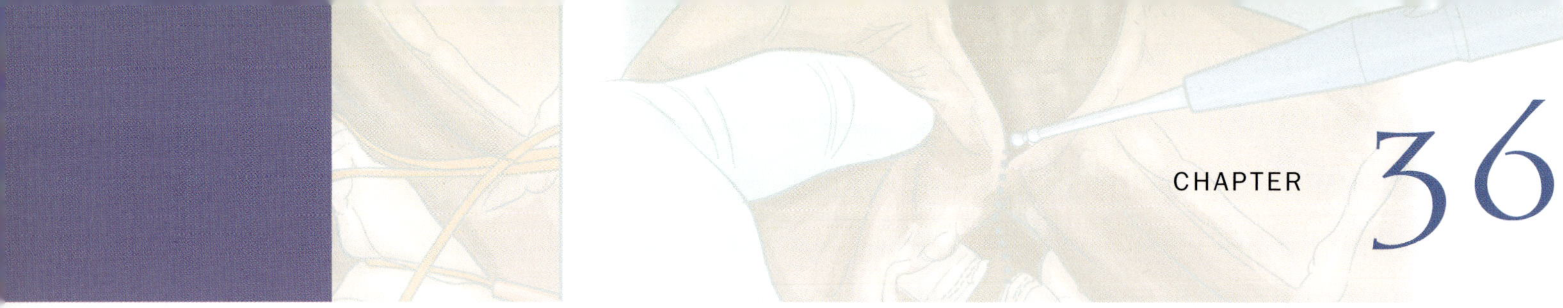

CHAPTER 36

Right and Left Trisectionectomies

Jacques Belghiti, MD, and Olivier Scatton, MD, PhD

I. SPECIAL PREOPERATIVE PREPARATION

- *Understanding nomenclature*: The internal architecture of the liver described by Couinaud includes eight segments supplied by a portal triad with a branch of the portal vein and hepatic artery and drained by a branch of the hepatic duct. The left and the right branch of both portal trunk and hepatic artery supply four segments, delimiting the left liver (segments I to IV) and the right liver (segments V to VIII). The four sectors are delimited by the three main hepatic veins, including respectively the left sector (segments II and III), the left median sector (segments I and IV), the right paramedian sector (segments V and VIII), and the right posterior sector (segments VI and VII). According to the new classification proposed by the International Hepato-Pancreato-Biliary Association in 2000, right trisectionectomy, also called extended right hepatectomy, includes resection of segments IV, V, VI, VII, and VIII, whereas left trisectionectomy, also termed extended left hepatectomy, includes resection of segments II, III, IV, V, and VIII. If necessary, segment I can be resected as well in either of these techniques (Fig. 36-1). Although both techniques have their particularities, they share median hepatic vein resection and leave a single hepatic vein to ensure liver remnant venous outflow.
- Both right and left trisectionectomy are major liver resections that require preoperative liver function, resectability, and future liver remnant (FLR) volume assessment. Liver biological test (international normalized ratio [INR], bilirubin blood level, and sometimes indocyanine green clearance) should be performed preoperatively. Computed tomography scan with vascular reconstruction and liver volume measurement (total and FLR volume) is the preferred imaging modality to evaluate resectability, to anticipate FLR volume, and to evaluate the vascular relationship between the tumor and hepatic vessels. Magnetic resonance imaging is mainly used to characterize the tumor and/or to evaluate biliary tract involvement.
- The main complications to be expected and tracked down after such liver resections are postoperative liver insufficiency and biliary strictures or leakages. These complications are related to the large volume of resected liver parenchyma (extended liver resection) and to the biliary hilar plate dissection, which might impair biliary vascularization.
- The patient's vascular venous anatomy should be assessed in order to plan the need for vascular isolation techniques and to anticipate potential venous reconstruction. Hepatic vascular exclusion could be required because of a close relationship between the tumor and the inferior vena cava. Last, in both right and left trisectionectomy, the future remnant is drained by a single hepatic vein. A venous reconstruction could be required to ensure good venous outflow and avoid FLR congestion. Remnant left liver fixation in an anatomical position is then required to avoid remnant liver congestion.
- If FLR is estimated to be too small (less than 30% for normal liver and 40% for underlying liver disease), a preoperative portal vein embolization (PVE) can be performed in order to induce FLR hypertrophy. However, PVE needs to be performed only when patients are being considered for right trisectionectomy. PVE is rarely necessary before left trisectionectomy because the right posterior sector typically constitutes about 30% of the total liver volume and its natural position ensures an excellent outflow though the right hepatic vein.
- A modern approach is to perform extended resection without mobilization of the liver (anterior approach) and avoid vascular clamping of the small remnant liver. The hanging maneuver can be used in either of these resections. If necessary, an ipsilateral clamping of the resected liver is preferred, and pedicular intermittent clamping has been shown to be the best-tolerated clamping modality.

II. OPERATIVE TECHNIQUE

- In this chapter, we describe separately the technical aspects of both right and left trisectionectomy without hepatic vascular exclusion and without hepatic mobilization (anterior approach).

Position and Incision

- The patient is in a supine position with the left arm placed away from the body. A bilateral subcostal incision is usual, but a J-shaped incision can also be used.

Main Dissection

Hanging Maneuver

- The hanging maneuver can be applied for both right and left trisectionectomies. In the case of right trisectionectomy, the tape is placed between the left and the median hepatic veins. It is placed between the median and the right hepatic vein if a left trisectionectomy is to be performed. Hanging maneuver dissection starts on the right side of the middle and left hepatic vein common trunk. The anterior leaf of the coronary ligament and anterior part of the right triangular ligament are opened, and the space between the right and the median hepatic vein is dissected. Dissection of the suprahepatic vena cava safely starts with a large and smooth dissector. The inferior vena cava is dissected above the origin of the right renal vein. Usually one or two short Spiegel veins need to be ligated to avoid bleeding when performing the hanging maneuver. Then, scissors are passed along the avascular plan between the liver and the retrohepatic vena cava, toward the previously dissected space (Fig. 36-2). An aortic clamp replaces the scissors in order to grab the tape and pull it through the avascular space of the retrohepatic vena cava (Fig. 36-3). A 10 mm-wide soft, silicon multitubular drain is used as the tape. This latter

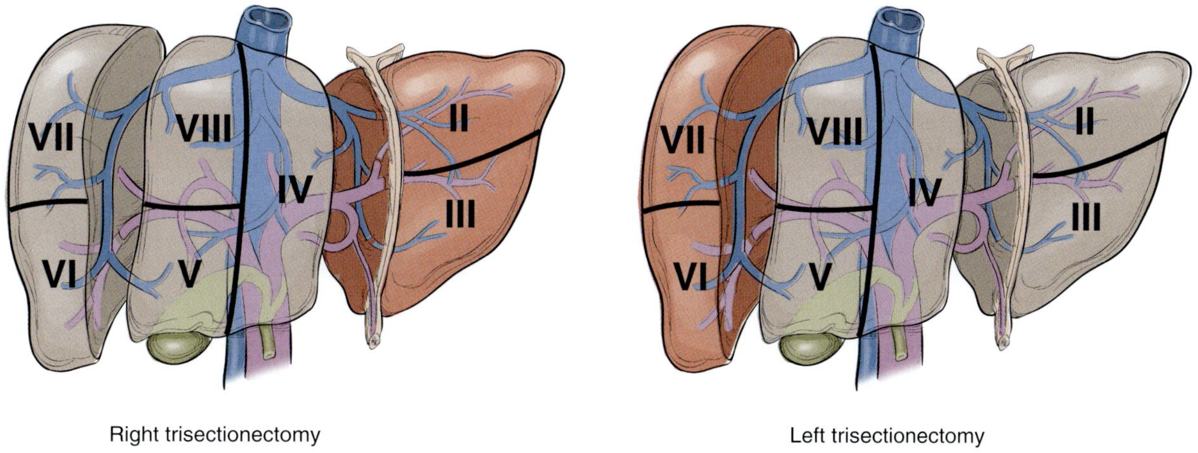

Figure 36-1.

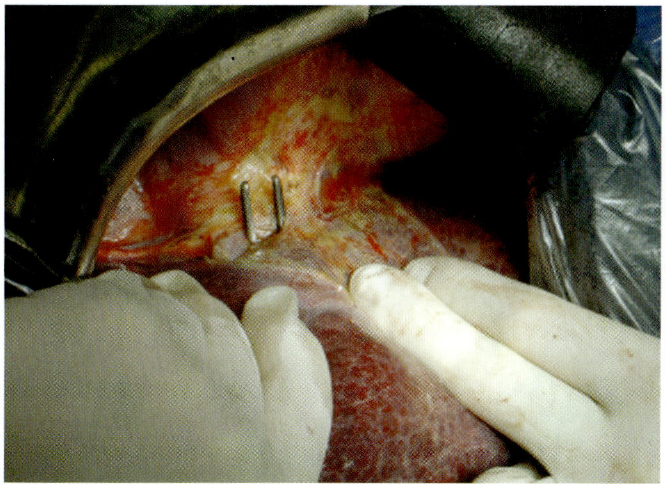

Figure 36-2.

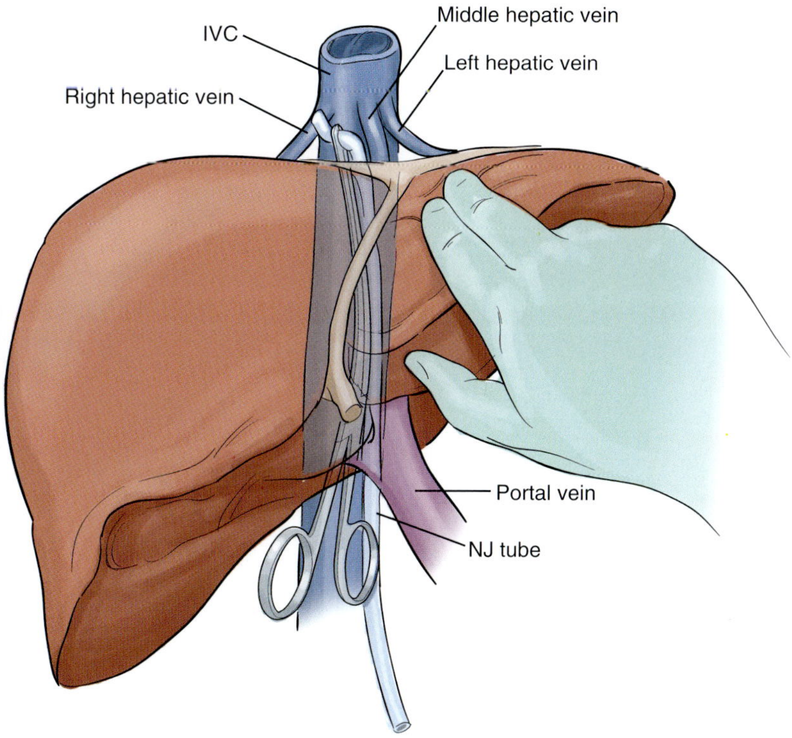

Figure 36-3. *IVC,* Inferior vena cava.

maneuver allows "suspension" of the liver during the transection. In the case of right trisectionectomy, parenchymal transection is begun near the middle and left hepatic vein confluence in order to switch the tape from the right to the left side to the middle hepatic vein (Fig. 36-4). When segment I is preserved, the tape is placed in front of segment I (Fig. 36-5).

Hilar Dissection and Parenchymal Transection for Right Trisectionectomy

- Hepatectomy starts with hilar dissection. Cholecystectomy is performed and a tube is placed in the cystic duct in order to check the absence of biliary leak with blue dye injection through the cystic duct drain. This drain is removed before abdominal closure, and the cystic duct is closed with a 4-0 polydioxanone surgical suture. Vascular anatomy is defined using intraoperative ultrasound. The first step of the procedure is dividing the right vascular pedicle in order to minimize blood loss and to ensure a good exposition of the left hilar plate, that is, to minimize the risk of left pedicle injury. The right biliary duct, hepatic artery, and portal vein are identified. Before any vascular ligation, the right hepatic artery and right portal vein are clamped, and the left portal and arterial inflows are checked to see that they are satisfactory. The right hepatic artery and right portal vein are divided (Fig. 36-6). An eventual overlying bridge of parenchyma between segments IV and III is divided.
- The second important step is to perform the segment IV devascularization and resection. To achieve this goal, the right side of the round ligament is dissected from its inferior to its superior part. Step by step, portal and arterial pedicles to segment IV are identified and ligated on the right side of the round ligament which is retracted upwards (see Fig. 36-6).

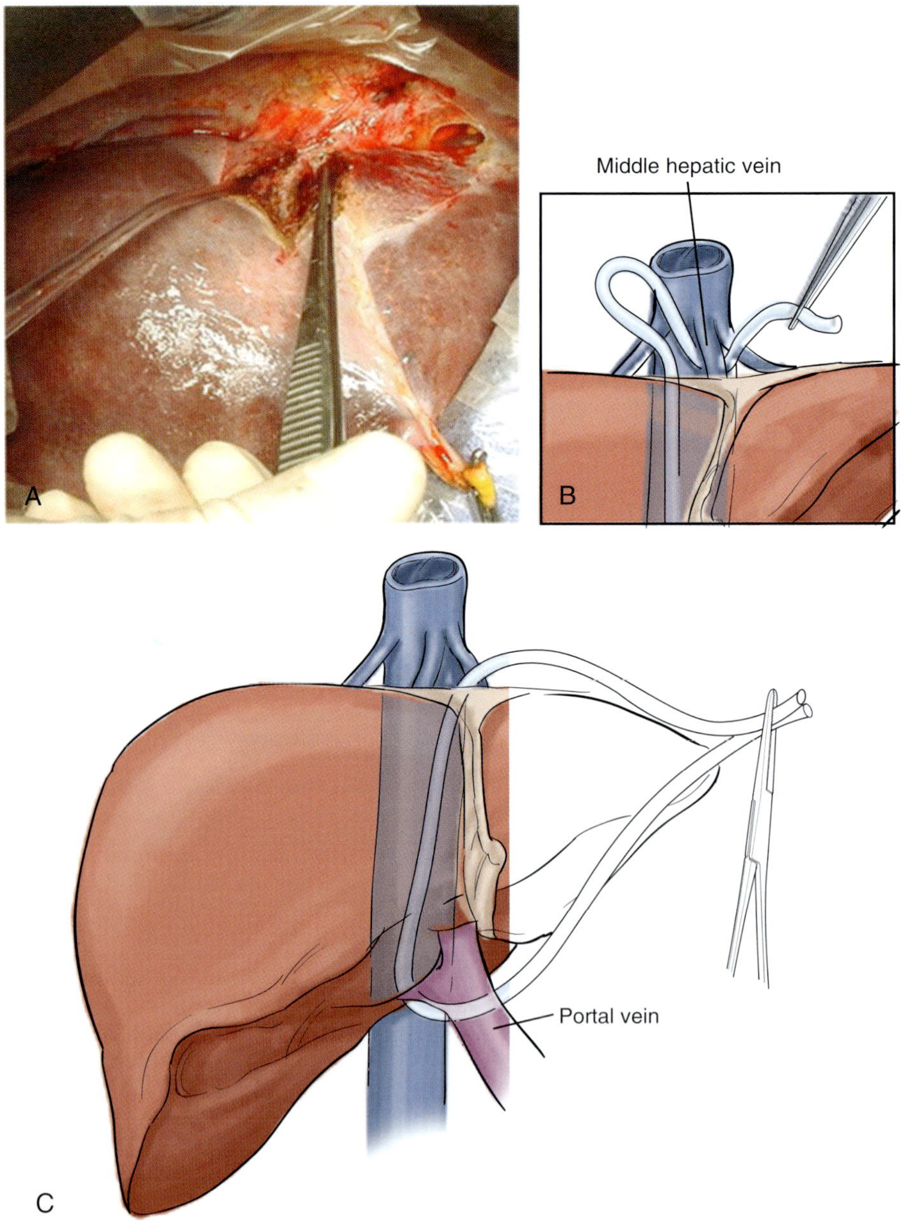

Figure 36-4.

- Parenchymal transection is performed with or without pedicle clamping using clamp fracture or ultrasonic dissector (Dissectron, Satelec Medical, Mérignac, France). The hanging tape is used to raise the transection plane and safely meet the middle hepatic vein. Biliostasis and hemostasis are performed using irrigated bipolar coagulation or ligation.
- The dissection proceeds with the ultrasonic dissector beneath the hilar plate and left bile duct. The dissection continues along the hilar plate, and the right hepatic duct is identified and cut.
- The parenchymal transection is completed when the hanging tape is seen. When parenchymal transection is achieved, the median hepatic vein is controlled and divided using either running suture or a vascular stapler. The right hepatic vein also is divided. The final step of the procedure involves the section of the right hepatic ligament. To avoid left hepatic vein kinking and venous outflow obstruction, it is mandatory to replace the remnant liver in the anatomic position using the round ligament.

Hilar Dissection and Parenchymal Transection for Left Trisectionectomy

- This operation is technically demanding. Hepatectomy starts with a hilar dissection with the intent to divide the left pedicle early. Cholecystectomy is performed, and a tube is placed in the common bile duct through the cystic duct. The left hepatic artery and left portal vein are controlled, taped, and divided. Contralateral vascular inflows are checked before any vascular ligation. The left bile duct is

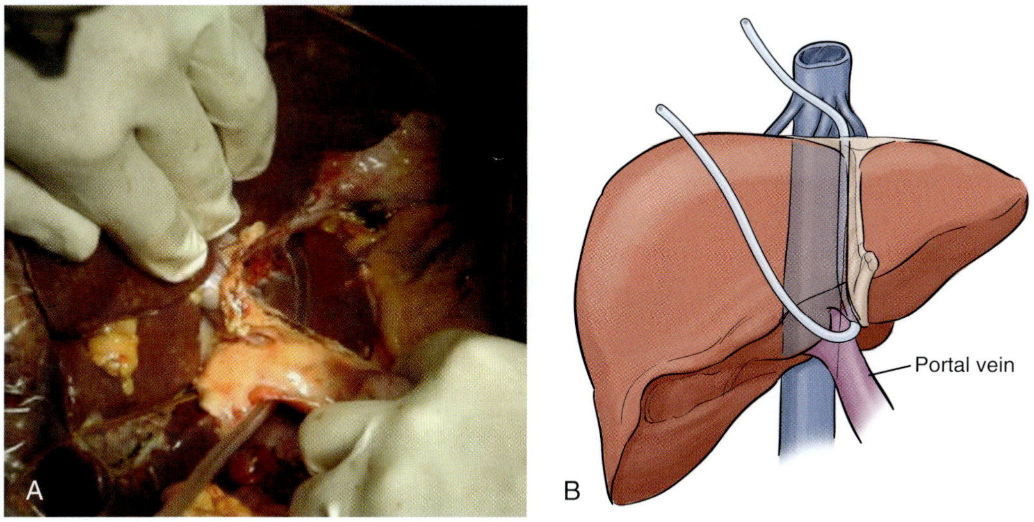

Figure 36-5.

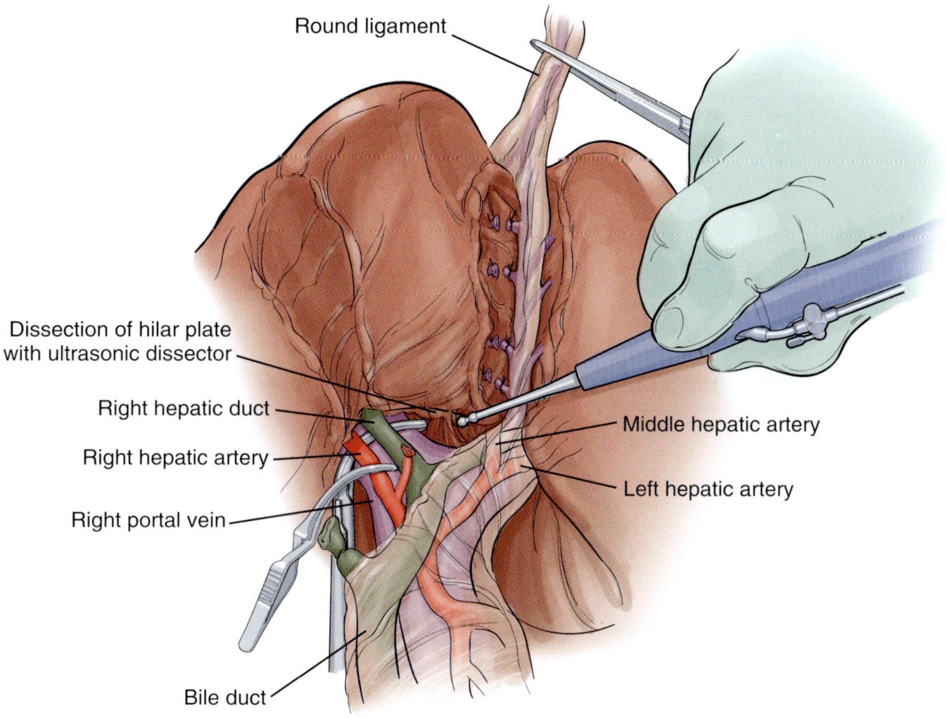

Figure 36-6.

cut. Using the ultrasonic dissector, the right portal pedicle is skeletonized from the left to the right so that the right anterior pedicle can be identified. This latter is clamped, and ultrasound is used to check the good vascularization of the posterolateral section. The right anterior pedicle is then ligated and divided, if this latter control is satisfactory. If control of the right anterior pedicle cannot be achieved safely, it may be divided after subtotal parenchymal transection. However, the right posterolateral pedicle should be identified before the right anterior pedicle section, irrespective of the technique used. Liver parenchyma transection starts on the left side of the right hepatic vein. In this view, intraoperative ultrasound is a helpful tool. Liver transection is then completed along the line of ischemic demarcation between right posterior and right anterior sectors (Fig. 36-7).

- Parenchymal transection is performed using ultrasonic dissector. Hemostasis and biliostasis are performed using irrigated bipolar forceps. Elements larger than 3 mm are ligated or clipped. Transection is completed when the hanging tape is reached (Fig. 36-8). The Arantius ligament is divided, allowing

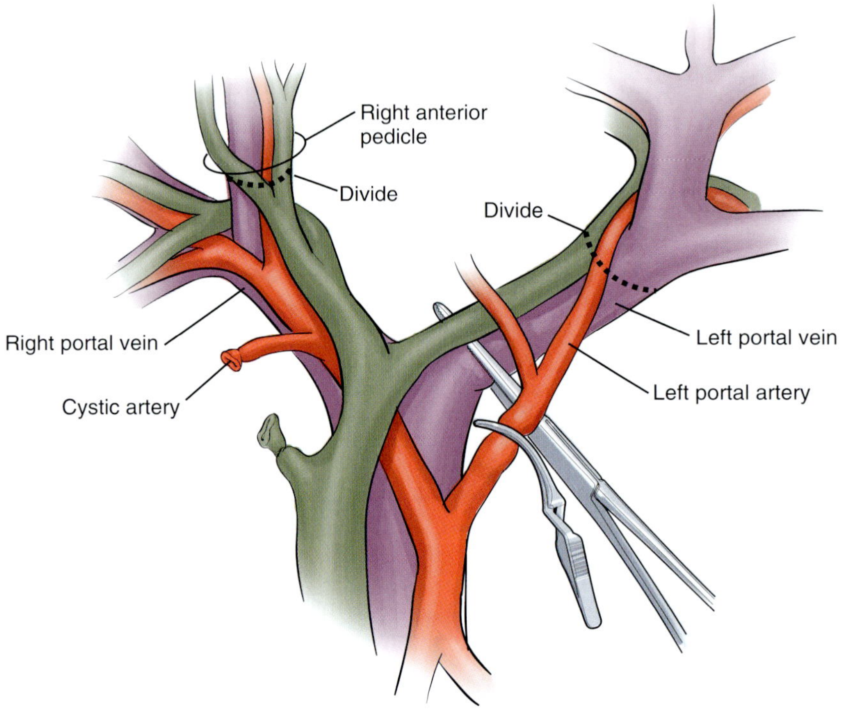

Figure 36-7.

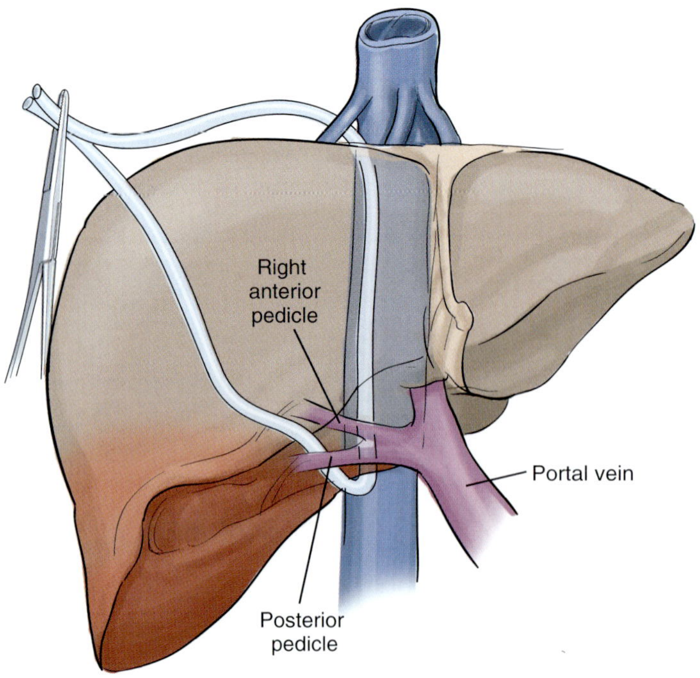

Figure 36-8.

the separation of segment I and the left liver. Finally, the inferior part of the tape is moved to the left to encircle the left and median hepatic vein common trunk. These two veins are divided and closed using running suture or vascular stapler.
- A cholangiogram is performed using the tube initially introduced in the cystic duct. This tube could be left in the common bile duct in order to detect or treat an eventual postoperative biliary complication.

Closure

- The J-incision is closed by approximating the midline linea alba with 1-0 monofilament suture, and the horizontal portion where the muscles of the anterior abdominal wall were divided is closed in layers with the same suture material. A bilateral subcostal incision is closed in layers with 1-0 monofilament suture. Skin is approximated with staples.

III. ALTERNATIVE TECHNICAL APPROACHES (PRO/CON) AND PEARLS

- For those who do not wish to use the liver hanging maneuver, the right lobe of the liver is mobilized by division of the right triangular ligament. The small venous tributaries draining into the inferior vena cava are divided between hemoclips. Larger veins are ligated with 3-0 silk. The Makuuchi ligament is divided, and this provides access to the right hepatic vein. The hilar pedicle dissection is performed by the Glisson technique to isolate the right liver segment IVA and IVB pedicle, which is then transected with a linear endovascular stapler.
- To increase safety for novices to the liver hanging maneuver, the retrohepatic dissection anterior to the inferior vena cava can be performed with use of the choledochoscope to allow visualization of the retrohepatic plane.

IV. SPECIAL POSTOPERATIVE CARE

- If the liver remnant volume is inadequately judged, postoperative liver failure can result. Thus the importance of liver volumetry and the use of portal vein embolization cannot be stressed too much.
- Appropriate precautions are taken to minimize or prevent the occurrence of general postoperative complications such as pneumonia, thrombotic events, and cardiac events.
- Liver-specific complications such as bile leak and liver failure, particularly in patients with cirrhosis and following massive (50% to 60%) resection, must be anticipated. In the event of liver impairment, particular attention is paid to avoiding hepatotoxic drugs, and the transplantation service should be engaged. Patients with cirrhosis also are at risk for developing portal vein thrombosis, and clinicians should be alerted to this event if persistent abdominal pain occurs with elevation of liver function tests. Duplex ultrasound of the liver is obtained, and if thrombosis is detected, anticoagulation is started.
- If the INR is elevated, the patient may require administration of vitamin K and/or fresh frozen plasma depending on the degree of INR elevation and associated drop in hematocrit.
- Epidural or patient-controlled analgesia is routinely instituted to ensure adequate pain control.

SUGGESTED READINGS

Blumgart LH, Belghiti J: Liver resections for benign disease and for liver and biliary tumors. In Blumgart LH, editor: *Surgery of the liver, biliary tract and pancreas*, ed 4, Philadelphia, 2007, Saunders, p 1341.

Kim SH, Park SJ, Lee S, et al: Various liver resections using hanging maneuver by three Glisson's pedicles and three hepatic veins, *Ann Surg* 245:201, 2007.

Ogata S, Belghiti J, Varma D, et al: Two hundred liver hanging maneuvers for major hepatectomy. A single-center experience, *Ann Surg* 245:31, 2007.

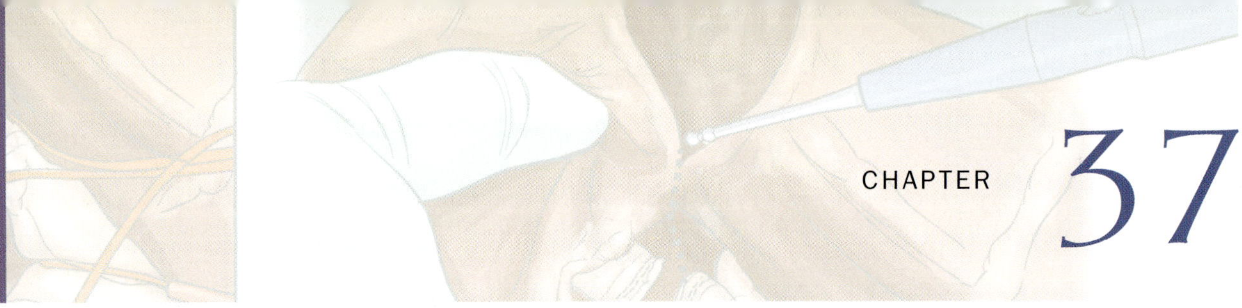

CHAPTER 37

Resection of the Caudate Lobe

Ho-Seong Han, MD, PhD

I. SPECIAL PREOPERATIVE PREPARATION

- The caudate lobe (segments I and/or IX) of the liver is surgically difficult to approach because of its deep location in the hepatic parenchyma. This lobe is surrounded by the confluence of the left and middle hepatic veins, the porta hepatis, the ligamentum venosum, and the inferior vena cava (IVC). Therefore, isolated caudate lobectomy is a challenging technical procedure even for experienced hepatic surgeons (Fig. 37-1).
- Several techniques, from limited to extended resection, have been reported for resecting the caudate lobe, including isolated caudate lobectomy and combined resection with other type of liver resection (partial hepatectomy with caudate lobectomy, hemihepatectomy with caudate lobectomy, etc.).
- There are various techniques for combined hepatectomy, but this technique can be modified from isolated caudate lobectomy. Therefore, the techniques for isolated caudate lobectomy are described in this chapter.
- The caudate lobe is generally divided into three regions: the Spiegel lobe, the caudate process, and the paracaval portion. The anatomy of the paracaval portion is the liver parenchyma that is ventral to the right side of the IVC and between the Spiegel lobe and the right lobe just inferior to the middle hepatic vein (Couinaud segment IX) (see Fig. 37-1).
- Four approaches to isolated caudate lobectomy have been described: the left, right, and anterior transparenchymal approaches, and the technique using the hanging maneuver. The former two techniques require mobilization of the right and left liver, respectively—except when the tumor is small, in which case a simple tumorectomy is possible without mobilizing other parts of the liver. This mobilization may not create a problem in noncirrhotic patients with normal liver function; however, in cirrhotic patients, transection of the liver ligaments and the peritoneum, which are thickened with dilated venous and lymphatic vessels, causes significant bleeding and loss of fluid before any parenchymal transection has begun. The anterior approach has the drawback of unnecessary parenchymal transection. These limitations can be avoided by a technique using the hanging maneuver. There have been several recent reports of caudate lobectomy with the laparoscopic approach. Although laparoscopic caudate lobectomy is complicated, it is feasible to perform by the left approach in selected patients with small tumors in the Spiegel lobe.

II. OPERATIVE TECHNIQUE: THE LEFT APPROACH FOR SPIEGEL LOBE RESECTION

- When small tumors are limited to the left part of the caudate lobe (the Spiegel lobe), a left approach is preferable.

Position

- The patient is placed in the supine position.

Incision

- A midline or bilateral subcostal incision is used, according to the preference of the surgeon.
- When large tumors are encountered, via the right approach or the anterior transparenchymal approach, a J-incision may be necessary.

Main Dissection

- The first step of the left approach for the caudate lobectomy is to inspect and palpate the caudate lobe by entering the lesser sac.
- The left lateral section of the liver is mobilized. After dissection of the left triangular ligament, the lesser omentum is resected. During excision of the lesser omentum, caution should be used not to injure the left hepatic artery that originates from the left gastric artery.
- The mobilized left lateral section is gently retracted to the right side to expose the Spiegel lobe. All the short hepatic veins draining from the caudate lobe to the IVC are isolated and ligated (Fig. 37-2). The caudate lobe is mobilized ventrally from the left side of the IVC, proceeding from the caudal portion of the IVC to the cranial direction. The short hepatic veins should be ligated with transfixing sutures.

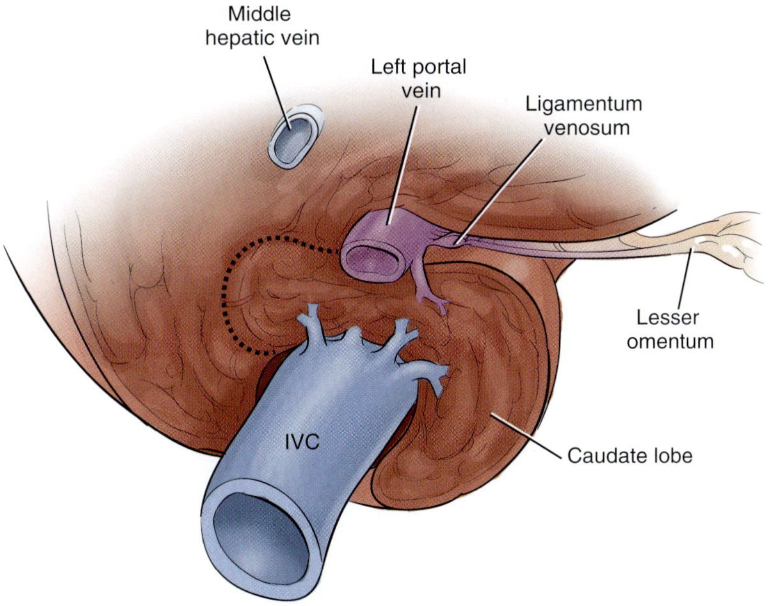

Figure 37-1. *IVC,* Inferior vena cava.

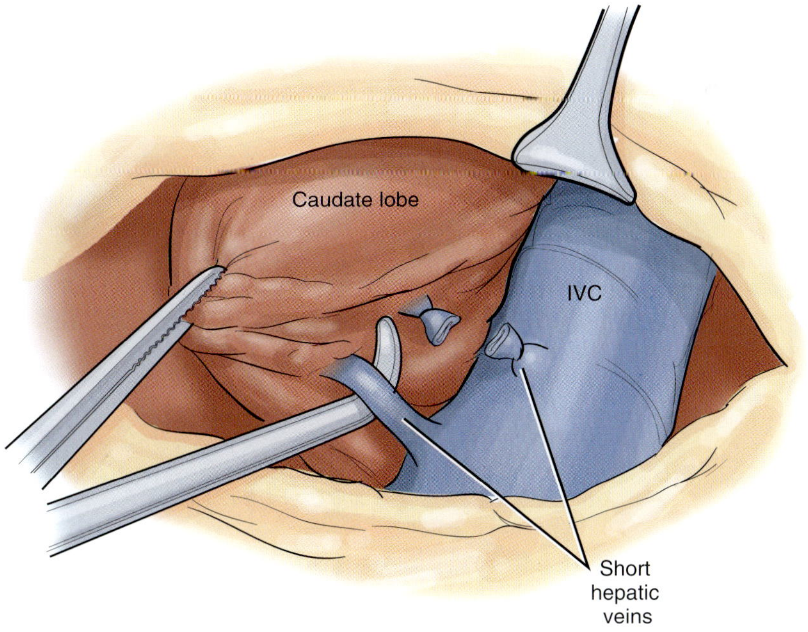

Figure 37-2. *IVC,* Inferior vena cava.

- The Arantius duct can be transected near the left portal vein to create a good view for the subsequent hepatectomy. The caudate lobe is retracted to facilitate good exposure of the transection plane (Fig. 37-3).
- After this is achieved, the liver resection is started. The Glisson pedicle and the vascular structures are isolated and ligated during transection. For complete Spiegel lobe resection, the transection may continue until the left and middle hepatic veins are reached (Fig. 37-4).

Closure

- The midline incision is closed by approximating the linea alba with 1-0 monofilament suture. The subcostal incision is closed in layers by approximating the layers of the anterior abdominal muscles with 1-0 monofilament suture.

III. OPERATIVE TECHNIQUE: THE RIGHT APPROACH

- When tumors arise from an area beneath the main portal bifurcation extend into the caudate process, or spread from both the caudate process and paracaval portion, a right approach can be selected, although this operation is technically challenging.

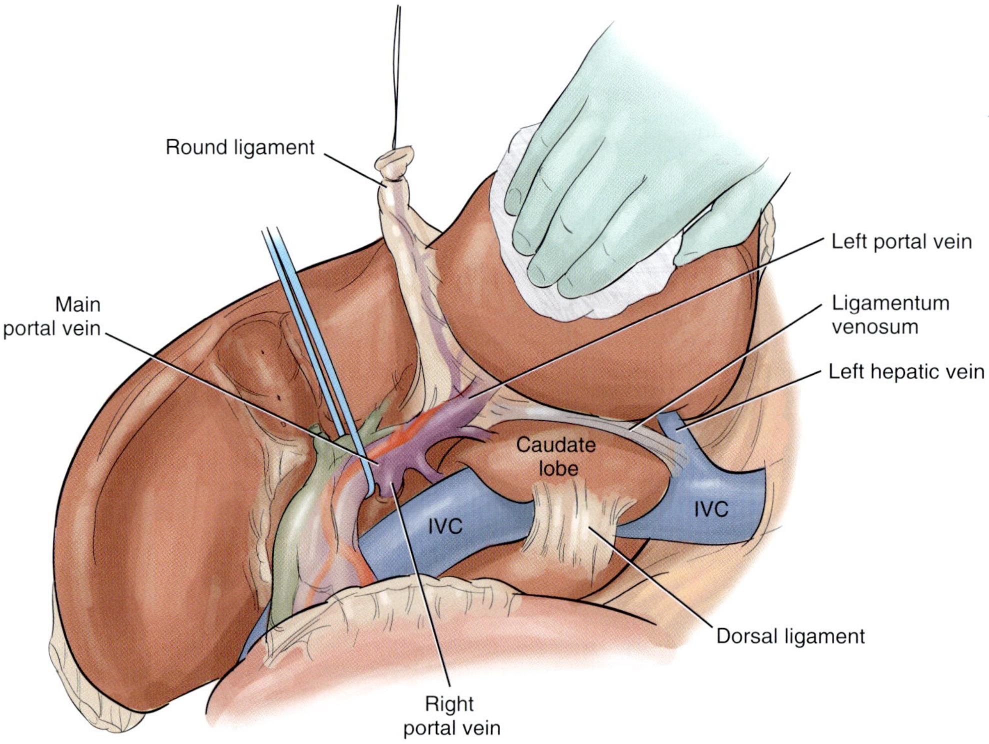

Figure 37-3. *IVC,* Inferior vena cava.

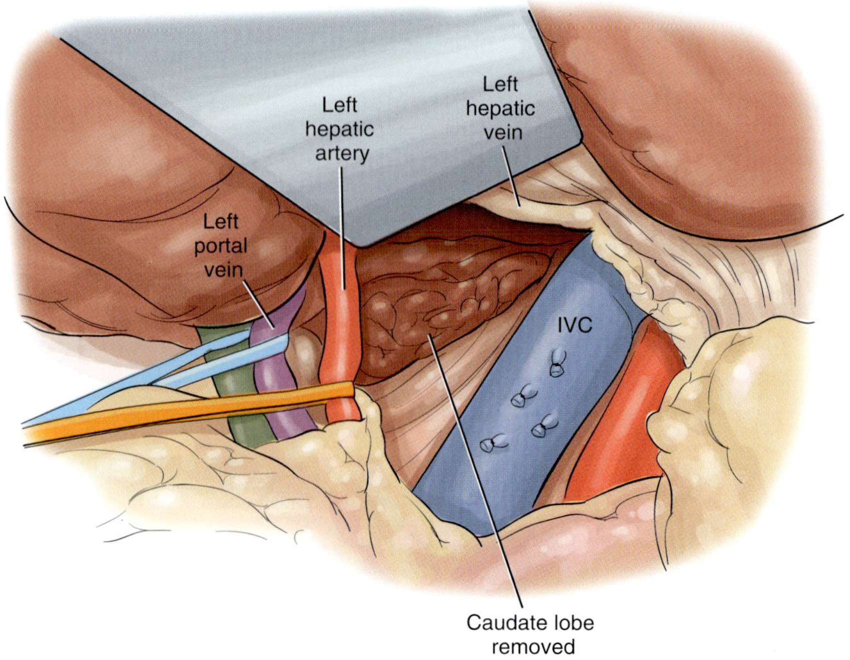

Figure 37-4. *IVC,* Inferior vena cava.

Position

- The patient is placed in the supine position.

Incision

- A midline or bilateral subcostal incision is used, according to the preference of the surgeon.
- When large tumors are encountered, via the right approach or the anterior transparenchymal approach, a J-incision may be necessary.

Main Dissection

- The approach to the caudate lobe from the right side involves initial complete mobilization of the right liver by division of its peritoneal attachments. The right lobe is retracted toward the left, and the short hepatic veins are isolated and ligated. The right liver is mobilized from below to upward, with division of all veins until the major hepatic trunks are reached.
- During dissection of the short hepatic veins, it is easy to extend over the anterior surface of the IVC to the left side until the caudate lobe is completely mobilized and freed from the IVC (Fig. 37-5).
- A total caudate lobectomy can require the injection of a dye, such as indigo blue, into the portal vein branches to exactly define the limits of the caudate lobe, particularly those of the paracaval portion. Clamping the right posterior Glisson pedicle can be helpful to identify the demarcation line of the paracaval portion.
- The portal branches to the caudate lobe are ligated and dissected from the right side of the hilum. All the Glisson and biliary branches from the right hilum, which drain the process portion of the caudate lobe, are ligated and dissected, and the surgeon proceeds with the dissection toward the cranial direction. The transection continues until major hepatic trunks are visualized. Pringle's maneuver, with cycles of 10 minutes of ischemia and 5 minutes of reperfusion, can be used throughout the liver resection.

Closure

- The midline incision is closed by approximating the linea alba with 1-0 monofilament suture. The subcostal incision is closed in layers by approximating the layers of the anterior abdominal muscles with 1-0 monofilament suture.

IV. OPERATIVE TECHNIQUE: THE ANTERIOR TRANSPARENCHYMAL APPROACH

- The anterior transhepatic approach is rarely required, but it is a potentially curative surgical option for a tumor in the paracaval portion of the caudate lobe.

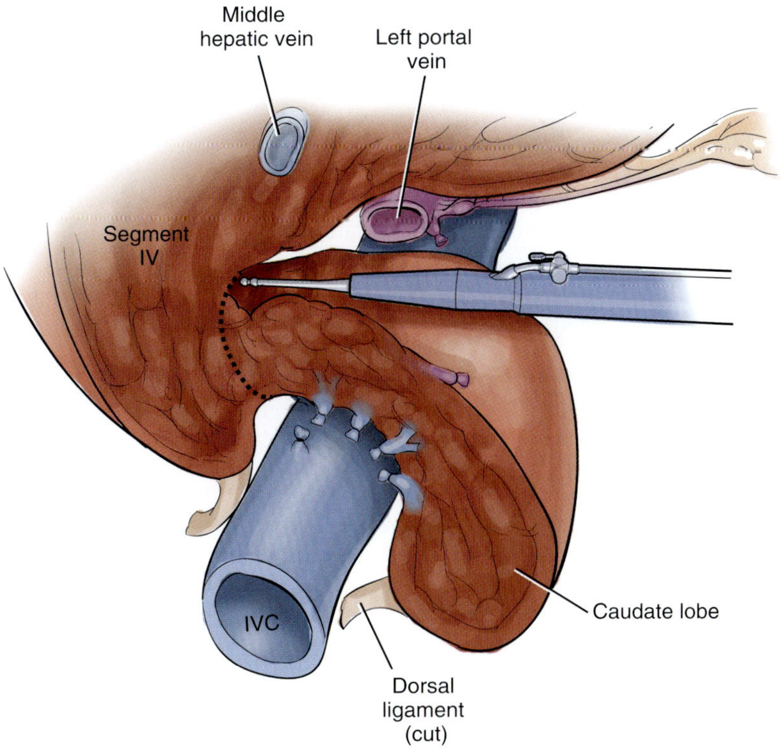

Figure 37-5. *IVC,* Inferior vena cava.

Position

- The patient is placed in the supine position.

Incision

- A midline or bilateral subcostal incision is used according to the preference of the surgeon.
- When large tumors are encountered, via the right approach or the anterior transparenchymal approach, a J-incision may be necessary.

Main Dissection

- After cholecystectomy, the right lobe is mobilized from the retroperitoneum and the IVC by ligating and dissecting the short hepatic veins cranially. The right hepatic vein is securely isolated after division of the vena cava ligament.
- On the left side, after dissecting and bending up the lateral section and dividing the ligamentum venosum at the junction of the left hepatic vein, the Spiegel lobe is separated from the IVC. The trunk of the left and middle hepatic veins are taped for safety. The liver is completely separated from the IVC, except for the major hepatic veins.
- Before liver transection, the outline of the caudate process and the paracaval portion against the posterior segment is identified by a counterstaining technique or clamping the right Glisson pedicle. Under the Pringle maneuver, transection is performed along the left side of the middle hepatic vein, opening the interlobar plane and exposing the anteromedial surface of the paracaval portion and the hilar plate.
- The paracaval portion is detached from the hilar plate by ligating and dividing the caudate portal branches. The transection proceeds in two directions: to the left side toward the sulcus of the ligamentum venosum, and to the right side just behind the middle hepatic vein. On the left side, after dividing the ligamentum venosum and the Spiegel branches from the portal vein, the Spiegel lobe is liberated from the left lobe.
- On the right side, the hilar plate is exposed up to the bifurcation of the anterior and posterior Glisson pedicles. With the right lobe bent medially, liver transection is conducted from the border of the posterior section and the caudate process to expose the dorsal surface of the middle hepatic vein. The resection is complete when the major hepatic trunks are visualized.

Closure

- The midline incision is closed by approximating the linea alba with 1-0 monofilament suture. The subcostal incision is closed in layers by approximating the layers of the anterior abdominal muscles with 1-0 monofilament suture.

V. ALTERNATIVE TECHNICAL APPROACHES (PRO/CON) AND PEARLS

Isolated Caudate Lobectomy Using the Hanging Maneuver

Indication

- Isolated caudate lobectomy using the hanging maneuver is most appropriate when complete caudate lobectomy is necessary. This applies especially to patients with chronic hepatitis and cirrhosis, regardless of tumor size, if the tumor is confined to the caudate lobe without involvement of the major hepatic vascular structures, and if the resection margin is adequate, because much more liver parenchyma can be preserved.

Operative Procedure

- Two tunnelings are required in this maneuver. One is retrohepatic tunneling on the IVC, and the other is caudal tunneling to the common trunk of the left and middle hepatic veins (Fig. 37-6). The former is a blind dissection, but can be performed safely by a strict positioning of the clamp on the anteromedian surface of the IVC between the right and middle hepatic veins. The latter can be performed safely by dividing the ligamentum venosum and dissecting behind the common trunk of the left and middle hepatic veins toward the space previously cleared between the right and middle hepatic veins.
- The transection plane of the right side of the caudate lobe is determined by the location of the tumor and the adequate resection margin, with both ends of the tape pulled up in the proper alignment for the transection plane to include the tumor. The hepatic parenchymal dissection begins from the caudal part of the caudate lobe, if necessary, using the Pringle maneuver, and continues cephalad along the tape. The parenchymal transection is conducted to reach the posterior surface of the right Glisson pedicle.
- Pulling up both ends of the tape plays an important role in lifting the liver. The posterior surface of the caudate lobe is dissected and separated from the IVC without compression or retraction of the other parts of the liver. The exposed short hepatic veins draining directly into the IVC are ligated and divided individually. Pulling both ends of the tape anteroinferiorly facilitates exposure of the deeper part of the parenchyma. The hepatic parenchymal dissection continues cephalad along the tape to the upper border of the caudate lobe.

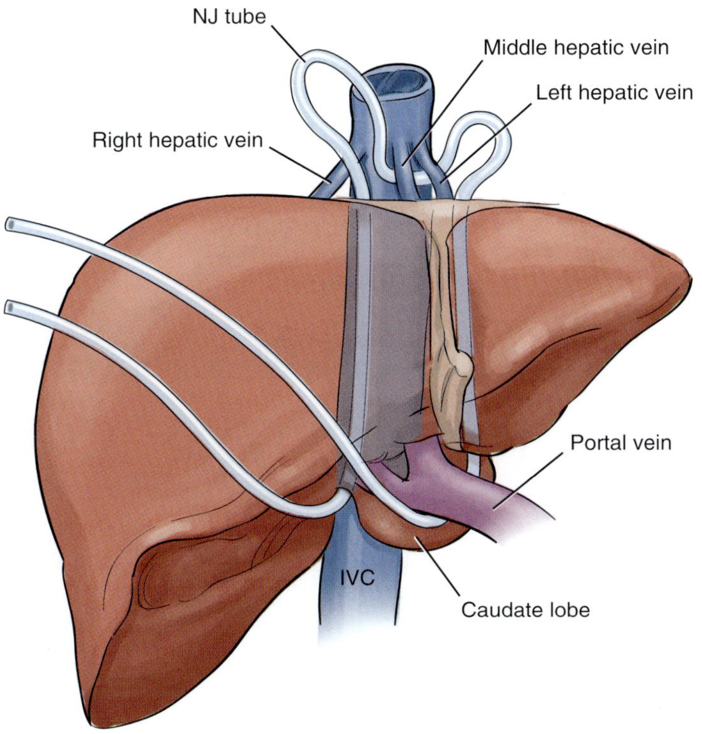

Figure 37-6. *IVC,* Inferior vena cava; *NJ,* nasojejunal. *(Redrawn from Kim SH, Park SJ, Lee SA, et al: Isolated caudate lobectomy using the hanging maneuver,* Surgery *139:847–850, 2006, Fig. 1, B.)*

- When the transection line meets the posterior surface of the hepatic hilum, all the branches of both the right and left Glisson pedicles that supply the caudate lobe are ligated and divided in the dorsal portion of the hepatic hilum. The parenchymal transection continues cephalad, directed toward the tape; when the transection meets the tape, the common trunk of the left and middle hepatic veins are seen.

Laparoscopic Caudate Lobectomy

Indication

- Although laparoscopic caudate lobectomy is complicated, it is feasible in select patients by the left approach, and especially in patients with small tumors located in the Spiegel lobe.

Operative Procedure

- For isolated caudate resection, the patient is placed in the 30-degree reverse Trendelenburg position with the legs apart. The surgeon stands between the legs of the patient.
- The first procedure is complete mobilization of the left hemiliver. The caudate lobe is then retracted ventrally from the IVC, and the small hepatic veins from the caudate lobe to the IVC are isolated and divided.
- After completing mobilization of the caudate lobe, parenchymal transection is performed while maintaining the medial traction of the caudate lobe. The small glissonian, vascular, or biliary tributaries to the caudate lobe, which are encountered during transection, are isolated, clipped, and divided (see Fig. 37-5).

VI. SPECIAL POSTOPERATIVE CARE

- Appropriate precautions are taken to minimize or prevent the occurrence of general postoperative complications such as pneumonia, thrombotic events, and cardiac events.
- Liver-specific complications, such as bile leak and liver failure, particularly in patients with cirrhosis and following massive (50% to 60%) resection, must be anticipated. In the event of liver impairment, particular attention is given to avoid hepatotoxic drugs, and the transplantation service should be engaged. Patients with cirrhosis are also at risk for developing portal vein thrombosis, and clinicians should be alerted if persistent abdominal pain occurs with elevation of liver function tests. A duplex ultrasound scan of the liver is obtained, and if thrombosis is detected, anticoagulation is started.
- If the international normalized ratio is elevated, the patient may require administration of vitamin K and/or fresh frozen plasma, depending on the degree of elevation and the associated drop in hematocrit.
- Epidural or patient-controlled analgesia is routinely instituted to ensure adequate pain control.

SUGGESTED READINGS

Chaib E, Ribeiro MA Jr, Silva Fde S, et al: Caudate lobectomy: tumor location, topographic classification, and technique using right- and left-sided approaches to the liver, *Am J Surg* 196:245–251, 2008.

Han HS, Cho JY, Yoon YS: Techniques for performing laparoscopic liver resection in various hepatic locations, *J Hepatobiliary Pancreat Surg* 16:427–432, 2009.

Kim SH, Park SJ, Lee SA, et al: Isolated caudate lobectomy using the hanging maneuver, *Surgery* 139:847–850, 2006.

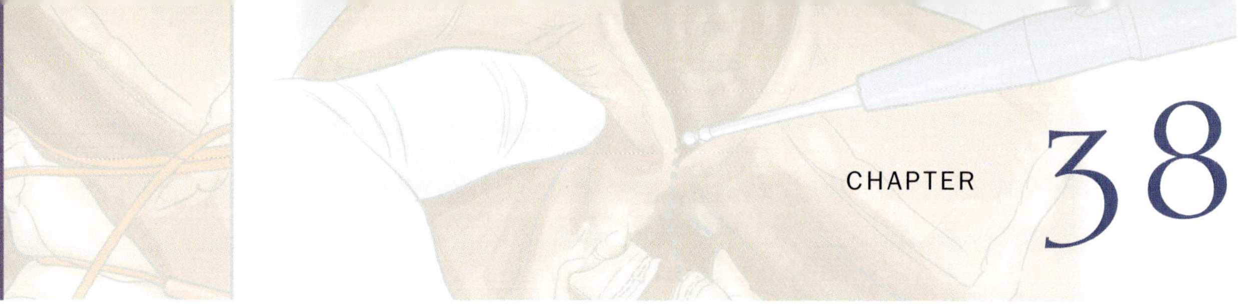

CHAPTER 38

Hepatectomy with Inferior Vena Cava Resection and Reconstruction

Kristin L. Mekeel, MD, FACS, and Alan W. Hemming, MD, MSc, FRCSC, FACS

I. SPECIAL PREOPERATIVE PREPARATION

- Patients who have aggressive local hepatic malignancy invading or encasing the inferior vena cava (IVC) but do not have extrahepatic or metastatic disease are candidates. Long-term survival should not be significantly different from that of similar patients with no involvement of the hepatic vasculature. This includes intrahepatic cholangiocarcinomas, sarcomas, hepatocellular carcinoma, and selected cases of metastatic colorectal cancer and benign diseases.
- Careful patient selection is paramount to ensure that the possible benefits outweigh the risks of surgery, and patients must be counseled appropriately. Patients with significant comorbidities, in particular renal insufficiency or cardiac dysfunction, are poor candidates for combined resection of the IVC and liver.
- Tumors involving or encasing the IVC may require total vascular isolation of the liver, controlling both inflow and outflow, and cold-perfusion in situ and ex vivo techniques may also be necessary. The availability of venovenous bypass and vascular grafts required should be assessed during the preoperative planning of the procedure.
- As with any hepatic malignancy, complete tumor staging is mandatory. This includes dedicated hepatic imaging as well as detection and staging of extrahepatic disease.
- Hepatic imaging should include both vascular and volumetric assessment, using computed tomography or magnetic resonance imaging. Assessment of the location of the liver tumor in relation to the vascular structures (Figs. 38-1 and 38-2) is critical to plan the course of the operation, including need for clamping, volume loading, cold perfusion, venovenous bypass, and vascular grafts. Major venous tributaries that may need to be preserved should be identified to provide outflow for the remnant liver.
- In standard liver resection, a liver remnant volume of 25% or more is acceptable for proceeding to resection. In cases where major vascular resection is being considered, a liver remnant of 40% is optimal because of the additional ischemic insult to the liver during resection and vascular reconstruction. If the liver remnant is less than 40%, preoperative portal vein embolization of the portion of the liver to be resected should be considered to increase the liver volume 4 to 6 weeks before resection.

II. OPERATIVE TECHNIQUE

Position

- The patient is placed in the supine position. Depending on choice of retractor, the patient's arms can be tucked or left out.
- For cases that require venovenous bypass or median sternotomy, the patient should be prepped from the groin bilaterally to the chest.

Anesthesia

- The anesthesia team should have experience in liver surgery. An internal jugular cordis should be placed in expectation of the conversion to a cannula for use in venovenous bypass. Monitoring of central venous pressure (CVP) is mandatory, and potentially Swan-Ganz catheter monitoring may be beneficial. Large-bore peripheral or rapid-inflow catheters should be placed for volume loading and blood product transfusion.

- During hepatic parenchymal transection without vascular exclusion, CVP should be kept at or below 5 cm H_2O blood loss. Volume loading will be necessary after transection but before caval clamping, to decrease the risk of significant hemodynamic instability.

Incision

- Various incisions are used and generally involve some variation of a bilateral subcostal incision with or without a midline extension. Alternatively, a midline incision with a right extension parallel to the costal margin (hockey stick incision) can be used (Fig. 38-3). The midline incision can be extended to a sternotomy to improve access to the suprahepatic IVC.

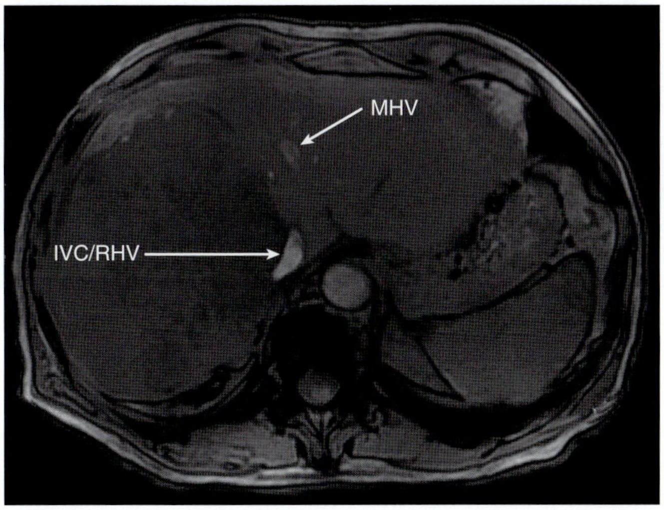

Figure 38-1. *IVC,* Inferior vena cava; *MHV,* middle hepatic vein; *RHV,* right hepatic vein.

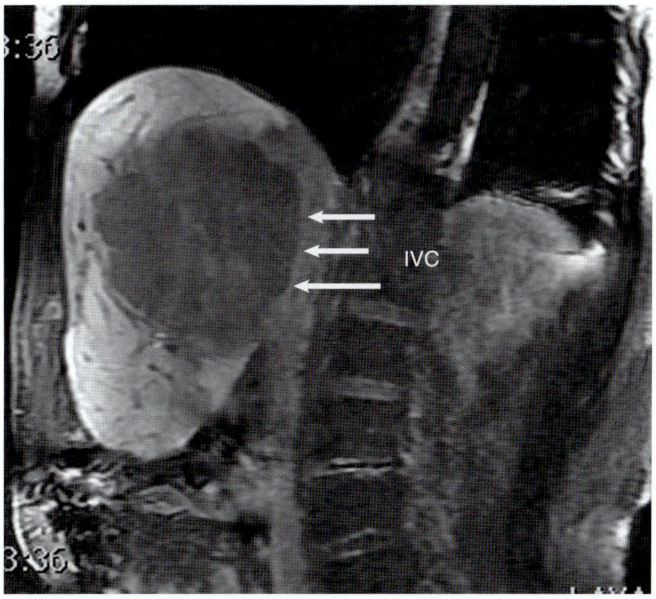

Figure 38-2. *IVC,* Inferior vena cava.

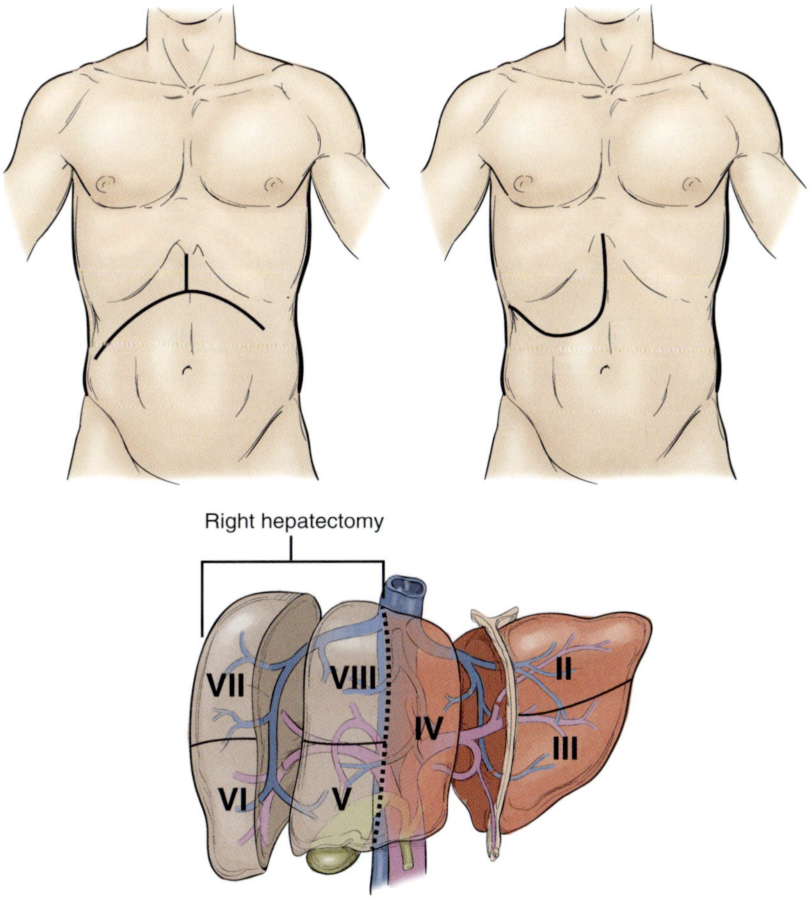

Figure 38-3.

Main Dissection

Initial dissection

- The abdomen must be assessed for extrahepatic disease that would preclude resection, including lymph node metastases.
- The liver is mobilized by dividing the right and left triangular ligaments as well as the gastrohepatic omentum. Care must be taken to identify and preserve replaced hepatic arterial inflow to the planned liver remnant.
- Intraoperative ultrasound should be used to stage and reassess tumor size and relationship to the major vascular structures. Resectability and need for vascular grafts can be determined at this time.
- The liver is mobilized as much as possible off of the IVC without broaching tumor planes.
- The portal structures to the side of the liver to be resected are divided either individually and extrahepatically in the porta hepatis, or en bloc via an extra-glissonian approach (Fig. 38-4, *inset*).
- The hepatic parenchyma is divided as much as possible toward the IVC under low-CVP conditions (see Fig. 38-4). If possible, the entire hepatic parenchyma is divided before the placement of clamps on the IVC.

Techniques for Vascular Control

- In many cases when only a small portion of the vena cava is involved, a side-biting vascular clamp may be used without interruption of the venous return (Fig. 38-5).
- If clamps can be placed above and below the area of tumor involvement inferior to the hepatic vein takeoff , then inflow occlusion is not necessary, and the liver can continue to be perfused (Fig. 38-6). The tumor can be removed en bloc with the liver and IVC, exposing the vena cava for reconstruction.

Total Vascular Isolation

Indications

- Indications for total vascular isolation (TVI) include resection of tumors involving the retrohepatic IVC or hepatic veins at the level of the hepatic veins as they enter the IVC. TVI allows control over the inflow (portal vein and hepatic artery) and outflow (suprahepatic and infrahepatic IVC) of the liver and provides proximal and distal control of the area of the IVC around the hepatic veins to allow resection and reconstruction (Fig. 38-7). Control of the IVC alone in this area does not stop blood flow through the liver, and portal venous and hepatic arterial inflow control is also required.

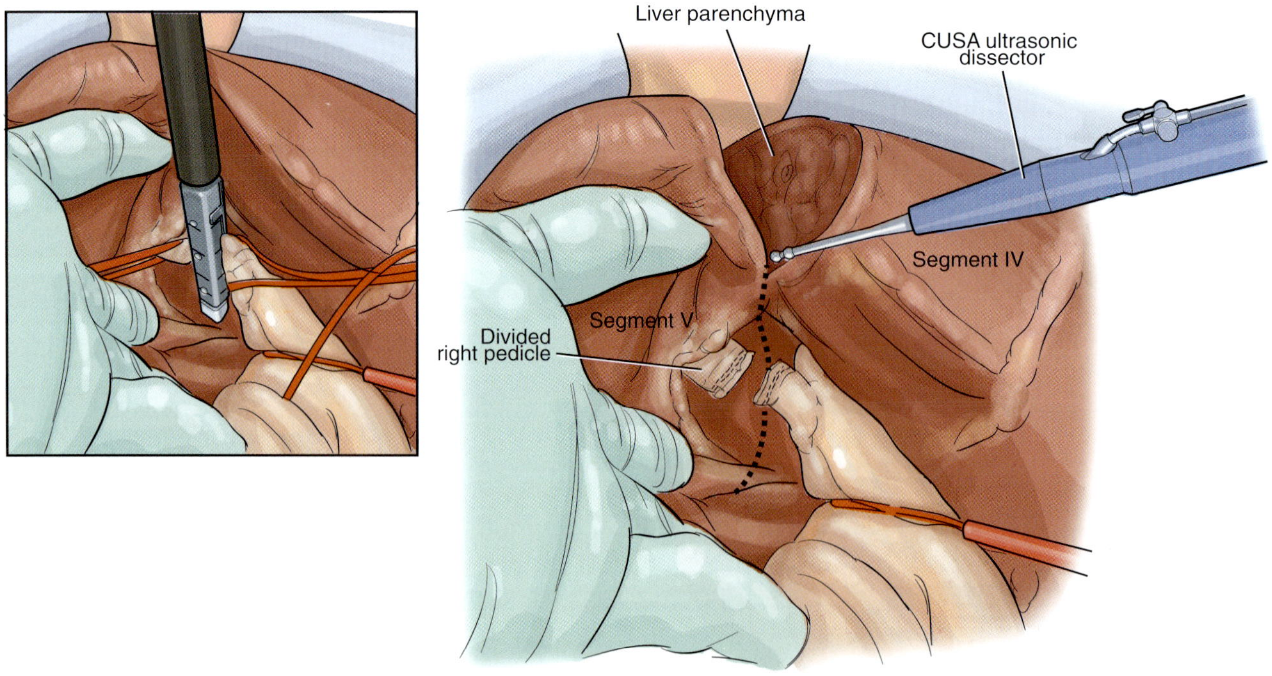

Figure 38-4. *CUSA*, Cavitron Ultrasonic Surgical Aspirator (Tyco Healthcare, Mansfield, Mass.)

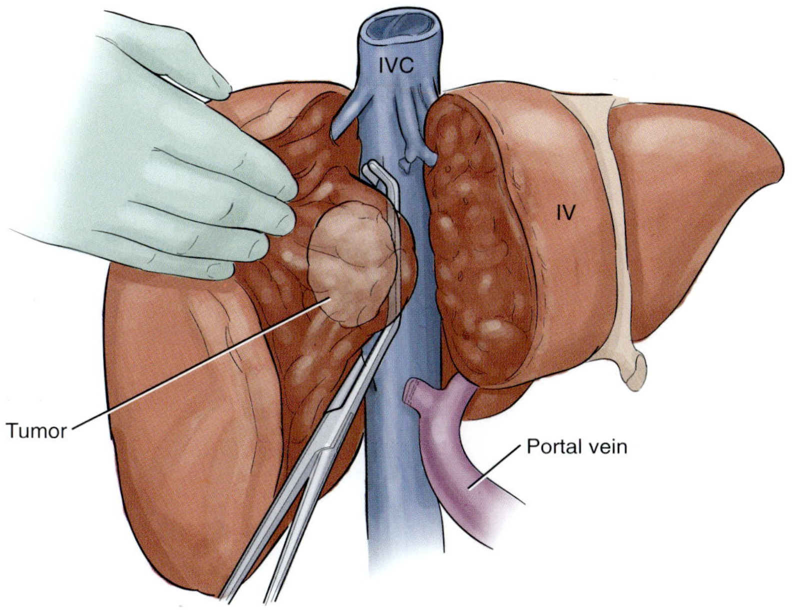

Figure 38-5. *IVC,* Inferior vena cava.

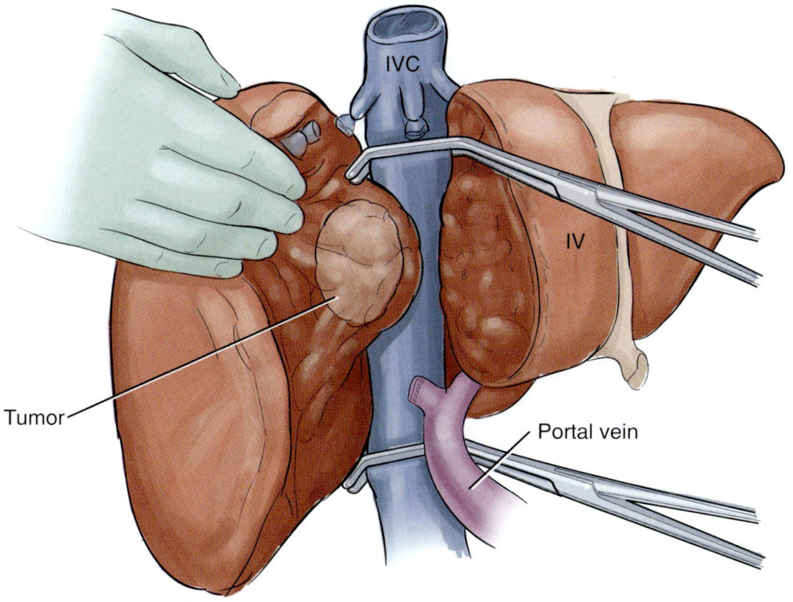

Figure 38-6. *IVC,* Inferior vena cava.

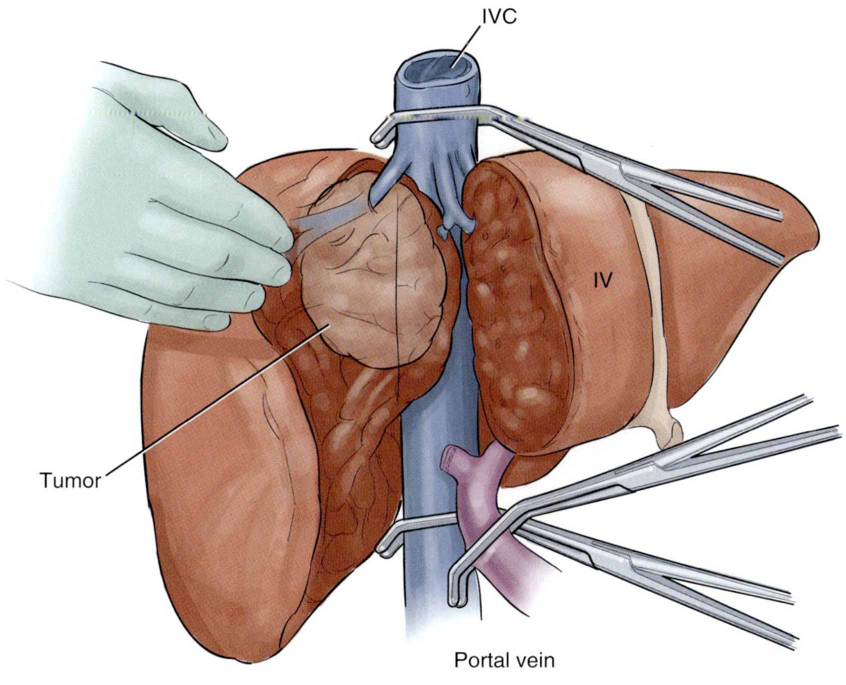

Figure 38-7. *IVC,* Inferior vena cava.

Technique

- A substantial portion or all of parenchymal transection and mobilization of the liver from the vena cava can be completed before instituting total vascular isolation (Fig. 38-8).
- After parenchymal transection is complete, inflow occlusion, if used during hepatic parenchymal transection, can be released, and the patient should be volume loaded.
- Clamps are placed in the following order: on the infrahepatic vena cava, portal vein, hepatic artery (or both of the latter together), and suprahepatic vena cava. Hemodynamic stability is assessed before resecting the IVC. If the patient is unable to tolerate TVI, then venovenous bypass will be required. The majority of patients will tolerate TVI with gentle volume loading. The vena cava is resected en bloc with the tumor (Fig. 38-9, *A* and *B*) and reconstructed as outlined later.

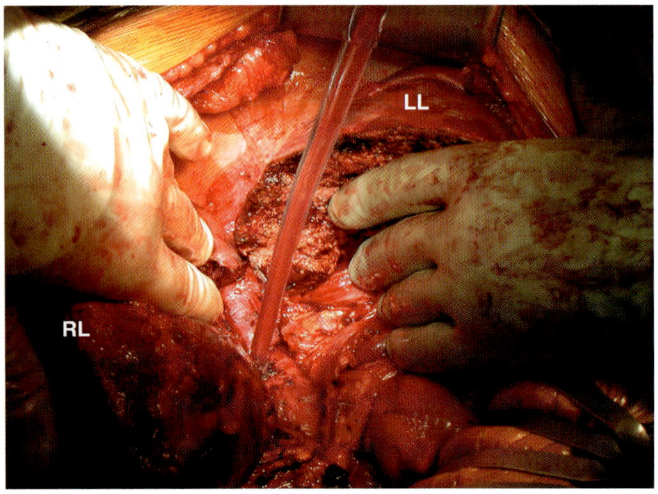

Figure 38-8. *LL,* Left lobe; *RL,* right lobe.

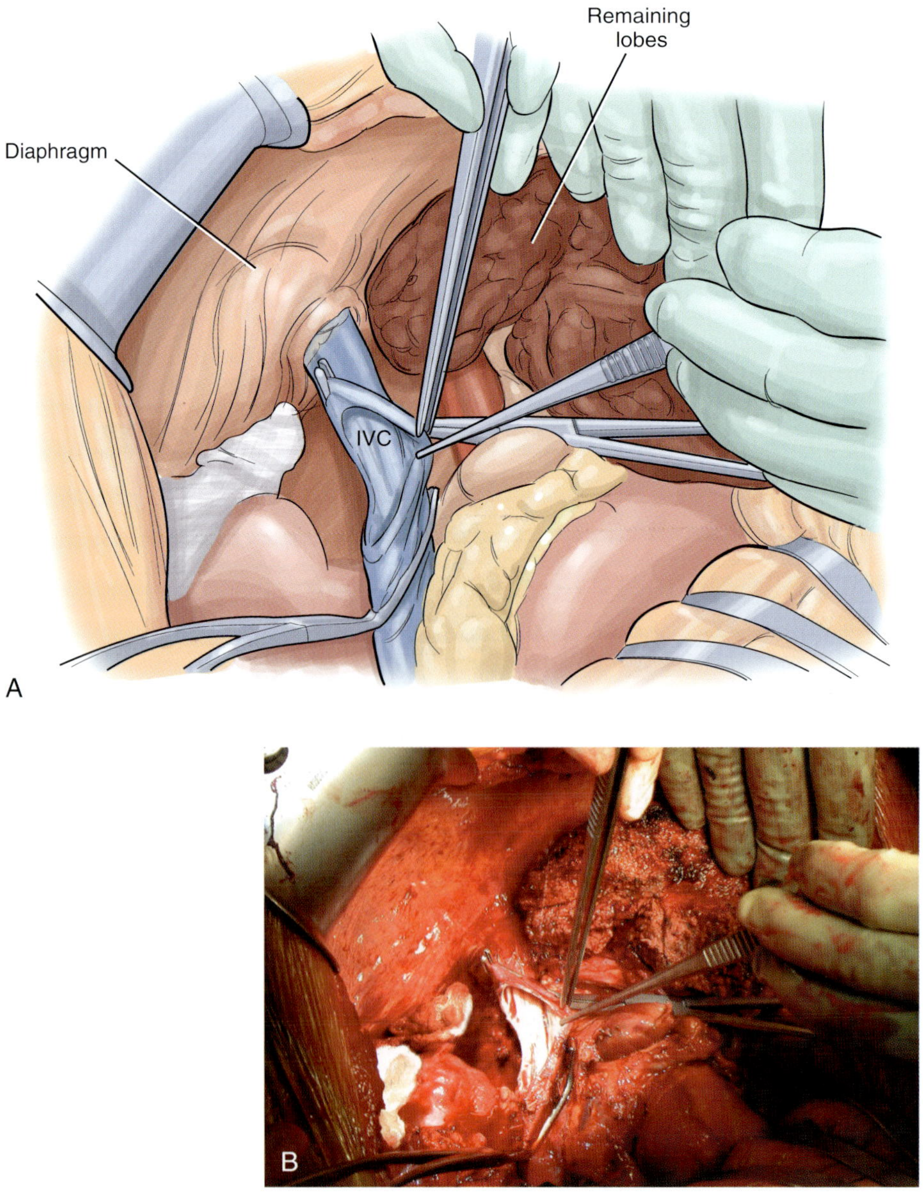

Figure 38-9. *IVC,* Inferior vena cava.

- The infrahepatic and suprahepatic vena caval clamps are released first, to control any bleeding from the vena caval anastomosis and allow assessment of bleeding from the cut surface of the liver. The portal and hepatic arterial clamps are removed.

Techniques for Reconstruction

- *Primary repair:* if only a small portion of the caval wall is involved and will be narrowed by less than 50%, it can be resected and repaired primarily with 4-0 Prolene suture.
- *Patch:* if the defect is larger than can be repaired primarily, a patch of autologous vein, bovine pericardium, or Gore-Tex can be used. Hepatic veins can be patched or reconstructed with autologous vein. Saphenous vein, superficial femoral vein, internal jugular vein, left renal vein, and cryopreserved vein grafts all have been used. Segments of uninvolved hepatic vein from the side of the liver resected can be salvaged as well.
- *Interposition graft:* A ringed 20-mm Gore-Tex tube graft is used to replace the segment of retrohepatic IVC, sewn using a running 3-0 or 4-0 Prolene suture (Figs. 38-10, 38-11, and 38-12).

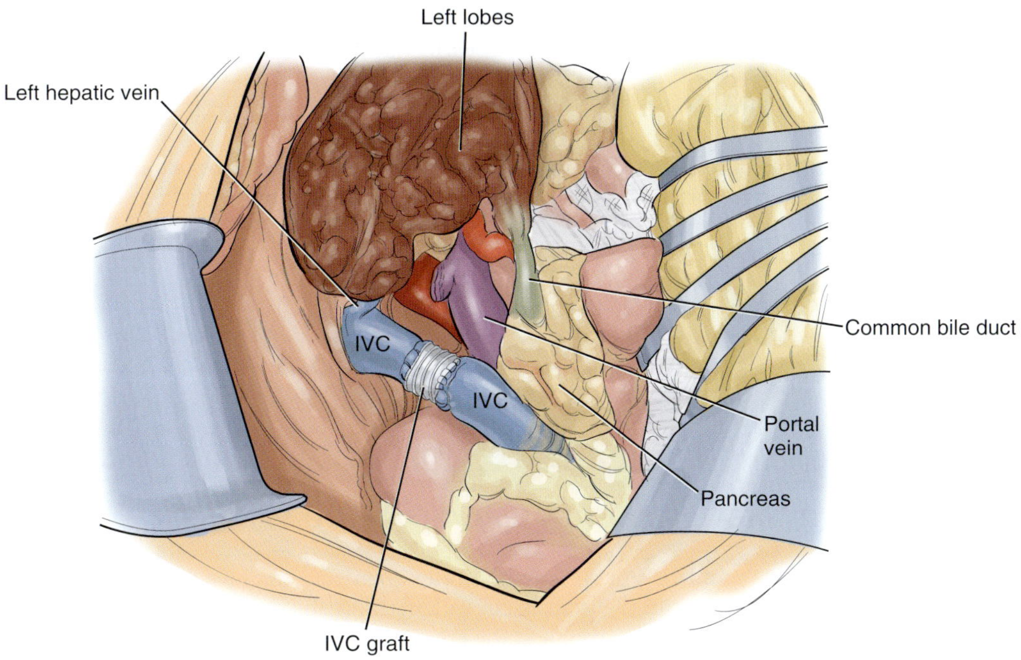

Figure 38-10. *IVC,* Inferior vena cava.

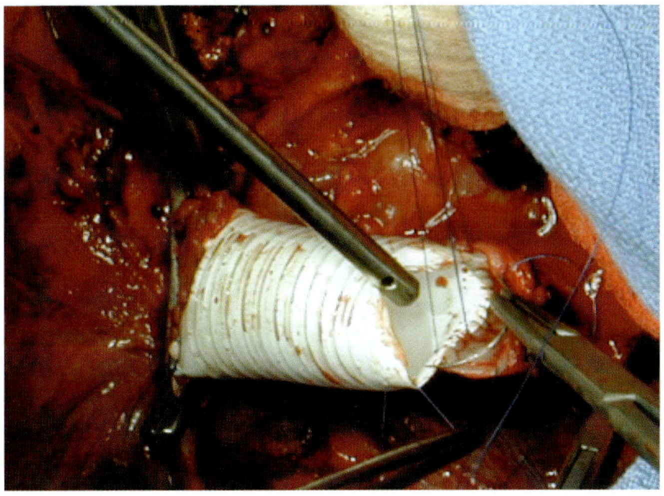

Figure 38-11.

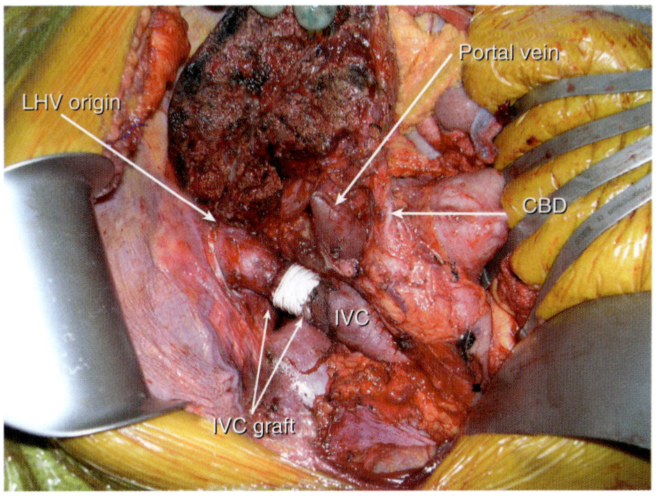

Figure 38-12. *CBD,* Common bile duct; *IVC,* inferior vena cava; *LHV,* left hepatic vein.

Advanced Caval Resection Techniques

Cold Perfusion

- In situ hypothermic perfusion describes the cold perfusion of the liver through the portal vein, and resection continues through standard techniques. The suprahepatic IVC can also be divided in the so-called ante situm procedure, rotating the liver forward to allow access to the retrohepatic vena cava and hepatic vein confluence.
- Indications include single hepatic vein or IVC reconstruction that would require more than 1 hour of total vascular isolation, or in an injured/marginal liver that may require hypothermic perfusion of the liver to allow subsequent complex hepatic resection and vascular reconstruction.

Technique

- As discussed previously, the majority of parenchymal transections can be performed without inflow occlusion, and total vascular isolation is applied to divide and reconstruct the vascular structures only.
- Portal vein dissection is carried into the hilum, past the bifurcation, and the cannula is placed into the ipsilateral portal vein of the side to be resected but directed into the contralateral portal vein (it can be placed in the main portal vein, which necessitates repair afterward).
- Volume load and clamps are placed on the infrahepatic vena cava in the following order: portal vein, hepatic artery, and suprahepatic vena cava.
- A venotomy is made in the vena cava, and cold perfusion is commenced with one of the standard organ preservation solutions (University of Wisconsin [UW] or histidine-tryptophan-ketoglutarate [HTK]). The IVC is then resected with the tumor. Reconstruction (outlined previously) can then be completed in a bloodless field with less time pressure than when normothermic.
- Before anastomotic completion, the liver is flushed with cold 5% albumin, and then portal and hepatic arterial flow is reestablished.
- The portal cannula is then removed, and the defect and the IVC venotomy (if separate from the resection site) are closed.
- The suprahepatic clamp is removed first to assess the integrity of the venous reconstruction and to stop any surface bleeding. Portal and hepatic arterial flow is then reestablished, and the patient is decannulated.

Closure

- If a Gore-Tex tube graft has been used, the omentum is mobilized and the graft wrapped with omentum.
- A Silastic drain connected to closed suction is placed in the resection bed. Fascia and skin are closed in standard fashion

III. ALTERNATIVE TECHNICAL APPROACHES (PRO/CON) AND PEARLS

- Ringed Gore-Tex grafts should be cut to length shorter than one might expect. The superior caval anastomosis is performed first, and the graft is cut to length. Grafts cut to fit the apparent defect will be too long once the retractors are removed and the area is not distracted and under tension. Parachuting the back wall down on the Gore-Tex graft allows the graft to be cut shorter than the apparent defect but still be performed without undue tension and match the defect appropriately.
- Cold perfusion can be with either HTK solution or UW solution. Although the author prefers to perform cold perfusion with as much of the liver divided as possible before perfusion, an alternative technique is to cold perfuse at the initiation of liver transection. This is particularly helpful for tumors that abut long stretches of major intrahepatic hepatic veins.
- For cold perfusion techniques, the liver can be flushed with a cold flush of 5% albumin or Ringer lactate before reperfusion, or warm flushed with blood to wash the preservation solution out of the liver and prevent hyperkalemia.
- When reimplanting hepatic veins into a ringed Gore-Tex graft, it is important to make a larger opening in the Gore-Tex than one might expect and to triangulate the anastomosis to prevent anastomotic stricture.
- During resection of any tumor that obstructs outflow and mandates one of the foregoing techniques, care must be taken not to injure the liver during the initial mobilization, as a small breach of the liver capsule in a congested liver can lead to massive bleeding. Large tumors of the right lobe may require an anterior approach, without mobilization of the right triangular ligament until after the division of the hepatic parenchyma.
- An alternative method can be performed in cases that have complex hepatic vein involvement without IVC involvement with tumor that preserves the IVC and uses a temporary portacaval shunt to decompress the gut during the anhepatic phase. This option avoids bypass, but it can be used only when there is no IVC involvement and when the IVC can be preserved in situ.

IV. SPECIAL POSTOPERATIVE CARE

- Postoperative care is similar for combined liver and caval resection whether performed warm or cold. Day 1 transaminases in the 200 to 1000 IU/L range are standard, but return to near normal by 1 week.
- Hyperbilirubinemia is common and seems to vary inversely with the size of the liver remnant. Hyperbilirubinemia alone is not a cause for concern if other markers of liver function are improving. An early sign that the autograft is functioning is the return of lactate levels to baseline in the first 12 to 24 hours after surgery.
- Maintenance of coagulation parameters, in particular prothrombin time or international normalized ratio (INR), suggests recovery of liver function. Fresh frozen plasma is given only if there is ongoing bleeding or if the INR rises above 2.0.
- Narcotic use must be minimized. Resecting 50% or more of the liver and inducing ischemic injury to the remnant reduces the ability to metabolize narcotics. A standard dose of narcotics may result in profound depression of the level of consciousness with subsequent disastrous sequelae such as aspiration.
- Hypophosphatemia can occur between postoperative days 1 and 3 as the liver regenerates. It may be profound and require constant intravenous replacement.
- With the volume loading that is required with caval clamping, it is common to have a patient mobilize the additional fluid in postoperative days 3-5. Careful volume management, including judicious use of diuretics, may be required.
- Without much evidence as to its effectiveness, we have used low-dose intravenous heparin (500 units/hr) perioperatively with long-term low-dose aspirin for patients with Gore-Tex grafts. This is maintained for life, although there are no data to confirm the need for long-term anticoagulation.

SUGGESTED READINGS

Azoulay D, Andreani P, Maggi U, et al: Combined liver resection and reconstruction of the supra-renal vena cava: the Paul Brousse experience, *Ann Surg* 244:80–88, 2006.

Hemming AW, Reed AI, Langham MR Jr, et al: Combined resection of the liver and inferior vena cava for hepatic malignancy, *Ann Surg* 239:712–719; discussion 719–721, 2004.

Sarmiento JM, Bower TC, Cherry KJ, et al: Is combined partial hepatectomy with segmental resection of the inferior vena cava justified for malignancy? *Arch Surg* 138:624–630, discussion 630–631, 2003.

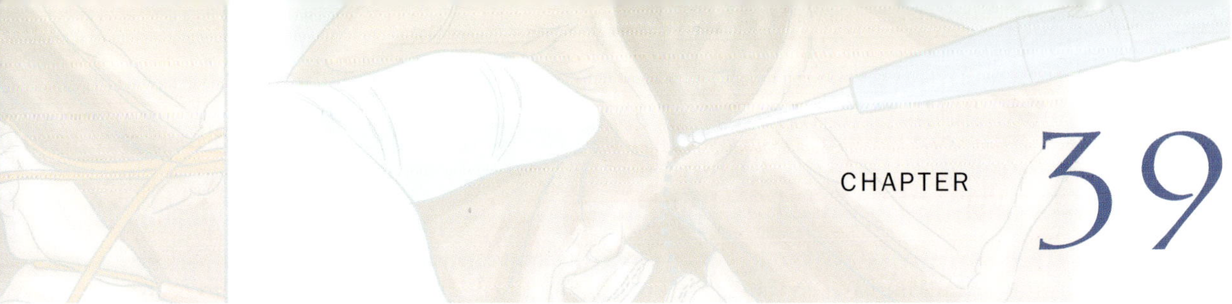

CHAPTER 39

Transverse Hepatectomy

Vijay P. Khatri, MBChB, FACS, and Ferenc Jakab, MD, PhD, DMSc

I. SPECIAL PREOPERATIVE PREPARATION

- Pretreatment radiologic imaging, particularly a four-phase liver computed tomography (CT) scan or a liver magnetic resonance imaging scan, provides valuable information regarding the extent of the primary or malignant disease and the presence of satellite lesions. Such imaging also allows the surgeon to judge the extent of the resection needed to achieve a negative margin resection while leaving a functional residual liver with intact vascular inflow and outflow. It is also important to assess whether there is direct involvement of the inferior vena cava and hepatic venous confluence that precludes resection without necessitating venous outflow resection and reconstruction (Figs. 39-1 and 39-2).
- Using an existing formula to calculate total liver volume and with the assistance of the three-dimensional CT scan, the functional residual liver volume can be calculated. If it is determined that the functional residual volume is inadequate to prevent postoperative hepatic failure, portal vein embolization is employed. At present portal vein embolization should be considered when a major hepatic resection is estimated to leave less than 25% of the functional residual volume in patients with a normal liver and less than 40% functional residual volume for those with compromised liver function (cirrhosis or postchemotherapy steatohepatitis).
- Preoperative discussion with the anesthesiologist ensures that a lower central venous pressure technique is employed. This preoperative discussion, in combination with inflow occlusion during parenchymal transection, results in significantly less hemorrhage and consequently reduced morbidity and mortality.
- In the case of suspected hepatocellular carcinoma, tissue diagnosis is not necessary when there is a history of cirrhosis or a hepatic lesion with an associated elevated alpha-fetoprotein level. This is also true for hepatic colorectal metastases which, given a history of a high-risk colorectal cancer and hypoattenuated liver lesions in the presence of an elevated carcinoembryonic antigen level, precludes the need for a tissue diagnosis.
- It is appropriate in the case of hepatic resection for metastatic disease to obtain a staging CT positron emission tomography scan to exclude extrahepatic disease, particularly in the case of colorectal metastases.
- For a patient with cirrhosis, a detailed history to determine the Childs-Pugh criteria and the Model for End-Stage Liver Disease (MELD) score is valuable in forming a preoperative judgment of mortality and morbidity.
- The main indication for transverse hepatectomy is the presence of hepatocellular carcinoma, gallbladder cancer, or colorectal metastases in segments IVB, V, or VI.

II. OPERATIVE TECHNIQUE

Position

- The patient is placed in the supine position. The patient undergoes anesthesia with endotracheal intubation. A central venous catheter is necessary to facilitate lower central venous pressure anesthesia. The patient's lower chest and abdomen are then prepped and draped in a sterile manner.

Incision

- A subcostal incision is made from the edge of the left costal margin extending one finger breadth along the right costal margin. If necessary, the incision can be extended obliquely along the sixth intercostal space to provide better exposure. Alternatively, a J-incision can be used (Fig. 39-3).

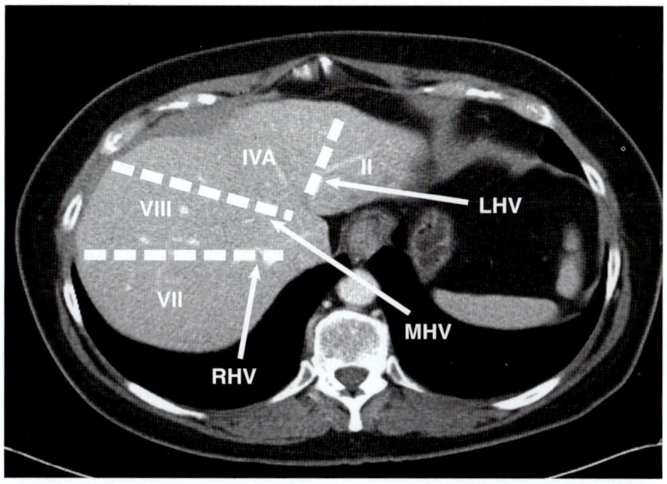

Figure 39-1. Cross-sectional image showing the right, middle, and left hepatic veins used to designate the Couinaud segmentation. *LHV,* Left hepatic vein; *MHV,* middle hepatic vein; *RHV,* right hepatic vein.

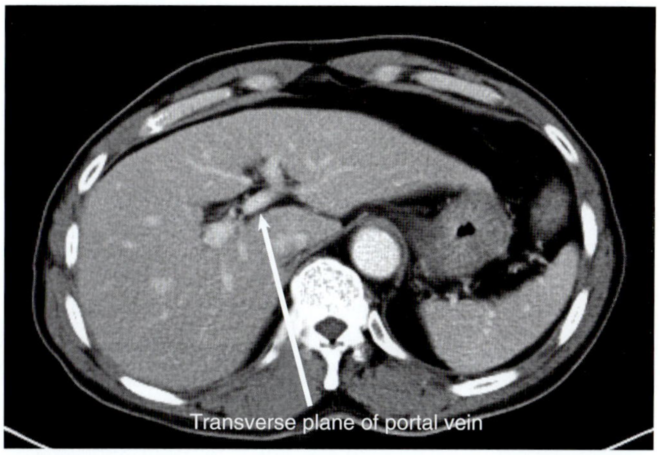

Figure 39-2. Cross-sectional computed tomography scan of the liver at the level of the portal vein bifurcation section.

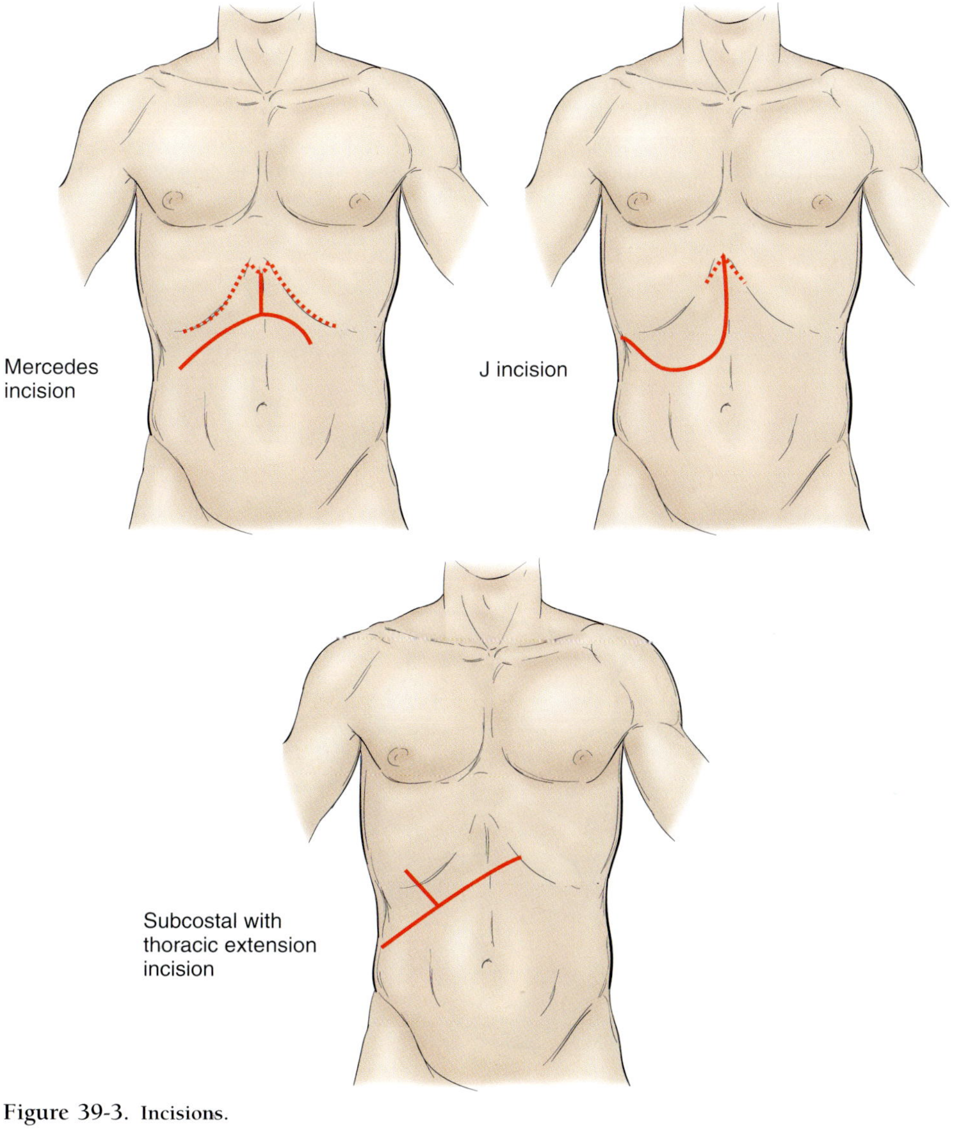

Figure 39-3. Incisions.

Main Dissection

- First the ligamentum teres is divided between clamps and ligated with 0-0 silk. The falciform ligament is then divided with electrocautery and separated from the attachments to the abdominal wall. This allows upper retraction of the costal margins using a Thompson retractor without risk of causing inadvertent capsule tear. Any additional adhesions to the liver are also carefully divided at this point with electrocautery to avoid any tears in the liver capsule during mobilization.
- Next, a thorough evaluation of the intraabdominal cavity is performed to exclude the presence of extrahepatic disease, with particular attention given to the peritoneal lining and lymph nodes in the hepatic portal. In the absence of extrahepatic disease, the liver is carefully evaluated with ultrasound scan to determine the relationship of the tumor to the major intrahepatic vasculature and also to exclude the presence of additional lesions that could alter the operative approach (Fig. 39-4).
- For a transverse hepatectomy, segments IVB, V, and VI are removed. To facilitate the resection, the right triangular ligament is divided, which allows rotation of the right liver medially to expose the inferior vena cava. If an inferior right hepatic vein is present, it is isolated, ligated in continuity with 2-0 silk, and divided. In addition, small multiple venous branches entering the inferior vena cava are also controlled with hemoclips and divided at this point.
- Using ultrasound scan, the proposed plane of parenchymal transection for the transverse hepatectomy is evaluated. A determination is made as to whether immobilization of the liver and the inferior vena cava is adequate to allow safe transection.
- Attention is directed toward the hilum, where the flimsy lesser omentum is divided and a vessel loop placed around the porta hepatis in the event inflow clamping is required (Fig. 39-5). If selective right liver inflow clamping is necessary, the right portal pedicle is also isolated.
- Next, the round ligament is followed toward the umbilical fissure, where the liver tissue between segments III and IV might need to be divided. On the right side of the umbilical fissure, the first pedicle encountered is for segment IVB, which is carefully isolated (Fig. 39-6). It can then be controlled with a vascular clamp to visualize the area of devascularization to ensure that it does supply segment IVB. This pedicle is then transected with an endovascular 2.0 linear stapler.
- The portal pedicles to segments V and VI are fairly deep and usually difficult to dissect from the hilum. They are approached in the traditional fashion of intraparenchymal isolation and division.

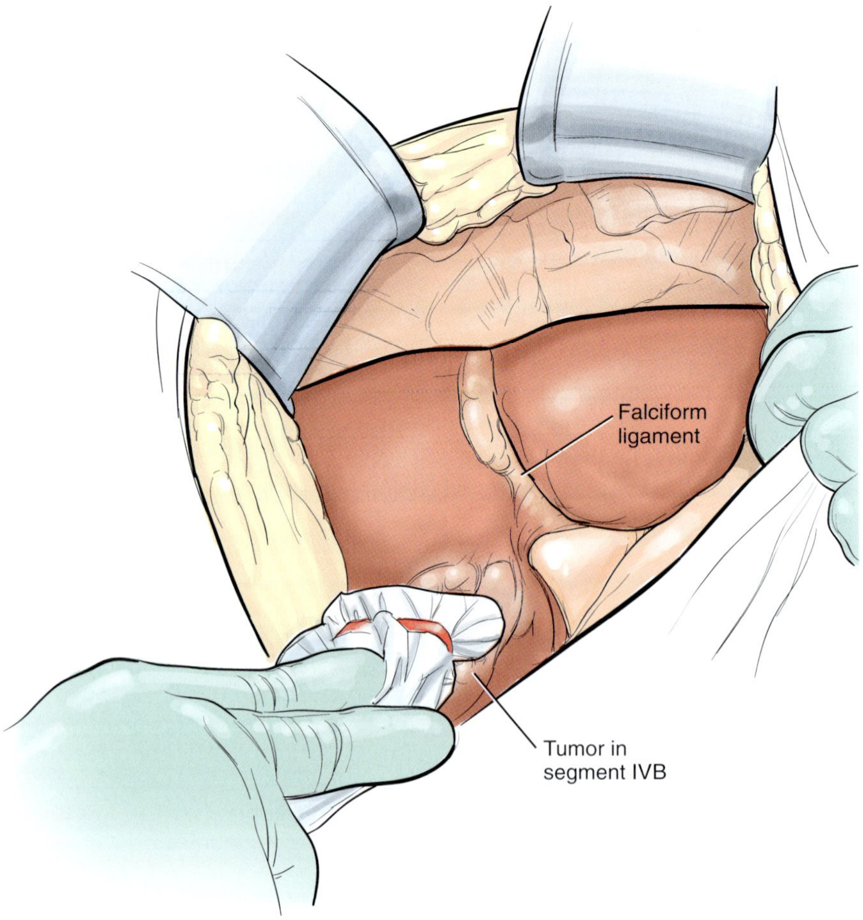

Figure 39-4.

- The transverse plane is identified with the ultrasound scan, further ensuring that there is an adequate margin. The proposed plane of transection is marked with electrocautery. With intermittent portal triad clamping, the liver parenchyma can be transected by kellyclassis. Branches of the middle and right hepatic veins (as previously identified by ultrasound scan) are controlled either by dividing and ligating with 2-0 silk or with the use of endovascular 2.0 linear staplers.
- If necessary, the portal triad can be clamped during the transection phase intermittently. The ablated liver tissue can then be divided with Kelly clamps. The portal pedicles to segments V and VI are isolated, and vessel loops are placed around them.

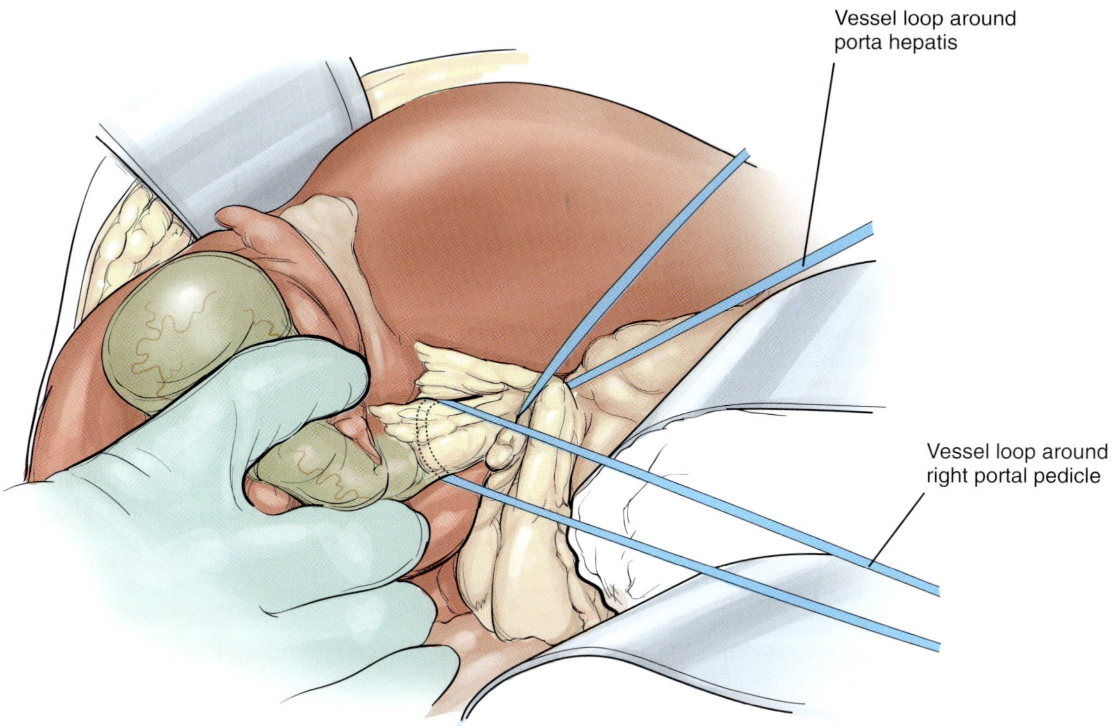

Figure 39-5.

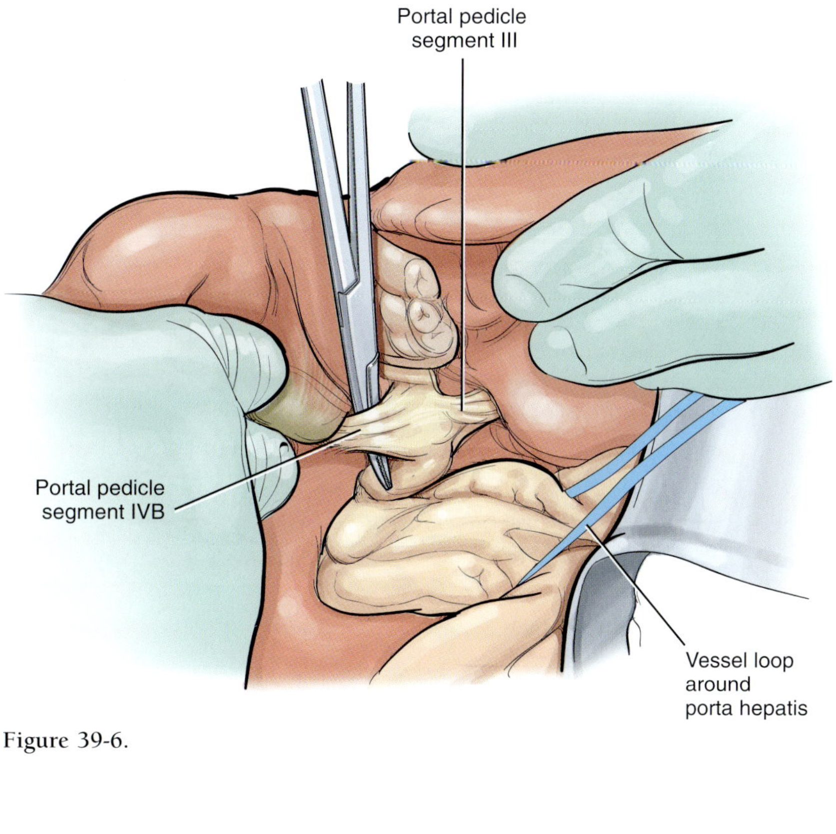

Figure 39-6.

- The portal pedicles to segments V and VI are then transected with a linear endovascular 2.5 stapler (Fig. 39-7).
- The remaining transverse plane is divided, and resection is completed by transecting segment IVB just at the right side of the falciform ligament. Care should be taken not to damage the ascending portion of the left portal vein, which can be identified with ultrasound.
- Once the transection plane is completely divided, the liver surface can be slowly coagulated. Any large bleeding veins can be controlled with 3-0 or 4-0 monofilament suture. The surface is inspected for bile leak, which is hemoclipped or suture ligated with 4-0 polypropylene. The surface can be treated with Bioglue.
- Ultrasound can be used to confirm adequate flow to the remaining liver segments.
- The right upper quadrant is irrigated, and a Jackson-Pratt drain is placed.

Closure

- Anterior abdominal wall muscles are approximated in layers with 1-0 monofilament absorbable suture. The skin is approximated with staples.

III. ALTERNATIVE TECHNICAL APPROACHES (PRO/CON) AND PEARLS

- Various different incisions can be used, including a "Mercedes incision" (a rooftop with a midline extension) and a J-shaped incision.
- With ultrasound guidance, the transverse plane is sequentially ablated with use of the InLine bipolar radiofrequency device (Resect Medical Inc., Fremont, Calif.) (Fig. 39-8). This greatly facilitates parenchymal division by minimizing blood loss.
- New energy devices are being used for hepatic resection when the parenchymal transection must proceed without full inflow control. These include the 10-mm LigaSure. Often in areas where it is difficult to obtain exposure, the vessels can be controlled with the linear endovascular stapler.

IV. SPECIAL POSTOPERATIVE CARE

- Appropriate precautions are taken to minimize or prevent the occurrence of general postoperative complications such as pneumonia, and thrombotic and cardiac events.

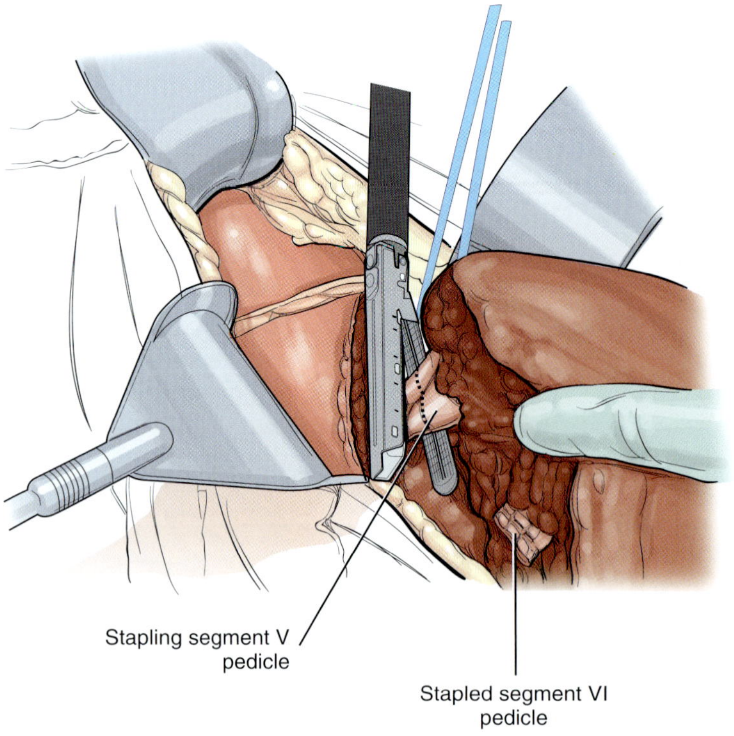

Figure 39-7.

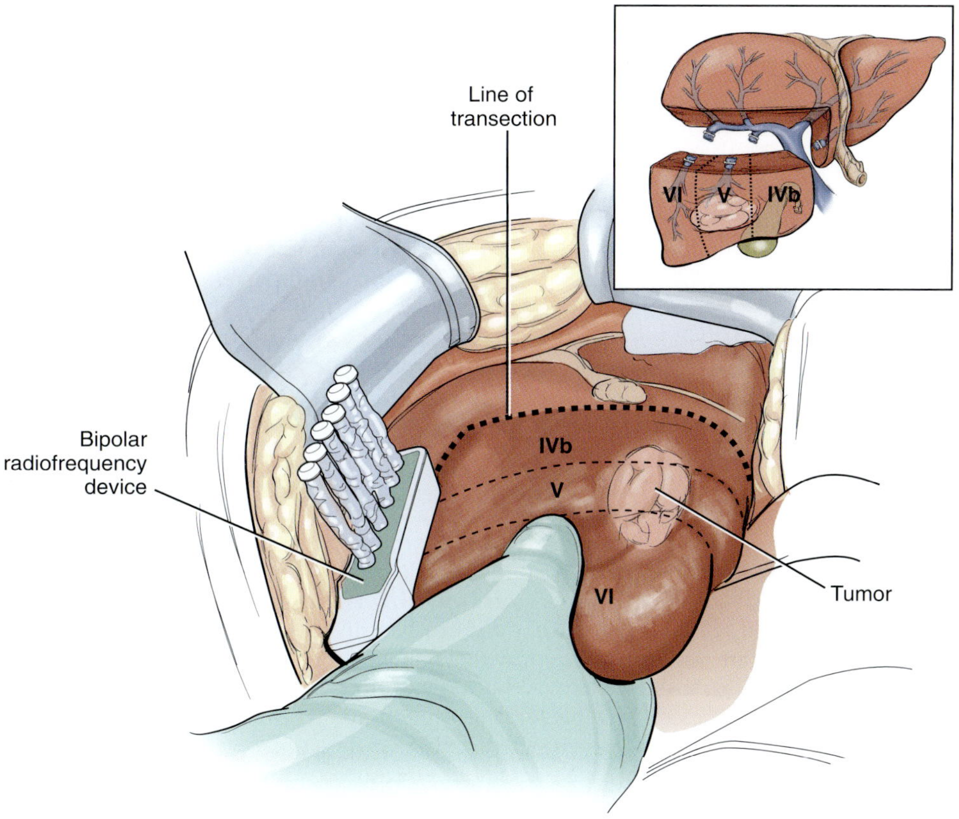

Figure 39-8.

- Liver-specific complications such as bile leak and liver failure must be anticipated, particularly in patients with cirrhosis and following massive (50% to 60%) resection. In the event of liver impairment, particular attention is given to avoid hepatotoxic drugs, and the transplantation service is contacted. Patients with cirrhosis are also at risk for developing portal vein thrombosis, and clinicians should be alerted if persistent abdominal pain occurs with elevation of liver function tests. A duplex ultrasound scan of the liver is obtained, and if thrombosis is detected, anticoagulation is started.
- If the international normalized ratio (INR) is elevated, the patient may require administration of vitamin K and/or fresh frozen plasma, depending on the degree of INR elevation and the associated drop in hematocrit.
- Epidural or patient-controlled analgesia is routinely instituted to ensure adequate pain control.

SUGGESTED READINGS

Jakab F, Brçzda E: Transverse hepatectomy in surgical treatment of gallbladder carcinoma, *Acta Chir Hung* 36:143–144, 1997.
Johnson LB, Kuo PC, Plotkin JS: Transverse hepatectomy for symptomatic polycystic liver disease, *Liver* 19:526–528, 1999.
Sugarbaker PH: En bloc resection of hepatic segments 4B, 5 and 6 by transverse hepatectomy, *Surg Gynecol Obstet* 170:250–252, 1990.

CHAPTER 40

Mesohepatectomy

Vijay P. Khatri, MBChB, FACS, and Mark S. Roh, MD, MMM

I. SPECIAL PREOPERATIVE PREPARATION

- Pretreatment radiologic imaging, particularly a four-phase liver computed tomography (CT) scan or a liver magnetic resonance imaging scan, provides valuable information regarding the extent of the primary or malignant disease. It also allows the surgeon to judge the extent of the resection needed to achieve a negative margin resection while leaving a functional residual liver with intact vascular inflow and outflow. It is also important to assess whether there is direct involvement of the inferior vena cava and hepatic venous confluence that would preclude resection without necessitating venous out-flow resection and reconstruction (Figs. 40-1 and 40-2).
- Using an existing formula to calculate total liver volume and with the assistance of the three-dimensional CT scan, the functional residual liver volume is calculated. If the functional residual volume is inadequate to prevent postoperative hepatic failure, portal vein embolization is employed. At present, portal vein embolization should be considered when a major hepatic resection is estimated to leave less than 25% of the functional residual volume in patients with normal liver and less than 40% functional residual volume for those with compromised liver function.
- Preoperative discussion with the anesthesiologist ensures that a lower central venous pressure technique is employed. The preop discussion, in combination with portal pedicle occlusion during parenchymal transection, results in significantly less hemorrhage and consequently reduced morbidity and mortality.
- In the case of suspected hepatocellular carcinoma, tissue diagnosis is not necessary with a history of cirrhosis or a hepatic lesion with an associated elevated alpha-fetoprotein level. This is also true for hepatic colorectal metastases which, in a patient with a history of high-risk colorectal cancer and hypoattenuated liver lesions in the presence of an elevated carcinoembryonic antigen level, would preclude the need for a tissue diagnosis.
- It is appropriate in the case of hepatic resection for metastatic disease to obtain a staging CT/positron emission tomography scan to exclude extrahepatic disease, particularly in the case of colorectal metastases.
- For patients with cirrhosis, a detailed evaluation to determine the Childs-Pugh criteria and the Model for End-Stage Liver Disease (MELD) score is valuable in determining preoperative mortality and morbidity.

II. OPERATIVE TECHNIQUE

Position

- The patient is placed in the supine position. The patient undergoes anesthesia with endotracheal intubation. A central venous catheter is necessary to facilitate lower central venous pressure anesthesia. The patient's lower chest and abdomen are then prepped and draped in a sterile manner.

Incision

- A subcostal incision is made from the edge of the left costal margin extending one finger breadth along the right costal margin (Fig. 40-3). If necessary, the incision can be extended obliquely along the sixth intercostal space to provide better exposure. Other common incisions used are the bilateral subcostal incision with a midline extension (Mercedes incision) or the J-shaped incision (see Fig. 40-3).

Main Dissection

- First the ligamentum teres is divided between clamps and ligated with 0-0 silk. The falciform ligament is then divided with electrocautery and separated from the attachments to the abdominal wall. This allows upper retraction of the costal margins using a Thompson retractor without risk of causing

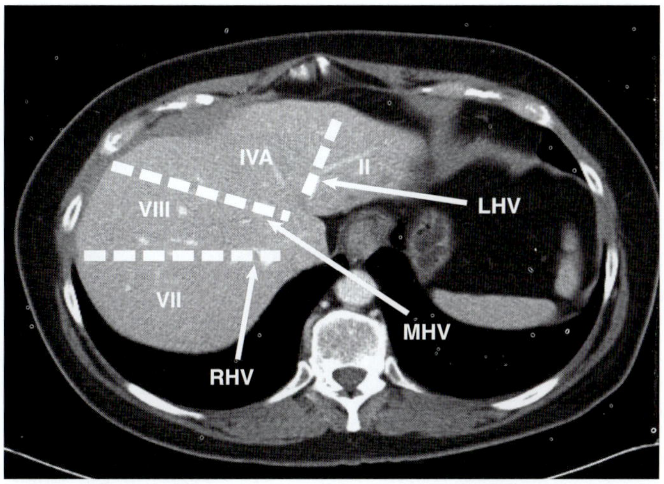

Figure 40-1. Cross-sectional image showing the right (*RHV*), middle (*MHV*), and left (*LHV*) hepatic veins used to designate the Couinaud segmentation.

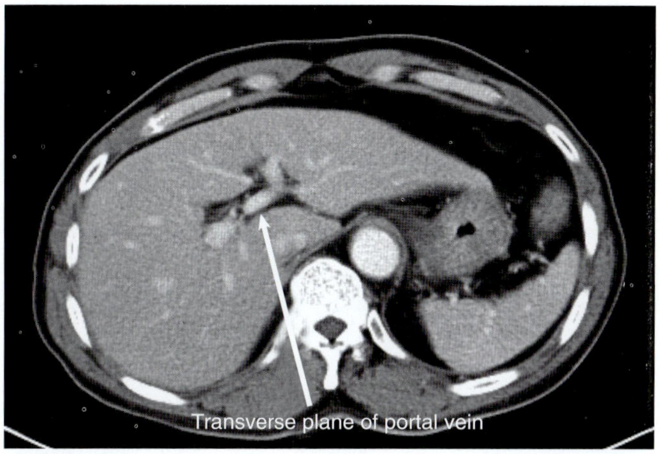

Figure 40-2. Cross-sectional computed tomography scan of liver at the level of the portal vein bifurcation section.

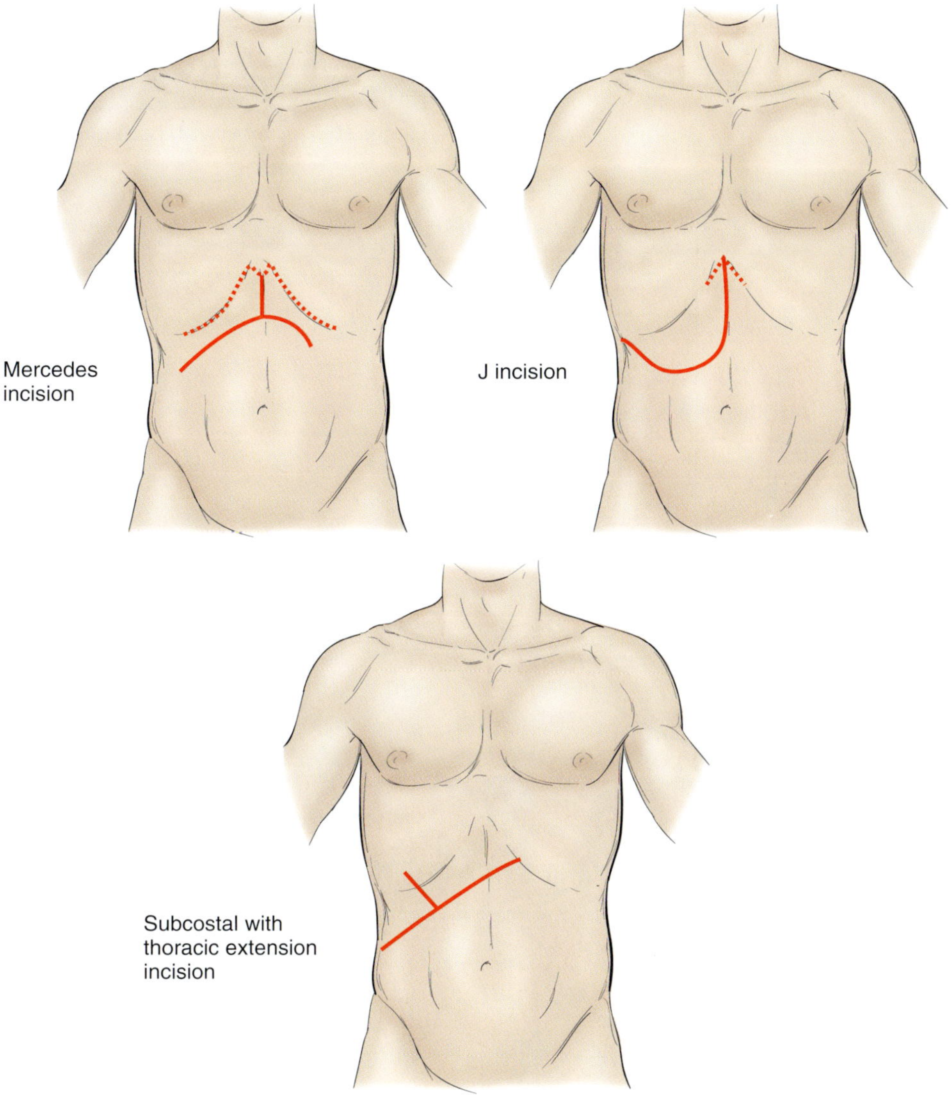

Figure 40-3.

inadvertent capsule tear (Fig. 40-4). Any additional adhesions to the liver are also carefully divided at this point with electrocautery to avoid any tears in the liver capsule during mobilization.

- Next, a thorough evaluation of the intraabdominal cavity is performed to exclude the presence of extrahepatic disease, with particular attention paid to the peritoneal lining and lymph nodes in the hepatic portal. In the absence of extrahepatic disease, the liver is carefully evaluated with ultrasound scan to determine the relationship of the tumor to the major intrahepatic vasculature and to exclude the presence of additional lesions that would alter the operative approach (Fig. 40-5).
- For mesohepatectomy, segments IV, V, and VIII are removed (Fig. 40-6). First the falciform ligament is divided, and this division proceeds superiorly, where its two leaves are divided with electrocautery to begin exposing the inferior vena cava. The liver is further mobilized by dividing the right and left triangular ligament.
- The dense fibrinous tissue surrounding the suprahepatic cava is carefully divided to expose the middle hepatic vein and its junction with the left hepatic vein.

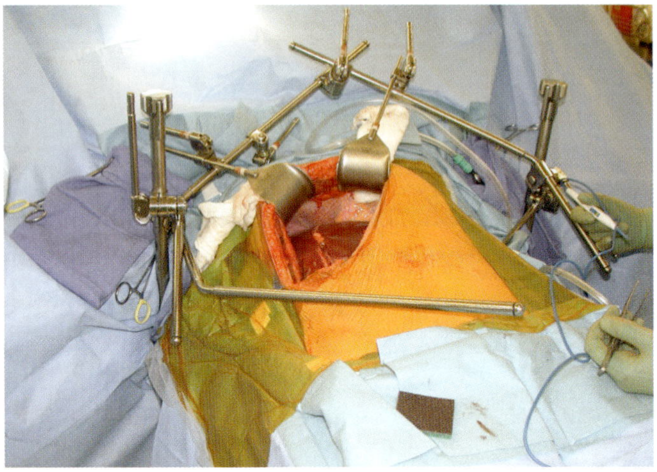

Figure 40-4.

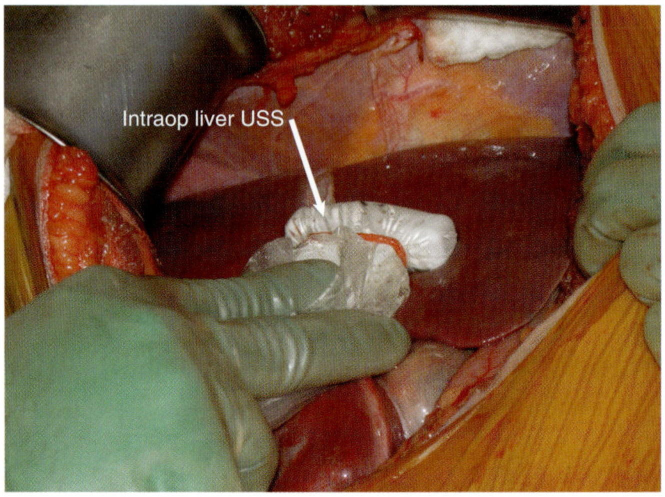

Figure 40-5. *Intraop liver USS,* Intraoperative liver ultrasound scan.

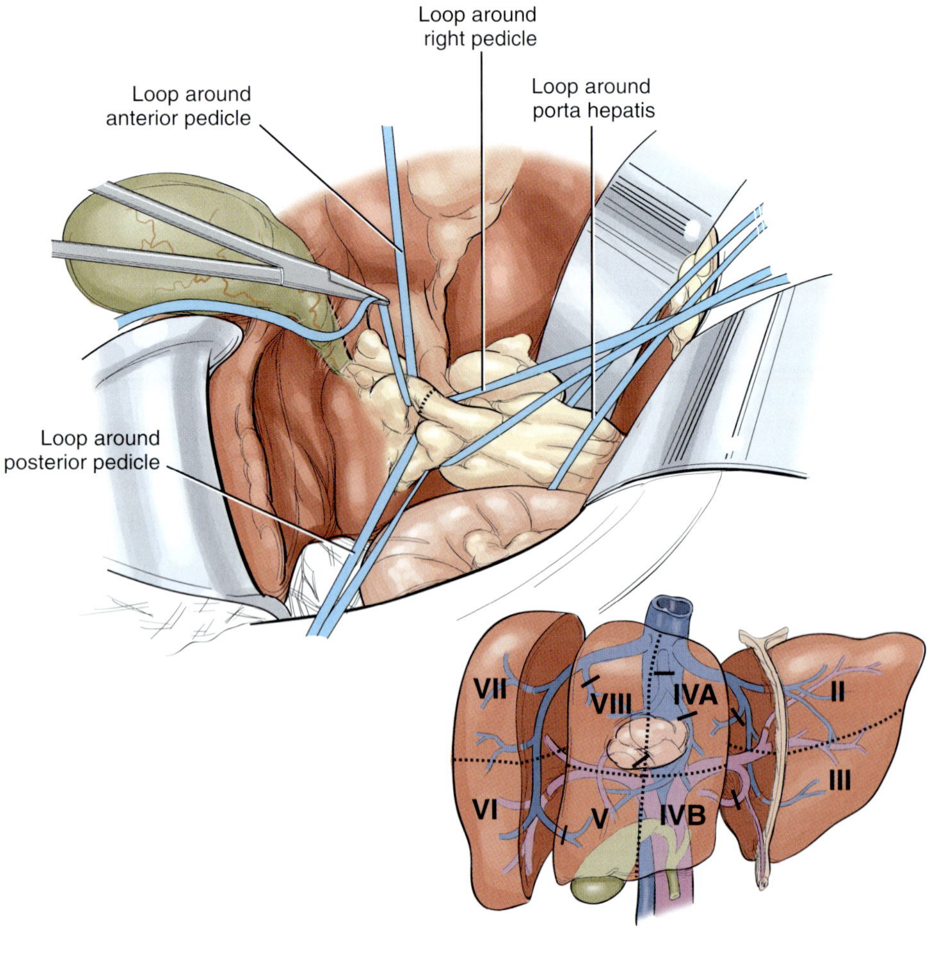

Figure 40-6. Bars mark transected vessels.

- Attention is directed toward the hilum for the hilar dissection; the incisions necessary to perform glissonian pedicle dissection are shown in Figure 40-7. The round ligament is followed to the umbilical fissure, where the liver tissue between segment III and IV might need to be divided. On the right side of the umbilical fissure, the first pedicle encountered is for segment IVB, which is carefully isolated (Fig. 40-8). It is then controlled by a vascular clamp to visualize the area of devascularization to ensure

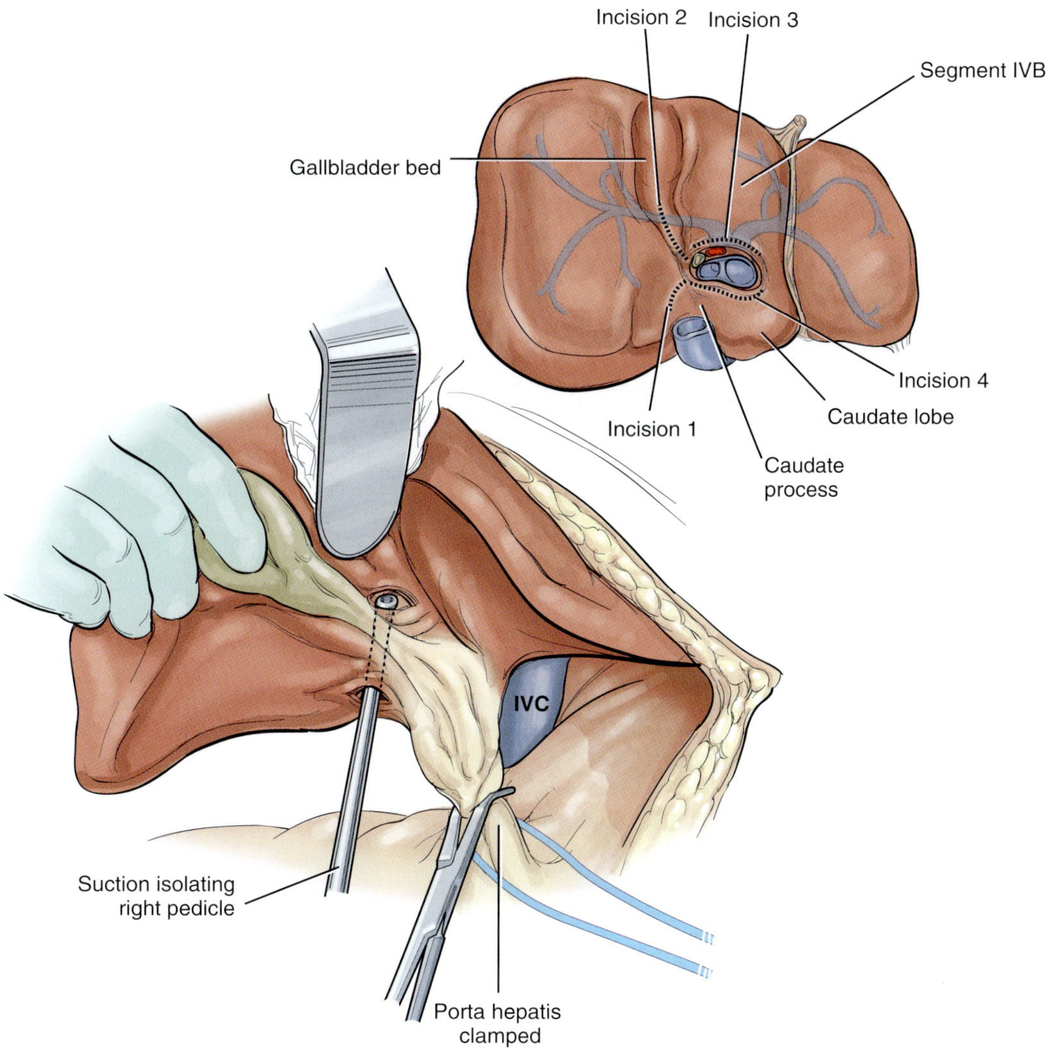

Figure 40-7. *IVC,* Inferior vena cava.

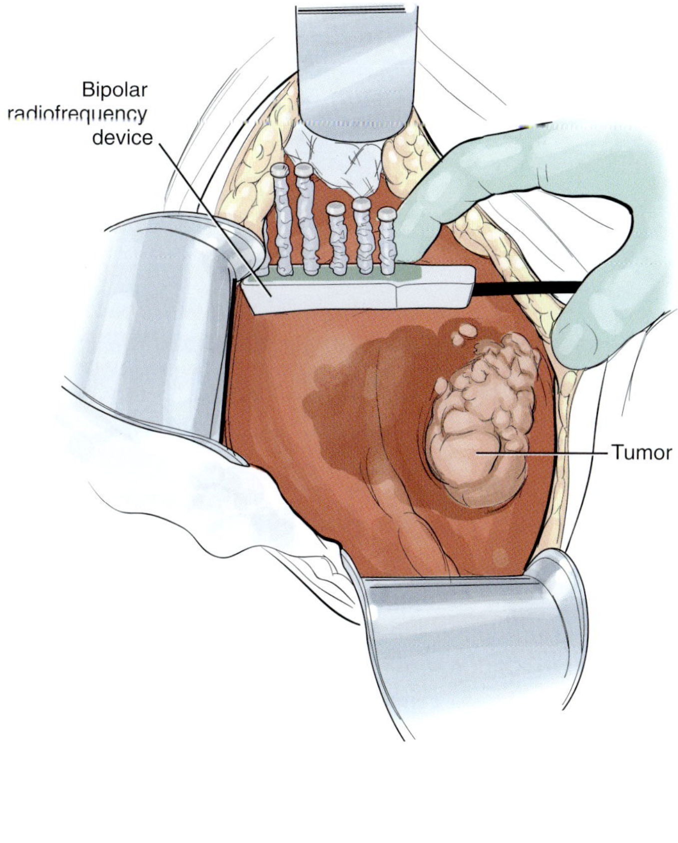

Figure 40-8.

that it supplies segment IVB. This pedicle is then transected with an endovascular 2.0 linear stapler. In a similar fashion, the portal pedicle to segment IVA is isolated and transected with an endovascular 2.0 linear stapler.

- Attention is directed to the hilum, where the lesser omentum is divided and a vessel loop is placed around the portal pedicle. Before beginning the portal dissection, the preoperative CT scan is reviewed to examine the portal vein anatomy, particularly the manner in which it divides into the left and the right (and subsequently anterior and posterior pedicle) and if there are variations to note.
- Next, the gallbladder is removed.
- The portal pedicle is then clamped (Pringle maneuver) and the liver parenchyma anterior (base of segment IVB) and posterior (caudate process) to the hepatic portal is incised to isolate the right portal pedicle (see Fig. 40-7). This pedicle is then further dissected peripherally to identify and isolate the anterior and posterior portal pedicle (see Fig. 40-6). After completion of this dissection, the portal pedicle is unclamped, and any bleeding from the parenchyma is controlled.
- The anterior pedicle is clamped with a soft vascular clamp to confirm devascularization of the sector to be resected. After this confirmation, the anterior pedicle is transected with an endovascular 2.5 linear stapler.
- Intraoperative ultrasound scan is used to ensure that an adequate margin can be achieved. The proposed plane of transection is marked with electrocautery.
- With intermittent portal triad clamping, the liver parenchyma can be transected by kellyclassis. As branches of the hepatic vein are encountered, they are isolated and transected with an endovascular 2.0 linear stapler.
- If the pedicles to segment IV were not divided at the outset, these can be carefully isolated while avoiding injury to the ascending left portal vein after the parenchyma has been divided (Fig. 40-9).
- During transection at the right side of the falciform ligament, care should be taken not to damage the ascending portion of the left portal vein, which can be identified with ultrasound.
- Superiorly, dissection in the middle hepatic vein is isolated before it joins the left hepatic vein. The middle hepatic vein is then transected with a linear endovascular 2.0 stapler or divided between clamps and sutured with 3-0 polypropylene.
- Once the transection plane is completely divided, the liver surface is slowly coagulated. Any large bleeding veins are controlled with either 3-0 or 4-0 monofilament suture. The surface is inspected for any bile leak, which is either hemoclipped or suture ligated with 4-0 polypropylene. The surface can be treated with Bioglue (Fig. 40-10).
- Ultrasound is used to confirm adequate flow to the remaining liver segments.
- The right upper quadrant is irrigated, and a Jackson-Pratt drain is placed.

Closure

- Muscles of the anterior abdominal wall are approximated in layers with 1-0 monofilament absorbable suture. The skin is approximated with staples.

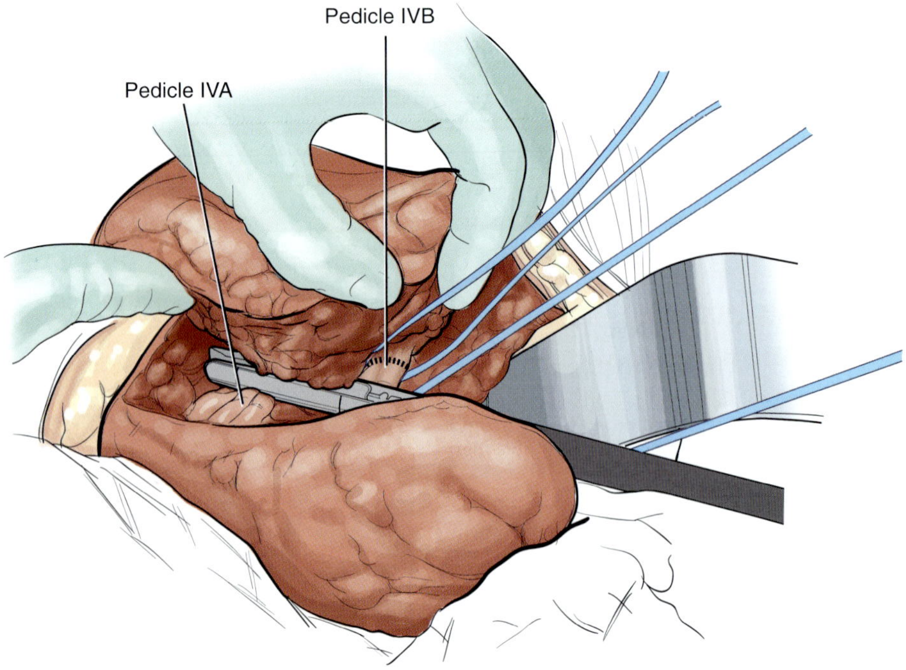

Figure 40-9.

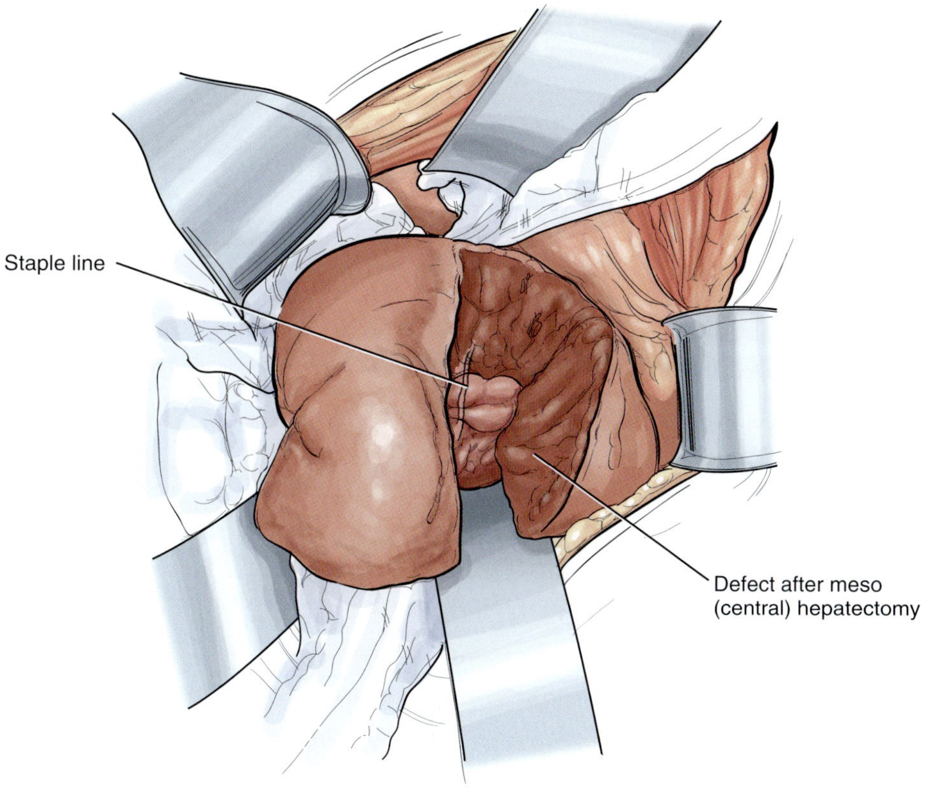

Figure 40-10.

III. ALTERNATIVE TECHNICAL APPROACHES (PRO/CON) AND PEARLS

- Various incisions can be used, including a "Mercedes" incision (a rooftop with a midline extension) and a J-shaped incision.
- Radiofrequency-assisted parenchymal transection can be performed. With ultrasound guidance, the transverse plane can be sequentially ablated with use of the InLine bipolar radiofrequency device (see Fig. 40-8). This greatly facilitates the parenchymal division by minimizing blood loss.
- New energy devices are being used for hepatic resection when the parenchymal transection must proceed without full inflow control. These include the 10-mm LigaSure. In difficult areas where it is not easy to obtain exposure, the vessels are often controlled with the linear endovascular stapler.

IV. SPECIAL POSTOPERATIVE CARE

- Appropriate precautions are taken to minimize or prevent the occurrence of general postoperative complications such as pneumonia and thrombotic and cardiac events.
- Liver-specific complications such as bile leak and liver failure must be anticipated, particularly in patients with cirrhosis and following massive (50% to 60%) resection. In the event of liver impairment, particular attention is given to avoid hepatotoxic drugs, and the transplantation service will be contacted. Patients with cirrhosis are also at risk for developing portal vein thrombosis, and clinicians should be alerted if persistent abdominal pain occurs with elevation of liver function tests. A duplex ultrasound scan of the liver is obtained, and if thrombosis is detected, anticoagulation is started.
- If the international normalized ratio (INR) is elevated, the patient may require administration of vitamin K and/or fresh frozen plasma, depending on the degree of INR elevation and the associated drop in hematocrit.
- Epidural or patient-controlled analgesia is routinely instituted to ensure adequate pain control.

SUGGESTED READINGS

Machado MA, Herman P, Machado MC: Intrahepatic Glissonian approach for pedicle control during anatomic mesohepatectomy, *Surgery* 141:533–537, 2007.

Mehrabi A, Mood ZA, Roshanaei N, et al: Mesohepatectomy as an option for the treatment of central liver tumors, *J Am Coll Surg* 207:499–509, 2008.

Scudamore CH, Buczkowski AK, Shayan H, et al: Mesohepatectomy, *Am J Surg* 179:356–360, 2000.

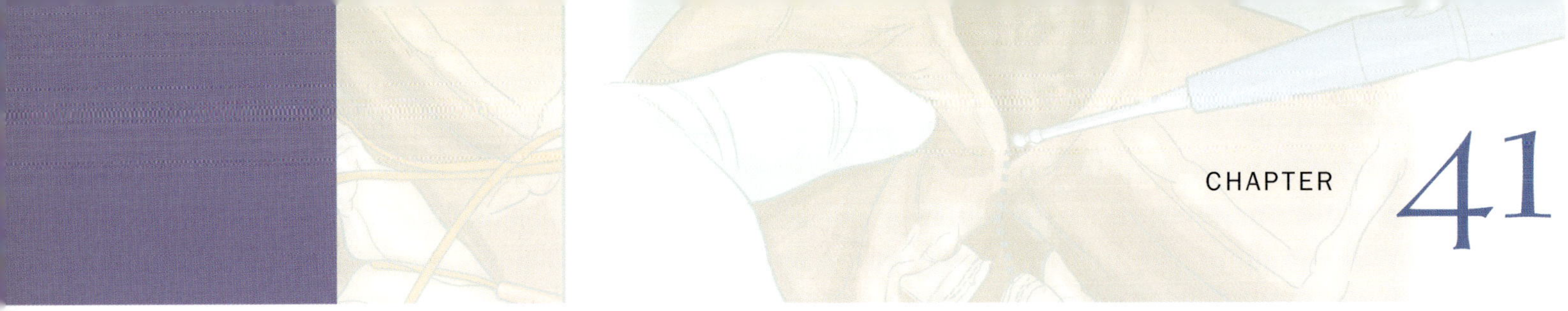

CHAPTER 41

Liver Segmentectomies

Guido Torzilli, MD, PhD, and Henri Bismuth, MD, FACS(Hon)

I. SPECIAL PREOPERATIVE PREPARATION

Patient Selection

- Patients with hepatocellular carcinoma (HCC) in the cirrhotic liver are selected for surgery based on the presence or absence of ascites, total serum bilirubin level, no extrahepatic tumoral spread, and technical feasibility. Patients with other neoplastic focal liver lesions are selected for surgery based on the technical feasibility, regardless of the size or number of metastases. The technical feasibility is based on the requirement that, once the entire tumor has been removed, there must be enough residual liver volume with optimal blood inflow, blood outflow, and biliary drainage.

Preoperative Imaging

- Preoperative imaging workup consists of abdominal ultrasound, and spiral computed tomography (CT) or magnetic resonance imaging (MRI) for every patient. As well as being the preferred method for screening at-risk populations and generally the diagnostic method that allows the first detection of the disease, ultrasound is also used by surgeons as a complementary method to CT and/or MRI to better decide what surgical strategy to adopt. Spiral CT is the preferred method for defining the tumor relationship with intrahepatic vascular structures, whereas MRI is the most sensitive for nodule detection and differentiation, benefitting from the use of superparamagnetic contrast agents. Intraoperative ultrasonography (IOUS) with and without intravenous contrast enhancement (CEIOUS) is also performed to more precisely define the liver involvement by the tumor.

II. OPERATIVE TECHNIQUE

Position

- The patient is placed in the supine position with the arms 90 degrees laterally abducted from the body. The drape-free area is limited from cranial to caudal by the intermammary line and a line parallel to the umbilical line but located 2 to 3 cm below; laterally, the drape-free area should be limited from right to left by the right posterior axillary line and the left anterior axillary line (Fig. 41-1).

Incision

- Two types of incision can be selected: the subcostal incision and the J-shaped incision (Fig. 41-2, *A* and *B*). Each has the horizontal portion running 3 to 4 cm above the umbilical line.

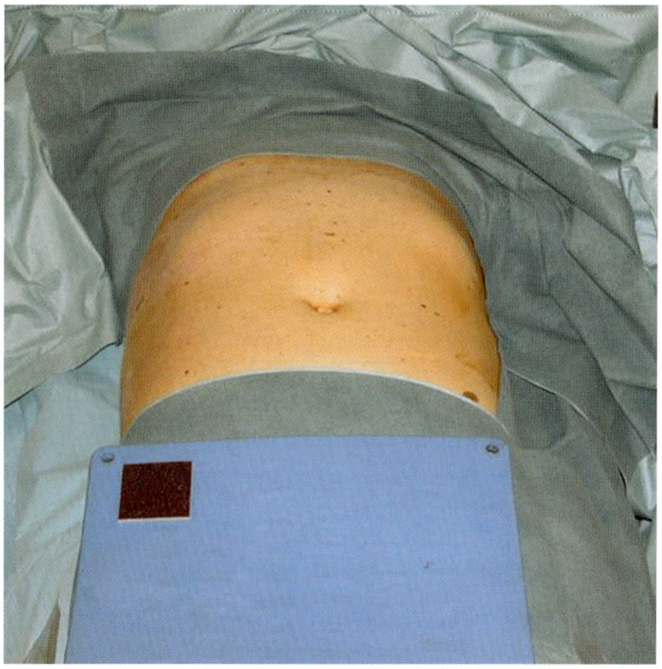

Figure 41-1.

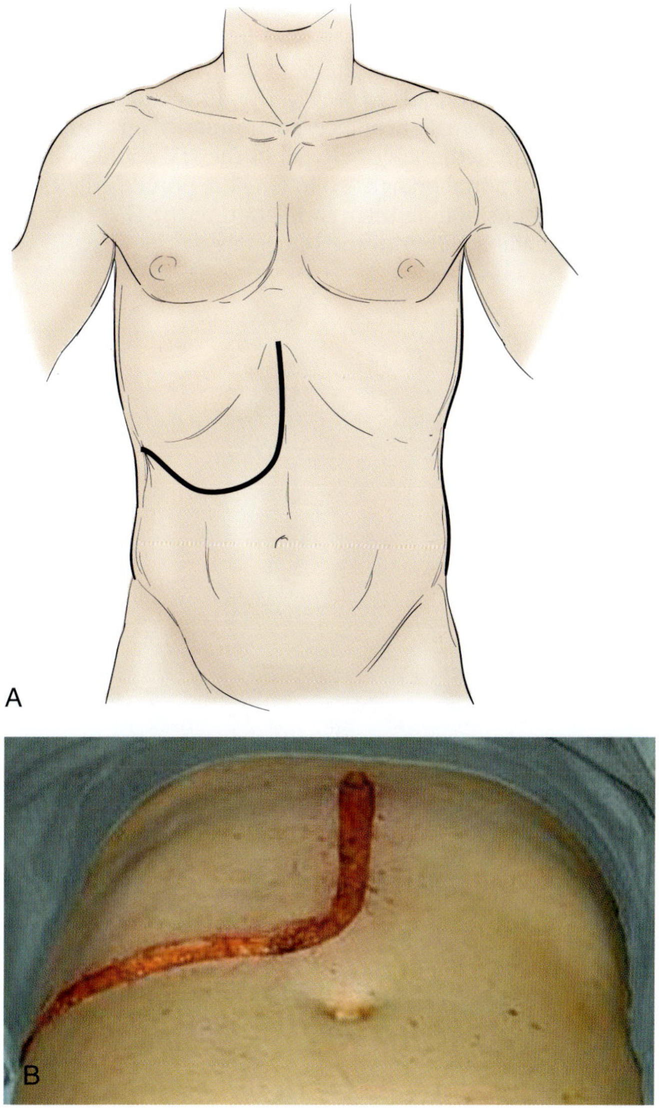

Figure 41-2.

- The operative field is constantly maintained by special retractors (Kent, Takasago, Tokyo) (Fig. 41-3).
- The xiphoid process is routinely removed.
- If the lesion is located in segment II, III, or IV, an inverted T-shape abdominal incision is selected.
- If the tumor to be resected is located in the paracaval portion and/or in the caudate process of segment I or in segments IV superior, VII, or VIII, close to the hepatocaval junction (last 4 cm of each hepatic vein), the thoracic cavity may need to be opened. Opening the chest is carried out through the ninth intercostal arch, prolonging the skin incision up to the anterior axillary line and the intercostal incision to the posterior one.

Main Dissection

- After the abdominal cavity is entered, liver mobilization dividing the round and falciform ligaments and division of eventual adhesions to free the anterosuperior and inferior surfaces of the liver is carried out. IOUS is performed at this time.

Intraoperative Ultrasonography

- By pulling the round ligament, the liver surface is widely exposed, and following the portal branches and the hepatic veins (HVs), the liver can be studied in its entirety. The probe is managed using enough pressure to ensure good contact with the liver surface but without compressing the intrahepatic vascular structures and in particular the HV. The three main hepatic veins are readily identified at their junction with the inferior vena cava (IVC). The probe is positioned at this level and tilted upward once the confluence of the HVs into the IVC is recognized. Then, gently withdrawing the probe, the HV paths are traced into the liver. HVs appear as echo-free zones in the liver parenchyma; the vessel wall appears as a thin hyper-echogenic line or is undetectable (Fig. 41-4). HV wall thickness can be greater in the cirrhotic liver and its lumen thinner as a function of the hard stiffness of the organ (Fig. 41-5).
- The portal vein branches can be followed by positioning the probe horizontally above segment IV inferior to visualize the first-order bifurcation; the first-, second-, and third-order portal branches can then be followed with the probe. Because of the existence of the Glisson capsule, the portal pedicles, which run together with the arteries and the bile ducts, have thicker-walled vessels compared with the HVs, and for this reason they appear at IOUS as echo-free zones surrounded by a thicker hyperechogenic layer (see Fig. 41-4). The other parallel thinner vascular structures that are visible are the arteries and the bile ducts of the glissonian triad. However, the distinction between HV and portal branches should be based not merely on their appearance but primarily on their anatomy. Indeed, in the cirrhotic liver, as previously mentioned, the vessel wall of the HV could be thicker and not immediately differentiable from a peripheral portal branch. Following the portal pedicles at the sectional, segmental, and subsegmental levels, and positioning them in relation to the HVs, it is possible to precisely define the segmental and subsegmental location of the IOUS target.

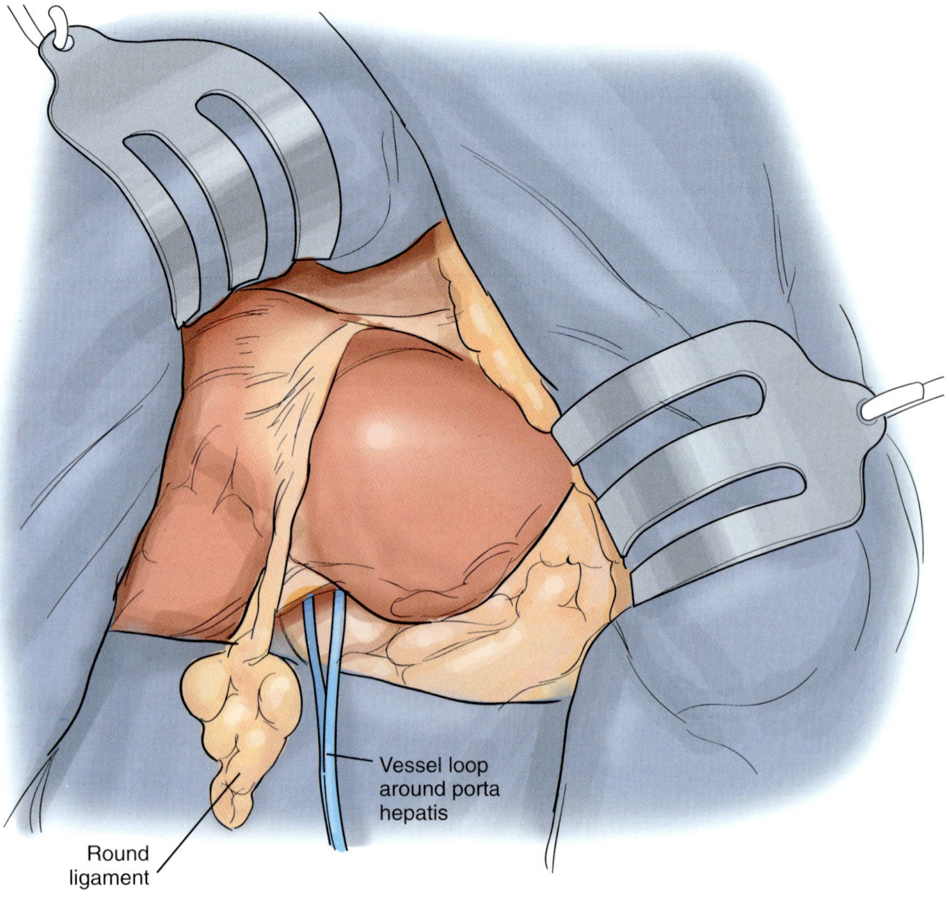

Figure 41-3.

Definition of the Surgical Strategy

- The proper surgical strategy is defined based on the IOUS findings concerning the relationship between the tumor and the portal branches and HVs. The relationships and related surgical strategies are classified as follows:
  - ▲ Portal branch (type A) or HV (type 1) in contact with a capsulated HCC without vessel wall discontinuation at IOUS: vascular resection is not associated; only enucleation at the level of the vascular contact is performed (Fig. 41-6, *A*).

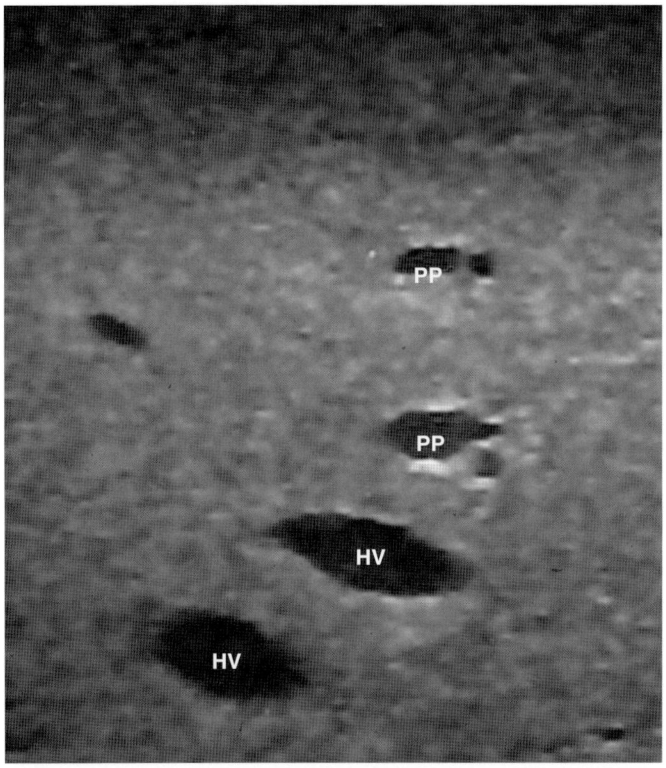

Figure 41-4. The portal pedicle (*PP*) and the hepatic vein (*HV*) have different wall thickness at intraoperative ultrasound. In addition, the PP is represented by at least two holes representing the artery and the portal vein, or three, including the bile duct—always for the first- and second-order branches, and when dilated in the case of more peripheral PPs such as those shown in the figure.

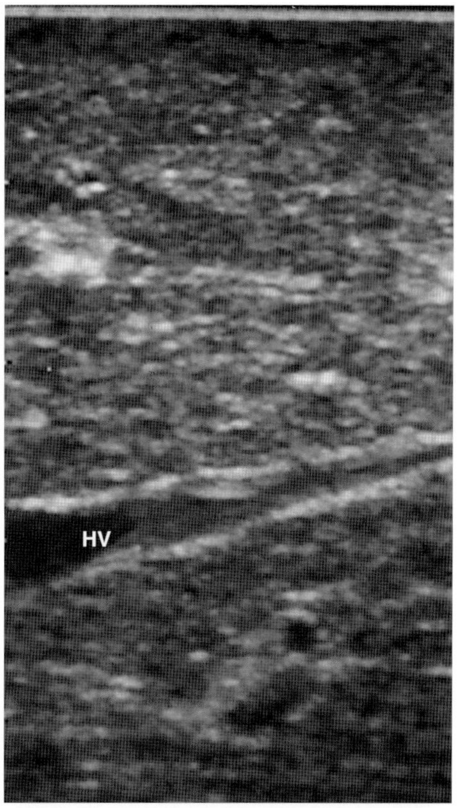

Figure 41-5. Hepatic vein (*HV*) has a thickened wall in cirrhotic liver at intraoperative ultrasound.

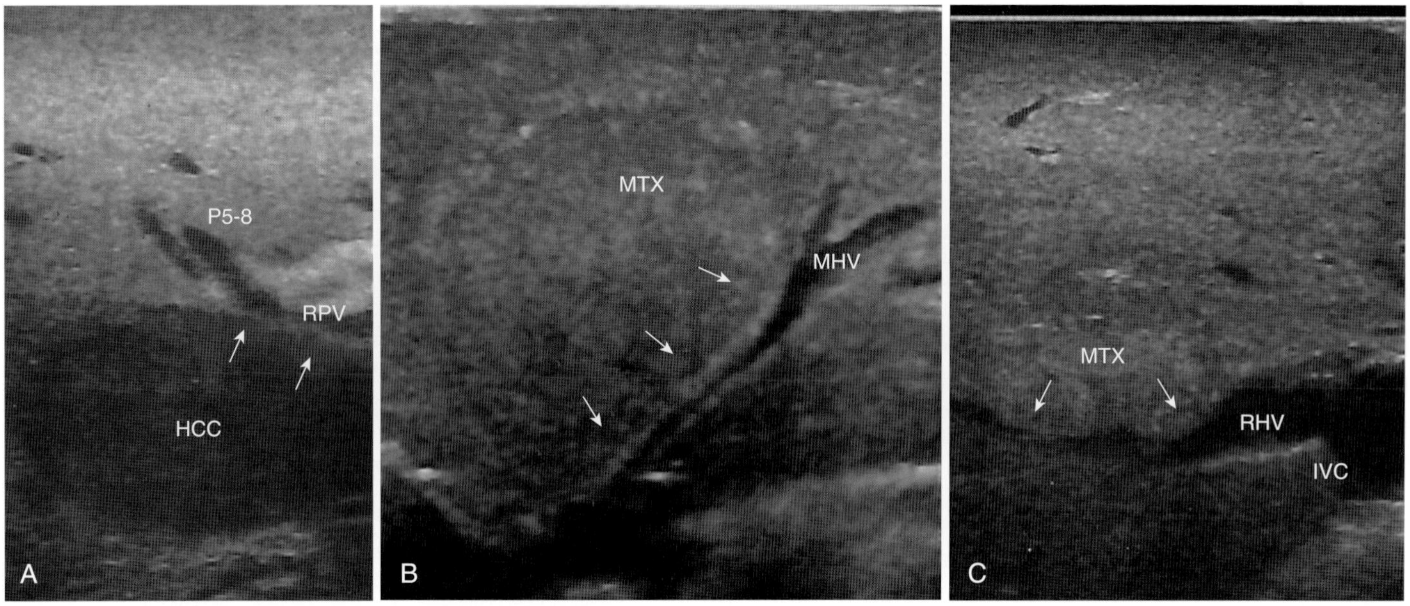

Figure 41-6. **A,** This patient had a hepatocellular carcinoma (*HCC*) located in the paracaval portion of segment I in contact with the right portal vein (*RPV*), with no sign at intraoperative ultrasound (IOUS) of direct infiltration; *arrows* indicate the contact with the vessel wall (hyperechogenic line), which appears intact. The operation consisted of a segment I segmentectomy. *P5-8*, Portal branch to segments V and VIII. **B,** Colorectal cancer liver metastasis (*MTX*) at IOUS, showing its contact without invasion (*arrows*) with the wall of the middle hepatic vein (*MHV*) close to its confluence with the inferior vena cava. The operation consisted of segment IV superior and segment VIII segmentectomy, including resection of the MHV. **C,** IOUS image of a colorectal cancer liver metastasis (*MTX*) invading the wall (*arrows*) of the right hepatic vein (*RHV*) close to its confluence with the inferior vena cava (*IVC*). The operation consisted of segments VII and VIII segmentectomy including resection of the RHV.

- ▲ Portal branch (type B) or hepatic vein (type 2) separated by any ultrasonographically visible layer of liver parenchyma (even if thinner than 5 mm) from a colorectal cancer (CRC) liver metastasis: vascular resection is not associated.
- ▲ Portal branch (type C) or hepatic vein (type 3) in contact with an HCC with undefined margins without vessel wall discontinuation at IOUS: vascular resection is associated.
- ▲ Portal branch (type D) or hepatic vein (type 4) in contact with a CRC liver metastasis without vessel wall discontinuation at IOUS: vascular resection is associated (see Fig. 41-6, *B*).
- ▲ Portal branch or hepatic vein in contact with an HCC (type E1/5a) or CRC liver metastasis (type E2/5b) with vessel wall discontinuation at IOUS: vascular resection is associated (see Fig. 41-6, *C*).
- ▲ Portal branch (type F) in contact with an HCC or CRC liver metastasis with or without vessel wall discontinuation but with proximal bile duct dilation at IOUS: vascular resection is associated.

- Extension of the hepatectomy is always considered for parenchyma fed by an infiltrated portal branch (types 3 through 6). Inversely, in the case of infiltration of a hepatic vein, an extension of the resection to the whole liver parenchyma theoretically drained by this vein is considered only if there are no accessory hepatic veins at IOUS (Fig. 41-7) and if color-Doppler IOUS shows hepatofugal blood flow in the feeding portal branch once the hepatic vein is clamped.

Demarcation of the Resected Area

- As a general principle, to carry out a limited segmental or subsegmental resection, the surgeon should plan (with the aid of IOUS) the resection area, dissection plane, and the result of the planned resection before starting the liver dissection. The aim is to obtain a regular and relatively flat cut surface, which is at lower risk of leaving undisclosed bleeding sources and biliary leaks.
- After the identification of the tumor, under IOUS control the surgeon can use electrocautery to mark the border of the lesion on the surface of the liver just above the nodule. To perform this maneuver, the flat, thin tip of the electrocautery is positioned between the probe and the liver surface. This maneuver results in a shadow in the IOUS that runs deeply just below the electrocautery (Fig. 41-8, *A* and *B*). This technique makes it possible to define the position of the electrocautery with the tumor edge and consequently to mark with the electrocautery the nodule profile on the liver surface and to select the safer edge for the incision. The adequacy of the marked edge can be further checked with

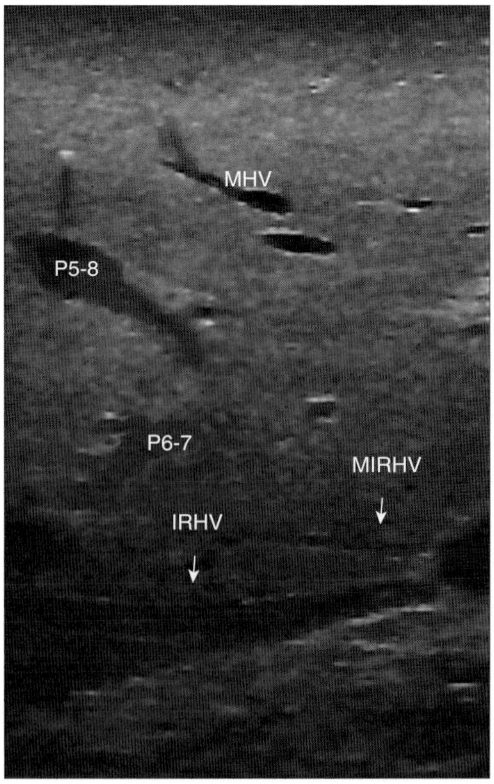

Figure 41-7. At intraoperative ultrasound, an inferior right hepatic vein (*IRHV*) and a middle inferior right hepatic vein (*MIRHV*) are visible (*arrows*) flowing into the inferior vena cava: these vessels typically run behind the first- and second-order right portal pedicles. *MHV,* Middle hepatic vein; *P5-8,* portal branch to segments V and VIII; *P6-7,* portal branch to segments VI and VII.

IOUS, because the air trapped between the probe and the irregular surface of the demarcation line drawn with the electrocautery on the liver surface can be visualized at IOUS.

- Another way to draw the tumor edge precisely on the liver surface with the aid of IOUS is using the fingertips (Fig. 41-9). With the probe positioned on the liver surface, the surgeon uses a fingertip to push on the opposite side, and the liver's profile is visualized at IOUS. As a result, the relationship between the fingertip and the tumor edge can be precisely estimated and the resection area can be marked on both liver surfaces.

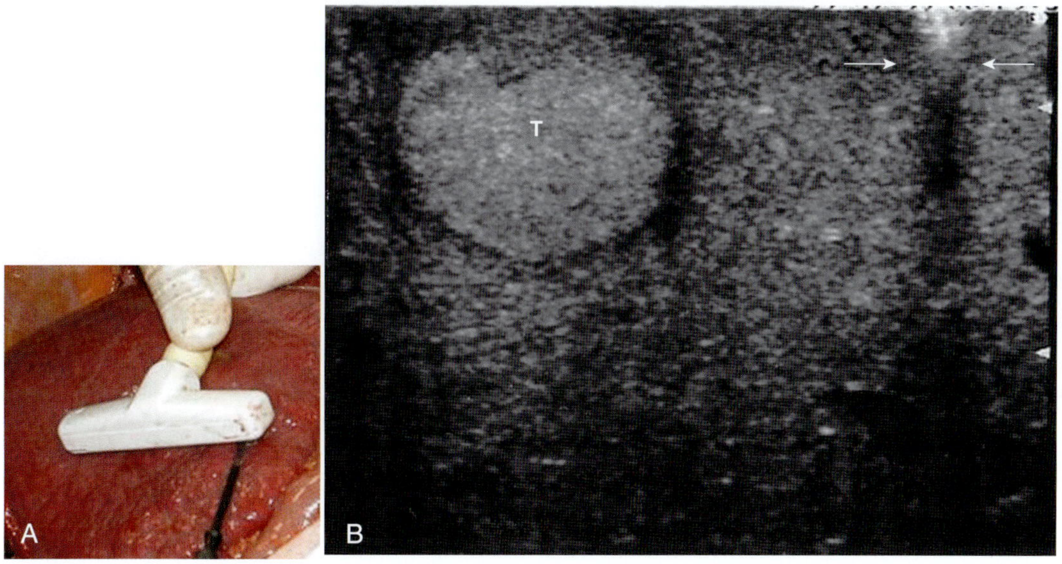

Figure 41-8. **A,** The electrocautery positioned between the liver surface and the probe. **B,** On intraoperative ultrasound, the electrocautery generates a shadow (*arrows*), which can be related to the tumor burden (*T*), and as a consequence the optimal resection area can be defined.

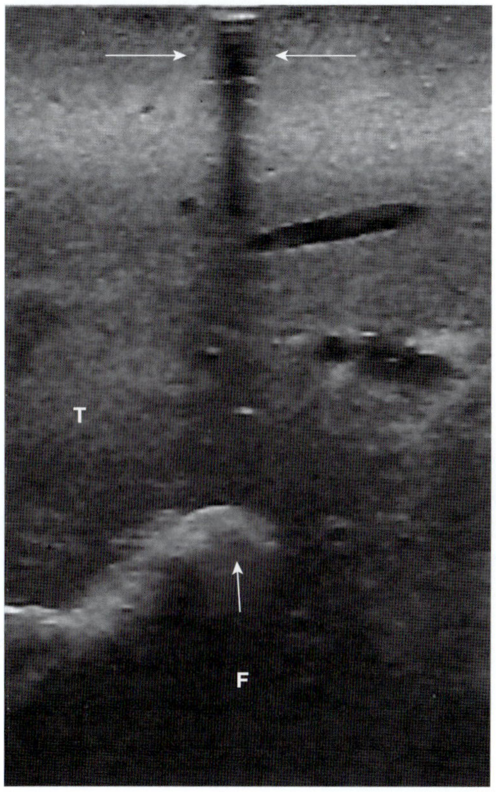

Figure 41-9. On intraoperative ultrasound, the electrocautery generates a vertical shadow (*horizontal arrows*), and the surgeon's finger is positioned on the opposite side of the liver (*F*) allowing the surgeon to draw an ideal plane for dissection that correspond to the vertical shadows. *T,* Tumor.

Preparation for Liver Dissection

- This maneuver and the previously described definition of the resective area by means of IOUS are carried out almost simultaneously.
- For right-sided segmentectomies or subsegmentectomies, the bare area is dissected and the right hemiliver is mobilized until the surgeon's left hand is positioned behind the hemiliver, supporting it, and is passing over the resection area established by means of IOUS as described earlier (Fig. 41-10). Therefore, a slight mobilization of the right hemiliver just dividing the triangular ligament and part of the bare area is accomplished for lesions located in segments V, VI, and VII inferior. Conversely, the right side of the retrohepatic IVC is reached for lesions located in segments VII and VIII ventral. If the lesion is located in segment VII superior or VIII dorsal, which means close to the hepatocaval confluence (last 4 cm), but is not in contact with the HVs, the retrohepatic caval ligament is not divided and only the space between the right hepatic vein (RHV) and the middle hepatic vein is slightly dissected to allow fingertip insertion. The RHV caval confluence is recognized following the trajectory of the right inferior phrenic vein, which flows into the RHV at this level and is a constant landmark (Fig. 41-11). Thus the second and third fingertips of the operating surgeon's left hand are positioned around the extrahepatic RHV, and the proper positioning is checked by ultrasound. IOUS with the aid of color Doppler allows the surgeon to check the proper and effective clamping of the extrahepatic RHV (Fig. 41-12, *A* and *B*). If confirmed, liver resection is started, with confidence that back-flow bleeding can be controlled just by finger compression of the RHV confluence.
- If the lesion is still right-sided but in contact with an HV at its caval confluence or is involving the paracaval portion of segment I, liver mobilization includes division of the retrohepatic caval ligament and exposure of the retrohepatic IVC until the area to be resected is under control of the surgeon's left hand. This means having the fingertips over the most distal portion of the planned dissection plane.
- For segment II and III segmentectomies or subsegmentectomies, the left triangular ligament and the left coronary ligament are divided, and the left lobe is handled with the surgeon's left hand.
- For lesions located at segment IV superior at the hepatocaval junction, the mobilization combines the procedure described for lesions at segments VII inferior and VIII ventral and the procedure for lesions in the left lobe.

Dissection

- The liver transection is carried out under warm ischemia. For this purpose, the Pringle maneuver is carried out with 15 minutes of clamping and 5 minutes of interval.
- The operating surgeon carries out the parenchymal dissection by Kelly crush-clamping and bipolar electrocautery for vessel coagulation using the right hand, while the first assistant ligates each vessel thicker than 2 mm with thin (3-0) sutures and the second assistant takes care of the suction. The left hand of the surgeon is supporting the liver, allowing control of the back-flow bleeding by pushing up

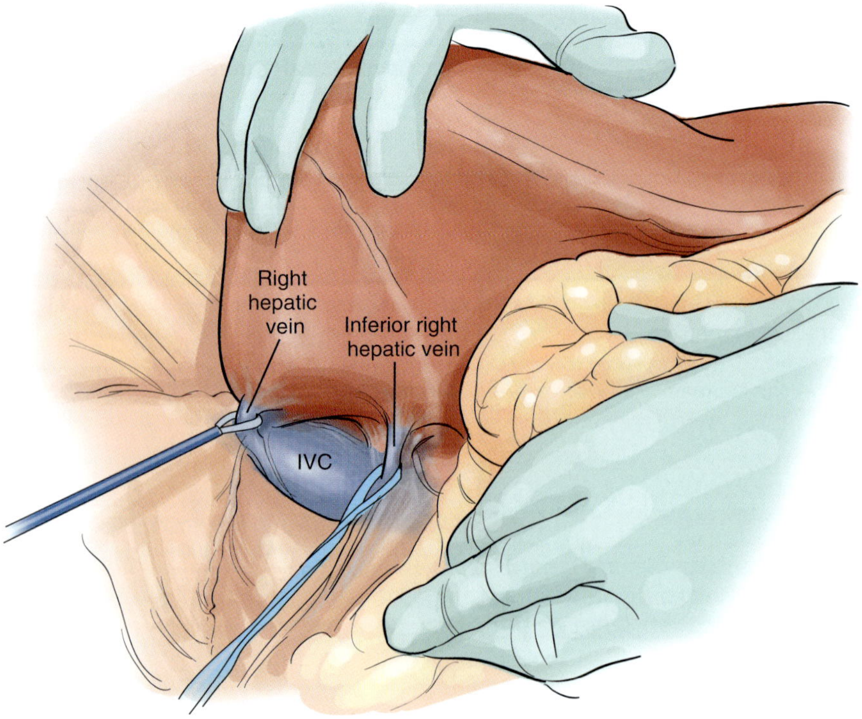

Figure 41-10. *IVC*, Inferior vena cava.

the liver when needed. Similarly, always with the purpose of controlling the back-flow bleeding, the HVs are clamped bluntly using the fingertips, which have been previously positioned (see previous section) with the aid of color Doppler IOUS, only for the time needed to achieve hemostasis by ligation or suture of the damaged vessel along the dissection line.

Closure

- The cut surface of the liver is secured by 2-0 or 3-0 sutures, electrocautery, fibrillar oxidated regenerated cellulose (Fibrillar Tabotamp, Ethicon, Somerville, N.J.), and fibrin glue (Tissucol, Baxter Healthcare, Deerfield, Ill., or Quixil, Ethicon). Repeated lavage of the abdominal cavity with sterile hypothermic

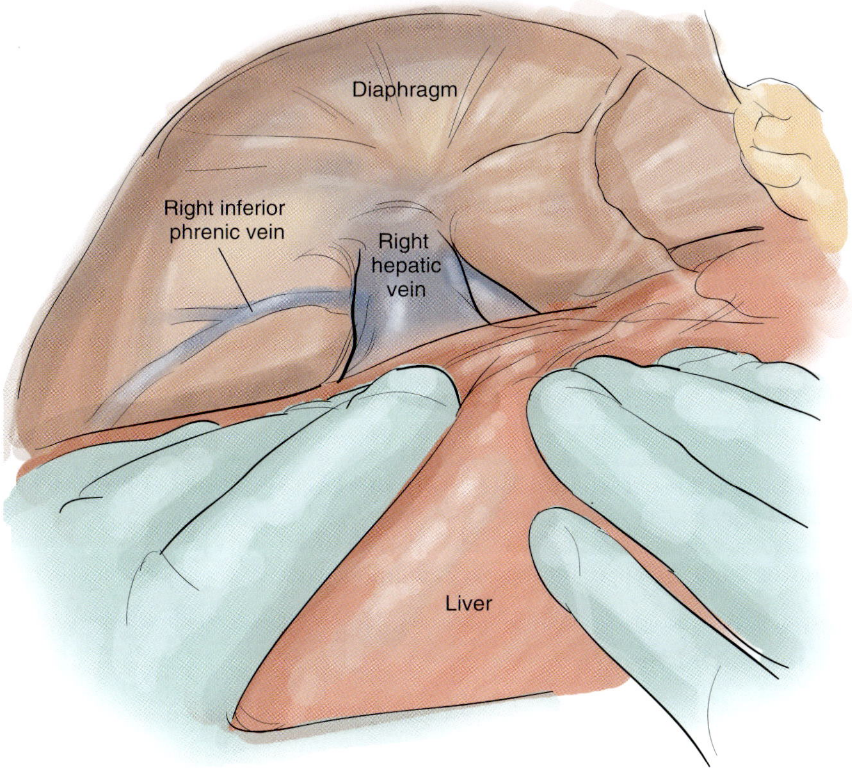

Figure 41-11.

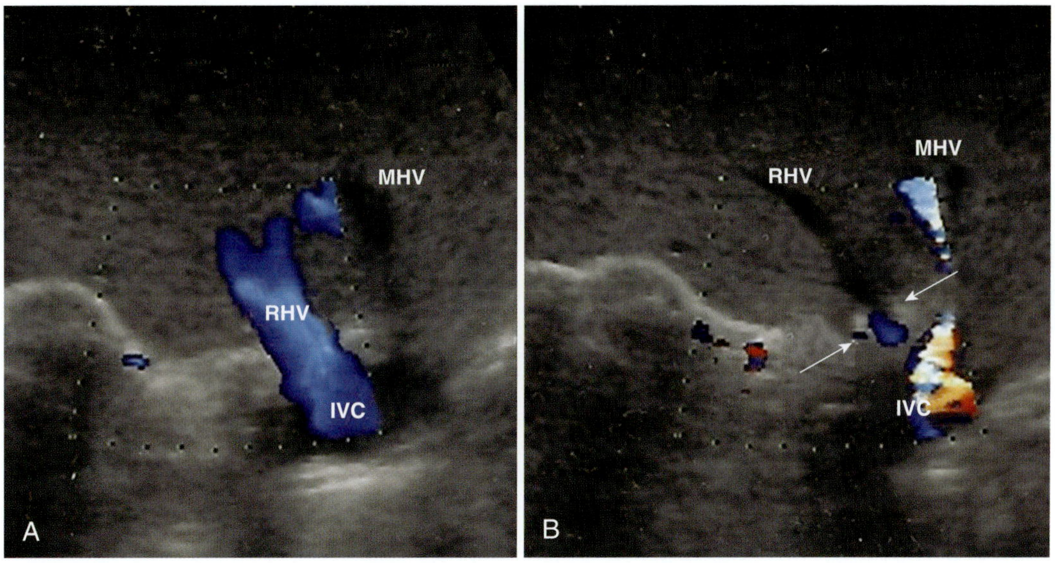

Figure 41-12. **A,** On color Doppler intraoperative ultrasound (IOUS), the right hepatic vein (*RHV*) is visualized with its blood flow (*blue color*). **B,** The surgeon's fingertips bluntly compress the RHV (*arrows*), and the temporary occlusion of the vessel is confirmed at color Doppler IOUS by the absence of blood flow (*no color*). *IVC,* Inferior vena cava; *MHV,* middle hepatic vein.

saline is performed. To rule out bile leakage, a careful examination of the resection area is done. Once hemostasis and biliostasis are achieved, wound closure begins. Closed suction drains are always left in the peritoneal cavity with the tip facing the cut surface of the liver. A chest drain is placed in the case of thoracophrenolaparotomy. Closure is carried out using absorbable sutures.

Intraoperative Management

- Blood loss and ascites production during the operation are balanced by infusing 10% to 20% more fresh frozen plasma than the volume of blood lost. Intraoperative blood transfusions are given only if the hematocrit is below 30%. The amount of sodium infused is restricted, because the sodium concentration of fresh frozen plasma is high. To ensure a total fluid infusion volume of 4 to 4.5 mL/kg/hr, equal volumes of crystalloid and 5% glucose solution are administered.
- The level of anesthesia is maintained by general and epidural anesthesia thereby reducing the quantity of inhalation agents and intravenous drugs. A muscle relaxant is also administered and the respiratory tidal volume is reduced to around 60% just before starting liver dissection to reduce the thoracic and central venous pressure (0 to 4 cm H_2O) and consequently, the back-flow bleeding from the HVs and/or their tributaries. Hydrocortisone (100 mg) is injected intravenously before starting vascular occlusion to protect the liver during warm ischemia.

III. ALTERNATIVE TECHNICAL APPROACHES (PRO/CON) AND PEARLS

- For CEIOUS, 2.4 to 4.8 mL of sulfur hexafluoride microbubbles (SonoVue, Bracco Imaging, Milan) are injected intravenously through a peripheral vein by the anesthesiologist when requested by the surgeon. This method allows better differentiation for new nodules detected in the cirrhotic liver by IOUS, of which only 30% are generally overt HCC. In the case of patients who undergo resections for liver metastases from CRC, CEIOUS significantly improves nodule detection. In summary, CEIOUS is adopted if new lesions are detected at IOUS in connection with surgery for HCC. CEIOUS is always carried out in patients operated on for liver metastases.
- Instead of marking the resection area based on the tumor site and its relationship to the intrahepatic vascular structures, both checked in real time with IOUS, it is possible to perform anatomic segmentectomies or subsegmentectomies by means of ultrasound-guided procedures. This policy is recommended in the case of resection for HCC, although its use is still controversial. Indeed, there are no truly randomized studies comparing anatomic and nonanatomic resections.

Puncture of the Portal Branch

- The portal branch feeding the tumor to be resected is punctured under IOUS guidance, through a freehand technique or with a proper device. Then 3 to 5 mL of indigo carmine dye is injected into the vessel. The stained area becomes evident on the liver surface and is marked with the electrocautery. If the nodule is located between two adjacent segments, two portal branches afferent to the area must be punctured and injected. In this case, the deepest and most dorsal vessel must be punctured first to prevent the air bubbles contained in the dye from disturbing the ultrasonographic detection and puncture of the other branch. The portal branch is punctured 1 to 2 cm distally from its origin to avoid dye reflux, and the direction and velocity of the infusion are controlled at IOUS. To prolong the staining, the hepatic artery at the hilum is clamped before portal branch puncture. When there are numerous and thin vessels to be punctured, or in the case of tumor thrombus in the segmental portal branch of the segment to be removed, the dye is injected in the portal branches afferent to the adjacent segment: this is the so-called counterstaining technique.

Hooking of the Portal Branch

- The segmental portal branches to segment IV are generally divided in two groups: those for the superior and those for the inferior portion. However, the most common branching pattern can be recognized in just half of cases. These branches, rather than being punctured under IOUS guidance, can be approached by dissecting the umbilical portion. Once exposed, the vessel can be encircled with a suture and pulled under IOUS control to verify whether it is the branch to segment IV inferior or not. The proper portal branch can then be ligated and divided. The discolored area that will appear on the liver surface should correspond to the segment IV inferior, which can be marked with electrocautery, after which the liver dissection proceeds. This is a peculiar application of the so-called hooking technique. Furthermore, the subsegment IV superior can be resected by clamping the portal branch to subsegment IV inferior, as it is identified with the previously described hooking technique. The discolored subsegment IV inferior caudally, the plan at IOUS, which includes the middle hepatic vein laterally and is marked by the falciform ligament medially, delimits the area to be resected.

Compression of the Portal Branch

- Subsegmental resections are feasible without clamping the hepatic artery and puncturing the feeding portal branches. Once the feeding portal branch has been identified at IOUS, it is compressed using the IOUS probe on one side of the liver lobe and the finger on the opposite side (Figs. 41-13 and 41-14). In this way, it is possible to induce a transient ischemia of the subsegmental portion of the liver distal to the compression site. This portion can be marked with the electrocautery; the

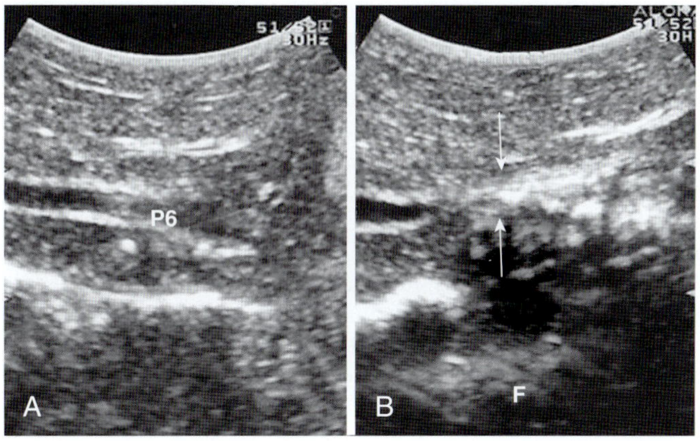

Figure 41-13. **A,** On intraoperative ultrasound, at *left* the portal branch to segment VI (*P6*) is visualized and the surgeon's finger is positioned (*arrow*), and at *right* P6 is compressed (*arrow*). **B,** Image shows how the compression is performed with the probe (*P*) and the finger (*F*).

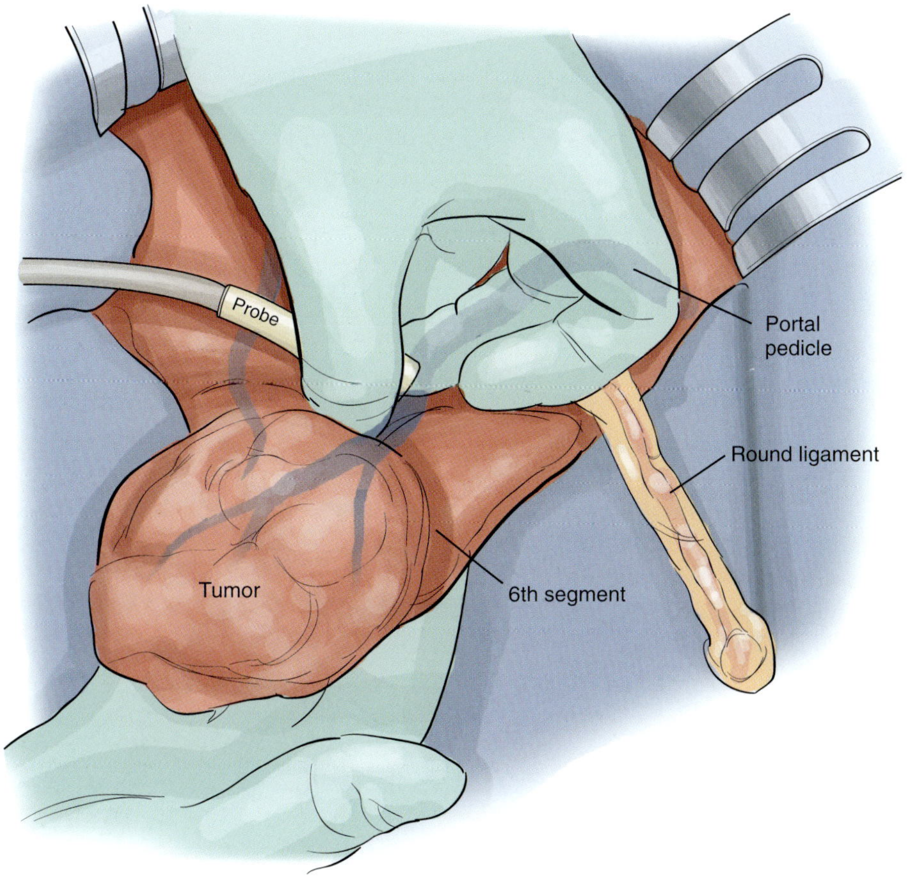

Figure 41-14.

compression is then released and the subsegmentectomy carried out (Fig. 41-15). This technique is simple, fast, noninvasive, and reversible. In addition, the possibility of modifying the site of compression and then the resection volume, allows the resection to be sized according to the tumor features and the status of the background liver. Together with the section IV subsegmentectomies, this operation represents an alternative to the puncture technique, which is less reproducible than these last two methods.

- IOUS allows following the dissection plane in real time, keeping it constantly in relation to the tumor edge, and then modifying its direction as necessary. This is because it is possible on the IOUS image to visualize the dissection plane, which appears as an echogenic line owing to the entrapment of air bubbles and clots between the faced cut surfaces (Fig. 41-16). If the dissection plane is not clearly visible, it can be better visualized by inserting gauze or specifically devised silicon gauze between the faced cut surfaces. These techniques allow the surgeon to keep the proper dissection plane. The artifacts that allow IOUS to show the dissection plane can mask structures such as portal branches that should be ligated or conversely respected. For this reason, to better visualize the targeted point where the portal branch is to be divided, the previously described hooking technique is used (Fig. 41-17, *A* and *B*). When the glissonian sheath is exposed and skeletonized, it is encircled with a stitch, which is visualized by IOUS as an echogenic spot with a posterior shadow. Under sonographic control, the stitch, hooking the exposed vessel, is gently pulled upward, which stretches the portal branch slightly. The traction point is demonstrated clearly by IOUS. If the exposed portal branch is not clearly visible because it has collapsed, the portal triad is unclamped to enable it to fill with blood, and then it is visualized better by IOUS. If the target site is correct, the portal branch is ligated and divided, and segmentectomy is completed under IOUS guidance.
- For both right- and left-sided segmentectomies, the fingertips of the left hand are positioned at the level where the dissection plane is to finish, to guide the surgeon while dissecting the liver in the proper trajectory.

IV. SPECIAL POSTOPERATIVE CARE

- Patients receive a total of about 40 to 45 mL/kg/day fluid by infusion. Glucose solution is given as a source of calories. Hydrocortisone is also given intravenously for 3 days postoperatively, and short-term

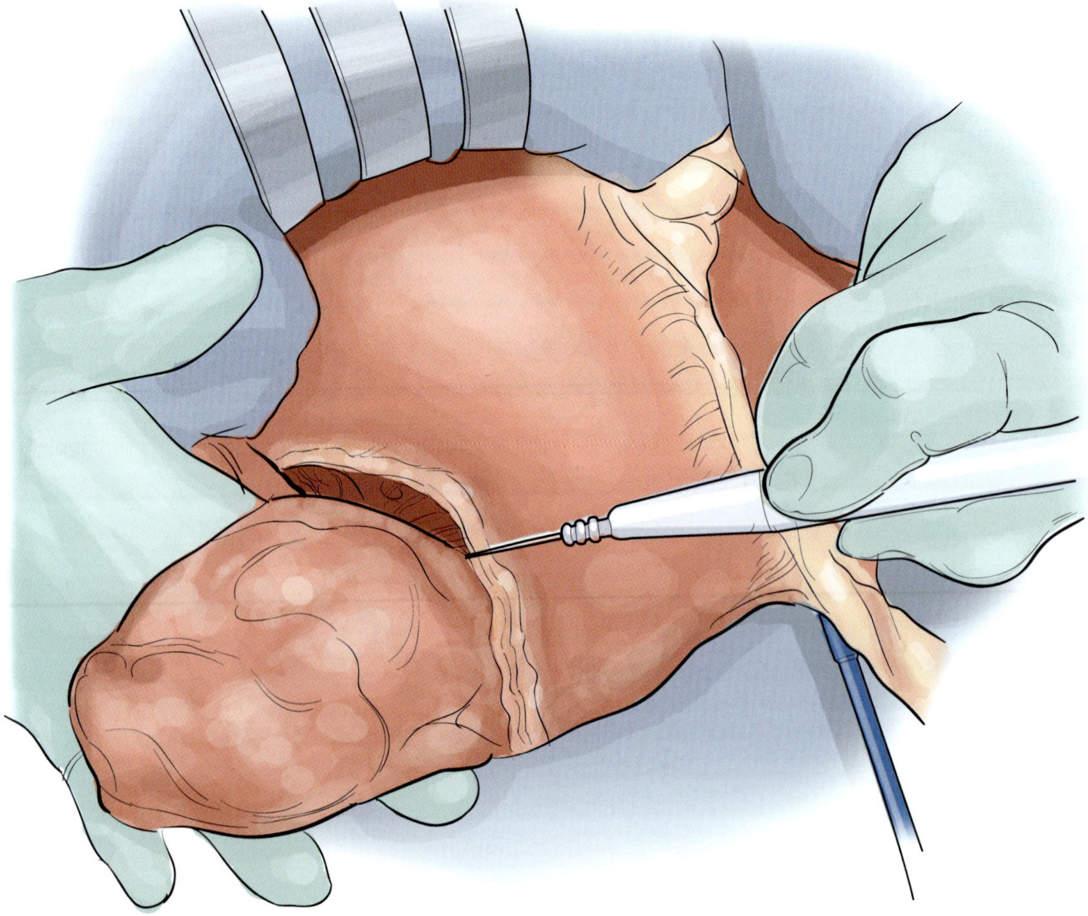

Figure 41-15.

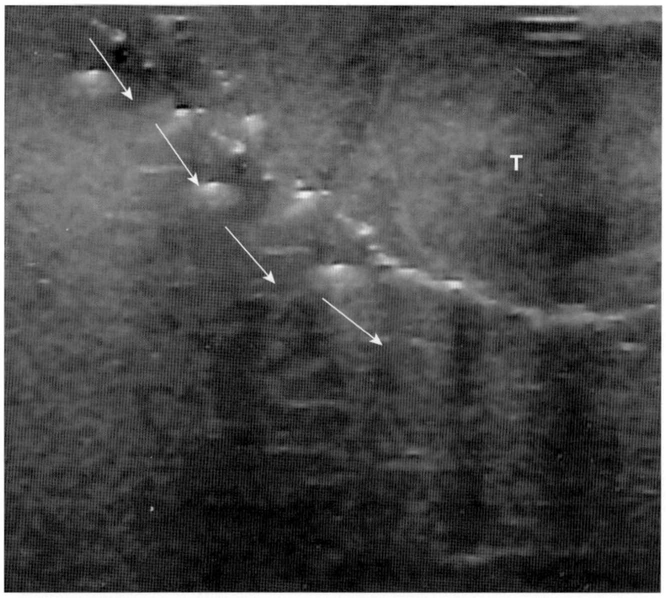

Figure 41-16. At intraoperative ultrasound the dissection line can be clearly visualized (*arrows*); it runs toward and under the tumor (*T*).

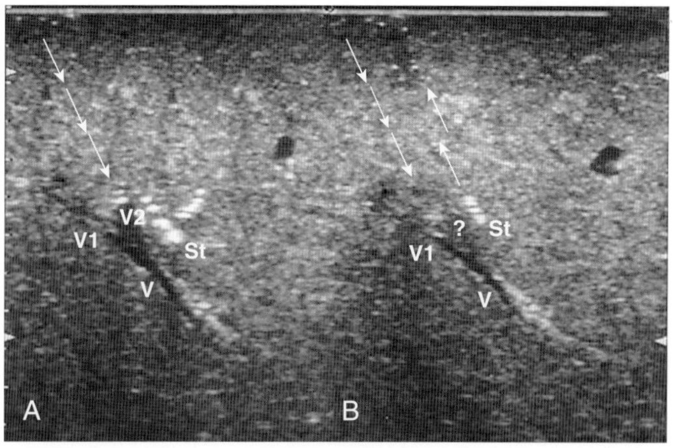

Figure 41-17. **A**, The vein (*V*) is achieved by the dissection line (*arrows*) at the level of its bifurcation in two veins *V1* and *V2*; one of the two veins is exposed on the cut surface, but whether it is V1 or V2 could be unclear. **B**, Once the exposed vein is encircled with a stitch, traction is applied (*arrows*) pulling up the stitch (*St*). V2 is no longer visible at this level (*?*), whereas V and V1 are still visible; therefore, it is certain that the encircled vessel is V2, and it is possible to spare or ligate it based on the surgical strategy.

antibiotic prophylaxis, omeprazole, and low-molecular-weight heparin are also administered. Appropriate oral intake is restored from postoperative day 3, but liquid oral intake is started on postoperative day 1.

- If the postoperative course is uneventful, the chest drain (if placed) is removed on postoperative day 3. The possibility of blood discharge in the drain is carefully checked, and an emergency laparotomy is performed if such discharge exceeds 100 mL/hr. Blood transfusions are administered only to patients with hematocrit values below 20% or in concomitance with symptoms of anemia. If no bile leakage is detected and the bilirubin concentration is less than that of the control on postoperative day 5, the drains are removed on postoperative day 7; conversely, the tube is maintained without closed suction until the bilirubin concentration is less than that in the previous control. Ultrasonography is performed on each patient after drain removal.

SUGGESTED READINGS

1. Torzilli G, Montorsi M, Del Fabbro D, et al: Ultrasonographically guided surgical approach to liver tumours involving the hepatic veins close to the caval confluence, *Br J Surg* 93:1238–1246, 2006.
2. Torzilli G, Montorsi M, Donadon M, et al: "Radical but conservative" is the main goal for ultrasonography-guided liver resection: prospective validation of this approach, *J Am Coll Surg* 201:517–528, 2005.
3. Torzilli G, Procopio F, Cimino M, et al: Anatomical segmental and subsegmental resection of the liver for hepatocellular carcinoma: a new approach by means of ultrasound-guided vessel compression, *Ann Surg* 251:229–235, 2010.

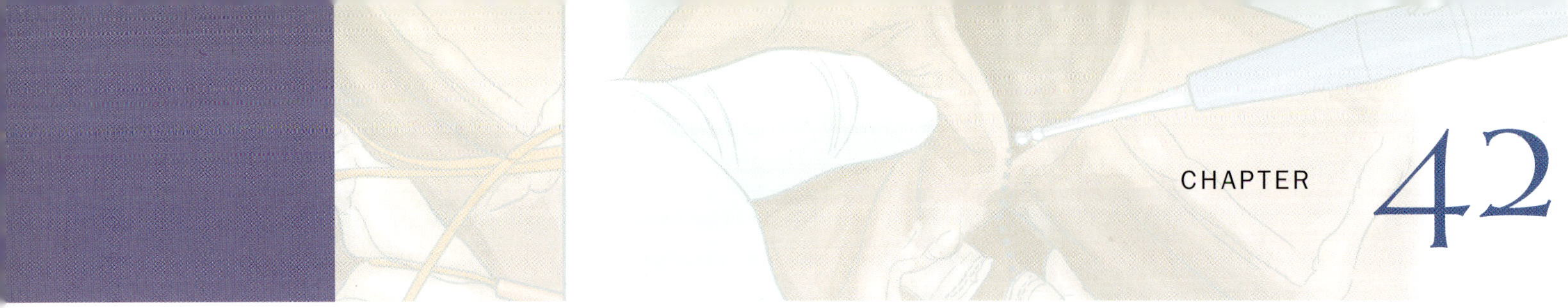

CHAPTER 42

Hepatic Artery Infusion Pump Placement

M. Margaret Kemeny, MD, FACS, and Anthony J. Froix, MD

I. SPECIAL PREOPERATIVE PREPARATION

- The architecture of the hepatic artery and its branches must be delineated before pump placement. This can be done by any means available. Thin-slice computed tomography (64 slice or higher) has made an arteriogram unnecessary. It can also delineate the liver metastases. The celiac axis and the common hepatic must be seen, along with the takeoff of the gastroduodenal artery (GDA) (Fig. 42-1). Care must be taken to define the left gastric artery, because there may be an accessory or replaced left hepatic artery arising from this artery. In addition, the superior mesenteric artery must be seen to rule out an accessory or replaced right hepatic artery. The relationship of the gastroduodenal artery takeoff and the bifurcation of the hepatic artery into the left and right branches is critical for pump placement. If the takeoff is at the same area as the bifurcation, making a trifurcation, the pump flow can sometimes go into one or the other branches and not equally into both. This is undesirable, and one of the hepatic artery branches needs to be ligated. The purpose is to have all of the arterial blood that flows into the liver pass by the pump catheter. Therefore all accessory or replaced branches must be ligated. This information must be known before pump placement.
- Other preoperative tests that can be useful include a positron emission tomography scan. This scan is the best tool available at present to identify metastases outside the liver. The pump is a treatment for patients with liver metastases. Because it is a regional treatment, metastases that are not in the liver would not benefit from a pump. Extrahepatic metastases should be identified because generally these are an exclusion criterion for pump placement.

II. OPERATIVE TECHNIQUE

Position

- The patient is placed on the operating table in the supine position. The lower chest, from below the nipples, and the entire abdomen are then prepped and draped. If the patient has an ostomy, it can be covered with a Tegaderm or other occlusive dressing. It is very important to have as little chance for contamination as possible, because if the pump becomes infected, it usually needs to be removed and cannot be replaced.

Incision

- Preoperative antibiotics should be given before the incision. Generally postoperative antibiotics should be continued to just before the patient's discharge to amplify the protection against a wound infection. The occurrence of a wound infection can be disastrous, because the pump pocket may get infected and result in removal of the pump.
- A midline incision is used from the xiphoid to the umbilicus. If a pump placement is being done in conjunction with a liver resection, then whatever incision is needed for the resection is appropriate (Fig. 42-2).

Main Dissection

Exploration

- Once the abdomen is entered, the liver should be examined to confirm preoperative findings of metastatic liver disease. If a liver biopsy is not available, it should be taken. The abdomen should be checked for extrahepatic metastatic disease. This includes palpating the colon and rectum, the retroperitoneal periaortic area, and, in women, the ovaries. If any extrahepatic disease is found, with the exception of a local recurrence, the use of a hepatic artery pump is of limited value.

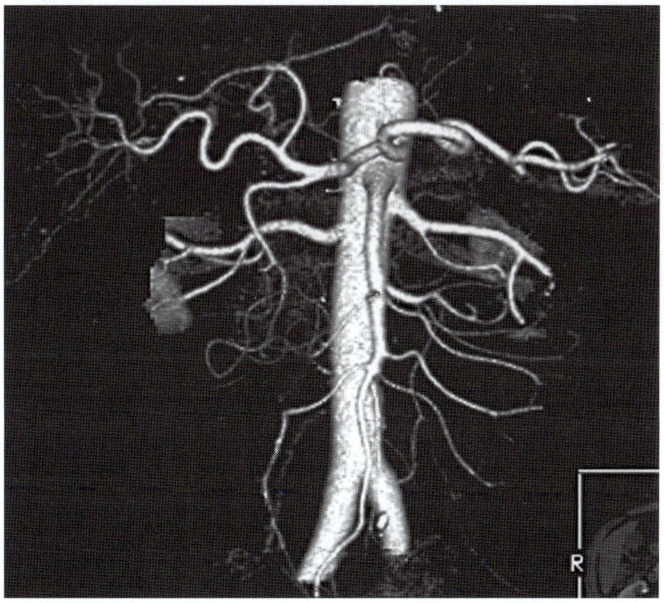

Figure 42-1.

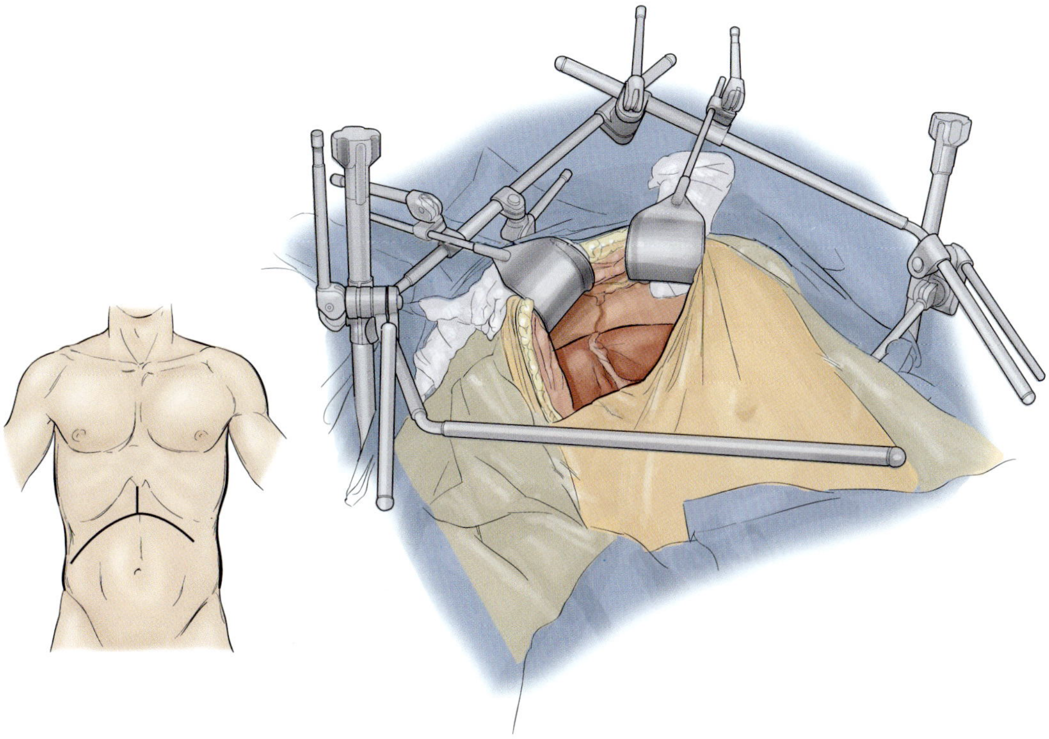

Figure 42-2.

The Portal Area

- The area of the porta hepatis needs to be examined for enlarged lymph nodes (Fig. 42-3). A manual palpation using a finger posteriorly into the foramen of Winslow is useful to appreciate enlarged nodes in the area of the porta hepatis. These nodes need to be excised and sent to pathology. If they are found to contain cancer, the use of the pump needs to be reconsidered.

Cholecystectomy

- A cholecystectomy is performed to avoid a chemical cholecystitis secondary to the chemotherapy given via the hepatic artery infusion pump. Because the cystic artery usually originates off the right hepatic artery, pump therapy will infuse the gallbladder with high doses of chemotherapy, which can cause necrosis of the mucosa of the gallbladder. To prevent this acalculous cholecystitis, the cholecystectomy is performed.

Preparation of the Gastroduodenal Artery

- The common hepatic artery should be identified. Careful dissection on the anterior aspect of this artery should take place to identify the takeoff of the GDA (Fig. 42-4). The preoperative radiologic pictures of the arteries should help to recognize the approximate area of this takeoff. The GDA should be skeletonized from its origin off the common hepatic artery, distally for approximately 2 cm. Care should be taken to ligate or cauterize any small lymphatics running along side of the GDA. The artery must be completely cleaned in all directions.

Dissection of the Hepatic Artery

- The common hepatic artery must be dissected out 2 cm proximal and distal to the GDA takeoff to the bifurcation into the left and right hepatics. The artery must be completely skeletonized so that any small branches are ligated or cauterized. The artery must be lifted to make sure there are no branches posteriorly. Using a vein retractor can help with this maneuver. Once the hepatic artery and the GDA are completely free, the area is ready for the pump implantation. If any branches are left, they can cause infusion of high-dose chemotherapy into the stomach, duodenum, or pancreas. This can result in a number of complications including duodenitis, gastritis, ulcerations, and pancreatitis.

Formation of the Subcutaneous Pocket for the Hepatic Artery Infusion Pump

- A subcutaneous pocket must be made for the pump placement (Fig. 42-5). The pump must be accessed percutaneously, similar to a long-term venous access port. It should not be placed so deeply that the

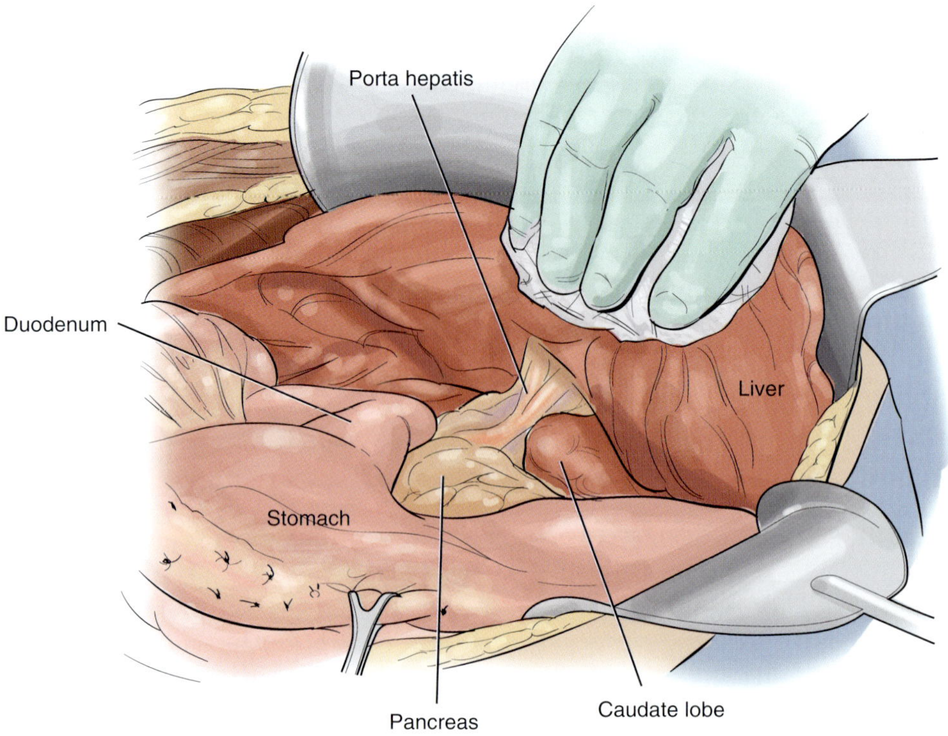

Figure 42-3.

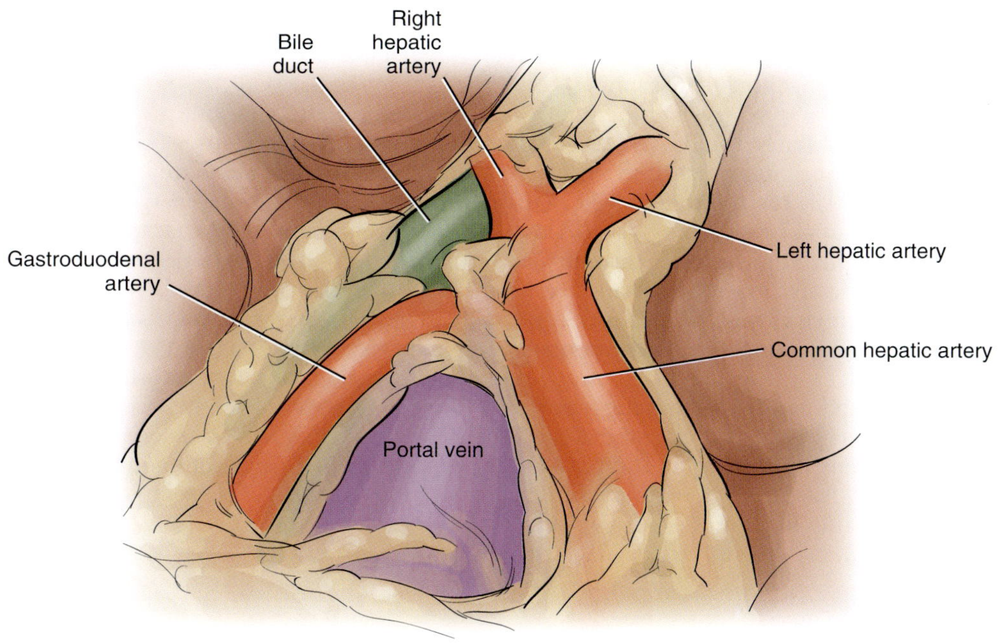

Figure 42-4.

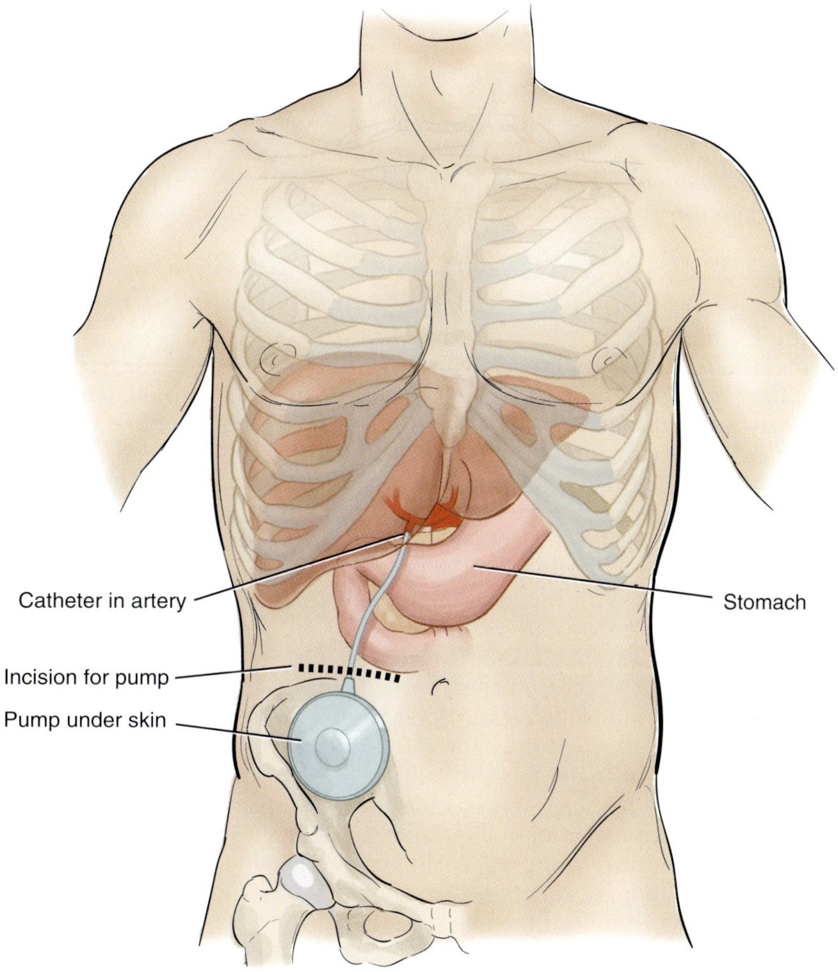

Figure 42-5.

needle cannot reach the pump. On the other hand, it should not be placed too superficially, because the pump can erode through the skin, especially in patients who are losing weight because of cancer cachexia. The left upper quadrant of the abdomen is preferable because it removes the pump from the area of the liver for subsequent scanning.

- If there is a colostomy on the left, the pump can be placed on the right, but it should be in the right lower quadrant of the abdomen, to prevent distortion on subsequent scans.
- The pocket is formed just anterior to the fascia. Three Kocher clamps are placed on the midline fascia on the left side. The top clamp is placed at the same level as the midcostal margin, and this serves as a marker of the upper end of the pocket. This allows the pump pocket to be fashioned below the ribs. If the pump is placed too high, it can rub against the ribs and cause the patient discomfort.
- The next two clamps are placed at approximately 3-cm intervals on the fascia below the first. Then tension is placed on the fascia with these three clamps, and the pump pocket is formed just anterior to the rectus abdominis fascia. This can be done with an electrocautery.
- All small bleeders must be cauterized. Any bleeding in the pocket can cause a postoperative hematoma in the pocket and make accessing the pump problematic.
- If the patient has a very thick abdominal wall, the pump pocket should be made more subcutaneous, instead of directly on the fascia. The pocket is made large enough to accommodate the pump when closed, and still leave enough of a rim of fascia to close the abdomen. The pump can be placed in the pocket temporarily to aid in the sizing of the pocket.

Priming the Pump

- Before the pump is placed in the patient, it must be primed in the operating room. The pump is placed on a sterile warmer, and 30 mL of warmed heparinized saline (1000 units/mL) is placed into the pump with a Huber needle (the noncoring needles). The pump catheter must be flushed. If it is a Codman pump, a special bolus needle is necessary for this.
- The pump must be kept on a warmer until there is a bead of fluid in the opening of the catheter. This signifies that the pump is working.
- If the pump is not primed, putting it into the artery may cause a back-flow of blood into the catheter and subsequent clotting of the catheter. Warming the pump sufficiently is a necessary step to prevent this.

Placement of the Pump into the Pocket

- Once the pump is primed and the pocket is made, the pump is placed into the pocket. A right-angle clamp is used to perforate the abdominal wall from the inside of the abdomen to the middle of the pump pocket. The catheter tip is placed into the jaws of the clamp and pulled into the abdomen. The pump is placed into the pocket so that it does not cool down while the catheter is being placed into the artery.

Insertion of the Catheter

- The catheter is cut at an oblique angle before insertion, leaving enough catheter distal to the first plastic ring to reach from the arteriotomy site to the opening of the GDA into the hepatic artery (Fig. 42-6). The GDA is then ligated distally with a 2-0 silk tie, and a clamp is placed on the silk to be able to put tension on the GDA. A vascular clamp is placed on the proximal GDA just at the takeoff of the GDA from the hepatic artery (see Fig. 42-6).
- Care should be taken not to include the hepatic artery with this clamp. The catheter should not extend into the hepatic artery; this helps prevent any future occlusion of the hepatic artery. An arteriotomy is then made in the GDA between the clamp and the ligature, but near the suture ligature. It is often simpler to use a Potts scissors for this arteriotomy rather than a no. 11 scalpel blade.
- The catheter is then fed into the GDA so that the tip of the catheter is flush with the opening of the GDA into the hepatic artery. If the catheter is placed so it is sitting in the GDA rather than being flush with the ostia, this might allow chemotherapy to pool in the GDA. The high concentration could cause a perforation in the GDA, with subsequent problems. On the other hand, if the catheter is placed too far into the hepatic artery, it may cause an occlusion of the hepatic artery. The small plastic vascular introducer is very helpful when guiding the catheter into the artery.
- Controlling the catheter with forceps, the vascular clamp is opened to allow the catheter to be pushed through. The clamp is then closed onto the catheter, holding it in place.
- The catheter is secured in place using a 2-0 silk ligature, tying knots proximal and distal to the most distal plastic ring of the pump catheter, which should be positioned at the arteriotomy of the GDA (Fig. 42-7). The vascular clamp can then be removed.
- The distal tie, which was previously placed on the GDA, is also tied around the catheter behind the middle plastic ring (see Fig. 42-7). If there are known accessory or replaced hepatic arteries, they should be ligated at this time. The catheter is then securely in place, and its stability can be tested by

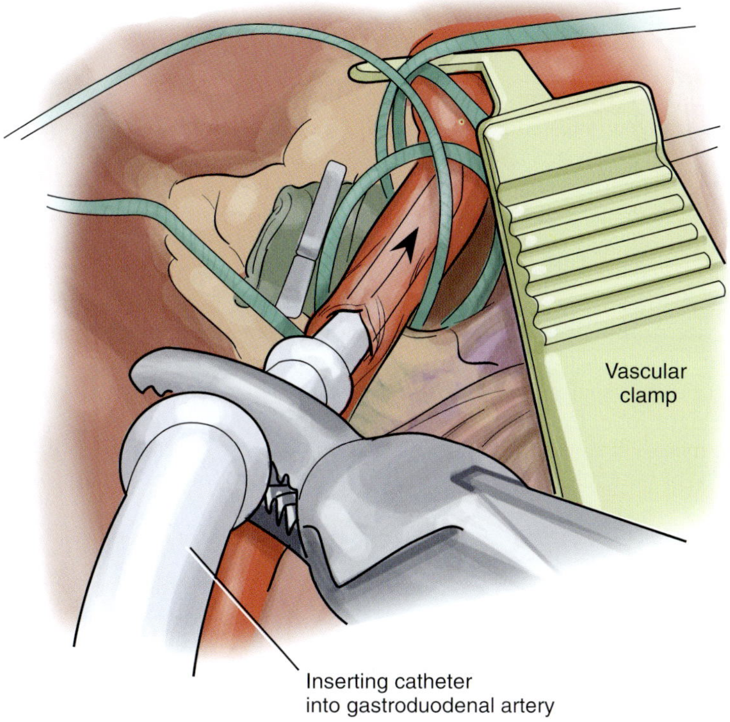

Figure 42-6.

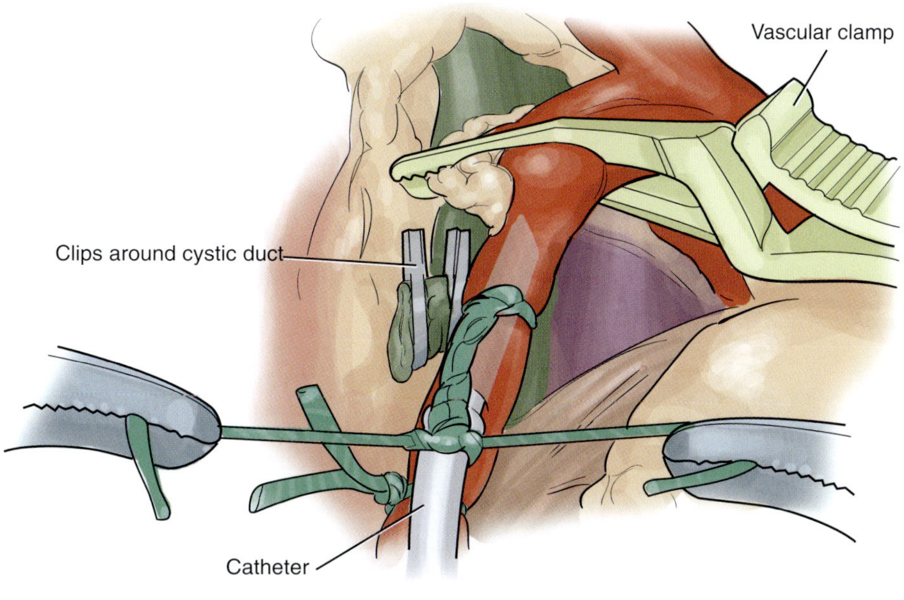

Figure 42-7.

tugging lightly on the catheter. There should be no bleeding or oozing at the entrance of the catheter into the artery (Fig. 42-8).

Testing the Hepatic Artery Infusion Pump Perfusion

- The pump perfusion pattern is tested by injecting fluorescein dye into the pump. The pump must be removed from the pocket. Before the dye is injected into the catheter (depending on the make of pump, this is via the side port or with a special bolus needle), the liver must be exposed so that both the left and right lobes can be seen, as well as the lesser curvature of the stomach. The lights in the operating room should be turned off, and only the Woods lamp should be illuminated.
- The dye is then injected followed by a 10-mL flush of heparin solution at 100 units/mL. The liver is inspected to make sure there is good perfusion of dye in both lobes. The stomach is also inspected to be sure the flow is not running retrograde into the stomach or duodenum. If there is no perfusion in one area of the liver, an accessory artery to that area must be identified and ligated. If the area is in the left lobe, the accessory usually runs in the gastrohepatic ligament above the area of the celiac axis. If the area is in the right lobe, the accessory runs behind the portal vein in the porta hepatis. If these are not ligated, the liver will not be perfused with chemotherapy in that area. If flow is seen into the duodenum, stomach, or pancreas, small collateral vessels coming off the hepatic artery must be identified and ligated.

Closure

- The pump is then replaced into the subcutaneous pocket. A 0-chromic suture is used to secure the pump to the fascia through the holes on the side of the pump (see Fig. 42-5). The pocket is then closed using 0-chromic interrupted sutures from the fascia below to the subcutaneous tissue above, making sure to leave enough fascia to close the midline wound securely. The sutures should be placed at overlapping intervals so that the pocket is watertight to prevent any wound problems affecting the pump pocket.
- We prefer interrupted sutures to close the abdomen. No drains are necessary.

III. ALTERNATIVE TECHNICAL APPROACHES (PRO/CON) AND PEARLS

- The procedure also can be approached laparoscopically or with robotic assistance. The Suggested Readings at the end of this chapter serve as a resource for readers. Surgeons, however, should have experience with complex laparoscopic procedures, a sound familiarity with open-pump placement technique, and knowledge of the biology of the disease to allow proper patient selection.

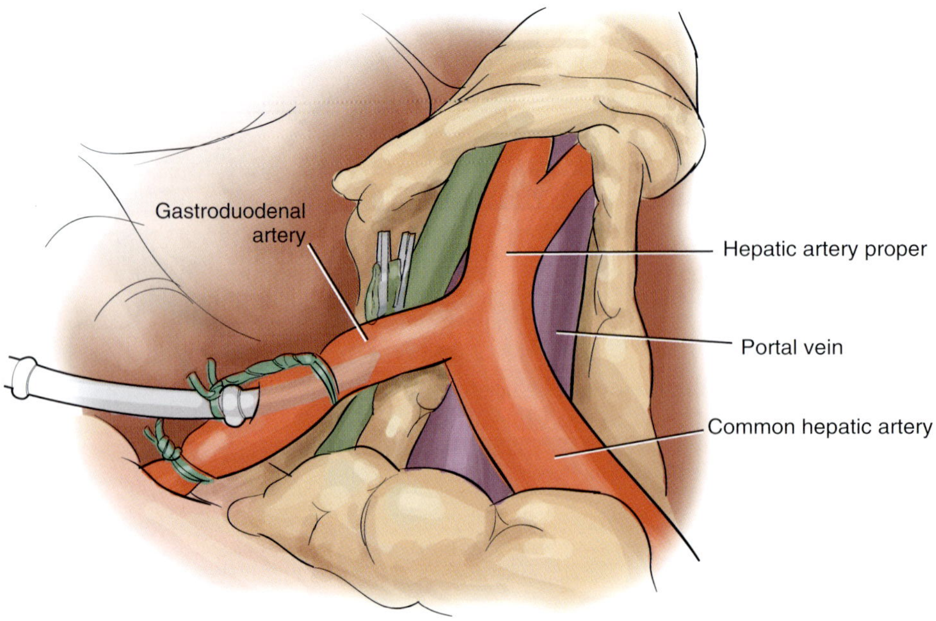

Figure 42-8.

- Patients who may not be surgical candidates may be considered for percutaneous placement of hepatic artery infusion pumps.
- To avoid misperfusion, it is important intraoperatively to recognize and ligate any accessory or replaced hepatic artery circulation. If for some reason these cannot be dealt with intraoperatively, then selective angioembolization can be performed postoperatively.
- The catheter should be placed to minimize turbulent flow and allow good runoff of the infused chemotherapeutic agent to ensure long-term patency of the catheter and the associated vessel.

IV. SPECIAL POSTOPERATIVE CARE

- Postoperative care is routine for abdominal procedures. Diet typically is started the night of the procedure. Perioperative intravenous antibiotics should be continued until the patient is discharged.

SUGGESTED READINGS

Kemeny M: Hepatic artery infusion of chemotherapy as a treatment for hepatic metastases from colorectal cancer, *Cancer J* 8:s82–s88, 2002.

Kemeny MM, Hogan JM, Goldberg DA, et al: Continuous hepatic artery infusion with an implantable pump: problems with hepatic artery anomalies, *Surgery* 99:501–504, 1986.

Kemeny NE, Kemeny MM, Lawrence TS: Liver metastases. In Abeloff MD, Armitage JO, Niederhuber JE, et al, editors: *Clinical oncology*, ed 3, New York, 2004, Churchill Livingstone, pp 1141–1178.

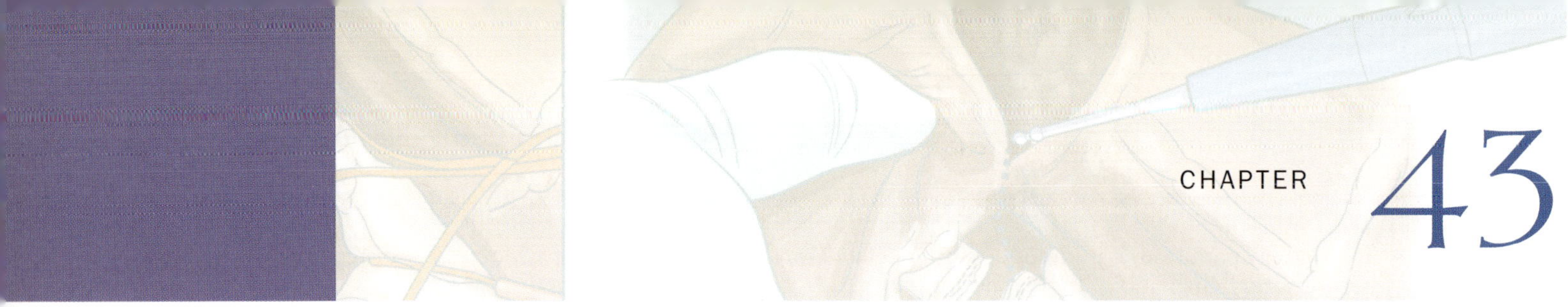

CHAPTER 43

Resection Hilar Cholangiocarcinoma with En Bloc Hepatectomy

Daniel Cherqui, MD, and Henri Bismuth, MD, FACS(Hon)

I. SPECIAL PREOPERATIVE PREPARATION

- Patients with obstructive jaundice and suspected hilar cholangiocarcinoma (HC) should be referred to a specialized center if possible before any invasive imaging or biliary drainage procedure is performed because such procedures may interfere with further staging or management of the disease.

Noninvasive Imaging

- Excellent imaging evaluation is required. Diagnosis is usually rather easy in the presence of jaundice and intrahepatic bile duct dilatation without an enlarged extrahepatic bile duct, typical of hilar bile duct obstruction. The tumor is usually small and infiltrative and may be difficult to individualize. The main goal of imaging is staging with special attention to the level of biliary obstruction (see Fig. 43-4) and the extension to hilar vascular structures (i.e., portal vein and hepatic artery).
- Ultrasound examination is usually the first examination showing bilateral intrahepatic bile duct dilatation above the hilar obstacle. The extrahepatic bile duct and gallbladder are not enlarged. Doppler examination of hilar vascular structures is useful.
- Dynamic postcontrast computed tomography (CT) scan confirms bile duct dilation, shows the level of obstruction, and assesses vascular structures and locoregional extension. The early arterial phase is used for arterial assessment. The venous phase is useful for portal evaluation and is the best phase for bile duct evaluation facilitated by portal enhancement (Fig. 43-1). New multidetector CT scans are of great value for vascular evaluation and reconstructions (Fig. 43-2, *A* and *B*). The tumor may be seen on the late vascular phase because of its dominant fibrous component. Volumetric evaluation of the liver is also required, including whole liver, right liver, left liver, and segment I volumes, allowing the surgeon to calculate the future liver remnant volume according to the planned procedure.
- Magnetic resonance imaging (MRI), especially with the advent of magnetic resonance cholangiography (MRCP), has been a major advance by providing excellent quality planar cholangiography and therefore accurately showing the level of obstruction (Fig. 43-3). Vascular and volumetric studies can also be performed by MRI, but these are challenged by the most recent multidetector CTs.
- At the present time, most experts recommend a combination of dynamic CT and MRCP for best assessment and decision making. This may also take into account local availability and expertise.

Invasive Procedures

- Diagnostic percutaneous transhepatic cholangiography (PTC) and endoscopic retrograde cholangiopancreatography (ERCP) should not be performed and have been replaced by CT and MRI. In addition, these procedures expose the patient to a risk of cholangitis (and also bile peritonitis and hemobilia for PTC) and therefore require biliary drainage of all opacified ducts during the same procedure. Early biliary drainage before complete imaging assessment should not be performed because it can interfere with staging and management. Therefore, PTC or ERCP should only performed after complete imaging evaluation and should be the first step of biliary drainage, if the latter is required.

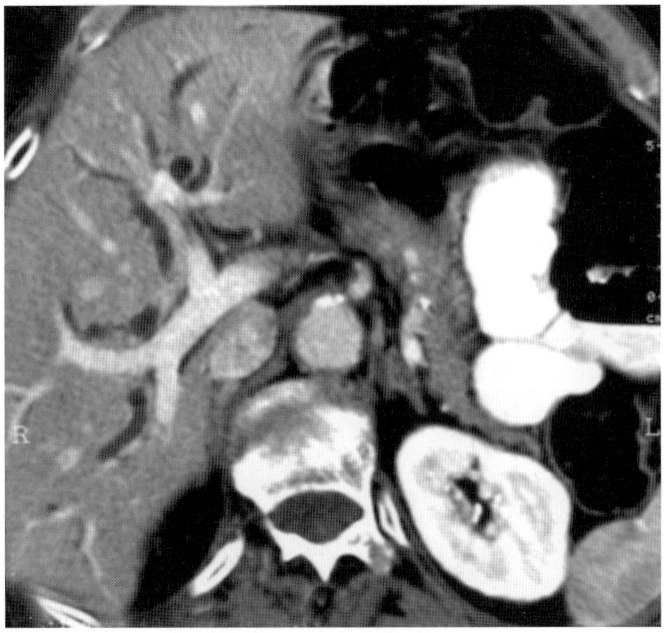

Figure 43-1. Type 2 operable hilar cholangiocarcinoma. Contrast-enhanced computed tomography showing dilated bile ducts, confluence separation without extension to secondary ducts, and no apparent vascular invasion.

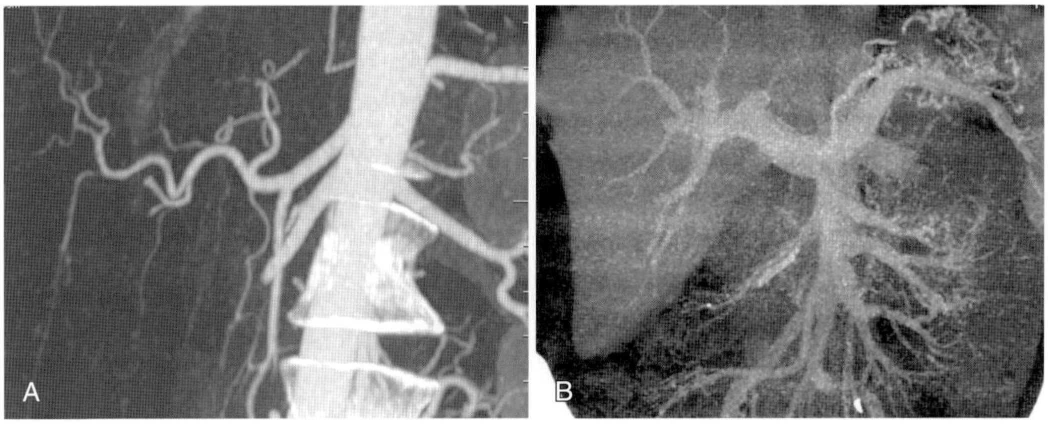

Figure 43-2. Computed tomography vascular reconstruction in an operable hilar cholangiocarcinoma. A, Arterial reconstruction showing no vascular encasement. **B,** Portal reconstruction showing left portal vein obstruction, which is not a contraindication to left hepatectomy.

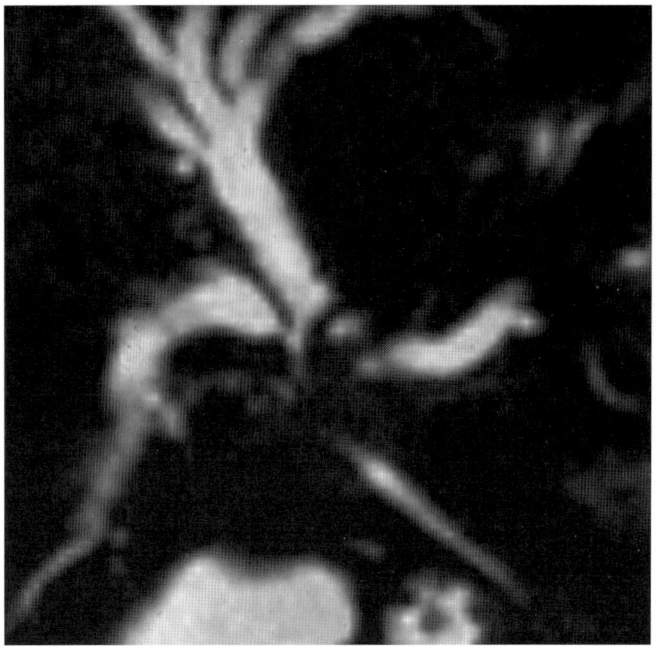

Figure 43-3. Magnetic resonance cholangiogram in an operable type 3a hilar cholangiocarcinoma. The tumor separates the biliary confluence and extends to the secondary ducts on the right. Indication for extended right hepatectomy.

- Celiac and mesenteric arteriography is no longer indicated as it has been replaced by CT or magnetic resonance angiograms.
- Endoscopic ultrasound is of limited value in hilar biliary obstruction and should be omitted.
- Tissue diagnosis is rarely available preoperatively because of the difficulty obtaining adequate samples. However, bile cytology or tumor brush biopsy samples obtained during biliary drainage procedures can be of value. This accounts for occasional resections of benign biliary strictures mimicking HC.

Resectability and Preparation for Surgery

- The level of biliary obstruction guides the type of resection according to the Bismuth classification (Fig. 43-4):
  - Type 1 (obstruction below the confluence) is rare and is treated by bile duct resection.
  - Type 2 (obstruction separating right and left biliary confluence without extension to secondary bile ducts) can theoretically be treated by bile duct resection in association with resection of segment I, but extended right hepatectomy is usually associated as it increases radicality and the rate of R0 resections.
  - Type 3 (obstruction separating right and left biliary confluence with extension to right, type 3a, or left, type 3b, secondary bile ducts) requires extended right or left hepatectomy, according to the side of biliary extension. In both cases segment I should be included in the resection. In type 3a, the most radical procedure is right hepatectomy extended to segments IV and I.
  - Type 4 (obstruction extending to both right and left secondary bile ducts) is theoretically a contraindication to resection and a marginal indication for liver transplantation. However, extended hepatectomies can occasionally be applied to these cases.
- Vascular invasion assessed as presented is probably the major limiting factor in resectability. It is marked by extrinsic vascular encasement seen as an irregular vessel caliber of the portal vein, hepatic artery, or their branches. Invasion of the main portal vein or common hepatic artery is a contraindication to resection (Fig. 43-5, *B*). Vascular invasion of the vascular branches ipsilateral to the biliary extension is not a contraindication to surgery. Vascular invasion of the vascular branches contralateral to the biliary extension is a contraindication to resection. Invasion of the portal or arterial bifurcation may be an indication for additional vascular resection and reconstruction in selected cases.
- Gross invasion of locoregional lymph nodes is as a contraindication to surgery when detected preoperatively (see Fig. 43-5, *A*).
- Distant metastases or peritoneal carcinomatosis are rarely detected preoperatively and are contraindications to surgery.
- Staging laparoscopy has not proved its efficacy in improving selection for resection and is not usually recommended.

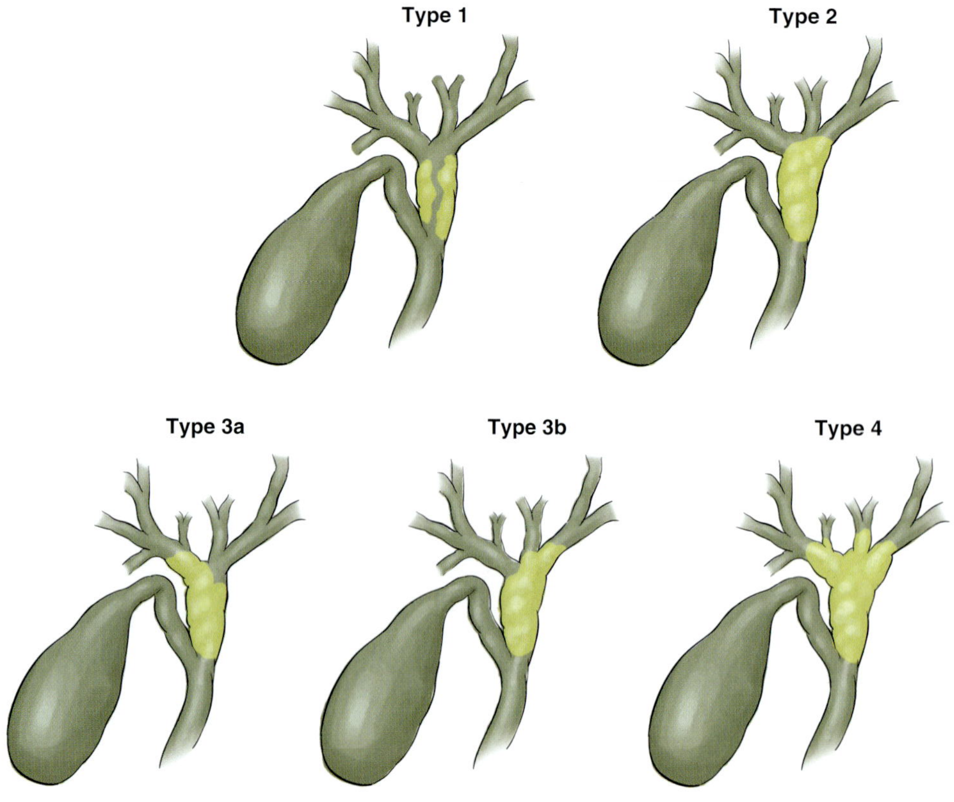

Figure 43-4.

Preoperative Biliary Drainage and Portal Vein Embolization

- The debate continues on the necessity of preoperative biliary drainage (PBD).
- Most authors recommend preoperative PBD in all patients with increased serum bilirubin to relieve the effect of biliary obstruction on the liver parenchyma associated with an increased risk of bleeding during transection and of postresection liver failure. Percutaneous or endoscopic drainage can be applied, depending on local availability and expertise. In cases where biliary confluence is separated, unilateral or bilateral drainage can be used. In case of unilateral drainage, the liver lobe to be spared during resection is the one that must be drained. However, all opacified segments of the liver must be drained to avoid cholangitis, the main complication of biliary drainage. Surgery is usually performed when serum bilirubin is less than 50 μmol/L.
- A smaller number of authors have a more selective approach to PBD, arguing that patients with recent jaundice and mild increased serum bilirubin (i.e., less than 150 to 200 μmol /L) can be operated without drainage, avoiding the risk of biliary superinfection and cholangitis. This is when the future liver remnant is sufficient, as is the case when unilateral liver atrophy is present and in the majority of left-sided resections (Fig. 43-6).
- Liver resection for HC removes functional parenchyma only because the tumor is small and located in the hilar bile ducts, not in the liver. Therefore, estimation of the future liver remnant is very important, and a 30% to 40% remnant is required. Smaller remnants are usually observed when an extended right hepatectomy is anticipated. In such cases, preoperative percutaneous portal vein embolization (PVE) of the right liver is recommended to increase the volume of the future remaining left lobe (Fig. 43-7). Rarely, PVE of the left liver in preparation for extended left hepatectomy is proposed. PVE should be always be preceded by PBD when jaundice is present. Surgery is usually performed 1 month after PVE.

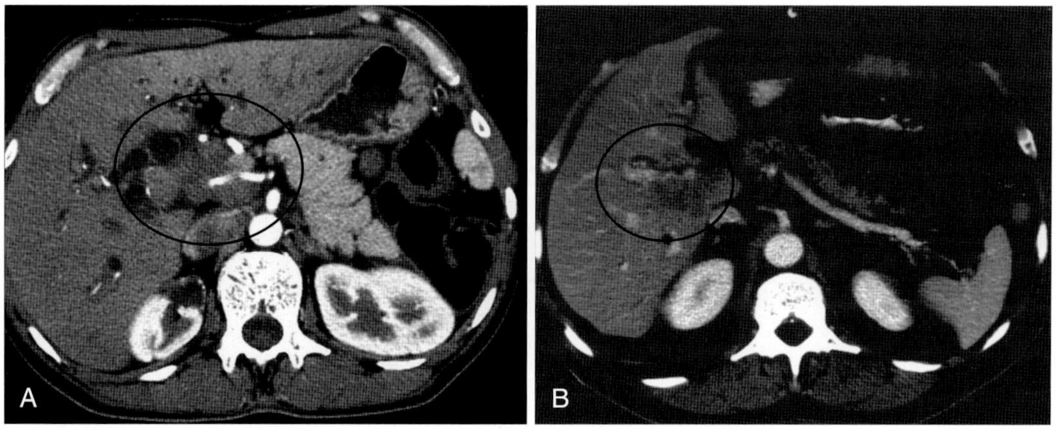

Figure 43-5. Inoperable hilar cholangiocarcinomas because of major lymph node metastases (**A**) and portal vein invasion (**B**).

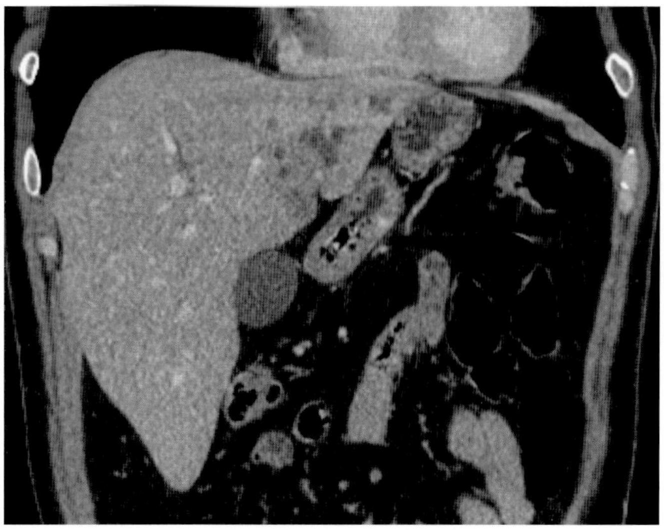

Figure 43-6. Type 3b hilar cholangiocarcinoma, Bile duct dilatation is more pronounced on the left side, and left liver is atrophic. Left hepatectomy without biliary drainage or portal vein embolization is possible.

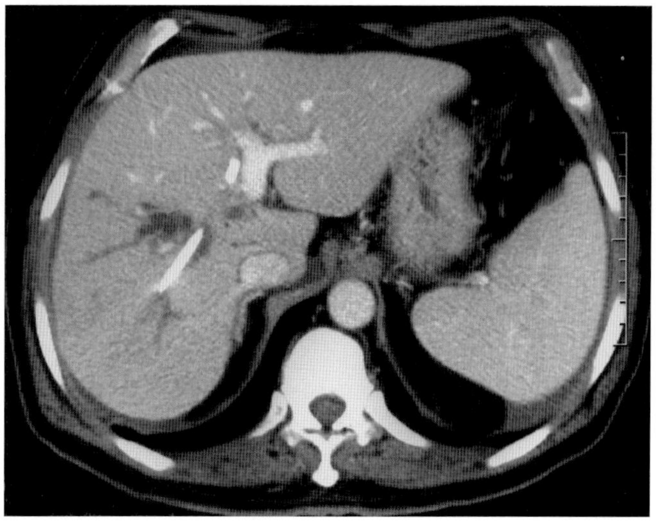

Figure 43-7. Type 3a hilar cholangiocarcinoma. Bilateral stents are in place, and portal vein embolization has resulted in hypertrophied left lobe.

II. OPERATIVE TECHNIQUE

- The principle of surgical treatment for HC is to obtain an R0 resection. This is achieved by en bloc extrahepatic bile duct and liver resection with hepatic pedicle lymphadenectomy. Because of specific biliary drainage of the caudate lobe at the level of the hilum, segment I should be included in the liver resection in all cases (Fig. 43-8). Biliary reconstruction is obtained by means of proximal bilioenteric anastomosis to a Roux-en-Y loop. One or several lobar, sectional, or even segmental bile ducts may be anastomosed to the bowel loop. When appropriate, additional vascular resections and reconstructions may be required (i.e., portal vein or hepatic artery bifurcation).
- Because of the infiltrative nature of HC, it is difficult to ascertain the quality of surgical margins macroscopically. Frozen sections are recommended to assess biliary or vascular surgical margins. However, these should only be done if their result will affect the surgical procedure.
- The side of the liver resection is in most instances decided on preoperative imaging, although intraoperative findings may occasionally result in a different procedure. The description of the procedure will include three parts: surgical exploration and pedicular dissection; liver resection; and biliary reconstruction.
- Although the quality of preoperative assessment has attained high accuracy with modern imaging, contraindications to resection may yet be found at surgery. These include peritoneal carcinomatosis, liver metastases, and encasement of the porta hepatis or celiac region by lymph node metastases. These should be confirmed by frozen section.

Position

- The patient is placed in supine position.

Incision

- The operation is started with a right subcostal incision. After contraindications to resection are eliminated, the incision is extended to a bilateral subcostal incision with midline extension to the xiphoid. A large incision is required for a safe procedure.

Main Dissection

Exploration and Pedicular Dissection

- The tumor may be visible at the liver hilus (at the reflection of the hilar plate with segment IV) as a small growth sometimes associated with peritoneal umbilication. In many instances the tumor is not visible but palpable. Occasionally, it is neither visible nor palpable, which remains consistent with the diagnosis. Intraoperative ultrasound is required for exploration, although its yield is reduced in the presence of biliary stents. It is used to assess biliary and vascular extensions.
- The size, color, and consistency of the liver are assessed, as well as the volume of the anticipated future liver remnant. In the absence of PBD, the liver is usually cholestatic (green) and firm, whereas it has a normal appearance when efficient PBD has been performed. When PVE has been performed, the embolized lobe should be hypotrophic while the spared lobe is enlarged.
- Intrahepatic biliary extension is very difficult to assess and a diagnosis relies mainly on preoperative imaging, palpation, and intraoperative ultrasound. Occasionally, transcystic or transhepatic intraoperative cholangiography can be used in patients without biliary stents in place.
- Exploration and dissection of the hepatoduodenal ligament is the next step. It is important to not perform any irreversible division before the possibility of resection is confirmed. The frequent presence of stents in the bile duct may help in their identification, although they may also interfere with tumor assessment. The gallbladder can be removed en bloc with the specimen, but cholecystectomy or simple cystic duct division help the dissection, provided these structures are at a distance from the tumorous area. The peritoneum is then incised behind the bile duct, exposing the portal vein which is encircled. An additional right hepatic artery originating from the superior mesenteric artery may be present and can be preserved at this stage. Dissection is continued to expose the arterial and portal bifurcations, and vascular invasion is assessed (Fig. 43-9).
- The surgeon must decide whether the tumor is resectable and the type of liver resection required according to the pre- and intraoperative exploration.

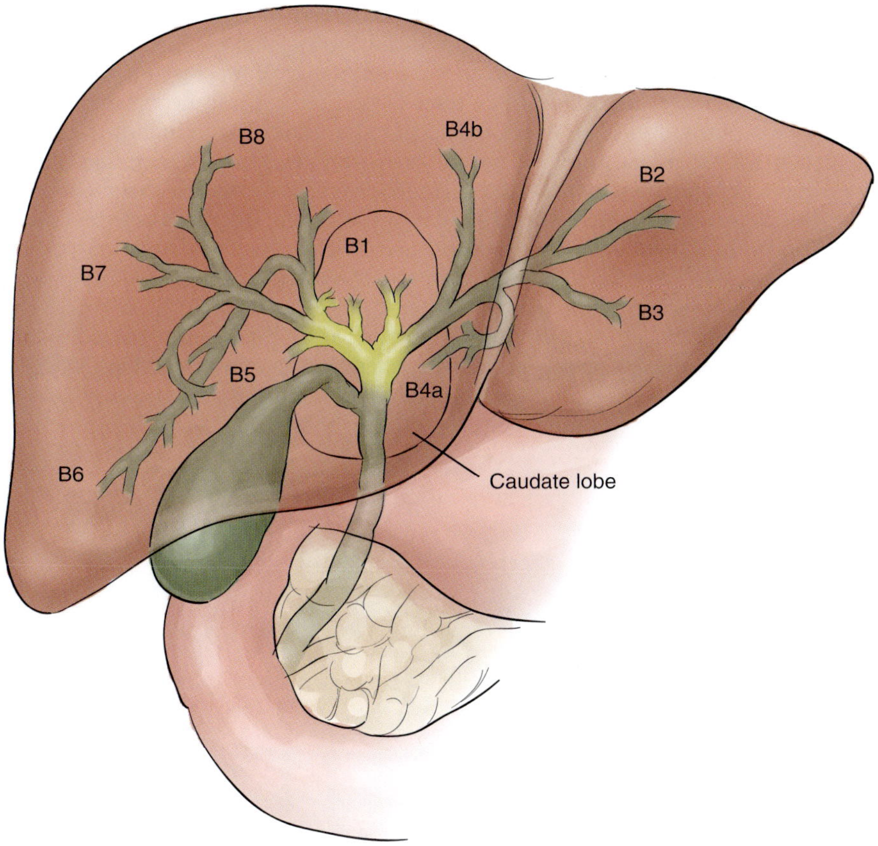

Figure 43-8.

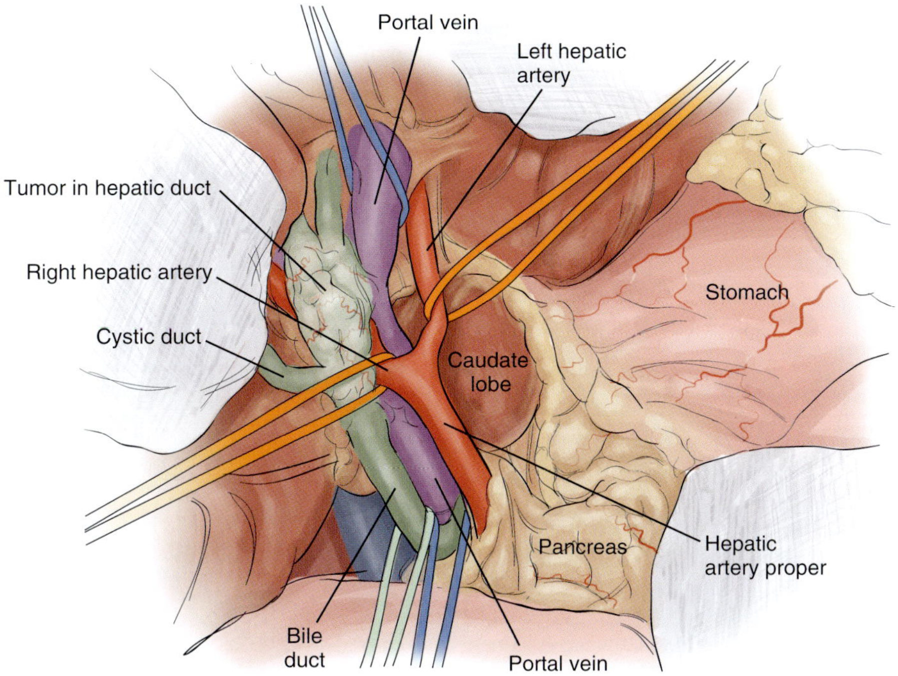

Figure 43-9.

- If the tumor is resectable, the common bile duct is divided just above the duodenum and a frozen section is done (Fig. 43-10). If positive, a more distal intrapancreatic bile duct division is performed or an associated pancreaticoduodenectomy may be required. When present, stents are removed, and bile samples are always sent for culture. Bile duct dissection is continued cranially for better exploration of the vascular structures (Fig. 43-11). The portal and arterial branches to the resected lobe are divided (right or left hepatic arterial and portal branches), thus devascularizing the lobe. In the case of extended right hepatectomy, pedicles to segment IV can be divided extrahepatically on the right side of the round ligament, at this stage, or later in the procedure, by a transparenchymal approach during transection. Inflow pedicles to segment I are divided flush with the left pedicle during right-sided resections, whereas they are included with the specimen during left-sided resections.
- Resection and reconstruction of the portal or arterial bifurcation may be required in about 10% of cases. The invaded segment of these vessels is resected to reach a healthy vascular wall on both sides, and the trunk is anastomosed to the branch destined to the preserved lobe using vascular suture techniques derived from partial graft liver transplantation (Fig. 43-12). In most cases a direct anastomosis is possible, although a graft may occasionally be required.

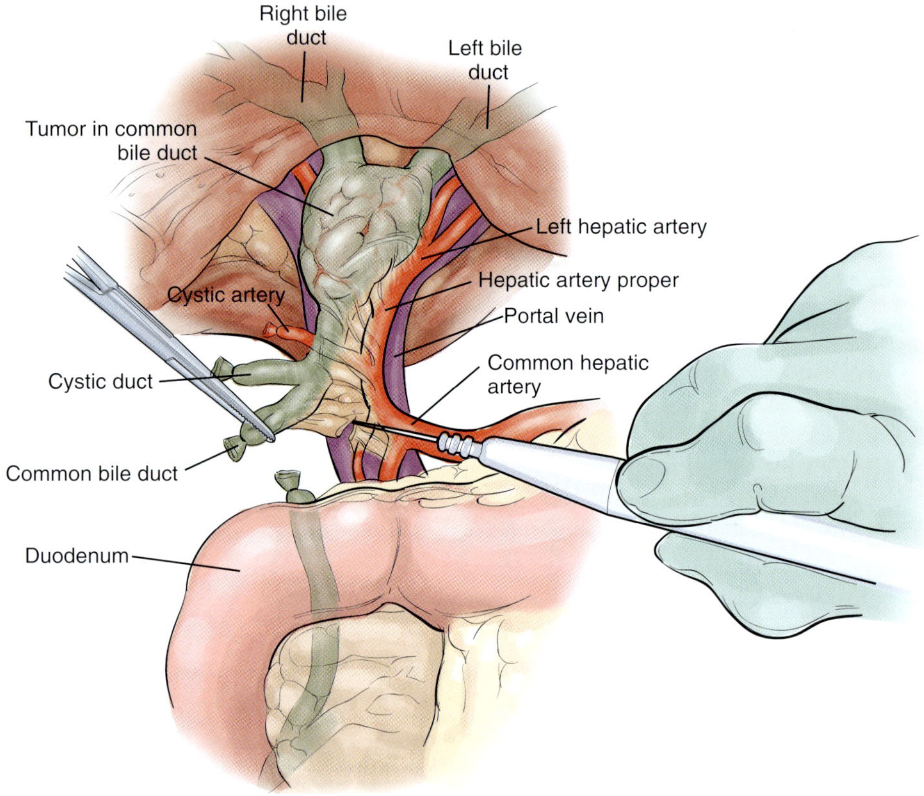

Figure 43-10.

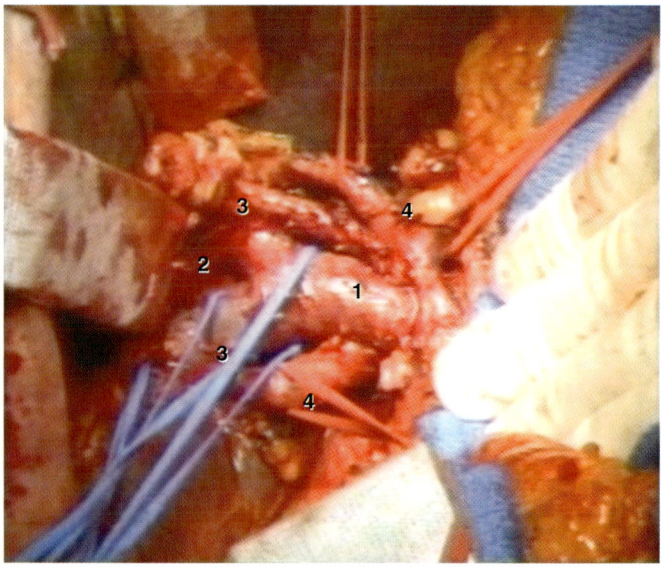

Figure 43-11. Retrograde dissection of the liver hilus after bile duct division with skeletonization of the portal trunk (*1*), bifurcation (*2*), and branches (*3*) and of arterial branches (*4*).

- To achieve the maximal biliary clearance margin, bile duct division is left for a later stage by a transparenchymal approach when transection has reached the bile duct level.
- Lymphadenectomy is also performed by skeletonizing the portal vein downward to the pancreas and the hepatic artery upward to the celiac axis. Retroperitoneal lymphadenectomy at the interaorticocaval and left renal vein regions may be associated (Fig. 43-13).

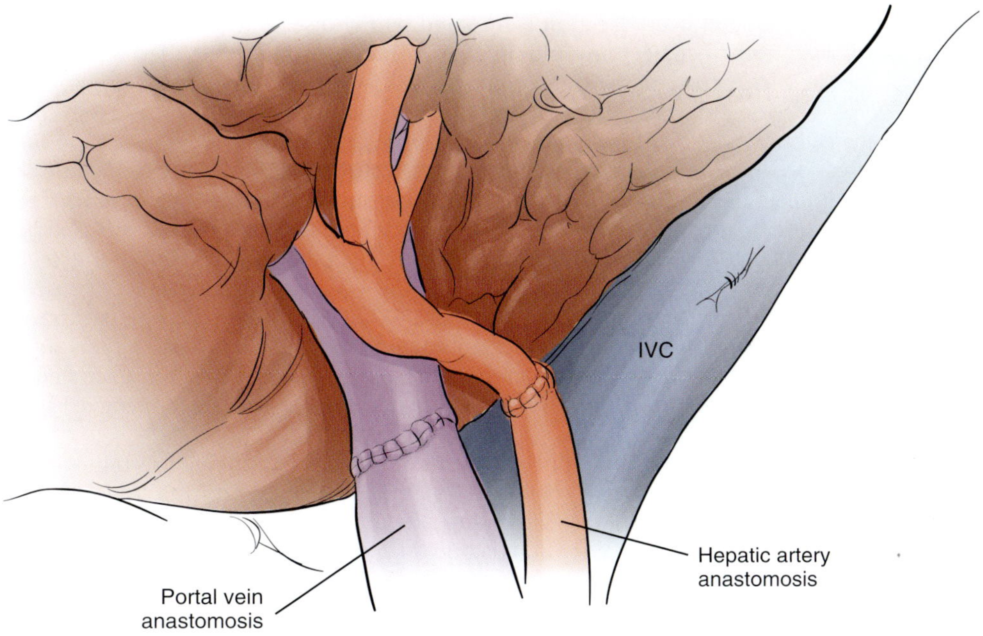

Figure 43-12. *IVC,* Inferior vena cava.

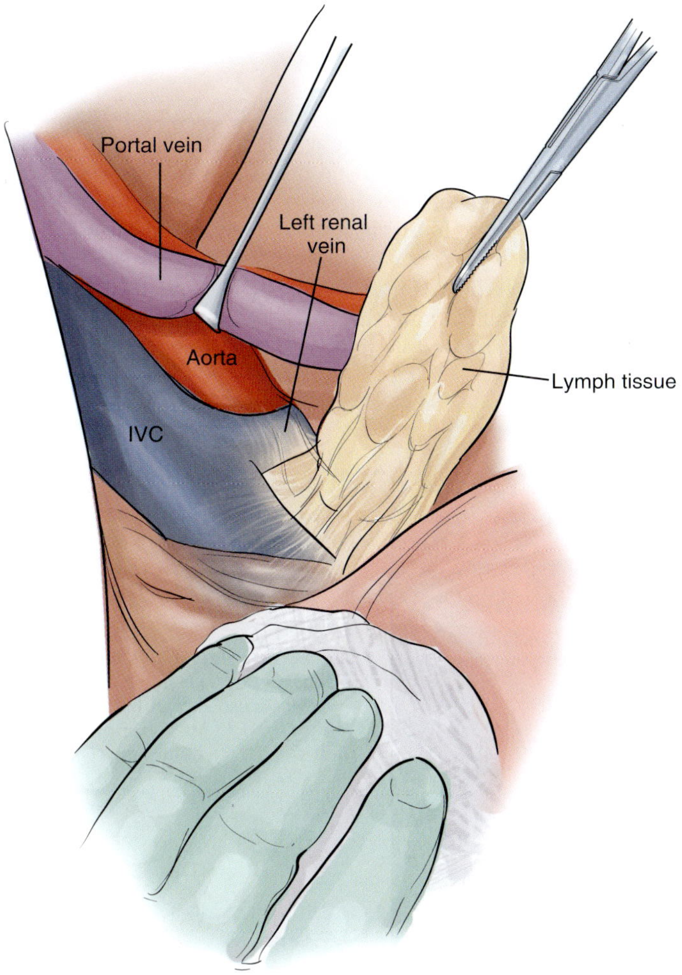

Figure 43-13. *IVC,* Inferior vena cava.

Liver Resection

- In the rare Bismuth type 1 tumors, bile duct resection alone may be sufficient. In the more typical Bismuth type 2 through 4 tumors, liver resection is required. In all cases, segment I should be removed because its bile ducts drain in the tumorous biliary confluence.
- In type 2 lesions, extended right hepatectomy (i.e., right hepatectomy plus segments I and IV) is the preferred option because the length of the left bile duct increases the chance of an R0 resection. However, this usually requires preoperative PVE to ensure a sufficient liver remnant volume.
- In type 3 lesions, the side of liver resection is imposed by the disease: extended right hepatectomy for type 3a lesions (i.e., right hepatectomy plus segments I and IV) and extended left hepatectomy for type 3b lesions (i.e., left hepatectomy plus segment I).
- Occasional type 4 lesions may be amenable to resection, but an R1 resection is more likely. In such cases, left hepatectomy extended to segments I, V, and VIII is an option.
- After hilar dissection, liver mobilization is performed. Because of the necessity to include segment I in the resection, complete mobilization of the caudate lobe from the inferior vena cava (IVC) is required. Right and left hepatic ligaments are divided. All accessory and spigelian hepatic veins are divided. Of note, when left hepatectomy is performed, the inferior right hepatic vein draining segment VI, if present, should be preserved. Complete separation of the IVC from the liver requires division of the retrocaval ligament on the right side of the retrohepatic IVC. On the left side, the peritoneal reflection between segment I and the right pillar of the diaphragm is divided to expose the left side of the retrocaval IVC. During caval dissection, the main hepatic veins are controlled and encircled. In the case of extended right hepatectomy, the right hepatic vein is divided at this stage using a vascular stapler (Fig. 43-14).
- Parenchymal transection is performed along ischemic margins determined by inflow division. Low central venous pressure anesthesia is recommended to reduce bleeding during transection. Because of previous extensive dissection and devascularization, pedicular clamping (i.e., the Pringle maneuver) may often be avoided. However, if even mild bleeding occurs, pedicular clamping is applied. Intermittent clamping is now the preferred technique (especially if the liver is cholestatic) with successive periods of 15-minute clamping and 5-minute revascularization. Pedicular clamping may be associated with clamping of the main hepatic veins to reduce back-flow bleeding, although low central venous pressure is usually sufficient. Total vascular exclusion (i.e., pedicular clamping combined with clamping of the IVC above and below the liver) is required in resection of HC.
- There are several transection techniques, but the one we recommend includes incision of the Glisson capsule with diathermy followed by parenchymal division with an ultrasonic aspirator or by Kelly clamp fracture. Vascular and biliary structures are treated with bipolar diathermy, clip, or ligatures, depending on their size.
- When transection has reached the Glisson sheath of the remaining portal pedicle, the intrahepatic bile duct is transected. This is a critical step because it will define the R quality of the resection. A frozen section should be performed only if a more distal bile duct division is possible, which is in fact rarely the case. Intrahepatic bile duct division may involve one or several bile ducts.
- After bile duct division, transection should be pursued up to the level of the main hepatic veins and should encompass segment I.
- In case of extended right hepatectomy (Fig. 43-15), the transection line moves to the left behind the left portal pedicle and head cranially along the Arantius fissure to include segment I. Care is taken to preserve the left portal pedicle. The middle hepatic vein in divided close to its end using a stapler or

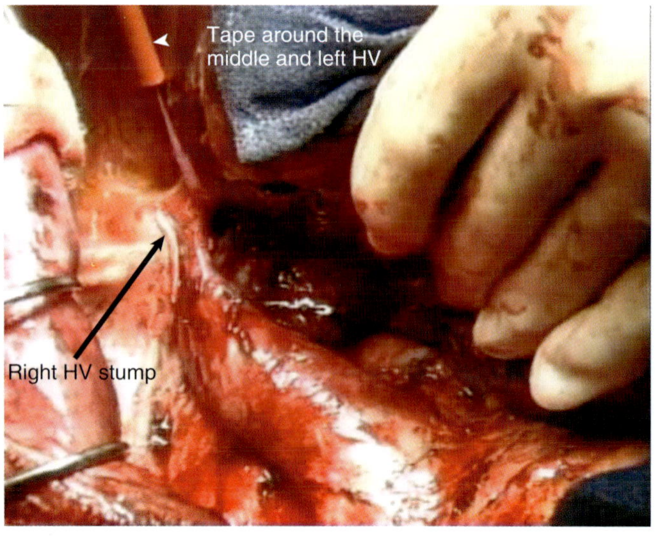

Figure 43-14. Mobilization of segment I from the inferior vena cava from the right side. The right hepatic vein has been divided with a stapler. *HV,* Hepatic vein.

over a clamp. The resection is concluded by division of the right hepatic vein using a stapler or over a clamp. The latter may also have been divided earlier in the procedure at the time of IVC dissection.

- In case of left-sided hepatectomy (Fig. 43-16), the transection line should continue directly to the midline of the IVC, thus including segment I. The transection line should progress along the exposed

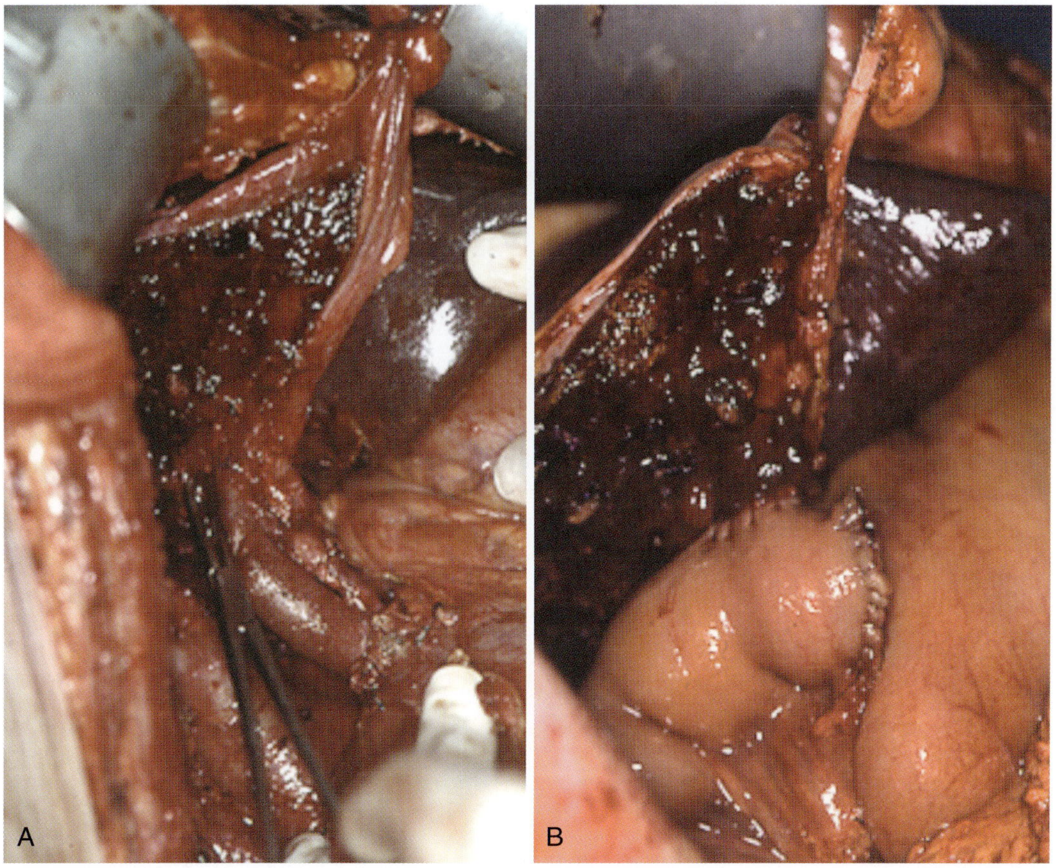

Figure 43-15. Extended right hepatectomy. View at the end of transection (**A**) and after Roux-en-Y hepaticojejunostomy (**B**).

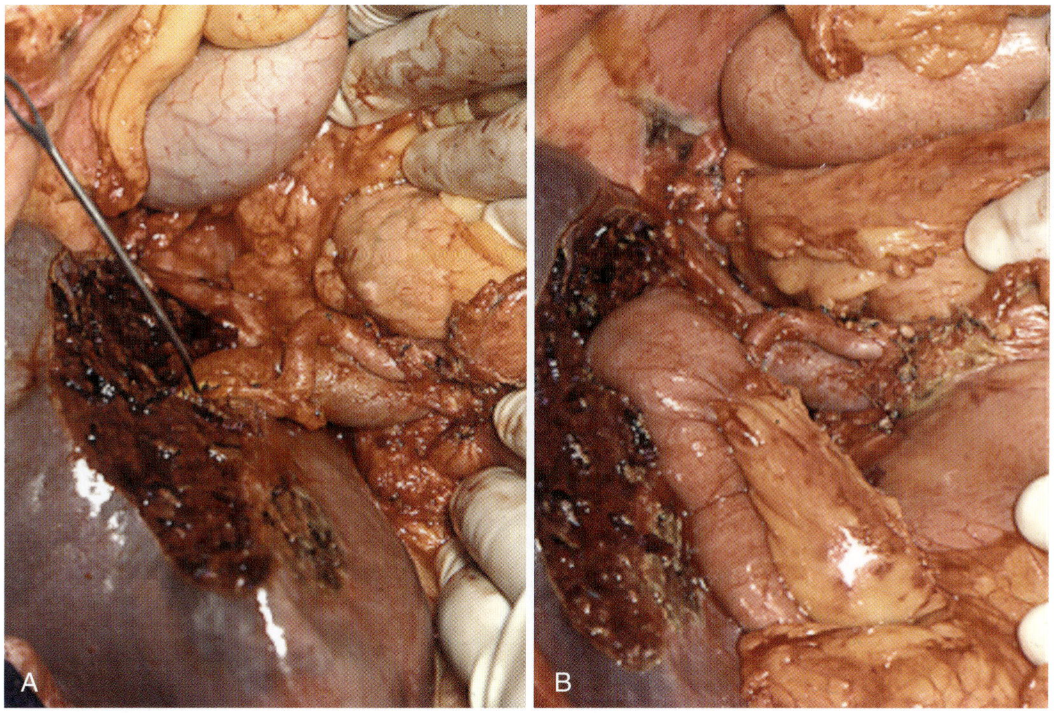

Figure 43-16. Extended left hepatectomy. View at the end of transection (**A**) and after Roux-en-Y hepaticojejunostomy (**B**).

left side of the middle hepatic vein, which should be preserved. Resection is concluded by division of the left hepatic vein with a stapler or over a clamp and is closed with a running 3-0 or 4-0 continuous suture.

Biliary Reconstruction

- Biliary reconstruction requires a Roux-en-Y loop with exclusion of 60 to 80 cm of bowel to avoid reflux cholangitis. The bowel loop is passed in a retrocolic fashion through the avascular area located just ventral of the head of the pancreas and duodenum.
- The bilioenteric anastomosis should include all the divided bile ducts exposed on the transection line. When several bile ducts are present and are close to one another, they can be joined in a single stoma by a series of interrupted 6-0 absorbable monofilament sutures. In other cases, several anastomoses are required. In right-sided hepatectomies, up to four bile may need to be reconstructed, whereas in left-sided resections, there are one or two bile ducts to reconstruct. The bilioenteric anastomoses are facilitated by the prior bile duct dilation, although PBD often has reduced the intrahepatic bile duct caliber (Fig. 43-17).
- End-to-side bilioenteric anastomosis is performed (see Figs. 43-15 and 43-16). Multiple anastomoses should be performed sequentially, from the deepest to the most superficial. Double-needled 6-0 absorbable monofilament is used. We favor continuous sutures for the posterior wall and interrupted sutures for the anterior wall. In difficult cases, it may be useful to place the anterior sutures on the biliary side before constructing the posterior wall and save them on rubber shut hemostats. The anterior sutures can then be easily passed on the bowel after the posterior wall has been completed.
- Some authors suggest that the surgeon stent the bilioenteric anastomosis. The stents are passed through the anastomoses after the posterior wall has been completed and are exteriorized through the bowel loop according to Volker. Such stents allow for postoperative choloangiograms or other manipulations in the event of complications.

Closure

- Before closing, transection surface hemostasis should be checked. Fibrin glue or topical hemostatic mesh can be placed on the raw surface.

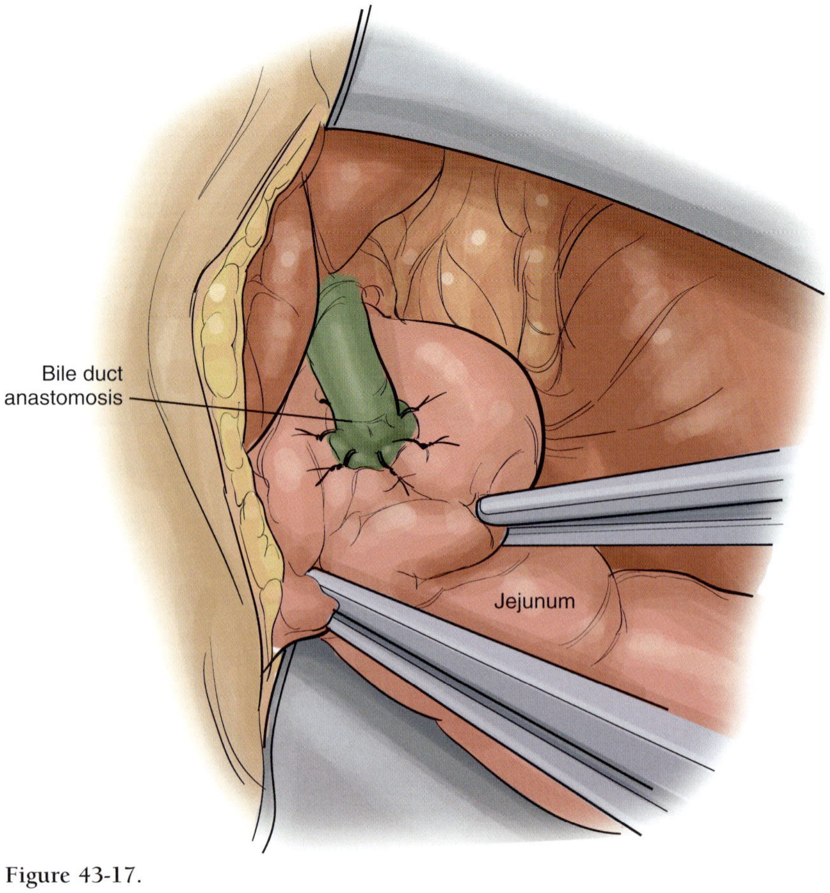

Figure 43-17.

- Because of the risk of bile leak, one large abdominal drain is placed close to, but not in contact with, the bilioenteric anastomoses.
- The abdomen is meticulously closed in layers using size 1 slowly absorbable sutures, and the skin is closed as usual.

III. ALTERNATIVE TECHNICAL APPROACHES (PRO/CON) AND PEARLS

Alternative Techniques

- *Anterior approach:* This approach consists of liver transection without prior mobilization. It has been initially proposed for large tumors when liver mobilization is difficult and hazardous. However, it has recently been shown to be associated with reduced blood loss and less ischemic injury to the remaining liver, even in small tumors. It is possible for most types of resections, including segment I. It requires particular expertise because the IVC and major hepatic veins are only controlled at the end of transection, and therefore the surgeon must have sufficient skill to avoid bleeding or deal with it if it occurs. We use it for large tumors but not for Klatskin tumors.
- *No-touch technique:* The portal bifurcation is often infiltrated with tumor in HC, but this cannot be assessed until this area has been removed. However, if infiltration is discovered at that stage, it is often too late because the tumorous invasion has been exposed and the peritoneum is contaminated with tumor cells. To avoid this, Neuhaus proposed avoiding dissection of the portal bifurcation (no touch) in cases requiring extended right hepatectomy. The portal trunk and the left portal branch are dissected and the portal bifurcation is systematically resected, followed by immediate end-to-end anastomosis of the divided portal vein to the stump of the left portal branch (Figs. 43-18

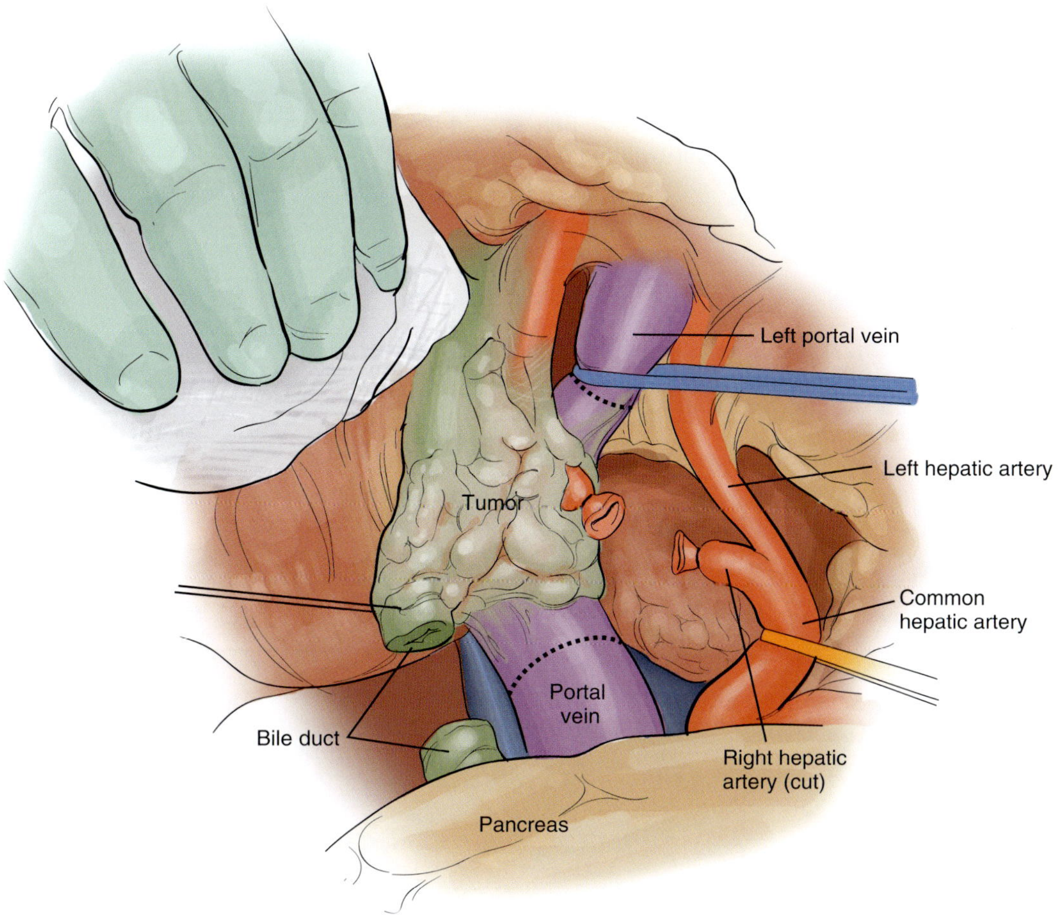

Figure 43-18.

and 43-19). According to Neuhaus, this technique is associated with a higher rate of R0 resections and better survival. Although this has not been confirmed by others, it is oncologically sound and can be recommended during extended right hepatectomies with a high suspicion of portal bifurcation invasion.

Pearls

- Excellent preoperative imaging is required, including MRCP and vascular reconstructions.
- Preparation for surgery with biliary drainage and portal vein embolization is often required.
- R0 resection is the goal of surgery.
- The keys to R0 resection are: (1) extensive hepatic pedicle dissection with vascular skeletonization and (2) liver resection including segment I.
- No irreversible vascular or biliary division should be made before resectability has been demonstrated.
- One must be prepared for vascular resection and microvascular reconstruction.
- Liver transection should be bloodless and the intermittent Pringle maneuver used when necessary.
- Proximal (intrahepatic) bile ducts are transected as high as possible in the liver during transection.
- Bilioenteric reconstruction includes all divided proximal bile ducts and should be performed meticulously.

IV. SPECIAL POSTOPERATIVE CARE

- Because of the magnitude of the procedure, patients should go to the intensive care unit until liver function has been restored. Although some Eastern studies have reported series of resections for HC without mortality, most Western studies still report a 5% to 10% mortality rate. Expert units using modern imaging and refined techniques should not observe a mortality above 5%. Morbidity rate is about 50% in Eastern and Western studies.
- The patient should be extubated as soon as possible. Prophylactic anticoagulants should not be started before prothrombin time is above 50% of normal. Prophylactic antibiotics should be continued for 48 hours if intraoperative bile culture is sterile. If bile culture is positive, antibiotics should be adapted and continued for 5 days. The nasogastric tube should be used for aspiration until gas is passed. Parenteral nutrition may be used until enteral feeding is resumed.
- Close patient monitoring is required for early diagnosis of complications.

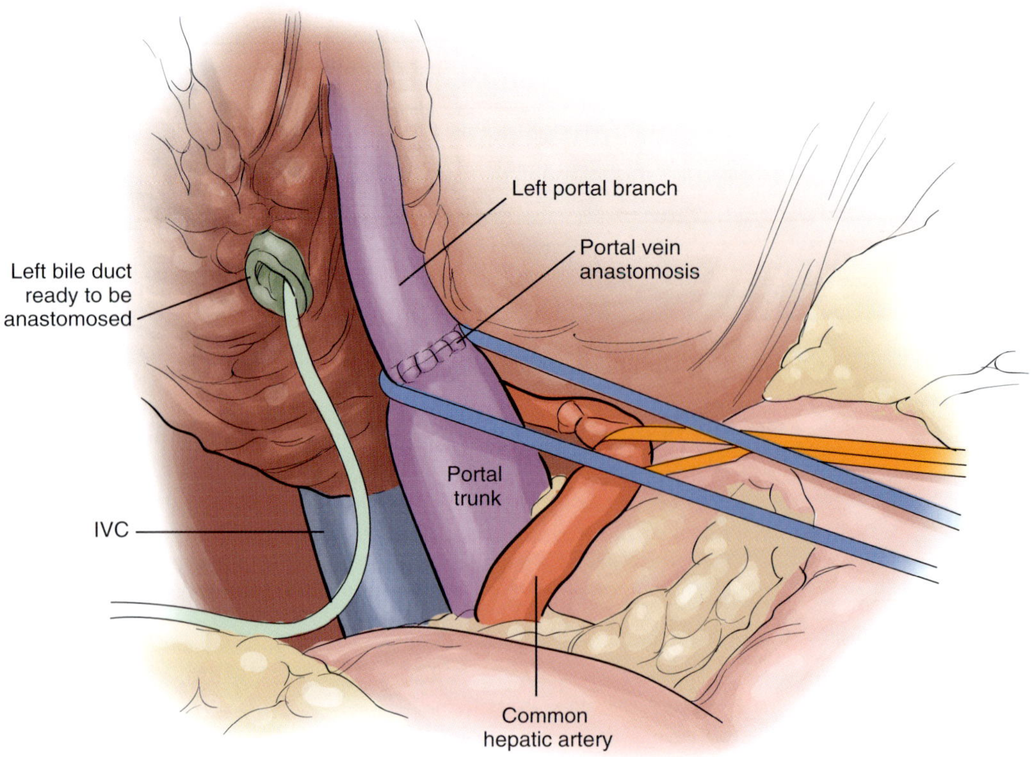

Figure 43-19. *IVC,* Inferior vena cava.

- The main complication during the first 24 hours is bleeding. Vital signs, abdominal drain output, and hemoglobin should be checked at regular intervals.
- Within the next few days, there is a risk of liver failure marked by prolonged prothrombin time, increase in bilirubin (or failure of bilirubin to decrease), and encephalopathy. There is no specific treatment, and it should improve within a few days.
- Bile leak should be screened. It can originate from the cut surface or from bilioenteric anastomosis failure. It can be externalized through the abdominal drain and heal spontaneously or result in a subphrenic collection that often becomes infected. In case of sepsis, abdominal CT is required, and any subphrenic collection must be drained percutaneously.
- Sepsis is favored by liver failure and operative complications. In turn, sepsis may aggravate liver failure and should be treated readily. Causes of sepsis include subphrenic collection with or without bile leak, cholangitis, anastomotic failure, pneumonia, wound infection, intravenous line infection, or urinary tract infection. All of these should be screened and treated.
- In most cases, patients can be discharged from the intensive care unit after 3 days and leave the hospital after 10 days.

SUGGESTED READINGS

Bismuth H, Corlette MB: Intrahepatic cholangioenteric anastomosis in carcinoma of the hilus of the liver, *Surg Gynecol Obstet* 140: 170–178, 1975.

Bismuth H, Nakache R, Diamond T: Management strategies in resection for hilar cholangiocarcinoma, *Ann Surg* 215:31–38, 1992.

Cherqui D, Benoist S, Malassagne B, et al: Major liver resection for carcinoma in jaundiced patients without preoperative biliary drainage, *Arch Surg* 135:302–308, 2000.

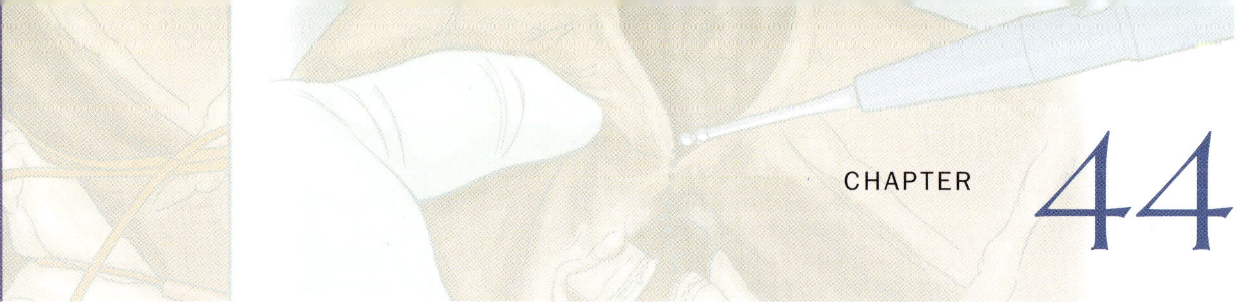

CHAPTER 44

Radical Cholecystectomy/ Liver Bed Resection with Regional Lymph Node Dissection

Keiji Sano, MD, and Masatoshi Makuuchi, MD, PhD

I. SPECIAL PREOPERATIVE PREPARATION

- The imaging diagnosis of gallbladder carcinoma must include ultrasonography (US) and computed tomography (CT).
- US provides the best assessment of gallstone existence. It may also have the advantages of diagnosing the depth of tumor extension into the gallbladder wall, as well as involvement of the adjacent vessels and organs such as the common bile duct, right hepatic artery, right portal vein, liver, duodenum, colon, and pancreas. Moreover, endoscopic US is more accurate in diagnosing such tumor extent.
- Dynamic contrast-enhanced CT is also one of the most accurate modalities for diagnosing and staging gallbladder carcinoma. Tumor involvement of the bile duct and the main hepatic artery is best assessed by the early phase of CT (Fig. 44-1, *A* and *B*) than by other modalities such as arteriography. CT is also accurate for discerning hepatic invasion (see Fig. 44-1, *A* and *B*) and liver metastasis. Lymph node involvement, peritoneal dissemination, and extensive involvement of the adjacent organs should also be assessed by CT (Fig. 44-2, *A* and *B*), but CT may be less accurate for hepatic and vessel invasions.
- Endoscopic retrograde cholangiopancreatography (ERCP) and magnetic resonance imaging can provide a reasonably accurate assessment of invasion to the bile duct. ERCP is more invasive but makes it possible to perform tissue diagnosis, such as cytologic examination of bile and brush and scrape biopsy from the bile duct and gallbladder. Angiography is also useful not only for diagnosing the depth of the tumor extent with encasement of arteries, but also for recognizing vascular anatomy, especially arterial anatomy in the hepatic hilum.
- When the tumor extension is limited to mucosa or muscularis propria, simple cholecystectomy, including laparoscopic cholecystectomy, is appropriate. When the tumor involves the common bile duct, extended right hepatectomy with extrahepatic bile duct resection should be planned to perform en bloc resection of the adjacent right hepatic artery and right portal vein.
- Liver bed resection with regional lymph node dissection is recommended when the tumor invades the subserosal layer or beyond, including direct invasion of the liver, duodenum, and colon. This operative procedure should be limited to patients without tumor involvement of the bile duct, especially without jaundice.
- The same preoperative bowel preparation as for colectomy is necessary, because gallbladder carcinoma can easily involve the adjacent transverse colon.
- For patients with possible bile duct involvement, preoperative portal vein embolization should be done 2 weeks before extended right hepatectomy to prevent postoperative liver failure. However, the diagnosis of bile duct involvement must be accurate, because a 2-week interval after the embolization may allow further growth of gallbladder carcinoma.

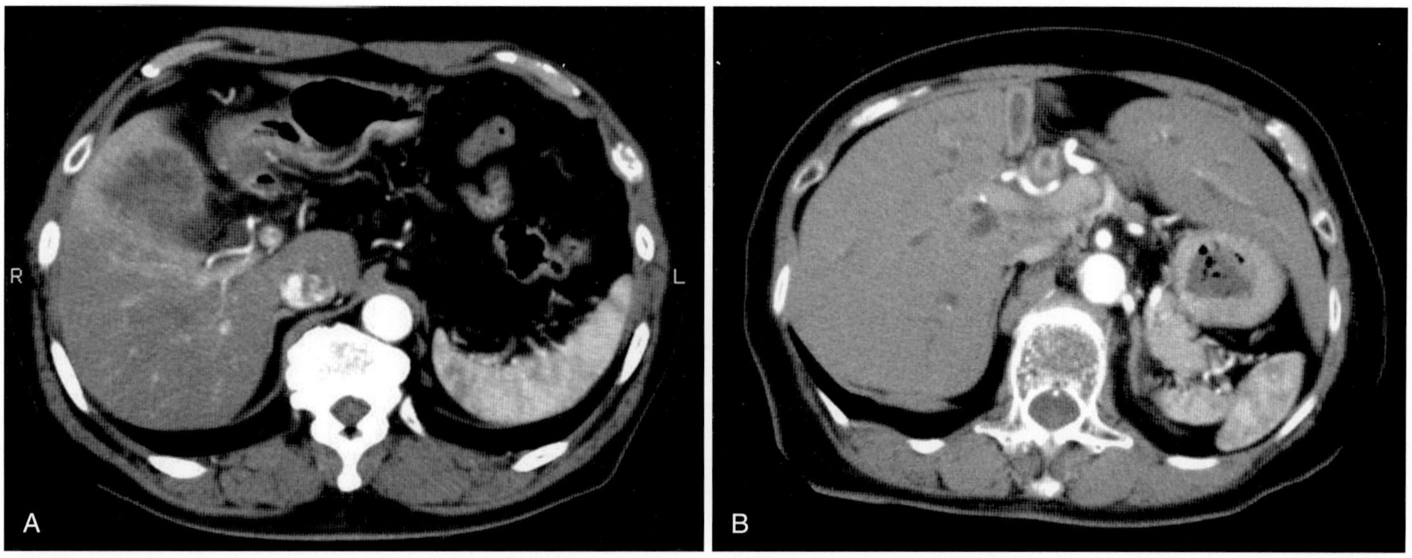

Figure 44-1. **A,** Early phase of dynamic contrast-enhanced computed tomography (CT) in patient with gallbladder carcinoma. Tumor in the fundus involves hepatic parenchyma. However, no involvement of the common hepatic duct or right hepatic artery is recognized. **B,** Early phase of dynamic contrast-enhanced CT in patients with hilar bile duct carcinoma involving right hepatic artery. Gallbladder wall is thickened with inflammation. Thick common hepatic duct is enhanced and the density of adjacent connective tissue is increased because of tumor involvement. The right hepatic artery runs through the high-density connective tissue, which suggests tumor involvement.

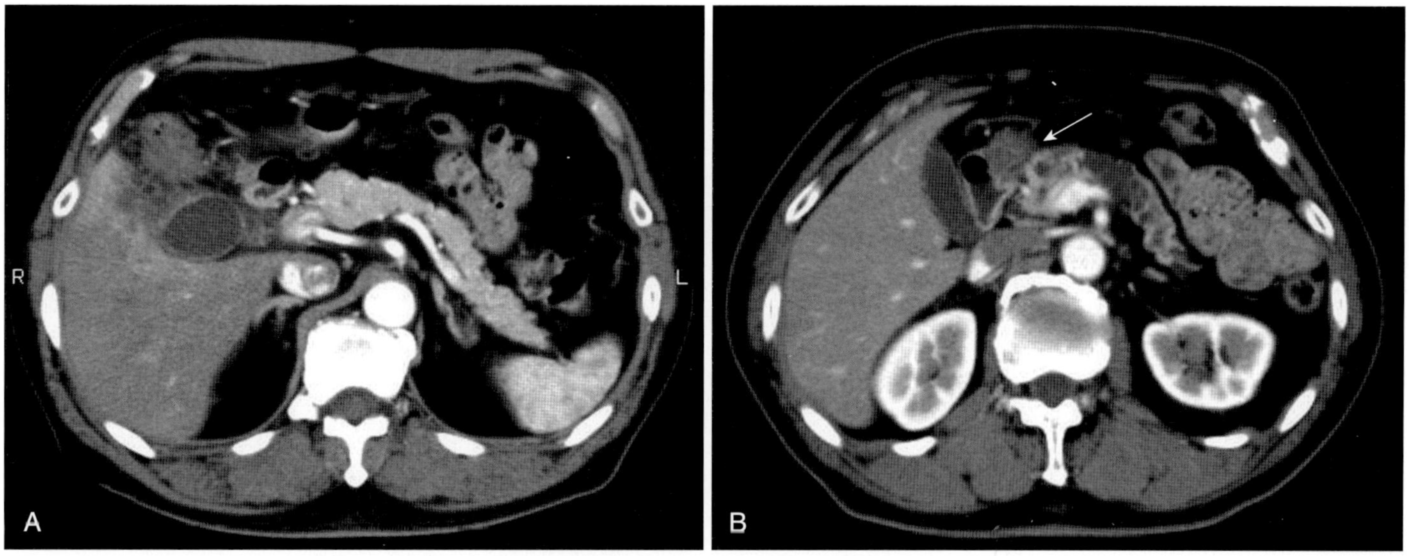

Figure 44-2. **Early phase of dynamic contrast-enhanced computed tomography in the same patient.** **A,** This slice provides findings of tumor extension to the body of the gallbladder and involvement of liver parenchyma and transverse colon. **B,** The cystic duct is enhanced, which suggests involvement of the cystic duct, but the common bile duct is not enhanced (*arrow*).

II. OPERATIVE TECHNIQUE

Position

- The supine position should be selected.

Incision

- Upper midline incision, right subcostal incision, Mayo-Robson incision, and J-incision are mainly used. Among these, the J-incision is recommended (Fig. 44-3). The classic J-incision includes thoracotomy in the ninth intercostal space, but in this procedure (liver bed resection), thoracotomy is unnecessary. Xyphoidectomy should be undergone.

Main Dissection

- First, the absence of peritoneal dissemination, distant lymph node involvement, and liver metastases is confirmed. Intraoperative ultrasound may provide better assessment for the diagnosis of lymph node involvement and hepatic metastasis than manual palpation. Also, bile duct involvement should be assessed by palpation and ultrasound.
- Once contraindication factors have been ruled out, the duodenum is extensively mobilized (Kocher maneuver). After palpation of the retroperitoneum to assess for metastatic nodes, lymph nodes on the dorsal side of the pancreas head are dissected. Meticulous dissection should be done to prevent injury to the pancreas parenchyma, which could cause leakage of pancreatic juice. The posterior superior pancreaticoduodenal artery and vein, which run on the dorsal surface of the pancreatic head, are exposed (Fig. 44-4).
- The distal common bile duct is divided just on the edge of the pancreas and is closed with a transfixing suture. The stump is submitted to frozen section. If the stump is diagnosed as positive for cancer pathologically, which is very rare, pancreaticoduodenectomy should be added afterward. A drainage tube (8-Fr) is inserted from the proximal stump of the distal common bile duct for biliary decompression during the operation.
- Dissection of the proper, left, and right hepatic arteries and main portal vein continues cephalad (Fig. 44-5). The common hepatic artery is also exposed after retropancreatic lymph node dissection. The

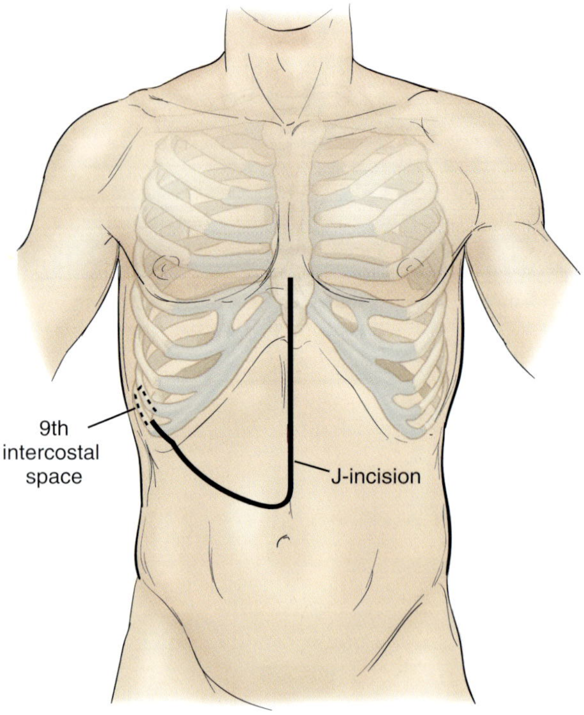

Figure 44-3.

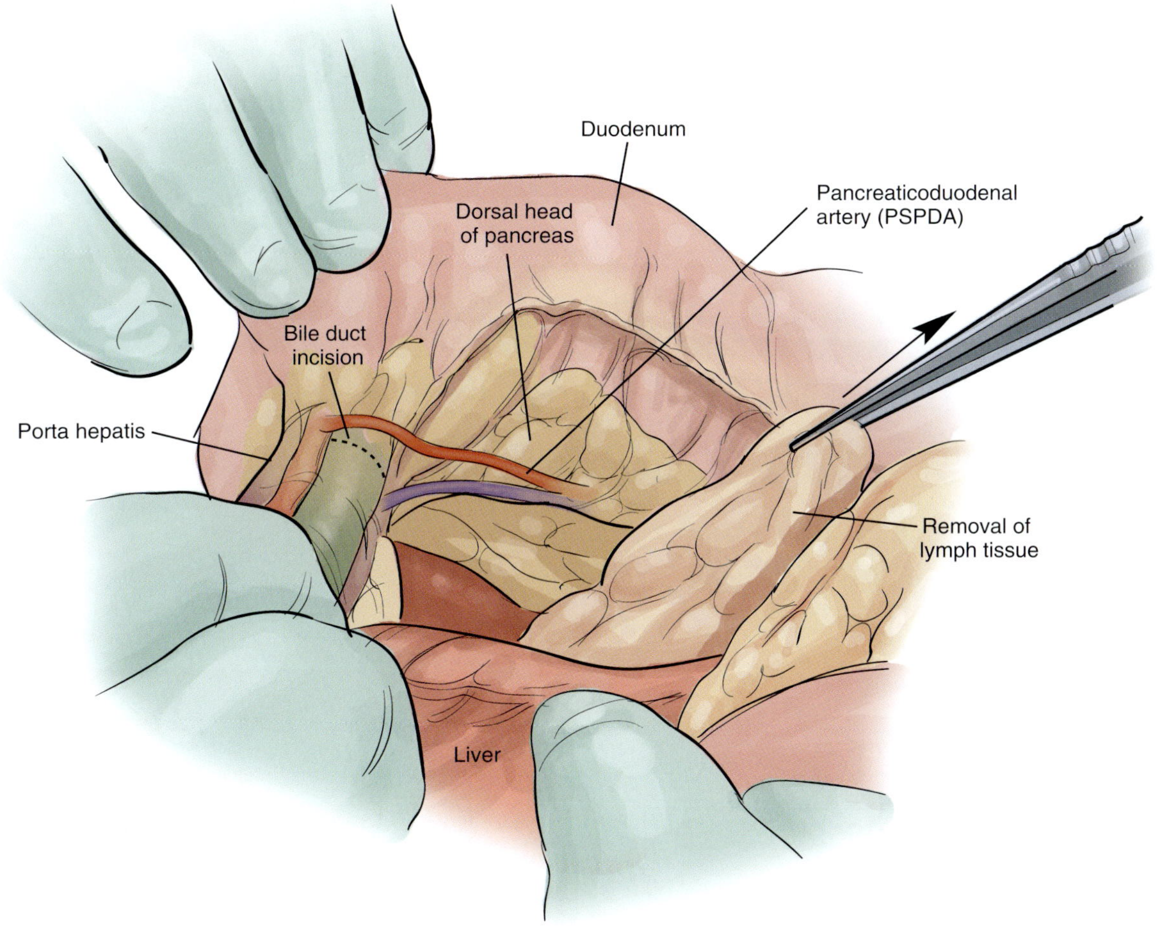

Figure 44-4.

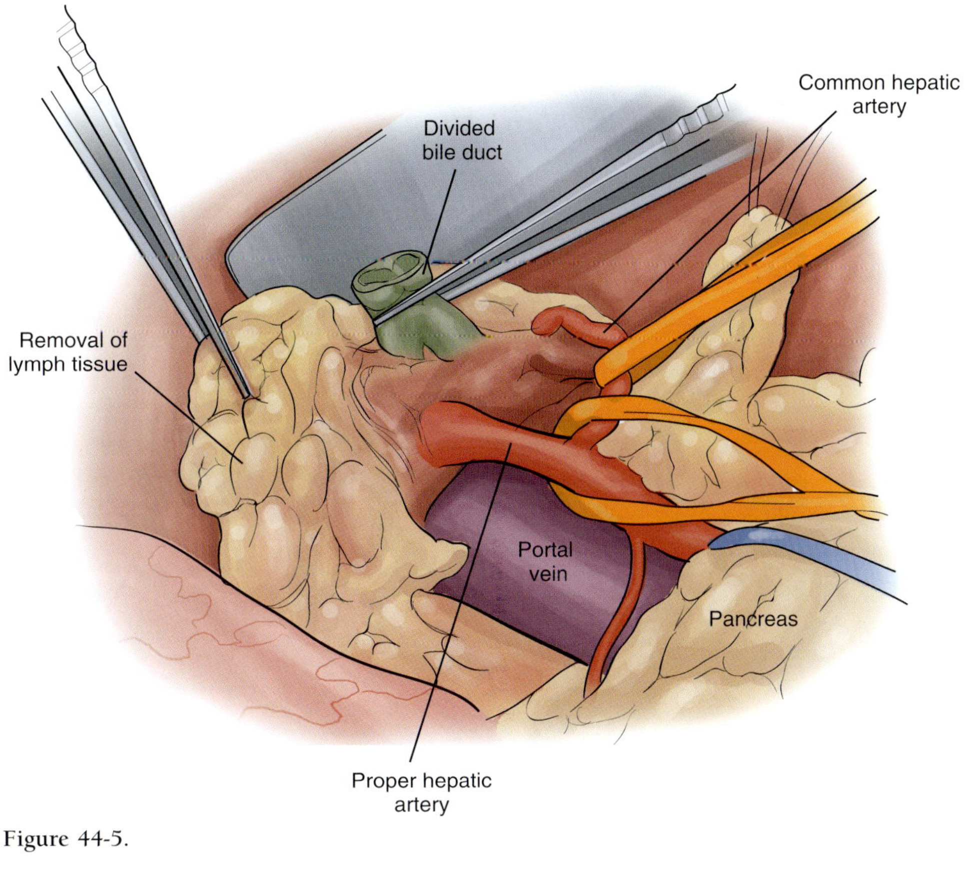

Figure 44-5.

right hepatic artery is exposed distally to the bifurcation of each anterior and posterior branch (Fig. 44-6, *A* and *B*).

- The hepatic parenchyma surrounding the gallbladder bed is divided under intermittent inflow occlusion (intermittent Pringle maneuver). Parenchymal division applying the crush clamping method proceeds along the line approximately 1 to 2 cm distant from the gallbladder bed or the tumor in the hepatic parenchyma (Fig. 44-7, *A* and *B*).

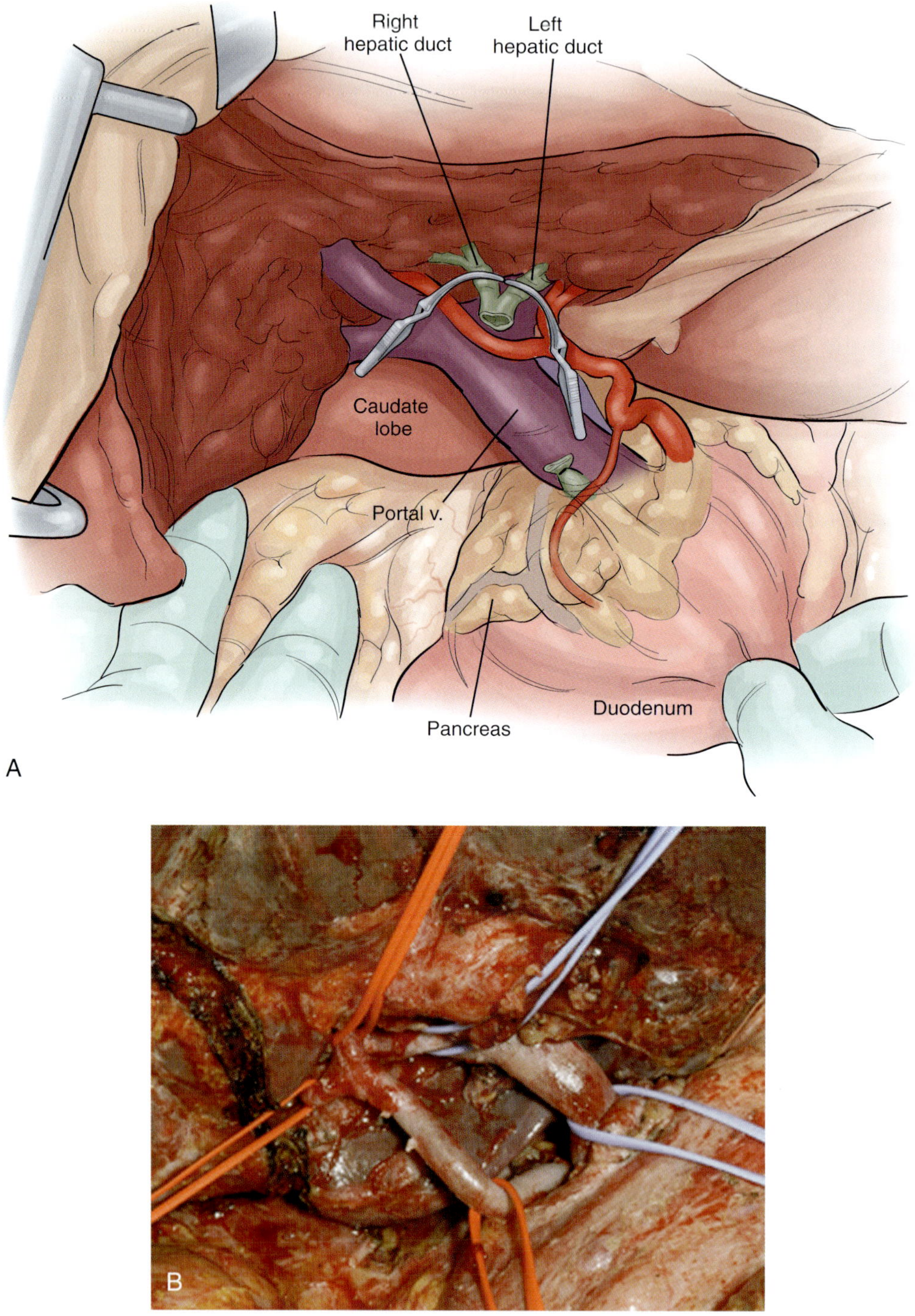

Figure 44-6.

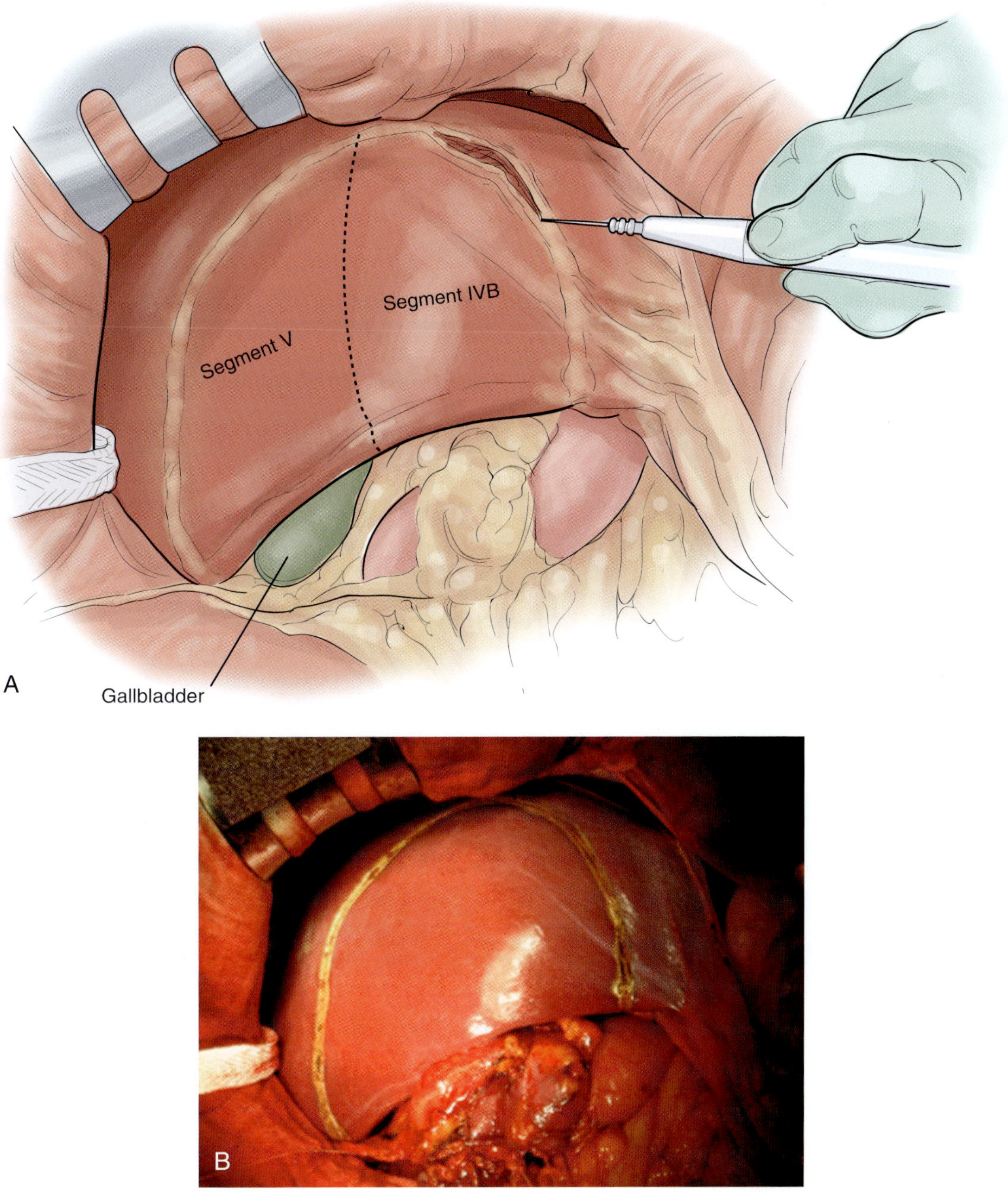

Figure 44-7.

- Hepatic transection is directed toward the hepatic hilum and the anterior portal pedicle just behind the gallbladder bed. The posterior portal pedicle in the Rouviere fissure is then exposed (Fig. 44-8). Intraoperative ultrasound plays another major role in guiding direction of hepatic division.
- When the two portal pedicles are exposed, hepatic division is finished, and the specimen is resected, dividing the proximal bile duct at the hilum (see Fig. 44-8, *A* and *B*). The proximal stump of the bile duct from the resected specimen should be submitted to frozen section to confirm that it is free of tumor invasion.
- For the biliary reconstruction, the jejunum is divided 40 cm distal from the ligament of Treitz. The distal jejunum is elevated through the retrocolic route. When the number of bile duct orifices is more than two, these orifices are combined to make one large orifice (Fig. 44-9).
- Anastomosis is performed in an end-to-side manner using 4-0 absorbable suture. After the posterior wall is sutured, short stent tubes are inserted and fixed by one of the posterior suture strings. After biliary reconstruction is completed, a jejunostomy tube is inserted from the proximal stump of the elevated jejunum for the decompression of the anastomosis.
- Jejunojejunostomy is carried out in an end-to-side manner 40 cm distal from the bilioenteric anastomosis.

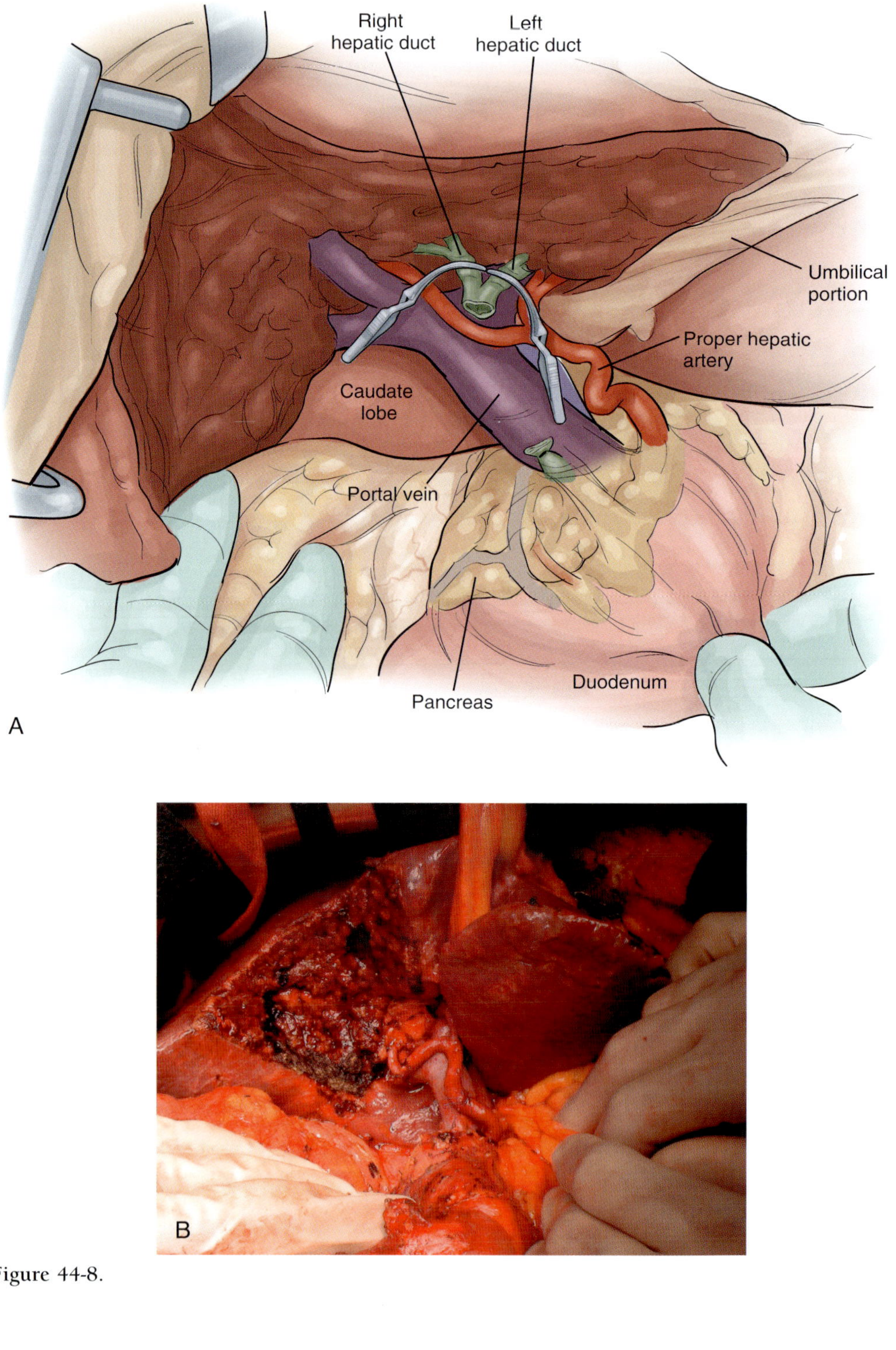

Figure 44-8.

Closure

- Complete hemostasis and no bile leakage should be confirmed after peritoneal lavage. Drainage tubes are inserted in the Winslow foramen and hepatic stump. The wound is closed in a layer-to-layer manner so as not to create dead space.

III. ALTERNATIVE TECHNICAL APPROACHES (PRO/CON) AND PEARLS

- When a large tumor involves the transverse colon, the approach to the hepatic hilum and evaluating the extent of tumor involvement of the duodenum, pancreas, bile duct, hepatic artery, or portal vein is impossible. Division of the involved colon before assessment of resectability should be considered. Even when the tumor proves to be too advanced for resection after exploration, the divided transverse colon can be left with the tumor by mucosectomy.
- The posterior superior pancreaticoduodenal artery originates from the gastroduodenal artery, and the posterior superior pancreaticoduodenal vein drains through the main portal vein. The artery usually runs on the ventral side of the bile duct, and the vein runs on the dorsal side. These vessels help in identifying distal common bile duct and dividing it as distally as possible.
- The common bile duct can be preserved when the bile duct is definitely free from tumor. Lymph nodes around the bile duct are dissected, and the confluence of the cystic duct is exposed. The cystic duct is dissected just on the confluence, and the stump is sent for frozen section. If the stump proves to be positive for cancer, a routine procedure with bile duct resection is selected. If not, regional lymphadenectomy is performed, preserving the common bile duct. The right hepatic duct is exposed in the ventral side of the right hepatic artery and right portal vein. Preservation of the common bile duct eliminates the need for bilioenteric anastomosis and can prevent postoperative reflux cholangitis. However, it would make resection of perineural invasion and lymphatic duct permeation less complete because of the preservation of the epicholedochal plexus. Therefore, use of this procedure should be limited to patients without lymph node involvement and infiltration to the hepatoduodenal ligament.

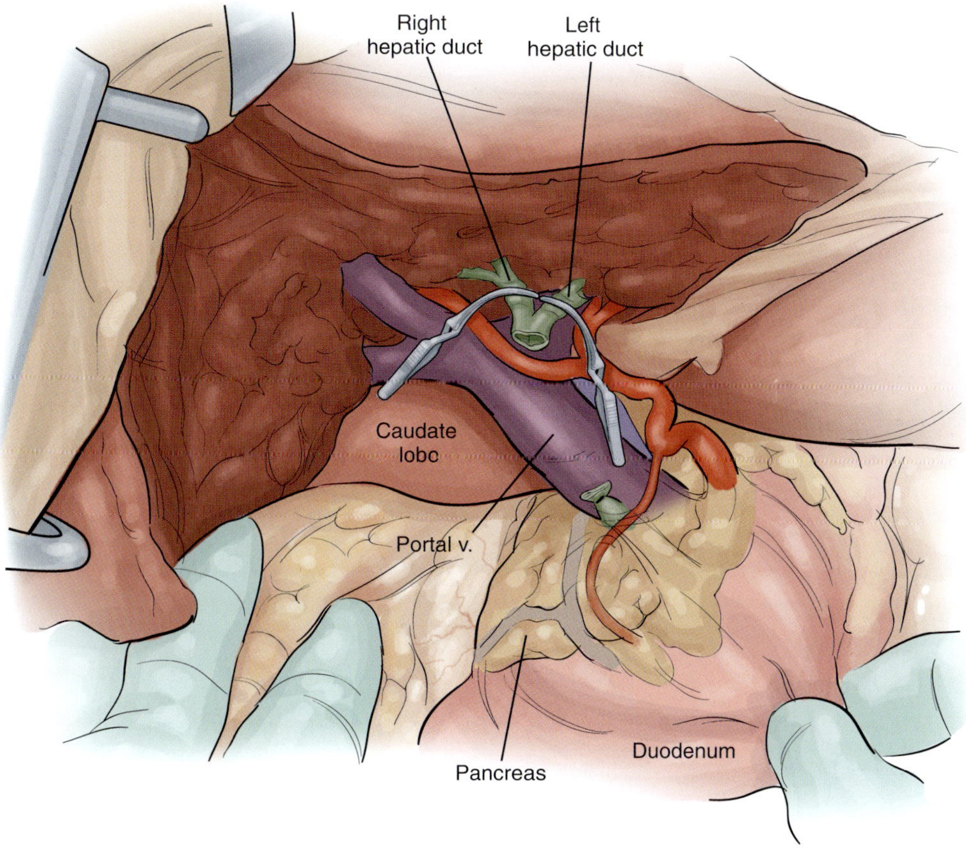

Figure 44-9.

IV. SPECIAL POSTOPERATIVE CARE

- Bleeding from the resected surface of the liver, bile leakage, and pancreatic juice leakage are major immediate complications after this procedure.
- Reoperation for hemostasis should be immediately performed when the amount of blood from the drainage tube exceeds 100 mL per hour. Bile leakage can be stopped conservatively by keeping the drainage tube inserted. Pancreatic juice leakage is a special postoperative complication after this procedure. The amylase concentration of drain discharge from the Winslow foramen should be examined, and if it is higher than the serum level, the drainage tube cannot be removed.
- Reflux cholangitis and ileus are two major late complications. The chief complaint of reflux cholangitis is high fever with shivering. Immediate administration of antibiotics will prevent liver abscess, and ultrasound examination must be done to check bile duct dilatation. When the thick bile duct is found with or without jaundice, drainage of the relevant bile duct should be performed without delay.
- When the common bile duct is preserved, biliary stricture is an additional late complication. One of the main reasons for the stricture is tumor recurrence. Another common reason is insufficiency of blood perfusion after dissection of the common bile duct. Resection of the common bile duct and hepaticojejunostomy should be performed for benign biliary stricture.

SUGGESTED READINGS

Kokudo N, Makuuchi M, Natori T, et al: Strategies for surgical treatment of gallbladder carcinoma based on information available before resection, *Arch Surg* 138:741–750, 2003.

Kosuge T, Sano K, Shimada K, et al: Should the bile duct be preserved or removed in radical surgery for gallbladder cancer? *Hepatol Gastroenterol* 46:2133–2137, 1999.

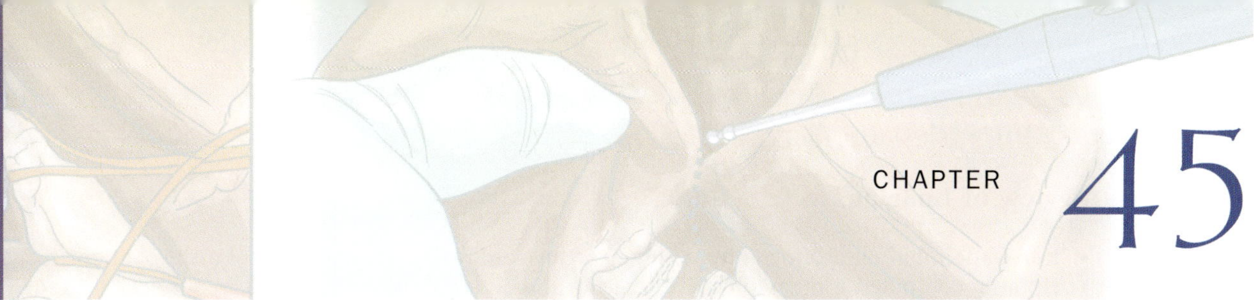

CHAPTER 45

Laparoscopic Approach to Hepatic Cysts

Fady K. Balaa, MD, and David A. Geller, MD

I. SPECIAL PREOPERATIVE PREPARATION

Differential Diagnosis

- Cystic lesions of the liver are a common occurance. These can be grouped as congenital or acquired hepatic cysts.
- The more common congenital hepatic cysts are often solitary cystic formations containing serous fluid. Most are lined by biliary epithelium. They can range in size from subcentimeter to greater than 20 cm. Giant hepatic cysts can cause attenuation and atrophy of adjacent hepatic parenchyma. Other common types of congenital hepatic cysts include polycystic liver disease, often in association with polycystic kidney disease.
- Acquired hepatic cysts include neoplastic cystadenoma and cystadenocarcinoma, traumatic pseudocysts, and infectious echinococcal cysts (Fig. 45-1).
- Many reports document the safety and efficacy of laparoscopic liver surgery, especially for treatment of simple hepatic cysts.

Operative Indications

- Most simple hepatic cysts are asymptomatic and can be observed. Occasionally they can cause enough pain to require surgical management.
- Other rare surgical indications include:
  - ▲ Hemorrhage
  - ▲ Infection
  - ▲ Obstructive jaundice

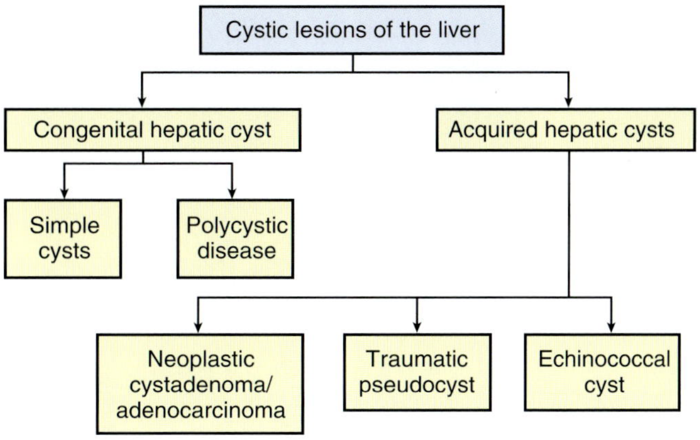

Figure 45-1.

Review of Imaging

- Transabdominal ultrasonography is sufficient for confirming the diagnosis of a simple hepatic cyst.
- Biphasic computed tomography (CT) scan of the abdomen is very helpful in surgical planning as it identifies:
  - ▲ Exact location of the cyst within the liver
  - ▲ Relationship of the cyst to major vasculature including hepatic and portal veins (Fig. 45-2, *A* and *B*)
  - ▲ Presence of associated hepatic parenchyma atrophy or biliary tract dilatation
  - ▲ Other intraabdominal pathology that can be the cause of presenting symptoms

Instruments

- 10-mm 30-degree telescope
- 5-mm 30-degree telescope
- Laparoscopic tissue graspers
- Laparoscopic flexible liver retractor
- Laparoscopic scissors
- Laparoscopic hook electrocautery
- Laparoscopic suction irrigation device
- 12-mm trocars (2)
- 5-mm trocar (2)
- Endo GIA linear stapling device
- Laparoscopic ultrasound
- Closing device

Anesthesia and Antibiotics

- Patients are admitted on the morning of surgery.
- General anesthesia is administered, avoiding nitrous products to minimize bowel distention.
- Ampicillin/sulbactam or first-generation cephalosporin is administered intravenously before skin incision.

Accessory Devices

- An orogastric tube is inserted after induction and is removed before reversal of anesthesia.
- A urinary catheter is inserted after induction and is removed in the operating room, or on the first postoperative day.
- Pneumatic compression stockings are placed before induction.

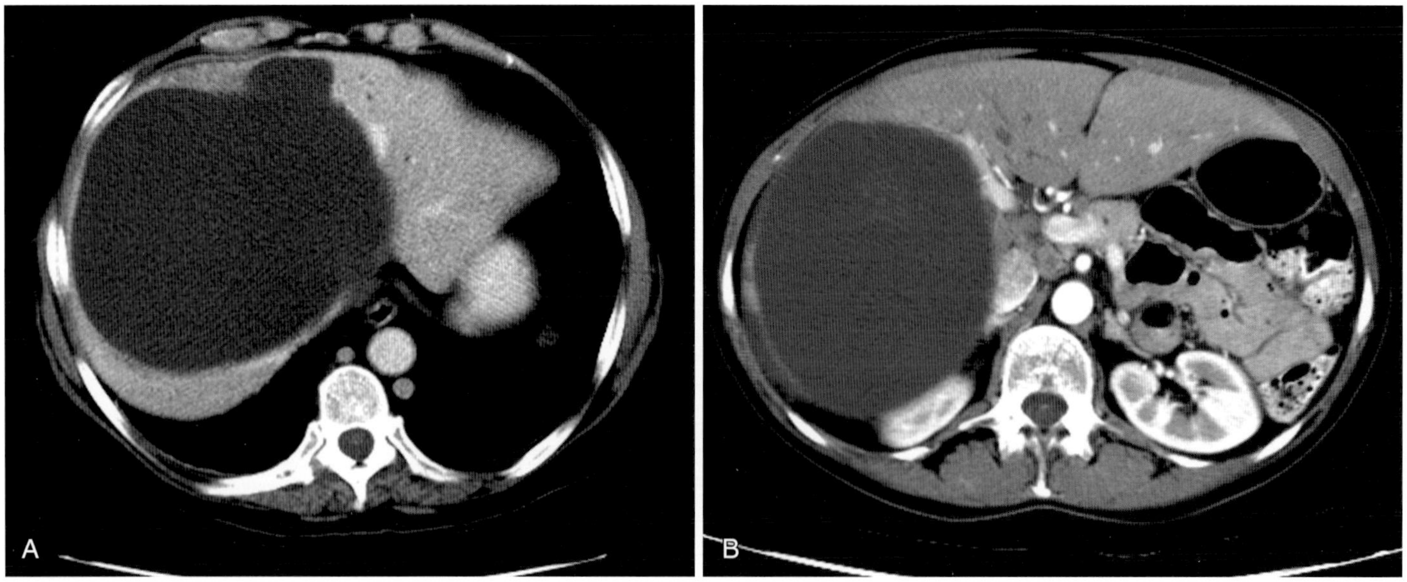

Figure 45-2. Computed tomography scans showing giant hepatic cysts and relation to major vessels.

II. OPERATIVE TECHNIQUE

Position

- The patient is placed in a supine position with arms well-padded and extended 60 degrees on each side.
- The patient is strapped to the table, and a footboard is placed to prevent movement during reverse Trendelenburg position.
- For right-sided lesions, the surgeon is on the patient's right side, and the assistant surgeon is on the patient's left side (Fig. 45-3).
- The scrub nurse is on the patient's left side.
- The two video monitors are at the head of the table above each shoulder.
- The ultrasound machine is on the patient's left side, immediately behind the assistant surgeon, and can be wheeled closer when needed.
- We prefer to feed the ultrasound image to the video monitors for picture-in-picture imaging.

Trocar Placement

- A total of four trocars are required.
- All trocar sites are preinjected with 0.5% bupivacaine.
- Open technique is used for first trocar placement in the supraumbilical space.
- Under direct visualization, the accessory trocars are placed as follows (with variation according to body habitus):
  - ▲ *Right lobe cysts* (Fig. 45-4):
    A 12-mm trocar in the right paramedian space midclavicular line; a 5-mm trocar in the right subcostal space anterior axillary line; and a 5-mm trocar in the midline subxiphoid space
  - ▲ *Left lobe cysts*: A 12-mm trocar in the left paramedian space midclavicular line; a 5-mm trocar in the left subcostal space anterior axillary line; and a 5-mm trocar in the right subcostal space midclavicular line

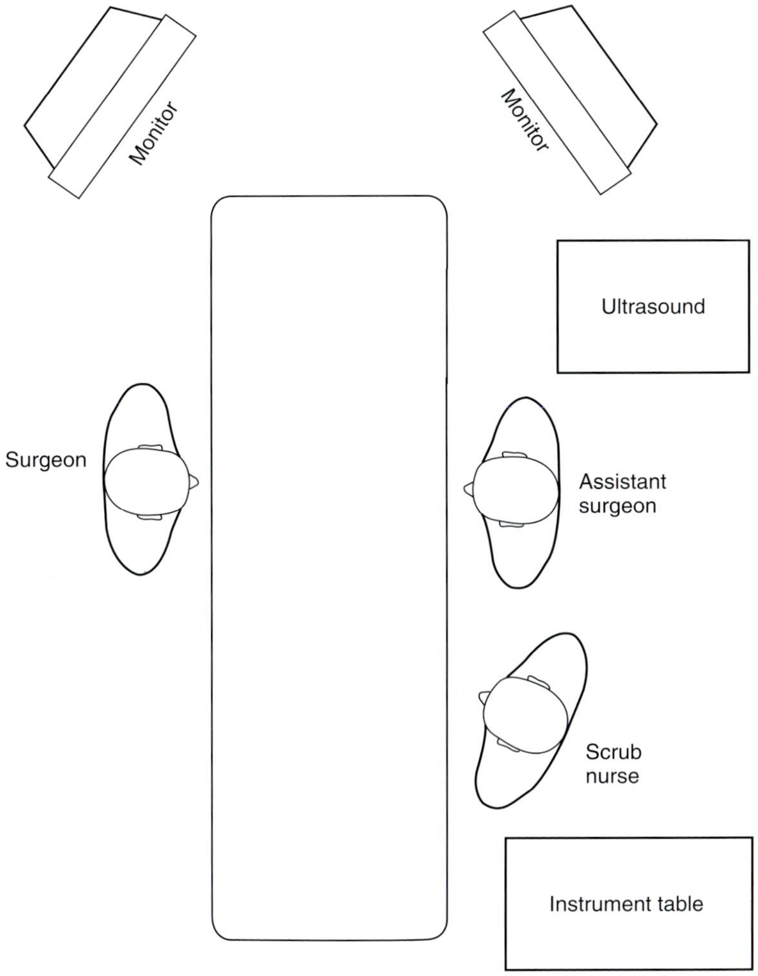

Figure 45-3.

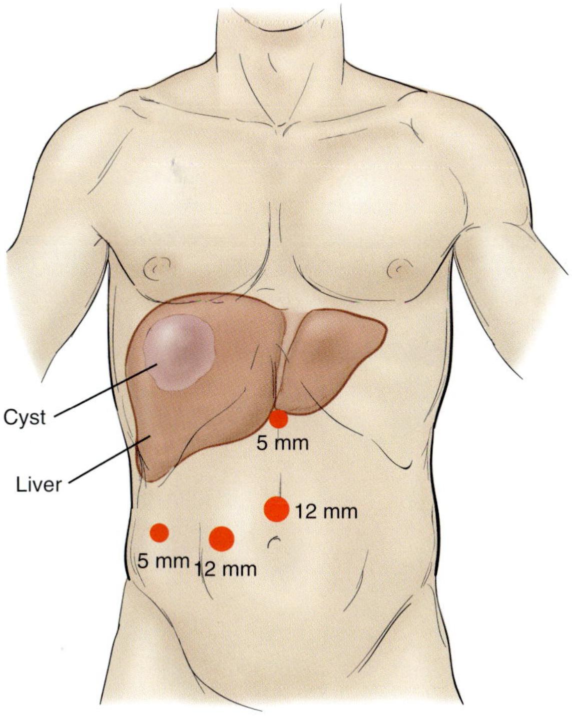

Figure 45-4.

Main Dissection

- The main goal of the procedure is to minimize recurrence by safely resecting the majority of the cyst wall. We routinely try to resect 70% to 80% of the cyst wall, leaving 20% to 30% that overlies either portal or hepatic veins.
- After pneumoperitoneum is established and trocars are placed, necessary adhesiolysis is performed (Fig. 45-5).
- For right-sided lesions, the flexible retractor is introduced through the subxiphoid port and used to retract the right lobe of the liver. The right lobe is then mobilized by division of the right triangular ligament. This is carried out using endoscopic scissors and hook electrocautery (see Fig. 45-5).
- In left-sided lesions, the left lobe of the liver is mobilized by dividing the falciform and left triangular ligaments. This is also carried out using endoscopic scissors and hook electrocautery.
- Laparoscopic liver ultrasound is performed to identify the relationship of the cyst wall to major vasculature.
- With the respective lobe well-mobilized, we prefer early incision of the cyst wall, and drainage of cyst contents using laparoscopic suction (Figs. 45-6 and 45-7). Cyst contents can either be clear serous fluid, or murky brown fluid resembling the consistency of motor fluid. The latter suggests the presence of a biliary communication. In such cases we search for the biliary leak and control it with laparoscopic suturing.
- The cyst wall is excised using a combination of endoscopic scissors, Endo GIA staplers (we prefer the white 2.5-mm load with roticulating 45-mm cartridge length), or other hemostatic devices (Figs. 45-8 and 45-9).
- The cyst wall is sent for frozen section analysis. In the unlikely event that quick section analysis documents the presence of a neoplastic cyst (cystadenoma or cystadenocarcinoma), we recommend conversion to an open procedure for formal hepatic resection.

Closure

- After the specimen is removed, we ensure adequate hemostasis at the cyst wall resection margin and absence of any biliary leak.
- A 10-Fr closed suction drain is introduced through the lateral 5-mm port and placed in the bed of the resection. A 4-0 nylon stitch is sutured but not tied at the skin level around the drain. This can be tied at the bedside when the drain is removed before discharge on postoperative day 1 or 2. The drain is anchored in place with 2-0 silk suture.
- Both 12-mm port sites are closed at the fascia with size 0 Vicryl.
- The skin is closed with 4-0 Vicryl stitch in a running subcuticular technique.

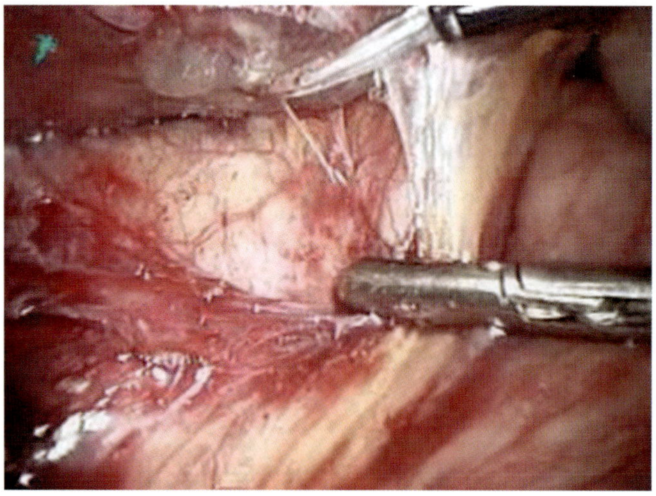

Figure 45-5.

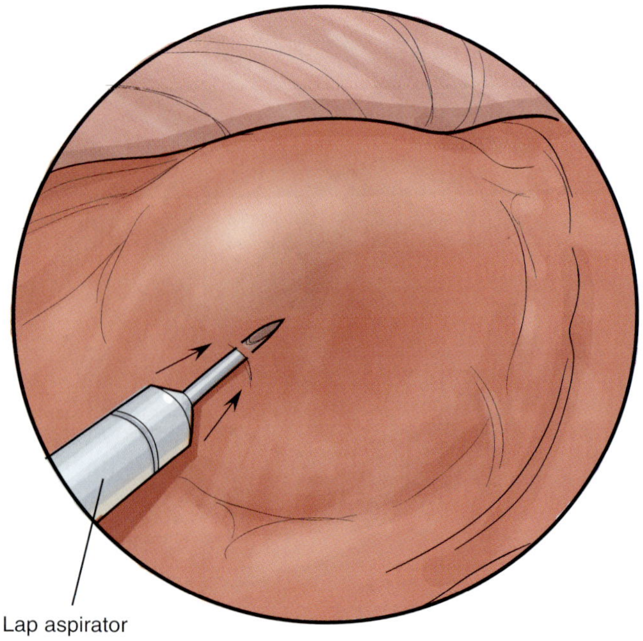

Figure 45-6.

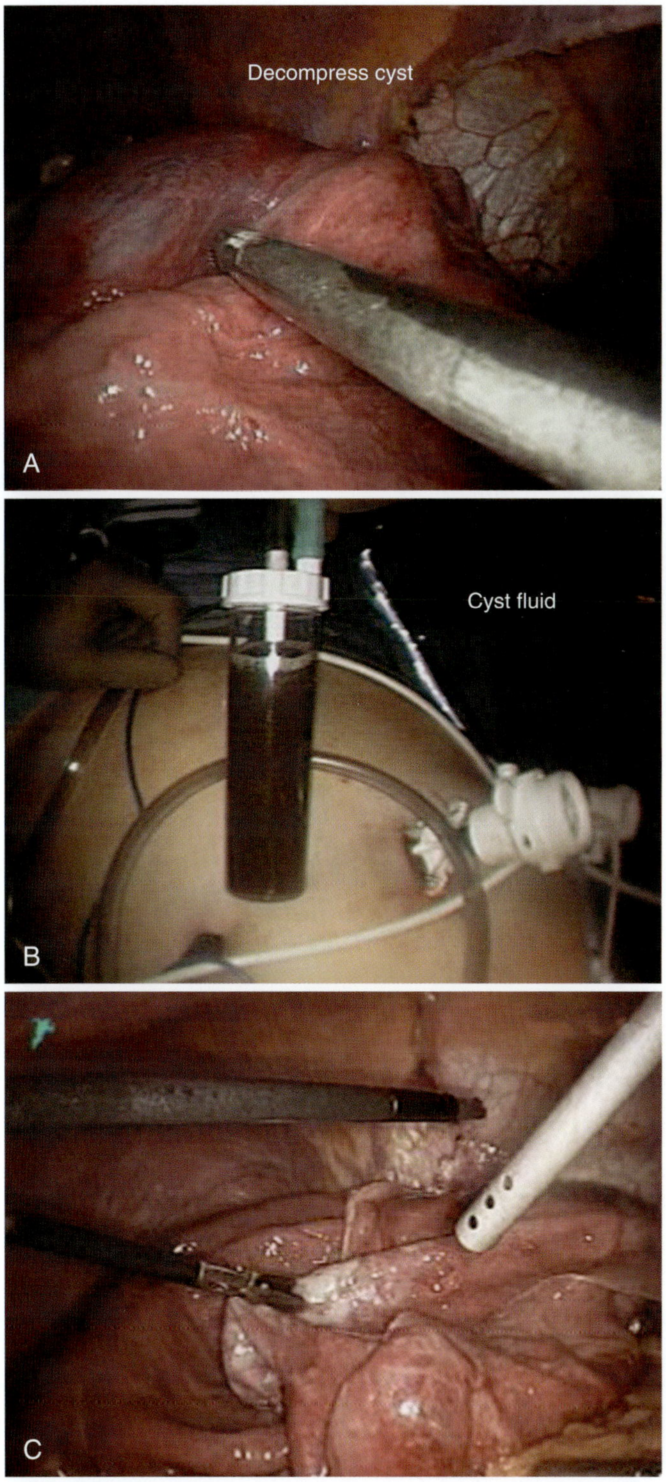

Figure 45-7.

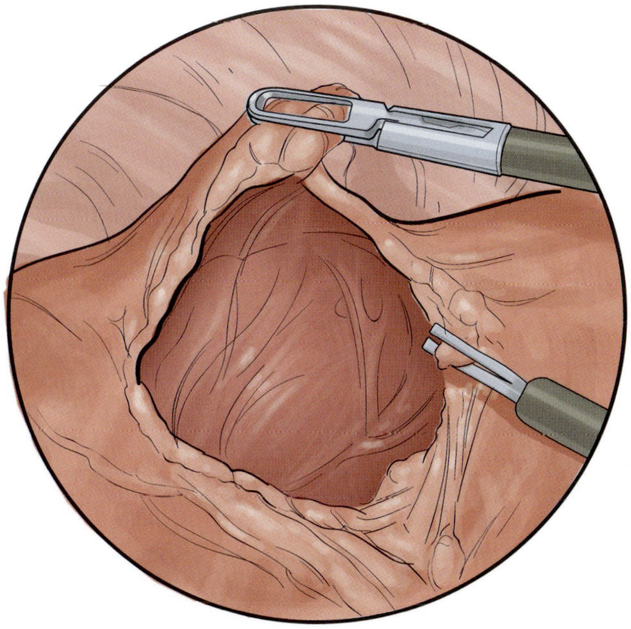
Figure 45-8.

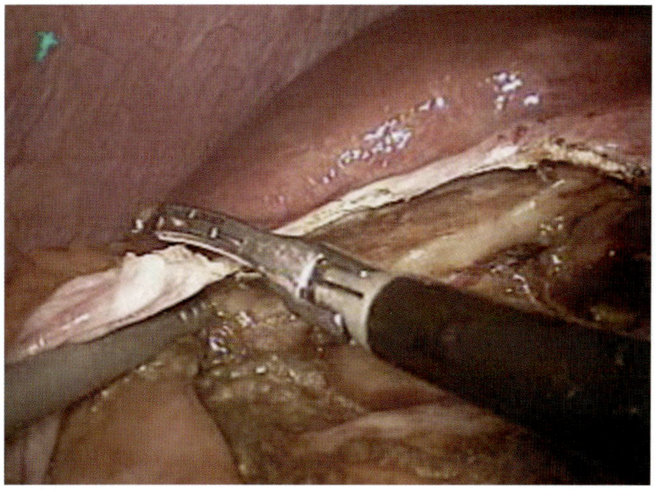
Figure 45-9.

III. ALTERNATIVE TECHNICAL APPROACHES (PRO/CON) AND PEARLS

Alternative Approaches

- These cysts can also be approached by laparotomy with a midline incision, or subcostal incision with midline extension. This approach is associated with increased morbidity, but it may be indicated if cystadenoma or cystadenocarcinoma is suspected.

Technical Pearls

- Early incision of the cyst wall facilitates manipulation of the liver and resection of the cyst.
- Once the cyst wall is opened and contents evacuated, the deep portal or hepatic veins that have been displaced by the expanding cyst can usually be visualized as a linear ridge just deep to the back wall of the cyst. These are soft and ballotable when probed with the laparoscopic instruments.
- It is best not to be overly aggressive and attempt to remove the entire cyst wall, because this can lead to torrential bleeding from the deep portal or hepatic veins.
- If the cyst content is bilious, an attempt should be made to identify and suture any active biliary leak along the residual back wall of the cyst.
- The side wall of the cyst can displace the liver parenchyma to the point where the liver might only be 1 cm thick adjacent to the cyst and requires parenchymal resection. When dividing the cyst wall in this region, it can be quite thick and hyperemic. We prefer to utilize the Endo GIA staplers that achieve hemostasis and also seal any crossing hypertrophied hepatic ducts.
- If too thick a bite is attempted with the stapler, the deep liver edge can crack or form a subcapsular hematoma. This can be controlled with the laparoscopic TissueLink devices (hook or floating ball).
- Although simple laparoscopic "marsupialization" with insertion of omentum into the opened cyst is described in the literature, we have found that this is associated with a high recurrence rate, and prefer to resect as much of the cyst wall (70% to 80%) as safely possible.
- Placement of a hand port for redo cyst excision cases should be considered.

IV. SPECIAL POSTOPERATIVE CARE

- Patients are typically discharged on the first postoperative day.
- Regular diet is resumed on the first postoperative day.
- Pain control is achieved with regular doses of antiinflammatory drugs with occasional oral narcotics.
- The closed suction drain is removed on the first postoperative day. In the event of either high-output drainage (more than 150 mL/24 hr) or bilious drainage, the patient is discharged home with the drain in place and follow-up assessment in 1 week. Patients are informed preoperatively regarding the possibility of 1 to 2 weeks with closed-suction drainage. In the rare event of a persistent bile leak, we advocate early endoscopic retrograde cholangiopancreatography and stenting.
- A follow-up CT scan of the abdomen checking for cyst recurrence is obtained at 1 year (Fig. 45-10, *A* and *B*).

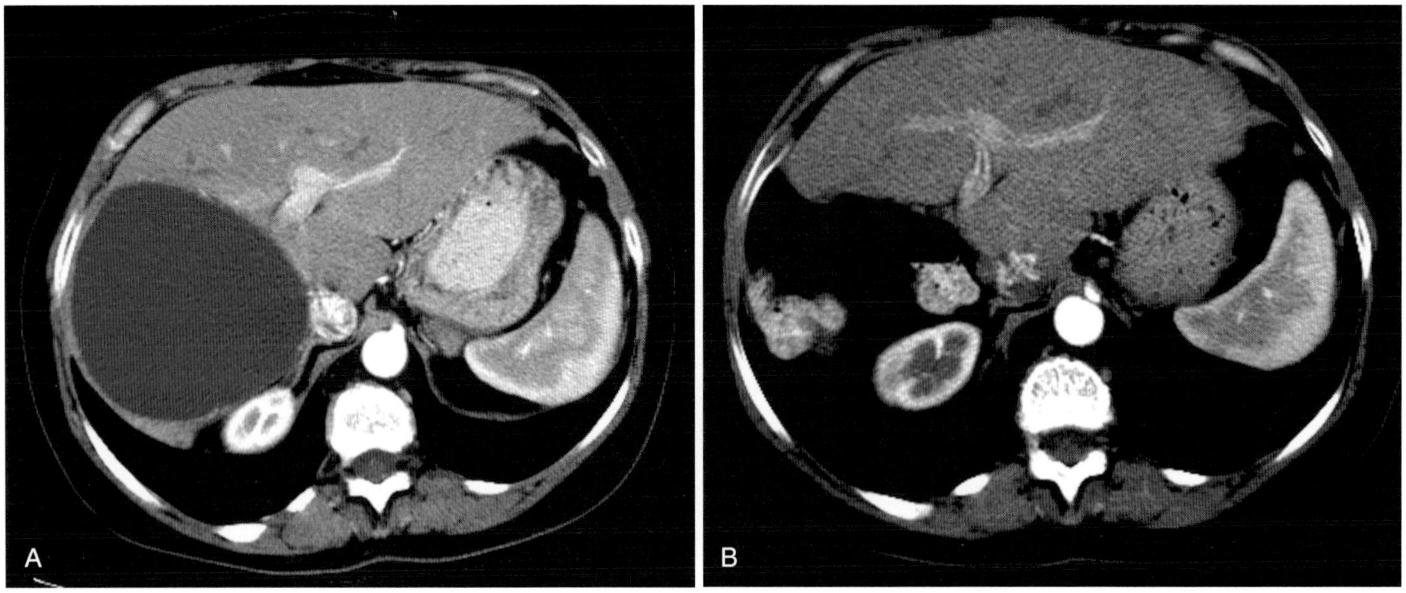

Figure 45-10. Follow-up computed tomography scan after resection of hepatic cyst.

SUGGESTED READINGS

Are C, Fong Y, Geller DA: Laparoscopic liver resections, *Adv Surg* 39:57–75, 2005.

Cappellani A, Zanghi A, DiVita M, Menzo E: Nonparasitic cysts of the liver: laparoscopic treatment and long-term results, *Ann Ital Chir* 73:85–88, 2002.

Tan YM, Chung A, Mack P, et al: Role of fenestration and resection for symptomatic solitary liver cysts, *ANZ J Surg* 75:577–580, 2005.

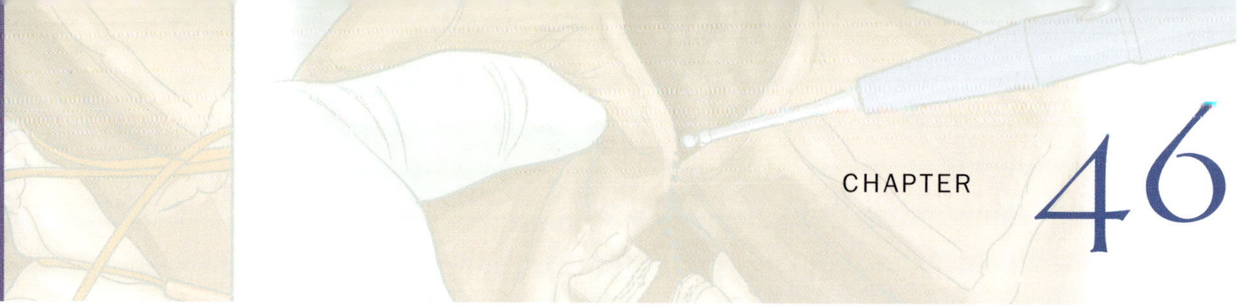

CHAPTER 46

Resection of Congenital Bile Duct Cysts

Jean-François Gigot, MD, PhD, FRCS, and Jean-Yves Mabrut, MD, PhD

I. SPECIAL PREOPERATIVE PREPARATION

- The management of a congenital bile duct cyst (BDC) is based on the site and anatomy of bile duct dilatation and the presence of coexistent hepatobiliary and pancreatic (HBP) disease. In general, the clinical presentation is more complicated in adults than in children, more often including cholangitis, pancreatitis, or malignancy. Previous cyst drainage operations, which should be avoided, can expose the patient to a greater risk of infection and cancer.
- The *Todani classification of BDC* (Fig. 46-1, *A*) has stratified the disease into five types, according to site, extent, and shape of cystic anomalies within the intra- and/or extrahepatic biliary tract. The present chapter focuses on Todani type I BDC, a fusiform or saccular dilatation of the extrahepatic biliary tract (Fig. 46-2), and on Todani type IV BDC, adding intrahepatic cystic dilatations to the extrahepatic cystic component encountered in Todani type I BDC (Fig. 46-3).
- The role of *preoperative imaging studies* is to define the type of BDC, to detect the presence and type of anomalous pancreaticobiliary ductal junction (see Fig. 46-2), and to exclude associated HBP complications, such as hepatic fibrosis or cirrhosis, ductal biliary or pancreatic ductal stones, or stricture. Because congenital BDC carries an increased age-related risk of malignancy, coexistent cancer must be ruled out by pre- and intraoperative studies.
- *Magnetic resonance cholangiography* is the gold standard noninvasive method to image the whole hepatobiliary and pancreatic system, to achieve an accurate diagnosis, to classify adequately the type of BDC, and to identify coexistent HBP diseases or complications. Endoscopic retrograde cholangiography is now employed only for therapeutic purposes, not diagnostically (Fig. 46-4).
- *Preoperative nonsurgical techniques* can be useful in preparation before surgery in cases of complicated BDC. Severe cholangitis from obstructive ductal stones should be treated by endoscopic extraction with nasobiliary drainage. Intrahepatic abscess (usually from cholangitis due to intrahepatic stones or biliary stricture) should be treated by percutaneous drainage procedures. Portal hypertension from hepatic cirrhosis owing to long-standing complicated BDC usually requires a portal decompression procedure before surgery for BDC, either by a transjugular intrahepatic portosystemic shunt or by a surgical splenorenal shunt, if a liver transplant is not required.
- Because of the usual complicated presentation of BDC in adults and the tendency for malignant degeneration, surgery is indicated in all patients, even if asymptomatic.
- The endpoint of surgical management of BDC includes complete cyst excision with cholecystectomy and restoration of bilioenteric continuity by an 80-cm Roux-en-Y hepaticojejunostomy with a mucosa-to-mucosa anastomosis on healthy noncystic biliary mucosa.
- *Preoperative patient preparation* is minimal for elective surgery of uncomplicated BDC. Absence of solid oral ingestion is required beginning the evening before surgery. Bowel preparation is not used. The procedure is conducted under the administration of antibiotic prophylaxis, or treatment in the case of superinfection.

II. OPERATIVE TECHNIQUE

Position

- The patient is placed in the supine position.

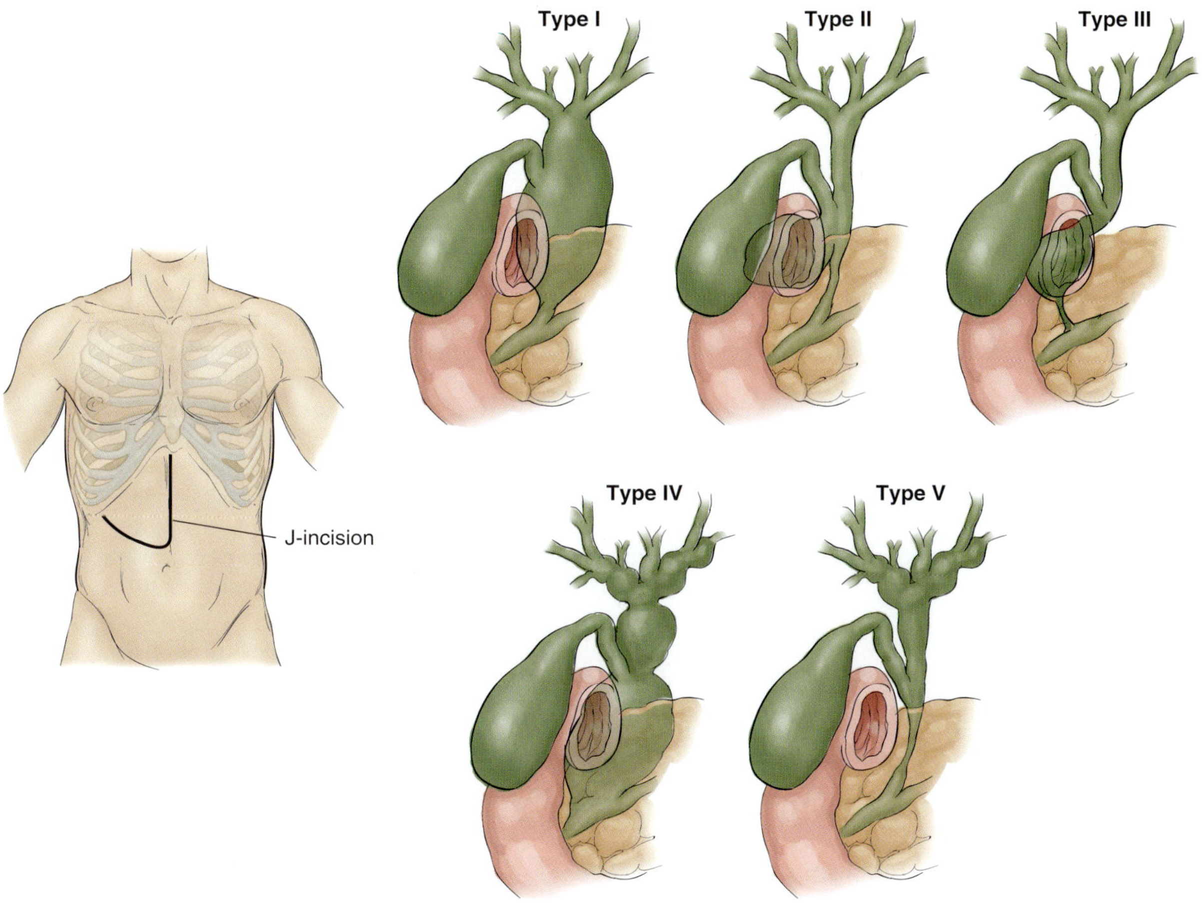

Figure 46-1.

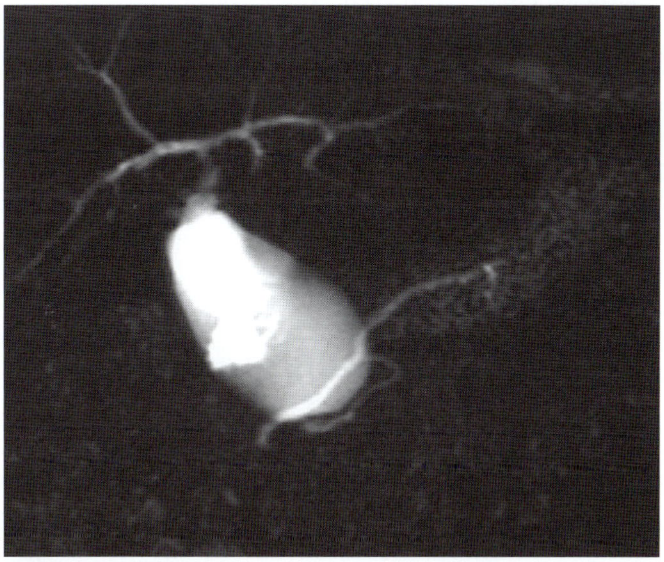

Figure 46-2. Magnetic resonance cholangiography of a Todani type I bile duct cyst, demonstrating distally the anomalous pancreaticobiliary junction and proximally the noncystic main biliary convergence.

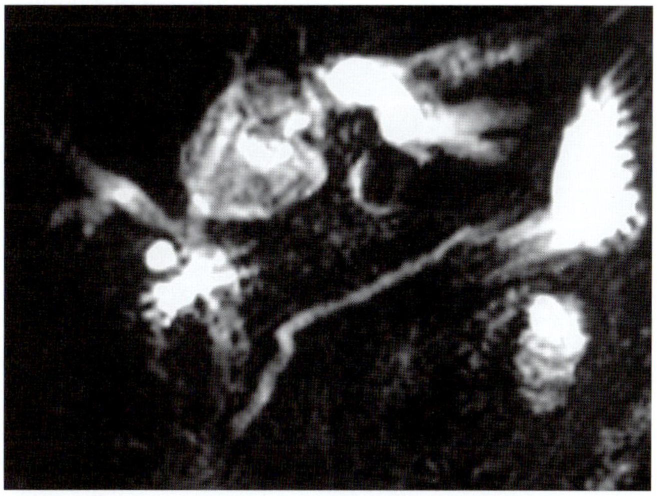

Figure 46-3. Magnetic resonance cholangiography of a Todani type IV bile duct cyst, associating with the extrahepatic component the presence of intrahepatic cystic dilatations.

Figure 46-4. Endoscopic retrograde cholangiopancreatography demonstrating the presence of a large obstructing intraductal stone in a long common channel. This was treated by endoscopic sphincterotomy and stone extraction.

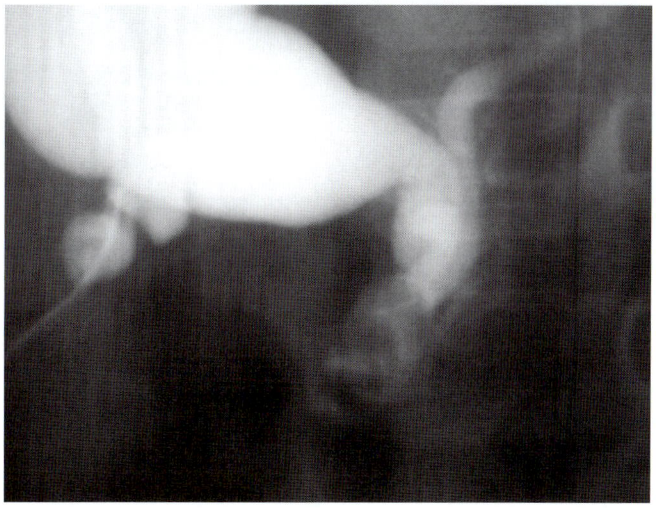

Incision

- A right subcostal, J-shaped, or upper midline incision can be used to achieve a vertical approach to the hepatoduodenal ligament (see Fig. 46-1, *B*). When an associated left hemihepatectomy is required, a bilateral subcostal incision can be necessary.

Main Dissection

- *Exposition of the cystic bile duct dilatation:* The cystic extrahepatic dilatation of the bile duct is the most anterior structure within the hepatoduodenal ligament (Fig. 46-5, *A* and *B*). Exposition and stretching of the hepatoduodenal ligament are achieved by proximal retraction of the quadrate lobe by an atraumatic retractor while the head of the pancreas is pulled downward by the assisting surgeon's hand. If the BDC is extremely large, the hepatic artery is usually pushed onto the left side.
- *Taking down a previous cyst-enterostomy:* When a previous cyst drainage procedure such as a cystoduodenostomy or a cystojejunostomy has been performed, the first step of the dissection consists of dissecting and taking down the cyst-enterostomy. The duodenum is carefully closed transversely in two layers by resorbable sutures. The existing Roux loop, sometimes too short, can be reused for the future anastomosis.
- *Intraoperative cholangiography (IOC):* Detailed imaging of the biliary and pancreatic ductal anatomy is achieved by IOC, paying particular attention to the proximal extent of BDC in relation to the common hepatic duct or the main biliary convergence (Fig. 46-6), to the distal intrapancreatic extent of BDC in relation to the pancreaticobiliary ductal junction, and to the presence of biliary and/or pancreatic intraductal stones, strictures, or cancer. IOC is usually superior to preoperative imaging studies for surgical decision making, and thus its routine use is recommended.
- *Dissection of the cystic bile duct dilatation:* The operation starts by cholecystectomy, keeping the cystic duct in continuity with the cystic dilatation (Fig. 46-7). The gallbladder is then retracted medially to approach, dissect, and mobilize the BDC into the hepatoduodenal ligament. The BDC is progressively sharply dissected from the hepatic artery and the portal vein, posteriorly to them. Partial decompression of the BDC by needle aspiration can be useful to facilitate the dissection (Fig. 46-8). Bile is taken for culture, cytology, and pancreatic enzyme determination. An attempt is made to encircle the BDC with a tape to facilitate further mobilization.

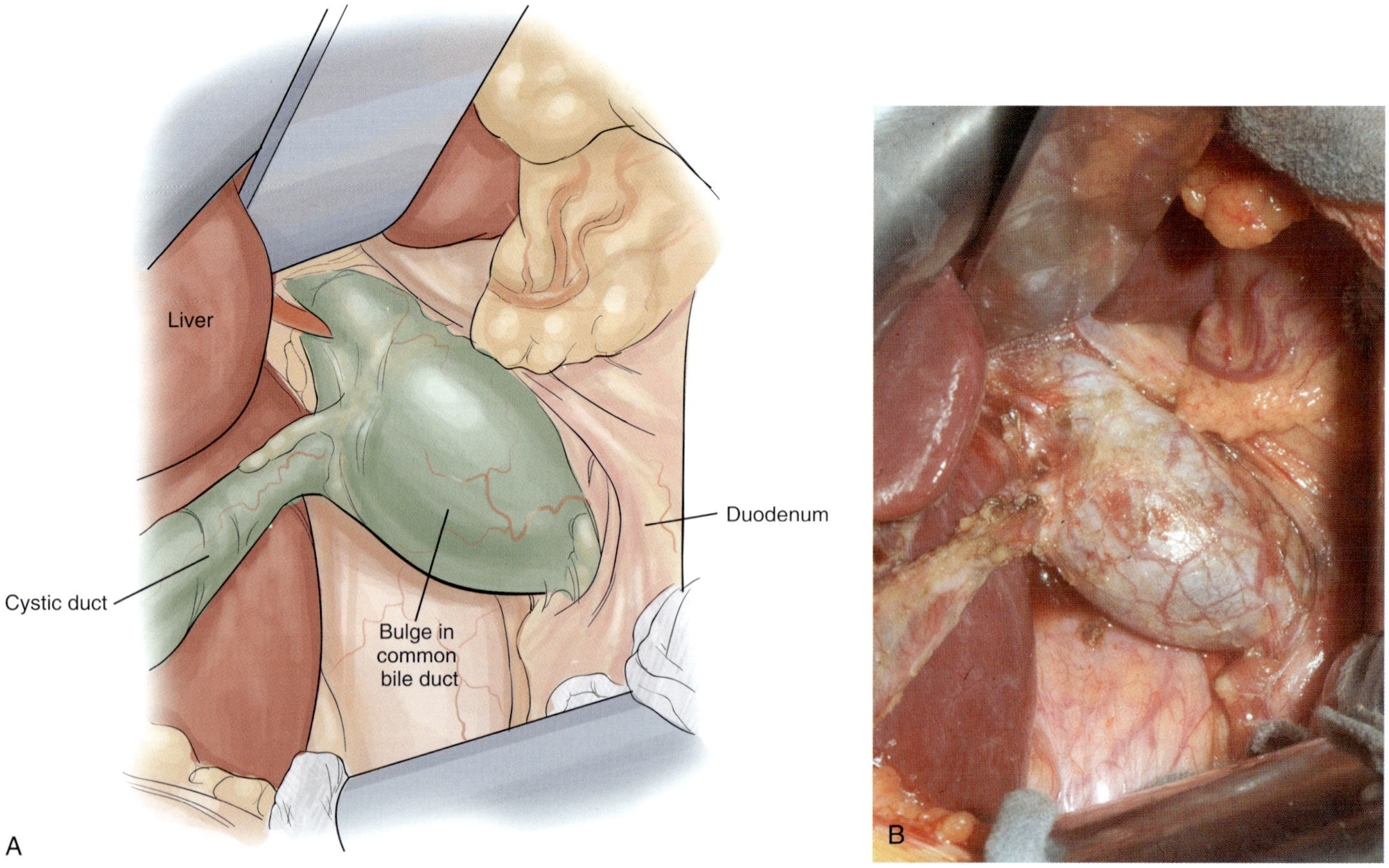

Figure 46-5. Operative view of the extrahepatic component of cystic dilatation as the most anterior structure within the hepatoduodenal ligament.

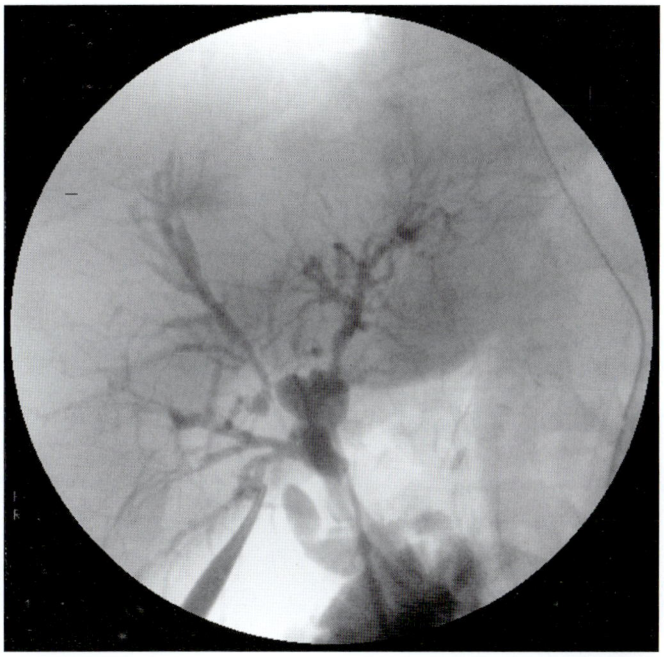

Figure 46-6. Intraoperative cholangiography demonstrating clearly that the extrahepatic component of the cystic disease is extending to the main biliary convergence and interrupting the secondary biliary divisions on the right side.

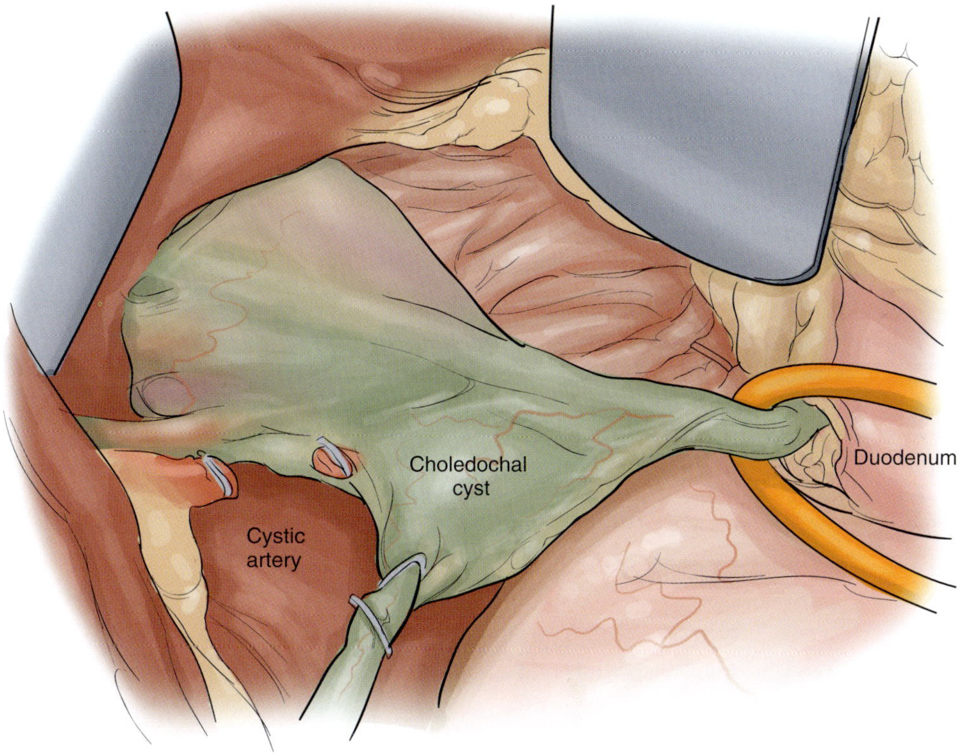

Figure 46-7.

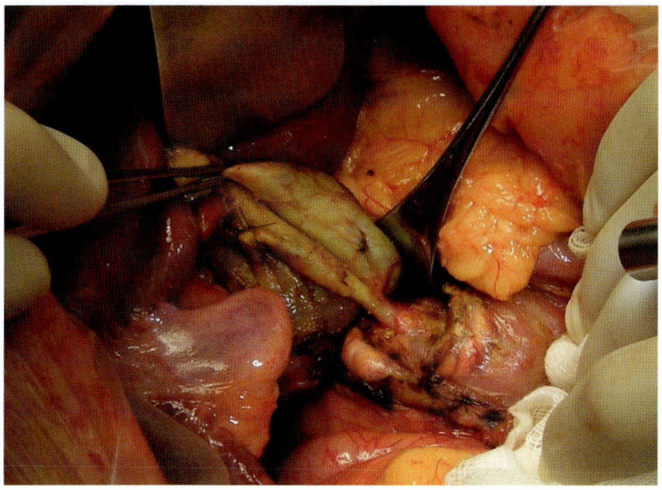

Figure 46-8. Operative view after complete dissection of a Todani type I bile duct cyst. The cyst is deflated by aspiration to facilitate the dissection. Distal bile duct cyst dissection in the pancreatic head is well-demonstrated down to the pancreaticobiliary junction.

- *Distal dissection within the pancreatic head:* The distal part of the BDC is usually entering the pancreatic head downward to the pancreaticobiliary ductal junction (see Figs. 46-7 and 46-8; Fig. 46-9). A gentle dissection of the cyst wall is undertaken from the pancreas, using small clips and avoiding entering the pancreatic parenchyma (see Fig. 46-9). Perioperative cholangioscopy is useful to exclude occult ductal stones in the pancreatic duct or the long common channel, requiring additional maneuvers of extraction or sphincterotomy. This phase of the dissection balances the risk of incomplete distal resection of BDC (with the potential for late complications or degeneration) against the risk of injuring the pancreatic ductal system by too extensive surgery. When the termination of the BDC has been carefully determined, it is closed by clips and suture ligation (Fig. 46-10).
- *Proximal dissection of BDC:* After having been distally transected, the BDC is dissected upward from the portal vein to the ductal confluence. Care is taken to transect the bile duct at a healthy portion with complete proximal removal of the cystic dilatation. More often, the transection takes place at the level

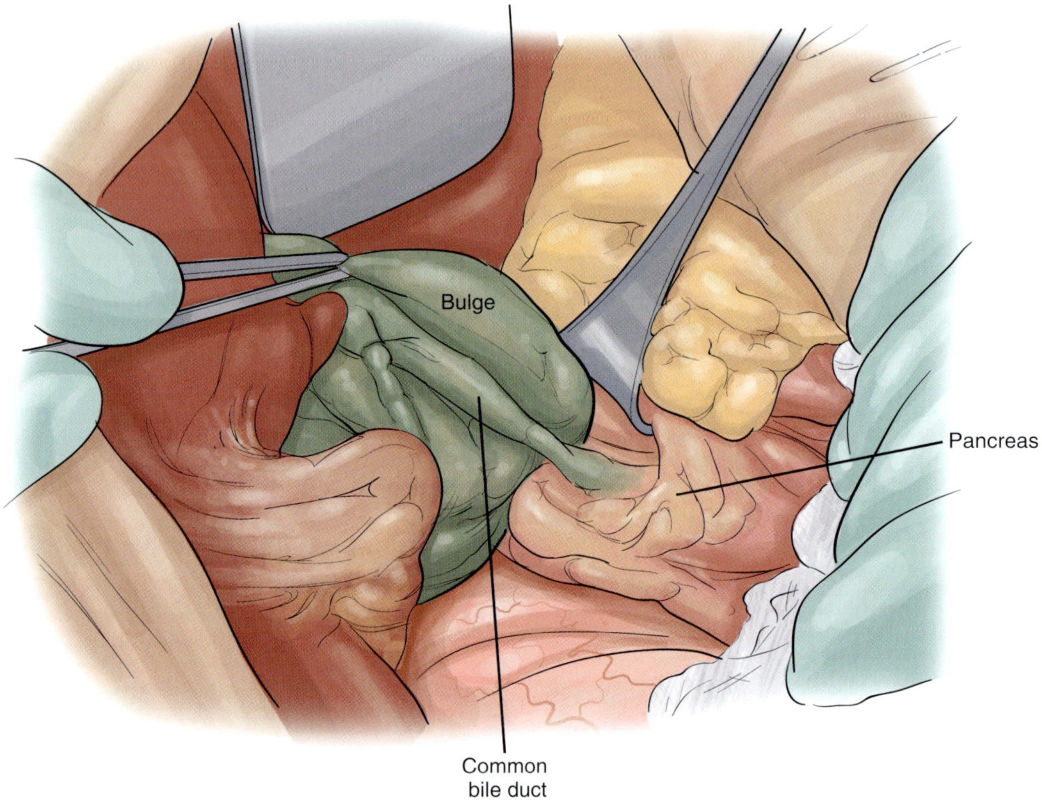

Figure 46-9.

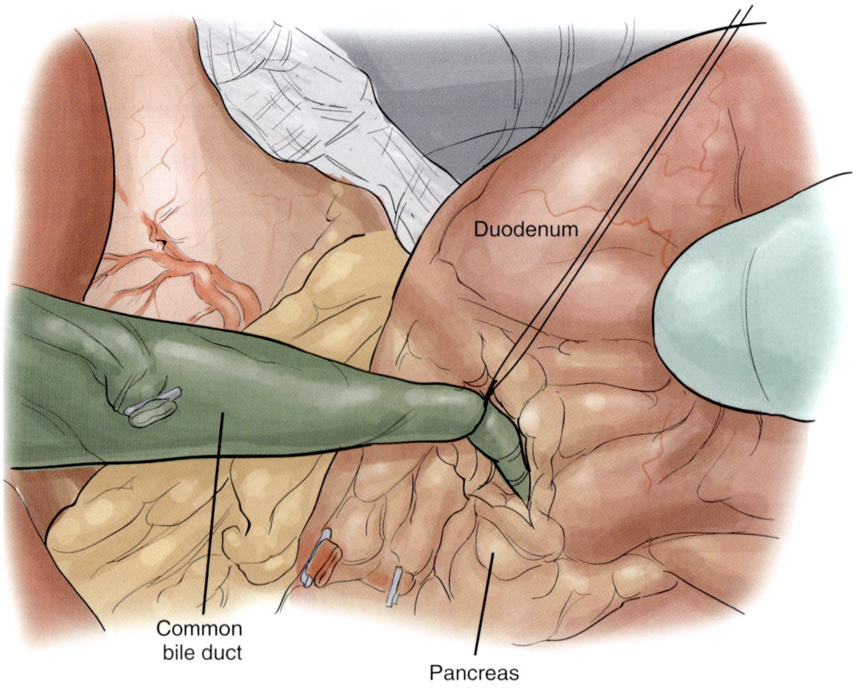

Figure 46-10.

of the main biliary convergence (Fig. 46-11). The presence of membranous proximal stricture should be excluded, and any stricture found should be resected. The cyst is removed and sent for frozen section examination to exclude occult malignancy.

- *Bilioenteric reconstruction:* Restoration of the bilioenteric flow is accomplished by constructing a wide mucosa-to-mucosa Roux-en-Y hepaticojejunostomy using 5-0 resorbable stitches. The most important feature of success is to perform the anastomosis on healthy, noncystic biliary tissues, so as to prevent late anastomotic stricture or malignancy. If the proximal bile duct is thin, a temporary transanastomotic Silastic splint can be used to control the permeability and watertightness of the anastomosis. End-to-side enteroenterostomy is performed 60 to 80 cm from the transmesocolic hepaticojejunal anastomosis (Fig. 46-12).

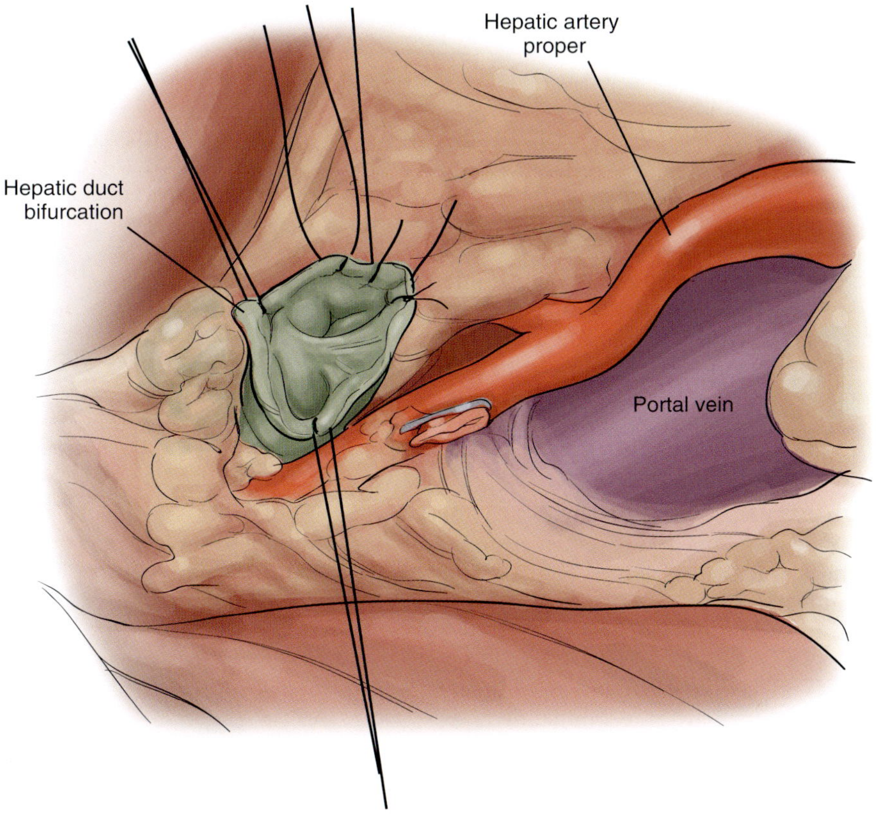

Figure 46-11.

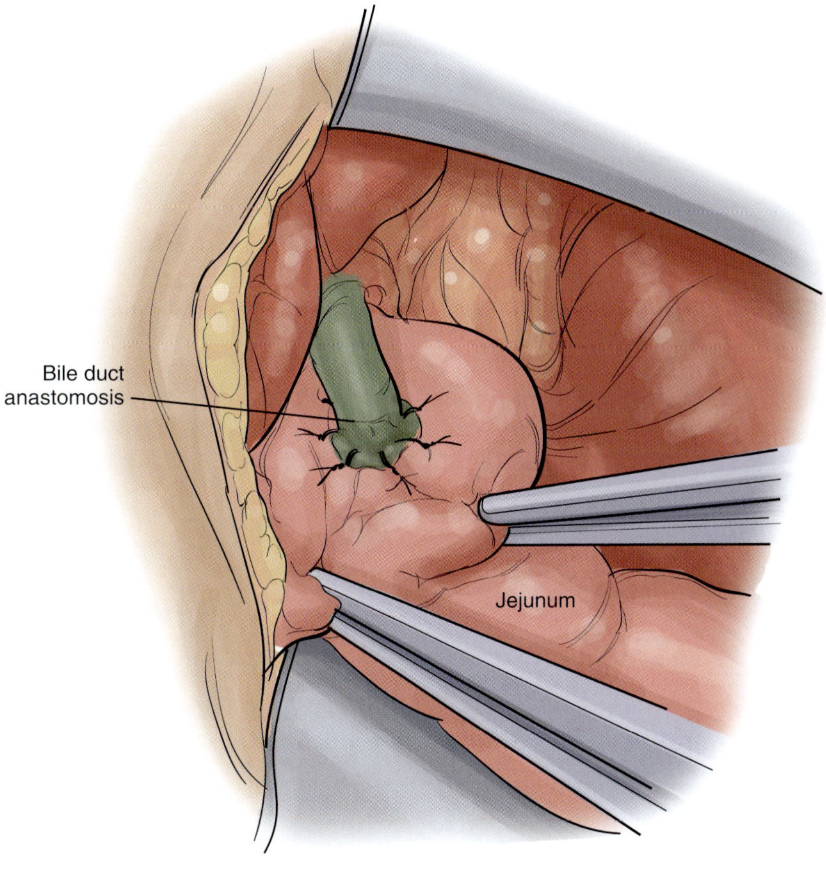

Figure 46-12.

- *Perioperative complications:* The most severe complications that occur during the surgical procedure include hepatic artery or portal vein injury during the difficult dissection of the BDC and pancreatic duct injury during the intrapancreatic dissection of a distal BDC. Great care should be taken not to overlook ductal strictures or anomalies and to accomplish total cyst excision, both distally and proximally.

Closure

- At the end of the procedure, a peritoneal drain is placed close to the site of the intrapancreatic dissection of BDC. The abdomen is then closed classically.

III. ALTERNATIVE TECHNICAL APPROACHES (PRO/CON) AND PEARLS

- In the case of inflamed BDC from recurrent cholangitis, significant pericholedochal hypervascularity can be present, making the dissection of the BDC more difficult. Some authors have suggested *conducting the dissection within the posterior BDC wall*, leaving in place a part of the posterior wall. However, because of the risk of occult malignancy, everything must be done to achieve total cyst excision.
- If the *main biliary convergence is involved* as a result of the cystic disease (see Fig. 46-6), dissection and excision of the ductal confluence should be done using an ultrasonic dissector to the point of the secondary biliary divisions bilaterally. A double hepaticojejunostomy is then constructed using 5-0 or 6-0 resorbable suture material and transanastomotic splinting (Fig. 46-13).
- In contrast with the classic hepaticojejunostomy, restoration of the bilioenteric flow is accomplished by constructing a *hepaticoduodenostomy*, a technique that gives easy access to intrahepatic bile ducts for long-term endoscopic assessment.
- If intrahepatic stones are present, intraoperative extraction with a flexible cholangioscope is recommended, sometimes assisted by intraductal intracorporeal shock wave lithotripsy.
- In case of a Todani type IV BDC, the extrahepatic component is treated as for a type I BDC. The management of the intrahepatic component remains controversial. In uncomplicated intrahepatic cystic dilatations, many authors favor a conservative approach. When constructing the hepaticojejunal anastomosis, we recommend creating a further percutaneous access to the Roux-en-Y loop by suturing the supramesocolic portion of the loop to the peritoneum using metallic pacemaker suture material, to identify the site of puncture (Fig. 46-14).
- In the case of a unilobar Todani type IV BDC complicated by intraductal strictures, stones, intrahepatic abscess, atrophy, or malignancy, hemihepatectomy is recommended.
- An increasing number of series of laparoscopic resections of Todani type I BDC have been reported in highly selected patients, mostly children. However, the ability of laparoscopy to achieve treatment goals for BDC remains questionable.

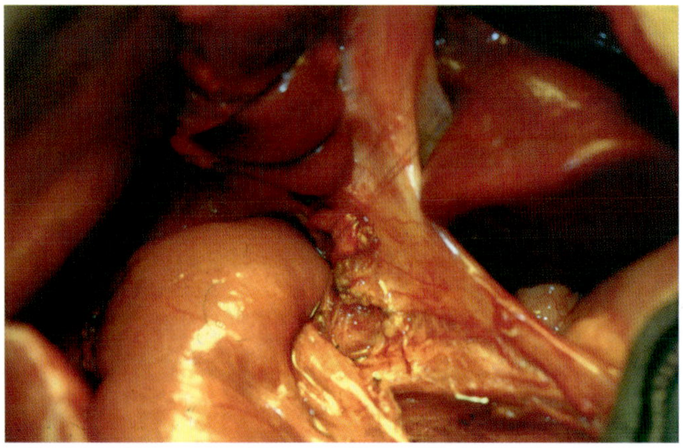

Figure 46-13. Operative view of the bilioenteric reconstruction through a Roux-en-Y hepaticojejunostomy for a complex form of bile duct cyst involving the main biliary convergence.

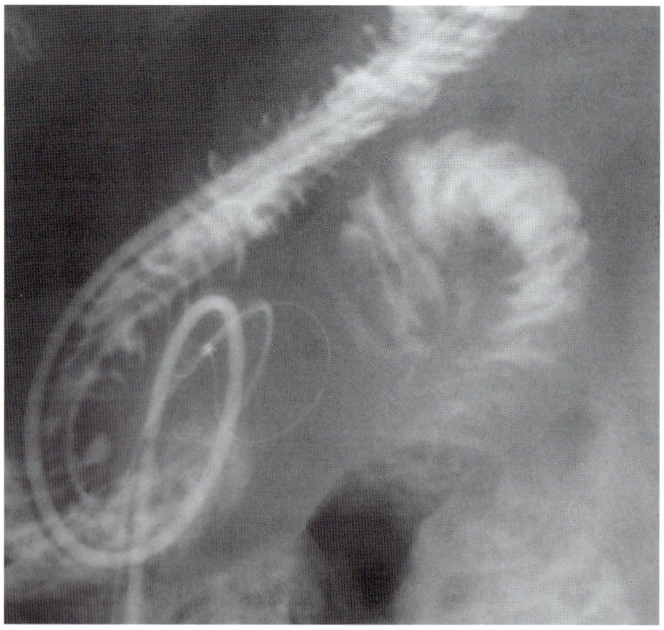

Figure 46-14. This postoperative cholangiography shows the Roux loop containing a transanastomotic Silastic drain that is exteriorized using the Volker technique with placement of a metallic ring at the site of transparietal exteriorization, to serve as a guide for future percutaneous approach to the Roux loop and the anastomosis.

IV. SPECIAL POSTOPERATIVE CARE

- The early postoperative complications that may be encountered with resection of BDC include bleeding, biliary leak, pancreatic fistula, collection, or abscess.
- Postoperative management includes perioperative antibiotics treatment and proton pump inhibitors. Liver function tests and pancreatic enzymes are regularly monitored.
- Postoperative pain control is achieved with a patient-controlled anesthesia pump for a few days and then by oral analgesics.
- Regular clinical assessment of peritoneal drains is made for blood, bile, or pancreatic juice.
- Careful long-term follow-up is required for patients who have undergone surgery for BDC because of the significant incidence of late complications, including anastomotic stricture, intrahepatic lithiasis, and metachronous cancer. Magnetic resonance cholangiography is recommended.

SUGGESTED READINGS

Gigot JF, Nagorney DM, Farnell MB, et al: Bile duct cysts: a changing spectrum of presentation, *J Hep Bil Pancr Surg* 405–411, 1996.
Lenriot JP, Gigot JF, Segol P, et al, and the French Association for Surgical Research: Bile duct cysts in adults: a multi-institutional retrospective study, *Ann Surg* 159–166, 1998.
Todani T, Watanabe Y, Narusue M, et al: Congenital bile duct cysts: classification, operative procedure and review of thirty-seven cases including cancer arising from choledochal cyst. *Am J Surg* 263–269, 1977.

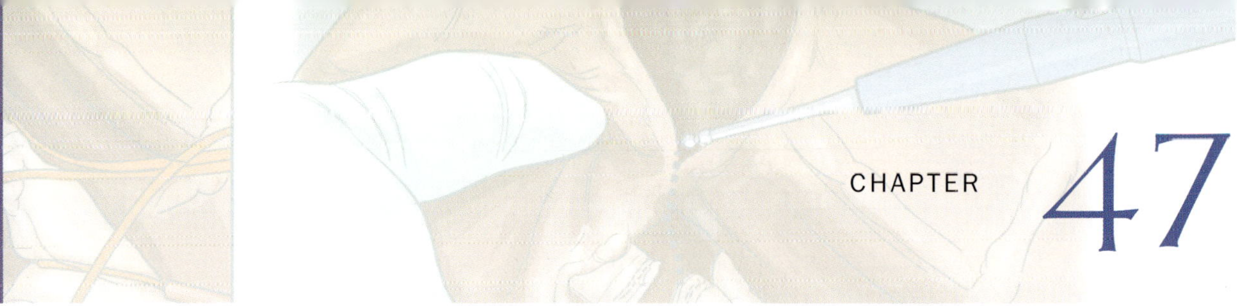

CHAPTER 47

Laparoscopic Left Lateral Hepatic Lobectomy

Jean-François Gigot, MD, PhD, FRCS, and Catherine Hubert, MD

I. SPECIAL PREOPERATIVE PREPARATION

- According to the Couinaud classification of liver anatomy (Fig. 47-1, *A*), resection of the left lateral liver lobe (segments II and III) is the most reproducible type of anatomic liver resection through a laparoscopic approach.
- The *basic conditions* for a surgeon to attempt laparoscopic liver surgery include significant experience in advanced laparoscopic techniques *and* in open liver surgery, the availability of adequate equipment and instrumentation, and the use of a meticulous surgical technique. The patient must be informed that conversion to an open approach is an option and indicates a sound surgical judgment concerning the safety of the procedure.
- *Routine preoperative patient evaluation* is based on assessment of the patient's operability by anesthetist consultation, clinical examination, biologic evaluation (liver function tests, renal function, hematologic and coagulation profile), and imaging studies.
- *Selection of patients* includes healthy people with an acceptable operative risk. Age is not a contraindication. In the absence of severe comorbidities, elderly patients are good candidates. Only very high-risk patients with cardiovascular compromise or with uncorrectable coagulating disorders should be excluded. In addition, decompensated liver cirrhosis and liver failure (Child class C) are contraindications, but this is also true for open liver resection. Finally, histories of repeated abdominal surgeries and repeat hepatectomies are strong limitations to this approach in the case of severe, dense intraperitoneal adhesions.
- *Disease selection* includes symptomatic or complicated benign liver tumors or hepatic malignancies, such as primary liver cancer or metastatic liver disease located within the left lateral lobe (Fig. 47-2). Imaging studies, such as spiral computed tomography or magnetic resonance imaging, are useful for tumor detection and staging and for determination of precise intrahepatic segmental location. Radiologic studies should exclude tumor extension within segment IV (requiring a left hemihepatectomy rather than a left lateral lobectomy) and close tumor contact or invasion to the proximal part of the left portal vein or the left suprahepatic caval junction, which could be a cause of conversion due to vascular injury during liver transection.
- *Preoperative patient preparation* is minimal for such minor liver resection. Absence of solid oral ingestion is required beginning the evening before surgery. Bowel preparation is not used. As for all types of liver resections, a blood transfusion is anticipated. All patients are booked for a short postoperative stay in the intensive care unit. When the procedure starts, antibiotic prophylaxis is administered.
- *Intraoperative patient monitoring* includes central venous and arterial pressure monitoring through central and an arterial lines, continuous electrocardiogram, pulse oximetry, end-tidal carbon dioxide monitoring, and esophageal stethoscope. As in open liver surgery, great care is taken to keep the central venous pressure below 5 cm H_2O, to decrease bleeding during liver transection from hepatic venous branches. In high-risk patients, transesophageal cardiac ultrasonography can be used. A nasogastric tube is routinely inserted to decompress the stomach, which improves visibility and access to the operative field and avoids stomach injury during trocar insertion and intraperitoneal instrument manipulation. Finally, bladder catheterization is used only if extraction of the surgical specimen through a suprapubic incision is planned.

II. OPERATIVE TECHNIQUE

Position

- The patient is placed in the supine position in the inverted-Y position with the lower limbs apart, the surgeon stands between the patient's legs and the assistants on both sides. The entire abdomen is scrubbed, including the suprapubic region. This prepares the surgeon for easy conversion to an open approach in case of uncontrollable bleeding and for access to the delivery site, using a previous appendectomy scar or an aesthetic suprapubic horizontal incision.
- The operative table is placed in a 30-degree reverse Trendelenburg position to improve exposure of the liver by pulling the intestine downward.

Incision

- Carbon dioxide pneumoperitoneum is created through a routine open Hasson technique and maintained between 12 and 14 mm Hg using a powerful high-flow insufflator. Four to five 10-mm trocars are used; a 12-mm trocar is exchanged at the end of liver transection to introduce the vascular endostapler. All working ports are placed under direct vision. The routine use of 10-mm trocars with 5-mm reducers allows easy optics and instrument exchange. Great care is taken during trocar positioning to achieve a triangulation technique so as to avoid a "knitting needle" effect of laparoscopic instruments.
- The position of the trocars is illustrated in Figure 47-1, *B*. A central trocar is inserted on the midline above the umbilicus for a 0-degree laparoscope. Two 10-mm working ports are placed on either side of the median trocar, laterally from the rectus muscle sheath. A subxiphoid trocar is placed on the left

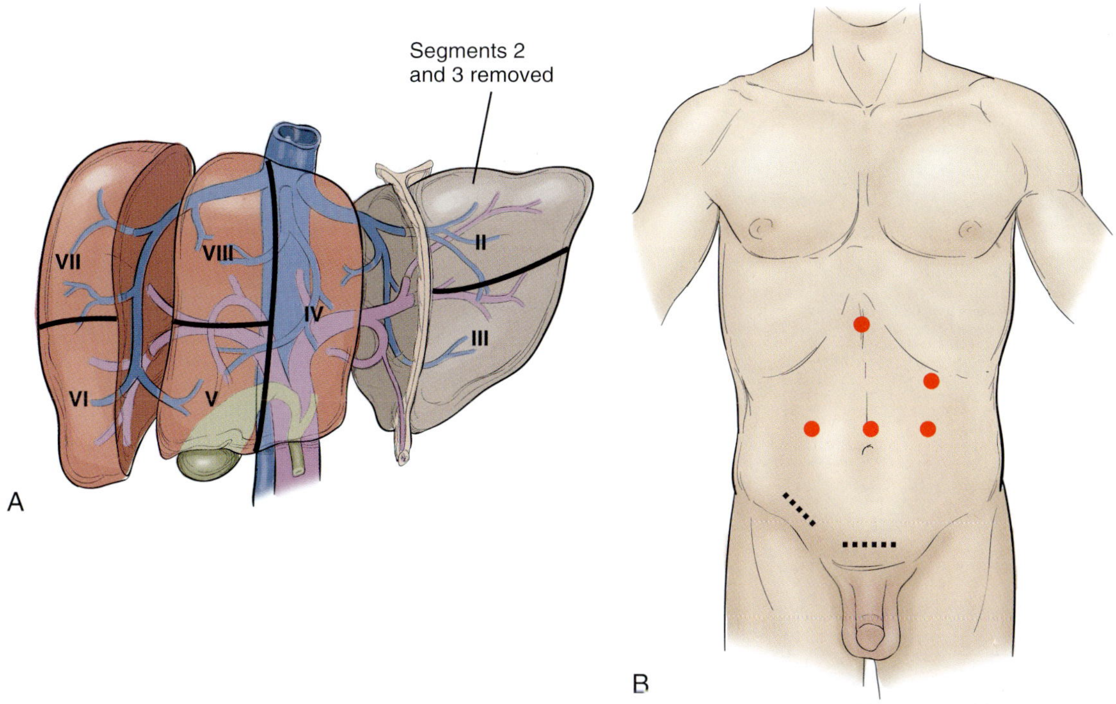

Figure 47-1.

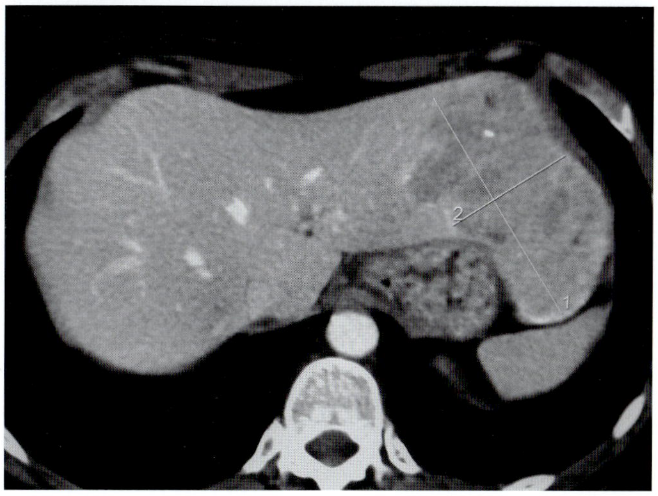

Figure 47-2. Axial cross-sectional magnetic resonance image showing a huge liver cell adenoma in the left lateral segments.

side of the falciform ligament to grasp the stump of the round ligament and pull it to the right side. The last trocar is placed along the left costal margin for liver wound opening by an atraumatic retractor.

Main Dissection

- *Peritoneal and liver exploration and staging:* When there is concern for liver malignancies, the operation starts with exploration of the whole peritoneal cavity searching for neoplastic deposits and malignancies of the liver by careful inspection and intraoperative ultrasonography (IOUS). The benefits of IOUS of the liver are multiple, including detection of occult tumor and precise determination of segmental tumor location and close tumor relationship with major vascular and/or biliary trunks. In the absence of manual palpation during a totally laparoscopic approach, IOUS is also useful to determine the amount of surgical margin around the tumor by mapping the future transection line with cautery on the liver surface.
- *Exposition of the liver:* A reverse Trendelenburg position of the operating table, dissection of perihepatic adhesions due to previous surgeries, and sequential division of the round ligament, the falciform ligament, and the left triangular ligament are all part of adequate liver exposure. Division of perihepatic ligaments is accomplished with scissors, cautery, or Harmonic shears.
- *Extrahepatic vascular control:* To access the vessels to the left lateral segments at the umbilical fissure, the bridge of liver parenchyma between segments IV and II is first divided by means of Harmonic shears (UltraCision, Ethicon Endosurgery, Cincinnati). Then the quadrate lobe is elevated and the inferior part of the left lobe is retracted to the left, both by the use of articulated soft retractors. The arterial and venous inflow vessels to segments III anteriorly (Fig. 47-3, *A* and *B*) and to segment II

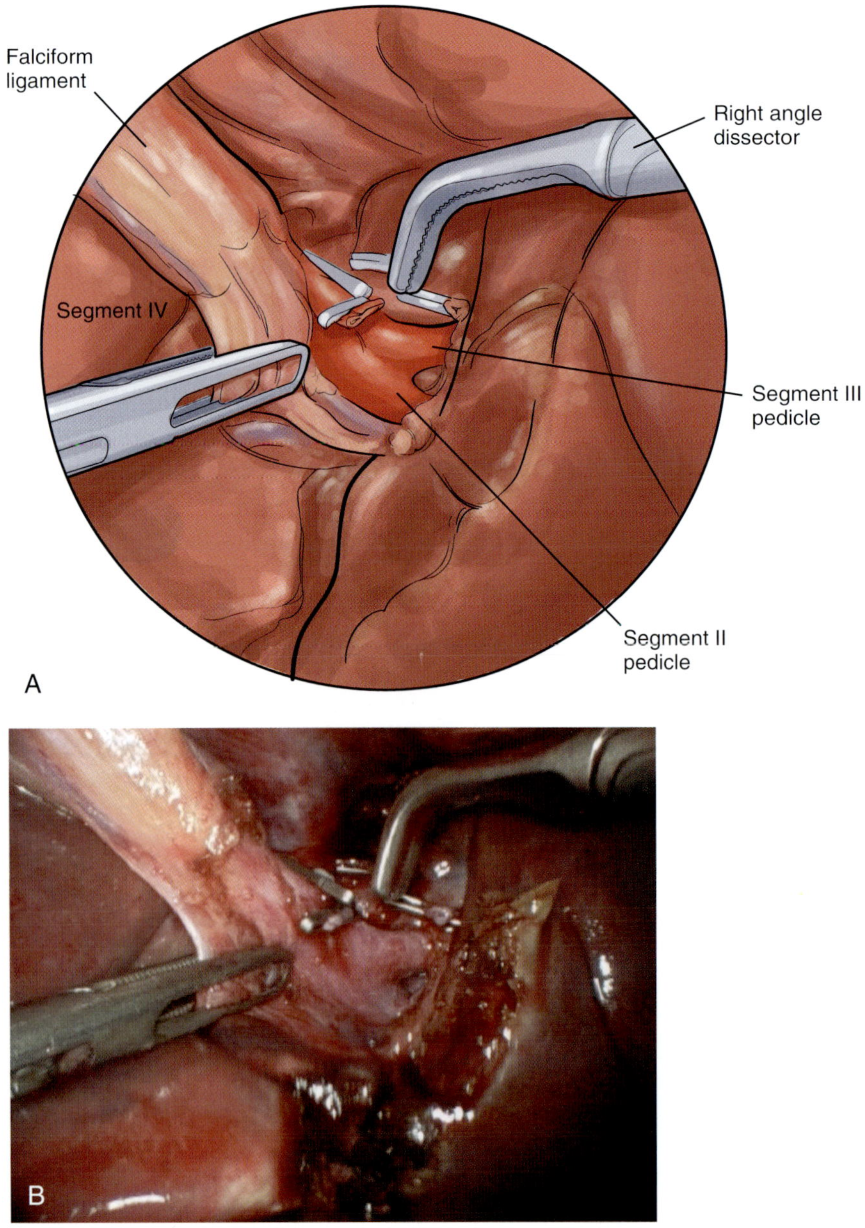

Figure 47-3. Extrahepatic control anteriorly of inflow vessels to segment III at the left of the Rex recess after having opened the umbilical fissure at the inferior surface of the liver by elevating and pulling segment IV to the right and the left liver lobe to the left with retractors.

posteriorly are sequentially gently dissected at the left side of the Rex recess (Fig. 47-4) with a hook dissector, scissors, or an ultrasonic dissector (CUSA, Valleylab, Boulder, Colo.). These vessels are clipped or secured by intraperitoneal ligation and divided with scissors. At this stage, dark discoloration of the left lateral segments is observed.

- *Transection of the liver:* Once the planned transection line has been marked on the liver surface with cautery after determination of the surgical margin by the IOUS or hand-assisted (HA) technique, the liver capsule is incised with Harmonic shears. Parenchymal transection is performed step by step with Harmonic shears (Fig. 47-5) for superficial or avascular parts of the liver, whereas deep

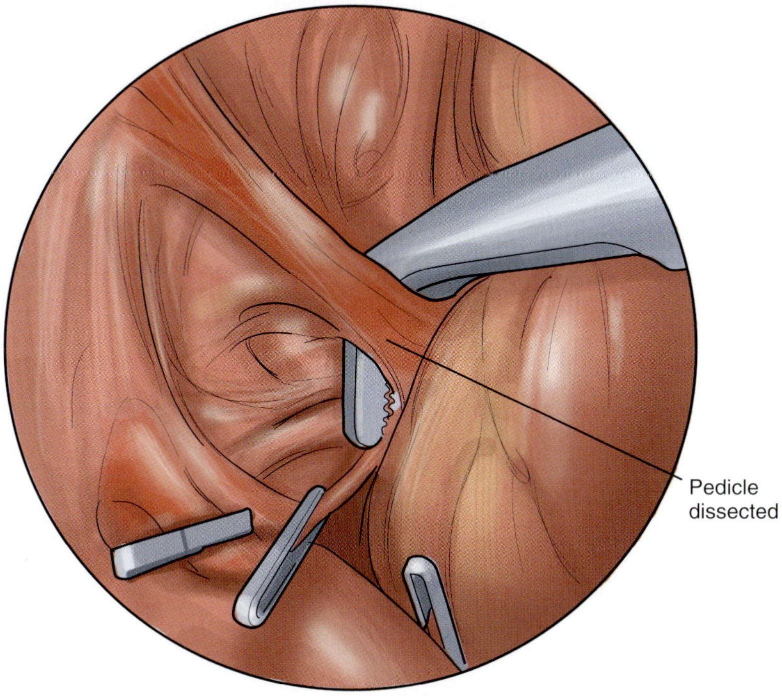

Figure 47-4.

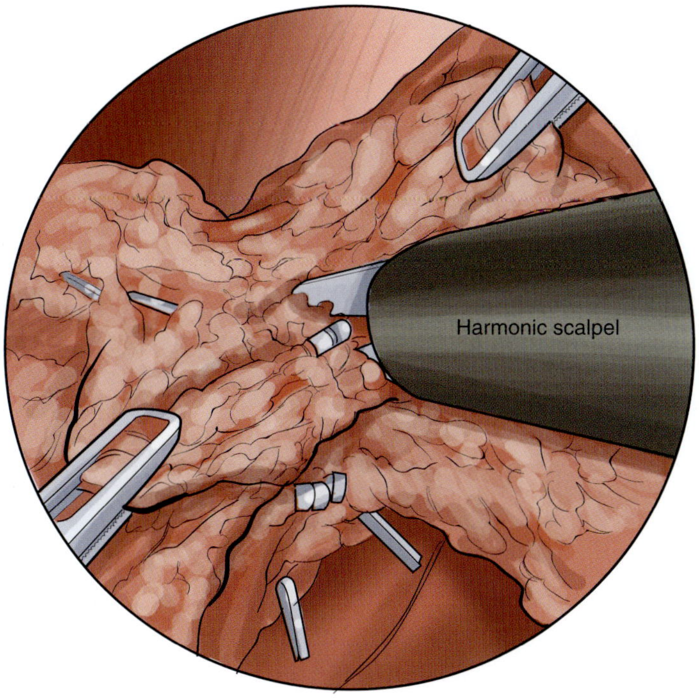

Figure 47-5.

intraparenchymal dissection is done with CUSA (Fig. 47-6) to gently skeletonize major vessels. These are then electively clipped and divided with scissors. Great care is taken to keep the transection line in the planned plane of liver transection and always to introduce the operating instruments in the line of this transection plane. When the dissection reaches the glissonian sheath inferiorly, great care is taken to double-clip the bile duct before dividing it with scissors. The liver transection is progressively pursued upward in the direction of the left hepatic junction, which can be identified by the IOUS or HA technique.

- *Intraparenchymal control of the left hepatic vein (LHV):* At this step of the procedure, there is a theoretical risk of gas embolism if a major injury occurs to the LHV junction during liver transection. For this reason, the pneumoperitoneum is reduced to 8 to 10 mm Hg, and the LHV and its branches are gently and carefully dissected using the CUSA or HA technique (Fig. 47-7). Once the LHV has been dissected, a linear vascular endostapler (Endopath, Ethicon Endosurgery) is introduced through a 12-mm port to safely divide this major vessel (see Fig. 47-7). This usually ends the phase of liver resection.
- *Extraction of the surgical specimen:* The specimen is placed into a resistant nylon bag (LapSac, Cook Surgical, Bloomington, Ind.) with a size adapted to the volume of the resected liver (Fig. 47-8). The specimen should be delivered in one piece without fragmentation, especially for liver malignancies. The bag is exteriorized through a previous appendectomy scar, a new horizontal suprapubic incision, or the incision used for the HA technique.
- *Management of the liver transection line:* When the surgical specimen has been extracted, the operative field is copiously irrigated and the hepatic transection line is carefully inspected for bleeding or bile leak. The transection line is vaporized with the argon beam coagulator (Birtcher Electrosurgical, Englewood, Colo.) (Fig. 47-9). During the use of the argon beam coagulator, great care is taken to avoid gas embolism from intraperitoneal overpressurization by leaving open a port valve. Additionally, the raw surface of the liver is covered with fibrin sealant (Tissucol, Immuno AG, Vienna Waref) and with hemostatic swabs (Surgicel, Ethicon Endosurgery) (Fig. 47-10).
- After careful hemostasis and biliostasis is obtained, a Jackson-Pratt or Silastic drain is placed through a trocar site close to the liver transection line.

Closure

- After delivery of the surgical specimen, the delivery incision is closed and the abdomen is reinflated to finish the laparoscopic procedure.
- After complete evacuation of the pneumoperitoneum, all trocar wounds are closed.

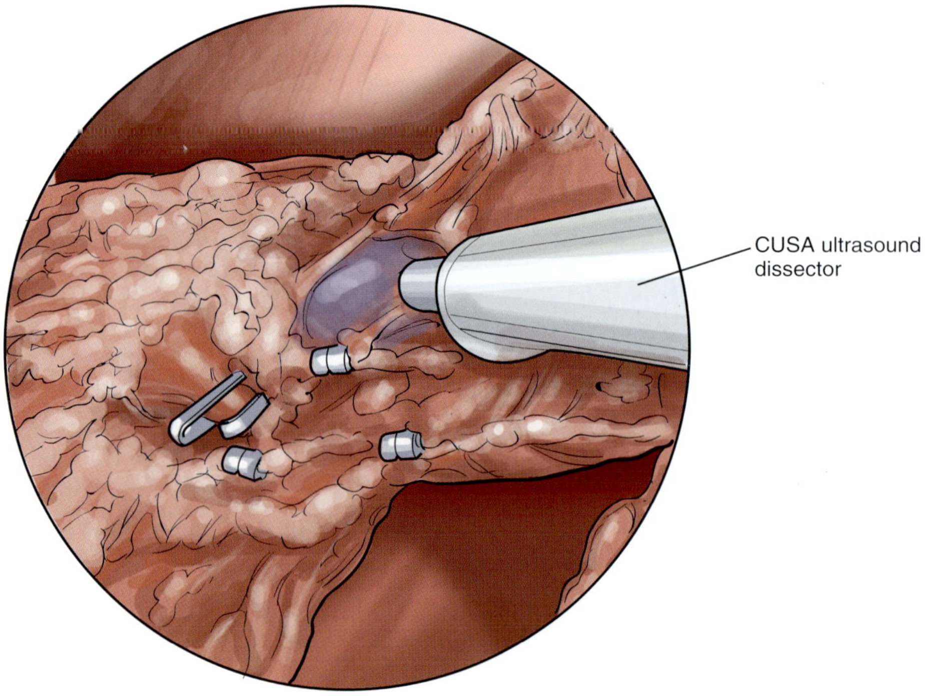

Figure 47-6. *CUSA,* Cavitron Ultrasonic Surgical Aspirator.

III. ALTERNATIVE TECHNICAL APPROACHES (PRO/CON) AND PEARLS

- *Dissection of the left suprahepatic junction* is usually not accomplished, the division of the falciform and the left triangular ligaments being pursued until the suprahepatic portion of the inferior vena cava is identified. However, some authors recommend careful dissection of the origin of the LHV (or the common left and middle HV in the case of a common trunk) to encircle the vessel with a sling and to obtain extrahepatic outflow control in case of HV injury. Because of the risk of injuring the HVs by this dissection at an early phase of the procedure, we do not use this particular technique.
- To achieve extrahepatic control of the liver inflow by *laparoscopic portal triad clamping*, some authors have also recommended beginning the procedure by encircling the hepatoduodenal ligament with a tape passed through a rubber drain to be used as a tourniquet. Intermittent or continuous clamping can be applied. However, with increasing surgical experience, the risk of severe bleeding is considered

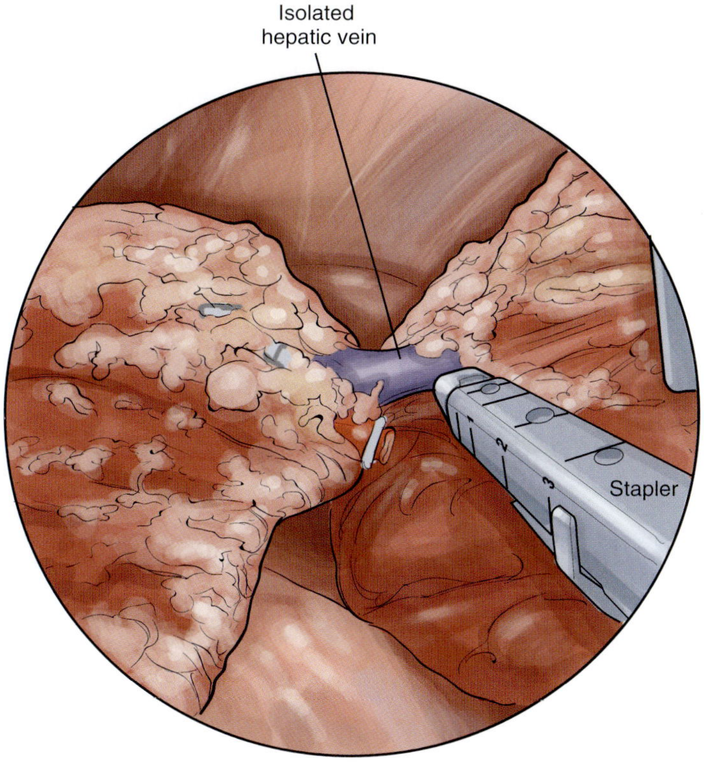

Figure 47-7.

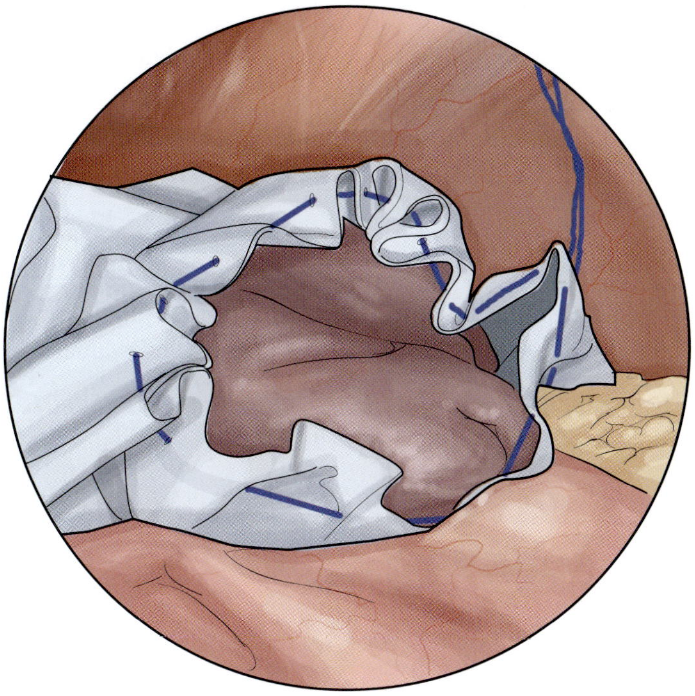

Figure 47-8.

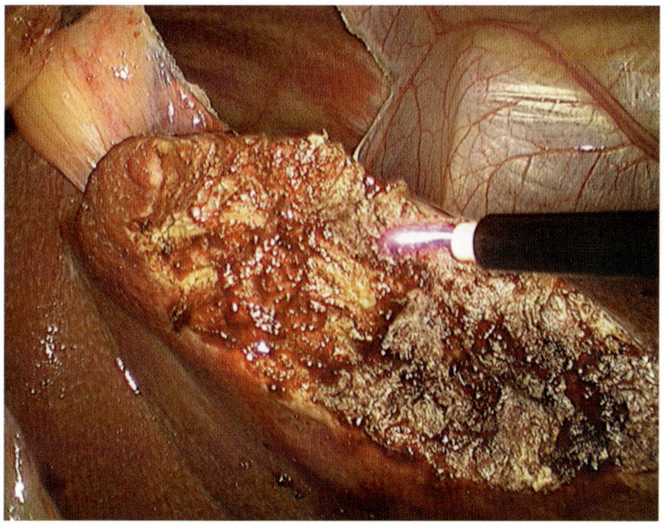

Figure 47-9. Hemostasis of the surgical transection line using an argon beam coagulator.

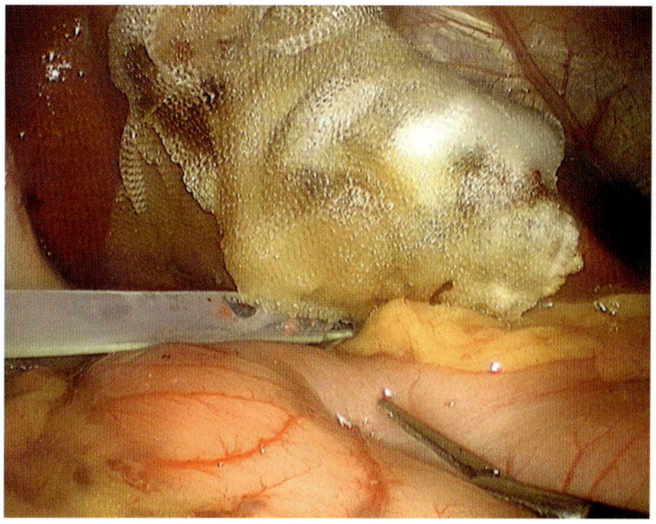

Figure 47-10. Intraperitoneal application of hemostatic swabs on and peritoneal drain close to the surgical transection line.

to be low for such a minor bisegmentectomy, and we have never required this maneuver in our experience. On the other hand, in the case of significant bleeding from inflow vessels, the Pringle maneuver can be achieved using a laparoscopic vascular clamp, providing that the pars flaccida has been incised to gain access around the hepatoduodenal ligament.

- Some surgeons do not advocate primary extrahepatic vascular control, as we do, but instead perform *en bloc parenchymal transection* and vascular division using an endovascular linear stapler without any preliminary inflow vessel dissection.
- Others have recently advocate the use of radiofrequency energy for parenchymal liver transection. In this technique, the transection plane is precoagulated 1 to 2 minutes using radiofrequency energy, and then parenchymal division is performed step by step using scissors within the precoagulated plane.
- The *HA technique* is considered to be useful in the early surgical experience with laparoscopic left lateral lobectomy, facilitating liver exposure and mobilization as well as parenchymal transection, to achieve easier vascular control (see Fig. 47-7) in case of bleeding, and to restore to the surgeon the tactile sensation lost during totally laparoscopic procedures, leading to a better determination of the peritumoral margin. The major advantage of the technique is to facilitate the extraction of the surgical specimen, especially for liver malignancies. However, a possible disadvantage is the decreased visibility of the operative field because of the space occupied by the surgeon's nondominant hand in the peritoneal cavity, if the "laparoscopic hand" is too close of the operative field and the laparoscope. To perform this technique, the HA device (HandPort System, Smith & Nephew, York, United Kingdom) is placed after the abdomen has been insufflated through an incision corresponding to the width of the surgeon's nondominant hand. Sites of insertion include an appendectomy scar, if present, or a right upper quadrant transverse incision.

IV. SPECIAL POSTOPERATIVE CARE

- The postoperative complications that may be encountered with laparoscopic left lateral lobectomy are the same as those for open surgery: bleeding, biliary leak, collection, or abscess. Incisional hernia is possible if fasciae around the 10-mm trocar sites are not closed, a point that is particularly important in obese patients.
- Postoperative management includes limited fluid and sodium administration, perioperative antibiotic treatment, proton pump inhibitors, and early mobilization and feeding. Liver function tests are regularly monitored.
- Postoperative pain control is achieved with a patient-controlled anesthesia pump for 1 to 2 days and then by oral analgesics.
- Regular clinical assessment of peritoneal drains is made for blood or bile.

SUGGESTED READINGS

Bismuth H: Surgical anatomy and anatomical surgery of the liver, *World J Surg* 6:3–9, 1982.

Couinaud C: *Le foie: etudes anatomiques et chirurgicales*, Paris, 1957, Masson.

Gigot JF, Glineur D, Azagra JS, et al: Laparoscopic liver resection for malignant liver tumors: preliminary results of a multicenter European study, *Ann Surg* 236:90–97, 2002.

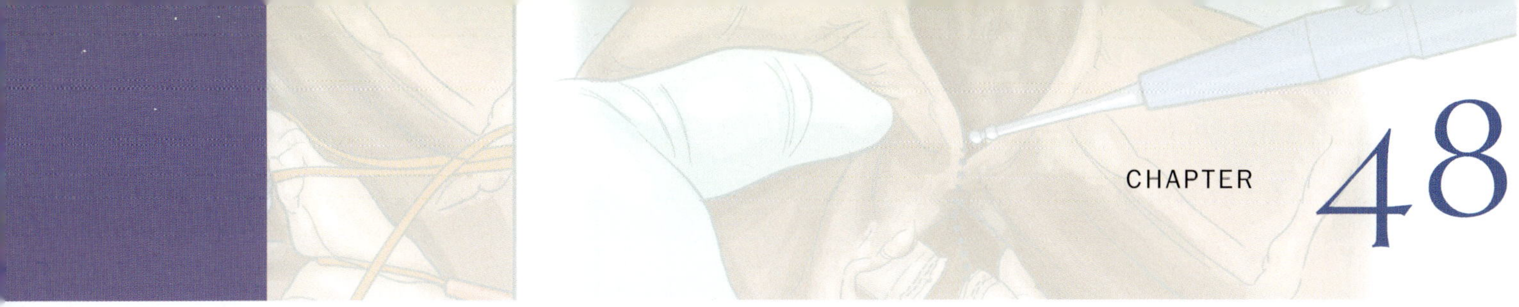

CHAPTER 48

Laparoscopic Common Bile Duct Exploration

Jason T. Wong, MD, FRCSC, and Demetrius E.M. Litwin, MD, MBA

I. SPECIAL PREOPERATIVE PREPARATION

Indications

- A common bile duct exploration (CBDE) is indicated in the presence of choledocholithiasis.
- Choledocholithiasis is suspected in patients with dermal or scleral icterus on physical examination, obstructive jaundice on laboratory studies, or biliary ductal dilatation on imaging studies. Its presence may be confirmed preoperatively by magnetic resonance cholangiopancreatography or endoscopic retrograde cholangiopancreatography (ERCP) or intraoperatively by cholangiogram.
- The ability to successfully explore the biliary tree laparoscopically may prevent an unplanned laparotomy and the attendant morbidity of a large incision or the risk of acute pancreatitis, duodenal perforation, or postsphincterotomy bleeding associated with ERCP.
- Laparoscopic CBDE also allows for clearance of the biliary tree when ERCP is unsuccessful. Duodenal diverticulum, prior gastric surgery (Roux-en-Y or Billroth II gastrojejunostomy), or large, numerous, or impacted stones may preclude successful ERCP.

Equipment

- Conventional laparoscopic equipment, including a CO_2 insufflator, light source, laparoscopic camera box, and monitors.
- Radiolucent operating table.
- Portable x-ray machine, preferably with fluoroscopic capabilities.
- Laparoscope: 5 or 10 mm; 0 , 30 , or 45 degree. We prefer the flexibility provided by an angled laparoscope.
- Laparoscopic instruments, including atraumatic graspers, dissectors, scissors, needle holders, cautery device (hook or spatula), and laparoscopic no. 11 blade (optional).
- Laparoscopic clip applier.
- Cholangiogram catheter.
- 3.5-mm sheath, 150-cm guidewire, balloon dilator, wire extraction baskets for choledochoscopy—these are often available as prepackaged laparoscopic CBD kits from various manufacturers.
- Flexible endoscope with outer diameter 3.2 mm or less (choledochoscope or ureteroscope)
- Protective x-ray/lead shielding for all operating room personnel

Preparation

- Pneumatic compression stockings for deep vein thrombosis prophylaxis.
- Foley catheter.
- Orogastric drainage tube.
- Broad-spectrum antibiotics before incision to cover gram-positive and -negative organisms.

II. OPERATIVE TECHNIQUE

Position

- The patient is positioned supine as for a cholecystectomy. The left arm is tucked at the side to facilitate entry of the C-arm and choledochoscopy equipment. The operating table should be positioned so that the C-arm can visualize the upper abdomen (see Fig. 48-1).
- The operating surgeon stands on the patient's left, and the assistant to the patient's right. If available, a second assistant can stand at the patient's lower left to operate the laparoscope.
- Once pneumoperitoneum is established, the patient is placed in reverse Trendelenburg position (head up) and is tilted toward the left.
- In Europe, it is common for the patient to be positioned in low lithotomy with the surgeon standing between the legs.

Trocar Placement

- The initial access port is periumbilical, with a 10-mm trocar. Access may be obtained by Veress needle or open Hasson technique, according to the surgeon's preference. This will serve as the main optical port. The abdomen should be insufflated to 15 mm Hg.
- In obese patients with a large pannus, a more appropriate port site may be above the umbilicus. In patients with hepatomegaly, the ports may need to be moved caudally.
- The remaining trocars should be inserted under laparoscopic visualization. Two 5-mm ports should be placed in the right upper quadrant and a third port in the subxiphoid region, to the right of the falciform ligament—this port may be 5 or 10 mm to accommodate the available clip applier (Fig. 48-1).
- In difficult cases, additional ports may be added as needed for retraction or assistance.

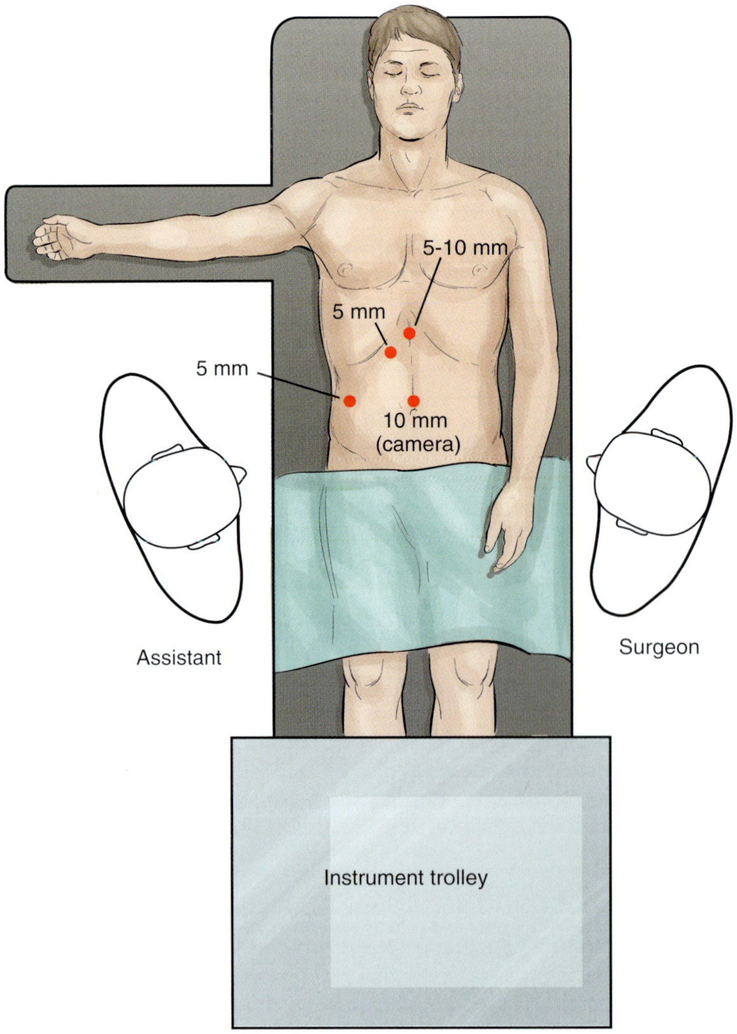

Figure 48-1.

Main Dissection

- As with a cholecystectomy, the fundus of the gallbladder is retracted cephalad by the assistant, using an atraumatic grasper from the most lateral right abdominal port. The Calot triangle is skeletonized, with clearance of the cystic duct and artery (Fig. 48-2).
- The cystic duct is ligated on the gallbladder with a surgical clip, and the duct is partially incised below this clip, allowing cannulation with the cholangiogram catheter. The catheter (usually a 4.0- to 4.5-Fr catheter designed for cholangiography) is introduced percutaneously through a 14-gauge intravenous catheter placed at the right costal margin (Fig. 48-3). The catheter may be held in place with a removable surgical clip or specialized clamp designed for this purpose (Olsen clamp, various manufacturers).

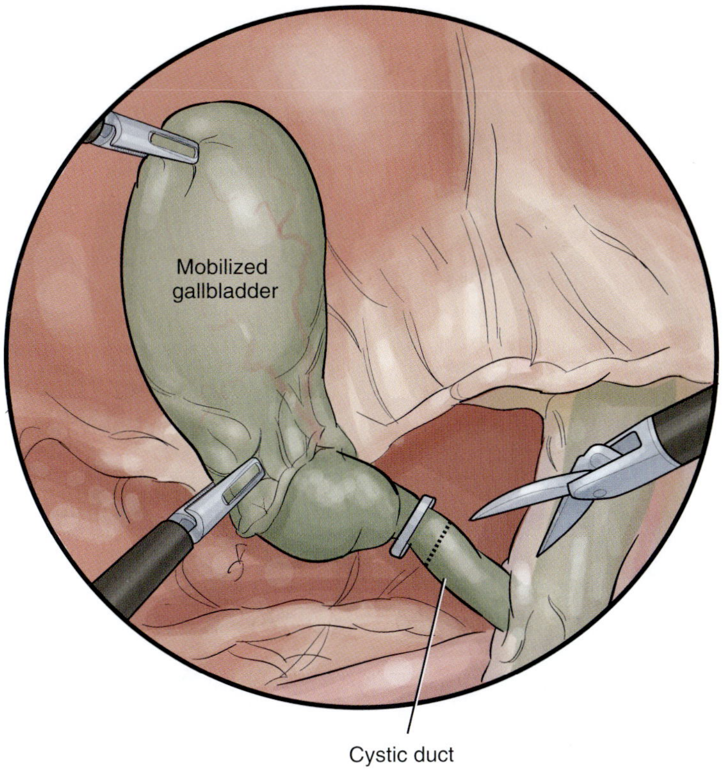

Figure 48-2.

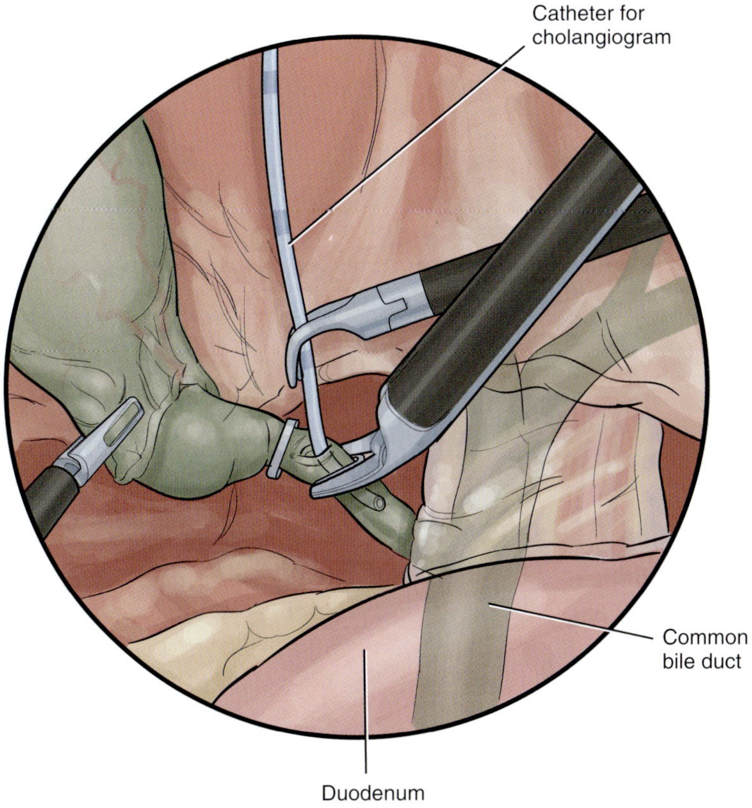

Figure 48-3.

- A cholangiogram is performed by injecting contrast dye into the duct. Care should be taken to flush all air bubbles from the syringe and cholangiogram catheter, because bubbles can be confused with calculi. We find fluoroscopy faster and more versatile than "flat plate" radiographs. The cholangiogram provides essential information about the duct anatomy and the number, presence, and position of the ductal stones (Fig. 48-4, *A*, *B*, and *C*).
- If the stones are small (less than 4 mm) and located in the CBD, the surgeon can attempt to flush them into the duodenum with sterile saline via the cholangiogram catheter and the intravenous administration of 1 mg of Glucagon.

Transcystic Fluoroscopic Wire Basket Exploration

- Small stones less than 4 mm that cannot be cleared by flushing the duct may be removed by transcystic wire extraction under fluoroscopy. A spiral (Dormia) or straight wire basket (Figs. 48-5 and 48-6) is introduced next to the cholangiogram catheter and advanced under fluoroscopic guidance through the ampulla of Vater, where it is opened. Additional contrast is injected, and the basket is withdrawn in a spinning motion until a stone is within the tines of the basket; the basket is closed around the stone and the stone and basket removed. The process is repeated until the duct is cleared; a completion cholangiogram is then performed.

Choledochoscopy

- Stones that cannot be flushed or removed by fluoroscopic basket will require choledochoscopy.
- The disposable devices for choledochoscopy—3.5-mm sheath, guidewire, balloon dilator, wire retrieval baskets—are available from various manufacturers, often combined in prepackaged kits. A flexible

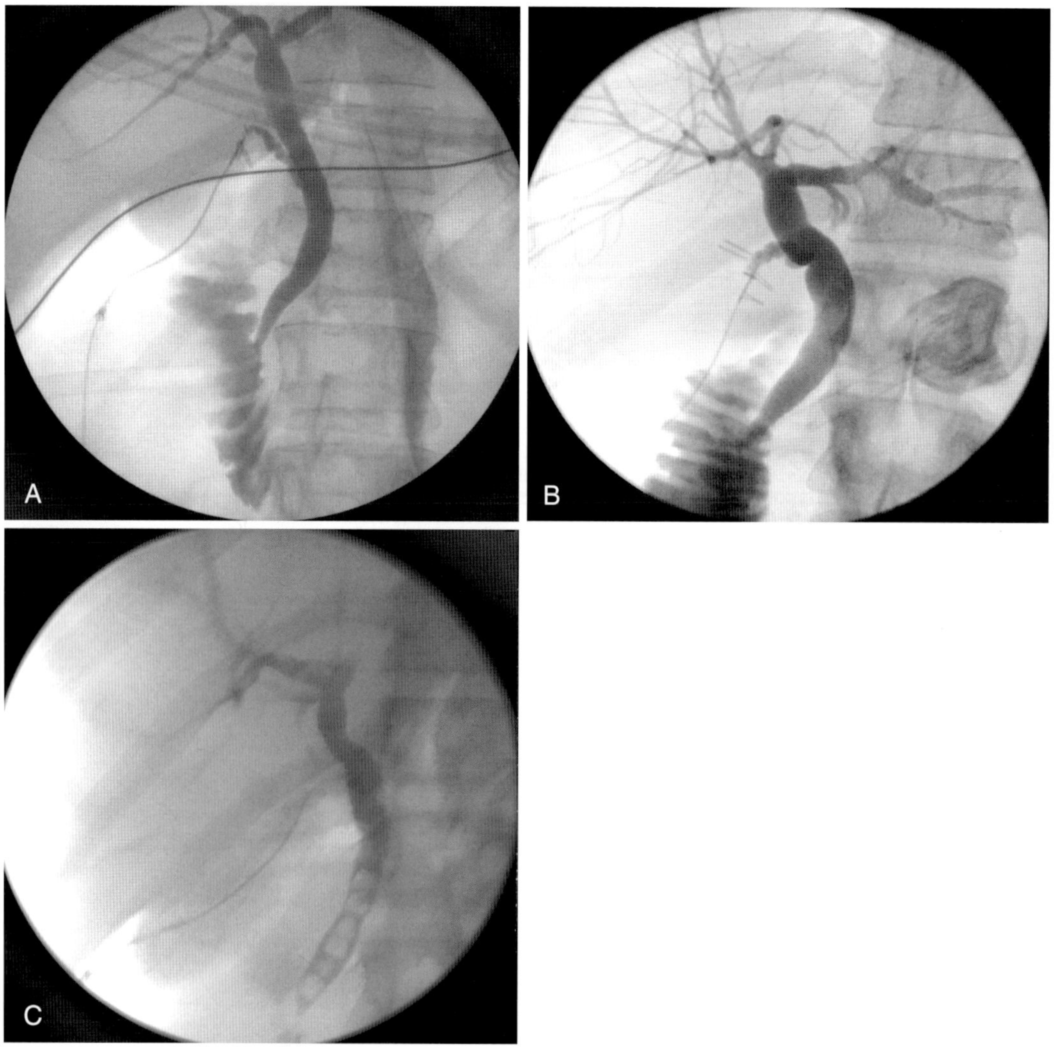

Figure 48-4. Cholangiograms. A, Normal; **B**, dilated; **C**, choledocholithiasis.

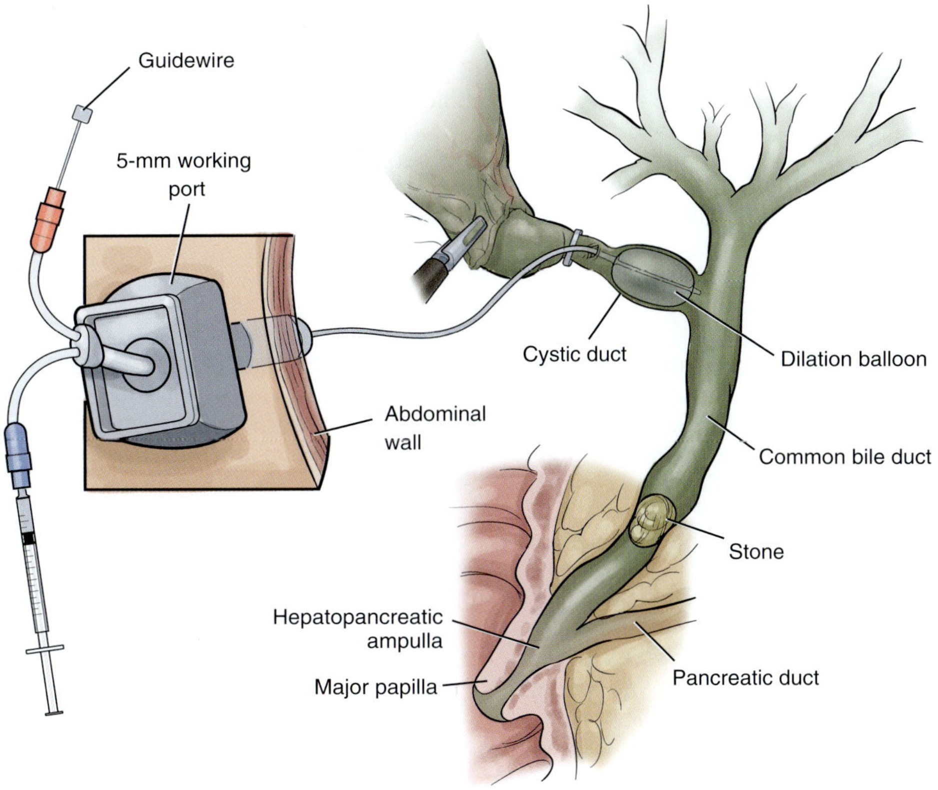

Figure 48-5.

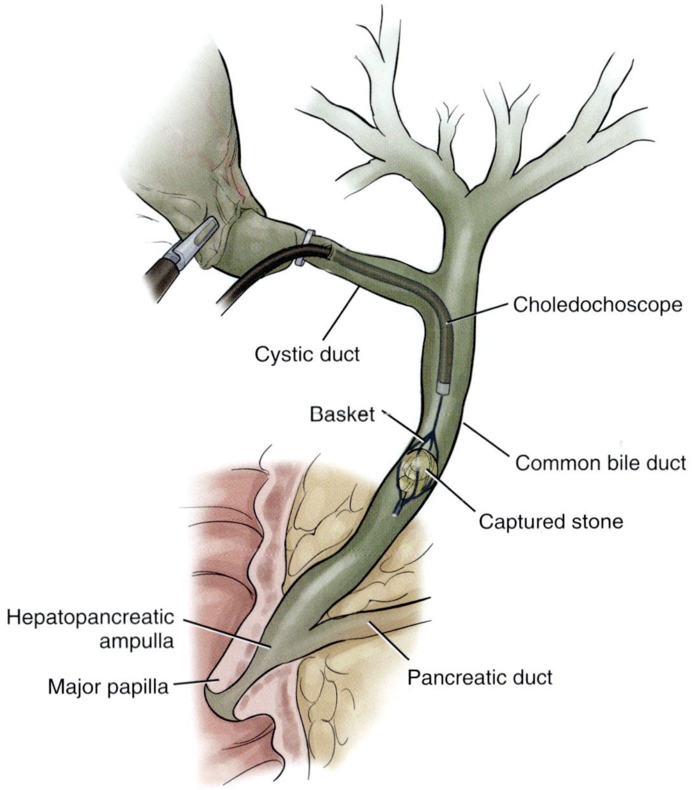

Figure 48-6.

endoscope—a choledochoscope or ureteroscope with a 2.7- to 3.2-mm outer diameter—is used (Fig. 48-7).

- Stones less than 1 cm in diameter in the CBD may be amenable to transcystic choledochoscopy. Where possible, this approach is preferred to avoid choledochotomy and T-tube insertion. Proximal stones (common hepatic duct or above) are difficult to access by the transcystic approach because of the acute angle at which the cystic duct joins the common hepatic duct. Cystic ducts inserting on the medial (left) side of the CBD can make for difficult transcystic exploration. Stones larger than 1 cm or exceeding the diameter of the dilated cystic duct may require a transcholedochal approach.

Transcystic Choledochoscopy

- A second cystic ductotomy near the CBD is often helpful, particularly if the cystic duct is long or the spiral valves prominent.
- The small caliber of the guidewire, balloon, and choledochoscope (outer diameter 3.2 mm) can create a substantial air leak if inserted though a 5-mm trocar. Therefore an introducer sheath is inserted percutaneously through a separate puncture below the right costal margin. A more lateral insertion site allows the choledochoscope to approach the porta hepatis obliquely, facilitating its entry into the cystic duct.
- Through the ductotomy, a guidewire is passed distally into the CBD. Over this guidewire, the balloon dilator is advanced into the cystic duct until the tip of the balloon enters the common duct. The balloon is then inflated according to the manufacturer's instructions, maintaining dilation for 2 minutes to facilitate instrumentation, choledochoscopy, and stone extraction (see Fig. 48-7).
- Next, the choledochoscope is passed over the guidewire and into the cystic duct. The irrigation port is opened, and the scope is advanced under video guidance into the CBD until the stones are visualized.
- Once the stones are seen, the wire basket (see Fig. 48-6) is moved into the duct in the closed position and advanced past the stone. The basket is opened and withdrawn until the stone is seen to be enclosed by the wires. The basket is then closed around the stone and the scope and basket withdrawn together to remove the stone from the duct. A separate pass is generally required for each stone to be extracted.
- Complete clearance of the distal CBD can be confirmed by passage of the choledochoscope, under direct vision, through the Ampulla and into the duodenum. However, if there is much resistance to the passage of the choledochoscope, this maneuver should be abandoned.
- Where possible, the scope is directed proximally into the common hepatic duct to look for stones. The acute angle of insertion of the cystic duct often makes this maneuver impossible. Duct clearance is confirmed by complete visualization of the biliary tree and by completion cholangiogram.

Transcholedochal Exploration

- A transcholedochal approach is indicated when the stones are large (greater than 1 cm) or proximal to the cystic duct insertion, when the cystic duct is narrow or brittle, or when a transcystic approach is unsuccessful.

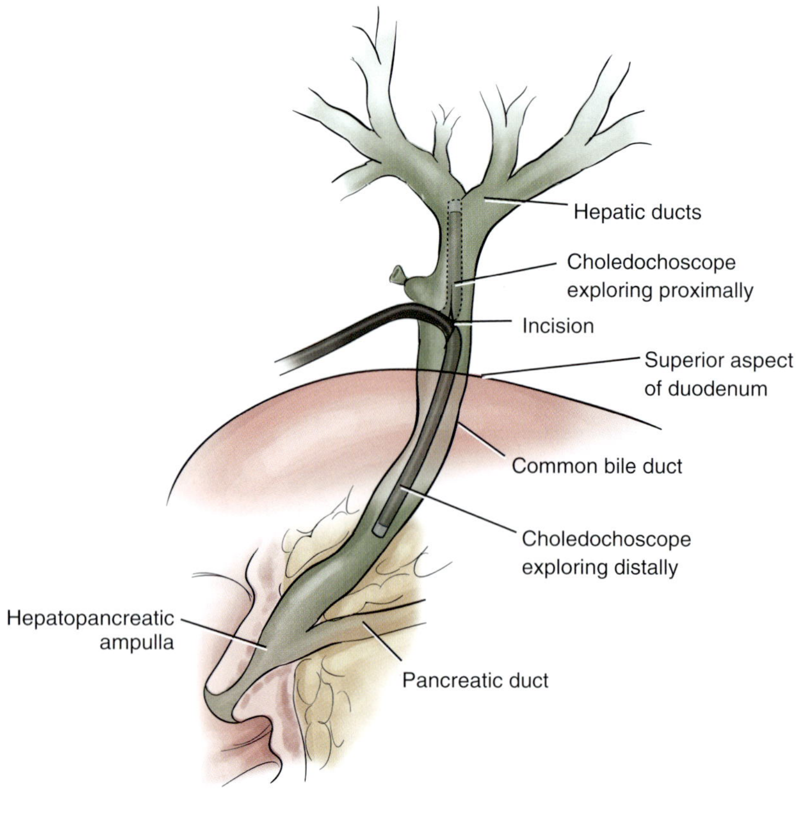

Figure 48-7.

- The CBD should be carefully exposed by dissecting the overlying adipose and lymphatic tissue medially. Electrocautery should be avoided, and the surgeon should attempt to minimize dissection to avoid devascularizing the CBD as this could lead to permanent stricture.
- It may be helpful to place long (30-inch) 3-0 stay sutures in the 10 and 2 o'clock positions on the CBD, on either side of the anticipated longitudinal ductotomy. The sutures are then brought through the abdominal wall with a suture passer to gently tent up the CBD. This is particularly useful if a laparoscopic no. 11 blade is used to open the duct, minimizing the risk of inadvertent portal vein injury.
- The CBD is opened longitudinally 1 to 2 cm above the superior aspect of the duodenum. The initial entry into the duct may be performed with laparoscopic scissors or a laparoscopic no. 11 blade and is extended 1 to 2 cm with the scissors. The low position of the choledochotomy allows choledochoduodenostomy, if indicated, and preserves the extrahepatic length of the bile duct in case of eventual stricture. Energy sources (electrocautery, ultrasonic dissection, etc.) should be avoided on the CBD.
- The choledochoscope is passed through the choledochotomy distally into the distal CBD and proximally into the hepatic ducts to ensure complete clearance of the biliary system. The 3.5-mm sheath is placed percutaneously under the right costal margin for the distal clearance; if the proximal duct is too difficult to access from this angle, the sheath may be placed in the lower abdomen or through the umbilical trocar (with the laparoscope moved to another port). Stone extraction is accomplished with wire baskets as described for transcystic ductal exploration. Once all known stones have been removed, the choledochoscope is again passed proximally and distally to ensure that there are no remaining stones.
- The T-tube is introduced from a lateral port site and placed through the ductotomy. The common bile ductotomy is closed with 3-0 absorbable suture distal to the T-tube until it is snug against the tube. Care must be taken not to incorporate the tubing into the duct closure.
- A closed suction drain is left in the Morrison pouch.

Closure

- The cystic duct, if small, can be closed primarily with surgical clips. Large ducts should be ligated with intracorporeal sutures or a pretied endoloop.
- The gallbladder is removed.
- The fascial defects of laparoscopic port sites 10 mm and larger should be closed.

III. ALTERNATIVE TECHNICAL APPROACHES (PRO/CON) AND PEARLS

- To allow clearance of small stones in the CBD, 1 mg of glucagon is administered intravenously, and the biliary system is flushed with several syringes of sterile saline via the cholangiogram catheter. A cholangiogram is then repeated to ensure clearance of the duct. If necessary, an additional 1 mg of glucagon may be administered, followed by further irrigation.
- Avoid use of a Fogarty catheter, which may displace the stone proximally into the common hepatic duct, where it is difficult to access without performing a choledochotomy.
- When using the choledochoscope, we find it useful to attach a separate video monitor for teaching purposes and improved ergonomics.
- If the laparoscopic CBD exploration is unsuccessful, one should proceed to either a postoperative ERCP or convert to an open CBD exploration. In situations where the ERCP is known to be difficult but an open procedure is not performed, the placement of a guidewire via the cystic duct or CBD through the Ampulla can greatly facilitate the subsequent performance of an ERCP, via a "rendezvous" technique.

IV. SPECIAL POSTOPERATIVE CARE

- On postoperative day 1, laboratory tests, including a CBC, amylase or lipase, and liver enzymes, should be obtained to rule out postoperative hemorrhage or pancreatitis. One should note that a moderate, transient leukocytosis is common after biliary manipulation and that signs of jaundice (i.e., elevated total bilirubin) may take a few days to resolve.
- When present, the T-tube should be left to gravity drainage. The patient may be discharged home with the tube in place, with instructions to monitor the output at home. Once the 24-hour output falls below 100 mL, a T-tube cholangiogram can be performed. If this demonstrates a nondilated, draining CBD, the T-tube can be clamped. After a minimum of 3 weeks, the tube can be removed.
- If the cholangiogram demonstrates persistent CBD stones, the tube should be left in place for 6 weeks, after which the tract may be instrumented by an interventional radiologist for stone extraction.

SUGGESTED READINGS

Parra-Membrives P, Díaz-Gómez D, Vilegas-Portero R, et al: Appropriate management of common bile duct stones: a RAND Corporation/UCLA Appropriateness Method statistical analysis, *Surg Endosc* 24:1187–1194, 2010. Review.

Rogers SJ, Cello JP, Horn JK, et al: Prospective randomized trial of LC+LCBDE vs ERCP/S+LC for common bile duct stone disease, *Arch Surg* 145:28–33, 2010.

Verbesey JE, Birkett DH: Common bile duct exploration for choledocholithiasis, *Surg Clin North America* 88:1315–1328, ix, 2008. Review.

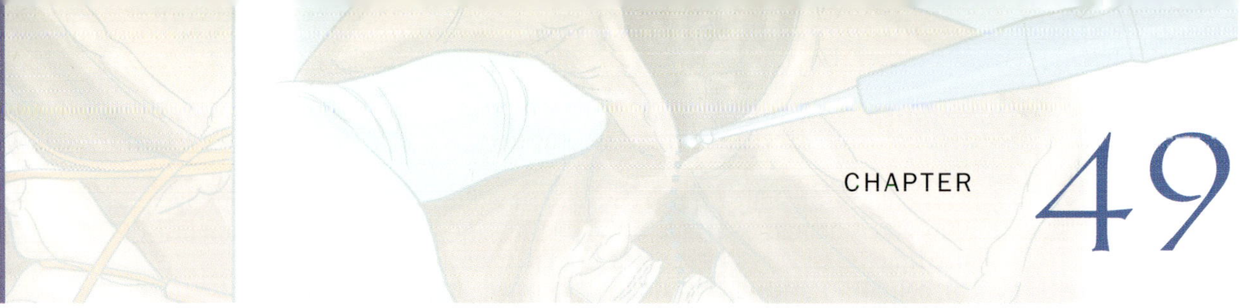

CHAPTER 49

Laparoscopic Radiofrequency Ablation of Liver Tumors

Fady K. Balaa, MD, and David A. Geller, MD

I. SPECIAL PREOPERATIVE PREPARATION

Therapeutic Principle

- A generator delivers high-frequency alternating current that moves from the tip of the electrode to the surrounding tissue (Fig. 49-1).
- Ionic agitation causes frictional heating, coagulation necrosis, and cell death in the ablation zone (see Figs. 49-8 and 49-9, later). The impedance (resistance to current flow) increase in the ablation zone is measured by the generator to signal completion of treatment. Temperature can also be measured to determine cell death.

Operative Indications

- Surgical resection remains the gold standard for the treatment of primary or metastatic liver cancers.
- Radiofrequency ablation (RFA) can expand operative indications:
  - ▲ Combine with major liver resection to clear all cancer
  - ▲ Bridge to transplantation for hepatocellular carcinoma
  - ▲ Treatment for hepatocellular carcinoma in patients who are not candidates for resection or transplantation
  - ▲ Second-line therapy for hepatic metastasis in patients who are not candidates for resection

Review of Imaging

- Biphasic computed tomography (CT) scan of the abdomen is mandatory in preoperative planning. It identifies:
  - ▲ Exact location of the lesion within the liver
  - ▲ Presence of multifocal disease
  - ▲ Relationship of the lesion to the major hepatic vasculature and biliary tree
  - ▲ Relationship of the lesion to the diaphragm and hollow viscus, including the gallbladder, duodenum, and colonic hepatic flexure
  - ▲ Location of collateral abdominal wall vessels in the cirrhotic patient with portal hypertension, thus facilitating safe trocar placement

Instruments

- 10-mm 30-degree telescope.
- 5-mm 30-degree telescope.
- Laparoscopic tissue graspers.
- Laparoscopic hook electrocautery.
- Laparoscopic suction irrigation device.
- 12-mm trocars (2).
- 5-mm trocar (1).
- Laparoscopic ultrasound (US).
- Closing device.
- Radiofrequency ablation generator. Currently there are three ablation systems available:
  - ▲ StarBurst devices (RITA Medical Systems, Mountain View, Calif.)
  - ▲ RF 3000 devices with LeVeen electrodes (Boston Scientific, Boston)
  - ▲ Cool-tip RF Tissue Ablation System (Valleylab, Boulder, Colo.)
- Radiofrequency ablation probes ranging from 2.0 to 5.0 cm in diameter (Fig. 49-2).

Anesthesia and Antibiotics

- General anesthesia is administered, avoiding nitrous products to minimize bowel distention.
- Ampicillin/sulbactam or first-generation cephalosporin is administered intravenously before skin incision.

Accessory Devices

- An orogastric tube is inserted after induction and is removed before reversal of anesthesia.
- A urinary catheter is inserted after induction and is removed in the operating room or on the first postoperative day.
- Pneumatic compression stockings are placed before induction.

II. OPERATIVE TECHNIQUE

Position

- The patient is placed in a supine position with arms well padded and extended 60 degrees to each side.
- The patient is strapped to the table, and a footboard is placed to prevent movement during reverse Trendelenburg position.
- Two video monitors are at the head of the table above each shoulder.
- The US machine is on the patient's left side.

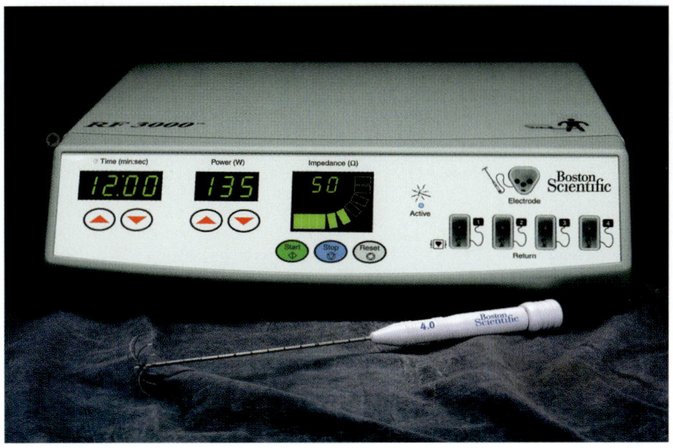

Figure 49-1.

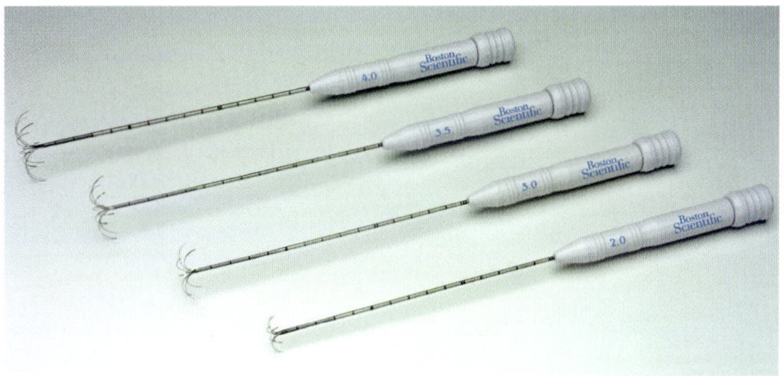

Figure 49-2.

- We prefer to feed the US image to the video monitors for picture-in-picture imaging.
- For right-sided lesions, the surgeon stands at the patient's right side, and the assistant surgeon stands at the patient's left side (Fig. 49-3).

Trocar Placement

- A total of three trocars are required. All trocar sites are preinjected with 0.5% bupivacaine.
- Open technique is used for first trocar placement in the supraumbilical space. If a recanalized umbilical vein is identified on preoperative CT scan, then the infraumbilical space is used for first trocar placement.
- Under direct visualization, the accessory trocars are placed as follows (with some variation according to the location of collateralizing abdominal wall veins as identified on CT scan and by transillumination):
  - ▲ *Right lobe and left medial segment lesions (segments IV to VIII)* (Fig. 49-4, *A* and *B*): 5-mm trocar in the right paramedian space midclavicular line; 12-mm trocar in the right subcostal space anterior axillary line
  - ▲ *Left lateral segment lesions (segments II and III)*: Mirror image of placement just described

Main Dissection

- The laparoscopic US probe is introduced through the right subcostal port, and a complete liver scan is performed. This identifies the lesion in question and rules out the presence of any other second lesions not seen on preoperative imaging (Fig. 49-5).
- The lesion to be ablated is brought into view and projected with picture-in-picture imaging (Fig. 49-6).

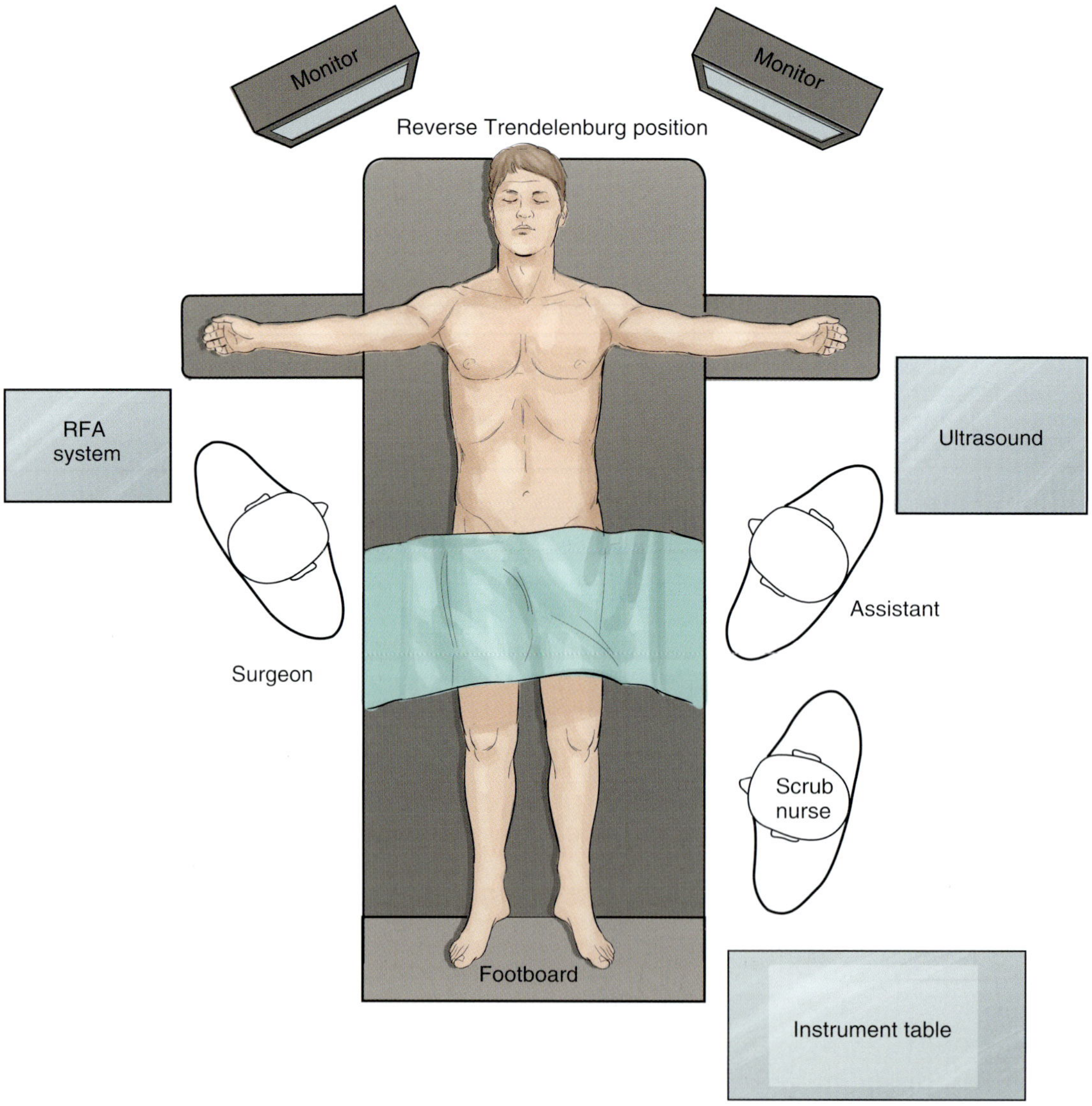

Figure 49-3.

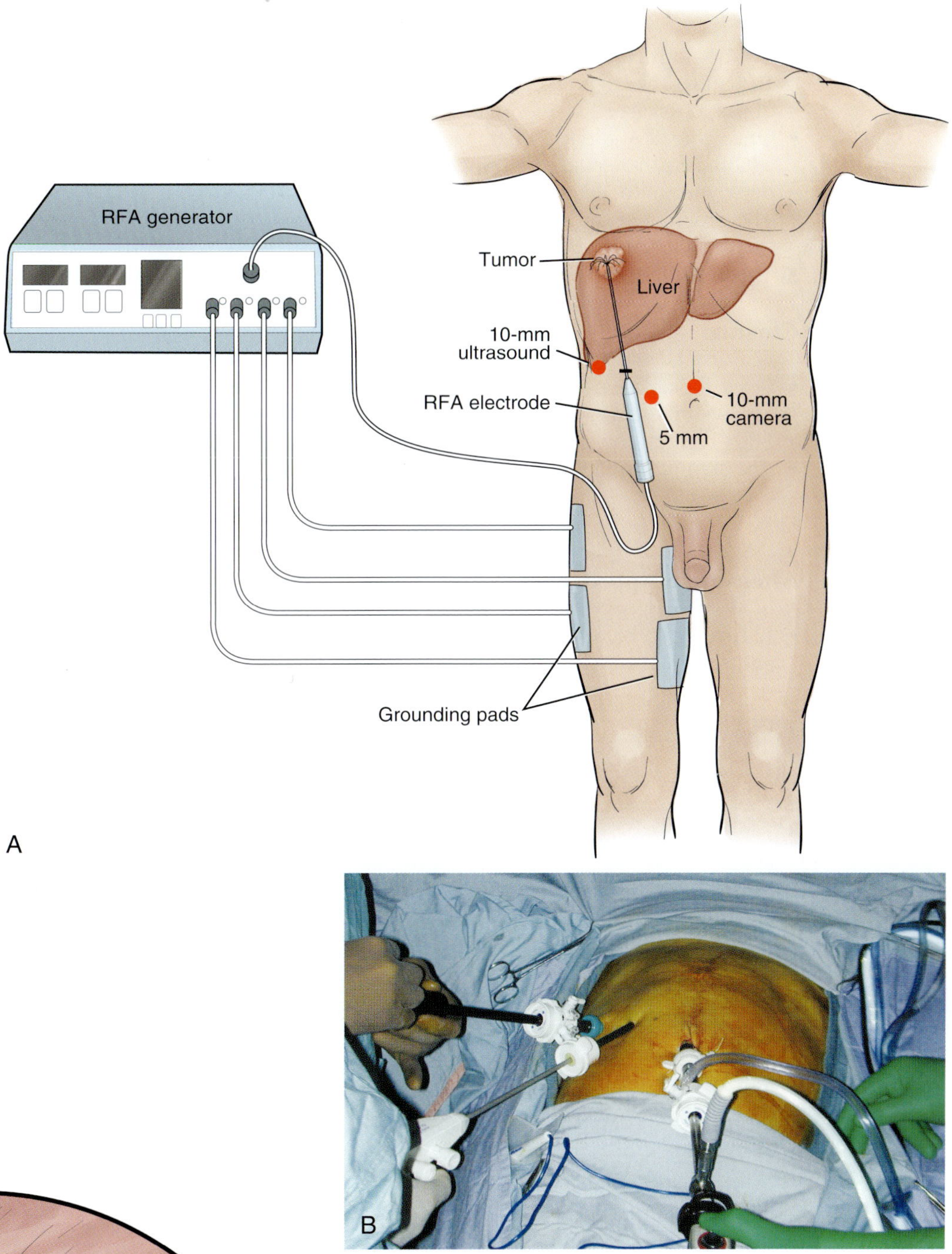

Figure 49-4. *RFA,* Radiofrequency ablation.

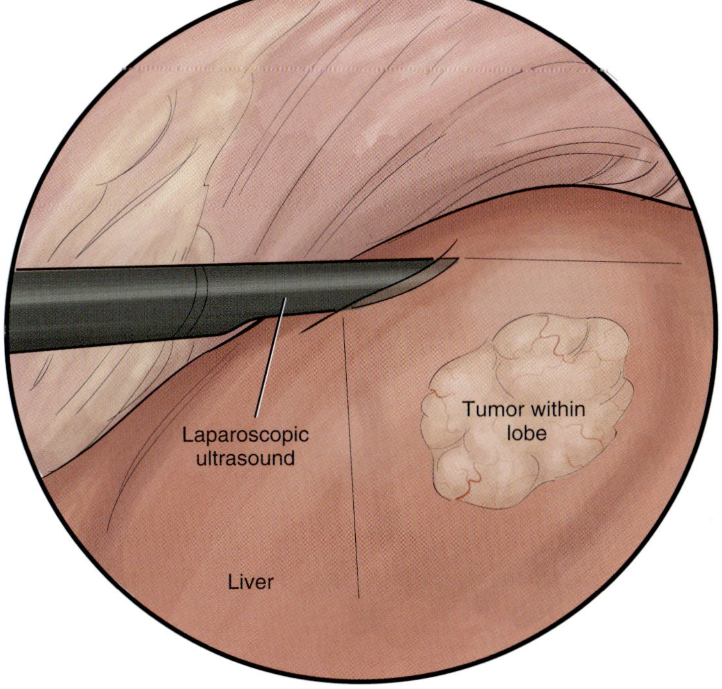

Figure 49-5.

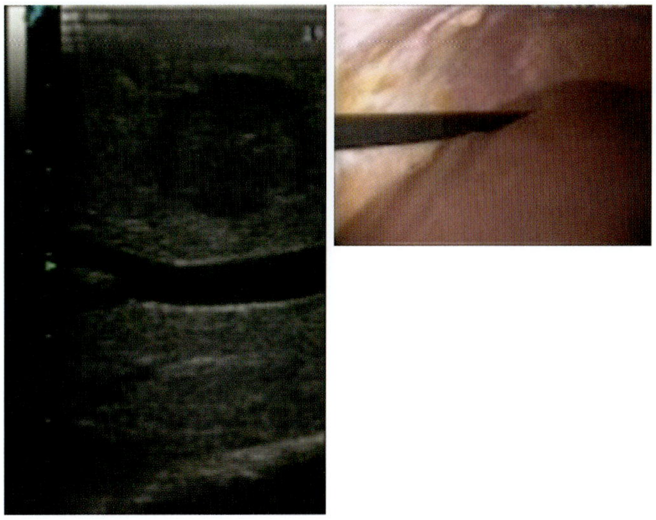

Figure 49-6.

- The appropriate-size RFA probe is introduced at the right subcostal space in a plane that is parallel to and under the US probe (Fig. 49-7, *A*). Under US visualization, the RFA probe is guided into the center of the lesion (see Fig. 49-7, *B*).
- Once the RFA probe is deployed, appropriate placement is confirmed by ensuring that the tines encompass the lesion in all three dimensions (X, Y, and Z planes). Larger lesions may require several deployments to ablate the entire mass.
- The progress of the ablation is monitored under US by visualizing the "outgassing" of nitrogen from thermally ablated cells (Figs. 49-8 and 49-9).
- The ablation is performed according to the specific algorithm for each device and probe used.

Closure

- Once the ablation is complete, the RFA probe is withdrawn, and the hook electrocautery is used to achieve hemostasis at the parenchyma puncture site. (Fig. 49-10).
- Both 12-mm port sites are closed at the fascia with size 0 Vicryl.
- The skin is closed with 4-0 Vicryl stitch in a running subcuticular technique.

III. ALTERNATIVE TECHNICAL APPROACHES (PRO/CON) AND PEARLS

Alternative Approaches

- RFA can also be performed by a percutaneous approach. This can be completed with local anesthetic and sedation, obviating the need for general anesthesia. For patients in whom adequate percutaneous

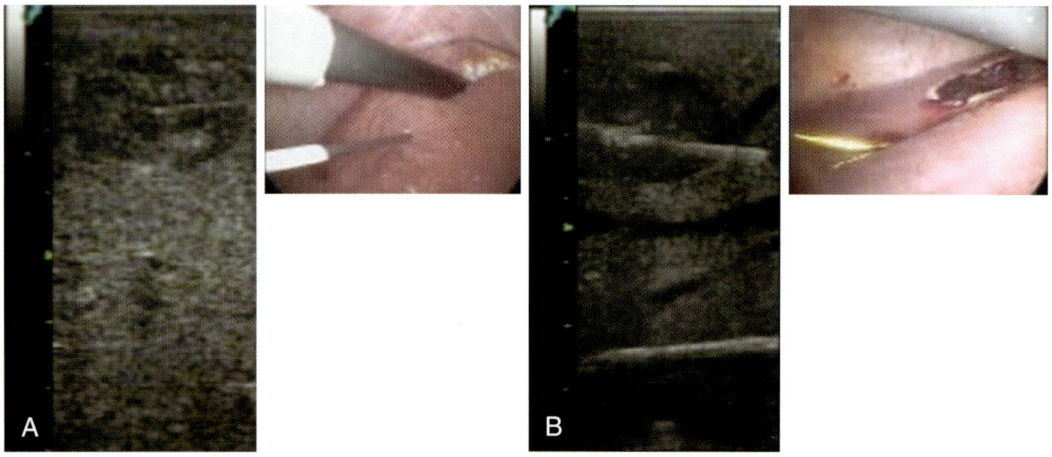

Figure 49-7.

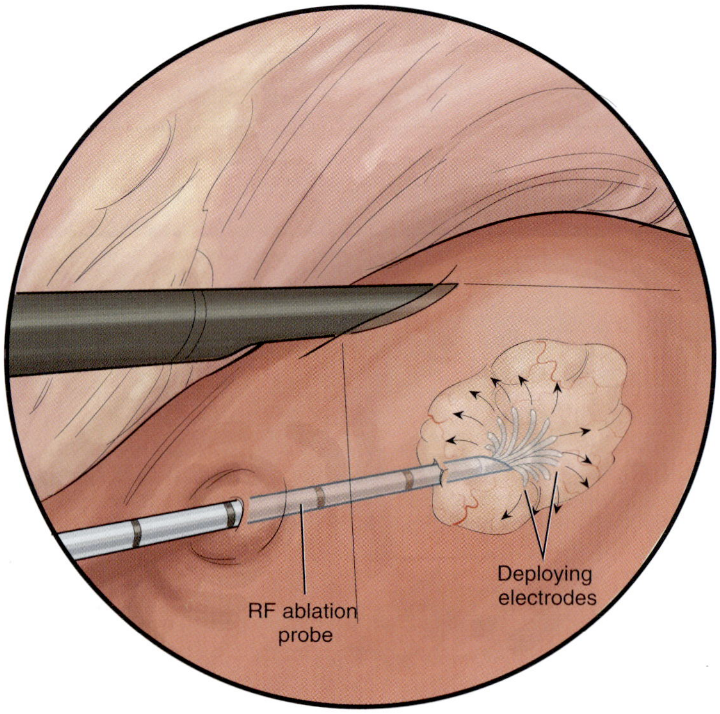

Figure 49-8. *RF,* Radiofrequency.

US localization is not feasible, laparoscopic RFA offers the advantage of superior visualization and targeting of the lesion.

Technical Pearls

- Any lesion in the liver that can be visualized by laparoscopic US can potentially be ablated. However, deep segment VII and VIII lesions are often challenging to localize by laparoscopic US. Central hilar lesions should be avoided because of the risk of bile duct injury.
- Whenever possible, the rigid laparoscopic US probe should be used.
- The RFA probe is targeted from a subcostal approach rather than an intercostal approach.
- An angiocatheter sheath is placed in the abdominal wall to cover the RFA probe and therefore minimize risk of tumor seeding.
- Experience in open liver US and open RFA is a prerequisite skill set before progressing to laparoscopic RFA.

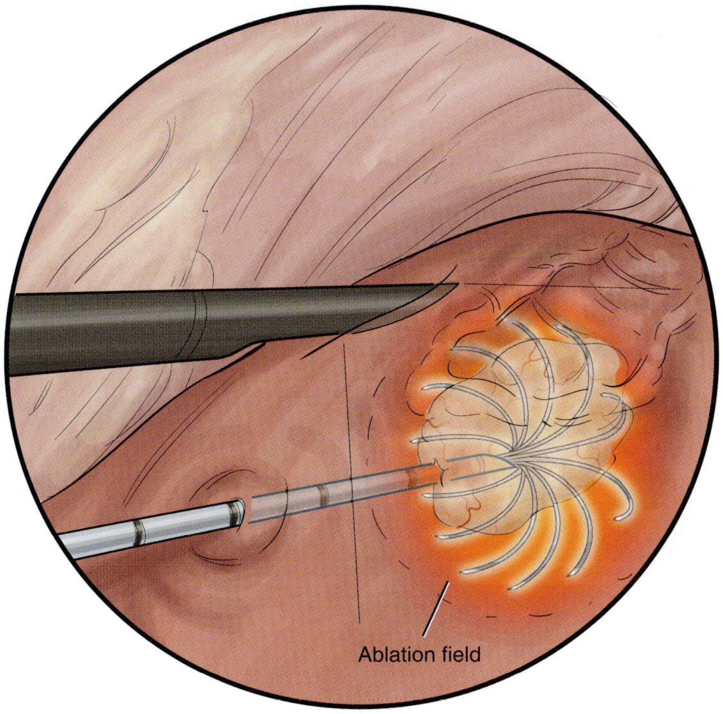

Figure 49-9.

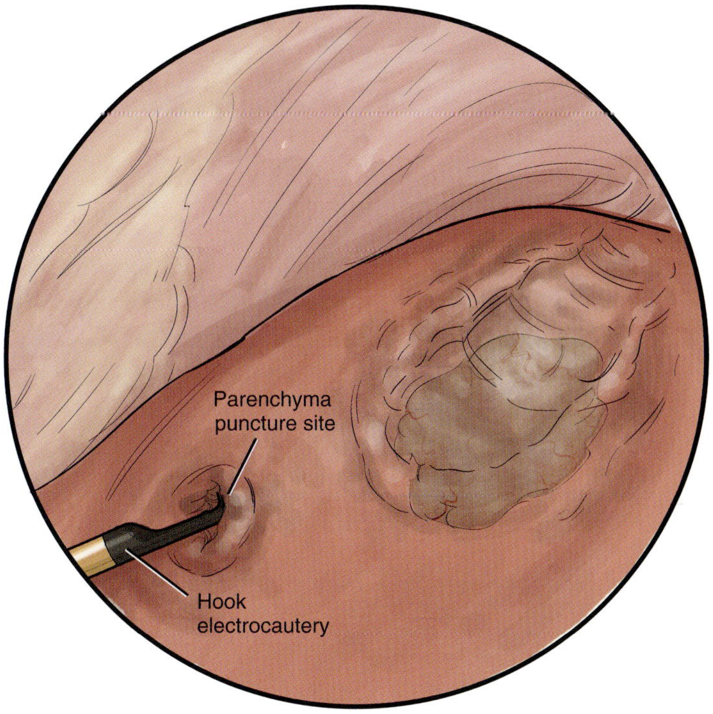

Figure 49-10.

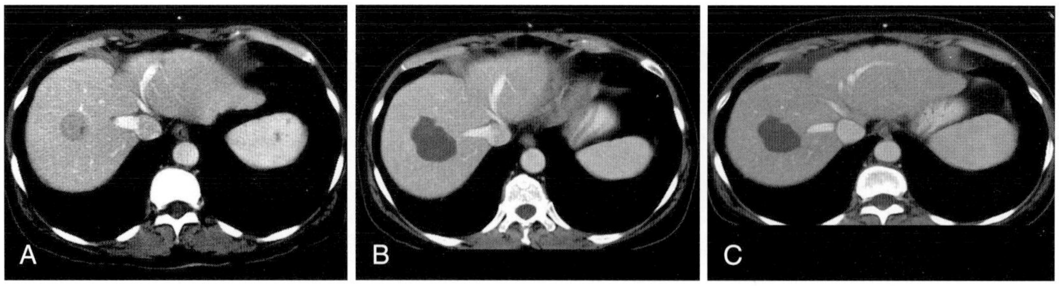

Figure 49-11.

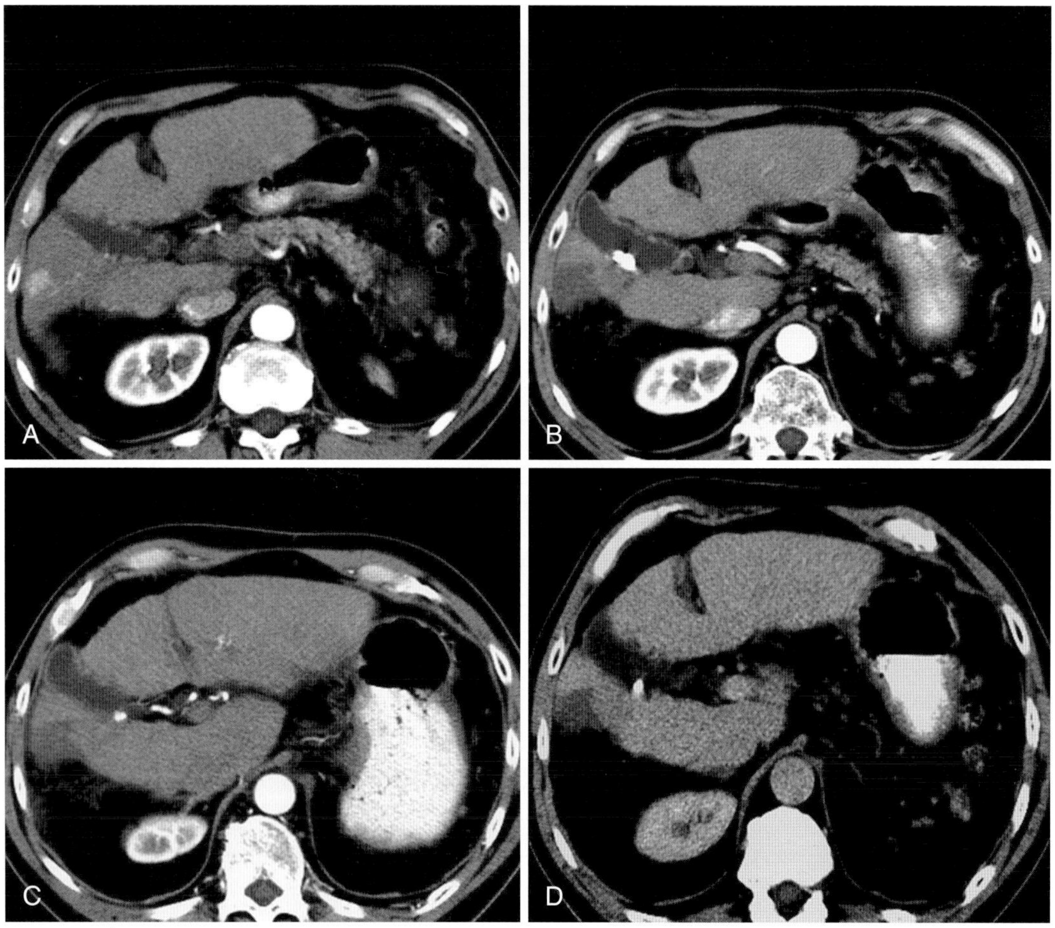

Figure 49-12.

IV. SPECIAL POSTOPERATIVE CARE

- On postoperative day 1, regular diet is resumed and patients are typically discharged.
- Pain control is achieved with antiinflammatory drugs and occasional oral narcotics.
- Follow-up surveillance CT scans and tumor markers are obtained at 3-month intervals to assess for recurrence (Figs. 49-11 and 49-12).

SUGGESTED READINGS

Berber E, Siperstein AE: Perioperative outcome after laparoscopic radiofrequency ablation of liver tumors: an analysis of 521 cases, *Surg Endosc* 21:613–618, 2007.

Curley SA, Marra P, Beaty K, et al: Early and late complications after radiofrequency ablation of malignant liver tumors in 608 patients, *Ann Surg* 239:450–458, 2004.

Mulier S, Ni Y, Jamart J, et al: Local recurrence after hepatic radiofrequency coagulation: multivariate meta-analysis and review of contributing factors, *Ann Surg* 242:158–171, 2005. Review.

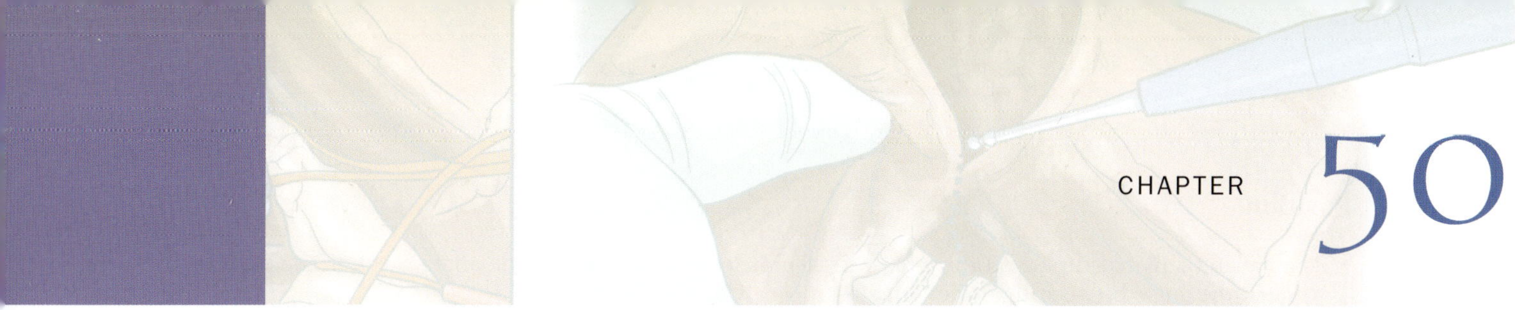

CHAPTER 50

Variceal Decompression: Distal Splenorenal, Portocaval, and Mesocaval Shunts

J. Michael Henderson, MBChB, FRCS

I. SPECIAL PREOPERATIVE PREPARATION

- Patients are considered for operative variceal decompression if they fail primary therapy for recurrent variceal bleeding with pharmacologic and endoscopic treatment. Approximately 15% of patients fail primary therapy and require decompression. The alternative to operative shunt for decompression is a transjugular intrahepatic portal systemic shunt.
- In reaching a decision as to the optimal approach for decompression, the liver disease, its severity, and technical factors for shunt need to be evaluated.
- The cause of the portal hypertension should be determined. Patients with a normal liver or good liver function are candidates for surgical shunts. Patients with advanced and progressive liver disease are not candidates for operative shunt, but must be considered for liver transplant. Those with poor liver function, and are not candidates for transplant, can only be decompressed using a transjugular intrahepatic portal systemic shunt.
- Assessment of liver function is primarily based on clinical grounds and blood tests. Clinical findings of jaundice, ascites, and encephalopathy suggest advanced liver disease and are factors that preclude patients from undergoing operative shunting. Blood tests with elevated bilirubin, low albumin, and prolonged prothrombin time support the diagnosis of advanced liver disease. It is only patients with no significant clinical signs of liver disease and normal blood tests who are candidates for decompressive shunt.
- The technical feasibility of performing an operative shunt is assessed with imaging studies of the portal venous system. Doppler ultrasound is adequate for most patients but may need to be augmented with angiography and venous phase imaging of the portal, superior mesenteric, and splenic veins. In the case of patients being considered for distal splenorenal shunt (DSRS), left renal venography should also be done, because 20% of the population have an abnormal (circumaortic) left renal vein.
- The operative methods for variceal decompression may be a total, partial, or selective shunt. This chapter addresses each of these options.

II. OPERATIVE TECHNIQUE: DISTAL SPLENORENAL SHUNT

- DSRS is a selective shunt that decompresses gastroesophageal varices through the spleen and splenic vein to the left renal vein. It maintains portal hypertension in the superior mesenteric and portal vein and therefore maintains portal perfusion to the cirrhotic liver. To perform this operation, the splenic vein and left renal vein must be patent in adequate apposition to each other, and the portal vein should show prograde portal flow to the liver on preoperative imaging.

Position

- The patient is placed supine on the table with slight elevation of the left side and a break in the table to open the angle between the lower left ribs and pelvis.

Incision

- A long left subcostal incision is made and extended across the right to include most of the right rectus muscle. A fixed retractor system that pulls upward on the left costal margin improves intraabdominal access.

Main Dissection

- The main dissection has two components: first, access to the splenic and renal veins that are going to be used for the shunt, and second, compartmentalization of the left upper quadrant, as the low-pressure variceal decompression compartment, from the right side and lower abdomen, which maintain portal hypertension.
- Initial access is gained to the lesser sac, as illustrated in Figure 50-1, by opening the gastrocolic omentum from the pylorus upward to the lowest short gastric veins. Any adhesions between the stomach and pancreas are taken down, and the stomach is retracted superiorly.
- Further access to the pancreas is gained by taking down the splenic flexure of the colon, retracting that inferiorly, and opening the plane between the splenic flexure and the posterior aspect of the pancreas. The peritoneum along the inferior border of the pancreas is then incised, as illustrated in Figure 50-1, to gain access to the posterior aspect of the pancreas.
- Dissection of the splenic vein is illustrated in Figure 50-2. Initially the splenic vein needs to be identified on the posterior surface of the pancreas, and this is easily done by palpation if the vein is not readily visible. The tissue overlying the splenic vein is incised, initially along its inferior margin, which is always devoid of feeding tributaries. Expose as much splenic vein as possible.
- The inferior mesenteric vein is the first significant vascular structure entering either the splenic vein (50%) or the superior mesenteric vein (50%) as one dissects from left to right along the pancreas. This should be identified and ligated, as shown in Figure 50-2. The "safe" plane of dissection is posteriorly, and the posterior aspects of the splenic and superior mesenteric veins can be opened with blunt dissection.
- The major and most difficult dissection for a DSRS is separating the small pancreatic tributaries to the splenic vein (Fig. 50-2). This involves delicate separation by opening the tissue in the line of these tributaries, and at right angles to the splenic vein. As these are serially identified, they are surrounded and ligated with 3-0 silk on the splenic vein with a small clip placed on the pancreas. As many of these small tributaries as possible should be identified and ligated as described. *Tip:* It is often better to hold this dissection until the left renal vein has been identified; see later discussion.
- The left renal vein is identified by initial palpation of the retroperitoneum to identify the aorta and superior mesenteric artery. The left renal vein passes between these two. The retroperitoneum is then opened, and with blunt dissection the left renal vein is identified. The left adrenal vein should be isolated and ligated to allow for full mobilization of the left renal vein. The left gonadal vein should be left intact, because it can serve as an additional useful outflow once the shunt has been created.

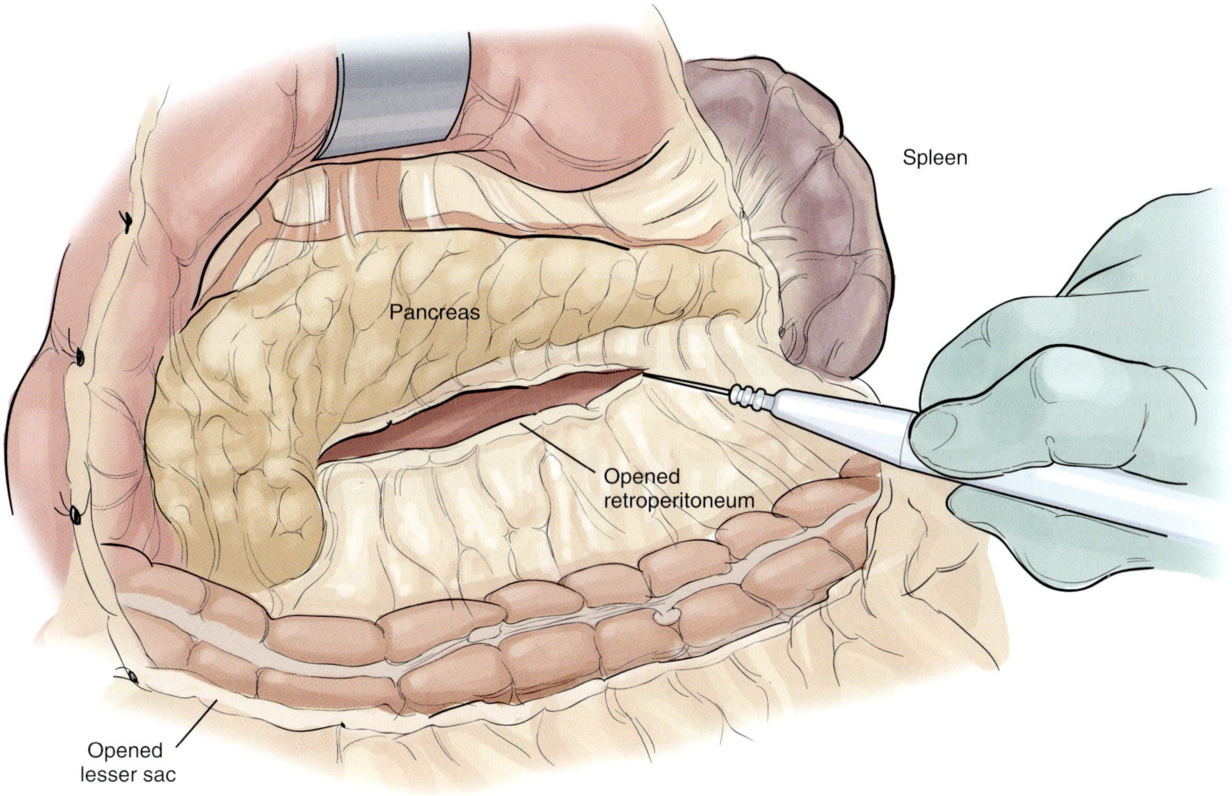

Figure 50-1.

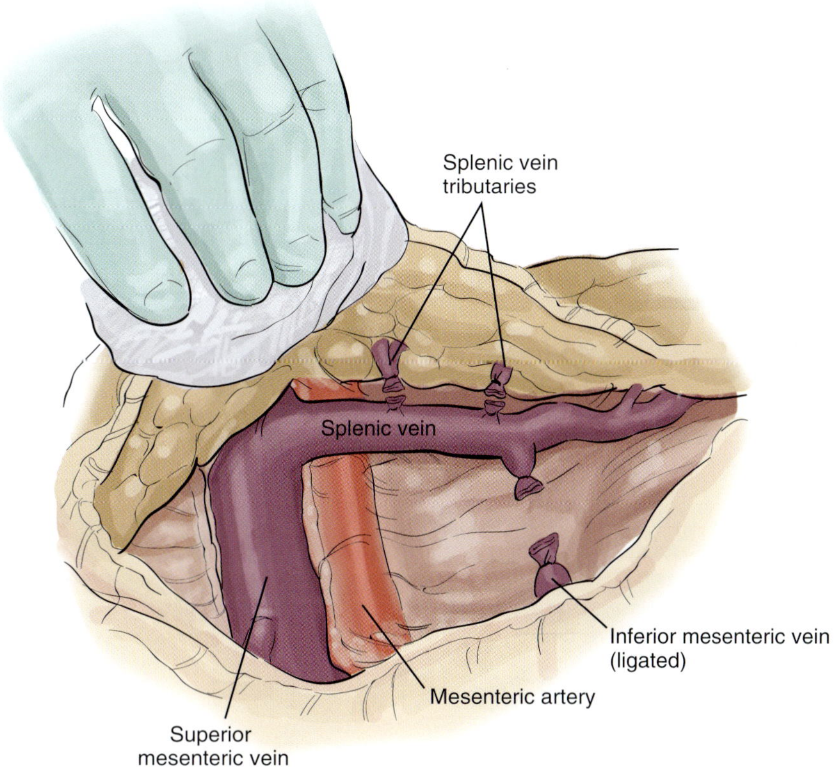

Figure 50-2.

Sufficient left renal vein must be mobilized to come up readily into a side-biting clamp, as in Figure 50-3.

- With the renal and splenic veins fully dissected, the junction of the splenic vein and superior mesenteric vein is ligated, and a large clip is placed behind the tie on the superior mesenteric vein junction. The splenic vein is divided, as shown in Figure 50-3, and is trimmed to an appropriate length to come down to the left renal vein without kinking.
- The anastomosis is fashioned as shown in Figure 50-3, with initial completion of the posterior layer by placing the two end stitches, bringing the left end needle into the lumen, and sewing the posterior wall on the inside. To complete the posterior layer, the needle is brought exteriorly and ligated at the right end of this anastomosis.
- The anterior layer of the anastomosis is completed with interrupted sutures to prevent purse-stringing of the anastomosis and allow subsequent growth, if necessary. The final phase of the operation is completion of the compartmentalization. It is important to identify the left gastric vein, preferably as it enters the splenic or portal vein, and clip it at this site. In addition, it should be ligated above the pancreas.
- Hemostasis is checked in all areas. On opening the shunt, the spleen should become softer and usually shrinks immediately by 10% to 20%.

Closure

- The abdomen is closed in two layers, without intraabdominal drainage.

Special Postoperative Care

- Because the majority of patients having DSRS have underlying cirrhosis as the cause of their portal hypertension, meticulous fluid management is key in postoperative care. The greatest risk to these patients is the development of ascites, fluid leak through the incision, and the development of infection. Careful perioperative fluid management, with "running the patient dry," is step 1. Continuing to restrict sodium (2 g sodium per day once patients are on a diet), and minimizing intravenous fluids

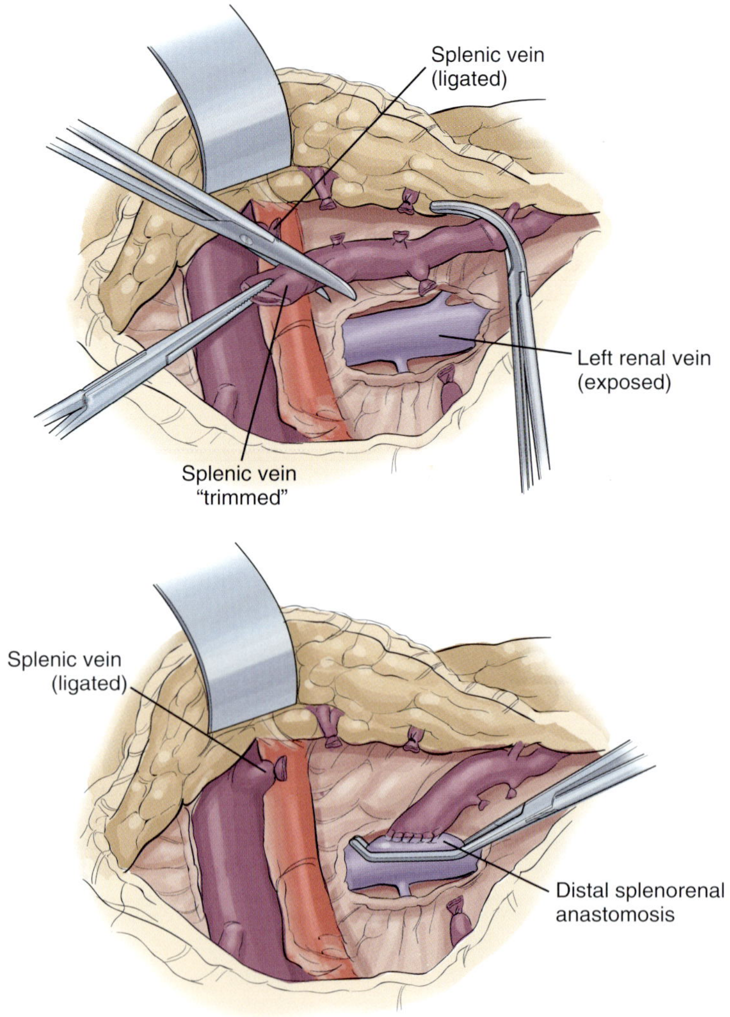

Figure 50-3.

postoperatively reduce the risk of developing ascites. In addition, dietary fat restriction to 30 g/day for 6 weeks will minimize the risk of chylous ascites, which can occur because of the many lymphatics divided around the left renal vein. Once patients are on adequate oral intake, spironolactone (100 mg/day) to reduce sodium reabsorption by the kidneys also minimizes the risk of ascites.

- Before hospital discharge, this author recommends catheterization of the distal splenorenal shunt from the groin to document patency and measure the gradient from the splenic vein to the left renal vein to the inferior vena cava. The gradient should be less than 10 mm Hg.

III. OPERATIVE TECHNIQUE: PORTACAVAL SHUNTS

- Portacaval shunts for variceal decompression fall into two categories: total and partial shunts. If the anastomosis is greater than 10 mm in size, all portal flow is diverted through the shunt; hence the nomenclature of a total portal systemic shunt. When the diameter is reduced to 8 mm in size and the pressure gradient is reduced to approximately 12 mm Hg, some prograde portal flow is maintained to the liver in 80% of patients, and this is considered a partial portal systemic shunt. Both are briefly illustrated here.

Position

- The patient is placed supine with the right side slightly elevated and the costal margin broken between the ribs and the pelvis.

Incision

- A long right subcostal incision is made. It may be extended across the midline if necessary for improved access. A fixed retractor system pulling up on the right costal margin improves access.

Main Dissection

- The main dissection for this operation is at the liver hilus. The cirrhotic liver is retracted superiorly, and the stomach and duodenum retracted to the left. Kocherization of the duodenum may be necessary to improve access to both the portal vein and the inferior vena cava.
- Initial dissection of the infrahepatic inferior vena cava is shown in Figure 50-4. This should be mobilized over sufficient length to allow it to be brought up toward the portal vein, which permits a direct vein-to-vein anastomosis if a total side-to-side portal systemic shunt is going to be performed.

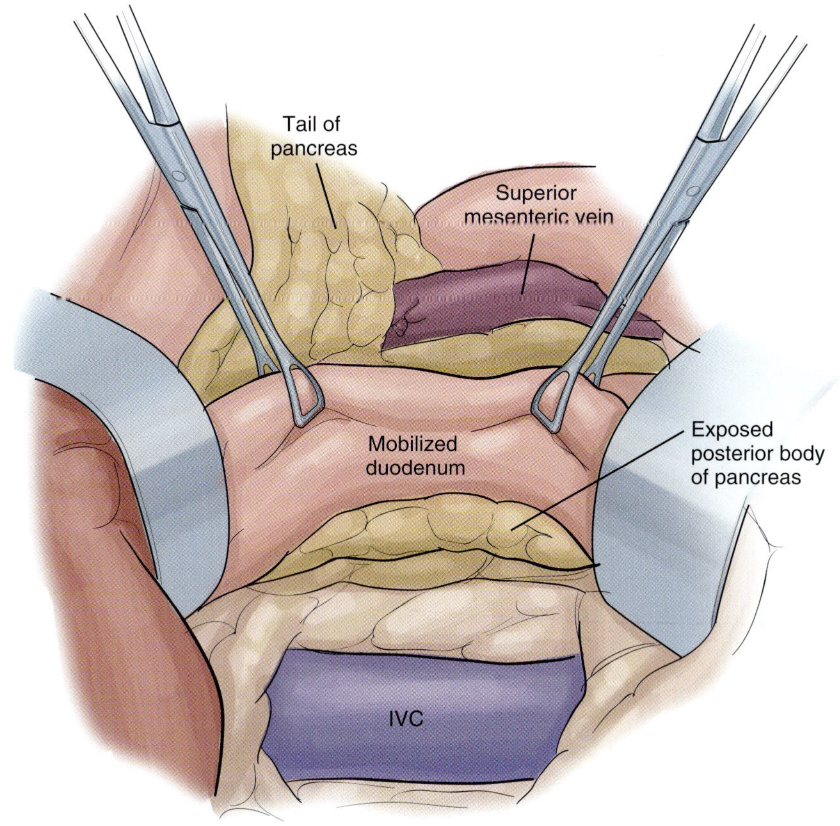

Figure 50-4. *IVC,* Inferior vena cava.

- Dissection of the portal vein in the hepatoduodenal ligament follows. The portal vein sits posteriorly, so the bile duct needs to be retracted to the left, the peritoneum incised posteriorly, and the portal vein identified. The portal vein is then freed from surrounding structures, as illustrated in Figure 50-5.
- Both the portal vein and the inferior vena cava should be fully mobilized, so that they can be approximated as illustrated.
- A side-to-side anastomosis is made, as illustrated in Figure 50-6. This figure shows a side-biting clamp on the inferior vena cava, and two small clamps on the isolated segment of the portal vein.
- Venotomies are made in both of these vessels, and they are approximated without tension.
- A side-to-side total portal portacaval shunt larger than 10 mm is constructed.
- With release of the clamps, any bleeding in the operative field rapidly stops as the portal pressure falls.

Operative Technique for 8-mm H-Graft Portacaval Shunt

- The dissection for this partial shunt is identical to that just described for total shunt.
- This operation places an 8-mm Teflon-reinforced graft between the inferior vena cava and the mobilized portal vein. The bevels at the two ends of the graft should be at 90 degrees to each other, such that the anastomoses at each end are approximately 1.5 cm in this 8-mm graft (Fig. 50-7).

Special Postoperative Care

- The postoperative management of patients undergoing total or partial portacaval shunt requires attention to detail, because most patients have cirrhosis. The advantage of a total shunt is that the patient will not develop ascites, because the hepatic sinusoids have been decompressed, in addition to variceal decompression. Patients with the 8-mm partial shunt have some risk of developing ascites because there is not a full sinusoidal decompression. These patients require appropriate fluid restriction and may require diuretics.
- As with distal splenorenal shunt, documentation of shunt patency before hospital discharge is advocated.

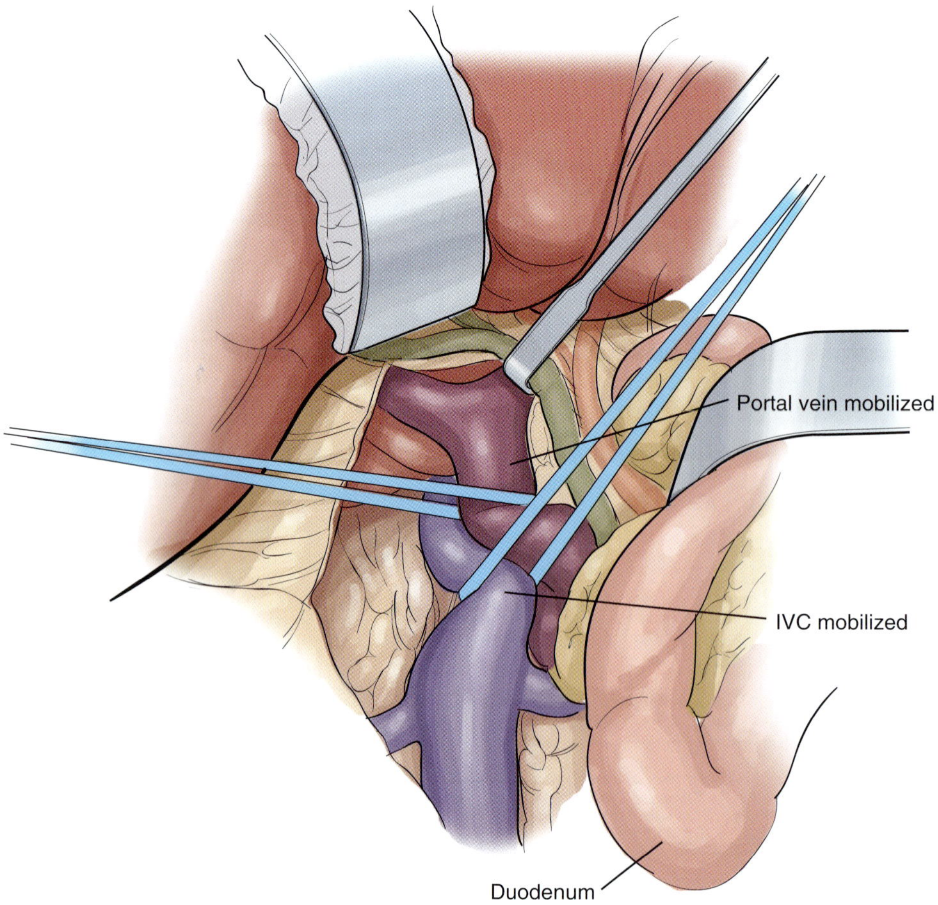

Figure 50-5. *IVC,* Inferior vena cava.

IV. OPERATIVE TECHNIQUE: MESOCAVAL INTERPOSITION SHUNT

- The third operative approach to variceal decompression is with an interposition mesocaval shunt. This operation takes the dissection away from the liver hilus, which may be an important factor if the patient is likely to come to subsequent liver transplant. This operation is done below the mesocolon with identification of the superior mesenteric vein and inferior vena cava. The difficulty of this operation is mobilizing the third portion of the duodenum sufficiently to satisfactorily interpose a graft between these two vessels.

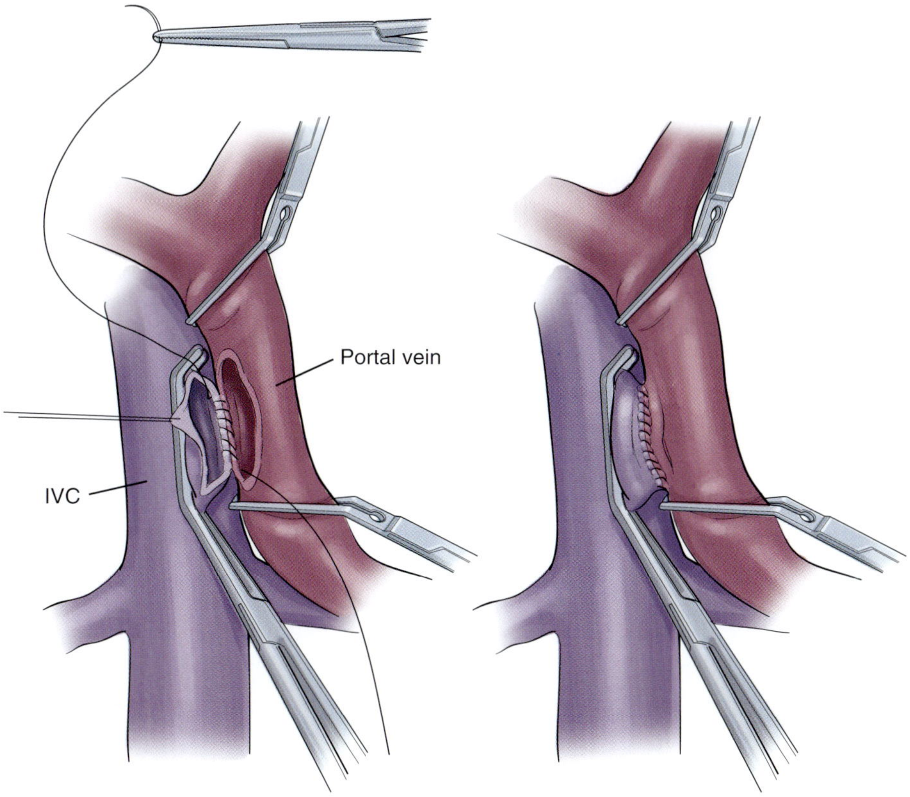

Figure 50-6. *IVC,* Inferior vena cava.

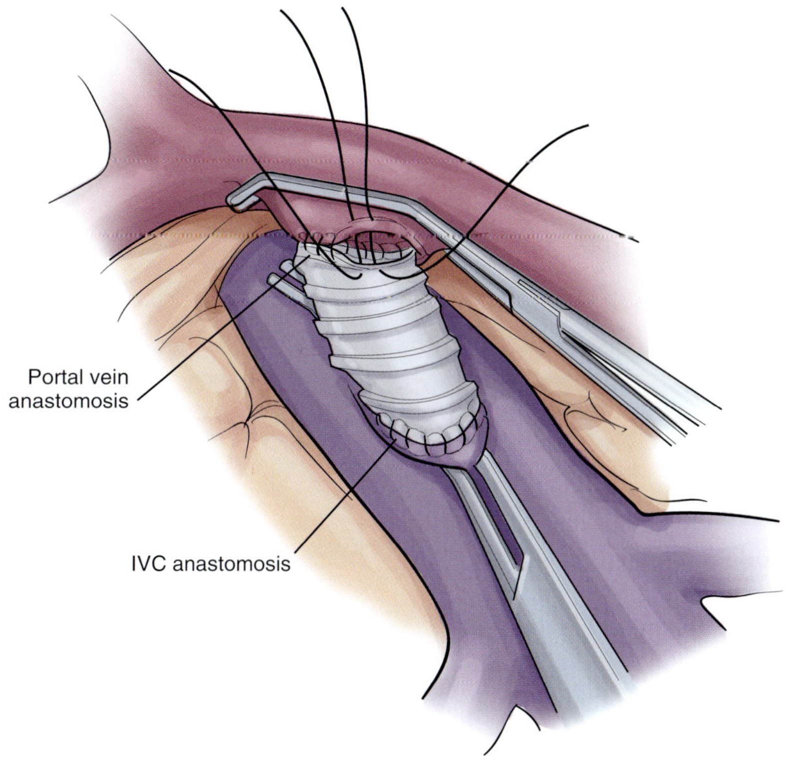

Figure 50-7. *IVC,* Inferior vena cava.

Position

- The patient is placed supine on the table.

Incision

- This operation may be performed through either a long midline incision or a right midtransverse abdominal incision.

Main Dissection

- Initial dissection is at the root of the mesocolon. The transverse colon is pulled anteriorly, and the peritoneum at its inferior margin is incised, following down the middle colic vein to the superior mesenteric vein.
- The superior mesenteric vein is identified and fully mobilized. This is most safely done on the right side of the superior mesenteric vein, but the entire vein needs to be surrounded to make for a subsequent safe anastomosis. At this point, the vein is passing in front of the third portion of the duodenum.
- The duodenum is stabilized with an extended Kocher maneuver, such that the third position can be displaced cranially.
- The inferior vena cava is then mobilized in the retroperitoneum. Sufficient inferior vena cava must be mobilized to allow it to be safely side-clamped for subsequent anastomosis. This is illustrated in Figure 50-4.
- The shunt is usually made with a reinforced Teflon graft. Alternatively, the internal jugular vein may be harvested from the patient and used for this shunt.
- The inferior vena caval anastomosis is first completed by side-biting the inferior vena cava and completing this anastomosis. Its patency and security are checked before continuing to the superior mesenteric vein anastomosis (Fig. 50-8).

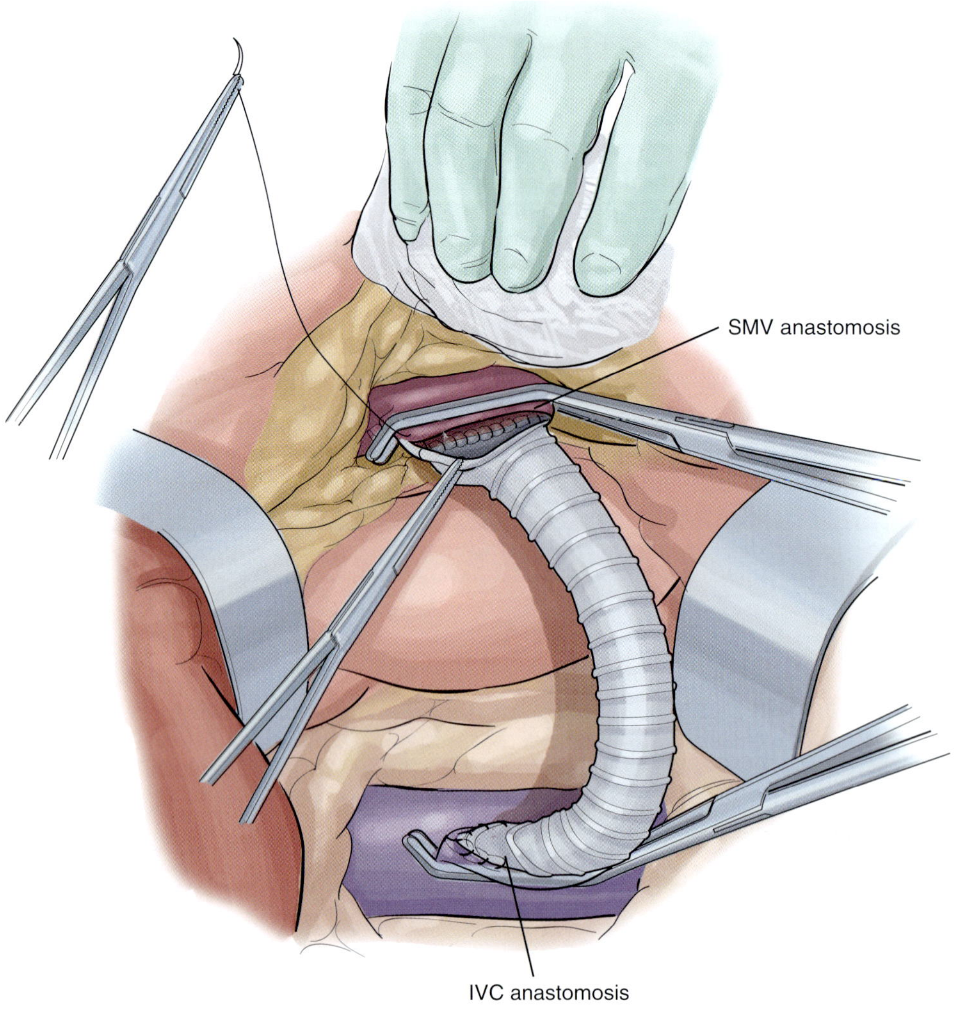

Figure 50-8. *IVC,* Inferior vena cava; *SMV,* superior mesenteric vein.

- The superior mesenteric vein anastomosis is completed with a side-biting clamp on the superior mesenteric vein, or alternatively, clamps or tape-tourniquet can be placed above and below the anastomotic site.
- The length of the shunt is dictated by the position and distance between these vessels and the relationship to the duodenum.
- Omentum, or fatty tissue in the root of the mesentery, can be placed between the graft and the duodenum to reduce the risk of graft erosion.
- The greater length of this prosthetic graft compared to that for an interposition portacaval shunt increases the risk of thrombosis for this procedure.

Special Postoperative Care

- This is similar to that already described for the other shunt procedures. Because most of the mesocaval shunts are larger, to lower the risk or thrombosis, they act as total portal systemic shunts, decompress the sinusoids, and therefore create a lower risk of ascites.
- Documenting patency of this shunt before hospital discharge is important because of its greater propensity for later thrombosis.

SELECTED READINGS

Henderson JM: Multidisciplinary approach to the management of portal hypertension. In Yeo CJ, Klein AS, editors: *Shackelford's surgery of the alimentary tract*, ed 6, Philadelphia, 2007, Saunders, pp 1751–1770.

Henderson JM, Boyer TD, Kutner MH, and the DIVERT Study Group: Distal splenorenal shunt vs. transjugular intrahepatic portal systemic shunt for variceal bleeding: a randomized trial, *Gastroenterology* 130:1643–1657, 2006.

Rosemurgy AS, Serafini FM, Zweibel BR, et al: Transjugular intrahepatic portosystemic shunt vs. small-diameter prosthetic H-graft portacaval shunt: extended follow-up of an expanded randomized prospective trial, *J Gastrointest Surg* 4:589–597, 2000.

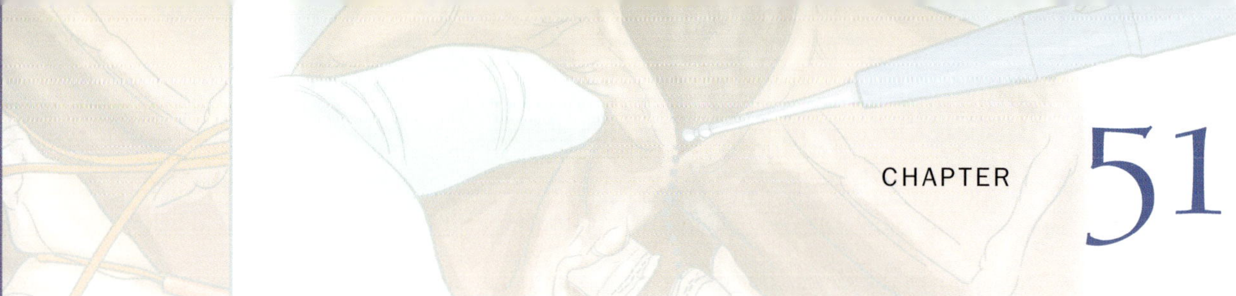

CHAPTER 51

Natural Orifice Transluminal Endoscopic Cholecystectomy

Ricardo Zorron, MD, MSC, PhD

I. SPECIAL PREOPERATIVE PREPARATION

- For natural orifice transluminal endoscopic surgery (NOTES) transvaginal cholecystectomy, patient selection is of great importance to avoid conversion to laparoscopic or open surgery, to reduce operative times, and to prevent complications. Candidates are women with mild disease, ideally with successful previous pregnancy and avoiding cases of jaundice, pancreatitis, or long-duration cholelithiasis. The ideal indication is mild symptomatic cholelithiasis or gallbladder polyp with surgical indication. Contraindications for the procedure include an intact hymen or pregnancy. Although intraoperative cholangiography is already possible for NOTES cases, patients with indications for common bile duct exploration should be preoperatively cleared by magnetic resonance imaging or preoperative endoscopic retrograde cholangiopancreatography.
- The size of the stones or polyps or a thickened and large gallbladder is not a contraindication for the transvaginal approach. On the contrary, this approach avoids larger laparoscopic extraction sites. Upper abdominal ultrasonography is the method of choice for diagnosis of biliary disease, although transvaginal ultrasonography is rarely used to access the pelvis to evaluate difficulties in vaginal NOTES access.
- In the case of previous hysterectomy, laparoscopic assistance using a 3- or 5-mm umbilical camera allows safety for the initial vaginal entrance and is highly recommended. Previous pelvic surgery usually does not represent an issue in accomplishing safe transvaginal access to the upper abdomen, and direct open access in the upper portion of the vagina is recommended.
- Preoperative gynecologic consultation is an important step in detecting preoperative vaginal infection and preventing issues as endometriosis.
- A multidisciplinary interventional team is required and is usually composed of a surgeon skilled in flexible endoscopy, a gastroenterologist/endoscopist, and a gynecologic surgeon. Previous consistent experience in performing the techniques in animals is highly recommended. Because natural orifice surgery is under clinical evaluation worldwide, each performing center must fulfill the local requirements for performance of NOTES techniques.

Special Equipment Needs

- A videoendoscopic set is needed for NOTES flexible cholecystectomy. Usually a single-channel gastroscope or colonoscope can be comfortably used, as shown in Figure 51-1. A full laparoscopic set and instruments should be available in case of conversion to laparoscopy or to allow laparoscopic assistance if needed.
- A laparoscopic insufflator with high flow rate is used to promote pneumoperitoneum with CO_2, to pressures of 8 to 14 mm Hg. The laparoscopic insufflator can be connected to one channel of the endoscope (in the case of a two-channel endoscope), but the rate of insufflation is usually low using

this method, and the insufflator becomes obstructed by fluid. An insufflation tube can be attached laterally to the endoscope, promoting safe CO_2 insufflation (Fig. 51-2), or through long laparoscopic transvaginal trocars. An umbilical Veress needle can alternatively be used, especially in cases of hybrid surgery.

- Direct ambient-air insufflation by the endoscope is prohibited, because the pressure cannot be controlled, easily leading to dangerous abdominal hypertension.
- The flexible endoscopic equipment suggested includes a disposable polypectomy snare, endoscopic monopolar scissors (Apollo Endosurgery, Austin, Tex.), and an insulation-tipped (IT) knife (Olympus, Tokyo). Disposable endoscopic clips are needed only for bleeding control and should be available. Rigid transvaginal equipment required includes two long laparoscopic 10-mm trocars (35 cm), long 5-mm scissors, a long 5-mm grasper, and a long 400-mm clip applier (each 60 cm, Karl Storz, Tuttlingen, Germany).

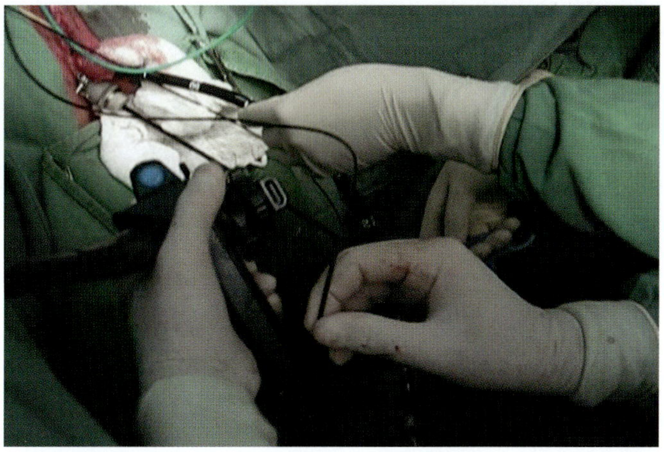

Figure 51-1.

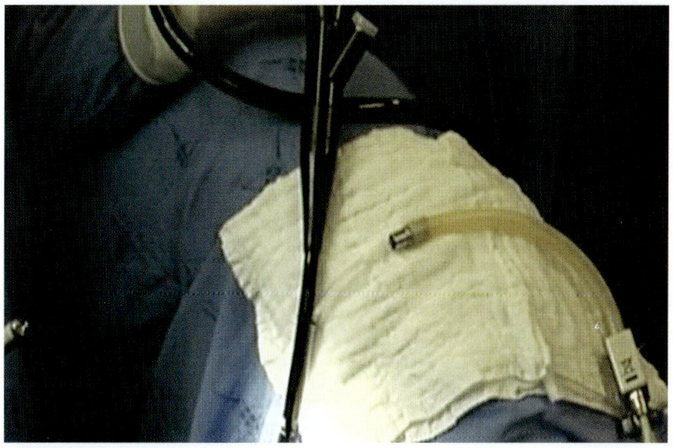

Figure 51-2.

- Figure 51-3 illustrates positioning of the surgeon and team. The arrangement of the endoscope and vaginal trocar is shown in Figure 51-4.

II. OPERATIVE TECHNIQUE

Position

- The patient is placed under general anesthesia and installed in a Lloyd-Davies position. Initially the inclination will be a full Trendelenburg position during the vaginal access dissection, evolving to a full anti-Trendelenburg inclination to perform gallbladder dissection (see Fig. 51-3).
- Disinfection of the vagina is achieved by topical povidone-iodine or chlorhexidine solution, and a urinary catheter is installed. Antibiotic prophylaxis is recommended, because total sterilization of the access site is not possible. Usually, a single intravenous bolus of either 2 g cephalexin or a combination of 500 mg metronidazole and 500 mg ciprofloxacin is given at the induction of anesthesia. The endoscopes have been previously sterilized by the ethylene oxide method, but some groups still prepare the endoscopes using a 2-hour immersion in glutaraldehyde or peracetic acid solution.

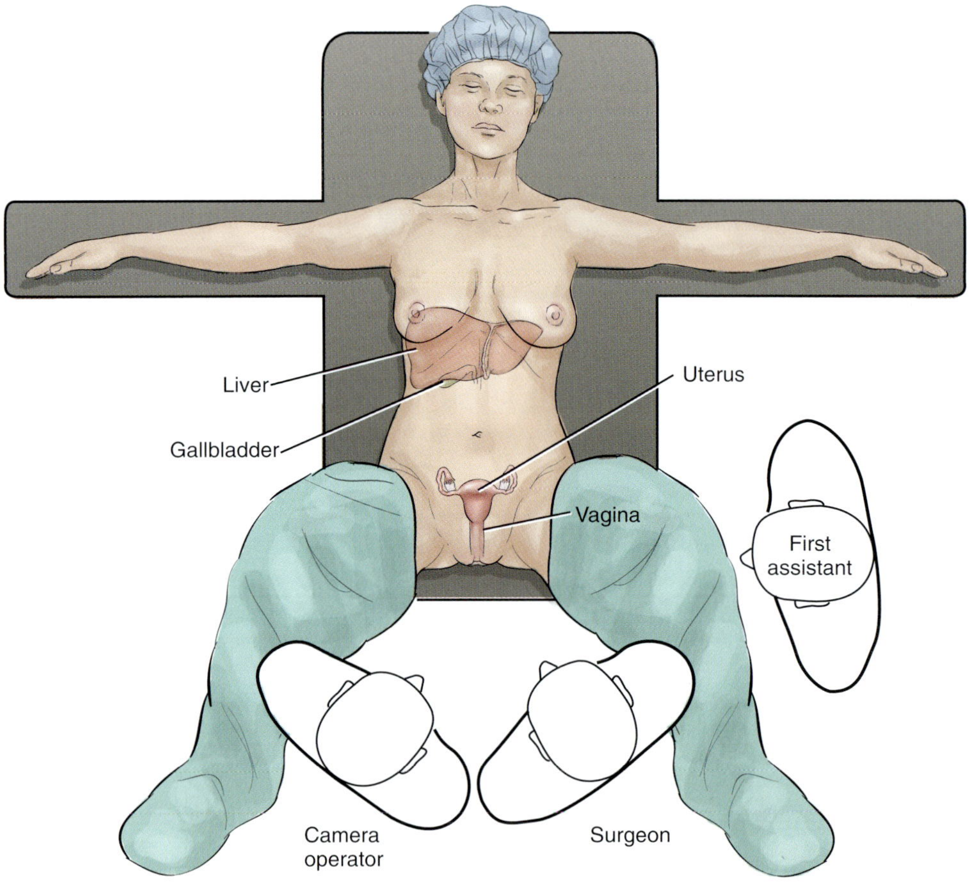

Figure 51-3.

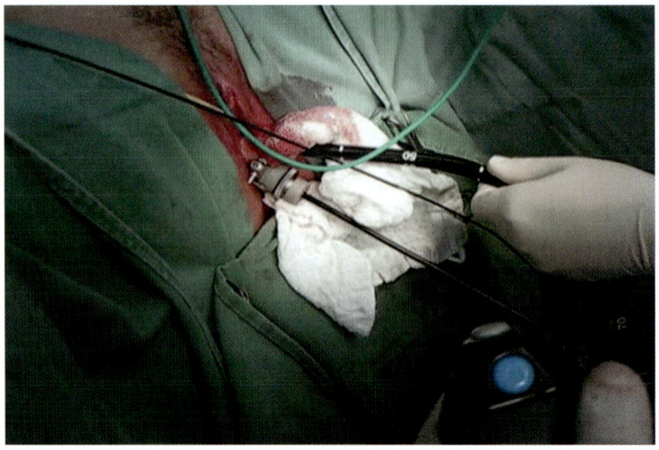

Figure 51-4.

Incision

Direct Access Visualization Method

- The posterior vaginal sac is opened under direct vision with conventional instruments and facilitates access to the peritoneal cavity. A Sims speculum is inserted in the vagina, and the posterior lip of the cervix is grasped with a Pozzi clamp (Fig. 51-5, *A*). The vaginal walls are retracted by two lateral retractors, and anterior traction is given to the cervix to stretch the posterior fornix. The vaginal mucosa in the posterior cul-de-sac is opened at the cervicovaginal junction by a semilunar 2.5-cm incision (see Fig. 51-5, *B*). The posterior margin is grasped by an Allis forceps, and sharp dissection is performed with scissors. The posterior cul-de-sac peritoneum is identified and opened. CO_2 is insufflated either through a tube parallel to the endoscope or by umbilical Veress needle. Insufflation through a working channel of the endoscope using a laparoscopic insufflator was used in early surgical experience but resulted in problems such as insufficient pressure and obstruction of the insufflation by water.

Laparoscopic Visualization Method of Access

- The surgeon stands between the patient's legs; the first and second assistants are on the left and right sides of the patient, respectively. In this setting, two visualization sets are used, one for the abdominal and the other for the transvaginal laparoscopic camera. The procedure starts with introduction of a Veress puncture through an incision in the umbilicus to avoid a visible scar. A 12 mm Hg pneumoperitoneum is then induced, and a 3- or 5-mm trocar and camera is installed in the umbilicus. A 12-mm trocar is inserted transvaginally and is substituted for the introduction of either a gastroscope or a colonoscope to inspect the abdominal cavity (Fig. 51-6). To avoid risk of injury to pelvic organs,

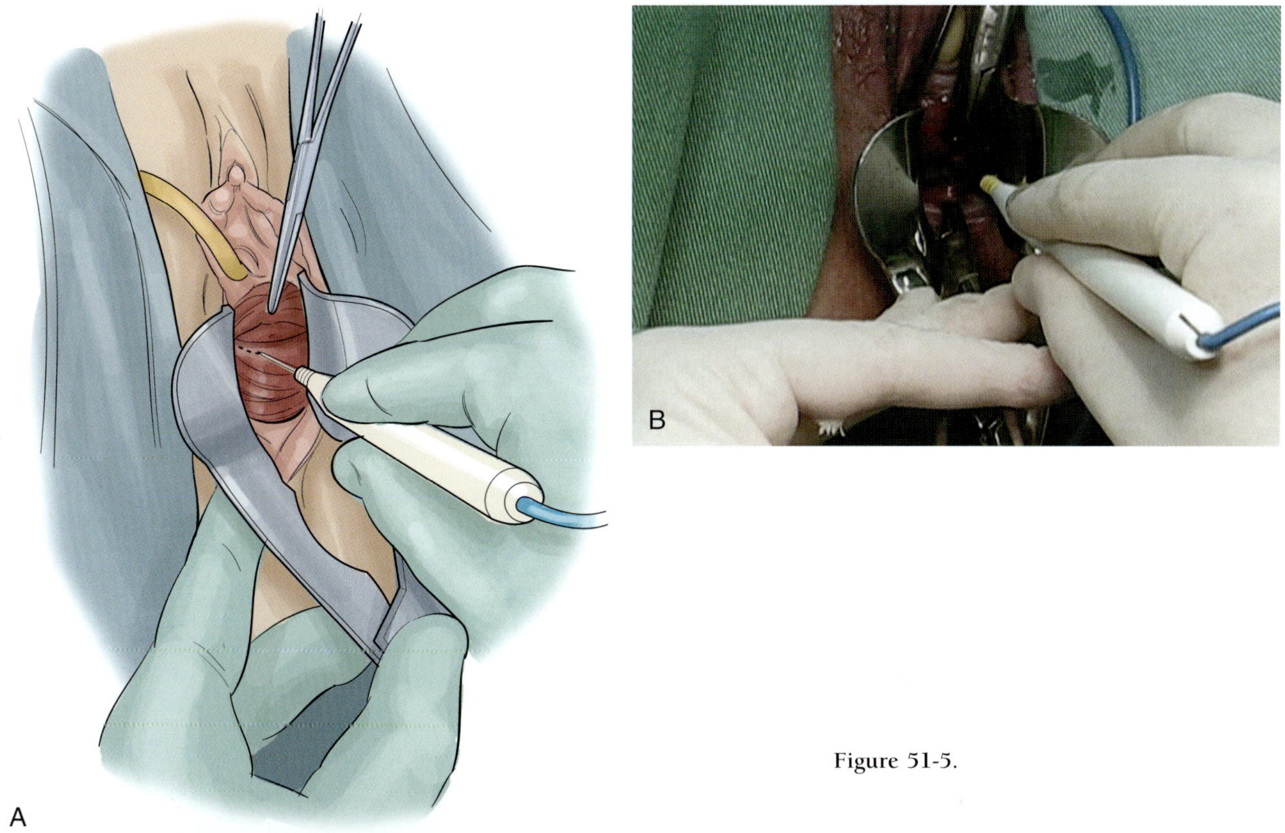

Figure 51-5.

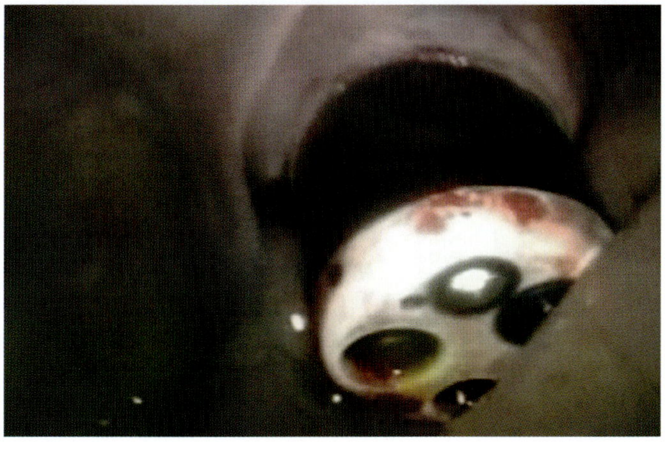

Figure 51-6.

a thorough examination of the pelvis is performed, looking for adhesions that might prohibit the transvaginal cul-de-sac puncture. In patients who have many adhesions within the pelvic organs, access will not be possible, and the procedure is converted to standard laparoscopy.

Main Dissection

- Parallel to the endoscope, another trocar (usually as long as a laparoscopic trocar used in obesity surgery, or longer) is inserted (Fig. 51-7) for retraction or for insertion of the long transvaginal laparoscopic clipator or scissors. This trocar can also be used for CO_2 insufflation.
- The technique starts as the vaginal long grasper catches the fundus of the gallbladder and provides distal retraction and good exposure of the bottom of the gallbladder (Fig. 51-8, *A*, *B*, and *C*).
- A 3-mm trocar is used for retraction in the umbilicus or right upper abdomen by minilaparoscopic graspers (Fig. 51-9, *A*). These graspers will work to better expose the Calot triangle, mimicking the "critical view," allowing dissection of lateral and medial aspects by the flexible endoscopic instruments.

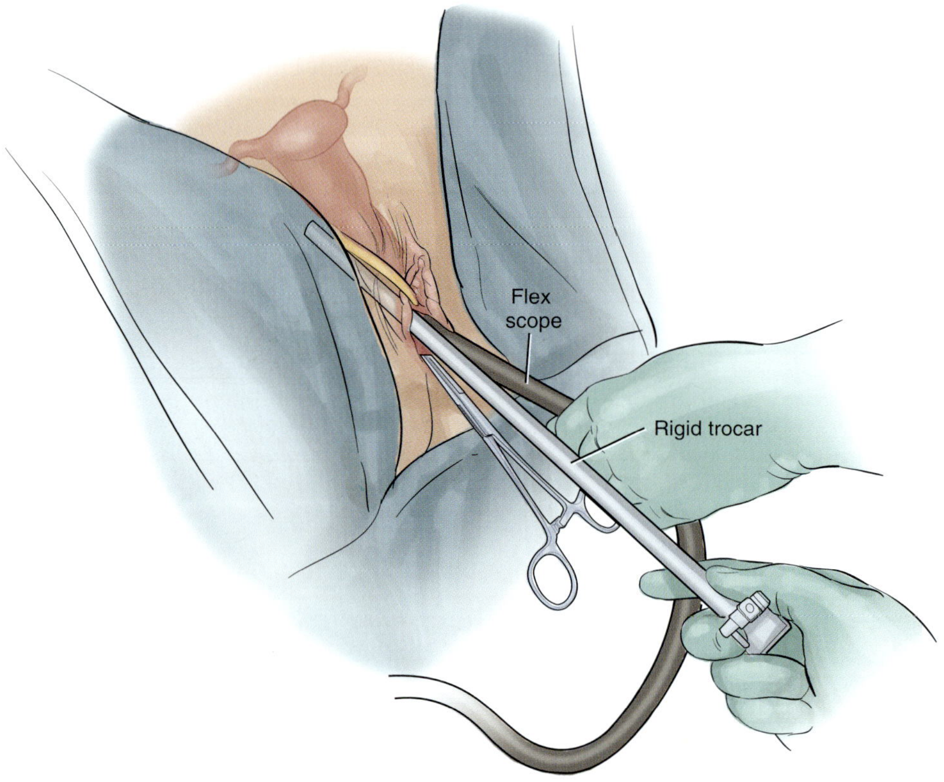

Figure 51-7.

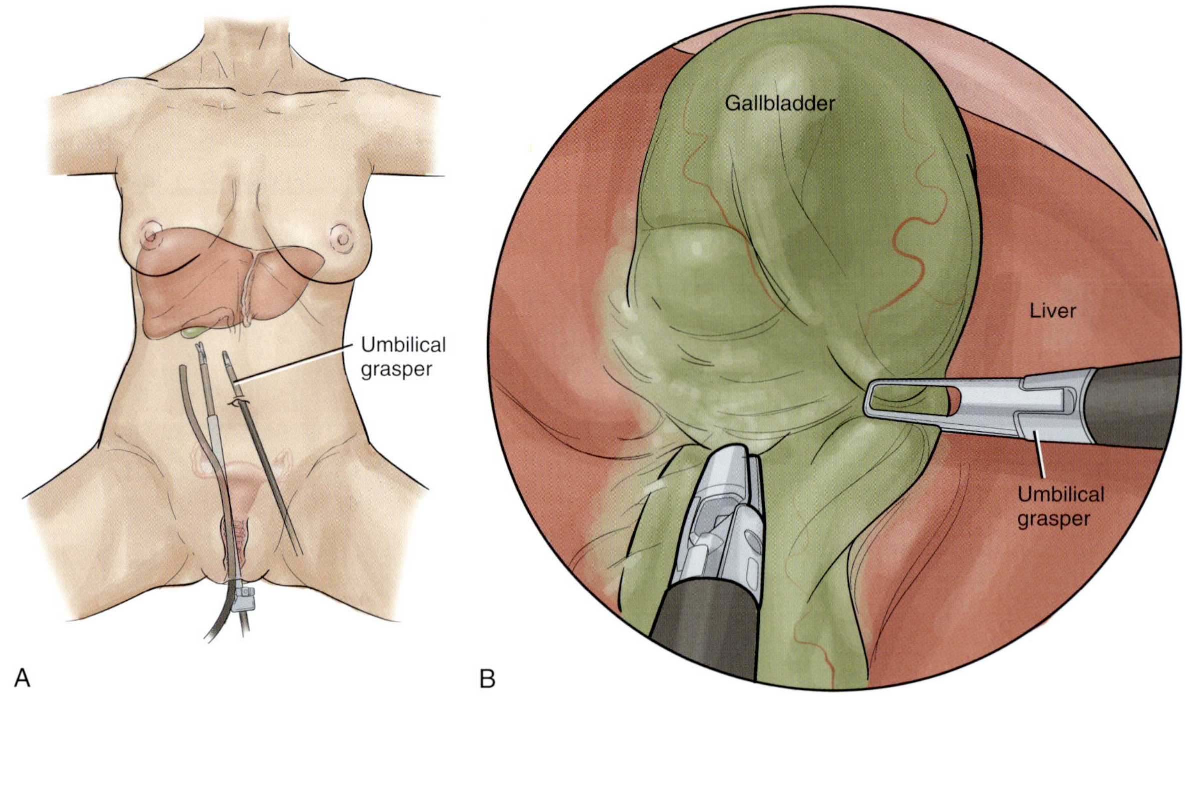

Figure 51-8.

- The peritoneum at the lateral and medial aspects is initially incised using flexible hot-biopsy forceps, an IT knife, a special monopolar probe (Karl Storz), or a polypectomy snare, and dissection of the cystic duct and artery is performed (see Fig. 51-9, *B*). One or two channels of the endoscope can be used.
- After full identification of the structures, the umbilical 3-mm grasper is repositioned to allow retraction of the gallbladder fundus. The cystic artery is usually electrocoagulated proximally to the gallbladder

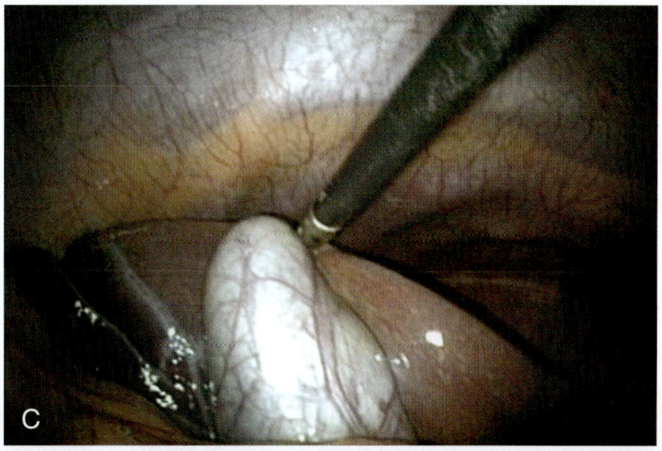

Figure 51-8, cont'd

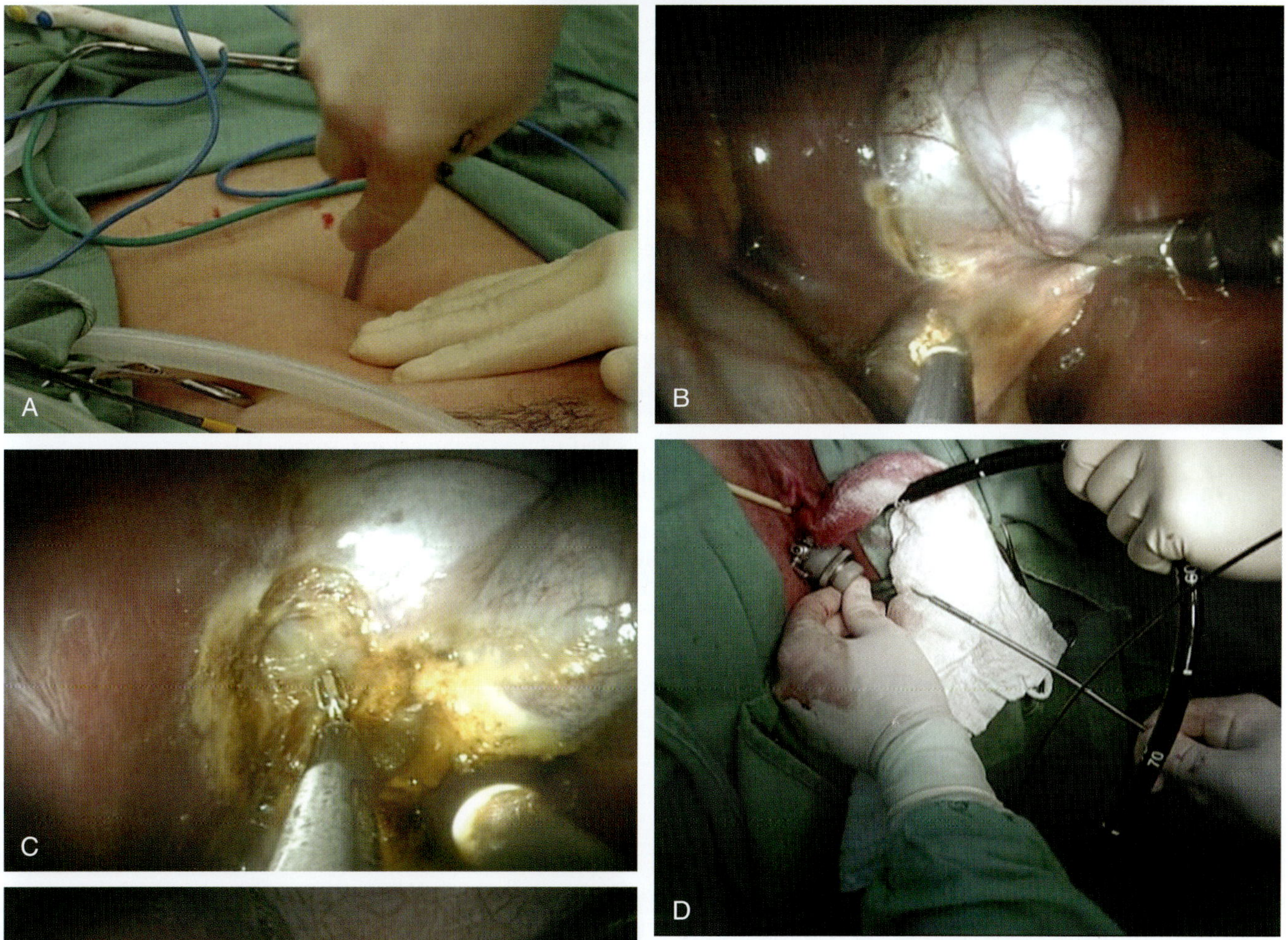

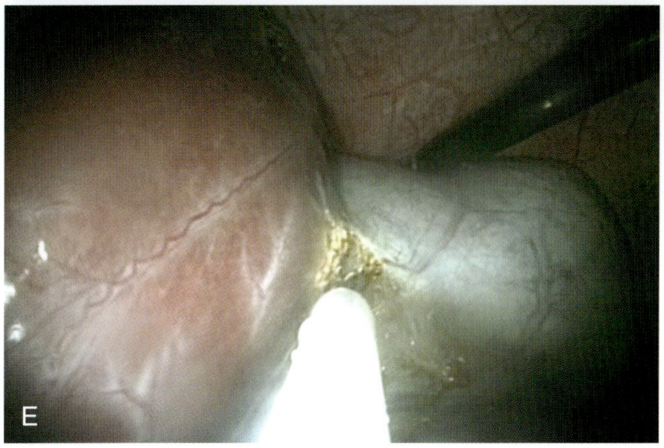

Figure 51-9.

using hot-biopsy forceps (see Fig. 51-9, *C*). Clipping of the cystic duct is performed using an especially long transvaginal clipator (Karl Storz) and cut with especially long transvaginal scissors (Karl Storz) (see Fig. 51-9, *D*).

- The gallbladder is then dissected from the liver bed using monopolar dissection (see Fig. 51-9, *E*).
- The specimen is captured and extracted transvaginally by a polypectomy snare (Fig. 51-10); visualization of the whole extraction is not necessary. Other graspers are not recommended for extraction, because the organ is often lost in the cavity, requiring time-consuming recovery of the specimen. To avoid stone spillage, extraction bags are used and inserted transvaginally to protect the exit, especially if the specimen was perforated during dissection.
- If the umbilical trocar is chosen for making the entire dissection, then vaginal access is used only for retraction, visualization, and specimen extraction. In this case, closure of the cystic duct is performed using either transumbilical externally tied polypropylene endoloops or laparoscopic clips.

Closure

- The vaginal wound is closed using absorbable running suture under direct vision (Fig. 51-11).

III. ALTERNATIVE TECHNICAL APPROACHES (PRO/CON) AND PEARLS

- Alternatively, a rigid long (obesity) laparoscopic optic (30 or 45 degrees) can be used instead of the flexible scope. In this variety of hybrid NOTES, all dissection, clipping, and cutting should be performed transumbilically (Fig. 51-12, *A*), which also shortens the operative time.
- Intraoperative cholangiography can be achieved in NOTES cases by directly puncturing the gallbladder or cystic duct percutaneously, or by installing a 5-mm trocar for manipulation during the procedure.
- Hybrid transvaginal surgery using laparoscopic assistance to achieve dissection, retraction, or visualization is the most common solution to overcoming NOTES issues, though it reduces the potential benefits of scarless surgery by having a trocar insertion.
- Totally NOTES cholecystectomy can be performed using the dual-scope method. Two endoscopes are inserted in the vaginal access, avoiding laparoscopic instruments (see Fig. 51-12, *B*). After retraction with the first endoscope, the second operating/visualization two-channel colonoscope is positioned about 4 to 5 cm from to the retracted gallbladder with the same orientation as the first endoscope. After orientation and after the endoscope has passed the pelvic organs, the position of the patient is changed to a reverse Trendelenburg position, allowing visualization of the upper abdomen. Dissection of the Calot triangle is performed using endoscopic instruments such as hot biopsy forceps, polypectomy snares, and endoscopic hooks. The cystic duct and artery are dissected and clipped using endoscopic clips, two proximal and one distal. After transection of the duct and artery with endoscopic scissors, the gallbladder is dissected from the liver bed using a polypectomy snare. This instrument is also used for vaginal extraction of the specimen. After delivery of the gallbladder, the pneumoperitoneum is aspirated before the second endoscope is removed.
- Another technique allowing total NOTES is the use of a specially designed vaginal port, performing the operation using all-transvaginal access for the endoscope and rigid instruments (see Fig. 51-12, *C*).

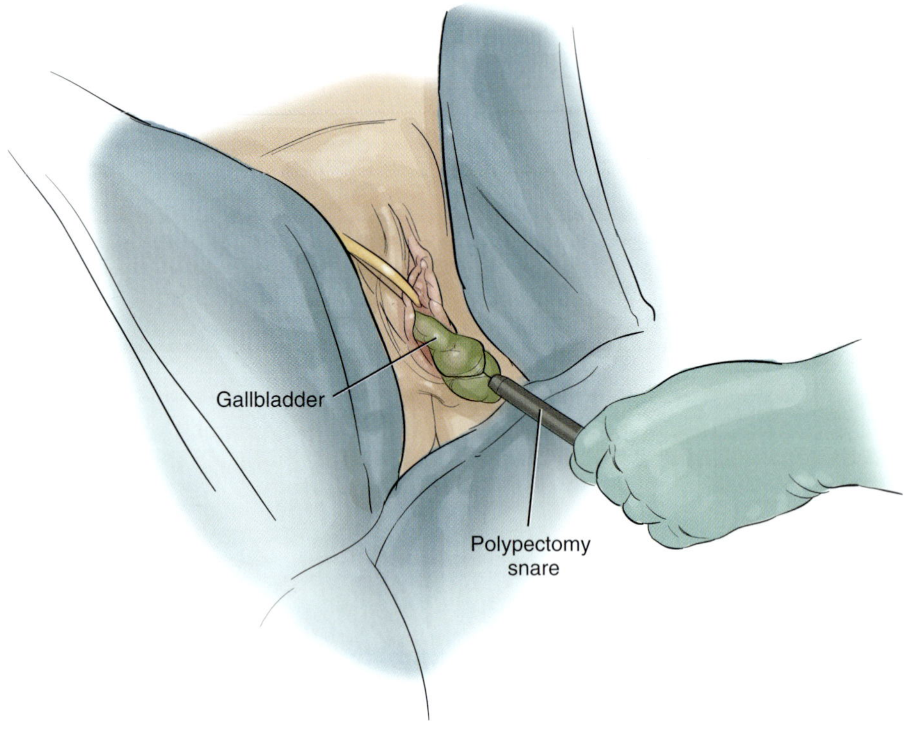

Figure 51-10.

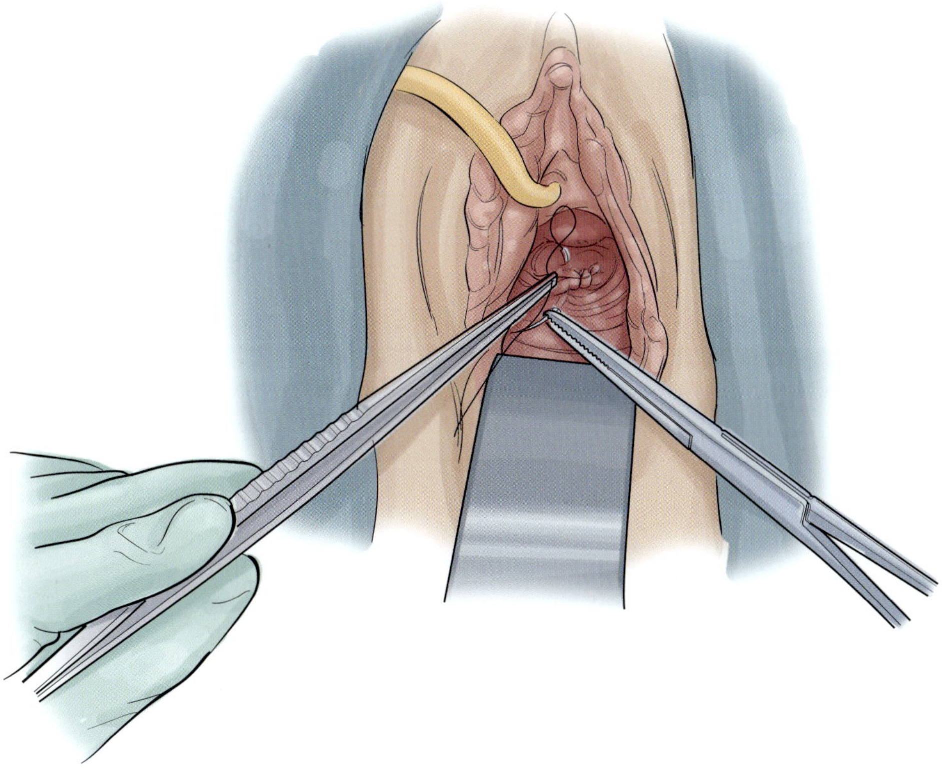

Figure 51-11.

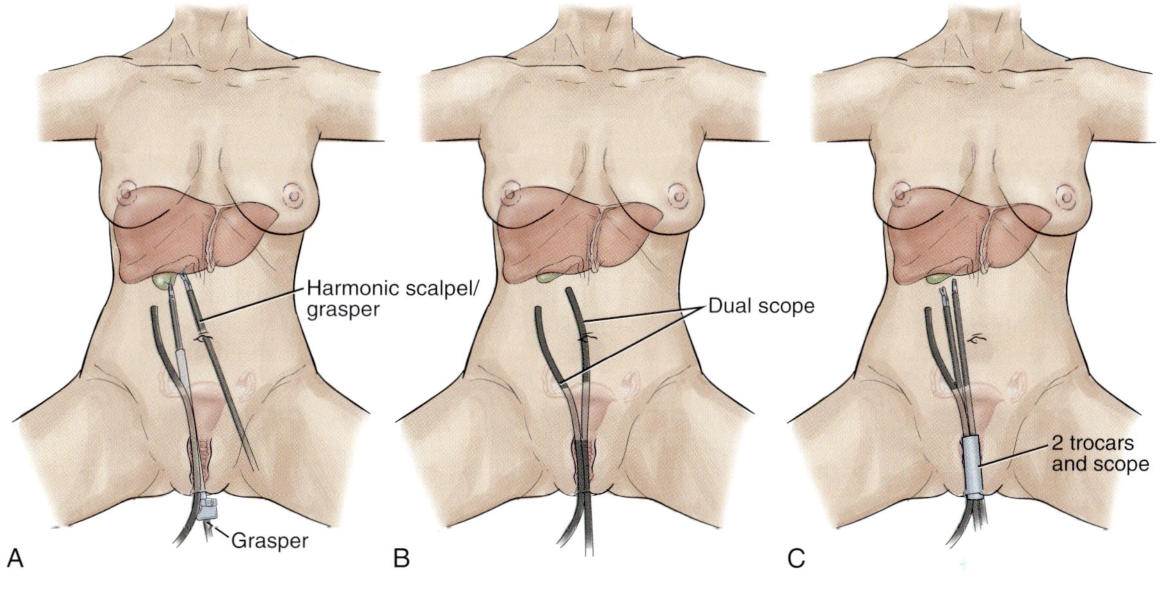

Figure 51-12.

IV. SPECIAL POSTOPERATIVE CARE

- Patients in whom this technique has been used are counseled to avoid sexual intercourse for 30 days. A postoperative gynecologic consultation is not necessary.
- If the total NOTES technique was employed, there are no physical restrictions after 24 hours postoperatively. A full diet is reintroduced in the first 48 hours. The vaginal absorbable sutures do not need to be monitored.
- The specific immediate postoperative complications that may be encountered with NOTES cholecystectomy are diffuse pelvic or upper abdominal pain. Biliary leak has been described in two cases in the literature and can be treated by nasobiliary drainage, drainage guided by computed tomography (CT), or laparoscopy. Delayed complications are dyspareunia, granuloma of the vaginal suture, and rarely pelvic abscess that can be managed conservatively with antibiotics, by CT-guided or laparoscopic drainage.

SUGGESTED READINGS

DeCarli L, Zorron R, Branco A, et al: New hybrid approach for NOTES transvaginal cholecystectomy: preliminary clinical experience, *Surg Innov* 16:181–186, 2009.

Zorron R: Techniques of transvaginal access for NOTES, *Tech Gastrointest Endosc* 11:75–83, 2009.

Zorron R, Maggioni LC, Pombo L, et al: NOTES transvaginal cholecystectomy: preliminary clinical application, *Surg Endosc* 22:542–547, 2008.

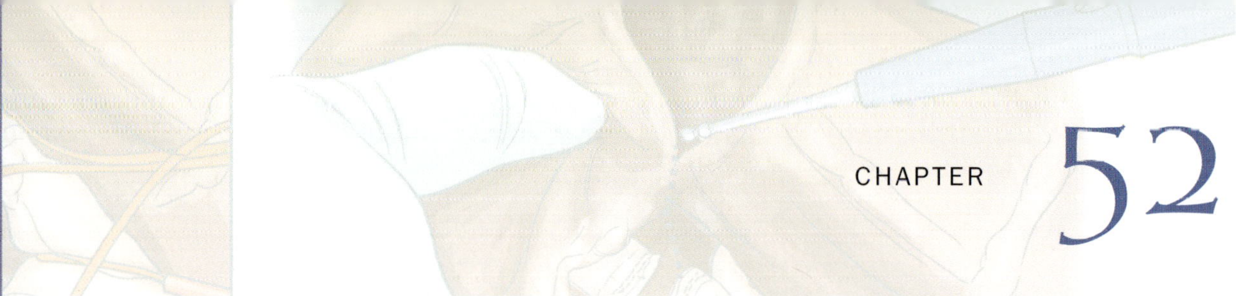

CHAPTER 52

Insertion of the Denver Peritoneovenous Shunt

Claudio Zanon, MD

I. SPECIAL PREOPERATIVE PREPARATION

- The Denver peritoneovenous shunt (PVS) is usually indicated for neoplastic refractory ascites and rarely for cirrhotic ascites. Pretreatment radiologic imaging provides useful information for defining the extent of the tumor and staging of the disease.
- The current imaging modes of choice are abdominal ultrasonography, as first proof of ascites, and a computed tomography (CT) scan to define the extent of the tumor and to ensure that no ascitic fluid is trapped. Only free ascitic fluid can be totally drained by the PVS. The CT scan gives a complete picture of tumoral stage, fluid distribution and volume in the abdominal cavity, and any possible metastasis into the lungs (Figs. 52-1 and 52-2). Magnetic resonance imaging and positron emission tomography are not usually required in the workup for PVS implantation as palliative treatment of a tumoral ascites.
- A chest radiograph is useful for showing signs of pulmonary area overload or myocardial dilatation due to cardiovascular insufficiency. The PVS can worsen subclinical lung edema.
- In patients with concomitant cirrhosis, esophagogastroduodenoscopy can disclose the possible presence of esophageal varices with hazard of forthcoming rupture. An overload of the pulmonary area caused by the shunted ascites can provoke a fatal hemorrhage owing to rupture of the varices.
- Preoperative ascitic fluid examination and blood tests are required. The PVS is not a useful option for patients with expected life less than 2 months, mucinous ascites, hemorrhagic ascites, or infected ascites with a white cell count of more than 500/mm^3. The PVS is likewise contraindicated for serum bilirubin of 3 mg/dL or higher and serious hemostatic disorders.
- In rare cases of uncertainty about the diagnosis of malignant effusion spread because of a negative result on cytologic examination of the ascitic fluid, a laparoscopic biopsy could be necessary. If the desirability of the PVS implant is confirmed, the PVS is introduced into the peritoneal space under the direct visual control of the laparoscope.
- A short-term antibiotic and low–molecular-weight heparin prophylaxis are recommended; mild coagulopathy is managed with fresh frozen plasma or platelets before the operation.
- I prefer the Denver PVS with a single- or double-miter valve pump chamber positioned under the skin, because its self-cleaning miter valve prevents occlusion of the system due to protein clots and cellular debris present in the neoplastic ascitic fluid. I never make use of the saphenous vein to introduce the Denver venous catheter because of the high rate of early occlusion of this device.
- The single-miter valve is preferable in clean, high-producing ascites, and the double-miter valve in ascites with clots and cellular debris and in chylous ascites.
- The Denver PVS can be positioned under local or general anesthesia according to the general conditions and the compliance of the patient. I usually prefer general anesthesia.

II. OPERATIVE TECHNIQUE

Position

- The following description is for a Denver system positioned in the right side (Fig. 52-3), but the same surgical steps are used for the left side.
- The patient is placed in supine position with the neck extended and the head turned left.

Incision

- Three incisions are required:
  - ▲ A longitudinal cervical incision of about 5 cm between the two clavicular insertions of the sternocleidomastoid muscle
  - ▲ A transverse abdominal incision of about 3 to 4 cm a few centimeters below the costal border
  - ▲ A transverse thoracic incision of 3 to 4 cm about 5 to 10 cm above the abdominal incision (see Fig. 52-3).

Main Dissection

- Exposure of the right internal jugular vein is the first step to avoid a peritoneal implantation of the Denver abdominal arm rendered useless by a venous thrombosis or venous anatomic anomalies. After

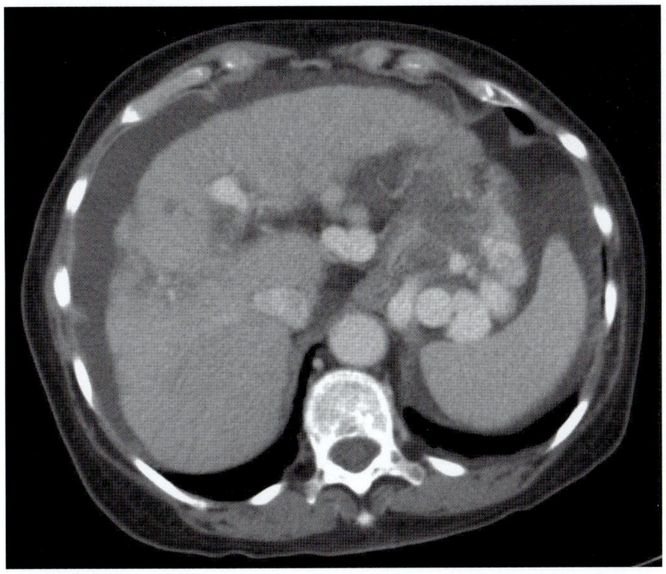

Figure 52-1. Cross-sectional image of the upper abdomen with an accumulation of free ascites around the cirrhotic liver and the spleen.

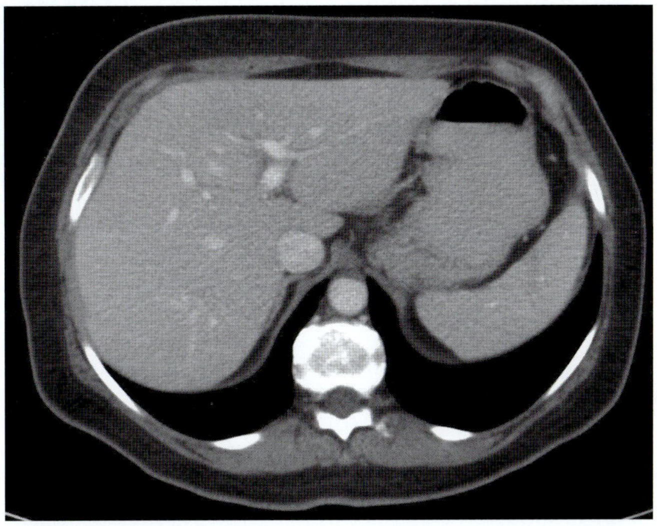

Figure 52-2. Cross-sectional image of the normal anatomy of the upper abdomen without ascitic fluid.

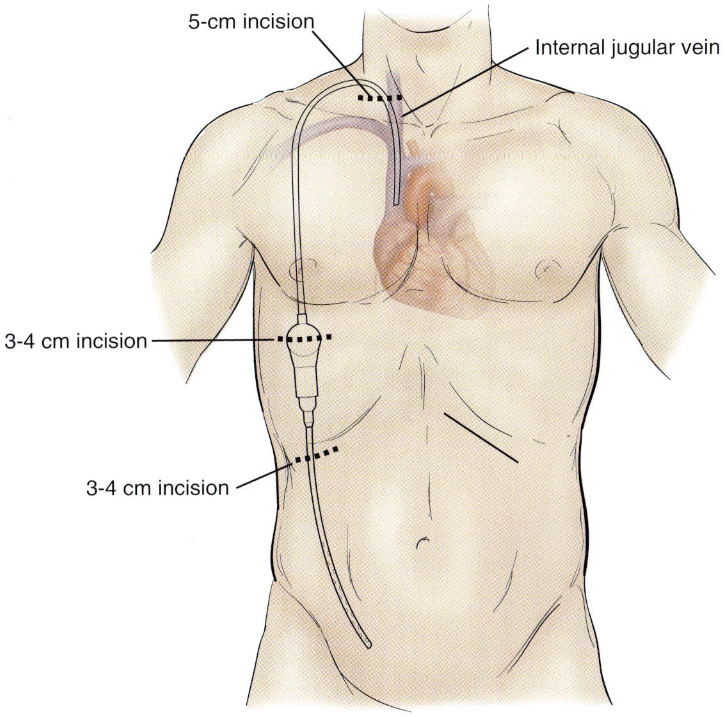

Figure 52-3.

incision of the platysma and of the superficial and middle cervical aponeurosis, the right internal jugular vein, next to the vagus nerve and the carotid artery, is exposed for 3 to 4 cm (Fig. 52-4).

- A few centimeters below the costal border, a transverse abdominal incision is made in the right upper abdominal site, the rectus abdominis aponeurosis is exposed, the rectus muscle fibers are split, and the peritoneal catheter is introduced into the abdominal cavity. A double purse-string suture is placed through the posterior rectus muscle aponeurosis and the peritoneum to ensure a watertight closure around the catheter (Fig. 52-5).
- After the catheter is positioned, the ascitic fluid is partially drained, leaving less than 1 liter in the peritoneal space to avoid possible heart overload and pulmonary edema. The catheter with its chamber valve is transported over the thorax (Fig. 52-6).

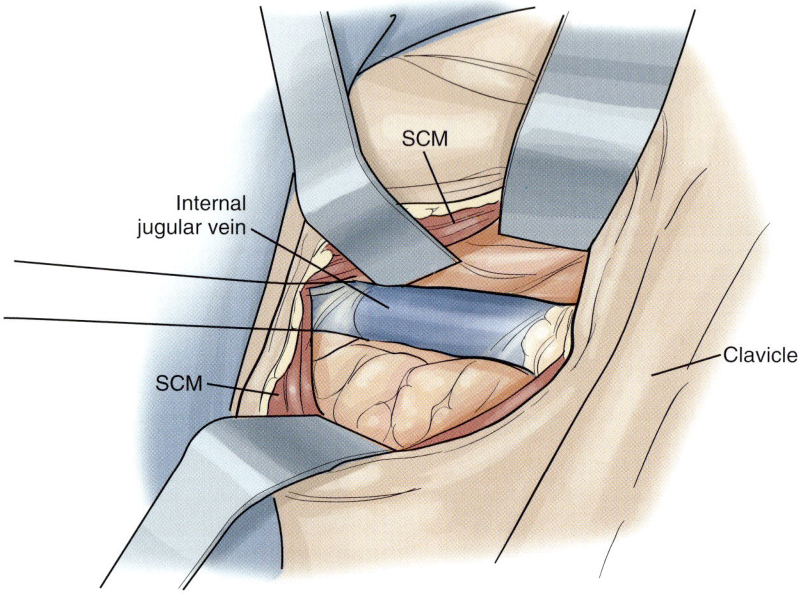

Figure 52-4. *SCM,* Sternocleidomastoid.

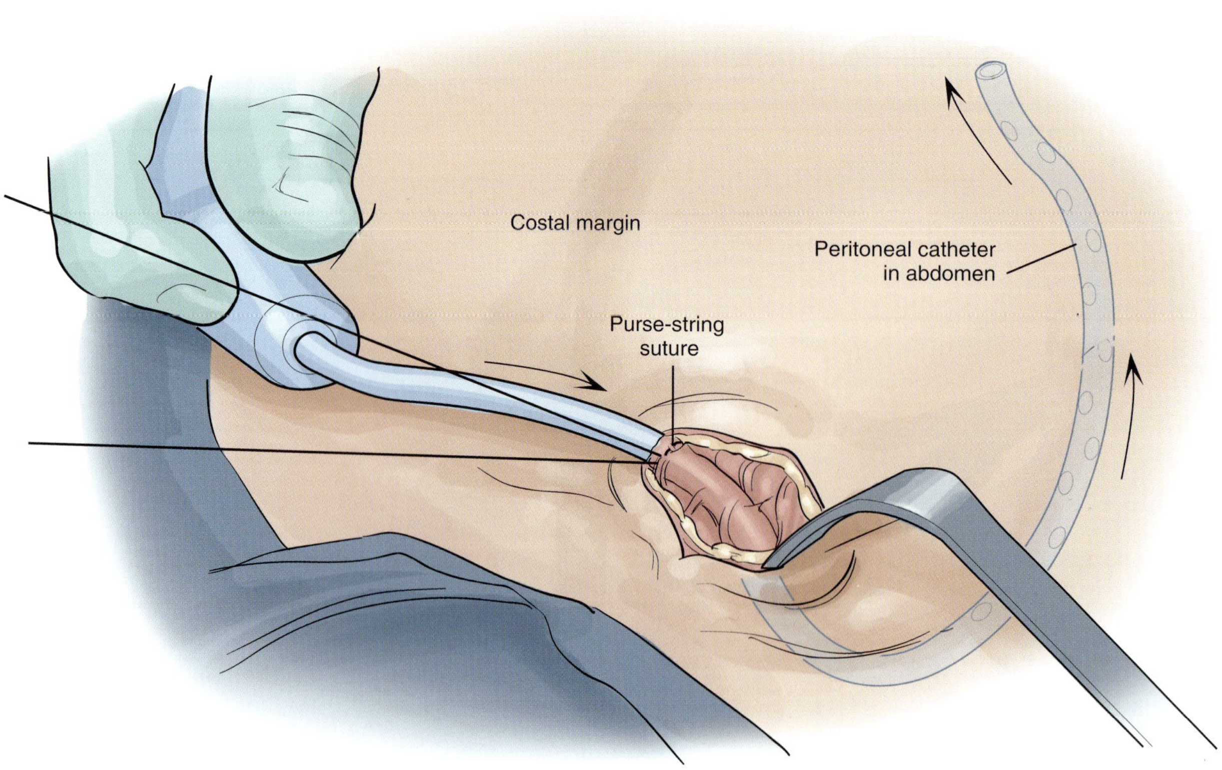

Figure 52-5.

- The venous end of the catheter is temporarily closed after the ascitic fluid has filled the Denver venous arm.
- A transverse thoracic incision is made 5 to 10 cm above the abdominal incision, and a subcutaneous pocket is created to position and to suture (four sutures through suitable holes) the pump chamber above the thoracic wall to give firm support for valve compression. The venous arm is tunneled subcutaneously, and the catheter end is transported to the cervical incision, close to the exposed jugular vein (Fig. 52-7).

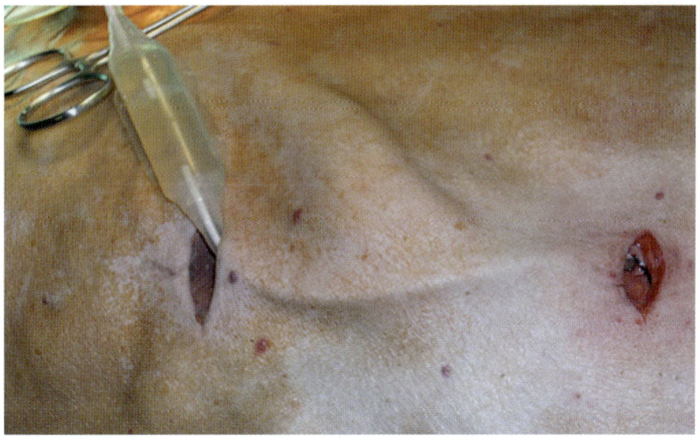

Figure 52-6.

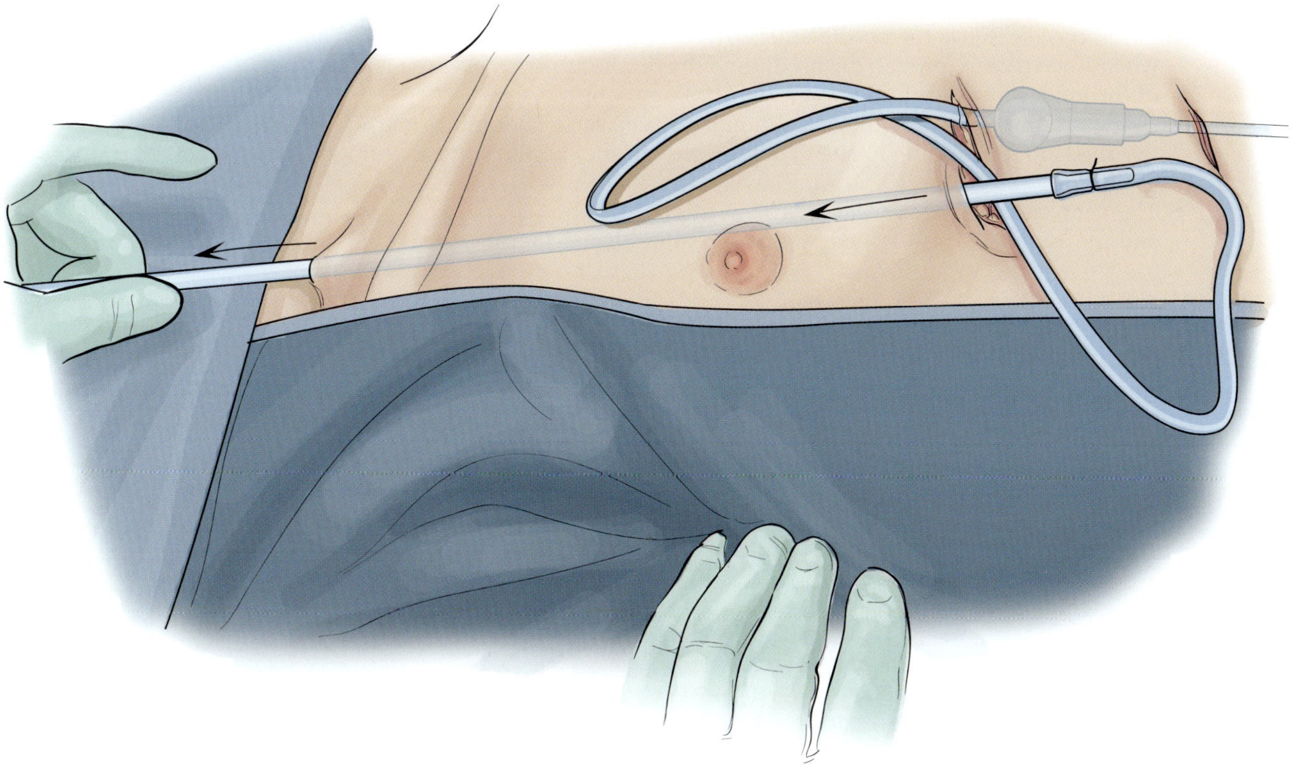

Figure 52-7.

- The jugular vein is interrupted before the Denver venous arm insertion point to prevent bleeding at the venous incision, and the catheter is blocked with a 2-0 silk suture (Fig. 52-8). After introduction of the catheter into the superior vena cava, the jugular vein is interrupted before the insertion point, and the catheter is blocked with a 2-0 silk suture. Venous collateral vessels supply the stopped right venous circulation from the head and the neck. A radiologic check verifies the correct position of the catheter in the innominate vein.

Closure

- Suturing the abdominal, thoracic, and cervical incisions with 2-0 nonabsorbable materials concludes the PVS implantation

III. ALTERNATIVE TECHNICAL APPROACHES (PRO/CON) AND PEARLS

- An alternative technical approach is the introduction of the Denver PVS using a peel-away set under fluoroscopic control. The kit includes the device, an 11.5-Fr diameter abdominal peel-away introducer, an 11.5-Fr diameter venous peel-away introducer, two guidewires, and an instrument to create the subcutaneous tunnels. This technique is less invasive, but often the introduction of the venous catheter of the valve into the subclavian vein is difficult because of the diameter of the catheter and the associated clavicular kinking.
- The following description is for a Denver system positioned in the right side (see Fig. 52-3), but, as noted previously, the same surgical steps are used for the left side.
- With the Denver peel-away set, local anesthesia is possible, if general conditions and the compliance of the patient permit.
- With this technique, implantation begins with the introduction of a guidewire into the right subclavian vein. The junction of the lateral third and the middle third of the clavicle just inferior to the clavicle in the "hollow space" is the preferred site. After an incision of 0.5 cm, a large-bore needle attached to a syringe is inserted just below the clavicle and over the first rib toward the suprasternal notch parallel to the clavicle. Once the needle enters the vein, a free flow of dark blood fills the syringe. The guidewire is then passed through the needle and the needle removed over the guidewire. The correct position of the guidewire is confirmed by means of fluoroscopy.
- A few centimeters below the costal border, a transverse abdominal incision of 2 to 3 cm is made in the right upper abdominal site. Through the needle, a guidewire is introduced into the abdominal cavity, followed by the 15.5-Fr peel-away.
- The peritoneal arm of the Denver PVS is introduced through the peel-away into the peritoneal cavity, and the ascitic fluid is drained, leaving no more than 1 liter of ascites (Fig. 52-9).

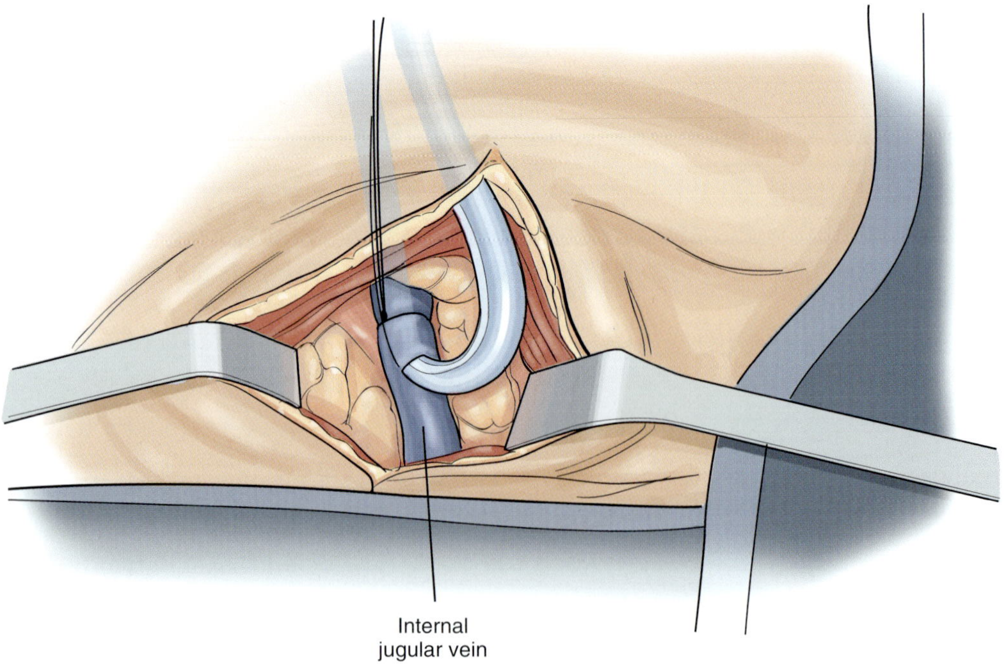

Figure 52-8.

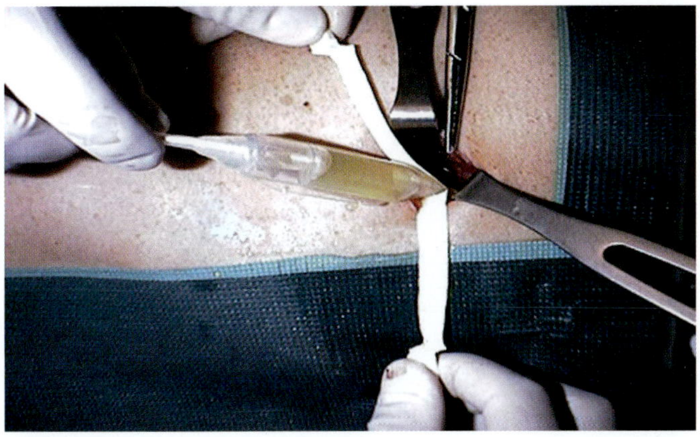

Figure 52-9.

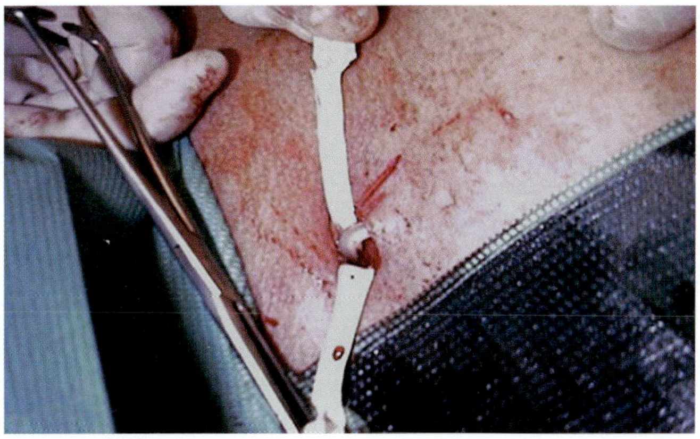

Figure 52-10.

- The tunnel and the subcutaneous pocket are created using the same procedure as in the open technique.
- The venous arm is tunnelized until it reaches the incision where the guidewire is inserted into the right subclavian vein.
- The cut venous arm is introduced into the superior cava vein through the 11.5-Fr venous peel-away inserted through the guidewire, which is then removed (Fig. 52-10).
- A radiologic check verifies the correct position of the catheter.

IV. SPECIAL POSTOPERATIVE CARE

- After the operation, diuretic therapy and a sitting position for the patient for 2 hours can prevent lung edema.
- Complete blood count, hemostatic and biochemical parameters, weight, abdominal girth, and ascites are monitored for at least 3 days. Mild hemostatic impairment is frequent, but overt disseminated intravascular coagulation is rare.
- For the patient's comfort, a tattoo is useful to help the patient or relatives localize the pump chamber for effective compression (20 pushes, three times daily). In the event of malfunction of the PVS owing to venous or peritoneal occlusion of the catheter (about 10% of cases in my experience), it is possible to remove a portion of the peritoneal or the venous arm, or the whole device, and to change them.
- Specific delayed complications that might be encountered include: clavicular kinking of the venous catheter introduced into the subclavian vein, with resulting difficult drainage of the ascitic fluid into the bloodstream; hepatic failure when the serum bilirubin cutoff is at or above 3 mg/dL; and pneumothorax during the puncture and the introduction of the guidewire into the subclavian vein.
- The postoperative death rate described in the literature is about 5%, but this can be improved by correctly selecting patients. Improved quality of life is registered in about 85% of patients.

SUGGESTED READINGS

Clara R, Righi D, Bortolini M, et al: Role of different techniques for the placement of Denver peritoneovenous shunt (PVS) in malignant ascites, *Surg Laparosc Endosc Percutan Tech* 14:222–225, 2004.

Sugawara S, Sone M, Arai Y, et al: Radiological insertion of Denver peritoneovenous shunts for malignant refractory ascites: a retrospective multicenter study (JIVROSG-0809), *Cardiovasc Intervent Radiol* 34:980–988, 2011.

White MA, Agle SC, Padia RK, Zervos EE: Denver peritoneovenous shunts for the management of malignant ascites: a review of the literature in the post LeVeen era, *Am Surg* 77:1070–1075, 2011.

SECTION VIII

Colorectal

CHAPTER 53

Restorative Proctocolectomy with J-Pouch Ileoanal Anastomosis

Sang W. Lee, MD, FACS, FASCRS, and Fabrizio Michelassi, MD, FACS

I. SPECIAL PREOPERATIVE PREPARATION

- The most common indications for restorative proctocolectomy (RP) are ulcerative colitis refractory to medical therapy and familial adenomatous polyposis.
- Contraindications to RP are patients with significant anal sphincter dysfunction and a history of surgery that removed a part or all of the sphincter muscles. A careful history focusing on fecal incontinence, physical examination, and, in certain cases, anal manometry are essential in determining baseline sphincter function.
- Other contraindications include a history of Crohn disease and carcinoma of the distal rectum.
- All patients should undergo mechanical bowel preparation before the operation. We do not use an oral antibiotic regimen.
- To ensure proper functioning of the stoma, potential sites should be determined before the operation.
- We recommend epidural anesthesia for postoperative pain management.
- We do not routinely use ureteral stents. Selective use of stents, especially in patients with a history of extensive surgery, may be prudent.

II. OPERATIVE TECHNIQUE

Position

- The patient is placed in the modified lithotomy position, and the arms are tucked to the sides. We use a gel pad underneath the patient and do not use a sandbag or tapes to secure patients onto the table. The patient is positioned with the buttocks overhanging just below the lower table break to allow access to the perineum for anastomosis and pelvic manipulations.
- Legs are placed in adjustable padded Yellofin stirrups. Pneumatic compression stockings are routinely used, and subcutaneous heparin and intravenous antibiotics are given preoperatively.
- Patients are placed in the modified lithotomy position. The flexion of the hips is kept at an angle less than 10 degrees to prevent instruments from abutting the thighs of the patient during transverse colon mobilization.

Incision

- A 10-mm camera port is placed in the supraumbilical position, and four additional 5-mm working ports are placed lateral to the rectus sheath as shown in Figure 53-1. Use of a 30-degree angled laparoscope can be helpful.

Main Dissection

- The procedure is broken into four phases: extended right colectomy, left colectomy, proctectomy, and ileal pouch formation and anastomosis.

Extended Right Colectomy

- The patient is placed in a neutral position with the right side of the body tilted upward. The terminal ileum is placed into the pelvis, and the rest of the small intestines are placed to the left side of the abdomen.
- The ileocolic pedicle is identified by gently retracting the ileocolic junction anteriorly and laterally. This maneuver places the ileocolic pedicle under tension as it crosses below the duodenal sweep. An avascular plane underneath the ileocolic vessels is developed by first scoring the mesentery inferior to the pedicle and then gently brushing the retroperitoneum away from the mesentery. The duodenal sweep just cephalad to the origin of the ileocolic vessels must be identified and carefully preserved. The ileocolic vessels are then divided using a 5-mm bipolar device (Fig. 53-2, *A* and *B*).
- Blunt dissection separating the retroperitoneum away from the mesentery is continued toward the hepatic flexure and laterally to the Toldt fascia.
- The transverse colon is retracted anteriorly, placing tension on the middle colic vessels. The peritoneum is gently scored transversely just distal to the origins of the middle colic vessels. In general, it is easier

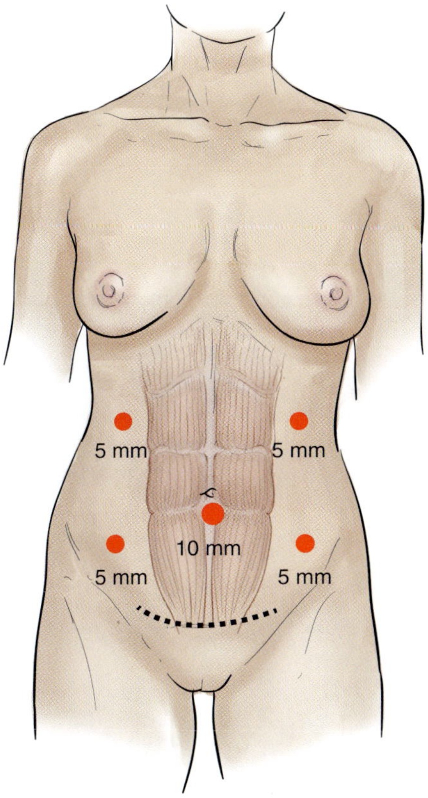

Figure 53-1.

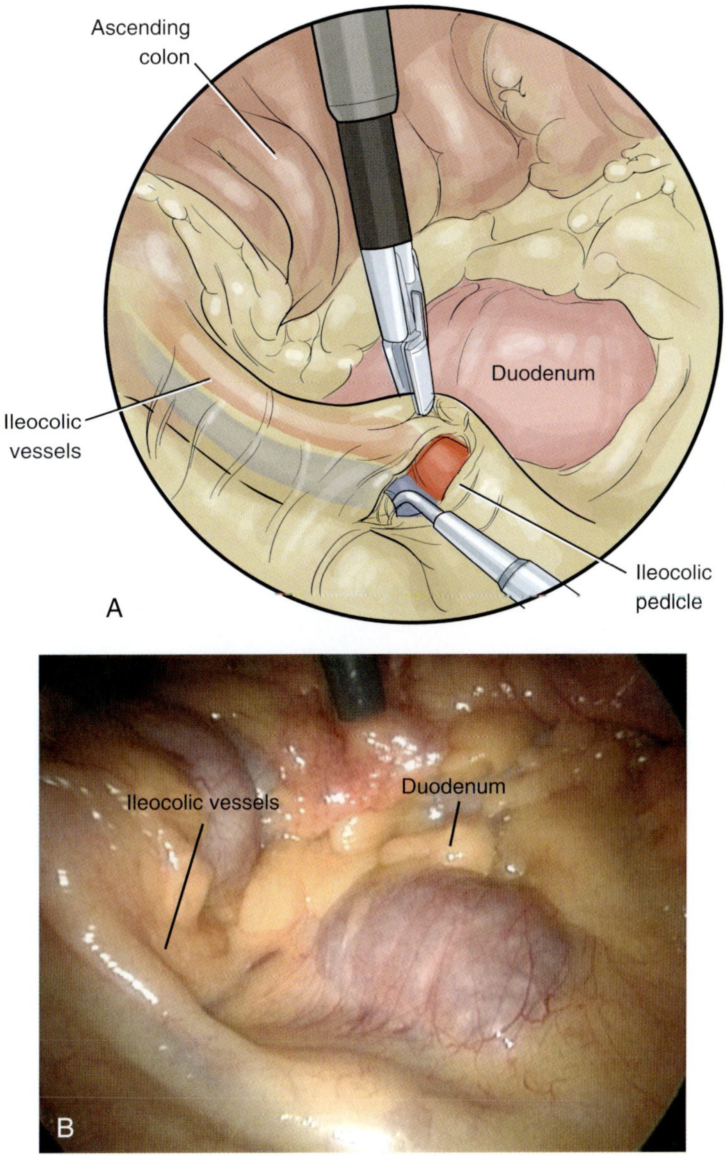

Figure 53-2.

to enter the proper plane by dissecting and dividing the left branch of the middle colic vessels first (Fig. 53-3, *A* and *B*).

- The greater omentum is transected from the proximal transverse colon using a bipolar device.
- The patient is placed in the steep Trendelenburg position, and the terminal ileum is retracted from the pelvis and into the upper abdomen. The retroperitoneal attachments of the terminal ileum and the cecum are divided by incising the peritoneum at the base of the appendix and the cecum. The attachments of the terminal ileal mesentery are divided upward to the duodenal sweep to maximize the reach of the ileal pouch.
- The lateral attachments of the right colon and the hepatic flexure are completely divided.

Left Colectomy

- The patient is placed in the steep Trendelenburg position with the left side tilted upward.
- The inferior mesenteric pedicle is identified and gently retracted anteriorly and laterally. The peritoneum is scored just dorsal to the pedicle of the inferior mesenteric artery (IMA) at the level of the sacral promontory and extended toward its origin, creating a wide window (Fig. 53-4, *A* and *B*).
- As dissection proceeds toward the origin of the IMA, the hypogastric nerves are identified and preserved. The retroperitoneum is then separated from the mesentery of the sigmoid colon using blunt dissection, and the ureter and gonadal vessels are identified.
- After the left ureter and gonadal vessels are dissected away from the left colon mesentery, the IMA and the inferior mesenteric vein are ligated separately using a bipolar device just distal to the origin of the left colic artery.
- Division of the IMA pedicle creates further access to the retroperitoneum. Blunt dissection over the Gerota fascia and laterally toward the Toldt fascia facilitates splenic flexure mobilization and prevents inadvertent dissection behind the kidney during lateral dissection.
- The greater omentum is then peeled off the transverse colon toward the distal transverse colon until dissection becomes difficult. It is very important to maintain proper tissue triangulation to avoid injury to the transverse colon. The Toldt fascia is divided, and the splenic flexure is completely mobilized.

Rectal Mobilization

- The monitors are repositioned near the foot of the table. A steep Trendelenburg position is maintained. The assistant standing to the left of the patient gently grasps the colon and rectum, retracting them out of the pelvis.
- The surgeon, dissecting from the right side, incises the peritoneum at the level of the sacral promontory into the pelvis. The rectum is mobilized, first posteriorly, then laterally, then anteriorly.

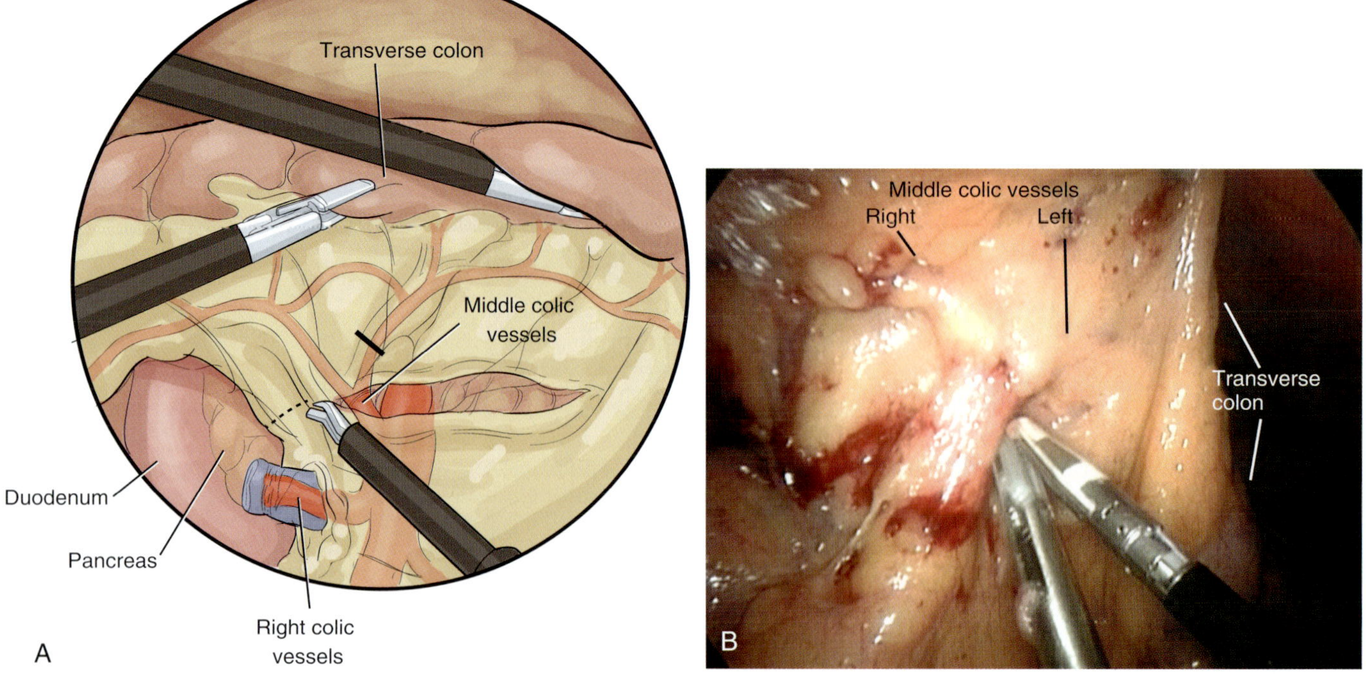

Figure 53-3.

- The initial dissection plane is similar to that of the total mesorectal dissection in which sharp dissection between the fascia propria of the rectum and the presacral fascia is performed (Fig. 53-5).
- After division of the Waldeyer fascia at the level of S2 and S3, posterior dissection is carried downward to the pelvic floor muscles.
- As the rectum is mobilized distally and laterally, further dissection is performed very close to the rectum to preserve the nervi erigentes.
- Peritoneal reflection is incised away from the colovesical fold onto the rectum, exposing the Denonvilliers fascia. Dissection is close to the rectum so that the periprostatic nerve plexus, seminal vesicles, and vaginal wall can be protected.
- Insertion of a double-gloved finger into the anus confirms the success of the dissection.

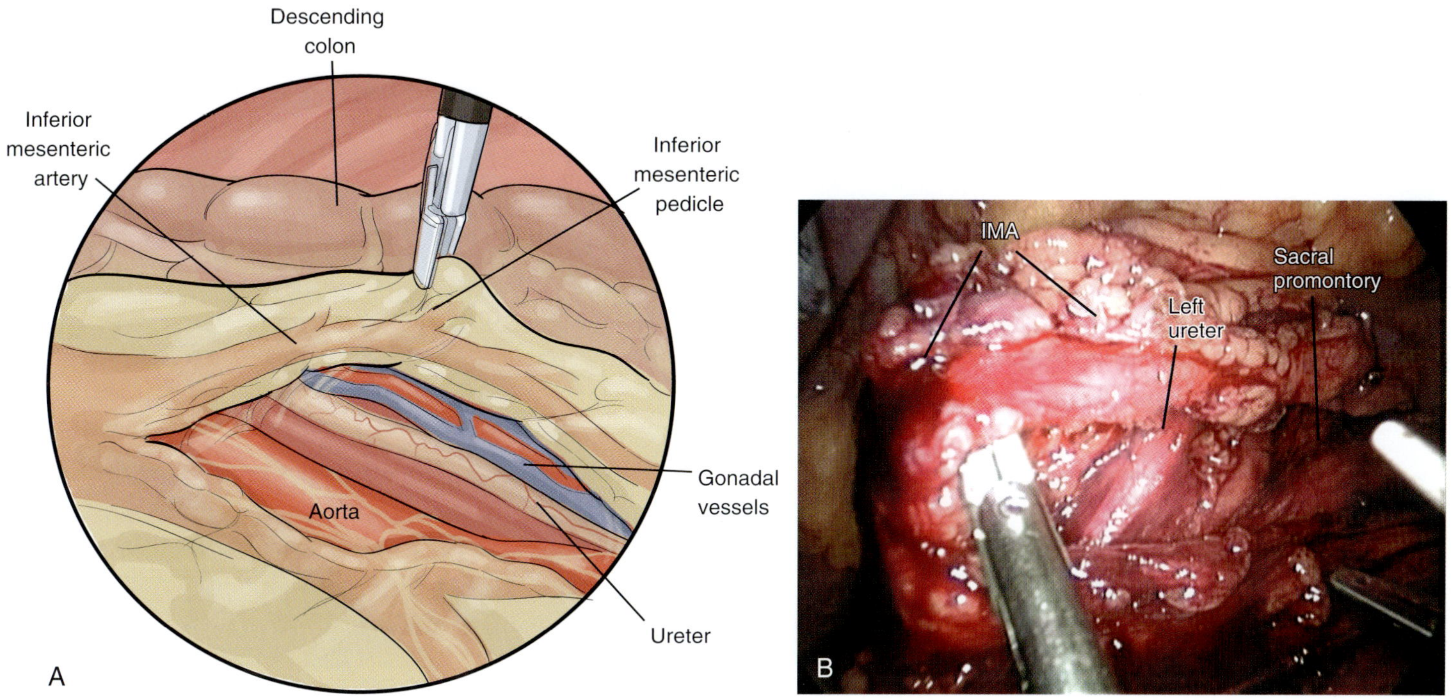

Figure 53-4. *IMA,* Inferior mesenteric artery.

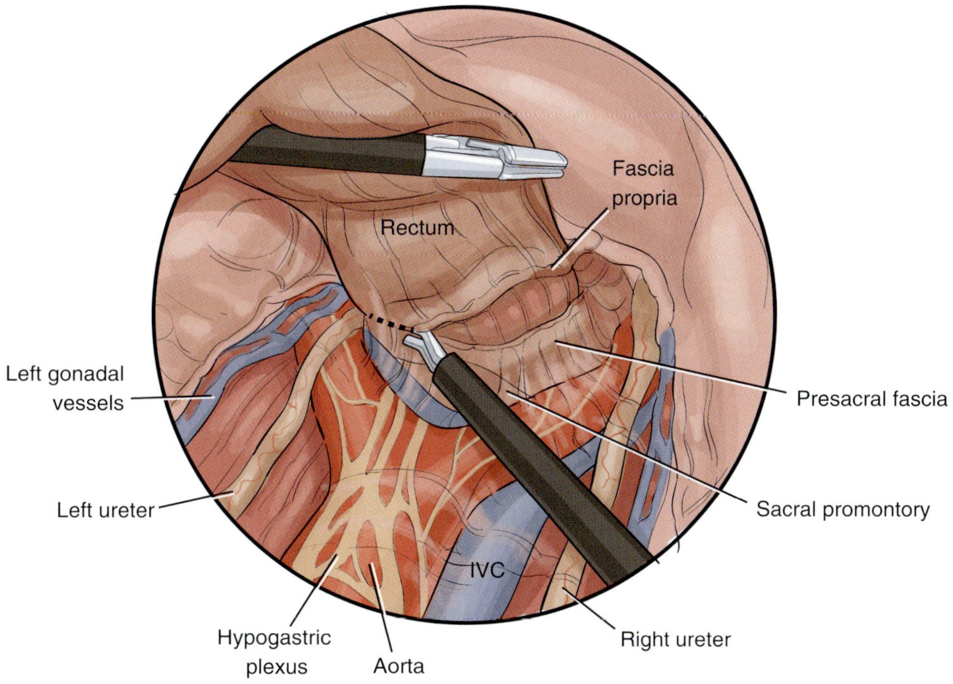

Figure 53-5. *IVC,* Inferior vena cava.

- Once the rectum is completely mobilized, the rectum can be transected with a laparoscopic stapler or an open thoracoabdominal (TA) stapler, or by mucosectomy from the perineal approach. We prefer creating a small Pfannenstiel incision for distal rectal stapling using a open TA stapler and specimen extraction.

Ileal J-Pouch Formation and Anastomosis

- Once the rectum is transected, the colon and the rectum are exteriorized through the Pfannenstiel incision. It is critical to maintain the proper orientation of the small bowel mesentery during extraction of the specimen. The terminal ileum is then divided from the colon.
- The J-pouch is created by folding the terminal ileum onto itself. The apex of the pouch is determined by placing the ileum over the pubis to identify the longest section of mesentery. Approximately a 2-cm longitudinal incision is made on the antimesenteric side of the terminal ileum at the apex of the pouch. Firing a series of 8-cm gastrointestinal anastomosis staples between the two limbs of the terminal ileum, a J-pouch at least 15 cm in length is created. The efferent limb of the pouch is closed using a TA stapler.
- An umbilical tape is placed around the afferent loop of the pouch, and the pouch is irrigated with saline and checked for leakage. Purse-string sutures are placed around the enterotomy site at the apex, and the anvil of an end-to-end anastomosis stapler is placed and secured (Fig. 53-6).
- Pneumoperitoneum can be reestablished by twisting the wound protector and clamping it at skin level. Before the anastomosis is performed, the orientation of the small intestines should be verified: the cut edge of the terminal ileal mesentery should be aligned straight on the right side, and there should be no small bowel loops trapped behind the terminal ileal mesentery.
- After performing the double-stapled anastomosis, an air leak test is performed, and a loop ileostomy is created at the preselected site in the right lower quadrant of the abdomen.

Closure

- The Pfannenstiel incision is closed in two layers. Fascial openings of trocar sites that are 1 cm or more in length are closed.

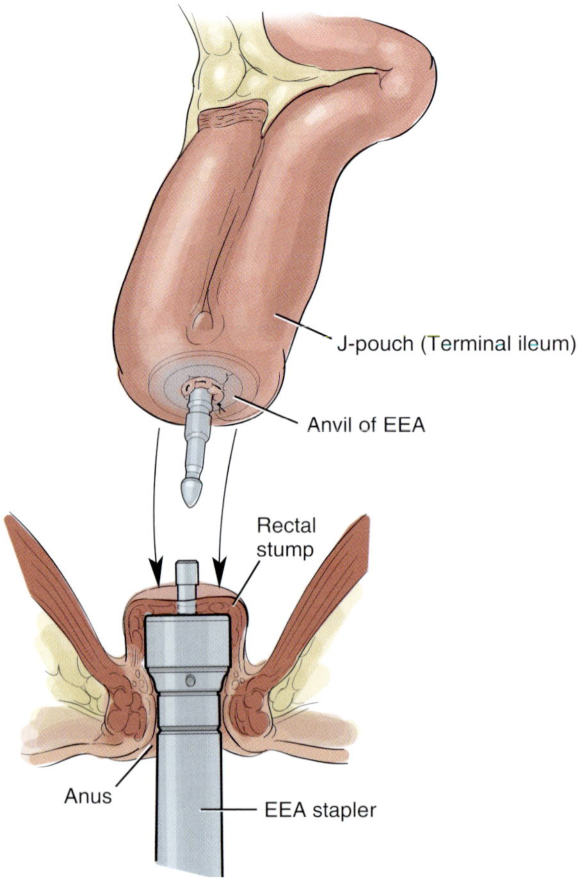

Figure 53-6. *EEA,* End-to-end anastomosis.

III. ALTERNATIVE TECHNICAL APPROACHES (PRO/CON) AND PEARLS

- In most elective settings, a laparoscopic approach can be considered. The surgeon must have extensive experience in performing laparoscopic segmental colectomies before attempting laparoscopic restorative proctocolectomy. Compared to open surgery, the laparoscopic approach results in longer operative time and better short-term outcomes, such as less pain, shorter length of stay, and quicker recovery.
- We find that a hand-assisted laparoscopic approach results in significantly decreased operative time with short-term outcomes equivalent to those for the "straight" laparoscopic approach.

Difficult-to-Reach Pouch

- A series of peritoneal incisions over the terminal ileal mesentery can increase the reach.
- Ileocolic artery ligation gives a length of 5 cm or more.
- Mobilization of the root of the mesentery beyond the fourth portion of the duodenum provides extra length.
- An S-pouch reaches 2 to 4 cm farther than a J-pouch.

IV. SPECIAL POSTOPERATIVE CARE

- Nasogastric tubes are not routinely used postoperatively.
- Clear liquids are usually started on postoperative day 1, and, if well tolerated, the patient is placed on a fiber-restricted diet.
- The Foley catheter is removed on postoperative day 4.
- Up to 30% of patients will develop pouchitis. A 1-week course of oral antibiotics is usually an effective treatment.
- Following a stapled anastomosis, the anal transition zone needs to be endoscopically surveyed and biopsied yearly for dysplasia and cancer. Up to 20% of patients who undergo mucosectomy and hand-sewn anastomosis can retain islets of rectal mucosa deep in the ileal pouch and are at risk of developing cancer. Routine follow-up of these patients is mandatory.

SUGGESTED READINGS

Fichera A, Silvestri MT, Hurst RD, et al: Laparoscopic restorative proctocolectomy with ileal pouch anal anastomosis: a comparative observational study on long-term functional results, *J Gastrointest Surg* 13:526–532, 2009.

Hurst RD, Michelassi F: Ileal-pouch anal restorative proctocolectomy for ulcerative colitis, *Adv Surg* 38:311–336, 2004. Review.

Reissman P, Salky BA, Pfeifer J, et al: Laparoscopic surgery in the management of inflammatory bowel disease, *Am J Surg* 171:47–50, discussion 50–51, 1996.

CHAPTER 54

Total Mesorectal Excision with Colonic J-Pouch Coloanal Reconstruction for Rectal Cancer

Brendan J. Moran, FRCSI, MCh, FRCS, and Richard J. Heald, OBE, MChir, FRCS

I. SPECIAL PREOPERATIVE PREPARATION

- The upper limit of the rectum is arbitrarily defined as within 15 cm from the anal verge. Measurement of the height of a rectal cancer should be performed using a rigid sigmoidoscope with the patient awake, usually in the left lateral position. A flexible instrument (e.g., colonoscope) may overestimate the distance from the anal verge.
- Clinical palpation of the rectum by an experienced rectal surgeon is mandatory to assess the extent, fixity, and relationship of low rectal cancers, generally defined as within 6 cm from the anal verge.
- Ideally the whole colon should be imaged by colonoscopy, barium enema, or computed tomography (CT) colonography.
- Colonoscopy under sedation may facilitate accurate assessment of low rectal cancer and may provide information similar to an examination under anesthetic.
- The focus of preoperative staging revolves around local staging and imaging for systemic disease. CT of the chest and abdomen provide optimal systemic staging. Local staging involves mandatory rectal examination and vaginal examination in females.
- Endoluminal ultrasound may help in staging early disease likely to be amenable to local excision (for example, uT1 very low in the rectum that could only be otherwise removed by abdominoperineal excision, or an early tumor in a patient with severe comorbidity).
- The focus of optimal staging in rectal cancer is the relationship of the primary tumor and any lymph nodes, or tumor deposits, to the mesorectal fascia—the proposed circumferential resection margin.
- Fine-slice surface coil magnetic resonance imaging provides optimal local staging of rectal cancer in relationship to the mesorectal margin and can help distinguish patients who can have surgery alone from those who require preoperative neoadjuvant treatment (Fig. 54-1).
- Optimal neoadjuvant therapy for patients with an involved or threatened mesorectal margin involves a combination of preoperative radiotherapy and chemotherapy, usually administered over a 6- to 8-week schedule, followed by a traditional delay of 6 to 8 weeks before surgical excision.
- Magnetic resonance images of low rectal cancer must be interpreted in light of clinical findings and repeat examination, and a second opinion may be helpful if there is a question regarding the feasibility of anterior resection (AR) or if an abdominoperineal excision (APE) is required. The decision whether an AR is possible needs to be made before chemoradiotherapy. Although "downstaging" and "downsizing" of a rectal cancer by chemoradiotherapy is common, the distal margin seldom recedes sufficiently to allow a change from APE to AR despite reports in the literature.

II. OPERATIVE TECHNIQUE

Practical Steps of the Operation

- The key principle is that dissection should proceed only in the perimesorectal tissue plane and leave intact:
  - ▲ The autonomic nerve plexuses
  - ▲ The nonvisceral presacral fat pad (when present)
  - ▲ The parietal sidewall fascia of the small pelvis
  - ▲ The hypogastric plexuses
  - ▲ The vesicles
  - ▲ The prostate in the male
  - ▲ The vagina in the female
- All surgery should be performed by sharp dissection with diathermy or scissors under direct vision and good light. Throughout, the assistants should provide three-directional traction and countertraction to open up the planes for the surgeon. Diathermy can only be used safely when the areolar tissue is on stretch. Compared with traditional methods of manual extraction, the difference in procedure time can be considerable. A careful total mesorectal excision (TME) plus pouch-to-anus reconstruction takes 3 to 5 hours depending on the patient's build and the particular cancer; a conventional APE is often completed in 1 hour.

Position

- The patient is placed in a modified Lloyd-Davies position, ensuring that all areas of pressure points are well padded.

Incision

- A long midline incision is made from the symphysis pubis to within a few centimeters of the xiphoid process (Fig. 54-2). If possible, at least 5 to 7 cm is best left at the top, as this facilitates packing away of the small intestine in the right upper quadrant. Some young women may prefer a suprapubic skin-crease incision combined with a vertical midline between the rectus muscles, and some surgeons may increasingly prefer to perform the abdominal part of the dissection by laparoscopy.

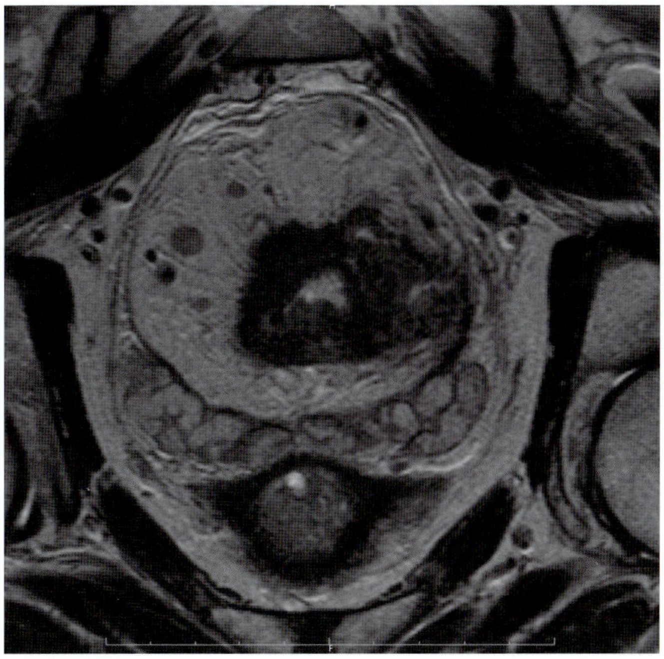

Figure 54-1.

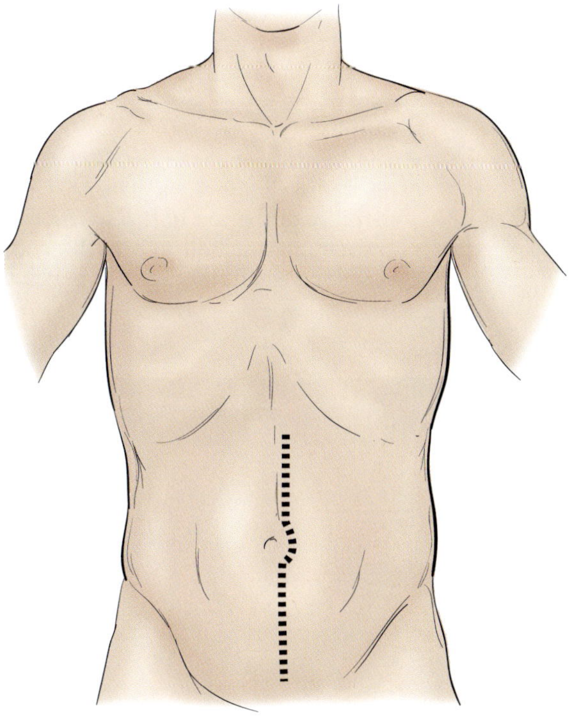

Figure 54-2.

Main Dissection

- *Laparoscopic anterior resection:* The authors suggest that only very experienced laparoscopic gastrointestinal surgeons should embark on the deep low dissection for cancer with sphincter preservation, and that special caution, if not total avoidance, is appropriate for very large cancers, especially in narrow male pelvises. The elevation of an intact mesorectal package, safely encompassing a large cancer, requires carefully applied but substantial upward traction, which is very difficult to achieve with laparoscopic instruments without risk of tearing the mesorectal surface. At present the authors counsel great caution with tumors larger than 7 cm. A further area of limitation is the cross-clamping and washout of the anorectal muscle tube beyond the cancer, for which laparoscopic instrumentation remains imperfect.
- *Manual palpation and inspection:* This must be thorough, with particular emphasis on liver and peritoneum. Careful assessment of the paraaortic nodes in the lesser sac is easy to forget. At this stage it is a good routine to review the CT and the colonoscopy report and to palpate the whole gastrointestinal tract carefully for synchronous primaries.
- *Retractors and packing:* Careful packing and retraction of the intestines upward and to the right is crucial to provide clear access to the pelvis. Adhesions in the right lower quadrant commonly require division.
- *Starting right—the pedicle package—the clue to the top of the "holy plane":* Starting correctly involves three-directional traction and countertraction between the colon and mesorectum and the retroperitoneum to identify the plane behind the back of the pedicle package and the gonadal vessels, ureter, and preaortic sympathetic nerves, all of which must be carefully preserved. The key to this phase is the recognition of the shiny fascia-covered surface of the back of the pedicle—like a shiny, tapering, longitudinal "sausage" with the inferior mesenteric vessels often visible within. This must be gently lifted forward to open up the plane. It is usual in open surgery to start on the left of the sigmoid mesocolon. It is equally satisfactory, as commonly performed in laparoscopic surgery, to start on the right. In either case the identification of the shiny fascial envelope, the "pedicle package," is crucial to properly entering into the pelvis.
- *High ligation of the inferior mesenteric vessels:* Adhesions between the sigmoid colon and the lateral peritoneal wall in the left lower quadrant need to be divided to allow easy grasp of the sigmoid colon (Fig. 54-3). With the pedicle package lifted gently forward, the dissection behind it can be extended up to its origin (Fig. 54-4). Separate high ligations of the inferior mesenteric artery and vein can be performed with the artery controlled by the left index finger and the thumb. The artery is taken 1 to 2 cm anterior to the aorta to spare the sympathetic nerve plexuses; the vein is divided several centimeters to the left of the artery above its last tributary and close to the pancreas. These two high ligations are an integral part of the otherwise avascular planes, which then need to be developed upward extensively for a full mobilization of the splenic flexure.
- The ascending left colic artery and either the accompanying inferior mesenteric vein or its last tributary from the left colon may also need to be divided separately to complete the vascular isolation of the specimen with full splenic flexure mobilization for ultralow pouch anastomosis.
- In a minority of cases, a particularly long and healthy sigmoid may obviate the need for this full mobilization process, which is not entirely without risk (e.g., to the spleen). Thus it is logical, if a decision is made to use such a long healthy sigmoid and thus avoid the splenic flexure, to ligate the inferior mesenteric artery just distal to the ascending left colic, which is essentially a part of its primary blood supply.
- *The "division of convenience" of the sigmoid colon:* The sigmoid mesentery and the sigmoid colon are divided well above the cancer. This is an important step in every cancer dissection, because optimal mobility of the top of the specimen facilitates gentle opening of the perimesorectal planes by traction and countertraction in any direction throughout the pelvic dissection. The division allows the best possible visualization of the pelvis with all of the gut to be retained to be drawn upward and to the right.

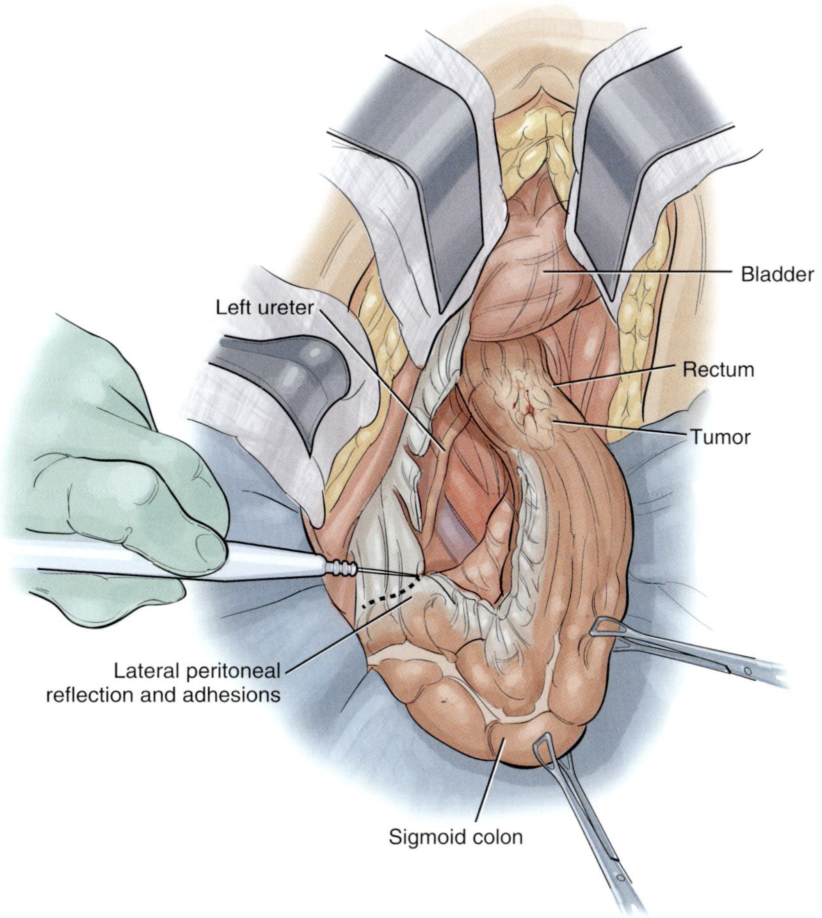

Figure 54-3.

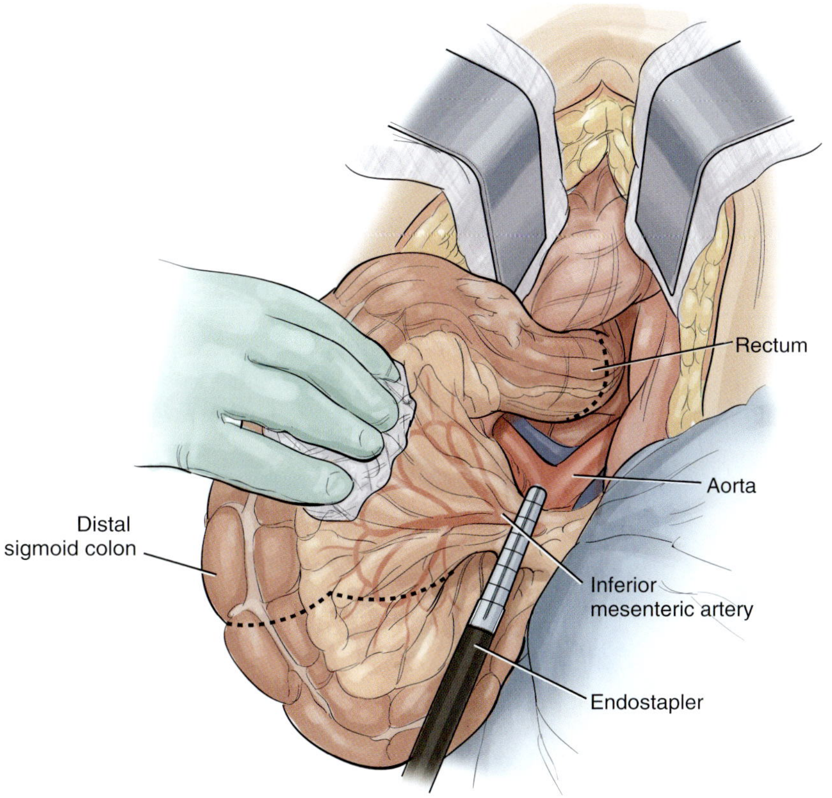

Figure 54-4.

- *Commencing the pelvic dissection:* The surgeon is now optimally placed to identify the key planes that must be developed circumferentially around the mesorectum. The surgeon starts at the back, lifting the rectosigmoid forward, and then follows identifiable areas of the "holy plane" at various points on the mesorectal circumference in a progressive manner (Fig. 54-5, *A* and *B*). If bleeding in one area is troublesome, it is sensible to tackle the opposite circumference so that pressure is applied while progress continues.
- *High posterior dissection:* The rectosigmoid is lifted carefully forward to identify the posterior embryologic plane—that is, the shiny posterior surface of the mesorectum within the bifurcation of the superior hypogastric plexus. This plane is extended downward toward and eventually beyond the tip of the coccyx, step by step as other sectors of the circumference are developed (Fig. 54-6). The rectosacral ligament or fascia may constitute an apparent barrier to downward progress in this plane posteriorly, requiring positive division with scissors or diathermy. Just in front of it, within the mesorectum, the superior rectal vessels can often be seen through the back of the mesorectal fascia, and around them cancerous nodes are likely to occur only millimeters away. This poses one of the greatest dangers of blunt manual extraction or of any haste or roughness, because the rectosacral ligament may be stronger than the surface fascia over the nodes. Thus, tearing into the lymphatic field by the inserted hand becomes a risk. Sharp dissection under direct vision is crucial. A further safety factor in positively identifying the holy plane posteriorly in front of the presacral fat pad (when present) is that one avoids the risk of tearing thin-walled presacral veins. These will never become a problem if the correct plane is followed and tearing is avoided; if veins are torn, a small pack and a considerable period of anterior dissection will provide the safest way forward.
- *Pelvic sidewall dissection:* This involves forward extension of the plane around to the sides, gently easing the adherent hypogastric nerves laterally off the mesorectal surface under direct vision (see Fig. 54-5, *A*). The freedom to lift the divided rectosigmoid forward often means that the tangentially running hypogastric nerves are first positively identified at this stage, the superior hypogastric plexus only becoming obvious proximal to the nerves after they have been dissected away from the mesorectal surface on each side. These nerves are far more important than proviously thought because they subserve many of the functions of orgasm in both sexes, whereas the inferior, more distal plexus is necessary for the more obvious parasympathetic function of erection.
- The so-called lateral ligaments are approached as the holy plane is followed downward toward the vesicles, with the expanding plexiform band of inferior hypogastric plexus outside it but increasingly adherent to it. There is no actual ligament, but there is an area of adherence between mesorectum medially and plexus laterally: small branches of nerves and vessels penetrate through, but none generally reaches more than 1 to 2 mm in diameter. The key nerves entering this flattened band are largely sympathetic hypogastric nerves curving distally from the superior plexuses and the "erigent" parasympathetic nerves coming forward to it from behind. These arise from the front of the roots of the sacral plexus (especially S3, out of sight behind the parietal sidewall fascia). This fascia is quite robust laterally, and the surgeon will note that he or she usually cannot even see the internal iliac vessels, which are outside it. Posteriorly, these "erigent pillars" from the front of the sacral plexus near its S3 root may also be invisible outside the parietal fascia, though medial to the primary branches of the internal iliac vessels.
- A little way forward, but well behind the vesicles, the erigent pillars pierce the fascia to join the plexus and often contribute nerve branches to the mesorectum and rectum. These "neural T junctions" are the nearest structures to "lateral ligaments" that the most attentive surgeon will find with precise dissection. The surgeon dissecting perfectly between the mesorectum and the inferior hypogastric plexus discovers nothing more than one or two tiny vessels that require no more than a touch of diathermy. "Coning in" compromises the oncologic quality of the block dissection, because it implies that part of the distal mesorectum is being left in the pelvis. A more distal vessel from the prostatic branch or from the pelvic floor is often found later and lower down, where it can cause troublesome bleeding. The surgeon should attempt to dissect at this point of adherence precisely between the outer aspect of the mesorectum and the triangulated neural band of nerve plexus that should be left intact. This technique is referred to as "mesorectal fat surface dissection," where no actual loose areolar tissue exists in the areas where mesorectum and plexus are adherent. The final specimen will often lack the shiny fascial covering this area.

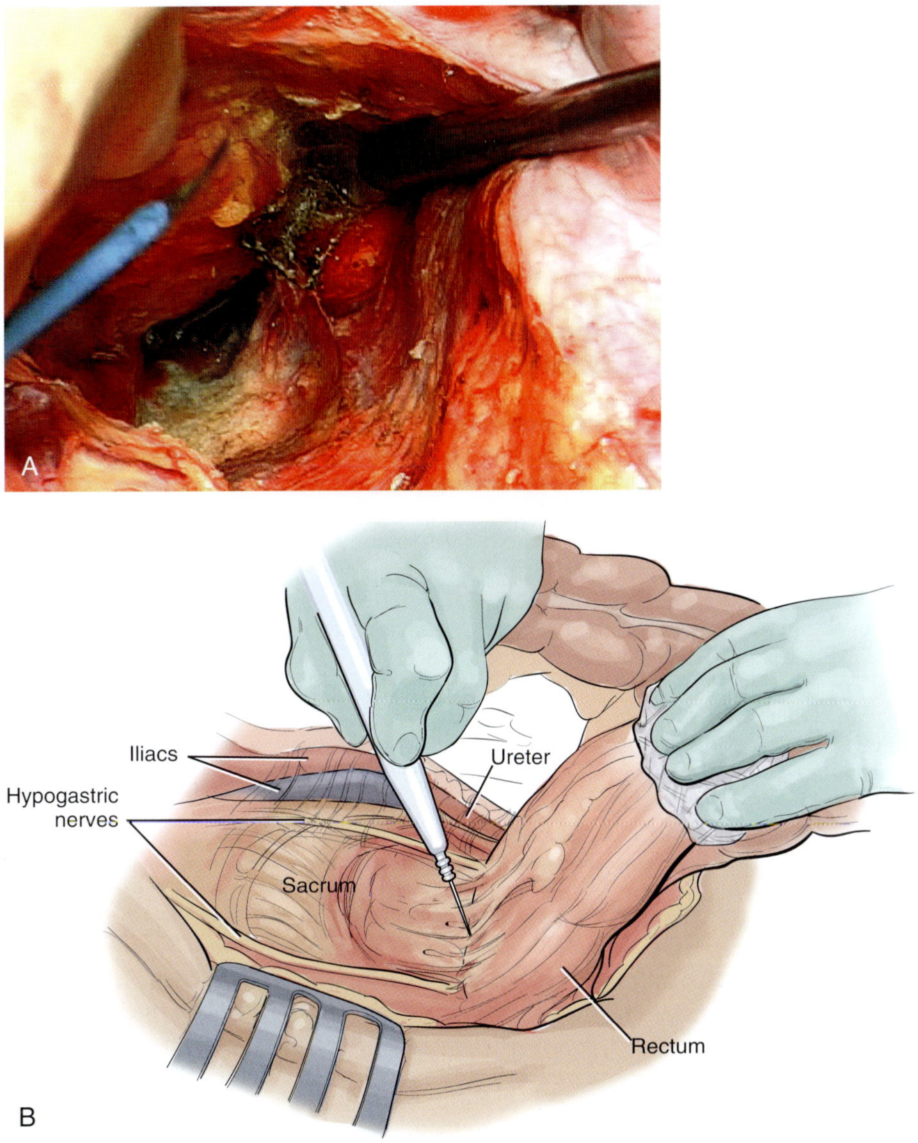

Figure 54-5.

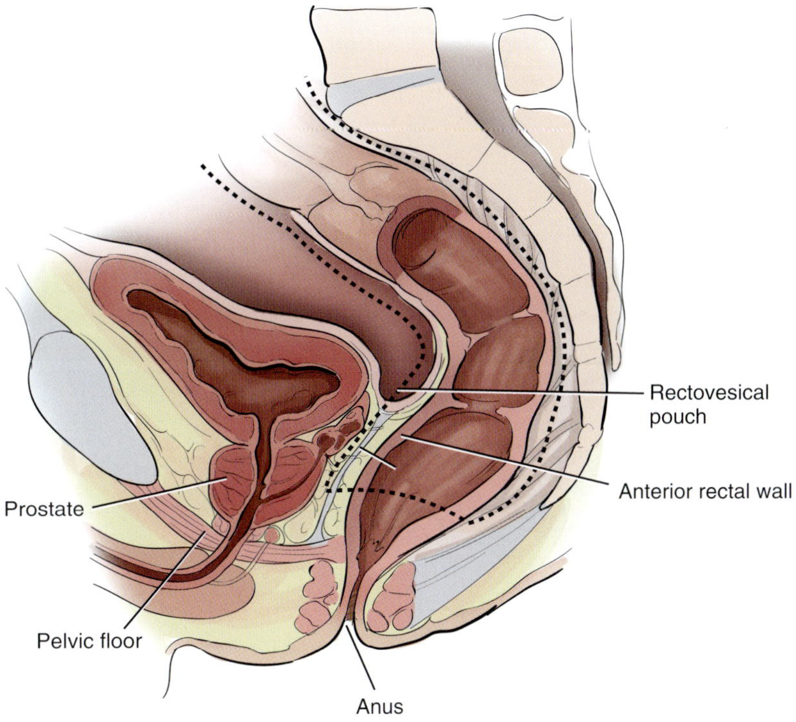

Figure 54-6.

- *The anterior dissection—Denonvilliers fascia* (Fig. 54-7): Dissection anterolaterally and anteriorly following the correct plane forward encompasses the peritoneal reflection that remains on the specimen and thus allows positive identification of the backs of the seminal vesicles. Forceful forward retraction on these with a St. Mark retractor will facilitate the development of the areolar space between the vesicles and the smooth front of the mesorectal specimen. We call this smooth surface that is generally adherent to the mesorectum the *Denonvilliers fascia* or *rectogenital septum* (see Fig. 54-7). As the surgeon works distally, there is a point where this fascia must be divided transversely as it becomes adherent to the posterior capsule of the prostate. Particular care is necessary during this step to avoid damage to the neurovascular bundles, which are converging medially.
- Hand in hand with this anterior dissection is the development of the lateral sidewall dissection. The dissection of the rectoprostatic interface is a major current challenge in technical surgery, both open and laparoscopic.
- The parasympathetic erigent nerves form posteroanterior lateral "pillars" on the pelvic sidewall. Cadaver dissections have led us to be taught that the pelvic parasympathetic outflow is tripartite S2-3-4. However, to the surgeon there is no doubt that a recognizable landmark is often a single or bifid "pillar" comprising a nerve root arising from the front of the S3 component of the main sacral plexus, which is out of sight posteriorly (Fig. 54-8). Possibly, the pillarlike appearance is in part a result of the forcible forward traction on the prostate and bladder making it difficult to visualize the structures during an open operation, and this tends to bow the nerves medially and thus make them stand out. This retraction does not occur to the same extent in a laparoscopic operation, which may account for the higher incidence of nerve damage reported from one center. These pillars and the hypogastric plexuses curve medially toward the back of the prostate, where they form the neurovascular bundles of Walsh, which taper toward the urethra at the apex of the prostate. Here they become the erectile nerves of the corpora cavernosa. The pillars or roots arise outside the parietal fascia that they penetrate obliquely at the point of adherence to the anterolateral aspect of the mesorectum. Further forward and more medially, as stated earlier, a "slice of prostate" may cause impotence.
- *Dissection of the most distal mesorectum:* The anatomy of the insertion of the mesorectal "package" into the pelvic floor becomes difficult for the surgeon to grasp because of its inaccessibility behind the vesicles and prostate and behind the vagina in the female. A clear three-dimensional perception of the now globular bilobed mesorectum in the depth of the pelvis and the surrounding neural lamella is the most elusive and challenging conceptual acquisition for the aspiring rectal cancer surgeon. Careful pursuit of the plane at this level eventually liberates the mesorectal package and leads the surgeon down to a clean muscle tube. Although crossed by a few small arteries and veins from the puborectal sling and some slips of sphincter muscle, the holy plane here becomes the intersphincteric plane, which is familiar to proctologists from a different view—a tube of red skeletal muscle outside a tube of whiter smooth muscle within.
- *Management of the anorectum distal to the cancer-stapling techniques:* In more than 90% of rectal cancers, it is technically feasible, though not necessarily optimal in terms of future function, to extend the dissection down to a clean muscle tube where a cross-clamp may be applied with a "finger and thumb" clearance beyond the lowest edge of the cancer. This is a difficult and challenging moment, requiring

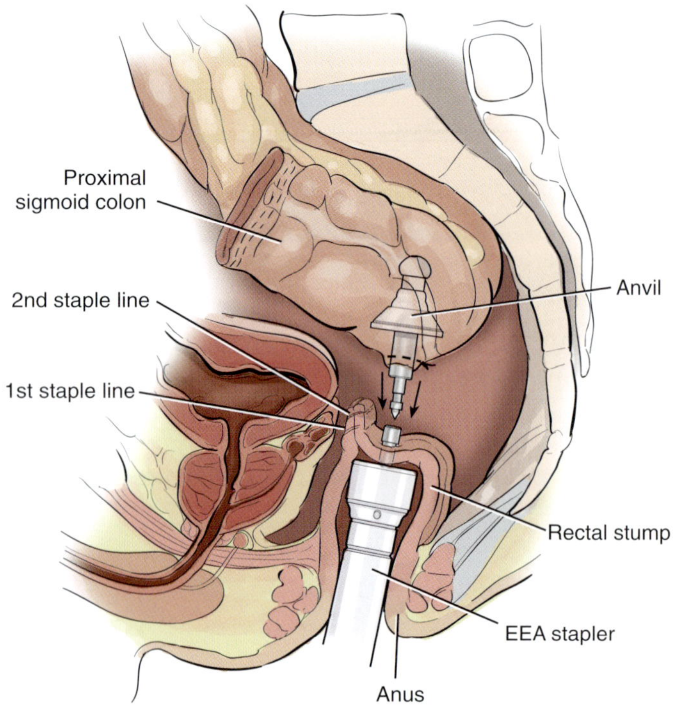

Figure 54-7.

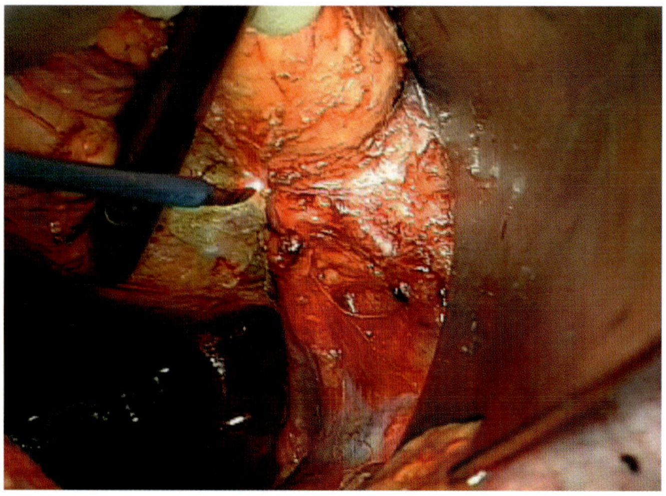

Figure 54-8.

both skill and experience. We have developed a preference for the use of the long linear stapler in place of the 90-degree clamp (the Moran triple stapling technique: see Fig. 54-9, *A* and *B*). The first TA-45, TA-30, or PI-30 (Tyco Healthcare, Norwalk, Conn.) staple line seals the muscle tube so that the anorectal lumen beyond can be washed out with water as a tumoricidal solution. The risk of incorporating viable exfoliated intraluminal cells in the second staple line is thus eliminated, and the second TA-45 or TA-30 is fired through the washed bowel while the anatomy is distorted by upward traction on the first (specimen-sealing) stapler. This process, in our view, justifies the cost of a second stapler because of the greater security against spillage of potentially malignant bowel contents. Only this washed staple line remains within the patient.

- The first of these two linear staple lines should be safely clear of the palpable distal edge of the cancer. This is usually, though not invariably, the microscopic edge. Downward spread along the muscle tube is not a significant factor in recurrence—a 2-cm clearance is more than adequate, and 1 cm plus the "doughnut" is acceptable.
- *The colon pouch—coloplasty or side-to-end?* Several variations of pouch construction are available. Typically, a GIA-60 is inserted 5 cm from the end of the fully mobilized colon to create a J-pouch. The anvil of the CEEA-31 staple anvil is inserted into the same colotomy, which is "purse stringed" around the shaft with size 00 Surgipro. The body of the circular stapler, usually the CEEA-31, is inserted from below transanally (Fig. 54-10). It is essential with ultralow anastomoses to be certain that only the internal sphincter is "purse stringed" into the instrument. Thus it must be confirmed that only one

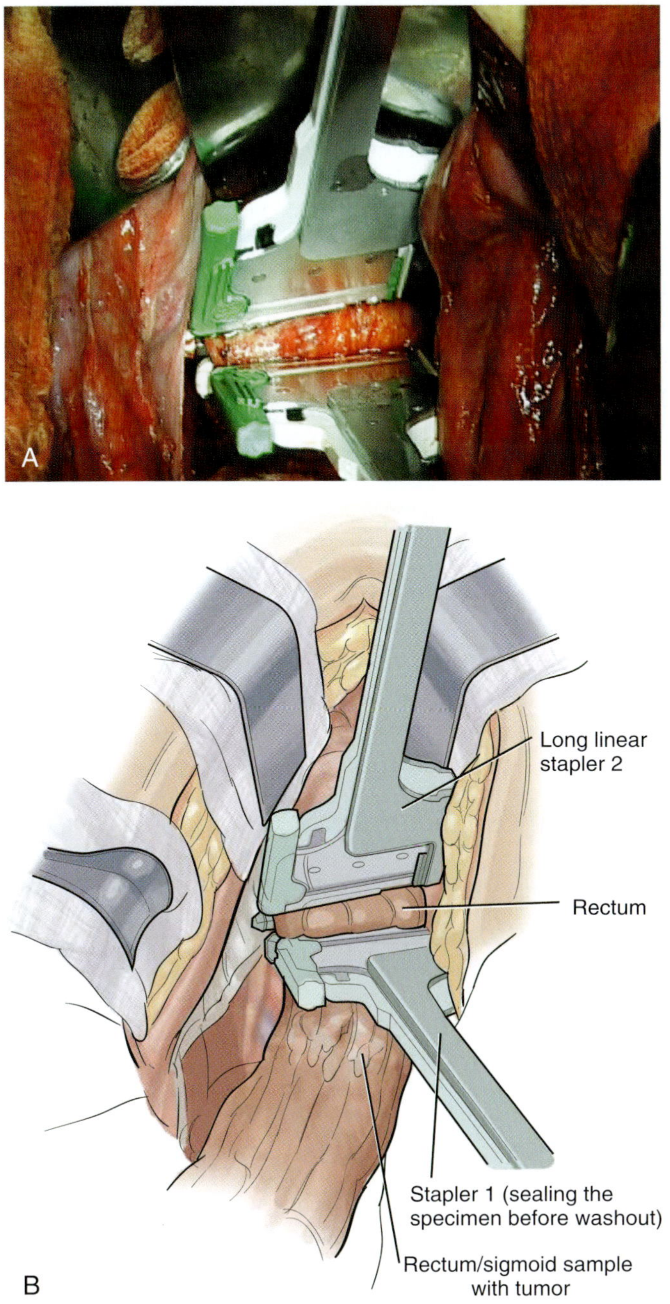

Figure 54-9.

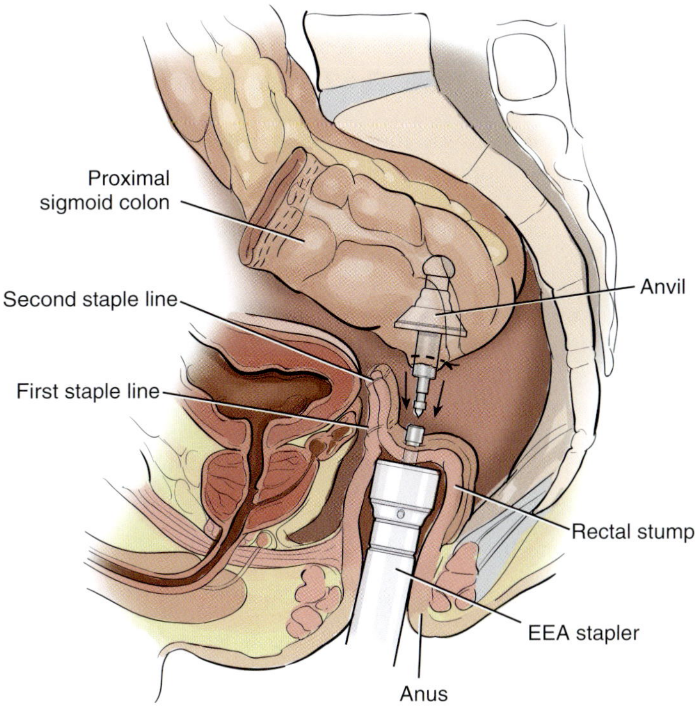

Figure 54-10. *EEA*, End-to-end anastomosis.

thickness of muscle can be felt around the periphery of the cartridge. Adequate length from the splenic flexure mobilization is essential for the pouch to lie without tension in the hollow of the sacrum, and a demonstrably pulsatile blood supply is the essence of success.

Closure

- The midline incision is closed by approximating the linea alba with 1-0 monofilament suture. Skin is approximated with staples.
- Two low-suction Abdovac drains are used for 48 hours, unless there is copious drainage, in which case they may need to be left intact longer. The objective is to avoid hematoma in the hollow of the sacrum, which can become infected, form an abscess, and point into the bowel at or near the anastomosis—thus creating a "late leak" around 10 to 20 days later.

III. ALTERNATIVE TECHNICAL APPROACHES (PRO/CON) AND PEARLS

Technical Pearls

- Four great principles apply throughout:
  - Precise dissection under direct vision—never "blind"
  - Traction and countertraction to open the holy plane
  - Circumferential dissection: first here, then there, never for too long on one area
  - Gentle surface protection with gauze swabs to avoid tearing

Partial Mesorectal Excision (High Anterior Resection and Mesorectal Transection)

- Below which level, or at what height of tumor above the anal verge, does TME become necessary? Height measurement, by general agreement, is the distance from the anal verge in the conscious patient using a rigid sigmoidoscope. It has long been convention and, a very sound rule, borrowed from German surgical practice, that a minimum of 5 cm of mesentery should always be excised both proximal and distal to any colorectal cancer. Although muscle tube margin may safely be reduced to 1 cm in the interest of anal conservation, we have always believed that, if less than a TME is contemplated, a minimum of 5 cm of mesorectum distal to the lower edge of the cancer must be dissected in the perimesorectal plane. If, therefore, after initial mobilization there is a clear 5 cm of mesorectum, then tapering into the mesentery, in the interest of making a more minor operation and a higher anastomosis, becomes acceptable.
- The operation then becomes perimesorectal mobilization, mesorectal transection, anterior resection, and primary anastomosis for rectal cancers, generally those above 12 cm. Either 5 cm of mesorectum distal to the tumor or the whole mesorectum must be removed intact, with the same preoccupation with clear circumferential margins.

TME Plus: The Levators, Ischiorectal Fossa, and Perianal Skin

- Recently much energy has been focused on methods of improving the abdominoperineal operation. Applying the principles of histopathologic audit, Quirke has drawn attention to the unacceptable frequency (in Britain and Scandinavia at any rate) of margin involvement by cancer, and many authors have drawn attention to poorer results than after anterior resection. Several principles for improvement have been highlighted.
- Extra care should be taken to perform the perimesorectal dissection that is inherent in TME—at least as far distally as the origin of the levator muscles from the obturator internus muscles (midpelvis). A disk of levators should be incorporated, therefore avoiding the lowermost holy plane dissection (i.e., dissection in the lowest part of the plane where it is in contact with the levators). In this way a more cylindrical and wider clearance may be achieved and the commonly observed "waist" on the specimen avoided. Ideally an intact "levator-wrap" covers the most vulnerable part of the specimen—the point of insertion on the anorectal muscle tube into the skeletal puborectal sling.

The Prone Jackknife Position for the Perineal Dissection

- The views into the pelvis from below are considered by many surgeons to be superior to those in the conventional steep Trendelenburg position. In particular, spectacular access is provided if the coccyx is excised with the cancer. In some cases even the lowest part of the sacrum may be excised with the coccyx. A line between the two palpable notches avoids the sacroiliac joints and the important nerve roots.

Starting the Operation from Below

- Although the approach is not widely accepted, there are some advantages in commencing the operation from below with the patient in the prone jackknife position. This is particularly true if there are likely to be major problems with the abdominal surgery—as, for example, when performing APE for a local recurrence after AR.

The Posterior Vaginal Wall

- Bimanual examination via the rectum and the vagina in the anesthetized patient is essential. If there is free mobility of the cancer on the posterior vaginal wall, then it need *not* be excised. If the cancer is tethered over a small area, a disk of vagina may be taken with the tumor, or in a case that requires APE, because of proximity to the sphincters, all or most of the posterior wall from the perianal skin upward may need to be removed. We now perform this once-standard procedure only when there appears no alternative because of the anterior extension of the cancer, as ultimate vaginal function may be much impaired. When it does have to be excised, it is not essential for the vagina to be resutured, though its long-term function must be in some doubt.

Other Organs Occasionally Requiring en Bloc Removal on Account of Direct Invasion

- Seminal vesicles
- One or both ureters
- Ileum
- The folded-over sigmoid
- One or both hypogastric plexuses
- Parts of the neural lamella
- Appendix
- Uterus, ovaries, and adnexal structures
- Bladder wall

IV. SPECIAL POSTOPERATIVE CARE

- Essentially the lower anterior resection operation is managed similarly to any other major gastrointestinal abdominal operation.
- The special risks specific to the anastomosis below about 6 cm from the anal verge is anastomotic leakage. Rullier (1998) has shown that risks of such leakage are 6 to 8 times higher when the anastomosis is situated below 6 cm from the anal verge. For this reason, most patients undergoing TME for middle or low rectal cancer who have had an anastomosis tend to receive a prophylactic defunctioning stoma.
- The most commonly chosen stoma is a loop ileostomy, although the authors see some advantages in using the rather old-fashioned loop right transverse colostomy. These advantages include the fact that the stoma is in the supracolic compartment and has much less colon intervening between it and the anastomosis.
- Although full bowel preparation is still recommended for rectal cancer operations, there is always a risk of residual stool within the colon, and this "backlog" will be less with a right transverse colostomy. The risk of colonic peristalsis leading to a significant fecal leak through an anastomotic weakness will be correspondingly less.
- Furthermore, the right transverse colostomy, being in the supracolic compartment drawn through the omentum, will have virtually no long-term risk of adhesions.
- Nevertheless, most authorities prefer the ease of the loop ileostomy. Provided the anastomosis is thus protected, the management of the patient is in virtually no way different from that for any major abdominal surgery.
- One or two low-tension suction drains are usually inserted into the pelvis to remove any potential hematoma, and these are generally removed at 48 hours unless there is prolonged drainage that may demand their presence for a longer period.

SUGGESTED READINGS

Holm T, Ljung A, Hèggmark T, et al: Extended abdominoperineal resection with gluteus maximus flap reconstruction of the pelvic floor for rectal cancer, *Br J Surg* 94:232–238, 2007.

MERCURY Study Group: Diagnostic accuracy of preoperative magnetic resonance imaging in predicting curative resection of rectal cancer: prospective observational study, *BMJ* 333:779, 2006.

Quirke P: Training and quality assurance for rectal cancer: 20 years of data is enough, *Lancet Oncol* 4:695–702, 2003.

CHAPTER 55

Laparoscopic Abdominoperineal Resection of the Rectum

K. Thomas Moesta, MD, PhD, and Ferdinand Köckerling, MD, PhD

I. SPECIAL PREOPERATIVE PREPARATION

- Digital examination, rigid rectoscopy, and eventually endosonography establish the need for abdominoperineal excision in rectal cancer, in accordance with national or local guidelines and policies.
- Appropriate imaging studies should have carefully ruled out liver metastases, because no manual exploration of the liver is possible by the laparoscopic approach.
- The lateral margins in cancers of the lower third of the rectum are best described by magnetic resonance imaging (MRI) and endorectal ultrasound. Any infiltration of the levator muscles should be documented and accounted for in surgical planning. Large cancers extending from the mid to lower third of the rectum are poor candidates for the laparoscopic approach.
- In male patients, infiltration of the prostate should be ruled out preoperatively by MRI, endo-MRI, or endosonography.
- In female patients, gynecologic evaluation should be carried out in tumors located within the ventral circumference of the rectum. Although a small excision of the dorsal wall of the vagina is no obstacle to the laparoscopic technique, more extended vaginoplastic procedures may require an open access through the abdomen.
- No bowel preparation is required for abdominoperineal excisions.
- The terminal colostomy position should be identified and labeled preoperatively in upright and standing positions by a stoma nurse or by the surgeon.

II. OPERATIVE TECHNIQUE

Position

- Patients are positioned in an overextended supine lithotomy position. For the perineal part of the procedure, repositioning with elevated legs is required. Both positions should be tested before sterile draping.
- Shoulder and pelvis supports can be used to safely realize extreme table positions. However, compression injuries have been reported as a consequence of such restraints. With growing surgical experience in the field, extreme positions become unnecessary. In our practice, additional patient supports are not used.
- Special care is required to protect the patient's legs. Extensive cushioning of the calves will protect the peroneal nerves from direct pressure even if several table repositionings are required. Furthermore, a prolonged Trendelenburg position may lead to inadequate arterial perfusion and eventually to an ischemia-induced compartment syndrome. This rare but sometimes severe complication can be avoided by a low position of the leg restraints, almost overextending the hip, and, of course, by avoiding very

prolonged and extreme Trendelenburg positions. If the perineal part of the excision takes more than 1 hour, measures should be taken to prevent ischemic damage to the elevated limbs.
- The right arm is positioned alongside the body to allow surgeon and camera operator to stand at the right side of the patient. The assistant stands at the left side of the patient.

Trocar Placement

- A four-trocar technique is used (Fig. 55-1).
- The camera trocar is inserted above and to the right of the umbilicus using an open access technique. All other trocars are placed after transillumination and under direct visualization, all lateral to the epigastric vessels.
- The further three trocars are positioned as follows: one in the left and two in the right lower abdomen. The trocars, including the camera trocar, form a rough semicircle open to the pelvis. The lower right trocar is later used to introduce the linear stapling device and thus should be appropriately sized (usually 12 or 13 mm). The left trocar should be centered within the predefined terminal colostomy position. All other trocars can be 5 mm in diameter.

Main Dissection

- Laparoscopic rectal surgery should be restricted to surgeons already experienced in laparoscopic colonic resections. Of course, those surgeons will continue to use their preferred approach to trocar positioning and mobilization of the sigmoid. In contrast to sigmoid or rectosigmoid resections, however, mobilization of the splenic flexure is usually not necessary. Here, for the sake of clarity, we describe our preferred variant.
- The first step of every procedure is an abdominal exploration to exclude secondary malignancies and hepatic or peritoneal metastases.
- The pelvis is exposed by retracting the small bowel toward the right upper abdomen, with the patient in Trendelenburg position with right inclination.
- The female pelvis is exposed by elevating the uterus and fallopian tubes to the anterior abdominal wall by a transcutaneous suture (straight needle).
- The sigmoid colon is mobilized starting laterally. The Gerota fascia is identified, and the preparation is continued until the left ureter has been safely identified down to the common iliac vessels (Fig. 55-2).

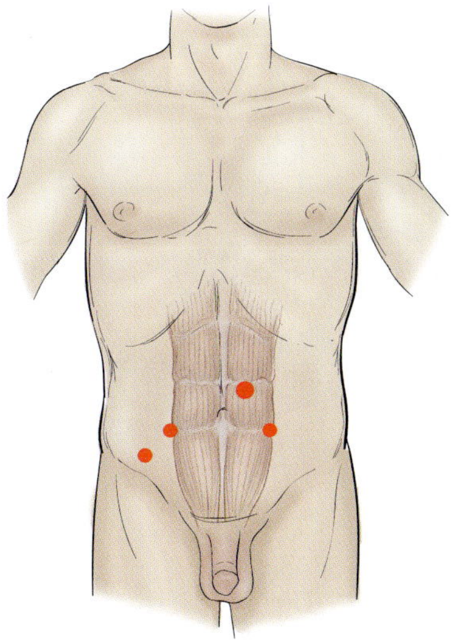

Figure 55-1.

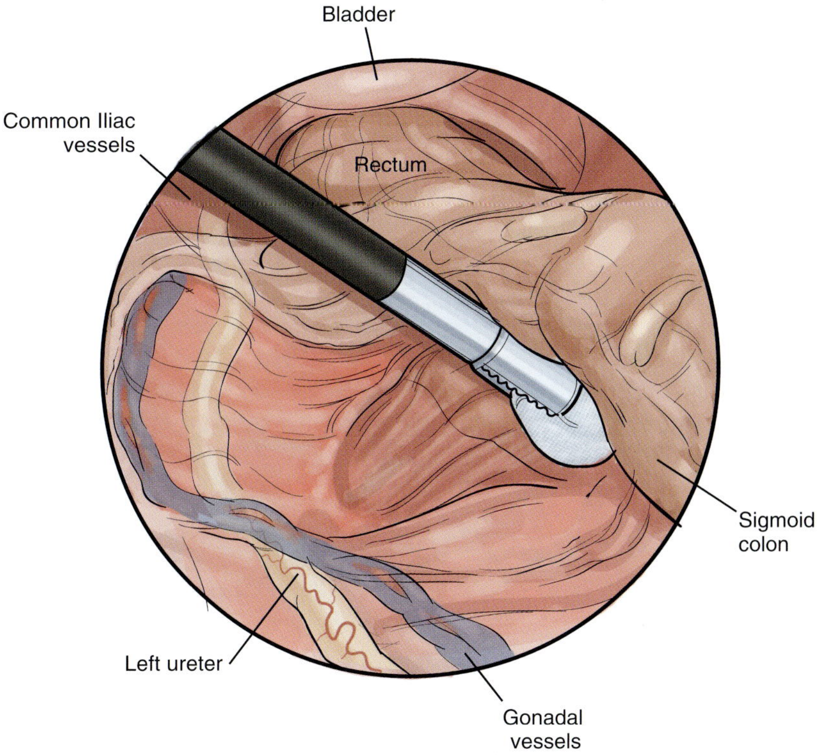

Figure 55-2.

- The peritoneum at the pelvic inlet is opened (Fig. 55-3). To ascertain the correct access to the retro rectal cleavage plane between the mesorectal and the pelvic fascia containing the hypogastric nerves, the assistant and the surgeon must take care to fully elongate and elevate the rectum with graspers. Slightly below the promontory, the avascular zone between visceral and parietal peritoneum is easily identified. This part of the preparation can be performed by electrocautery or ultrasonic dissection devices.
- The opening of the retrorectal cleavage plane is performed predominantly by blunt dissection using swabs or by blunt ultrasonic dissection. Extensive electrocautery should be avoided to safely preserve the autonomic innervation of the pelvic organs.
- The rectal mobilization dorsally should be conducted downward to the pelvic floor (Fig. 55-4). Strictly following the mesorectal fascia from back to front, the lateral sympathetic nerves, the hypogastric nerves, and especially the hypogastric plexus should be carefully preserved. We prefer ultrasonic dissection devices, most of the time in the form of blunt dissection with closed jaws.

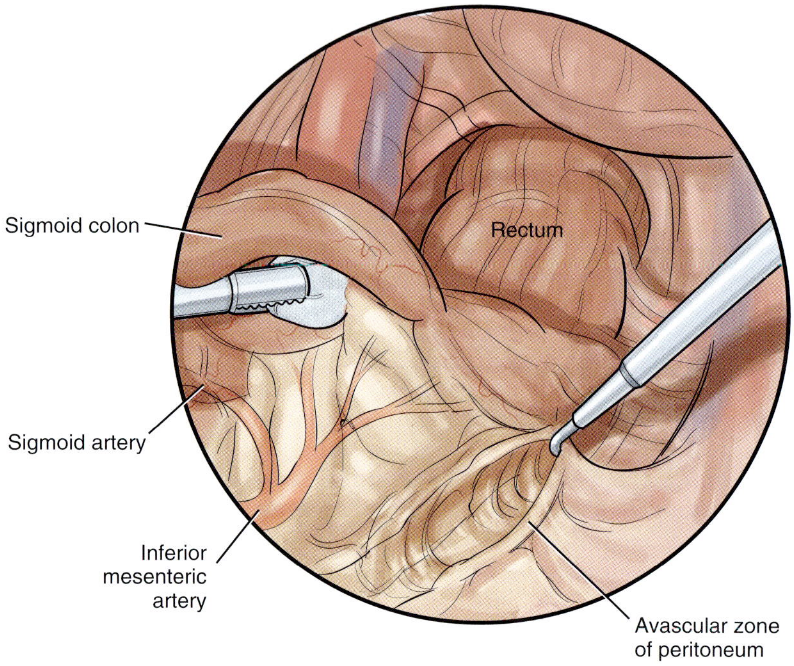

Figure 55-3.

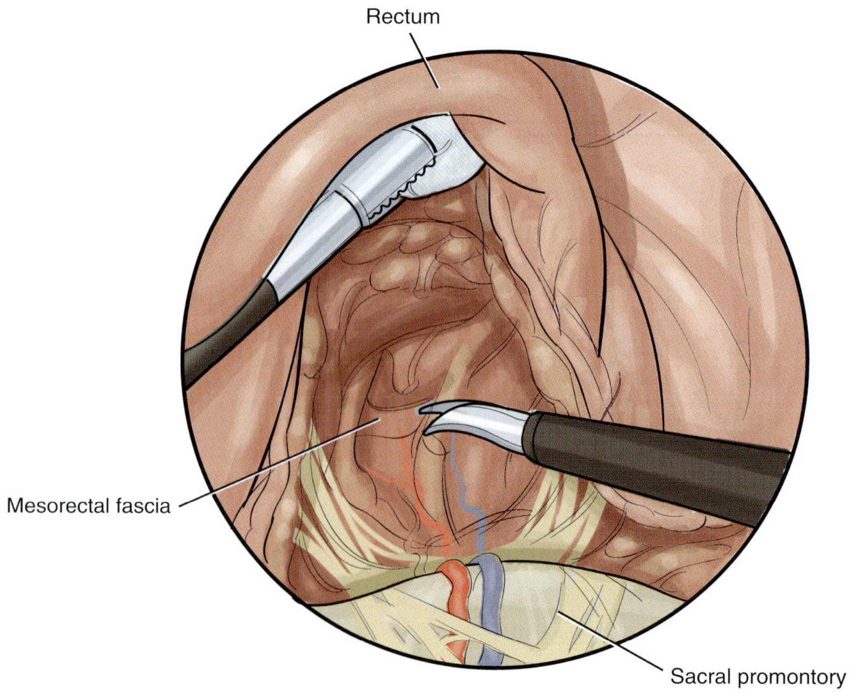

Figure 55-4.

- When the close connection between the mesorectum and hypogastric plexus is resolved, the rectum can be straightened considerably, allowing more space for all further dissection. Only then should anterior dissection be started (Fig. 55-5).
- Mesorectal dissection for tumors of the lower part of the rectum should always take into account the individual tumor position. In the presence of a regionally advanced tumor, proper soft tissue coverage of the lateral tumor borders can be ascertained only if the mesorectal dissection is not continued downward to the fat-free zone of the rectum. Instead, the pelvic insertions of the levator muscles are identified early, and the mesorectal dissection is stopped at this level. Using hemostatic devices such as an ultrasonic scalpel, the levator muscles can be divided at this point, greatly facilitating orientation for the perineal part of the operation.
- Only in uT1 or very early uT2 cancers is a more central division of the levator muscles permissible, enabling a more stable perineal wound closure.
- Anterior dissection in men is performed downward to below the prostate, even in the presence of anteriorly located cancers, as the laparoscopic view is usually better than the exposure from the perineum.
- Anterior dissection in women can be easier from the perineal approach, sometimes necessitating a pull-through of the specimen before the completion of the anterior dissection.
- After rectal mobilization, the presacral plane is followed proximally to expose the inferior mesenteric artery (IMA). Again, blunt dissection is used to carefully preserve the retroperitoneal nerves, which form the superior hypogastric plexus around the origin of the IMA.
- The IMA is isolated and divided 2 cm distal from its aortal origin. Again, care must be taken not to pull up the retroperitoneal layer (tent form) when isolating the vessel. For safe transection of the IMA, stable, bioresorbable clips are preferred. Alternatively, a vascular stapler may be applied. Electrocautery-based vessel sealing devices are also used; however, rare bleeding events have been reported after the use of this technique.

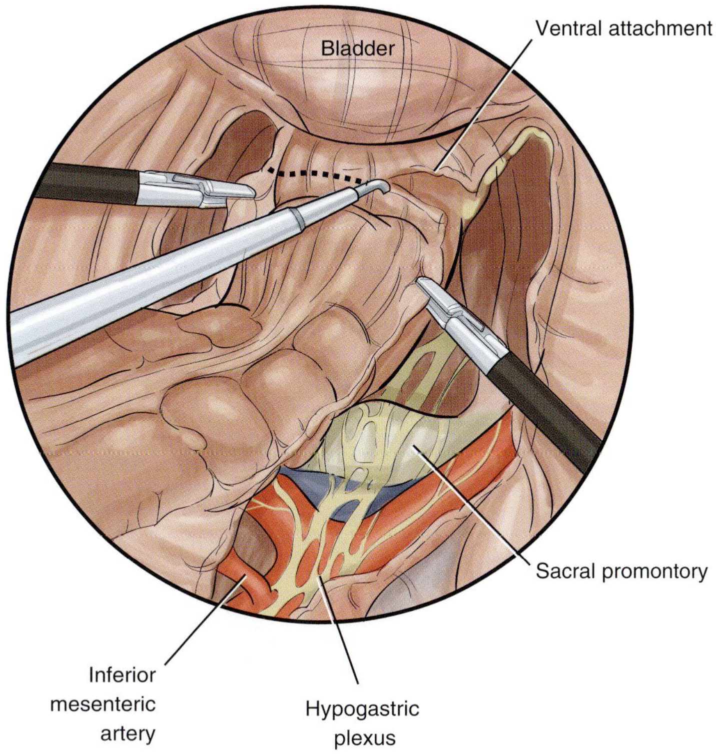

Figure 55-5.

- The colon is now divided at the descendosigmoidal junction using a linear stapling device (Fig. 55-6). The mesentery is dissected using hemostatic devices and or clips.
- The laparoscopic phase of the procedure is concluded by the creation of the terminal colostomy at the predefined position. With the distal end of the mobilized descending colon securely grasped by a forceps, a circular skin incision around the left-sided trocar is performed. With a nonmetallic instrument in place and the trocar retracted, the channel is easily enlarged on the fascial and muscular layers. The pneumoperitoneum is terminated, and the colon is pulled out to the colostomy site. Because of the potential contamination of the surgical field, the stoma is opened and formed only at the end of the procedure, with the colon held in place by soft graspers.
- The perineal phase is quite similar to the conventional procedure. Following perineal circumcision of the anus, the perianal fat is widely excised and the levator muscles are exposed (Fig. 55-7). Optimally this level is already partially transected from above, enabling proper orientation. Otherwise, the anococcygeal ligament may be divided first to gain access to the perineal cavity. A short reinstitution of the pneumoperitoneum can help to guide the dissection at this point. In all locally advanced tumor stages, the levator muscles should be resected at their lateral origin.
- In women, the anterior dissection can be facilitated by pulling the specimen out before completion of the anterior dissection.
- The perineal wound closure, if the levator muscles were excised, will join only the subcutaneous and the skin layer (Fig. 55-8). In those cases, additional omentoplasty should be performed.

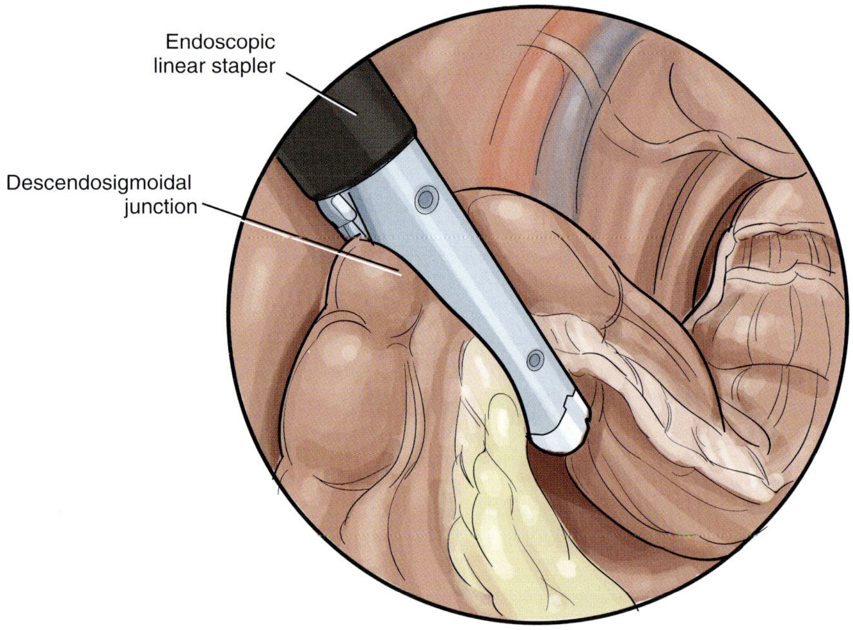

Figure 55-6.

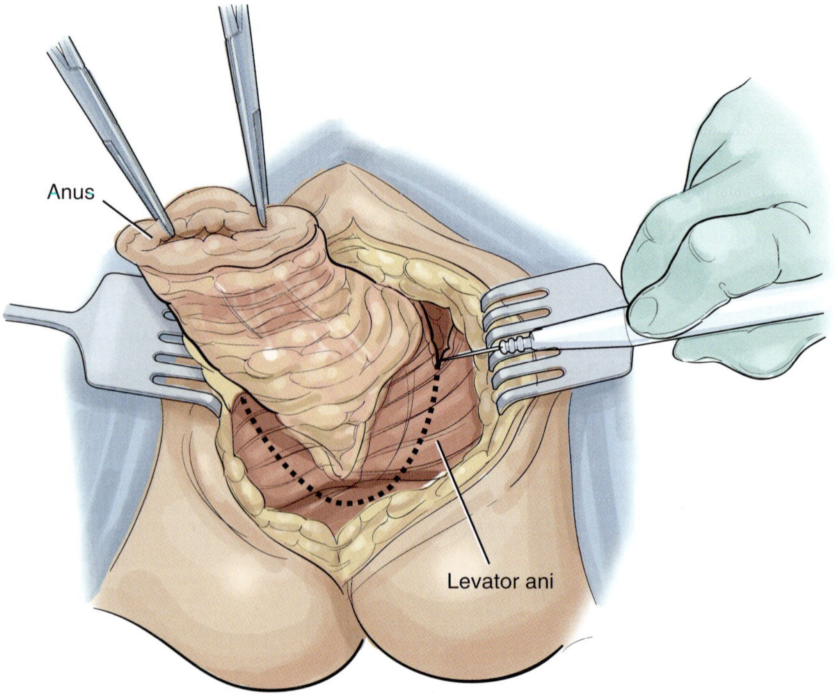

Figure 55-7.

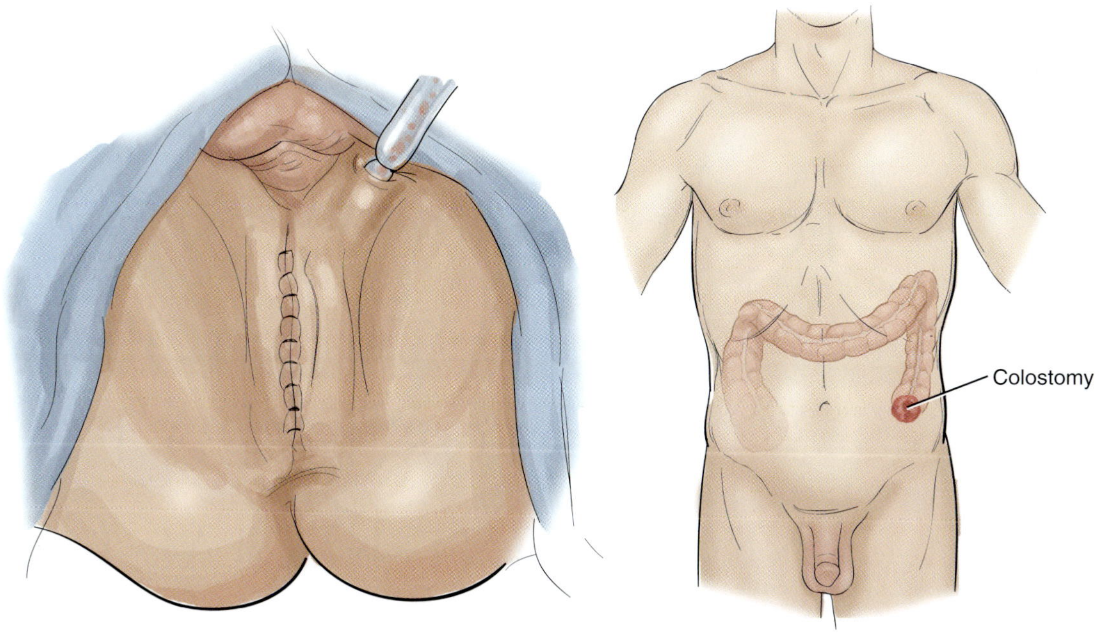

Figure 55-8.

III. ALTERNATIVE TECHNICAL APPROACHES (PRO/CON) AND PEARLS

Alternative Approaches

- Conventional abdominoperineal rectal resection should be considered in all advanced cases and in those with contraindications for the laparoscopic approach
- Depending on tumor stage and distance from the anocutaneous line, ultradeep intersphincteric resections can also be considered. Under favorable circumstances, these, too, are performed laparoscopically.

Pearls

- When beginning the dissection at the level of the sacral promontory, it is important to stay in the middle to identify the V shape created by the left and right pelvic nerves, which can be easily transected if the presacral dissection is begun without appropriate attention to the nerves. Often, following chemoradiation, these nerves are closely adherent to the rectal fascia proper. More distally, dissection needs to remain medial to the nerves to spare the pelvic ganglion at the lateral pelvic sidewall.
- For those inexperienced with laparoscopic rectal resection, or in cases in which bulky tumors have been treated with preoperative chemoradiation, it is often valuable to place ureteric stents.
- During the perineal dissection, to avoid injury to the urethra in men, it is important to identify the transverse perineal muscle and then stay dorsal to this muscle. The abdominal surgeon then directs the dissection from above while ensuring that the perineal surgeon stays dorsal to the level of the prostate gland.

IV. SPECIAL POSTOPERATIVE CARE

- Postoperative recovery is generally faster than that following an open procedure. No special measures are required; typically there is a rapid return to oral diet.

SUGGESTED READINGS

Ng SS, Leung KL, Lee JF, et al: Laparoscopic-assisted versus open abdominoperineal resection for low rectal cancer: a prospective randomized trial, *Ann Surg Oncol* 15:2418–2425, 2008.

Scheidbach H, Rose J, Huegel O, et al: Results of laparoscopic treatment of rectal cancer: analysis of 520 patients, *Tech Coloproctol* 8:s22–s24.

Scheidbach H, Schneider C, Konradt J, et al: Laparoscopic abdominoperineal resection and anterior resection with curative intent for carcinoma of the rectum, *Surg Endosc* 16:7–13, 2002.

CHAPTER 56

Total Pelvic Exenteration with Distal Sacrectomy for Fixed Locally Recurrent Rectal Cancer

Yoshihiro Moriya, MD, and Keisuke Uehara, MD

- By cause and growth pattern, locally recurrent rectal cancer is classified into three main categories: anastomotic and perianastomotic recurrence, perineal recurrence, and pelvic recurrence (Fig. 56-1, *A*, *B*, and *C*). By occupied site, pelvic recurrence is subdivided into anterior, lateral, and dorsal recurrences. For resecting the anterior pelvic recurrent tumor, the basic surgical procedure is total pelvic exenteration. In women, if there is no obvious bladder invasion, it is possible to preserve the urinary organs. Lateral pelvic recurrence occurs because of lateral lymph node metastasis after total mesorectal excision or insufficient dissection of lateral tumor margin. It begins to infiltrate the pelvic sidewall in its early stage. Dorsal pelvic recurrence is presacral extramural recurrence after abdominoperineal resection or low anterior resection that invades the pelvic wall. It also forms a fixed recurrent tumor from its early stage. The cause of this recurrence may be extramesenteric lymphatic spread, insufficient resection of the mesorectum, or a cut into the mesorectum during the initial operation. This pattern of recurrence is common.
- Once the diagnosis of locally recurrent rectal cancer is made, detailed studies should be conducted in terms of surgical indication from two aspects: (1) whether distant metastasis is present and (2) to what extent the tumor spreads within the pelvis. Extrapelvic disease is searched for by whole-body computed tomography (CT) scan. Magnetic resonance imaging (MRI) and fluorodeoxyglucose positron emission tomography (PET)-CT are also useful in detecting extrapelvic disease and distinguishing between recurrent disease and scar tissue. CT, MRI, and fluorodeoxyglucose PET-CT are useful in distinguishing between solitary and multifocal recurrences in the pelvis and between anterior organ involvement and dorsolateral pelvic wall involvement.
- Using pelvic CT, MRI, and/or PET-CT, the spread of recurrent tumor should be examined accurately (see Fig. 56-1, *A*, *B*, and *C*). For differential diagnosis between scar tissue and recurrent tumors, application of the following modalities is considered: (1) comparative evaluation of the results of a baseline CT performed within 6 months postoperatively with those of a pelvic CT performed over time, (2) MRI using gadolinium contrast material, and (3) functional imaging with PET-CT. However, it is not easy to diagnose recurrent tumors after radiation therapy. In such cases, CT-guided biopsy is performed to confirm recurrent tumors histologically.

I. SPECIAL PREOPERATIVE PREPARATION

- *Explanation for surgical procedures:* A patient should be well informed by the physician about procedures, invasiveness (expected operative time and blood loss), possible intraoperative incidents, postoperative complications and prognosis, and the fact that colostomy and urostomy will be made and consequently the patient must spend the rest of his or her life with double stomas, with loss of urination, defecation, and sexual functions after the operation. Surgeons do not persuade their patients to have this kind of major operation; they perform this operation only for those patients who understand the explanations just described and are willing to overcome their recurrent tumors. Patients and their families should understand this thoroughly.

- Site marking for stomas is performed in accordance with the criteria for stoma site marking established by the Cleveland Clinic. The site (1) should be via the rectus abdominis muscle route; (2) should be located below the umbilicus and at the top of the abdominal wall radius—in other words, in an area that the patient can check visually and easily manage the stoma; and (3) should not include bones such as the ilium or areas with wrinkles, scars, and/or wounds. The marking is performed by an enterostomal therapist.
- To prevent bacterial contamination during surgery, the entire contents of the intestine are removed preoperatively with purgatives and/or enema.
- Generally, this operation takes about 10 hours because quite a number of intraoperative procedures for freeing, ligation, anastomosis, hemostasis, and so forth are required to complete it successfully. It is necessary to perform each procedure accurately and carefully in accordance with basic technique. During management of the dorsal vein complex or internal iliac vessels and/or transection of the sacrum, a technical error can cause cumbersome bleeding. Furthermore, complications associated with urinary diversion should be avoided. If surgeons perform each procedure with appropriate surgical techniques, it is rare that severe complications occur during or after the operation.

II. OPERATIVE TECHNIQUE

- Total pelvic exenteration with distal sacrectomy (TPES) for primary pelvic malignancy is performed by first dividing loose connective tissues, such as the Retzius, obturator, and retrorectal spaces, and then dissecting along the parietal pelvic fascia. In recurrent cancer cases, however, those spaces disappear and are replaced by dense scar tissue, especially after radiotherapy (Fig. 56-2, *A* and *B*). Because of

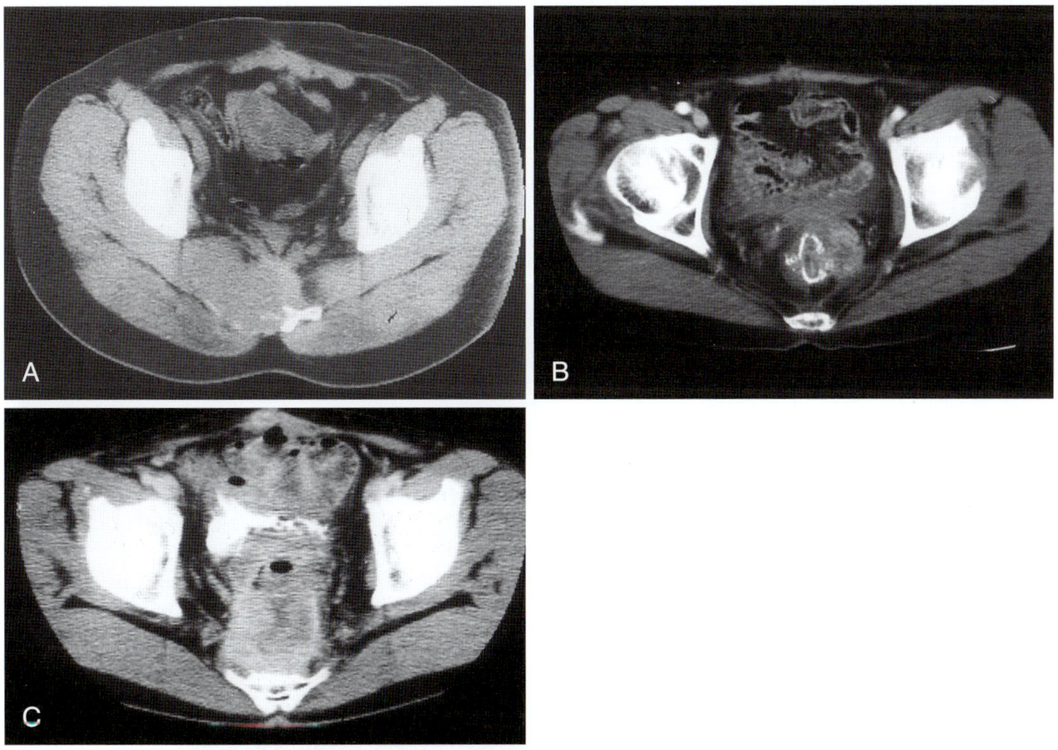

Figure 56-1.

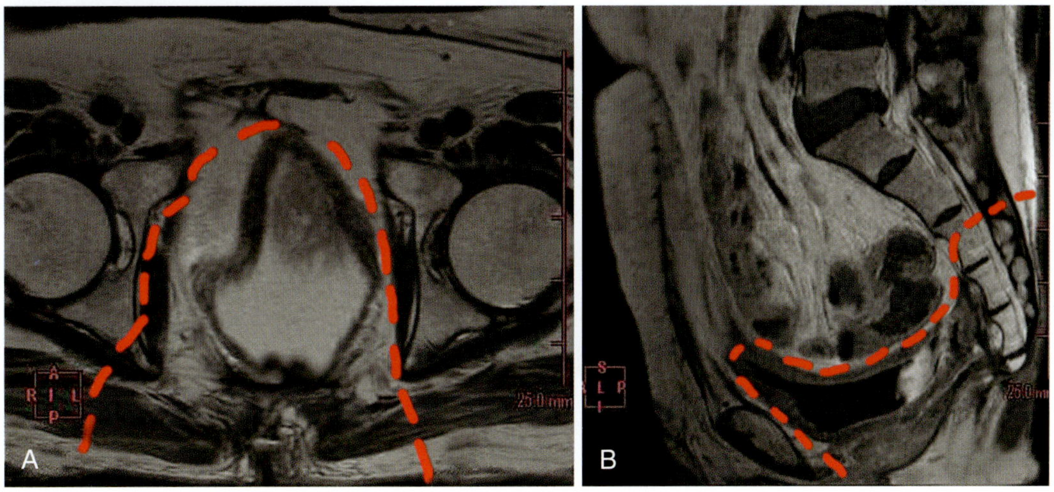

Figure 56-2.

this condition, TPES for fixed recurrent tumor is a challenging procedure. The operation is performed in the following order: abdominal, perineal, sacral, and second abdominal phase.

ABDOMINAL PHASE

Position

- The patient is placed in the lithotomy position using Levitator stirrups (Fig. 56-3). An intermittent massage apparatus is applied to the lower extremities to prevent deep vein thrombosis. The final confirmation of the extent of tumor in the pelvis including the perineum is conducted using a rectal digital examination. For female patients, vaginal examination is also conducted before vaginal irrigation. The patients is disinfected completely with povidone-iodine, including the area from the breast line to the middle of thigh, the lateral side area including posterior axillary line, and the perineal area including skin behind the coccygeus.

Incision

- A wide median incision is applied from the pubic bone to the xiphoid process.

Main Dissection

- After detaching adhesions caused by the initial surgery, the surgeon confirms the localization of the recurrent tumor within the pelvis and the absence of extrapelvic diseases such as hepatic metastasis, peritoneal deposits, and paraaortic lymph node metastasis. The surgeon then makes the final decision to proceed to TPES.
- First, the Retzius space is opened. The endopelvic fascia and puboprostatic ligaments can be identified bilaterally and divided using electrocautery to expose the levator ani muscle (Fig. 56-4). The dorsal vein complex together with the divided endopelvic fascia is bunched with the special forceps and doubly tied and divided.
- Next, the level of sacral amputation is determined. The anterior area from the aortic bifurcation to the sacral promontory is exposed to enter the anterior surface of the sacrum. The dissection is made using electrocautery downward to the distal sacrum, at which point sacral amputation is planned, while cutting off the thickened Waldeyer fascia with the presacral venous plexuses and scar tissue. During this process, some bleeding from the sacral vein complex occurs; however, hemostasis can be obtained using a combination of electrocautery and gauze packs. To minimize blood loss, the dissection layer is kept in the sacral periosteum. Entering into a shallower layer than the sacral periosteum can increase the chance of bleeding from the venous plexus.
- The next step is resection of the internal iliac vessels (Fig. 56-5). The area from the common iliac vessels (artery and vein) to the bifurcation between the internal and external iliac vessels is exposed. The internal iliac vessels are manipulated as follows. First the trunk of the internal iliac artery is doubly tied and divided at the distal portion after branching the superior gluteal artery. Second, several branches of the sacral nerve plexus that perforate the pelvic wall via crevices are divided. Finally, the trunk of the internal iliac vein is doubly tied and divided. Blood loss during TPES usually occurs from the venous plexus. Taking the appropriate steps to avoid congestion of the venous plexus at the earliest possible opportunity allows the operation to be performed with minimal blood loss from the venous

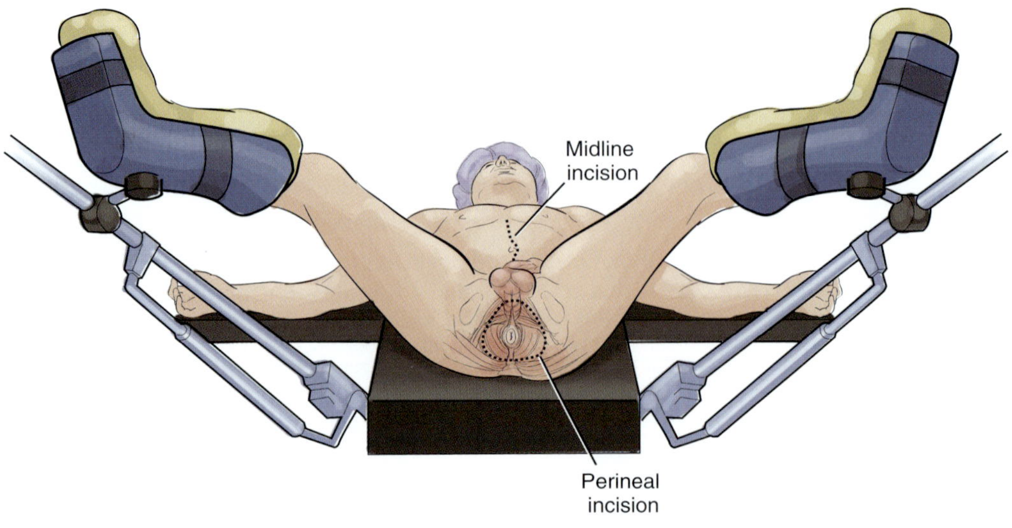

Figure 56-3.

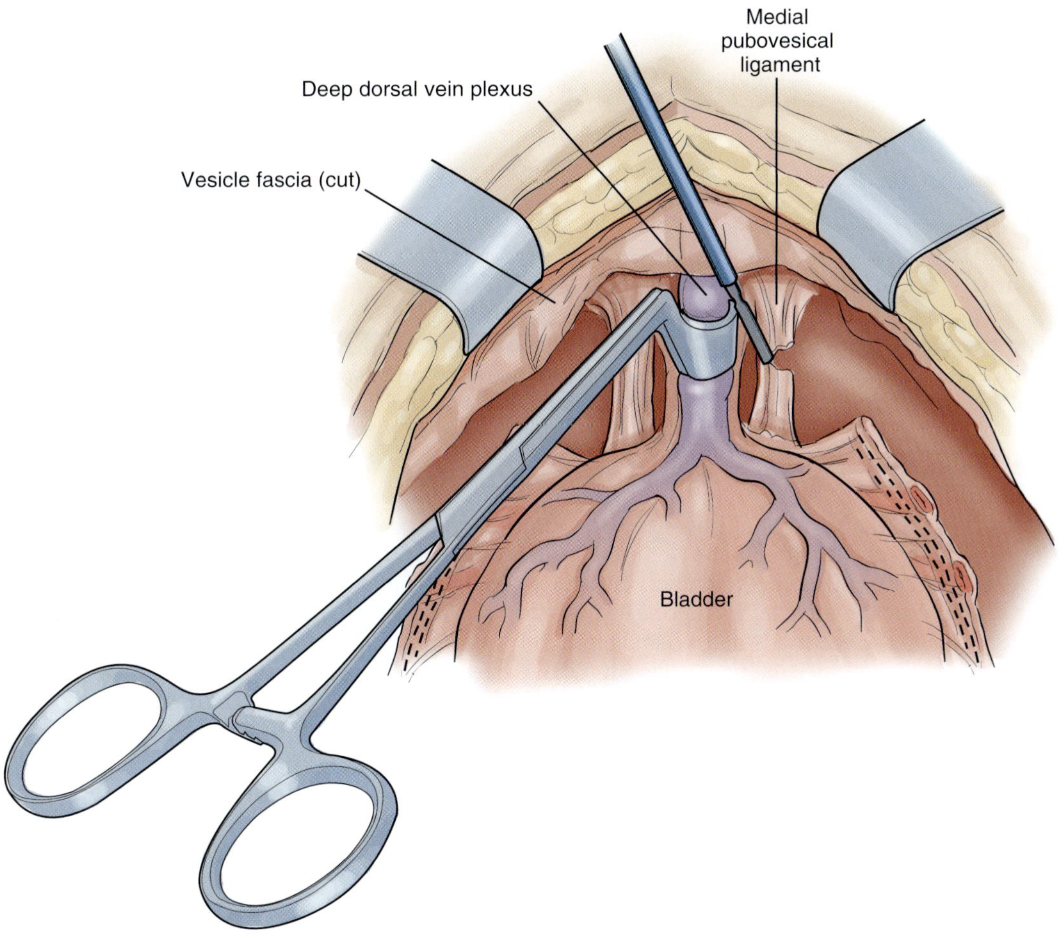

Figure 56-4.

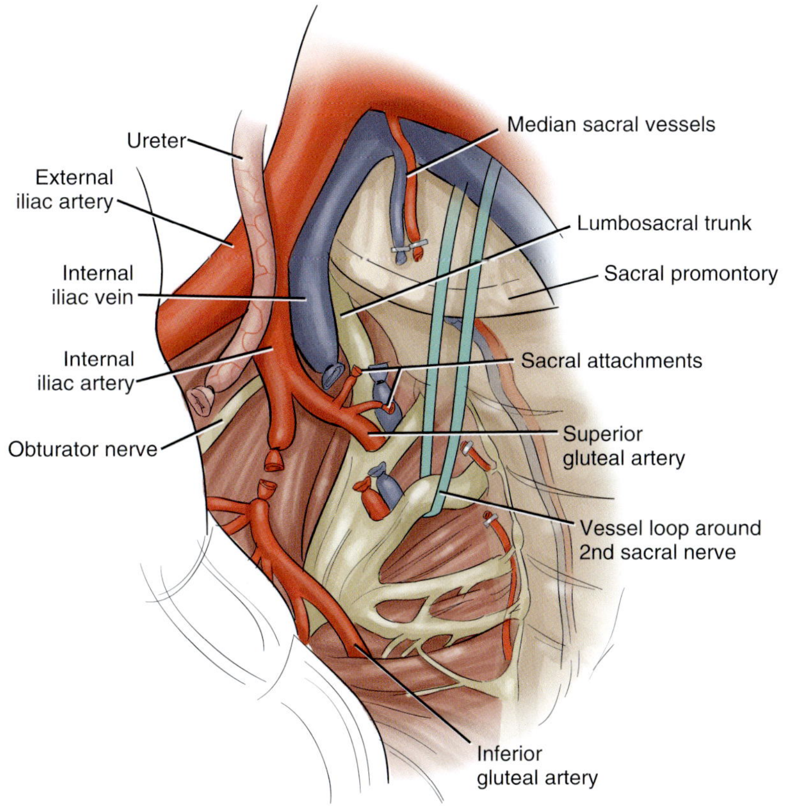

Figure 56-5.

plexus. Resection of the internal iliac veins is the most important part of this operation, and it requires advanced technical skills and careful maneuvers. Combined resection of the internal iliac vessels during the abdominal phase greatly contributes to reducing blood loss during sacrectomy.

- During dissection of the obturator space or when manipulating the internal iliac vessels while preserving the obturator nerve, components of the sacral nerve plexus, such as the lumbosacral nerve and S1 and S2 sacral nerves, can be identified. Marking the S2 sacral nerve with a rubber loop ensures precise recognition of sacral nerves during sacrectomy.

PERINEAL PHASE

Incision

- The scope of skin incision in the perineum is dependent on tumor invasion. If perineal invasion is not found, the skin incision for male patients is almost the same as for abdominoperineal resection, and that for female patients should include the anus and external genital organs.

Main Dissection

- At the level of the pelvic floor, the dissection range should be surrounded by the arcuate ligament, the inferior ramus of the pubic bone, the ischial tuberosity, and the edge of the gluteus maximus muscle (Fig. 56-6). The entire circumference should be freed, and after cutting of the urogenital diaphragm and the levator ani muscle, the perineal dissection is connected with the freed abdominal cavity. For male patients, the urethra is severed and closed in watertight fashion. At the time of perineal approach, ligation of bilateral internal iliac veins must have been completed; therefore, veins in the pelvic floor (e.g., the pudendal vein) are considerably congested, resulting in hemorrhage. For this reason, prompt implementation of perineal dissection is required.

SACRAL PHASE

Position

- The patient is placed in the prone position after temporary closure of the abdominal wound (Fig. 56-7). At that point, the padded operating frame for laminectomy is used to prevent an increase in abdominal or vertebral venous pressure. Bleeding caused by increased vertebral venous pressure makes sacral amputation complicated.

Incision

- The median incision is made approximately 20 cm longer from the posterior end of the perineal incision toward the head. The gluteus maximus muscle is detached from the sacrum so that the posterior surface of the sacrum can be exposed fully (Fig. 56-8).

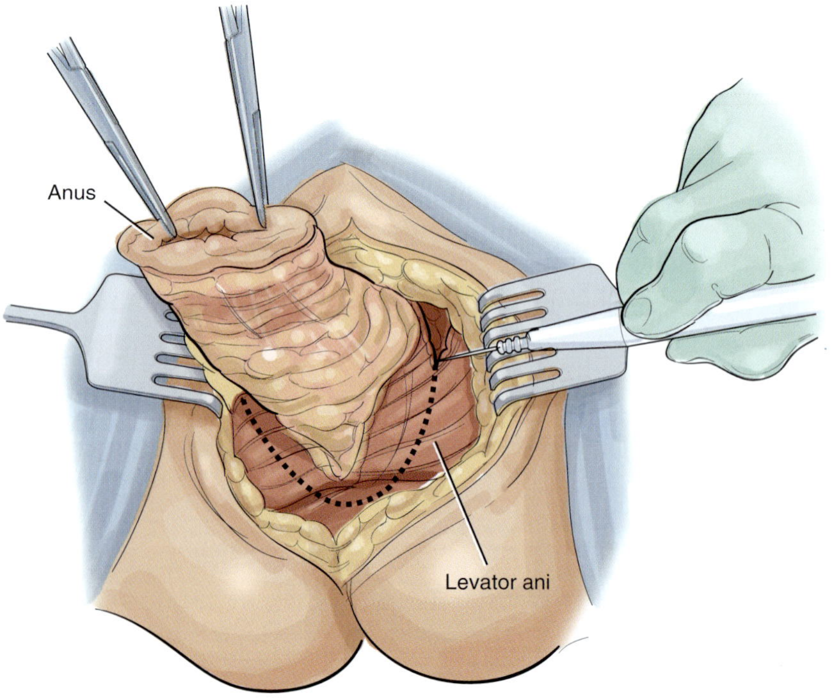

Figure 56-6.

Main Dissection

- The next step of this phase involves detaching the sacrotuberous and sacrospinous ligaments and piriform muscle that fix the sacrum. After dissection, these structures, the sciatic nerve, and a part of the sacral nerve plexus also can be checked (Fig. 56-9).

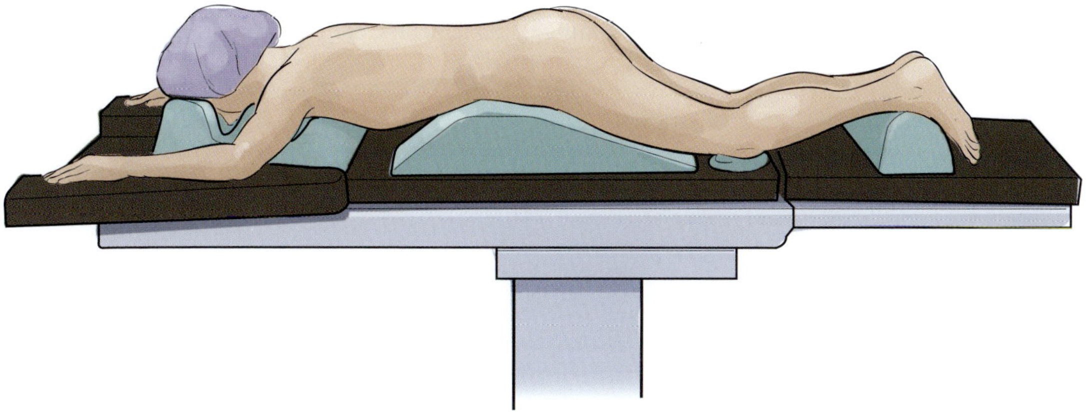

Figure 56-7.

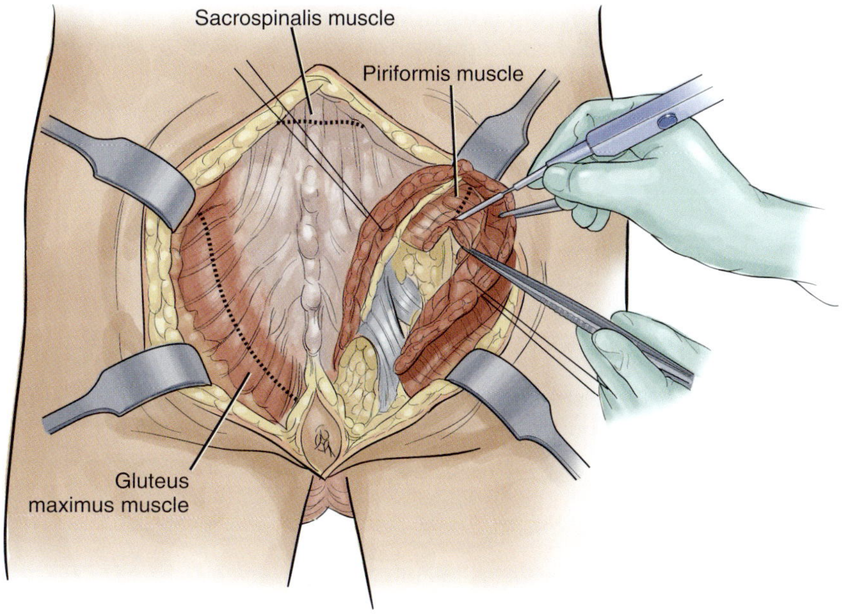

Figure 56-8.

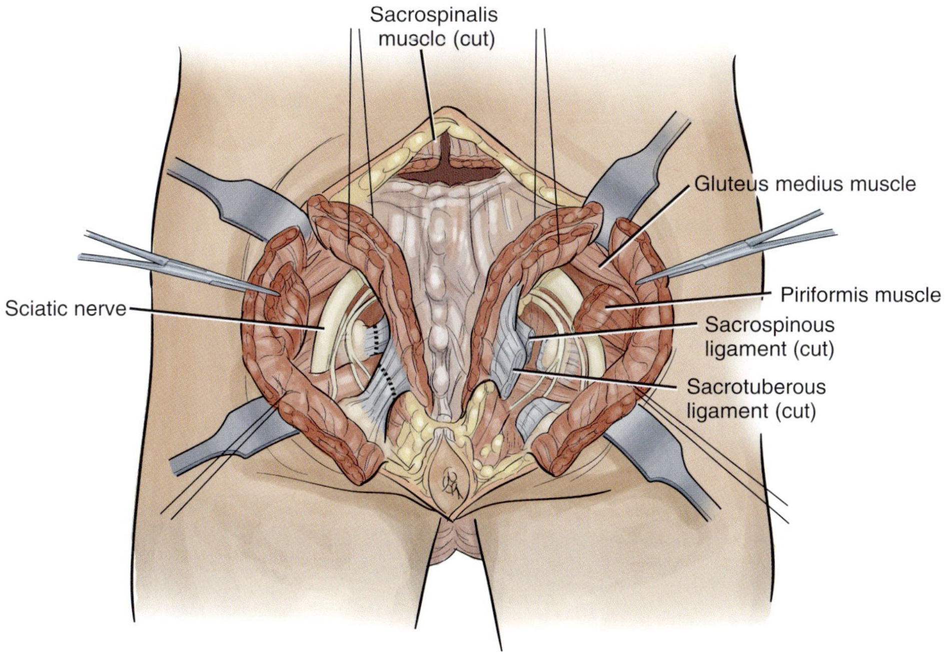

Figure 56-9.

- The surgeon inserts an index finger into the pelvic cavity from the lower edge of the sacroiliac joint and checks the dissected level of the anterior surface of the sacrum to determine the level of sacral amputation. After scraping of the medial sacral crest, laminectomy is performed and the root of the second sacral nerve is identified. The caudal end of the dura usually extends to around the lower edge of the S2 (Fig. 56-10). The dura and the cauda equina are tied and divided. The surgeon performs sacral amputation using chisel and hammer at a stretch. Hemostasis is performed quickly using electrocautery and bone wax (Fig. 56-11). In men, the urethra is closed tightly to prevent transurethral infection in the pelvis. The origin of the gluteus maximus muscle, the subcutis, and the skin are closed tightly layer by layer.

SECOND ABDOMINAL PHASE

Position

- The patient is placed in the supine position. Reconstruction of the urinary tract using ileal conduit and colostomy is performed (Fig. 56-12).

Main Dissection

- Mobilization of the right colon from the cecum to the hepatic flexure enables construction of a high urostoma. An ileoileostomy is lifted up above the pelvic brim and fixed to the mesentery so that it will not fall into the pelvic cavity. This procedure is invariably required to prevent anastomotic leakage secondarily caused by pelvic sepsis, especially after radiotherapy. If the greater omentum is long enough with favorable blood flow, omentoplasty into the pelvic cavity should be performed. In patients who underwent a wide resection of the perineal skin because of tumor invasion, reconstruction should be performed with a musculocutaneous flap.

Closure

- It is appropriate that gastrostomy be performed before closing the abdomen, because enteroparalysis continues for a while after TPES. A thick drain is placed in the pelvic cavity, and then the abdomen is closed in layer-by-layer fashion.
- The distal end of the conduit is brought out and sutured to the skin, producing a 5- to 10-mm nipple with buried, absorbable sutures. The colostomy is made.

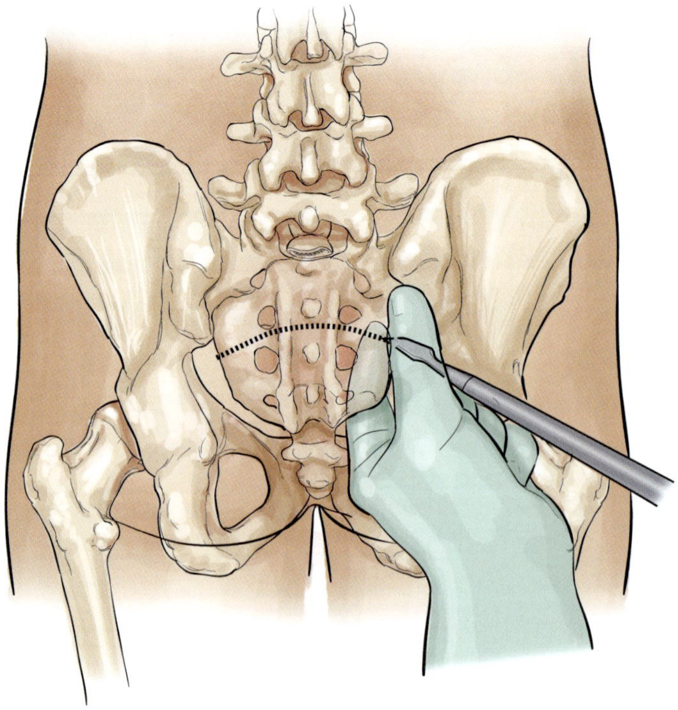

Figure 56-10.

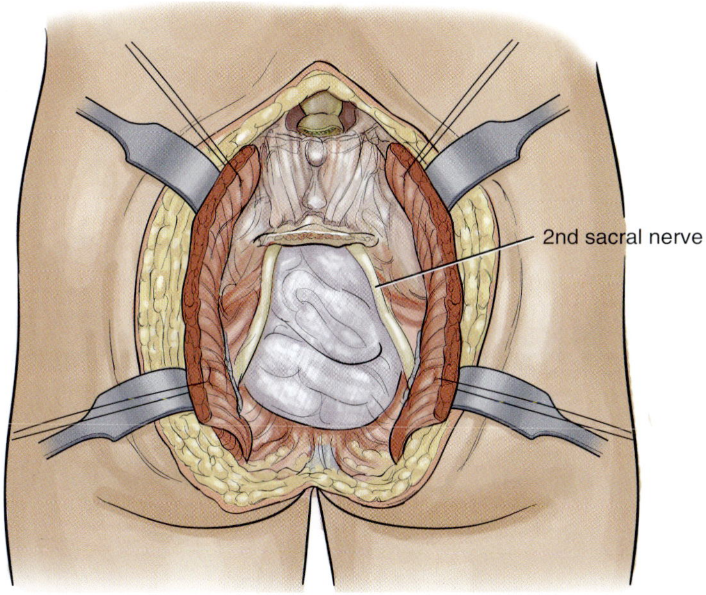

Figure 56-11.

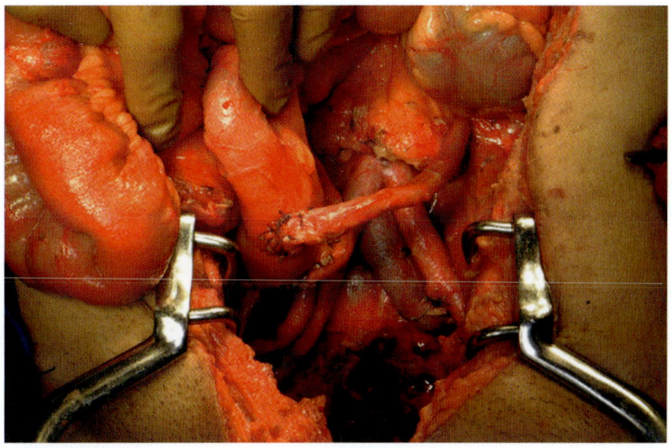

Figure 56-12.

III. ALTERNATIVE TECHNICAL APPROACHES (PRO/CON) AND PEARLS

- When surgical margins are proven to be positive for or very close to cancer intraoperatively, intraoperative radiotherapy should be considered.
- In controlling presacral venous hemorrhage during the sacral phase, a modified welding method using Surgicel absorbable hemostat is useful. After the bleeding point is occluded using Surgicel absorbable hemostat held by forceps, electrocautery is applied to the forceps to weld the bleeding site closed.
- During dissection of the obturator space, nerve block of the obturator nerve using lidocaine is helpful to prevent intraoperative reflex of the leg.

IV. SPECIAL POSTOPERATIVE CARE

- The specific and common postoperative complications that could be encountered after TPES are sacral wound dehiscence, pelvic sepsis, and urinary infection.
- Pelvic sepsis can cause secondary enteroperineal fistula, which is intractable and requires bypass surgery. Therefore open drainage of the perineal wound should be done without hesitation when pelvic sepsis is suspected, and daily irrigation of the pelvic space is needed.
- All patients have denervation pain around the buttocks lasting 2 to 6 months after TPES, and analgesic drugs are needed in spite of a lack of local recurrence.

SUGGESTED READINGS

Moriya Y, Akasu T, Fujita S, Yamamoto S: Total pelvic exenteration with distal sacrectomy for fixed recurrent rectal cancer in the pelvis, *Dis Colon Rectum* 47:2047–2053, 2004.

Wanebo HJ, Antoniuk P, Koness J, et al: Pelvic resection of recurrent rectal cancer, *Dis Colon Rectum* 42:1438–1448, 1999.

CHAPTER 57

Pelvic Exenteration: Total/Anterior/Posterior

Yoshihiro Moriya, MD, and Seiji Ishiguro, MD, PhD

I. SPECIAL PREOPERATIVE PREPARATION

Indications

- Pelvic exenteration is indicated for patients with a T4 intrapelvic malignancy that cannot be completely cured by partial resection of adjacent organs. In these cases, pelvic exenteration guarantees an R0 resection.
- The indications and the operative procedure vary by patient sex. For male patients, total pelvic exenteration (TPE) is indicated with rectal or sigmoid colon cancer invading the bladder, prostate, and/or seminal vesicle that cannot be cured by partial resection of these organs. The same applies for bladder or prostate cancer invading the rectum.
- On the other hand, the indication and operation technique for female patients are different from those for male patients. For patients with cancer of the female reproductive organs such as the uterus, ovary, or vagina, invading the bladder, anterior pelvic exenteration is indicated. In contrast, when invasion is directed posteriorly to the rectum, posterior pelvic exenteration is indicated (Fig. 57-1).
- TPE is indicated for female patients when the tumor is invading in both anterior and posterior directions when there is remaining tumor after radiotherapy. TPE is also indicated in the case of central recurrence in the stump of the vagina.
- Anterior pelvic exenteration requires urinary diversion, and posterior pelvic exenteration requires a colostomy. These two procedures can be performed successfully if the surgeon fully understands the procedures and techniques of TPE, which are explained in detail in this chapter.
- Pelvic exenteration is contraindicated for the following patients, in whom resection of the tumor by means of pelvic exenteration cannot result in an R0 resection: (1) patients with lymph node metastasis and/or peritoneal deposits outside the pelvis, (2) patients with distant metastasis in organs such as liver or lung, and (3) patients with edema in the lower extremities.

Preparation and Imaging

- Time and attention should be spent on obtaining informed consent for pelvic exenteration, when invasion of the tumor into surrounding structures is suspected (Fig. 57-2). Patients should be given a full explanation of the operative procedure and the consequences of urostomy or colostomy and function loss. Physicians should fully understand that they cannot simply select the best operative procedure without the patient's informed consent.
- Preoperative stoma site marking is especially important. In consideration of the patient's body shape and the presence or absence of operative scars, the site that the patient can care for the easiest should be determined. By determining the future stoma site in a seated position, attention is paid to skin grooves in abdominally obese patients (Fig. 57-3).
- A whole-body computed tomography scan is necessary to determine distant metastasis status and the extent of tumor in the pelvis. Positron emission tomography–computed tomography is also useful to check for distant metastasis.
- Magnetic resonance imaging is the most important imaging modality for the determination of the extent of tumor invasion (Fig. 57-4). Because this modality is excellent for creating an image of the iliac

vessels, it also provides information about the presence or absence of lateral lymph node metastasis. Gadolinium contrasts are useful in the differentiation among abscess, tumor invasion, or fibrosis.
- Ultrasonography has limited value for stenotic lesions or lesions in the middle and/or upper rectum. Further, the specificity of ultrasound is operator dependent and it lacks the ability to image the iliac vessels.

II. OPERATIVE TECHNIQUE

- TPE for primary pelvic malignancy is performed by first dividing loose connective tissues, such as the Retzius, obturator, and retrorectal spaces, and then dissecting along the parietal pelvic fascia. The operation is performed in the following order: abdominal, perineal, and second abdominal phase.

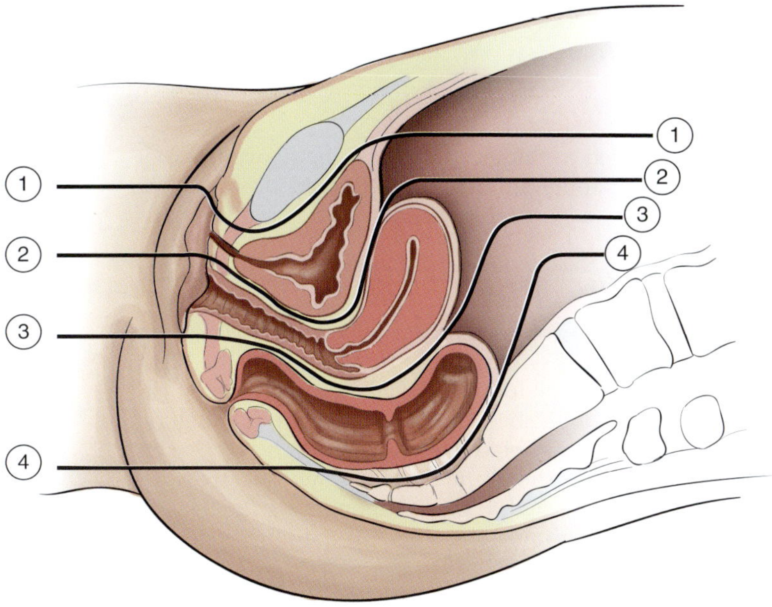

Figure 57-1.

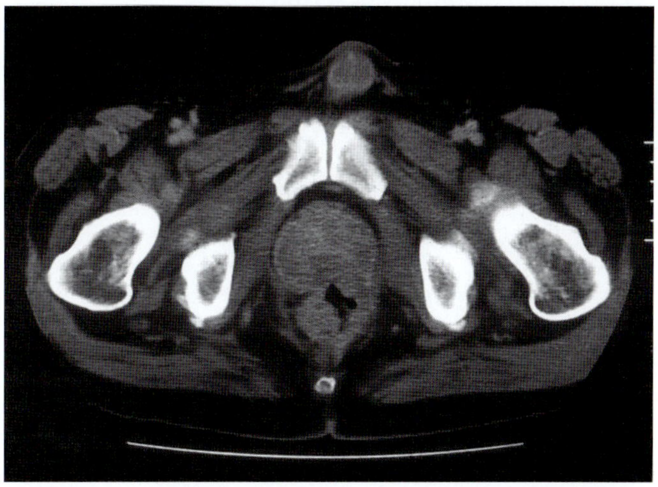

Figure 57-2. Computed tomography shows T4 rectal cancer that invades the prostate and right internal obturator muscle.

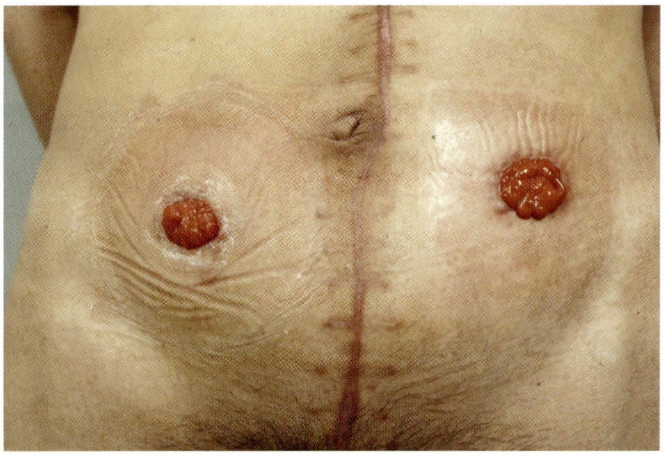

Figure 57-3.

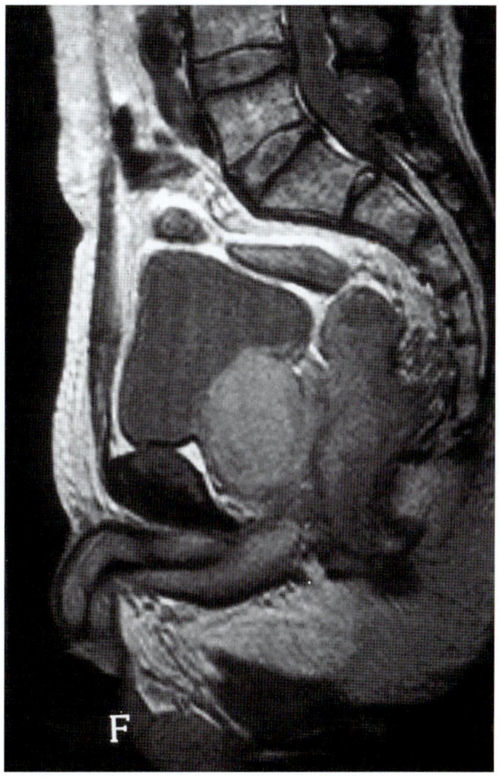

Figure 57-4. Magnetic resonance imaging shows T4 rectal cancer that widely invades the bladder.

Position

- The patient is placed in the lithotomy position using Levitator stirrups. Intermittent massage apparatus is applied to the lower limbs to prevent deep vein thrombosis (Fig. 57-5). The patient is disinfected completely with povidone-iodine, including the area from the breast line to the middle of the thigh, the lateral side area including the posterior axillary line, and the perineal area including skin behind the coccygeus.

ABDOMINAL PHASE

Incision

- After performing a wide midline incision, the surgeon confirms the localization of the tumor within the pelvis and the absence of extrapelvic diseases and then makes the final decision to proceed to TPE.

Main Dissection

- After the anterior surface of the abdominal aorta is exposed at the level of 2 to 3 cm above the root of the inferior mesenteric artery, paraaortic lymphadenectomy should be performed down to the abdominal aortic bifurcation. The inferior mesenteric artery is tied and divided at its origin during this dissection.
- For cutting the peritoneal leaf in the pelvis, a wide range of incision is made along the common iliac artery down to the external iliac artery (Fig. 57-6).
- *Freeing of the anterior aspect:* After opening the anterior space of the bladder or Retzius space, then continuing to separate loose connective tissues along the pubic symphysis by using scissors, the bilateral puboprostatic ligaments and dilated dorsal vein complex are found. After the puboprostatic ligaments are sharply divided, the dorsal vein complex is doubly tied and divided with a bunching technique, and the complex is separated downward below the pubic bone (Fig. 57-7).
- *Cutting the ureter:* Before cutting the ureter, the surgeon should make sure that the tumor is resectable. The division of the ureter is conducted below the pelvic brim. With regard to monitoring the urinary volume, it is enough to insert a single J-catheter into only the unilateral side. On the other side, the distal ureter is ligated.
- Performing lymphadenectomy around the common iliac vessels, the bifurcation of internal and external iliac artery is exposed, and the trunk of the internal iliac artery is tied twice and divided after branching the superior gluteal artery. With regard to the order of manipulation for the internal iliac venous system, the steps for tie and division of peripheral veins, including the obturator, inferior gluteal, and internal pudendal veins, should precede those for the trunk of the internal iliac vein.
- With the surgeon's left hand strongly displacing intrapelvic organs to the left, the right obturator fossa is opened widely. The vascular pedicles supplying the bladder are divided either between clamps or

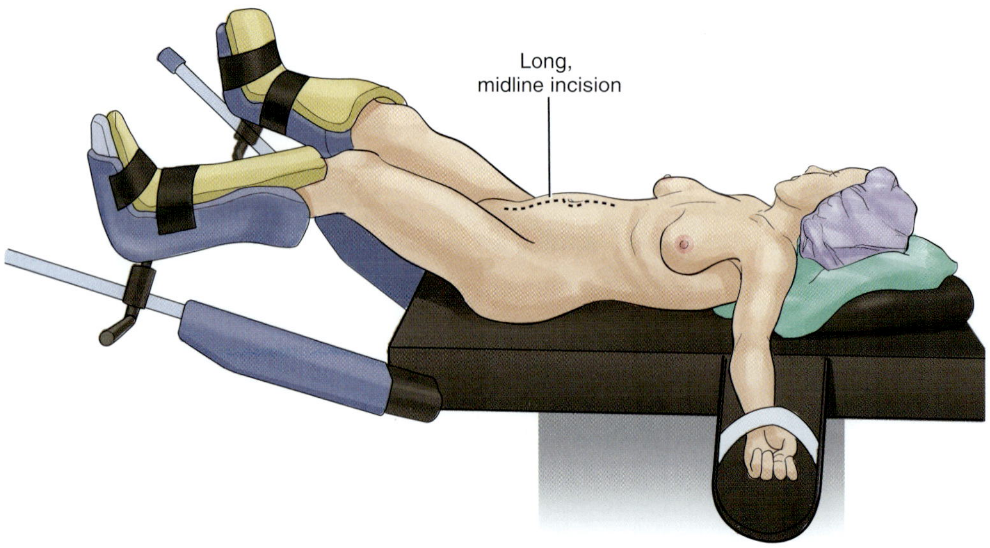

Figure 57-5.

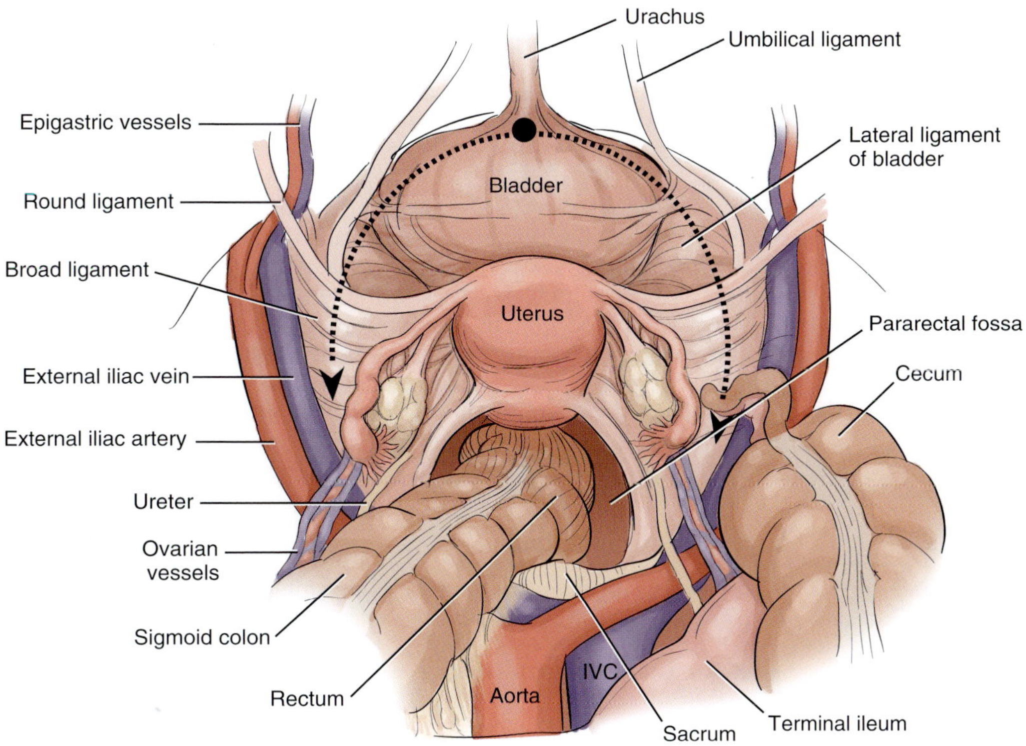

Figure 57-6. *IVC,* Inferior vena cava.

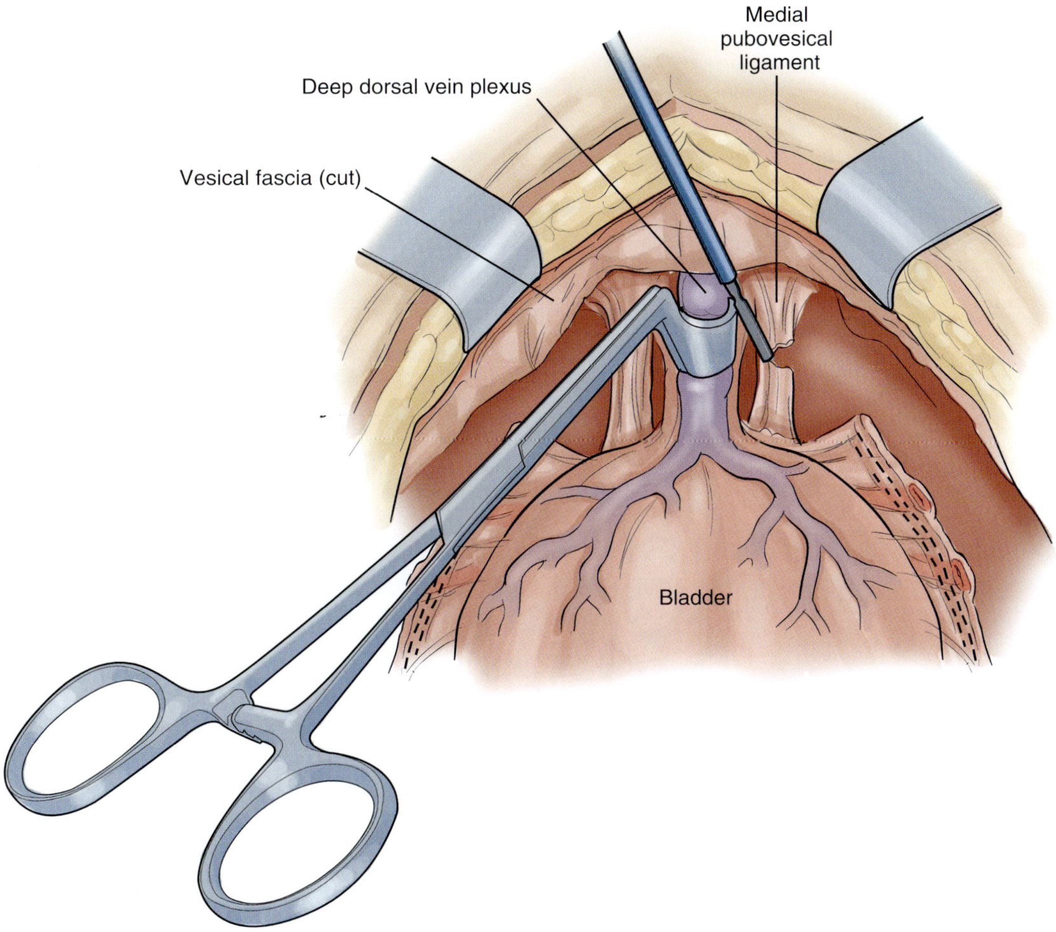

Figure 57-7.

with a linear vascular stapling device (Fig. 57-8). After identifying the obturator nerve and vessels, the nerve is elevated by a rubber loop and preserved, and the obturator vessels are severed at the level of the obturator foramen. The area posterior to the obturator fossa is then opened, and the sacral nerve plexuses, including the lumbosacral and S1 sacral nerves, are exposed. By implementing anatomic dissection of the peripheral vascular system of the internal iliac vessels, the obturator fossa has been cleaned of connective, adipose tissues, and lymph nodes en bloc while preserving the obturator nerve and sacral nerve plexus.

- *Freeing of the retrorectal space:* Blunt dissection of the presacral space should never be performed by the surgeon's hand because it may cause bleeding from the presacral venous plexus. By identifying the middle sacral vein under direct vision and sharply dividing loose connective tissue layers like peels of an onion between the visceral and parietal pelvic fasciae using long scissors and a long retractor, the freeing of the retrorectal space is completed from the promontory to the coccyx at a stretch (Fig. 57-9). During this freeing procedure, the surgeon should take care to not allow the freeing line to stray laterally from the middle sacral vein so to not damage the lateral sacral venous plexus. If bleeding from the presacral venous plexus occurs, the surgeon should grasp the bleeding point with forceps and then stop the bleeding by electrocautery. At this time, it is important to push the bleeding point toward the sacrum. Elevation of the point may result in greater damage to the venous plexus. If it is difficult to stop bleeding by this maneuver, the same hemostatic maneuver is repeated after weakening the force of bleeding by pressing the bleeding point with gauze.
- After the operative steps are completed for the dorsal vein complex anteriorly, the internal iliac vessels laterally, and the rectum posteriorly and any remaining stalks attaching the specimen to the pelvic wall are resected, the intrapelvic organs, including the internal iliac vessels and all lymph-connective tissues, become completely detached from the pelvic wall. At this time, only the continuity with the urethra and the muscle complex of the pelvic floor is preserved. After that, operative steps for the perineum are performed.
- In women, when total pelvic exenteration is undertaken, hysterectomy is performed in a standard fashion as described in Chapter 76. Once the urethra is divided, it provides access to the vagina, which is divided (Fig. 57-10).

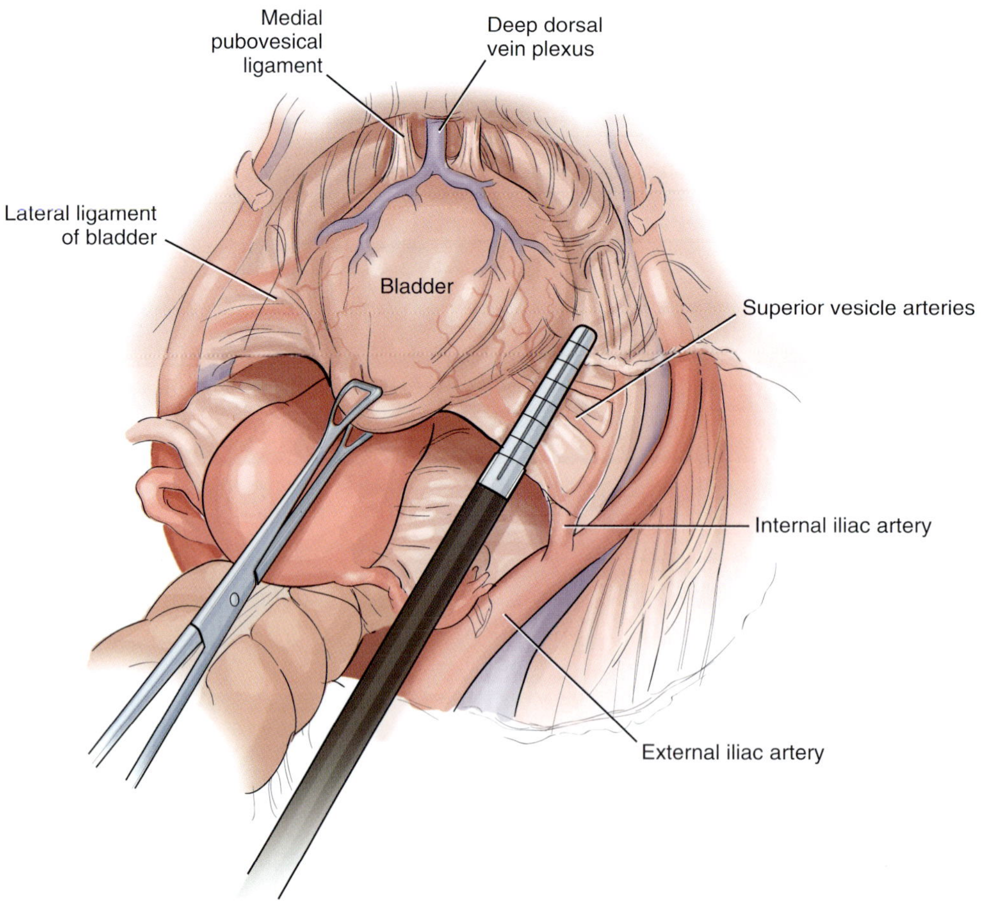

Figure 57-8.

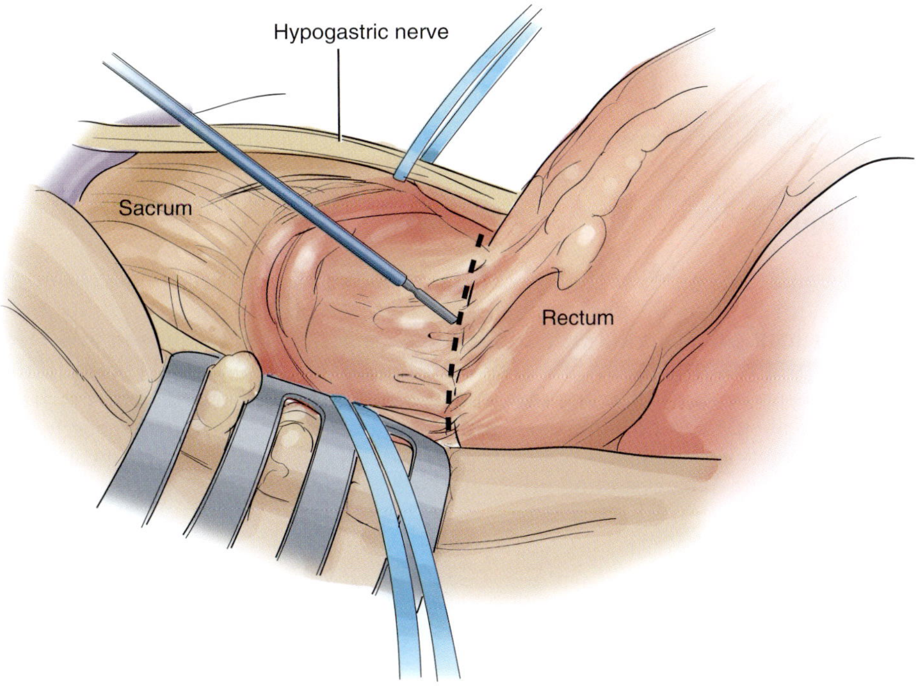

Figure 57-9.

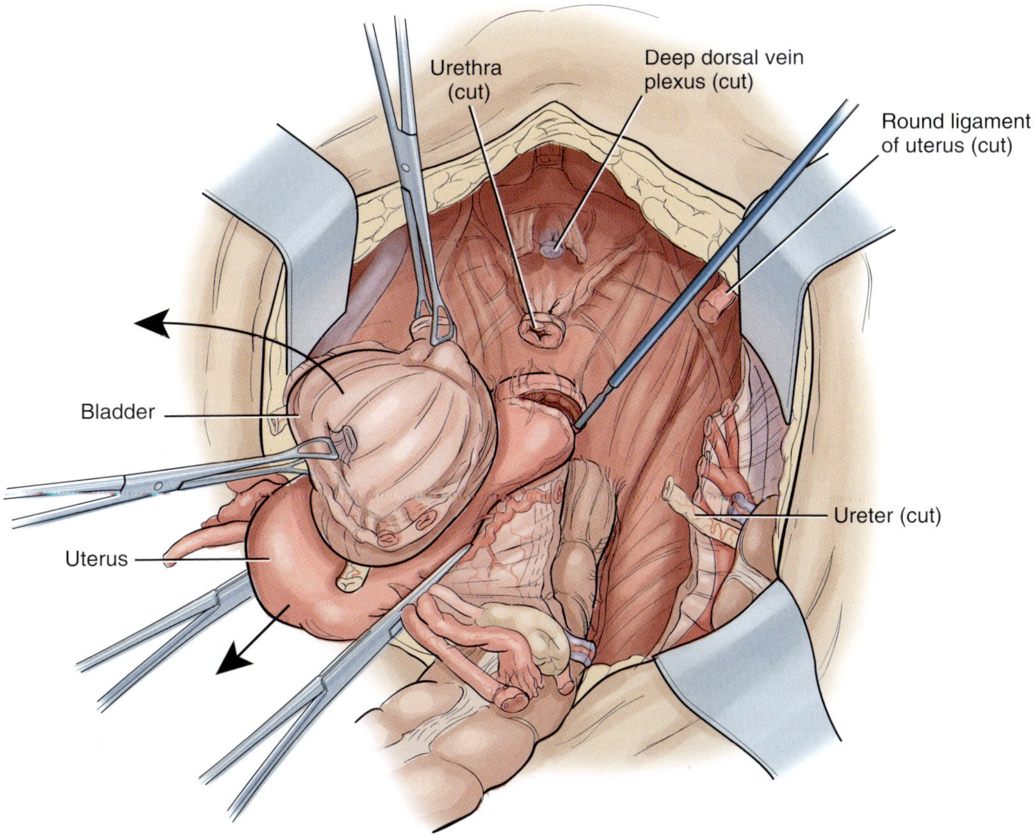

Figure 57-10.

PERINEAL PHASE

Incision

- The entire perineum and anus are circumscribed by an elliptical incision (Fig. 57-11).

Main Dissection

- Freeing of the muscle complex of the pelvic floor, including the urogenital diaphragm and levator ani muscle, is performed along the pubic arch and the gluteus maximus muscle. At this time, veins in the pelvic floor, including the perineal vein, can become congested. For this reason, it is possible to minimize bleeding by dividing the veins after ligation using 2-0 threads. For male patients, the urethra and corpus spongiosum penis are tied and divided. Just under the arcuate ligament attached to the pubic bone, the perineal side can be connected to the abdominal one to avoid damage to the dorsal vein complex. After anterior, lateral, and posterior dissection of the pelvic floor, perineal dissection is completed and the specimen can be removed (Fig. 57-12, *A* and *B*).

Closure

- The surgeon ensures that the urethra is closed in a watertight manner by absorbable threads. Insufficient closing of the urethral stump can cause transurethral infections in the pelvic dead space. The extent of perineal dissection varies depending on the patient's sex and the extent of tumor invasion. For female patients, the urethra and external genital organs are included in the extent of dissection. The perineal wound is closed in two layers, the subcutaneous adipose tissue layer and the cutaneous layer. If it is impossible to close the perineal skin primarily, it should be closed by using devices such as musculocutaneous flaps.

SECOND ABDOMINAL PHASE

Main Dissection

- There are several surgical procedures for urinary diversion: ileal conduit, Kock continent pouch, ureterocutaneostomy, etc. The ileal conduit diversion technique is considered to be the most reliable in terms of ease and long-term functional outcome.
- *Isolation of the ileal segment:* A 15-cm-long segment of pedunculated ileum, with good blood supply, located about 20 cm distal from the terminal ileum, is used as an ileal conduit. By observing branches

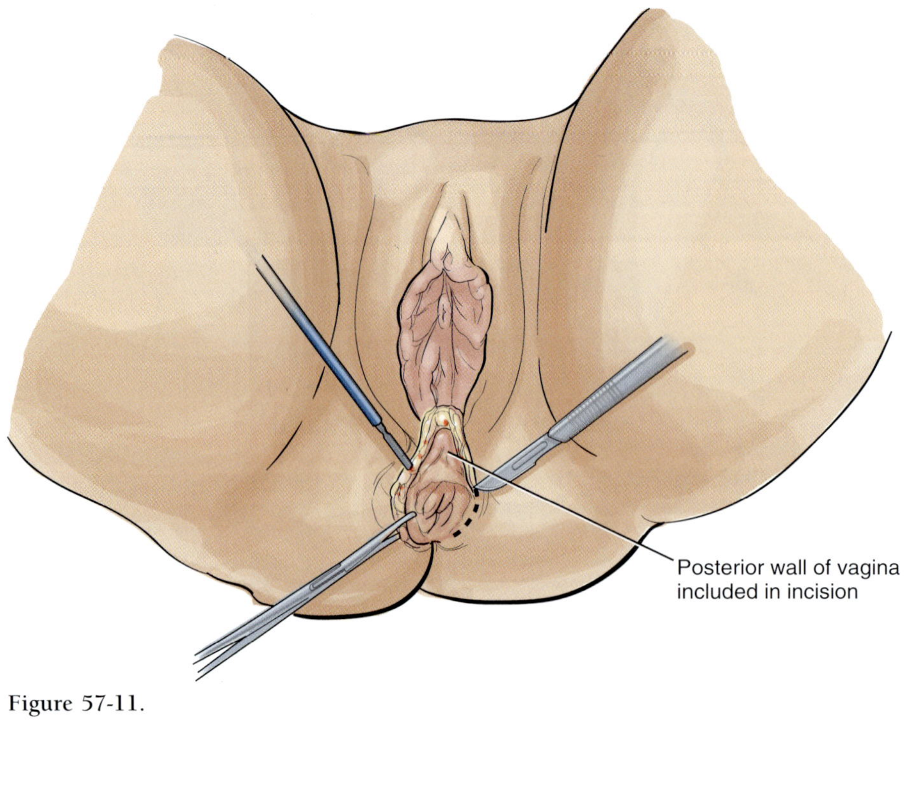

Figure 57-11.

of blood vessels in the mesentery with backlight, surgeons should make sure that there are two arteries in this segment. After insertion of a Foley catheter from the distal stump, the conduit is washed with physiologic saline. Placing the ileal conduit on the retroperitoneum, ileal continuity is established using a functional end-to-end anastomosis.

- *Ureteroileal anastomosis:* The anastomotic site for the left ureter is located 2 to 3 cm distant from the proximal stump of the segment. For the right ureter, it is located 3 to 4 cm right of the left ureter. After a single J ureteric stent is inserted into each ureter, the catheters are introduced into the conduit. The ureteroileal anastomosis is performed by interrupted one-layer suture, with eight stitches in total, using 5-0 Vicryl absorbable thread (Fig. 57-13).
- The right colon from the cecum to the hepatic flexure is mobilized to prevent tension on a pedicle of the ileal conduit. By attaching the ileal conduit to the retroperitoneum and peritoneum of the lateral abdominal wall with several stitches, the urostoma with a 5- to10-mm nipple is built above the skin level.

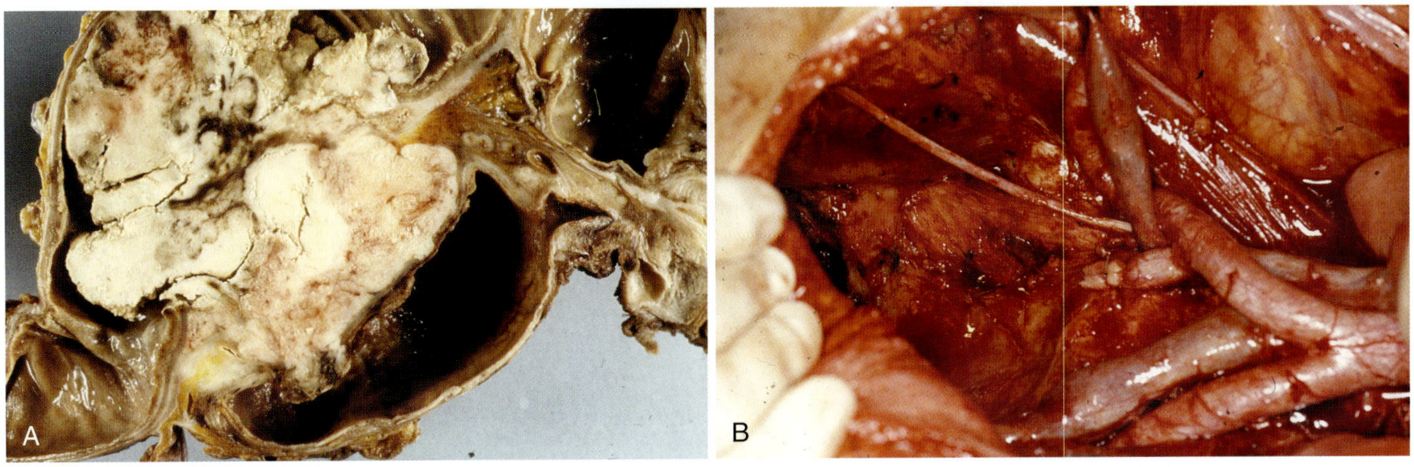

Figure 57-12. **A,** The resected specimen shows wide bladder invasion. **B,** Completion of total pelvic exenteration: skeletonized pelvis.

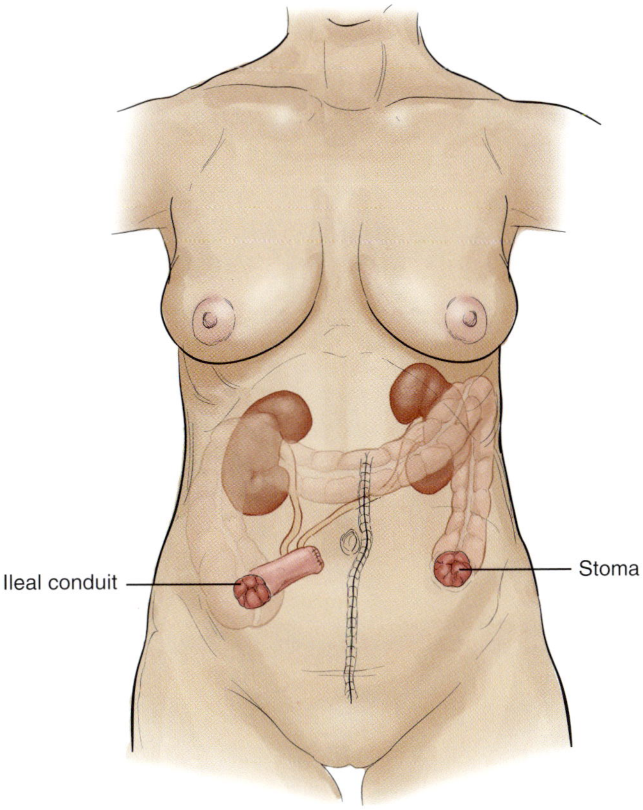

Figure 57-13.

Closure

- Pelvic sepsis is the most common postoperative complication. If the ileoileal anastomosis falls into the pelvis, pelvic sepsis can secondarily cause anastomotic leakage. For this reason, the anastomotic site should be attached to the mesentery above the pelvic brim with several stitches.
- If possible, a J-shaped omental flap is placed in the pelvis. Because enteroparalysis continues for a while after TPE, it is appropriate to perform gastrostomy before closing the abdomen to relieve patient discomfort and prevent pulmonary complications. The distal end of both conduit and sigmoid colon are brought out and sutured to the skin, producing a 5- to 10-mm nipple with buried, absorbable sutures. A thick 10-Fr drain is placed in the pelvis, and then the abdomen is closed using the layer-by-layer method.

III. ALTERNATIVE TECHNICAL APPROACHES (PRO/CON) AND PEARLS

- For patients with severe arteriosclerosis or those with less possibility of lateral sidewall lymph node metastasis (e.g., sigmoid/rectosigmoid colon cancer with massive involvement of the bladder), removal of the lymph nodes of the lateral pelvis can be omitted. Dissection is commenced at the aortic bifurcation and proceeds to the pelvis along the internal iliac artery, dissecting loose connective tissue between the internal iliac artery and pelvic plexus. The superior vesical artery, the middle rectal artery, and the inferior vesical artery accompanied by the similarly named veins are ligated and cut, and the pelvic floor is visualized medial to the pudendal vessels. This method is a safe and reliable alternative with fewer technical demands and less blood loss.
- High complication rates after construction of the ileal conduit in irradiated patients often have been attributed to postradiation fibrosis. Although use of the jejunum, which is outside the radiation field, is optimal, the possibility that it will lead to some metabolic complication should be kept in mind. As a simple and reliable alternative in patients with radiation damage in the distal ureter, the incontinent urinary diversion with cutaneous ureterostomy should be considered for safety. In patients with long life expectancy, creation of an orthotopic neobladder or a continent pouch is an attractive approach for improved quality of life.

IV. SPECIAL POSTOPERATIVE CARE

- Because loss of body fluid including lymph fluid through a drain is usually 500 mL/day or more, supplemental administration of blood products such as albumin is required.

SUGGESTED READINGS

Bricker EM: Substitution for the urinary bladder by the use of isolated ileal segment, *Surg Clin North Am* 36:1117–1130, 1956.
Lambrou N C, Pearson JM, Averette HE: Pelvic exenteration of gynecologic malignancy: indications, and technical and reconstructive considerations, *Surg Oncol Clin Am* 14:289–300, 2005.

CHAPTER 58

Laparoscopic Rectopexy for Rectal Prolapse

Ferdinand Köckerling, MD, PhD, and K. Thomas Moesta, MD, PhD

I. SPECIAL PREOPERATIVE PREPARATION

- Outer prolapse must be reducible on clinical examination.
- Nonreducible, chronic prolapse should not be treated by laparoscopic rectopexy but by extraabdominal procedures, that is, Delorme or Altemeier.
- Patients must be suitable for a prolonged laparoscopic procedure, with regard to general health status. Pronounced kyphosis, not uncommon in typically elderly women presenting with rectal prolapse, may represent an obstacle to an appropriate operative positioning.
- Manometry can be used to assure rectal continence. However, the prolapse leads to a distention of the anal sphincter, which is, at least in part, reversible after rectopexy. Thus, pathologic results are common and should not lead automatically to alter the concept of rectopexy in favor of definitive colostomy.
- Contrast enema serves to identify patients with a prolonged sigmoid colon, contributing to outlet obstruction in the presence of a deep peritoneal extension (cul-de-sac phenomenon; Fig. 58-1, *A*). If, in such a situation, rectopexy alone is performed, the procedure will lead to an accentuation of the angulation between the mobile sigmoid and the upper rectum fixed at the promontory, aggravating constipation. Therefore rectal prolapse in conjunction with an elongated sigmoid colon requires a resectional rectopexy.
- Colon transit time (Sitzmarker test) is useful to safely differentiate slow-transit constipation from rectal outlet syndrome. Slow-transit constipation may require more extensive colonic resections in combination with rectopexy.
- A balloon expulsion test can serve to objectively assess rectal outlet obstruction.
- Defecography is required to show intussusception and rectal outlet obstruction (see Fig. 58-1, *B*).

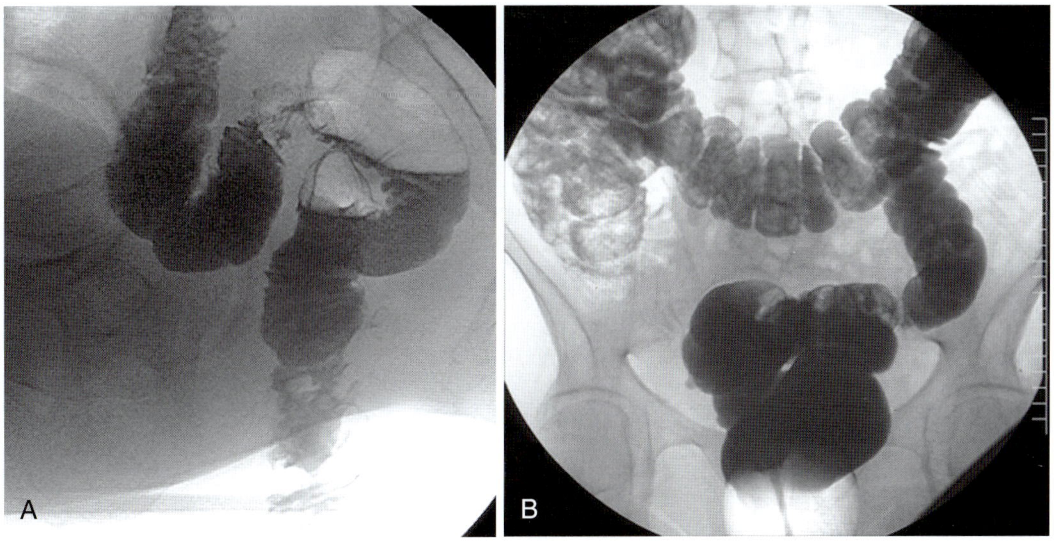

Figure 58-1. **A,** Barium enema of a patient with rectal prolapse with a clearly prolonged sigmoid colon. **B,** Defecography of the same patient revealing the prolapse and the interposition of the elongated sigmoid between vagina and rectum in the pathologically deepened rectouterine pouch.

- All of the above are required in the presence of a suspected internal prolapse if outlet obstruction is to be differentiated from constipation. In the presence of a full-layer rectal prolapse, defecography, manometry, and balloon expulsion tests may be impossible or of little additional diagnostic value. A contrast enema is, however, always performed to indicate whether a sigmoid resection is required in addition to rectopexy.

II. OPERATIVE TECHNIQUE

Position

- Patients are positioned in an overextended supine lithotomy position.
- Shoulder and pelvis supports may be used to safely realize extreme table positions; however, compression injuries have been reported as a consequence of such restraints. As surgeons gain more experience in the field, extreme positions may be unnecessary. In our practice, additional patient supports are not used.
- Special care is required in the protection of the patient's legs. Extensive cushioning of the calves should protect the peroneal nerves from direct pressure even if several table repositionings are required. Furthermore, a prolonged Trendelenburg position can lead to inadequate arterial perfusion and eventually to an ischemia-induced compartment syndrome. This rare but sometimes severe complication can be avoided by a low position of the leg restraints, almost overextending the hip, and, of course, by avoiding very prolonged and extreme Trendelenburg positions.
- The patient's right arm is positioned alongside the body to allow the surgeon and camera operator to stand at the right side of the patient. The assistant stands at the left side of the patient.

Trocar Placement

- A four- or five-trocar technique is used, depending on whether a sigmoid resection is performed in addition to the rectopexy (Fig. 58-2).
- The camera trocar is inserted above and to the right of the umbilicus using an open access technique. All other trocars are placed lateral to the epigastric vessels after transillumination and under direct visualization.
- In resectional rectopexy procedures, four trocars are positioned, two in the left and two in the right lower abdomen. Together with the camera trocar they form a rough semicircle open to the pelvis. The lower right trocar is later used to introduce the linear cutter and thus needs to have a 12-mm diameter; for the other trocars, a 5-mm diameter is sufficient.
- If rectopexy only is planned, the upper left trocar can be omitted, and all trocars may be 5 mm in diameter.

Main Dissection

- The first step of every procedure is an abdominal exploration to exclude relevant additional pathologies and to confirm, as far as possible, the preoperative assumptions as to the abdominal and pelvic

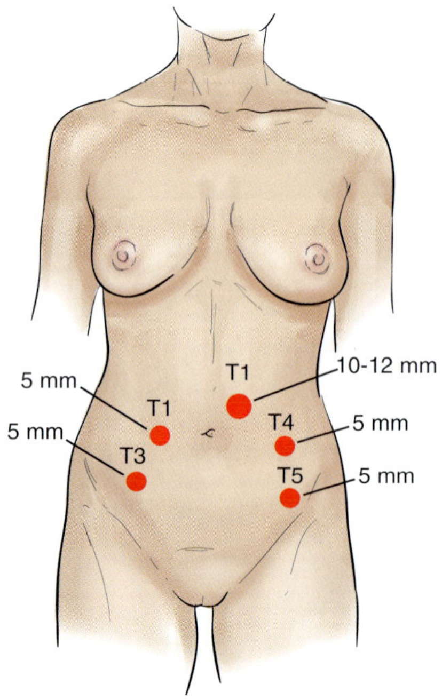

Figure 58-2.

pathologies leading to the patient's symptoms—that is, elongated sigmoid, deep rectouterine pouch, or mobile lateral ligaments.

- The female pelvis is exposed by elevating the uterus and the fallopian tubes to the anterior abdominal wall by a transcutaneous suture applied using a long, straight needle (Fig. 58-3).
- The peritoneum at the pelvic inlet is now opened (Fig. 58-4). To ascertain the correct access to the retrorectal cleavage plane between the mesorectal and the pelvic fascia containing the hypogastric nerves, the assistant and the surgeon must take care to fully elongate and elevate the rectum with graspers (Fig. 58-5). The ureter is also identified and preserved. Slightly below the promontory, the avascular zone between visceral and parietal peritoneum is easily identified. This part of the preparation is carried out by electrocautery or ultrasonic dissection devices (Fig. 58-6).

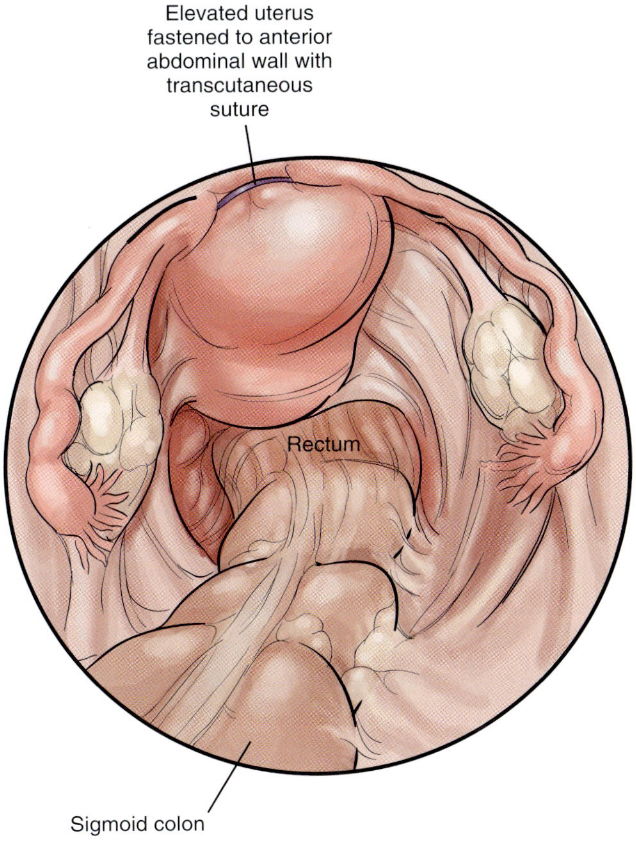

Figure 58-3.

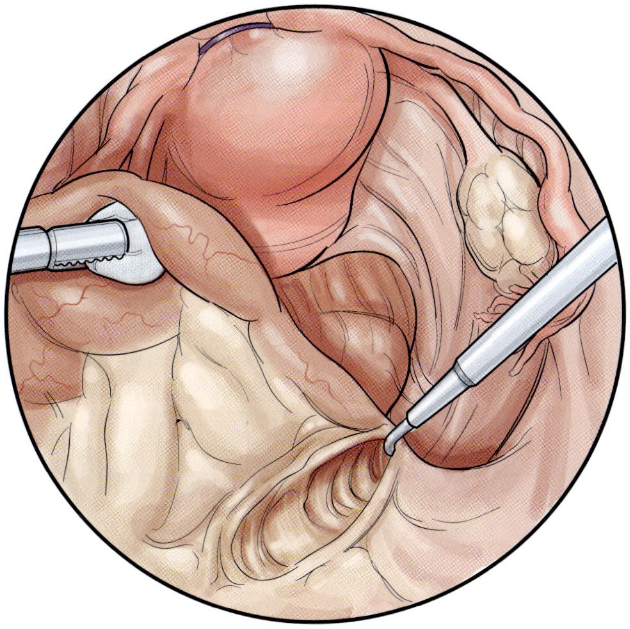

Figure 58-4.

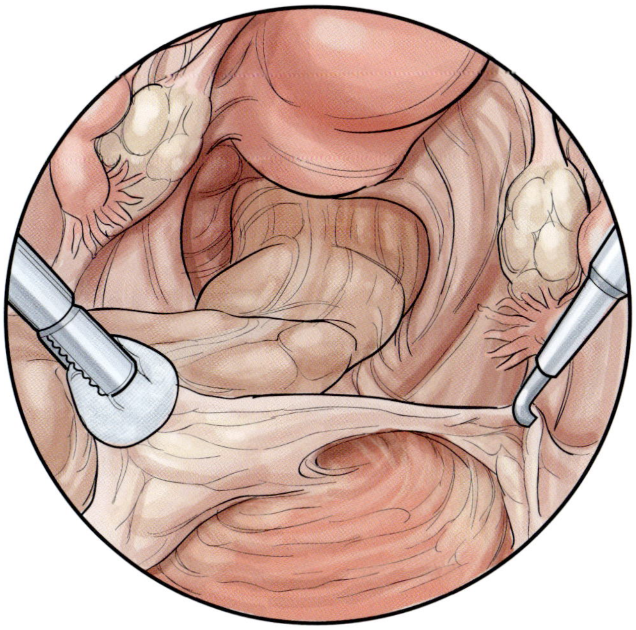

Figure 58-5.

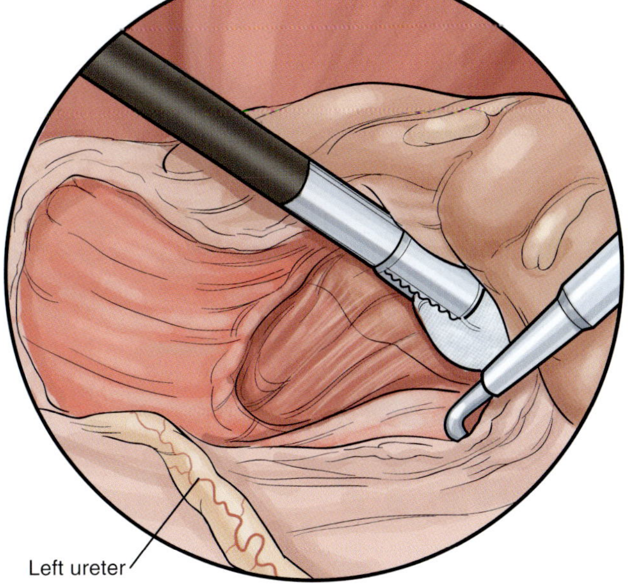

Figure 58-6.

- The opening of the retrorectal cleavage plane is performed predominantly by blunt dissection using swabs or by blunt ultrasonic dissection. Extensive electrocautery should be avoided to safely preserve the autonomic innervation of the pelvic organs.
- The rectal mobilization is carried out dorsally downward to the pelvic floor. Laterally, the mobilization should suffice to straighten the rectum, separating the mesorectal envelope from the "anchor points" at the level of the lower hypogastric plexus, taking care not to induce neural damage here. Carefully following the cleavage plane from back to front usually allows a very dry preparation without any requirement for electrocautery or clip placements.
- At the end of the mobilization, with the rectum extended by laparoscopic forceps, full reposition of an outer prolapse must be ascertained by inspection and eventually digital palpation of the anus.
- Rectopexy can now be performed with or without the use of alloplastic material. In the case of resectional rectopexy, the use of alloplastic material is contraindicated because of the risk of contamination and subsequent mesh infection. If only rectopexy is performed, we still favor the use of a mesh to enhance rectal fixation to the sacrum. Others have shown good results using suture rectopexy.
- A light polypropylene mesh of triangular shape, 11 cm long at the base, is prepared. Openings in the center of the mesh are cut away to facilitate secure fixation of the mesh to the presacral pelvic fascia by sutures or staples.
- The mesh is introduced through the camera trocar, if all other trocars are 5 mm in diameter.
- With the assistant lifting the mobilized rectum, the mesh is unfolded against the presacral fascia at the ventral surface of the sacrum, the base of the triangle at the level of the promontory. The mesh is fixed in place, preferably with sutures along the midline and at the base of the triangle, to the promontory (Fig. 58-7).

Closure

- The mobilized rectum is straightened and positioned against the securely fastened mesh. With the assistant holding the rectum in place, the surgeon wraps the mesh around the ventral surface of the rectum and fixes the mesh flaps to the rectal wall on both sides with three or four interrupted sutures. The mesh should not be circumferentially closed, but some 2 cm of the ventral circumference of the rectum should be left free to preserve elasticity and allow for peristalsis.
- The pelvic floor may be repaired by closing the peritoneal borders to both sides of the rectum, adding to the tension on the rectum and reducing the pathologically deepened rectouterine pouch.

III. ALTERNATIVE TECHNICAL APPROACHES (PRO/CON) AND PEARLS

- If sigmoid resection is to be combined with rectopexy, the sigmoid resection is performed after the mobilization of the rectum. Because a further fixation of the rectum is intended, the descending colon

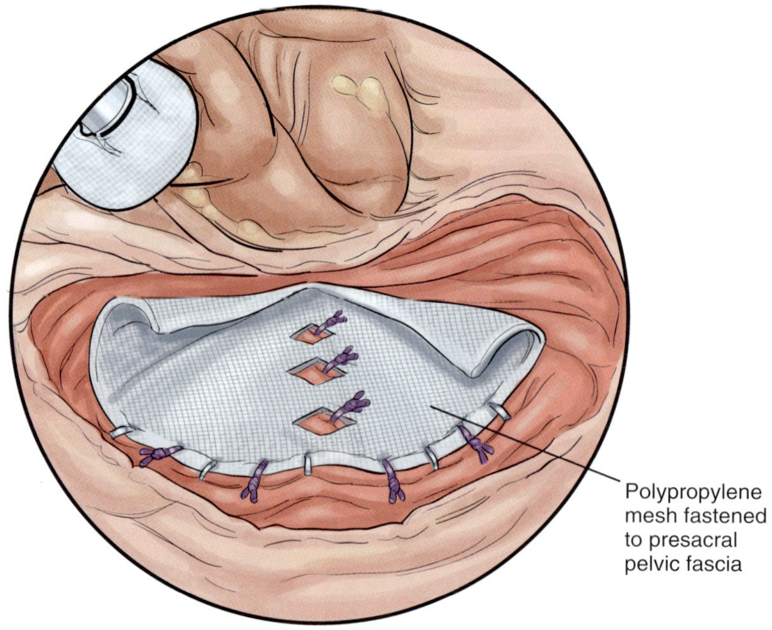

Figure 58-7.

and the splenic flexure are usually not mobilized. The division of the sigmoid mesentery is executed at midlevel, leaving the superior rectal artery and the left colonic artery intact. The sigmoid is extracted through a small (5 cm is usually sufficient) suprapubic midline or lower left-lateral incision, and a stapler descendorectostomy is performed using the usual double-stapling procedure.

- In cases with documented slow-transit constipation, left-sided hemicolectomy may be done in addition to rectopexy. In those cases the proximal resection line on the colon is chosen at the splenic flexure.

IV. SPECIAL POSTOPERATIVE CARE

- In cases of rectopexy alone, early mobilization and early enteral feeding are indicated.
- If colonic resection is performed as part of the procedure, postoperative care should follow hospital procedures for the appropriate colonic resection, without any adjustments for the rectopexy part of the procedure.
- Partial rectal incontinence is frequently observed and is usually due to the sphincter dilatation by the prolapse, becoming apparent only after the prolapse is corrected. Usually, there is considerable improvement in sphincter function over the first 3 months after the procedure.

SUGGESTED READINGS

Cadeddu F, Sileri P, Grande M, et al: Focus on abdominal rectopexy for full-thickness rectal prolapse: meta-analysis of literature, *Tech Coloproctol* 16:37–53, 2012.

Harmston C, Jones O: The evolution of laparoscopic surgery for rectal prolapse, *Int J Surg* 9:370–373, 2011. Review.

Rose J, Schneider C, Scheidbach H, et al: Laparoscopic treatment of rectal prolapse: experience gained in a prospective multicenter study, *Langenbecks Arch Surg* 387:130–137, 2002.

CHAPTER 59

Laparoscopic Colon Resection (Right, Left, Sigmoid)

Robert R. Cima, MD, MA, and John H. Pemberton, MD

I. SPECIAL PREOPERATIVE PREPARATION

- For any malignant colon lesion, a preoperative computed tomography scan should be obtained to assist in confirming localization of the lesion (if large enough to be seen) and to ensure that there is no invasion of adjacent organs, the abdominal wall, or retroperitoneal structures (Fig. 59-1, *A* and *B*).
- For polyps or smaller tumors, the colon lesion should be tattooed by endoscopic submucosal injection of India ink in four quadrants around the lesion. This will assist in the laparoscopic localization of the lesion.
- In cases of previous severe inflammatory processes involving the colon (i.e., complicated diverticulitis or Crohn disease) (Fig. 59-2) or reoperative surgery (i.e., recurrent Crohn disease at an ileocolonic anastomosis), ureteral stents should be placed to assist in ureter localization and identification of any intraoperative ureter injury.
- The operating room requirements for an efficient laparoscopic colon resection include:
  - An electronically controlled operating table with a significant range in side-to-side tilt and steep Trendelenburg and reverse Trendelenburg capability to facilitate the use of gravity to move the small intestine out of the way of dissection (Fig. 59-3).
  - A nonskid operating table surface to minimize patient movement on the table during the numerous position changes. This reduces the risk of the patient sliding off of the table, as well as the risk of shear injury to the patient's skin, which can predispose the patient to pressure-related skin breakdown. An alternative approach is to use a bean bag.
  - A minimum of three video monitors, ideally four, should be available for use during the case, with two positioned at the shoulders of the patient and one at the foot of the table.
  - Ideally all the equipment should be off the floor, attached to ceiling booms that permit easier movement of equipment during a procedure (Fig. 59-4, *A* and *B*).
- All patients need a padded chest strap placed, securing them to the table. If the patient is positioned supine on the operating table (ileal-cecal resections, right colectomy), ankle straps need to be used. For left-sided or rectal procedures, the patient's legs are placed in leg holders that allow the hips and thighs to be flat with respect to the abdomen but the lower legs to be positioned downward (i.e.,

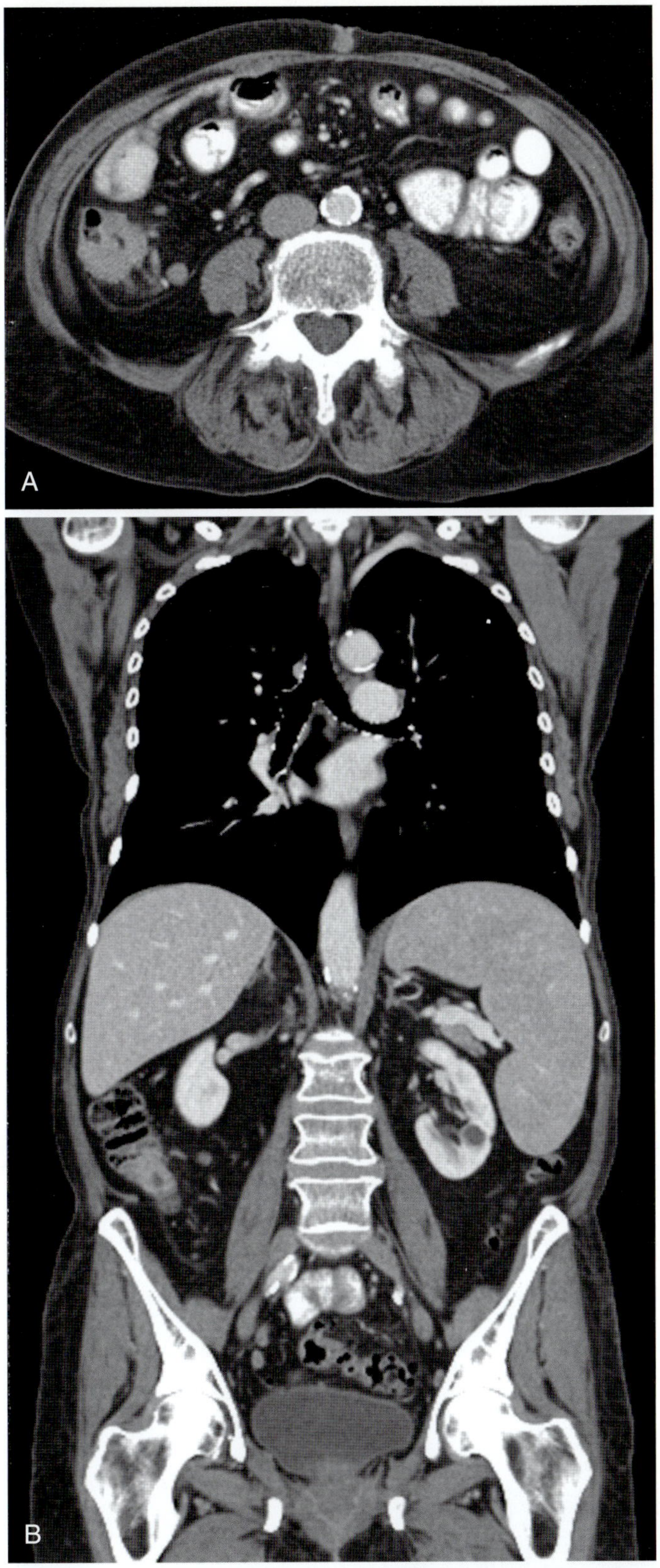

Figure 59-1. Right colon cancer with no evidence of invasion into nearby structures. This patient is a very good candidate for a laparoscopic approach.

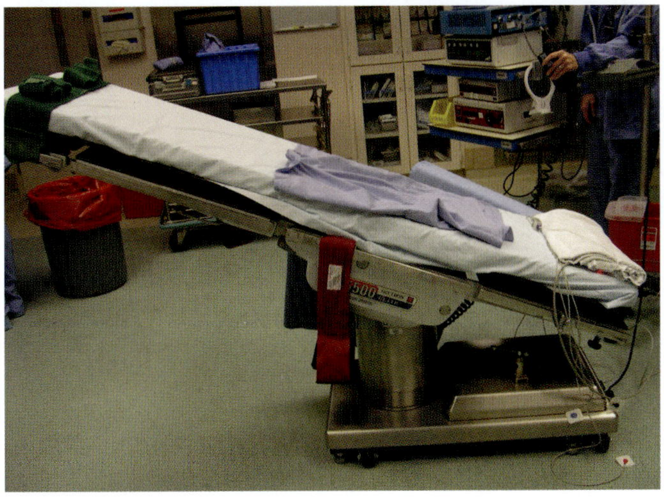

Figure 59-3. An operating table with electronic controls and a wide range of motion. Ankle straps are essential safety items.

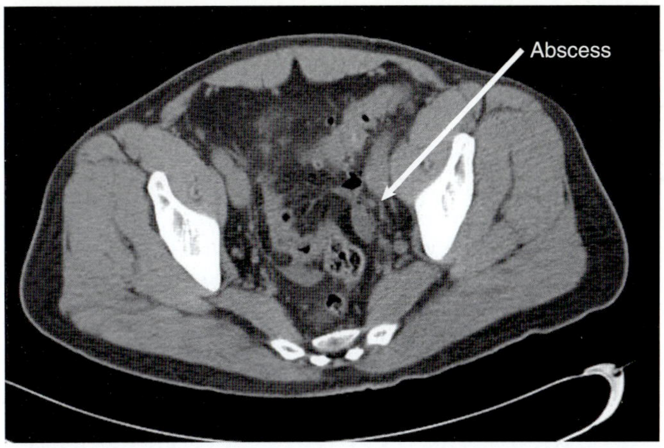

Figure 59-2. Perforated diverticulitis. This patient would certainly require preoperative ureteral stents, because the abscess involves the region where the left ureter resides.

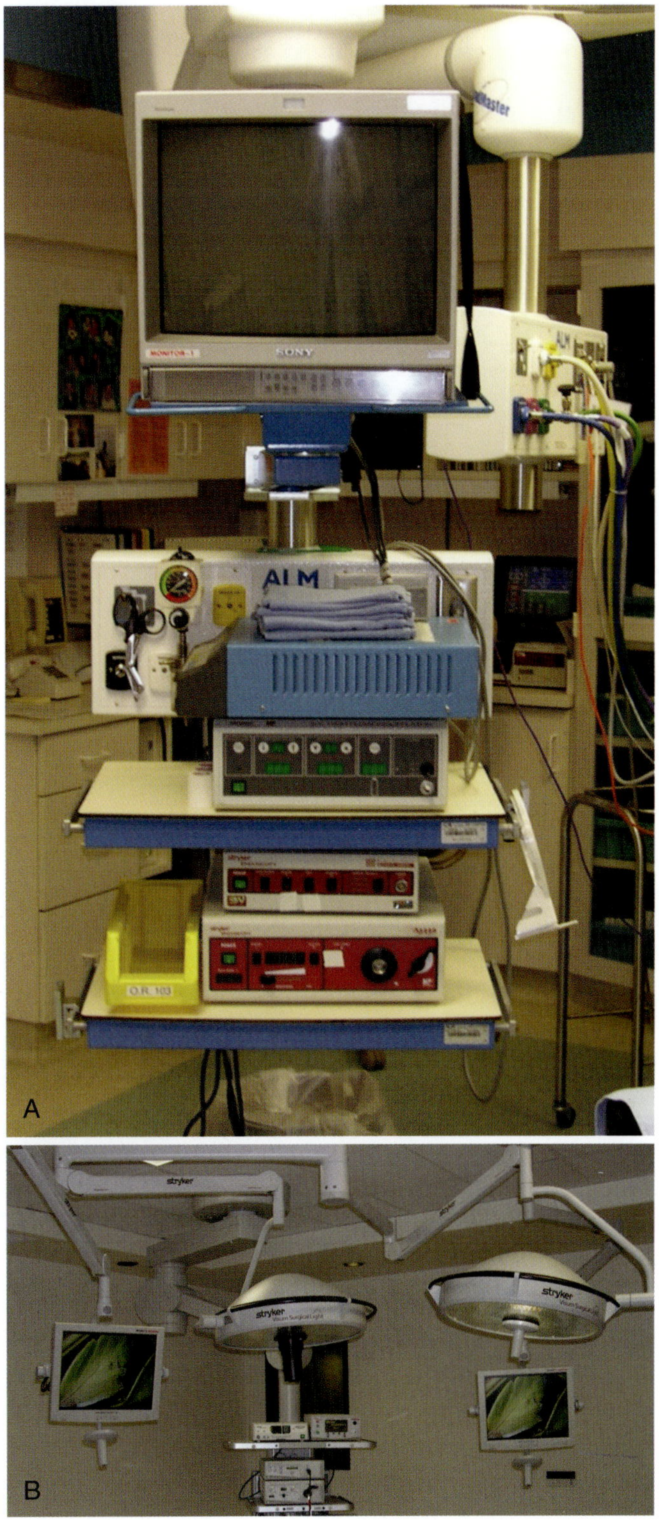

Figure 59-4. In order to maximize efficiency for laparoscopic colon procedures, all equipment and monitors should be on movable booms.

Yellofin Stirrups, Allen Medical Systems, Acton, Mass.) (Fig. 59-5). These leg holders minimize the chance of patient movement on the table during positioning changes as well as permitting access to the perineum for placement of a circular stapler or vaginal retractor/manipulator.

- We do not routinely use a mechanical bowel preparation, as it tends to cause bowel distention with liquid stool, which makes manipulation more difficult. Each patient receives one or two tap-water enemas the morning of the operation.

II. OPERATIVE TECHNIQUE: RIGHT-SIDED COLON RESECTION

LAPAROSCOPICALLY ASSISTED APPROACH

Position

- Thinner patients (body mass index less than 29) are positioned supine with arms padded and tucked at their sides. Heavier patients are positioned in the modified Lloyd-Davies position, also with their arms tucked. The advantage of using the modified Lloyd-Davies position in heavier patients is that the surgeon can stand between the legs to perform the hepatic flexure mobilization, which can be difficult from the patient's left side (Fig. 59-6, *A*).
- The surgeon and camera operator stand on the patient's left; the assistant is positioned on the right side of the table. The primary monitor is positioned over the patient's right shoulder, and the secondary monitor is by the right foot.

Trocar Placement

- An open technique is used for placement of the first trocar. A 1-cm incision is made in the midline above the umbilicus, and a 10/12-mm trocar is secured in the incision. After pneumoperitoneum is established, one 5-mm trocar is placed in the suprapubic region approximately 2 cm to the right of midline. Another 5-mm trocar is then placed 3 to 4 cm left of midline, halfway between the pubis and the 10/12-mm upper trocar. The camera is positioned in the upper trocar, whereas the surgeon's retracting instrument is in the left-sided trocar and the dissecting instrument (scissors) is in the lower trocar (see Fig. 59-6, *A*).
- The patient is positioned in steep Trendelenburg with maximal right-side elevation. This causes the small bowel to "fall out" of the pelvis and move to the left upper abdomen, facilitating mobilization of the terminal ileum and cecum.

Main Dissection

- The dissection begins by applying upward retraction of the terminal ileum/cecum toward the upper midabdomen (see Fig. 59-6, *B*; Fig. 59-7). Dissection of the retroperitoneum is performed up to the duodenum. Critical structures to identify and protect include the right ureter, gonadal vessels, iliac artery, vena cava, and duodenum (Fig. 59-8).

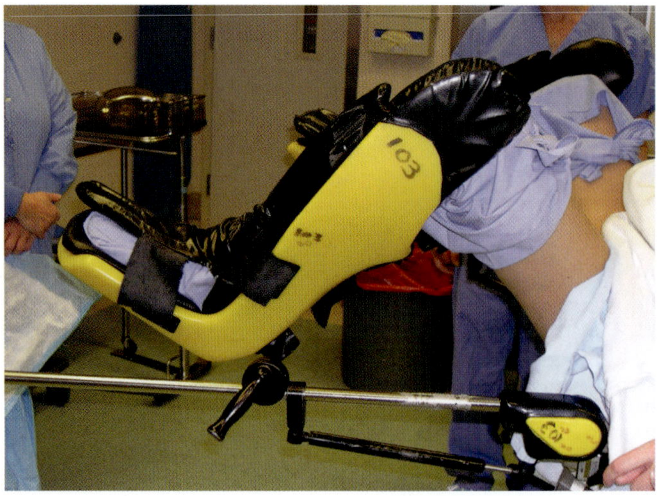

Figure 59-5. Appropriate leg support with multiposition capability is very helpful for left-sided procedures or for heavier patients, as it assists in preventing injury to the patient during position changes.

- The dissection of the colon from the retroperitoneum moves from lateral to medial and then back laterally while constant upward traction is applied.
- Once the duodenum is identified, the patient is repositioned into steep reverse Trendelenburg, maintaining maximal right side up, which causes the flexure to "fall down" toward the left lower abdomen.

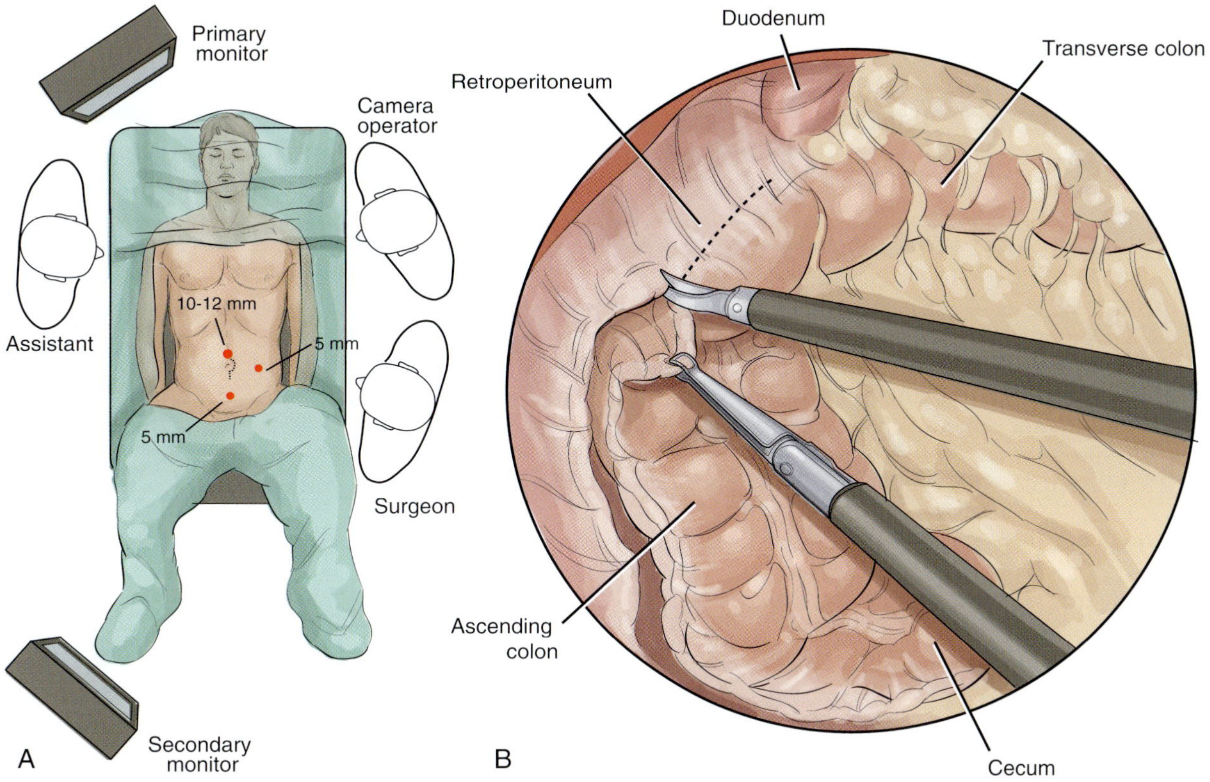

Figure 59-6.

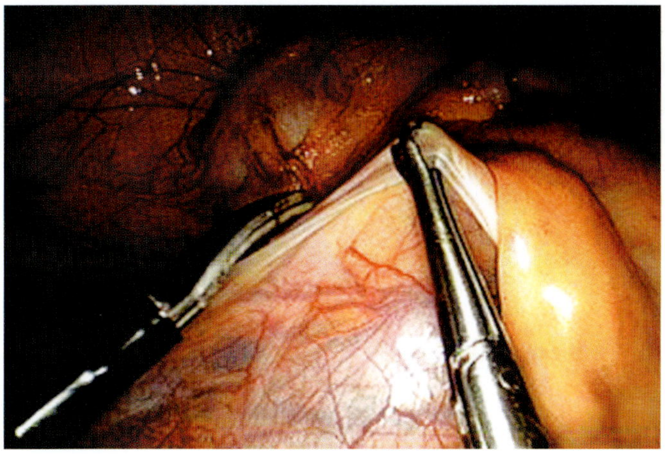

Figure 59-7.

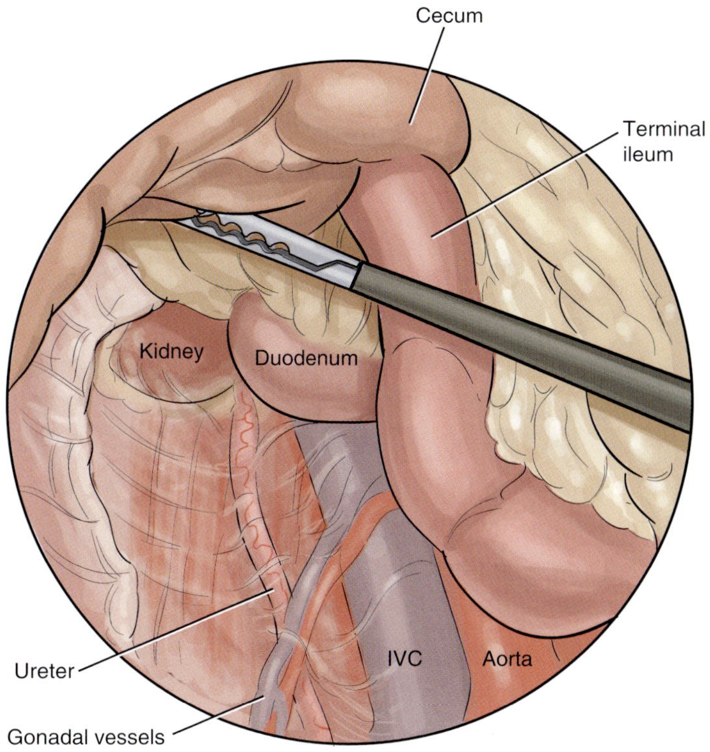

Figure 59-8. *IVC,* Inferior vena cava.

- The flexure is mobilized off of the duodenum from lateral to medial (Fig. 59-9). Once the flexure has been mobilized past the gallbladder, the colon can be exteriorized. In heavier patients, this portion of the procedure may be facilitated by having the surgeon move between the patient's legs and dissect from medial to lateral. Once the right colon has been mobilized past the gallbladder fossa and the small bowel mesentery upward near the origin of the superior mesenteric artery, the colon can be exteriorized through a small periumbilical incision (Fig. 59-10).
- A 5-cm incision is made starting at the upper trocar site. A wound protector is placed in the wound, and the colon is exteriorized. The mesentery is divided, and an anastomosis is performed (Fig. 59-11, *A* and *B*).

Closure

- The midline incision is closed with 1-0 monofilament suture. Because the incision is small, approximation is assisted if the patient remains relaxed. The skin is approximated with subcuticular 4-0 absorbable suture.

HAND-ASSISTED LAPAROSCOPIC APPROACH

- When using a hand-access device, the hand port is placed through a upper midline incision. Two 5-mm trocars are placed similar to a laparoscopically assisted (LA) right-sided resection as previously described. The surgeon stands on the patient's left and uses the right hand through the hand-access device to retract the right colon upward to the left.
- A 5-mm camera is placed through the right lower abdominal trocar while the dissecting scissors are used through the middle trocar.
- Once it is fully mobilized, the colon is extracted through the hand-access device.

III. OPERATIVE TECHNIQUE: LEFT-SIDED COLON RESECTION (LEFT AND SIGMOID COLON)

LAPAROSCOPICALLY ASSISTED APPROACH

Position

- The patient is placed in the modified Lloyd-Davies position with the arms tucked and is secured to the operating table by a chest strap.

Trocar Placement

- A 10- to 12-mm trocar is placed in the midline just above the umbilicus, using an open technique. One 5-mm trocar is placed in the midline 1 cm above the pubis. Another 5-mm trocar is placed between the supraumbilical and suprapubic trocars (Fig. 59-12, *A*).

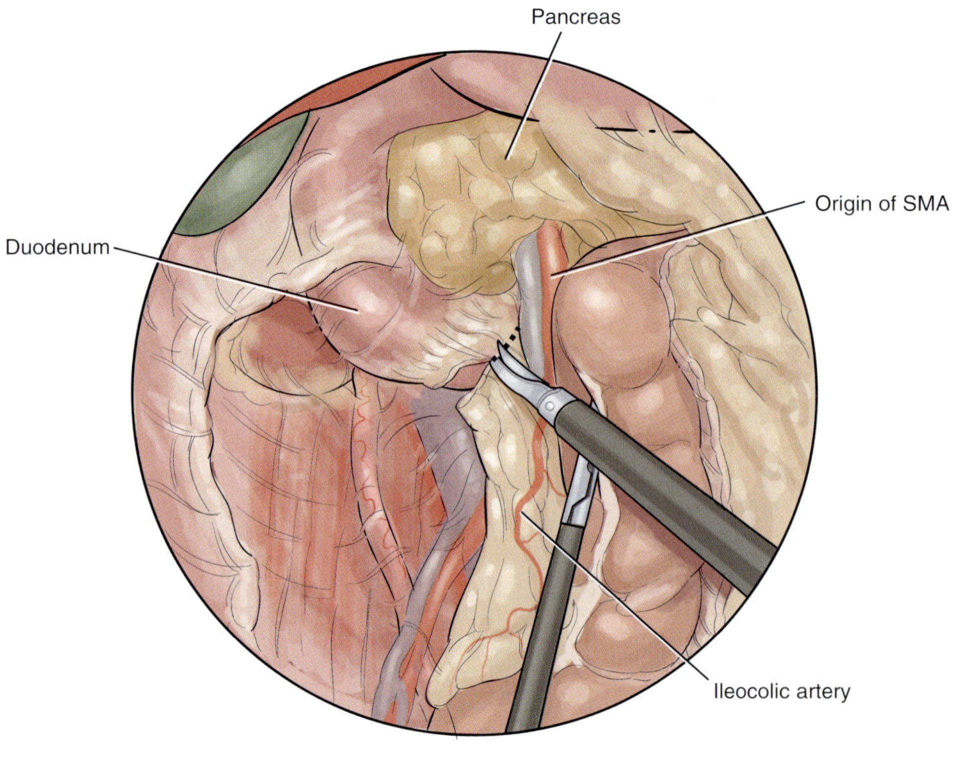

Figure 59-9. *SMA,* Superior mesenteric artery.

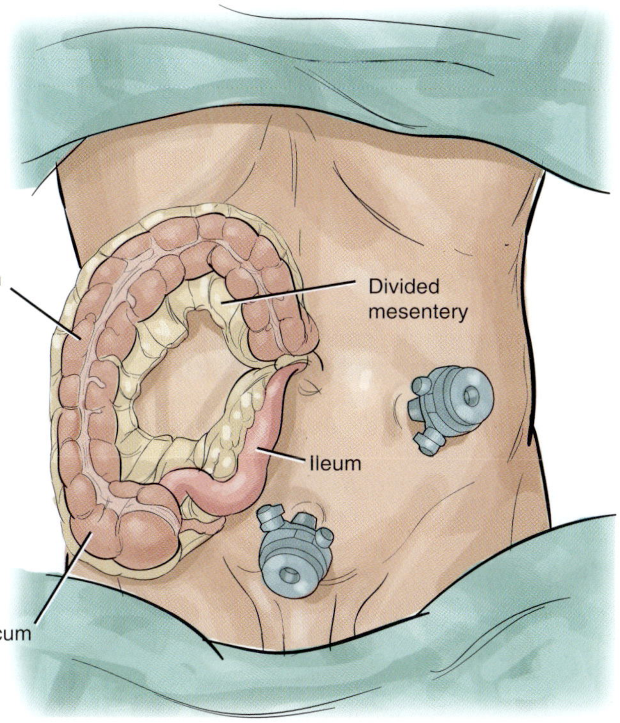

Figure 59-10.

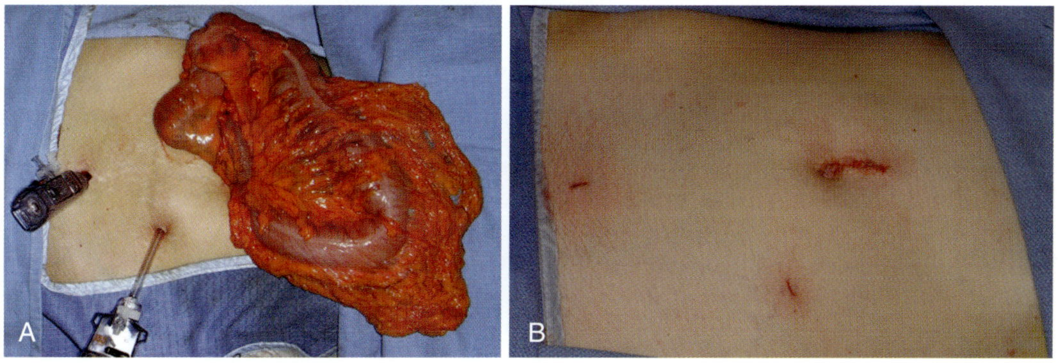

Figure 59-11. **A**, Photograph demonstrating how much colon can be brought out through a small incision if the colon is fully mobilized. **B**, End result of a laparoscopic right hemicolectomy.

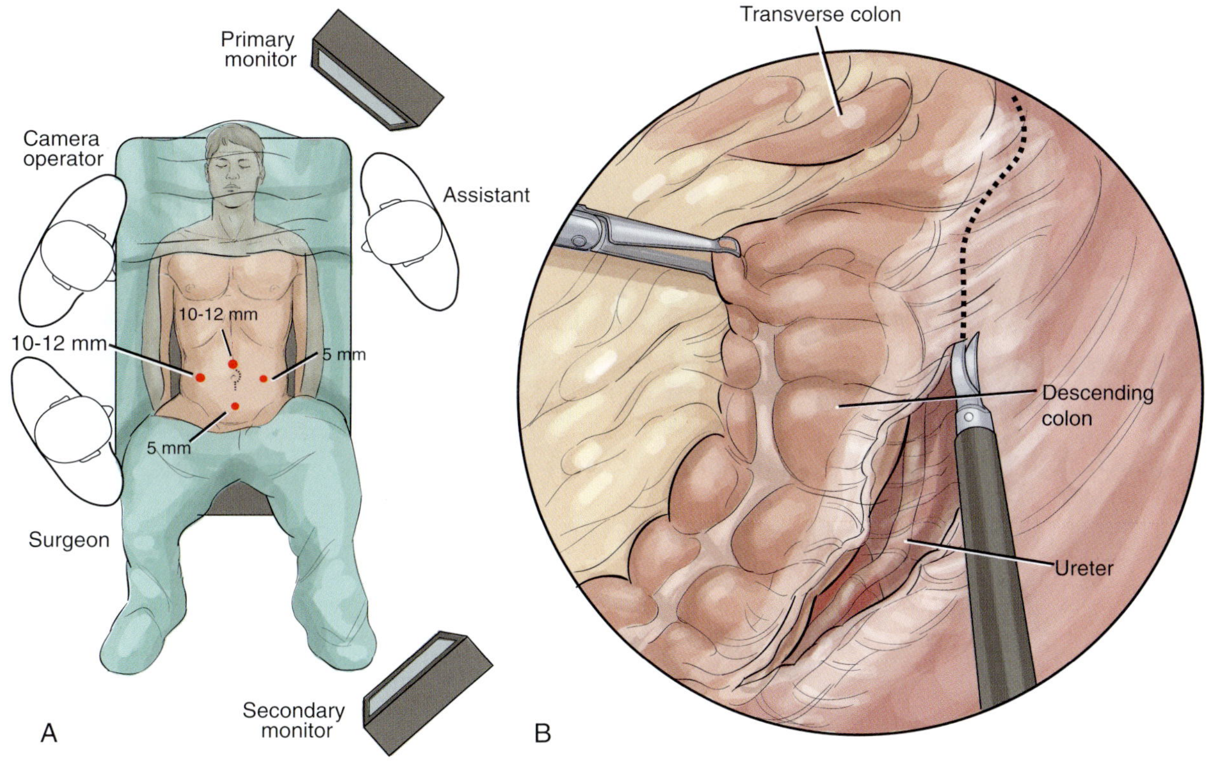

Figure 59-12.

- With the camera in the supraumbilical trocar and with the patient in steep Trendelenburg and maximal left side up, the surgeon standing on the patient's right side uses the midabdomen trocar for the retracting instrument and places the dissecting instrument in the suprapubic trocar.

Main Dissection

- The dissection begins at the pelvic brim and progresses upward along the descending colon (see Fig. 59-12, *B*).
- To mobilize the splenic flexure, the patient is repositioned in steep reverse Trendelenburg. The surgeon moves between the patient's legs (Fig. 59-13, *A*). Traction is applied downward toward the right lower quadrant to continue dissection around the flexure toward the mid-transverse colon.
- Often it is necessary to place another 5-mm trocar in the left midabdomen laterally, for the assistant from the patient's left side to retract the omentum upward and to the right to facilitate the dissection of the splenic flexure and distal transverse colon (see Fig. 59-13, *B*). This maneuver provides access into the lesser sac, which aids in splenic flexure mobilization.
- Our practice is to exteriorize the colon through a small low-midline or Pfannenstiel incision. Depending on the thickness of the patient's mesentery, the mesentery can be divided outside the abdomen or within the abdomen, making use of a 5-mm vessel sealing and cutting device (LigaSure, Valleylab, Boulder, Colo.) through the left lower quadrant trocar.

Closure

- The midline incision is closed with 1-0 monofilament suture. Because the incision is small, approximation is assisted if the patient remains relaxed. The skin is approximated with subcuticular 4-0 absorbable suture.

HAND-ASSISTED LAPAROSCOPIC APPROACH

- The patient is positioned in the modified Lloyd-Davies position with arms tucked at the sides.
- A small (7- to 8-cm) midline incision or Pfannenstiel incision is made 2 cm above the pubis (Fig. 59-14, *A*).
- A 5-mm trocar is placed in the midline just above the umbilicus for the camera, and another 5-mm trocar is placed in the left lower abdomen, 1.5 to 2 cm medial to the superior iliac spine.

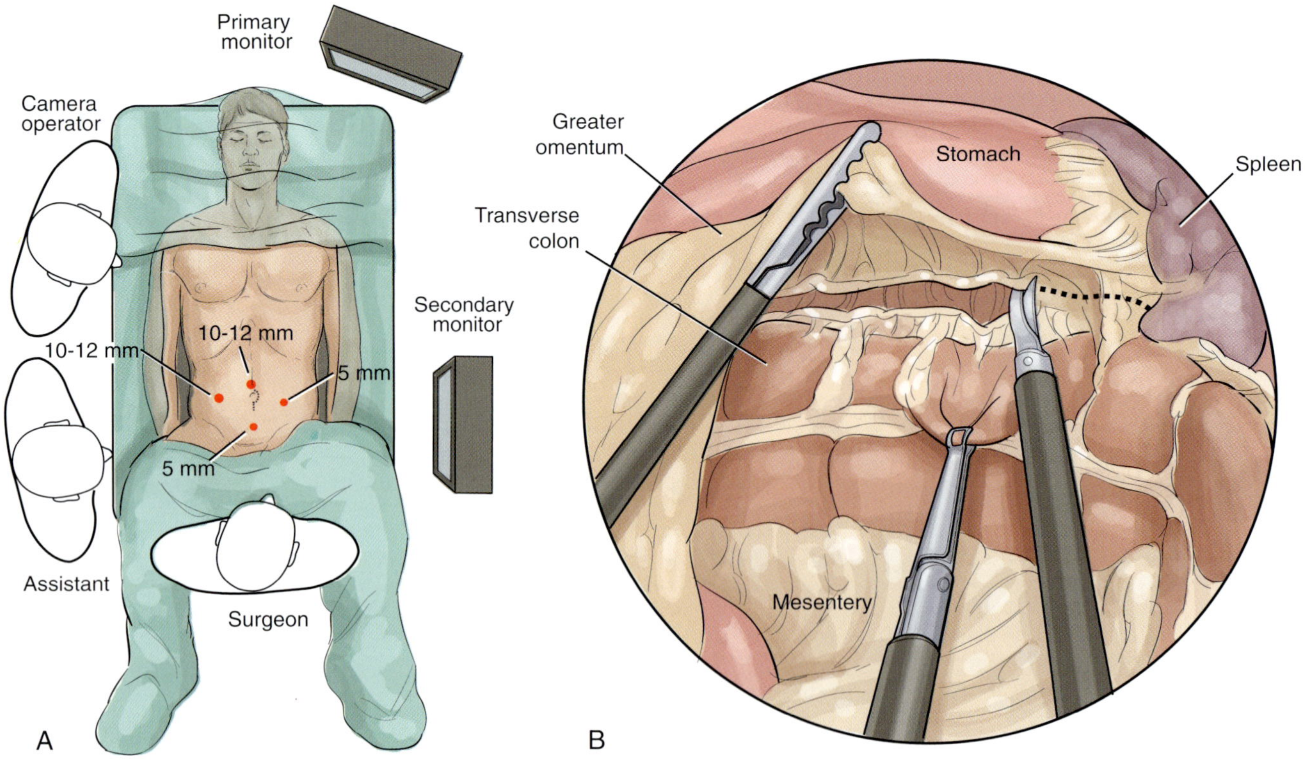

Figure 59-13.

- The surgeon stands between the patient's legs, with the camera operator on the patient's right side.
- The surgeon places the left hand into the abdomen and retracts the left colon toward the midline while dissecting with an electrified laparoscopic scissor through the left lower quadrant trocar (see Fig. 59-14, *B*; Fig. 59-15, *A*, *B*, and *C*).
- Initially, the patient is in steep Trendelenburg with the left side up, but as the dissection progresses upward toward the splenic flexure, the patient's position is changed to reverse Trendelenburg. This causes the splenic flexure to descend toward the surgeon's retracting hand.

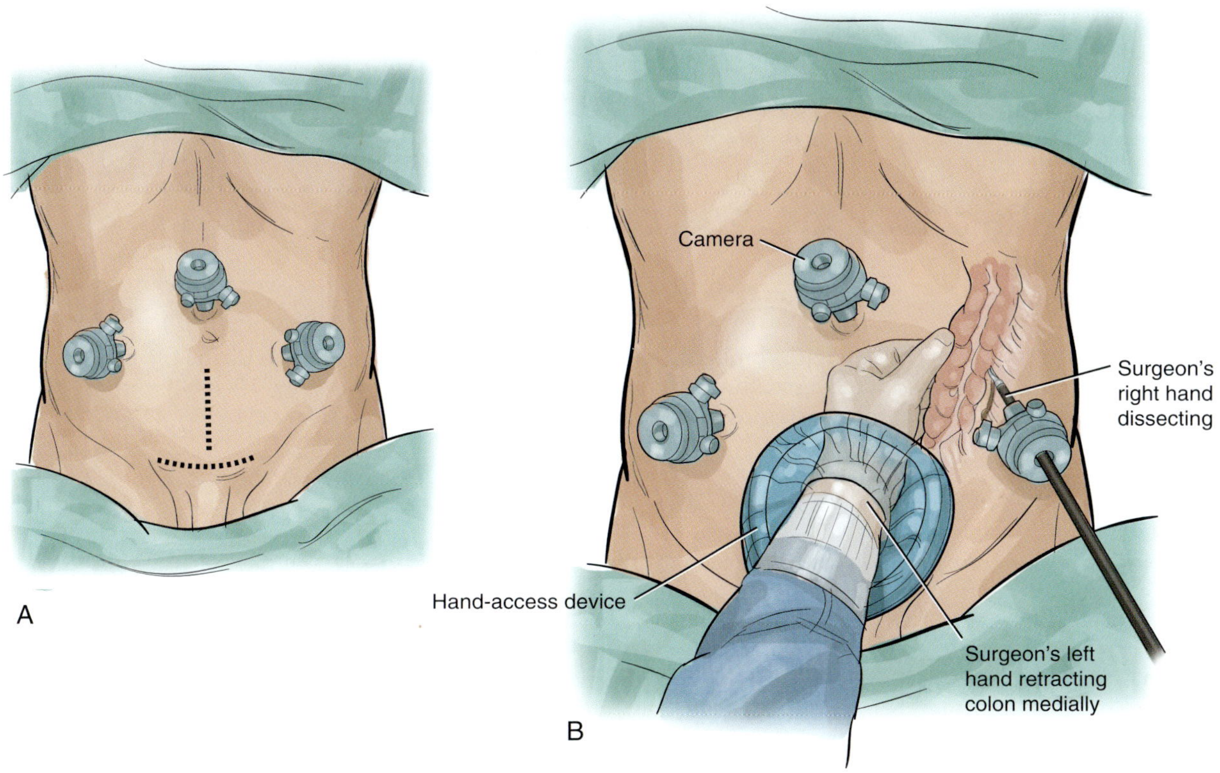

Figure 59-14.

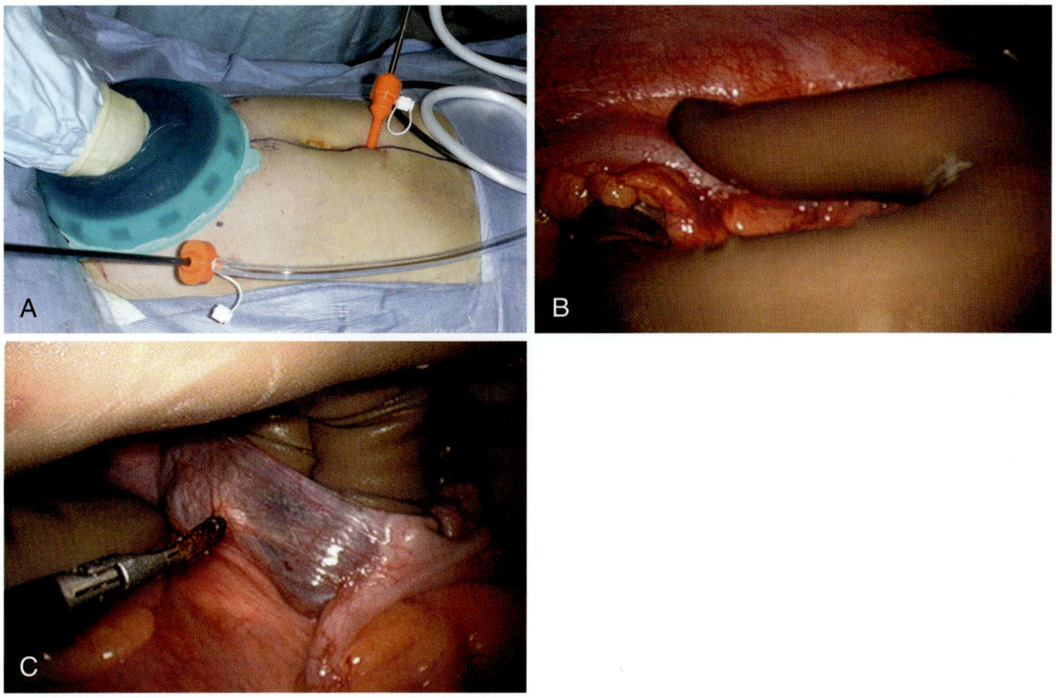

Figure 59-15. Hand-assisted laparoscopic left colon resection. A, Surgeon is between the patient's legs dissecting with the right hand while retracting the colon medially with the left hand. The camera is in the supraumbilical 5-mm trocar. **B,** The hand in the abdomen retracting the left colon medially. **C,** The surgeon's hand assisting in dissection of the pelvic sigmoid colon.

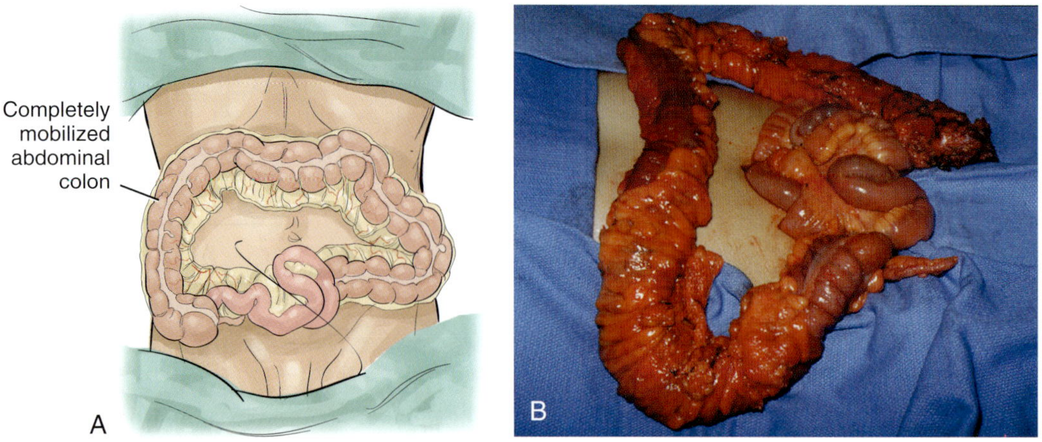

Figure 59-16. The completely mobilized abdominal colon brought out through the hand-access site.

- Once the colon is mobilized, it is brought out through the hand-access device to divide the mesentery, or a vessel-sealing device is used through the left lower quadrant trocar (Fig. 59-16, *A* and *B*). The bowel is divided, and the anastomosis is performed through the hand-access device.

IV. ALTERNATIVE TECHNICAL APPROACHES (PRO/CON) AND PEARLS

- Conversion from a laparoscopic approach to an open approach is associated with loss of the short-term clinical benefits of an LA approach and, in some studies, increased complications. Our practice is to convert from an LA to a hand-assisted laparoscopic approach, which retains the short-term benefits of the LA technique.
- In obese patients, it is more effective to move the placement of the trocars or hand-access device higher on the abdomen. This is most critical for hand-access device placement, as it is very difficult to have the device in the thickest part of the abdominal wall pannus.
- In a left-sided resection, if a temporary diverting ileostomy is planned, a 10- to 12-mm trocar can be placed in the planned stoma site in the right lower quadrant.

V. SPECIAL POSTOPERATIVE CARE

- Only oral gastric tubes are used during the operation, and they are removed at the end of the case.
- Intravenous fluids are minimized during the case and in the postoperative period. Fluid boluses are kept to a minimum, as increased total body water is associated with delayed return of bowel function and postoperative complications.
- Abdominal drains are rarely placed; if placed, they are removed early in the postoperative period.
- Urinary catheters are removed 24 hours after surgery for all laparoscopic abdominal colon procedures.
- All patients are started on a full liquid diet the morning after surgery. This is limited to less than 1 liter intake on postoperative day 1. If full liquids are tolerated, an unrestricted soft diet is begun on postoperative day 2.

SUGGESTED READINGS

Boller AM, Larson DW: Laparoscopic restorative proctocolectomy for ulcerative colitis, *J Gastrointest Surg* 11:3–7, 2007.

Marcello PW, Fleshman JW, Milsom JW, et al: Hand-assisted laparoscopic vs. laparoscopic colorectal surgery: a multicenter, prospective, randomized trial, *Dis Colon Rectum* 51:818–826, discussion 826–828, 2008.

Young-Fadok TM, Nelson H: Laparoscopic right colectomy: five-step procedure, *Dis Colon Rectum* 43:267–271, discussion 271–273, 2000.

CHAPTER 60

Surgical Procedures for Peritoneal Surface Malignancy

Paul H. Sugarbaker, MD, FACS, FRCS, and Lana Bijelic, MD, FACS

Background

Locations of Peritoneal Surface Malignancy

- Peritoneal surface malignancy tends to involve the visceral peritoneum in greatest volume at three definite sites. These are sites where the bowel is anchored to the retroperitoneum and peristalsis results in less motion of the visceral peritoneal surface.
- The rectosigmoid colon, as it comes up out of the pelvis, is a nonmobile portion of the bowel. Also, it is a dependent site, and therefore, it frequently requires resection. Usually a complete pelvic peritonectomy involves stripping of the abdominal sidewalls, the peritoneum overlying the bladder, the cul-de-sac, and the rectosigmoid colon.
- The ileocecal valve is another area where there is limited mobility. Resection of the terminal ileum and a small portion of the right colon is often necessary.
- A final site often requiring special attention is the antrum of the stomach. The antrum of the stomach is fixed to the retroperitoneum at the pylorus.
- Tumor coming into the foramen of Winslow accumulates in the subpyloric space and can cause intestinal obstruction as a result of gastric outlet obstruction. Occasionally, tumor in the lesser omentum will cause a confluence of disease on the lesser curvature of the stomach and encasement of the left gastric artery. Complete resection might require total gastrectomy, including the left gastric artery.

Electroevaporative Surgery

- To adequately perform cytoreductive surgery, the surgeon must use high-voltage electrosurgery. Peritonectomies and visceral resections using the traditional scissors and knife dissection will result in a large volume of small-vessel bleeding. Also, clean peritoneal surfaces devoid of cancer cells are less likely to occur with sharp dissection as compared to electrosurgical dissection. Electroevaporative surgery leaves a margin of heat necrosis that is devoid of viable malignant cells. Electroevaporation of tumor and normal tissue at the margins of resection minimizes the likelihood of persistent disease and also minimizes blood loss.
- The standard tool used to dissect tumor on peritoneal surfaces from the normal tissues is a 3-mm ball-tipped electrosurgical handpiece (Valleylab, Boulder, Colo.). The ball-tipped instrument is placed at the interface of tumor and normal tissues. The focal point for further dissection is placed on strong traction. The electrosurgical generator is used on pure cut at high voltage. The 3-mm ball-tipped electrode is used cautiously for tumor removal on tubular structures, especially the ureters, small bowel, and colon. Dissection of parietal peritoneal surfaces presents less risk for heat necrosis and fistula formation.
- Using ball-tipped electrosurgery on pure cut creates a large volume of plume because of the electroevaporation (carbonization) of tissue. To maintain visualization of the operative field and to preserve a smoke-free atmosphere, a smoke filtration unit is used (Stackhouse Associates, El Segundo, Calif.).

The vacuum tip is maintained 2 to 3 inches (5 to 7.5 cm) from the field of dissection whenever electrosurgery is in use.

- Extensive cytoreductions in the absence of perioperative intraperitoneal chemotherapy may actually harm patients in the long run rather than help them. Extensive removal of peritoneal surfaces without intraperitoneal chemotherapy allows tumor cells to become implanted within a deeper layer of the abdomen and pelvis. This can contribute to obstruction of vital structures such as the ureter or common bile duct. Also, deep involvement of the pelvic sidewall and tissues along the iliac vessels will occur.
- The surgeon who attempts to treat peritoneal surface malignancy must become thoroughly familiar with the techniques of intraoperative chemotherapy and early postoperative intraperitoneal chemotherapy.
- Complete cytoreduction, aggressive perioperative intraperitoneal chemotherapy, and proper patient selection are the three essential requirements of treatment for peritoneal surface malignancy.

I. SPECIAL PREOPERATIVE PREPARATION

- If the patient has received prior systemic chemotherapy, at least 1 month must pass between the last cycle of systemic chemotherapy and the cytoreduction. If prior treatment includes bevacizumab, then an 8-week interval is used. The patient is asked to identify a personal trainer to work with to maximize his or her general physical condition.
- A computed tomography scan with maximal oral and intravenous contrast is obtained within a few days before the cytoreductive procedure to rule out the interval development of systemic metastases and judge the rate of progression of the peritoneal metastases. A positron emission tomography–computed tomography scan is usually obtained on colon cancer patients who had lymph node positivity at the time of their primary colorectal cancer resection. A complete bowel prep is mandatory before cytoreductive surgery.

II. OPERATIVE TECHNIQUE

Position

- The patient is supine with the gluteal fold advanced to the end of the operating table to allow full access to the perineum during the surgical procedure (Fig. 60-1, *A*).
- This lithotomy position is achieved with the legs extended in St Mark's leg holders (AMSCO, Erie, Pa.). The weight of the legs must be directed to the soles of the feet by positioning the footrest so that minimal weight is on the calf muscle. Myonecrosis within the gastrocnemius muscle may occur unless the legs are protected by foam padding. The legs are surrounded by alternating-pressure boots (SCB Compression Boots, Kendall Co., Boston). These should be operative before the start of anesthesia for maximal protection against venothrombosis.
- A heating apparatus is placed over the chest and arms of the patient (Bair Hugger Upper Body Cover, Augustine Medical, Eden Prairie, Minn.) and also beneath the torso (Cincinnati Sub-Zero, Cincinnati).
- Abdominal skin is prepared from midchest to midthigh. The external genitalia are prepared in the male, and a vaginal preparation is used in females. The Foley catheter is placed in position. A Silastic 18-gauge nasogastric sump tube (Argyle Salem Sump Tube, Sherwood Medical, St. Louis) is inserted in the stomach and later confirmed to be positioned along the greater curvature of the stomach.

Construction of the Surgical Field to Provide Simultaneous Exposure of the Abdomen and Pelvis

- A self-retaining retractor (Thompson Surgical Instruments, Traverse City, Mich.) is positioned so that continuous retraction of all parts of the abdominal incision occurs (see Fig. 60-1, *B*). The retraction system must be securely anchored to the operating table to provide for continuous unencumbered visualization of the large operative field. Numerous pieces of surgical equipment are anchored to the self-retaining retractor outside of the bars used to hold rail clamps. Smoke evacuators are positioned superiorly and inferiorly to the field. The inferior smoke evacuator is a handheld tubing that is to be maintained approximately 5 cm from the electrosurgical clip by the scrub nurse. The clamp that secures the suction tubing makes this apparatus readily accessible. Without adequate smoke evacuation, there is dangerous environmental contamination from the electroevaporative surgery.
- The electrosurgical tip is a ball tip that allows contouring of the plane of dissection. The electrosurgery is used on pure cut at high voltage for dissection. When small bleeding points are encountered, high-voltage electrocoagulation is used. Abrasive pads are located at convenient sites on the right and left sides of the patient to allow rapid removal of tissue coagulant from the ball tip.

- Frequent irrigation of the operative field with a saline solution cools the tissues, irrigates away blood or blood products that may accumulate, and increases the conduction of the electrosurgical current.

Incision

- An incision starting above the xiphisternal junction to the pubis through the midline is constructed. An ellipse is created around the umbilicus to allow the peritoneal plane to be clearly exposed throughout the extent of the abdominal incision. Also, retaining the umbilicus leads to a high incidence of recurrence at this site. The fascia is divided through the linea alba from xiphoid bone to pubic bone. If there has been a prior midline abdominal incision, it is widely excised. Routinely, the xiphoid is completely resected at the xiphisternal junction as part of the specimen. With the fascia divided, the parietal peritoneum remains intact.

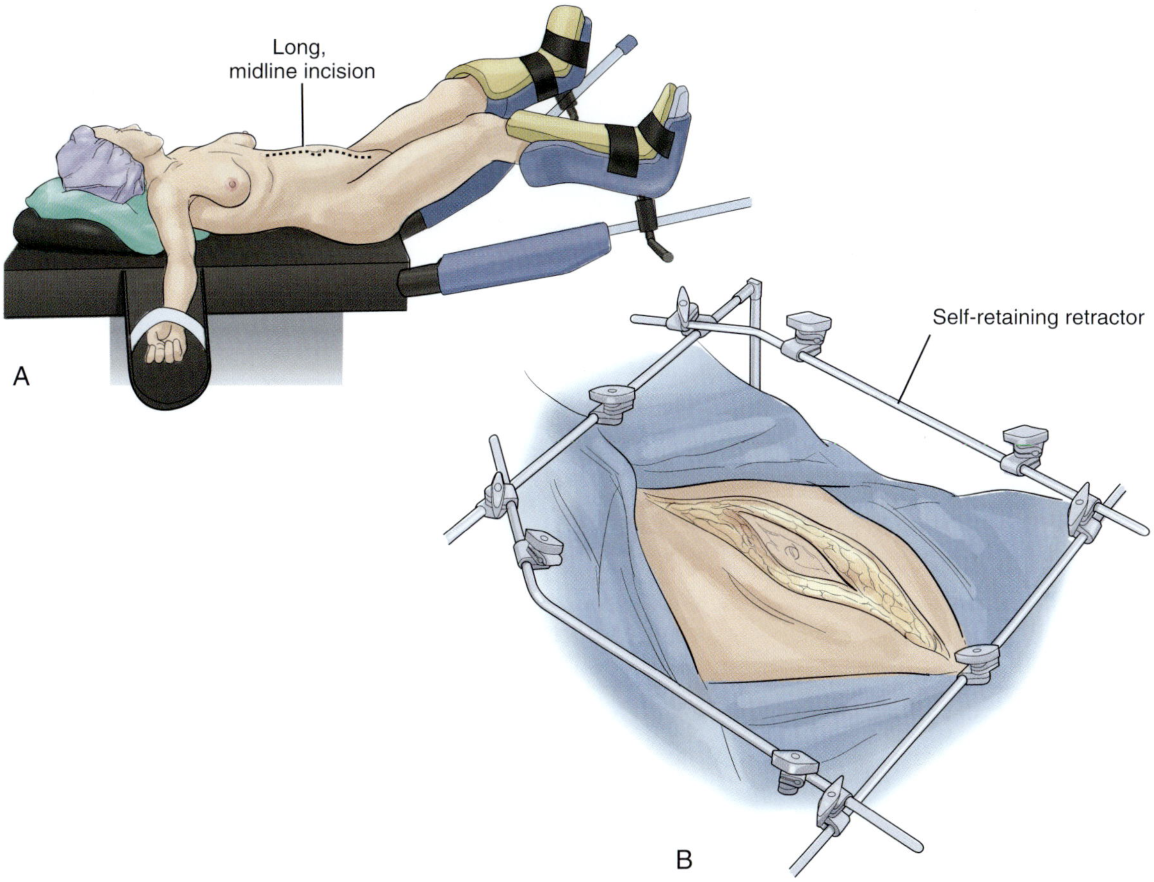

Figure 60-1.

Main Dissection

Parietal Peritoneal Stripping from the Anterior Abdominal Wall

- A single entry into the peritoneal cavity in the upper portion of the incision allows the surgeon to assess the requirement for a complete parietal peritonectomy (Fig. 60-2). If cancer nodules are palpated on the parietal peritoneum, a decision for a complete dissection is made. Except for the small defect in the peritoneum required for this peritoneal exploration, the remainder of the peritoneum is kept intact. Adair clamps are placed on the skin edge to provide broad traction along the complete line for tissue transection. The dissecting tool is the ball tip, and smoke evacuation is used continuously.

Stripping the Visceral Peritoneum from the Surface of the Bladder

- After generously dissecting the peritoneum on the right and left sides of the bladder, the apex of the bladder is localized and placed on strong traction using a Babcock clamp. The peritoneum with the underlying fatty tissues is stripped away from the surface of the bladder. Broad traction on the entire anterior parietal peritoneal surface and frequent saline irrigation reveal the point for tissue transection that is precisely located between the bladder musculature and its adherent fatty tissue. This dissection is continued inferiorly downward to the cervix in the female or to the seminal vesicles in the male. A continuous wide abdominal exposure is maintained through the use of a self-retaining retractor (Thompson Surgical Instruments).

Parietal Peritoneal Dissection to the Paracolic Sulcus and Beyond

- The self-retaining retraction system is steadily advanced progressively deeper into the abdominal cavity. This optimizes the broad traction at the point of dissection of the peritoneum and its underlying tissues. The peritoneum strips readily from the undersurface of the hemidiaphragm. It is most adherent directly

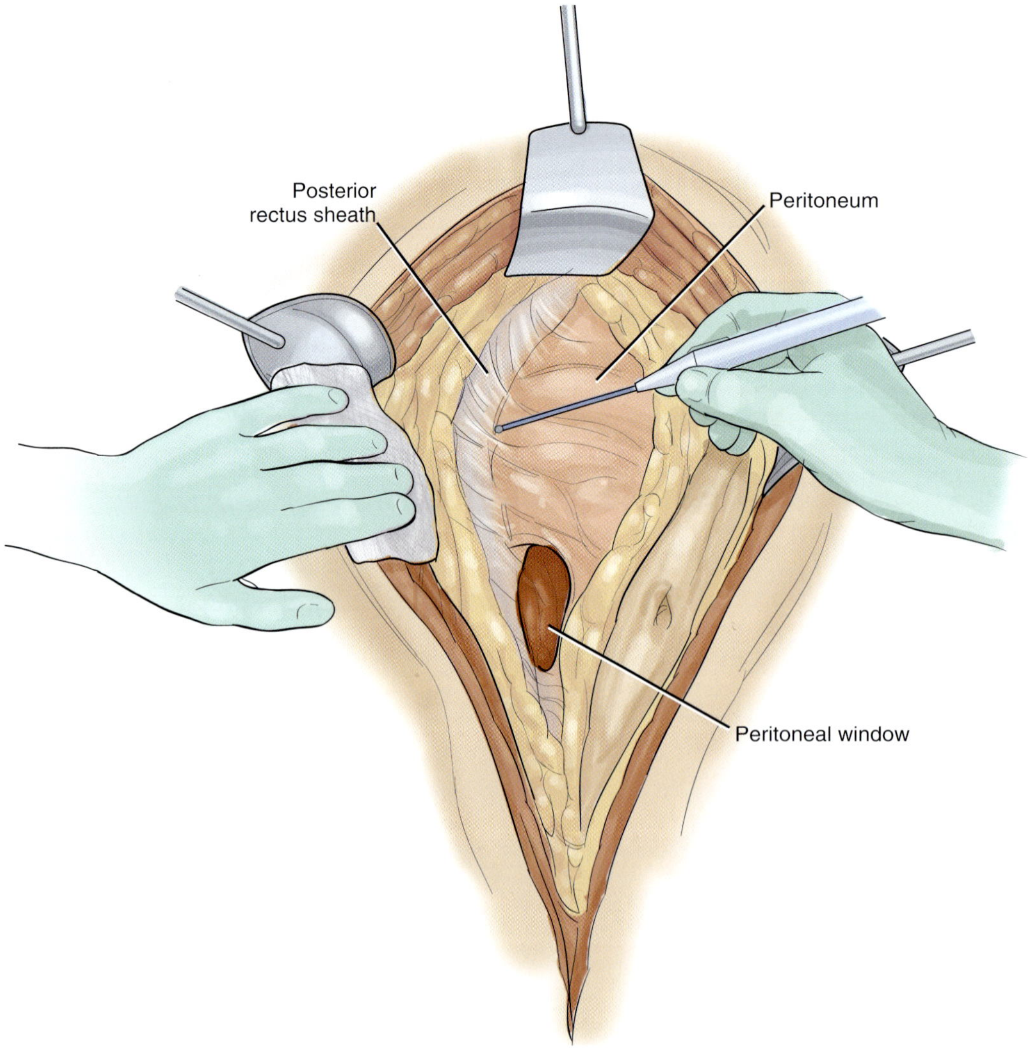

Figure 60-2.

overlying the transversus muscle. In some instances, blunt dissection from inferior to superior aspects of the abdominal wall facilitates clearing in this area. The dissection joins the right and left subphrenic peritonectomy superiorly and the complete pelvic peritonectomy inferiorly. As the dissection proceeds beyond the peritoneum overlying the paracolic sulcus (line of Toldt), the dissection proceeds more rapidly because of the loose connections of the peritoneum to the underlying fatty tissue at this anatomic site.

- Removal of this large peritoneal layer eradicates cancer implants from the posterior aspect of the anterior abdominal wall. Complete exploration of the abdomen and pelvis proceeds.

Peritoneal Stripping from beneath the Left Hemidiaphragm

- To begin peritonectomy of the left upper quadrant, the peritoneum is progressively stripped off the posterior rectus sheath. Broad traction must be exerted on the tumor specimen throughout the left upper quadrant. Strong traction combined with ball-tipped electrosurgical dissection allows separation of surface tumor from all normal tissue in the left upper quadrant, including the diaphragmatic muscle, the left adrenal gland, and the superior half of the perirenal fat. The splenic flexure of the colon is released from the peritoneum of the left abdominal gutter and moved medially.
- The dissection between diaphragm muscle and its peritoneal covering is performed with electroevaporative surgery, not by blunt dissection. Numerous blood vessels between the diaphragm muscle and its peritoneal surface are electrocoagulated before their transection, or unnecessary bleeding will occur as the divided blood vessel retracts into the muscle of the diaphragm. Tissues are dissected using ball-tipped electrosurgery on pure cut; all blood vessels are electrocoagulated before their division.

Greater Omentectomy and Splenectomy with Completion of the Left Subphrenic Peritonectomy

- To free the midabdomen of a large volume of tumor, the greater omentectomy-splenectomy is performed (Fig. 60-3). The greater omentum is elevated and then separated from the transverse colon using electrosurgery. This dissection continues beneath the peritoneum that covers the transverse

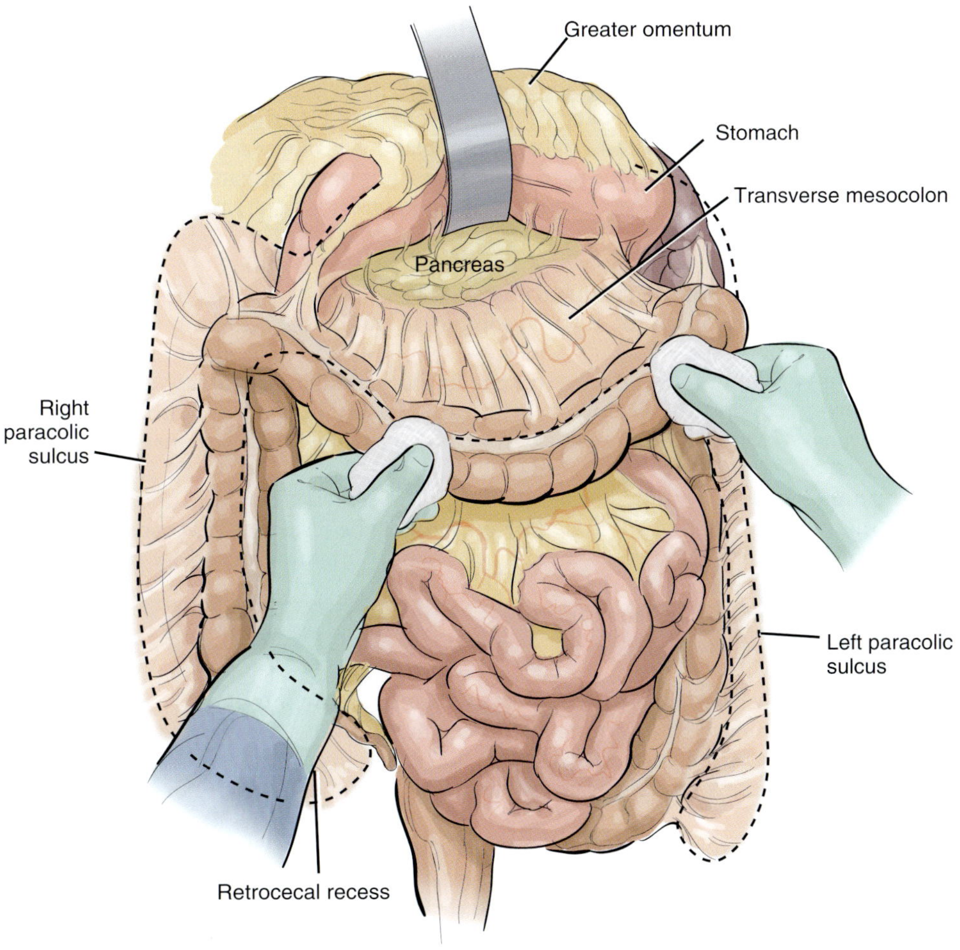

Figure 60-3.

mesocolon to expose the pancreas. The gastroepiploic vessels on the greater curvature of the stomach are clamped, ligated, and divided. Also, the short gastric vessels are transected. The mound of tumor that covers the spleen is identified. With traction on the spleen, the peritoneum anterior to the pancreas is stripped from the gland using electrosurgery. This freely exposes the splenic artery and vein at the tail of the pancreas. These vessels are ligated in continuity and proximally suture ligated. This allows the greater curvature of the stomach to be reflected to the right from the pylorus to the gastroesophageal junction.

- If clear access to the splenic vessels cannot be achieved by an anterior approach, they can be visualized posteriorly after completion of the left subphrenic stripping. Generous dissection posterior to the body of the pancreas allows its elevation without a crack in the pancreas capsule.
- When the upper-quadrant peritonectomy is completed, the stomach can be reflected medially. Numerous branches of the gastroepiploic arteries that have been ligated are evident. The left adrenal gland, pancreas, and left perirenal fatty tissue are visualized completely, as is the anterior peritoneal surface of the transverse mesocolon. The surgeon must avoid the main left gastric artery and its branches and the left gastric vein to preserve the sole remaining vascular supply to the stomach.

Peritoneal Stripping from beneath the Right Hemidiaphragm

- Peritoneum is stripped from the right posterior rectus sheath to begin the peritonectomy in the right upper quadrant of the abdomen. Strong traction on the specimen is used to elevate the hemidiaphragm into the operative field. Again, ball-tipped electrosurgery on pure cut is used to dissect at the interface of tumor and normal tissue. Coagulation current is used to divide the blood vessels as they are encountered and before they bleed.
- The stripping of the tumor from the undersurface of the diaphragm continues until the bare area of the liver is encountered. At that point, tumor on the superior surface of the liver is electroevaporated until the liver surface is cleared. With ball-tipped electrosurgical dissection, a thick layer of tumor is lifted off the dome of the liver by removing the Glisson capsule. Isolated patches of tumor on the liver surface are electroevaporated with the distal 2 cm of the ball tip bent and stripped of insulation ("hockey stick" configuration). Ball-tipped electrosurgery is used to extirpate tumor from attachments of the falciform ligament and round ligament.

Removal of an Envelope of Tumor from beneath the Right Hemidiaphragm, from the Right Subhepatic Space, and from the Surface of the Liver

- Tumor from beneath the right hemidiaphragm, the right subhepatic space, and the surface of the liver forms an envelope as it is removed en bloc (Fig. 60-4). The dissection is greatly facilitated if the tumor specimen can remain intact. The dissection continues laterally on the right to encounter the perirenal fat covering the right kidney. Also, the right adrenal gland is visualized and carefully avoided as tumor is stripped from the right subhepatic space. Care is taken not to traumatize the vena cava or to disrupt the caudate lobe veins that pass between the vena cava and segment I of the liver.

Completed Right Subphrenic Peritonectomy

- With strong upward traction on the right costal margin by the self-retaining retractor and medial displacement of the right liver, one can visualize the completed right subphrenic peritonectomy. The anterior branches of the phrenic artery and vein on the hemidiaphragm are visualized and preserved. The right hepatic vein and the vena cava below are exposed. The right subhepatic space, including the right adrenal gland and perirenal fat covering the right kidney, constitutes the base of the dissection.
- Frequently, tumor is densely adherent to the tendinous central portion of the left or right hemidiaphragm. If this occurs, the tissue infiltrated by tumor must be resected. This usually requires an elliptical excision of a central portion of the hemidiaphragm. It might be necessary on the right or the left but is more frequently needed on the right. The defect in the diaphragm is closed with interrupted sutures after the intraoperative chemotherapy is completed.

Cholecystectomy with Stripping of the Hepatoduodenal Ligament

- The gallbladder is removed in a routine fashion from its fundus toward the cystic artery and cystic duct. Blunt dissection of the base of the gallbladder away from the common duct and right hepatic artery distinguishes these structures from the surrounding tumor and fatty tissue. These structures are ligated and divided.
- To strip the peritoneum from the anterior aspect of the hepatoduodenal ligament, its peritoneal reflection to the liver surface is released. Special care is taken not to injure the left hepatic artery, which is usually the most superficial of the portal structures. The peritoneum is firmly grasped using a Russian forceps and peeled away from the common bile duct and hepatic artery. The gallbladder with

hepatoduodenal peritoneum is divided from the superior aspect of the first portion of the duodenum to release the specimen.

Circumferential Resection of the Hepatogastric Ligament and Lesser Omentum by Digital Dissection

- The triangular ligament of the left lobe of the liver is resected when performing the left subphrenic peritonectomy. This completed, the left lateral segment of the liver is retracted left to right to expose the hepatogastric ligament in its entirety. A circumferential release of this ligament from the fissure between liver segments II, III, and I, and from the arcade of right gastric artery to left gastric artery along the lesser curvature of the stomach, is required.
- After electrosurgically dividing the peritoneum on the lesser curvature of the stomach, digital dissection with extreme pressure from the surgeon's thumb and index finger separates lesser omental fat and tumor from the vascular arcade. As much as possible of the anterior vagus nerve is retained. The tumor and fatty tissue surrounding the right and left gastric arteries are split away from the vascular arcade. In this manner the specimen is centralized over the major branches of the left gastric artery. With strong traction on the specimen, the lesser omentum is released from the left gastric artery and vein.
- If an accessory left hepatic artery off the left gastric artery is present, it is resected with the lesser omentum specimen. This is done in preparation for resection of the peritoneal surfaces below this structure.

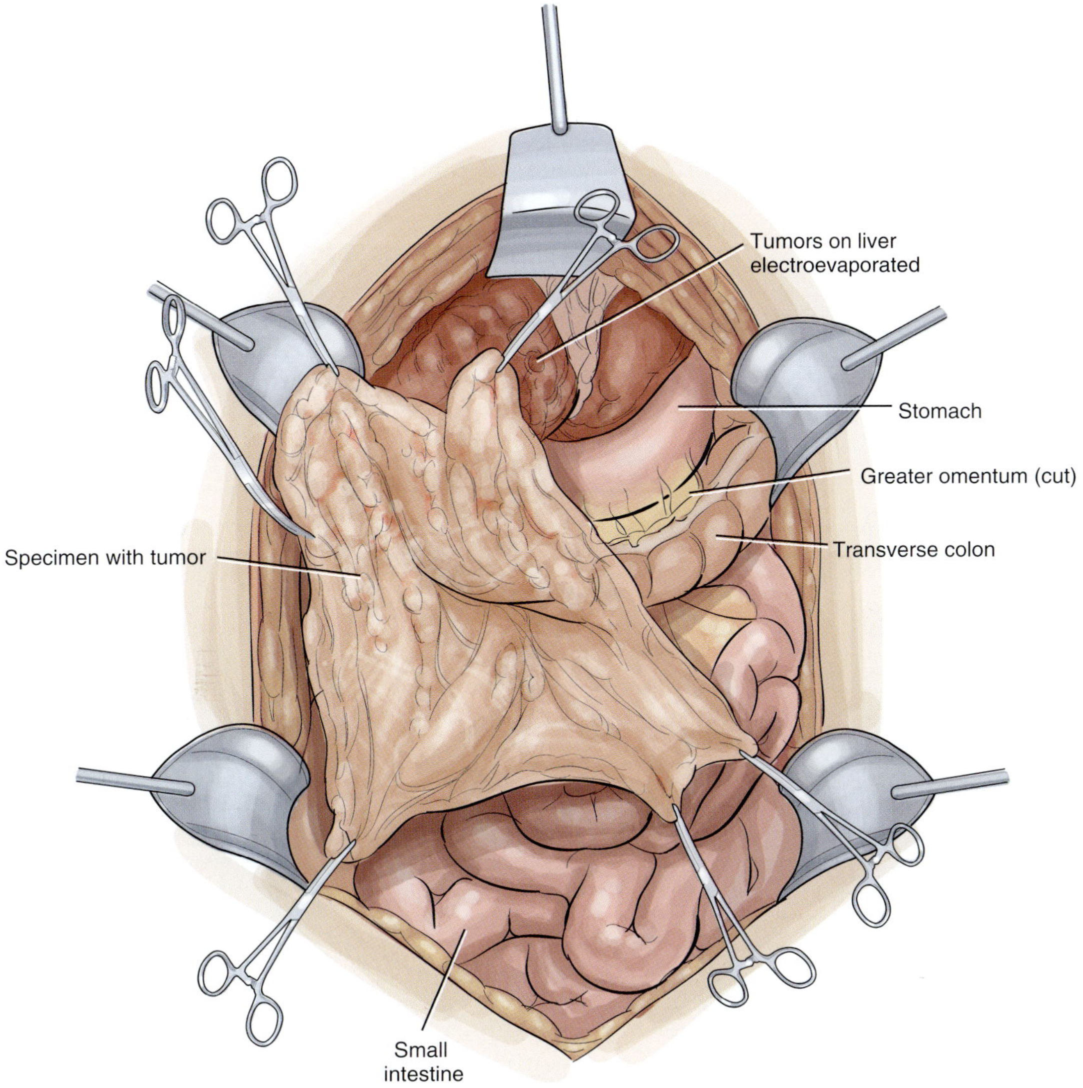

Figure 60-4.

Stripping of the Floor of the Omental Bursa

- A Deaver retractor or the assistant's fingertips beneath the left caudate lobe are positioned to expose the entire floor of the omental bursa (Fig. 60-5). Electroevaporation of tumor from the caudate process of the left caudate lobe of the liver might be necessary to achieve this exposure. Ball-tipped electrosurgery is used to cautiously divide the peritoneal reflection of liver onto the left side of the subhepatic vena cava.
- After the peritoneum is divided, Russian forceps assist in a blunt stripping of the peritoneum from the superior recess of the omental bursa, from the crus of the right hemidiaphragm, and from beneath the portal vein. Electroevaporation of tumor from the shelf of liver parenchyma beneath the portal vein and joining the right and left aspects of the caudate lobe might be required. Care is taken while stripping the floor of the omental bursa to remain superficial to the right phrenic artery.

Lesser Omentectomy and Omental Bursectomy Completed

- The tumor-bearing peritoneum is stripped from the posterior surface of the lower abdominal incision, exposing the rectus muscle while avoiding the deep epigastric vessels. The muscular surface of the bladder was exposed in a prior dissection. The stump of the urachus on the bladder is divided and elevated on a Babcock clamp as the leading point for this dissection. In the female, the round ligaments are divided as they enter the internal inguinal ring.

Resection of Rectosigmoid Colon, Uterus, and Cul-de-Sac of Douglas

- The peritoneal incision around the pelvis is completed, and it is connected to the dissection of the right and left paracolic sulcus. The right and left ureters are identified and preserved. In women, the right and left ovarian veins are ligated at the level of the lower pole of the kidney and divided. In the male, special care is taken to avoid the testicular vessels (Fig. 60-6).
- To begin the rectosigmoid colon resection, a linear stapler is used to divide the sigmoid colon just above the limits of the pelvic tumor; this is usually at the junction of the sigmoid and descending

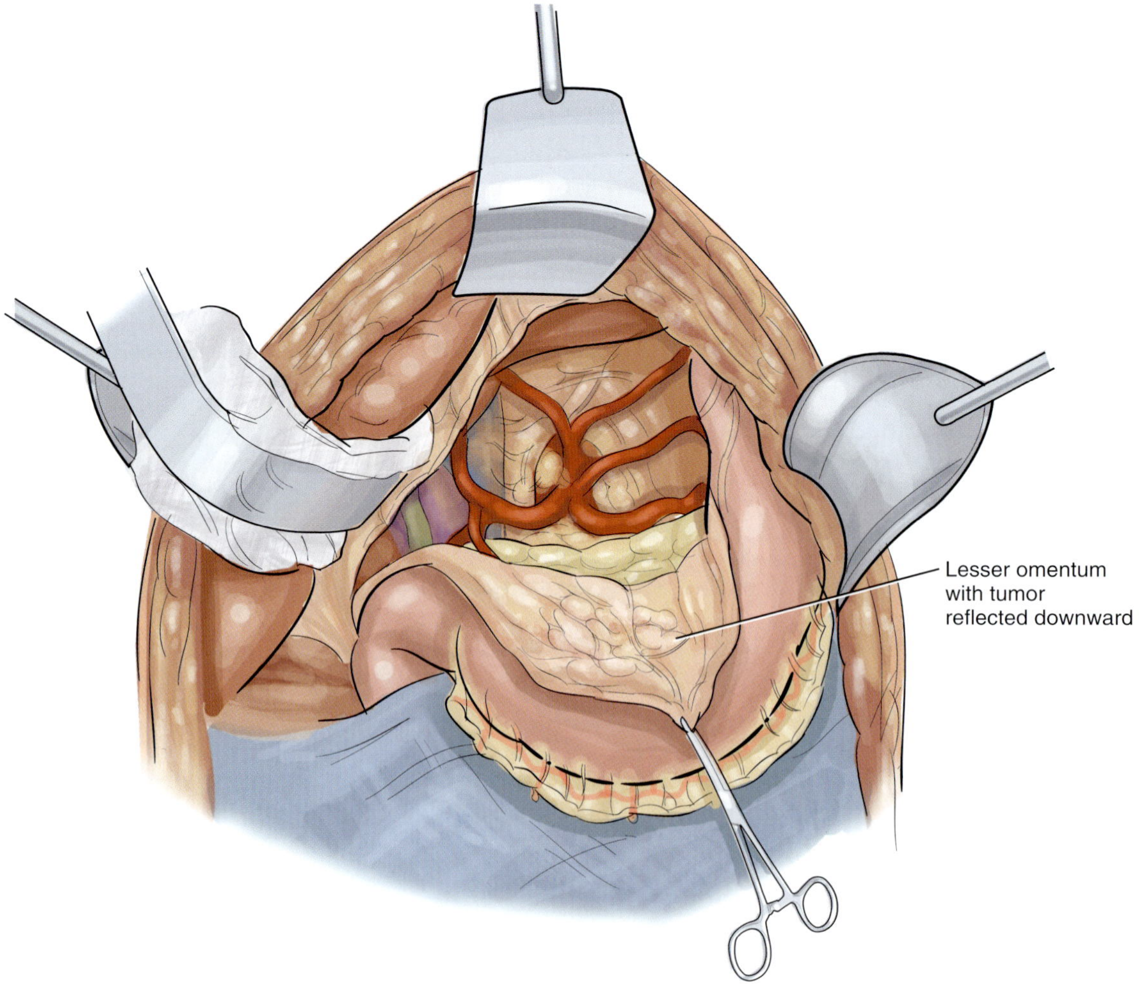

Figure 60-5.

colon. The vascular supply of the distal portion of the bowel is traced back to its origin on the aorta. The inferior mesenteric artery and vein are ligated, suture-ligated, and divided. This allows all the viscera, including the proximal descending colon, to be packed into the upper abdomen.

- Starting at the limits of the peritonectomy, the surgeon works in a centripetal fashion. Extraperitoneal ligation of the uterine arteries is performed just above the ureter and close to the base of the bladder. In women, the bladder is moved gently off the cervix, and the vagina is entered. The vaginal cuff anterior and posterior to the cervix is transected using ball-tipped electrosurgery, and the rectovaginal septum is entered. Ball-tipped electrosurgery is used to divide the perirectal fat beneath the peritoneal reflection. This ensures that all tumors that occupy the cul-de-sac are removed intact with the specimen. The rectal musculature is skeletonized using ball-tipped electrosurgery. Preservation of the lower half of the rectum will allow for a larger stool reservoir and diminish frequent bowel movements. A roticulator stapler (Autosuture, Norwalk, Conn.) is used to close the rectal stump, and the rectum is sharply divided above the staple line (see Fig. 60-6).

Left Colon Mobilization for a Tension-Free Low Colorectal Anastomosis

- A requirement for a complication-free low colorectal anastomosis is absence of tension on the staple line. Adequate mobilization of the entire left colon is needed, and several steps could be required to accomplish this.
- The inferior mesenteric artery is ligated on the aorta, and then its individual branches are resected as they arise from this vascular trunk. This is a Y-to-V transition that keeps the intermediate arcade intact.
- The inferior mesenteric vein is divided as it courses around the duodenum. The mesentery of the transverse colon and splenic flexure are completely elevated from the perirenal fat surrounding the left kidney.
- Taking care to avoid the left ureter, the surgeon divides the left colon mesentery from all its attachments. These maneuvers allow the junction of the sigmoid and descending colon to reach to the low rectum or anus for a tension-free anastomosis. Redundant descending colon should fall into the hollow of the sacrum. If further length is needed, the attachments of the first portion of the duodenum to the retroperitoneum are divided.

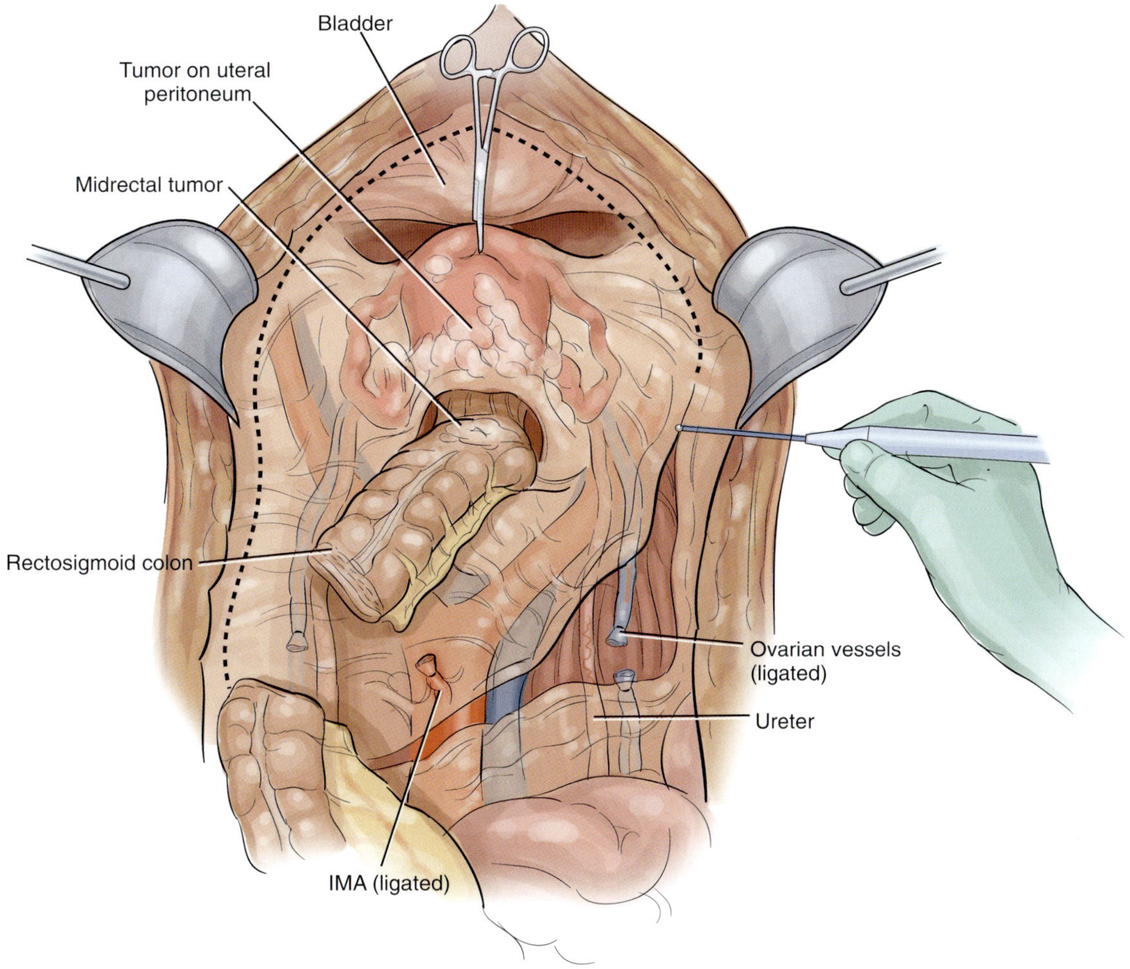

Figure 60-6. *IMA,* Inferior mesenteric artery.

- Attachments of the transverse mesocolon to the lower border of the pancreas are transected. This allows the transverse colon to course behind the duodenum on a straight path to the rectal stump.

Clearing the Small Bowel and Its Mesentery

- The electrosurgical techniques used in the peritonectomy procedures described earlier are not appropriate for the treatment of tumor nodules involving the small bowel. The high-voltage electrosurgical techniques using water cooling are appropriate for removal of cancer nodules on small-bowel mesentery but will cause significant heat damage to tubular structures such as the small bowel. Only limited use of electrosurgery on the small bowel is possible. Special techniques to resect tumor nodules and then partial- or full-thickness defects of the bowel wall created by removal of tumor nodules are described later.

Closure

- In females with a transection of the vagina, a loose suture repair must be performed before the intraperitoneal chemotherapy, or large-volume leakage may occur. This is the only suture repair performed before the intraperitoneal chemotherapy treatments. Four closed-suction drains are placed through the abdominal wall to lie in the right upper quadrant, left upper quadrant, right side of the pelvis, and left side of the pelvis. A Tenckhoff catheter is positioned within the midabdomen. All tubes and drains are secured at the skin with a purse-string stitch to prevent leakage of chemotherapy solution (Fig. 60-7).
- If hyperthermic intraoperative intraperitoneal chemotherapy is used, temperature probes are secured to the inflow catheter (Tenckhoff catheter) and to a remote site (see Fig. 60-7). The inflow catheter (maximal hyperthermia) may be placed at a site at high risk for cancer recurrence to maximize cytotoxicity at this site.
- Additional sutures are placed in the apex of the vagina. These sutures are left long so that they can be used to elevate the vaginal cuff and clearly expose the stump of the rectum. An anvil is placed in the distal colon with a purse-string suture; it is mated with the staple gun placed within the rectum. This completes the circular stapled colorectal anastomosis.

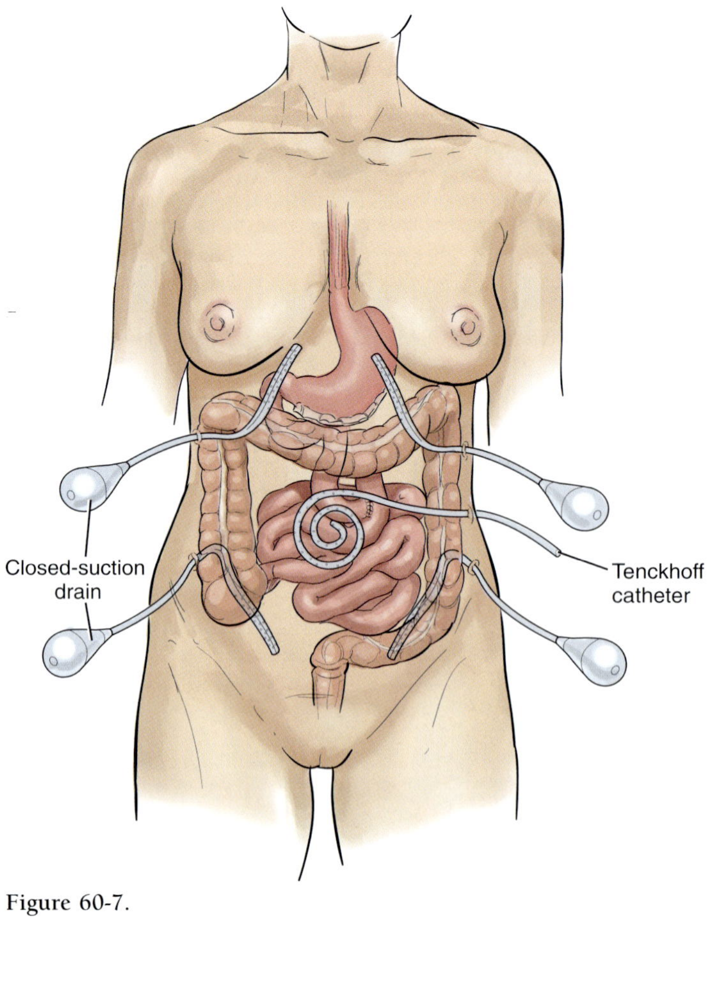

Figure 60-7.

III. ALTERNATIVE TECHNICAL APPROACHES (PRO/CON) AND PEARLS

Techniques Used in Cytoreduction of the Small Bowel

- Peritonectomy procedures have been most commonly used for cytoreduction of pseudomyxoma peritonei, but they also have been successfully applied to other tumors, especially colon cancer and diffuse malignant peritoneal mesothelioma. The histologic features and depth of invasion into the bowel wall of these tumors are not uniform. Based on the extent of the invasion, the size of the tumor nodule, and its anatomic location on the bowel wall, we classify small bowel involvement into five types:
  - *Type 1—Small or large noninvasive nodules*: The curved Mayo scissors are used to trim these noninvasive nodules from the surface of the small bowel. Larger nodules are frequently scissor dissected in a piecemeal fashion to avoid damage to the muscular portion of the bowel wall. There is usually no need for seromuscular repair or suture repair of the bowel surface.
  - *Type 2—Small invasive nodules on the antimesenteric portion of the small bowel*: These invasive nodules do not easily separate from the surface of the small bowel, and a partial-thickness resection of the seromuscular layer leaving mucosa and submucosa intact is required for their removal. This resection may be performed with frequent irrigation to cool the resection. Alternatively, scissors or knife dissection is used. The seromuscular layer is repaired by suture plication after intraoperative chemotherapy is completed.
  - *Type 3—Moderate-size invasive nodules on the antimesenteric portion of the small bowel*: Similar to small invasive nodules in this location, these nodules are removed by electrosurgery but require a full-thickness elliptical resection of the antimesenteric portion of the bowel wall. The closure is performed in two layers. The first layer is a full-thickness closure using absorbable sutures. One suture starts at each corner of the defect, and then the sutures are tied at the midportion of the closure. The hyperthermic intraoperative intraperitoneal chemotherapy is used before closing the defect with a second layer of nonabsorbable plication sutures.
  - *Type 4—Small invasive nodules at the junction of small bowel and mesentery*: These nodules can sometimes be removed by a localized removal with electrosurgery if sufficiently small and if the vascular supply to the segment of bowel is not compromised. A two-layer repair follows this localized resection. More often, these nodules are removed with a reduced incidence of fistula by a segmental resection with end-to-end anastomosis.
  - *Type 5—Large invasive nodules*: These lesions require a segmental resection with generous margins on the bowel wall and on the mesentery. The segment of small bowel and the mesentery to the anastomotic arch is resected. The bowel is divided using a linear cutter/stapler. After completion of the hyperthermic intraoperative intraperitoneal chemotherapy, a two-layer hand-sewn anastomosis is performed, remembering to close the mesentery.
- A right and left upper quadrant peritonectomy also is frequently required in appendiceal, colon, and ovarian cancer patients. Lymphatic lacunae (large peritoneal pores) exist on the undersurface of the diaphragm. These open lymphatic channels draw tumor cells to the superficial layer of the diaphragm's undersurface. These tumor cells then grow as a sheet of cancer adherent to the undersurface of the hemidiaphragm. As tumor beneath the diaphragm progresses, this malignancy may involve the dome of the right or left lobe of the liver. Complete removal of this tumor requires stripping of the undersurface of the diaphragm and a dissection of the Glisson capsule away from liver parenchyma.
- Greater omentectomy usually is combined with splenectomy to achieve a complete cytoreduction. Of course, if the spleen is free of tumor, it is left in situ. The same is true when performing a lesser omentectomy. If the gallbladder is not involved by tumor, it can be preserved.
- Perhaps the most difficult peritonectomy is the lesser omentectomy with stripping of the omental bursa. Vital structures here are of great density, and mistakes in dissection can lead to life-endangering hemorrhage or severe damage to the liver. The left hepatic artery is the most commonly traumatized vessel. Also, loss of the left gastric artery may result in the need for total gastrectomy. Ligation of the left gastric vein may cause gastric portal hypertension when all other venous drainage of the stomach is removed by dissection around this organ. The left hepatic vein or left inferior phrenic vein is thin walled and may be damaged inadvertently by sudden and unpredictable diaphragmatic contractions stimulated by electrosurgical dissection near the crus of the right hemidiaphragm.
- In some patients, the extent of damage to the anterior vagus nerve is difficult to assess. Sometimes, a pyloroplasty or gastrojejunostomy must be performed if the main trunk of the vagus nerve is divided. As a result of the anterior vagotomy, and in the absence of a gastric drainage procedure, gastric stasis can occur. Usually, if a generous pyloric outlet can be palpated through the stomach or if the nasogastric tube can be passed through the pyloric outlet, a gastric drainage procedure is unnecessary.
- An important advantage of the open technique for intraoperative intraperitoneal chemotherapy administration concerns the continued access to the bowel during the 90-minute irrigation. The majority of the small-bowel cytoreduction can be done while chemotherapy is being administered, and the reconstruction can be completed toward the end of the chemotherapy treatment to minimize cancer cells entrapped in small-bowel suture lines. In this way, the total length of the operation is significantly shortened, and the surfaces of the bowel that are being sutured are thoroughly washed with chemotherapy solution before closure.

- To assess the adequacy of a stapled colorectal anastomosis, the proximal and distal tissue rings are examined for completeness. Air is insufflated into the rectum with a water-filled pelvis to check for an airtight circle of staples. Two hands should easily pass beneath the reconstructed colon to ensure there is no tension on the stapled anastomosis. A rectal examination is done to check for staple-line bleeding at the anastomosis.

IV. SPECIAL POSTOPERATIVE CARE

- Postoperatively, if the patient is stable and the drainage from the closed-suction drains is serosanguineous (not gross blood), the patient is transferred to the surgical intensive care unit. The patient will be kept intubated for approximately 12 hours until hemodynamically stable and until swelling in and around the head and neck has at least in part resolved. It is unusual for patients to be maintained on mechanical ventilation for longer than 12 hours. After the first cycle of early postoperative intraperitoneal chemotherapy, the patient is transferred to the nursing unit, but telemetry is maintained during the 4 or 5 days required to administer early postoperative intraperitoneal chemotherapy.
- Chest tubes are removed when their drainage is less than 50 mL in 24 hours, and the same general rule is used for the closed-suction drains within the abdomen and the subcutaneous tissue. Patients are given prophylactic heparin after their bleeding and clotting parameters have returned to normal. Sequential compression devices are mandatory when the patient is in bed. Also, special exercises to encourage active motion of the lower extremities take place every 2 hours while the patient is awake. A family member remains in the patient's room around the clock for postoperative weeks 1 and 2. All patients are maintained on parenteral feeding until the nasogastric tube has been removed, usually on days 7 to 9. The diet is gradually augmented. One in 10 patients has a slow progression of oral intake and is required to leave the hospital on supplemental intravenous feeding.
- If an ostomy was performed, it is usually closed after the completion of systemic chemotherapy, but typically no sooner than 3 months postoperatively.
- Considering the technical differences between this technique and standard peritonectomy procedures, it may be appropriate to call this approach the "sixth peritonectomy procedure." Even though gastrointestinal complications continue to be an important source of postoperative morbidity, the rate of fistulas in our experience can be reduced to 3% with careful attention to the techniques for small-bowel cytoreduction.

SUGGESTED READINGS

Carmignani CP, Sugarbaker TA, Bromley CM, Sugarbaker PH: Intraperitoneal cancer dissemination: mechanisms of the patterns of spread, *Cancer Metastasis Rev* 22:465–472, 2003.

Sugarbaker PH: Peritonectomy procedures, *Ann Surg* 221:29–42, 1995.

Sugarbaker PH: Laser-mode electrosurgery. In Sugarbaker PH, editor: *Peritoneal carcinomatosis: principles of management*, Boston, 1996, Kluwer, pp 375–385.

SECTION IX

Lymph Node Dissections

CHAPTER 61

Radical Superficial and Deep Groin Dissection

Harald J.J. Hoekstra, MD, PhD, and Theo Wobbes, MD, PhD

I. SPECIAL PREOPERATIVE PREPARATION

- Immediate, prophylactic, or elective lymph node dissection has become an extremely uncommon surgical procedure in surgical oncology since the introduction of minimally invasive staging through a sentinel lymph node biopsy (SLNB). Indications for SLNB include melanoma; merkel cell carcinoma; and squamous cell carcinoma of the penis, vulva, and/or anal canal. A positive sentinel node in these patients will lead to a complete superficial groin dissection. When more nodes are involved, this procedure is followed by a deep groin dissection.
- The most important indication for a combined superficial and deep groin dissection is a therapeutic lymph node dissection with curative intent for proven lymph node metastases. The majority of these procedures are performed for melanoma (clinically stage III disease).
- Selection of patients for SLNB or therapeutic or palliative superficial and/or deep groin dissection is crucial.
- Ultrasonography of the groin and fine-needle aspiration (FNA) cytology of enlarged lymph nodes is of great value to avoid an SLNB and to plan immediately for a groin dissection. A palpable lymph node in the groin should always be cytologically investigated with FNA. In cases of negative cytology. an excisional biopsy is indicated, with or without frozen section, to confirm the diagnosis and allow the appropriate treatment to be performed. The FNA or biopsy site should be included in the definitive superficial groin dissection specimen.
- Clinically stage III melanoma patients should be staged using fluorodeoxyglucose–positron emission tomography to define the indication for a so-called curative or palliative superficial and deep groin dissection. Other diseases are appropriately staged with spiral computed tomography.
- Indications for deep groin dissection are based on preoperative imaging studies showing deep nodal involvement, gross disease in more than three nodes in the superficial lymph node dissection specimen, and/or metastatic disease in the Cloquet node.
- Superficial groin dissection involves the removal of the inguinal nodes. Deep groin dissection includes the removal of the parailiac and obturator nodes. A radical superficial and deep groin dissection includes the in-continuity resection of the superficial, iliac, and obturator nodes.

II. OPERATIVE TECHNIQUE

Position

- A groin dissection requires epidural, spinal, or general anesthesia. When a deep groin dissection is indicated, general anesthesia is required.
- The patient is placed in a supine position with the leg slightly abducted and flexed at the knee and externally rotated (slight frog-leg position) on the operating table (Fig. 61-1). A Foley catheter is placed. The entire limb, groin, and lower quadrant of the abdomen are prepared with antiseptic solution and draped.
- There is no routine use of perioperative antibiotics. The high rate of wound complications is more related to the surgical technique and less influenced by the use of antibiotics. There is one exception:

patients who undergo a completed lymphadenectomy after a positive SLNB have an increased risk for wound infection and therefore receive perioperative antibiotics.

Incision

- Groin dissections can be performed in two different ways: through one incision with an en bloc dissection of the superficial and deep nodes, or through two separate incisions with in-continuity of the superficial and deep nodal dissection (see Fig. 61-1).
- An oblique or transverse incision in the skin lines provides an inadequate exposure of the superficial and deep nodes and is not described in this chapter. A straight vertical or S-shaped incision with or without a skin ellipse and vertical transection of the inguinal ligament offers superior exposure of all nodes. The aim of a vertical incision instead of an oblique incision is to optimize the anatomic dissection and minimize damage to the lymphatic vessels and therefore decrease the risk of lymphedema. Excision of a skin ellipse guarantees a broad exposure and no prolonged skin traction, and undermining of the skin is unnecessary. When a previous transverse incision is used for the removal of a lymph node, the S-shaped incision and excision of a skin ellipse includes the previous biopsy site and guarantees an en bloc dissection. When no skin ellipse is excised, excision of skin flap edges is performed at the time of closure.
- A groin dissection can also be performed through two separate incisions above and below the groin. Particularly when preoperatively pathologic iliac lymph nodes are demonstrated (through positron emission tomography scan, spiral computed tomography, or magnetic resonance imaging), dissection through a separate pararectal incision should be contemplated because it may give a better opportunity to remove the lymph nodes more completely. The disadvantage of this technique is the in-continuity of the superficial and deep nodal dissection. However, two separate incisions leave the groin free to reduce the risk of wound infection, abdominal weakness, or hernia formation.
- There are no significant differences in complication rates between the two techniques. The most important prognostic factor for wound healing disturbances after groin dissection is the body mass index of the patient.
- Groin dissection wounds can in general be closed primarily. Sometimes a split-thickness skin graft is required, which can be applied on the mobilized sartorius muscle.

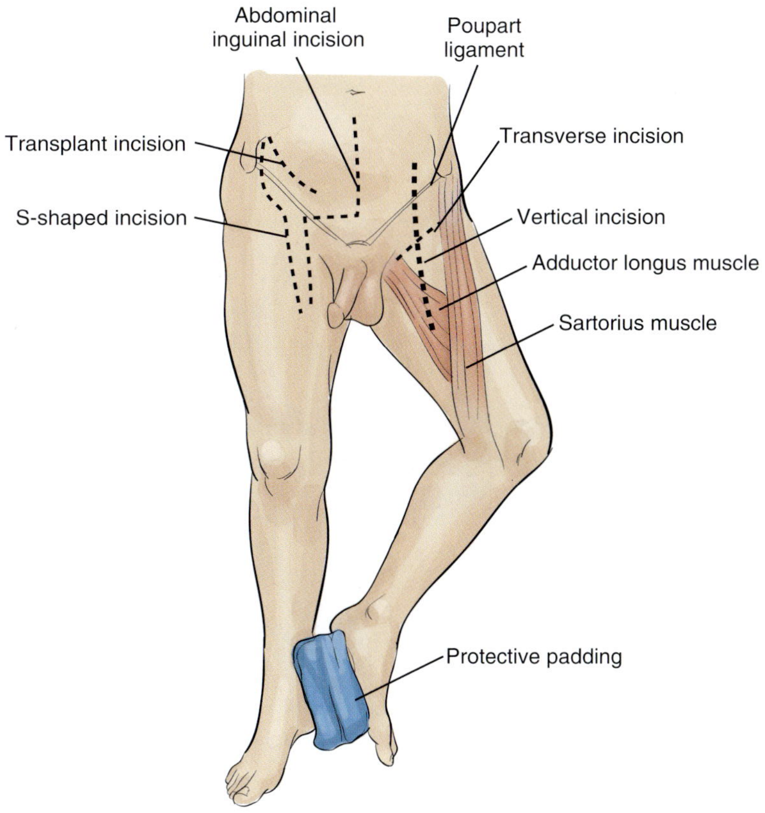

Figure 61-1.

MAIN DISSECTION

Superficial Groin Dissection

- An ellipse-shaped incision of the skin is begun cranially, 2 cm medial from the superior anterior iliac spine, slightly oblique to the midinguinal area, and then below the Poupart ligament vertically downward to the apex of the femoral triangle. The incision centers over the course of the lymphatic vessels and lymph nodes (see Fig. 61-1). The ellipse is 4 to 6 cm at its broadest point. Any scar tissue from previous lymph node excisions is included in the skin ellipse.
- The superficial dissection contains the subcutaneous fat and lymphatic tissue underneath the skin ellipse, limited by the external oblique fascia and inguinal ligament superiorly, the long adductor muscle medially, and the sartorius muscle laterally. The lymph nodes and adipose tissue are sharply dissected off the external oblique aponeurosis in continuity with the fascia of the adductor muscle and mobilized caudally and laterally (Fig. 61-2). Care should be taken in the male patient not to injure the spermatic cord. At the apex of the femoral triangle, the saphenous vein is divided (see Fig. 61-2). The femoral artery and femoral nerve now become visible, as well as the femoral vein on the dorsal side of the femoral artery (Fig. 61-3). With the dissection in the longitudinal plane of the femoral vessels and in continuity of the anterior half of the vascular sheath, the nodal tissue is taken to the fossa ovalis. The saphenous vein is suture ligated with nonabsorbable suture at the saphenofemoral junction. The distal femoral stump is clamped and carefully sutured, because the distal stump often retracts and begins bleeding. The sensory branches of the femoral nerve parallel and lateral to the femoral artery are identified. The motor branches are more deeply situated. The lateral part is now completed with dissection of the fascia of the sartorius muscle. The lateral femoral cutaneous nerve, supplying the skin of the lateral thigh, is identified and spared, whereas the accompanying small artery and vein are resected. The sensory femoral branches to the distal skin flaps are preserved unless suspicious lymph nodes are encountered. The superficial groin dissection is completed in front of the femoral vessels and medially below the Poupart ligament. When no in-continuity deep groin resection is performed, the medial portion of the Poupart ligament is sutured to the pectineal fascia to avoid a femoral hernia.
- The specimen is marked with small tags for histopathologic examination. The lymphatic tissue medial to the femoral vein at the superior aspect of the femoral canal is called the Cloquet or Rosenmuller node. The Cloquet node represents the leading lymph node into the pelvis from the inguinal basin and is sent as a separate specimen.

Deep Groin Dissection

- When a radical groin dissection is planned, the specimen is not divided at the femoral canal to ensure an en bloc groin dissection.
- The Poupart ligament is transected longitudinally 2 cm lateral to the neurovascular bundle by placing the index finger below the Poupart ligament and lateral to the femoral artery. The incision is extended through the internal oblique, transversus abdominis, and transversalis fascia (Fig. 61-4). The

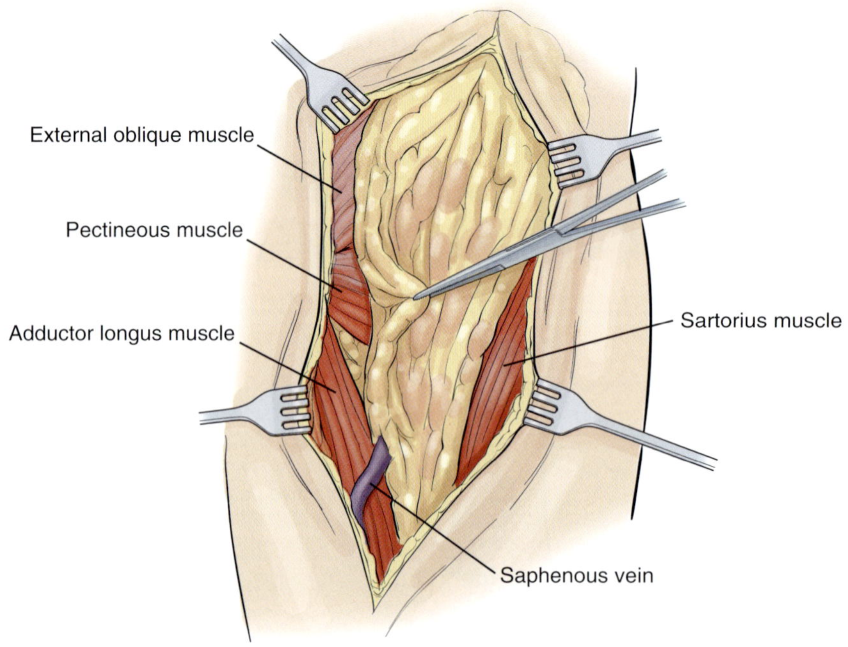

Figure 61-2.

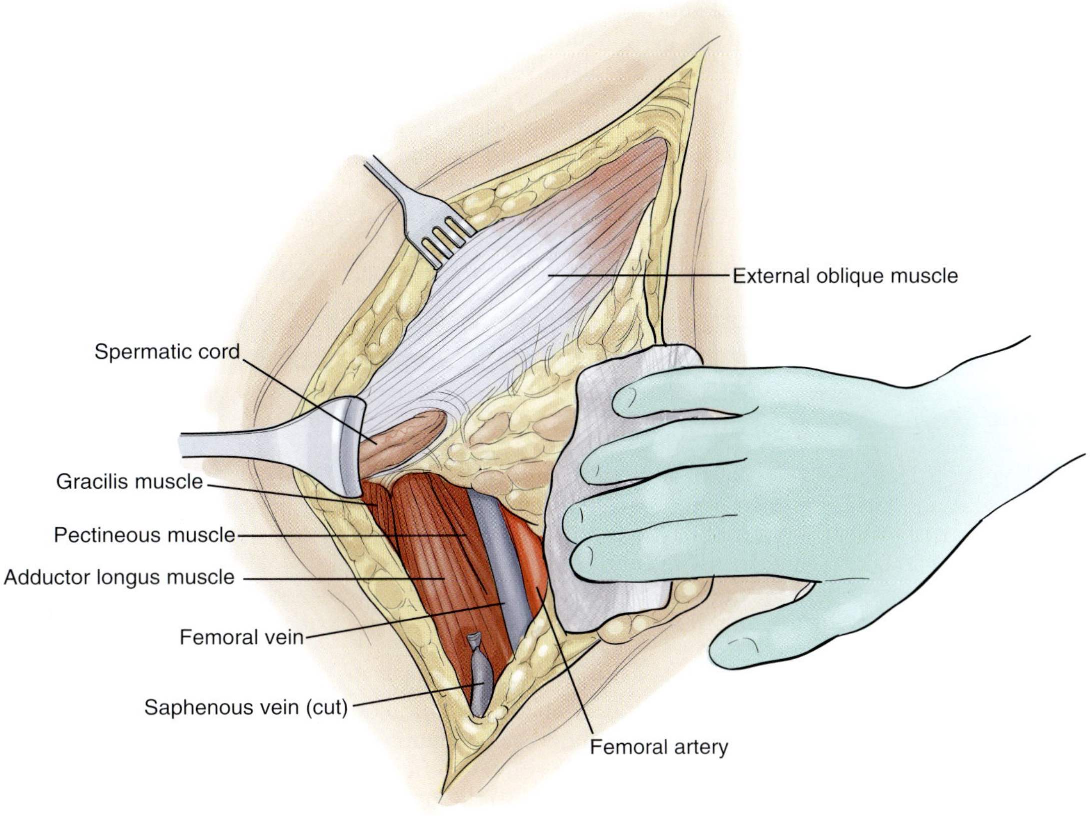

Figure 61-3.

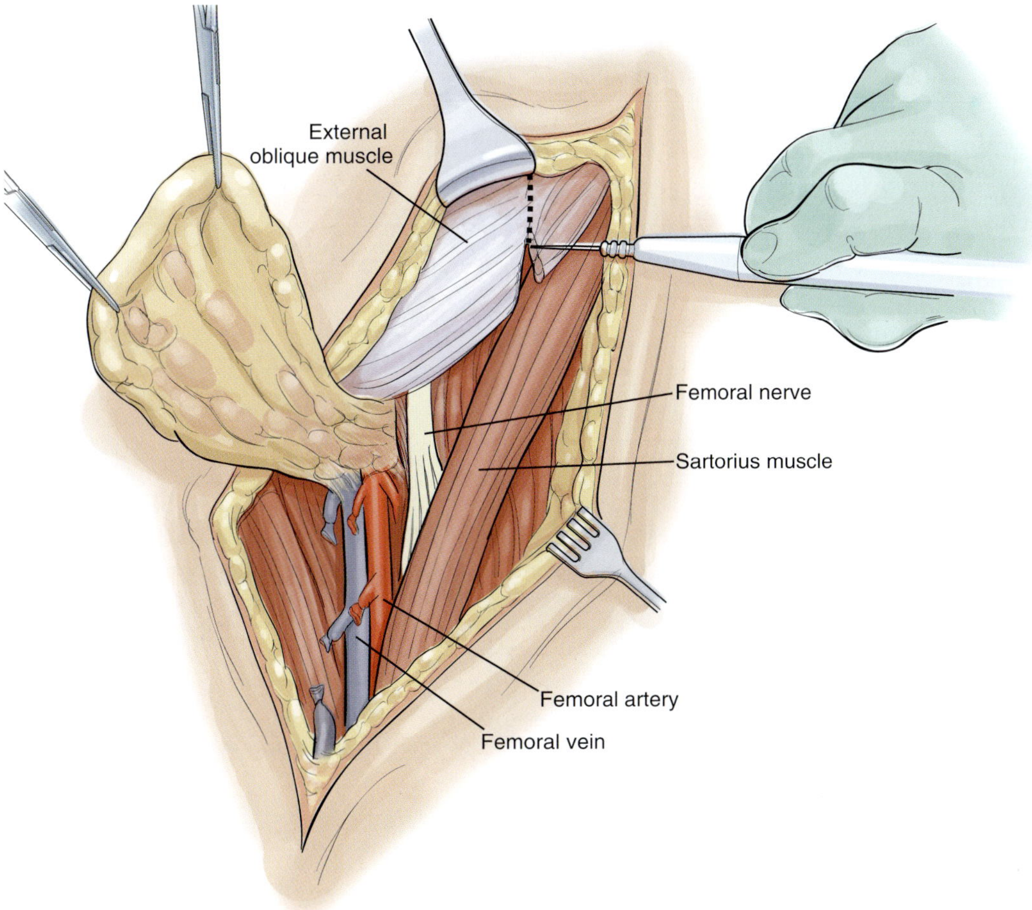

Figure 61-4.

peritoneum is bluntly displaced superiorly, and the retroperitoneal area with the iliac and obturator lymph nodes is exposed while the peritoneum is retracted. To obtain full access, the deep epigastric vessels should be divided (Fig. 61-5). The iliac lymph node dissection begins at the aortic bifurcation and is performed in front of the external iliac artery. The lateral border is the genitofemoral nerve (see Fig. 61-5). The medial border is the common femoral vein, and the dissection is performed from the level of the internal iliac artery caudally. The ureter is identified, and the dissection is continued medially along the obturator nerve (Fig. 61-6). In case of enhancement, the obturator nerve is resected en bloc with the specimen. The deep nodes are almost exclusively medial to the femoral vessels and cephalad to the fossa ovalis.

- The (en bloc) specimen is carefully marked for histopathologic examination, because deep nodal involvement has a more grave prognosis. The specimen is marked for the common iliac, internal iliac, obturator, and external iliac nodes with small tags.

Closure

- Following irrigation of the wound and meticulous hemostasis, the internal and external oblique and transverse abdominis muscles and Poupart ligament are closed with interrupted absorbable sutures. The Poupart ligament is sutured to the Cooper ligament medial to the femoral vessels and lateral to the iliac fascia, taking care that there is no pressure on the femoral vessels (Fig. 61-7).
- When two separate incisions are used, the wound is closed in a standard fashion with absorbable interrupted sutures for the muscles and a running suture for the external oblique fascia. The skin is closed with an intracutaneous suture or skin staples.
- The origin of the sartorius muscle is now divided at the level of the anterior iliac spine, and the lateral edge of the muscle is freed over a length of about 10 cm, taking care to avoid injury to the lateral femoral cutaneous nerve (see Fig. 61-7). The vascular bundles proximal to the sartorius muscle are preserved when possible. The sartorius muscle is rotated medially to cover the neurovascular femoral bundle and subsequently fixed with absorbable mattress sutures to the Poupart ligament and the fascia

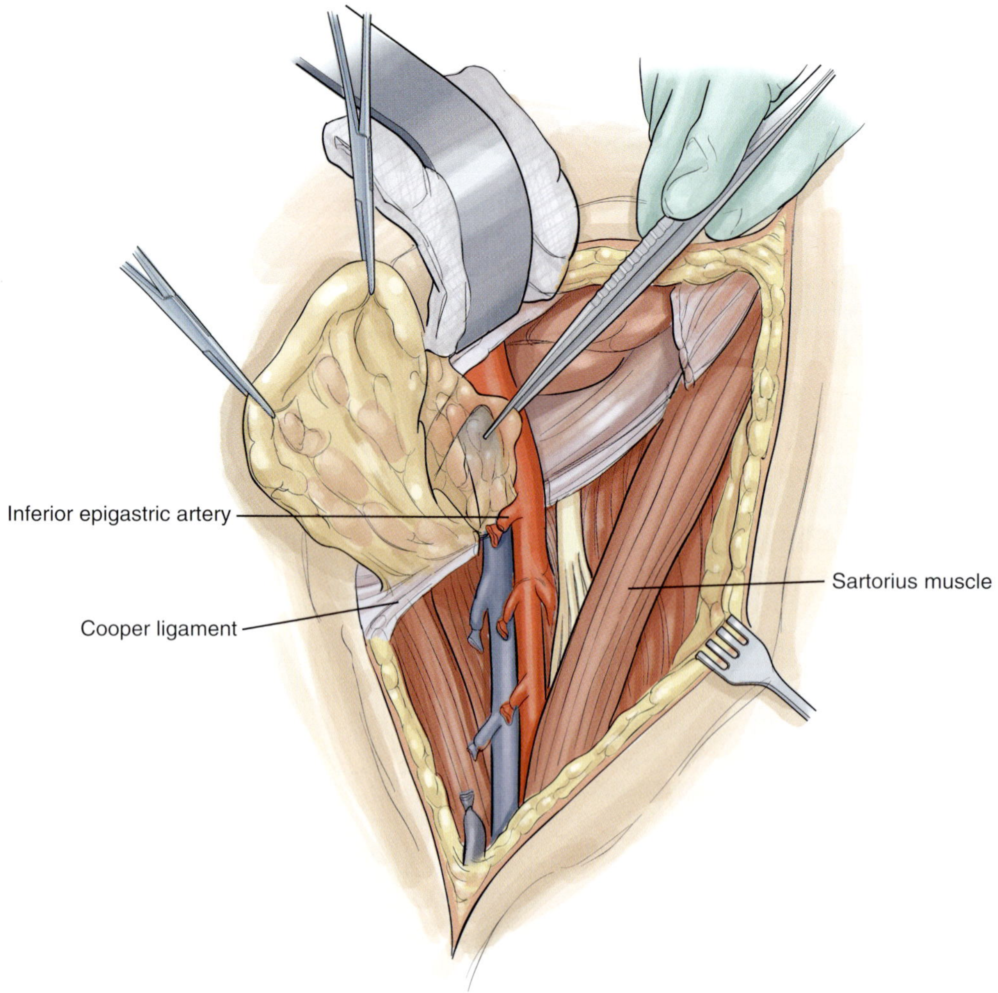

Figure 61-5.

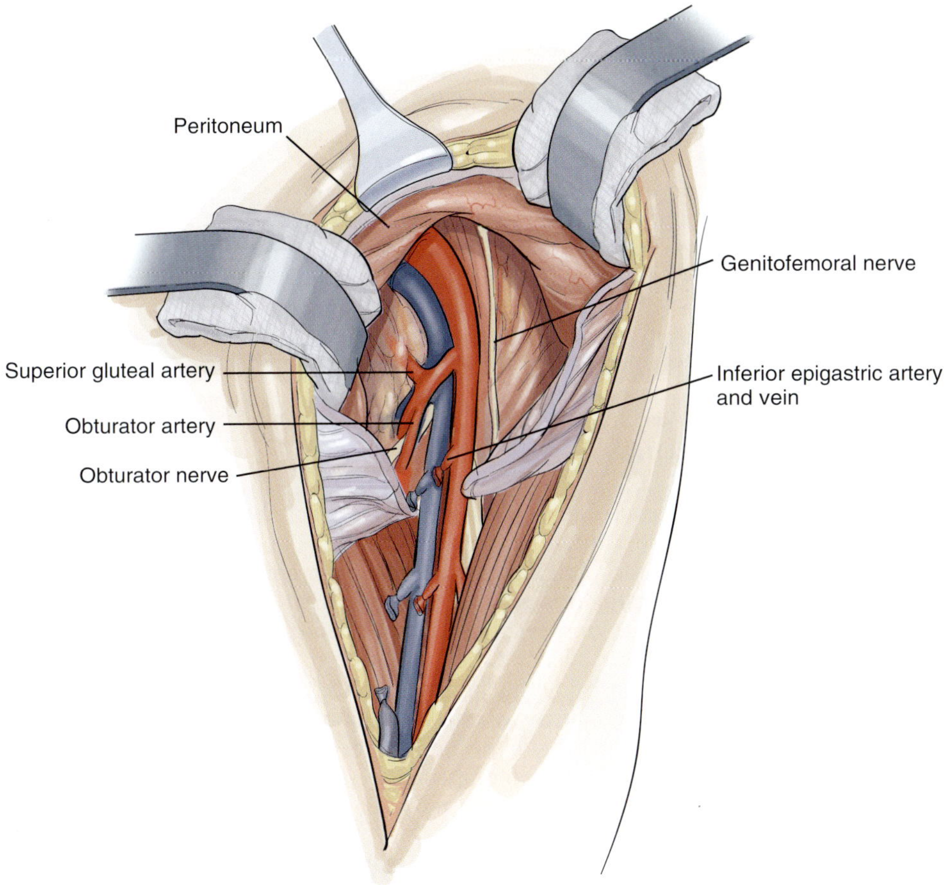

Figure 61-6.

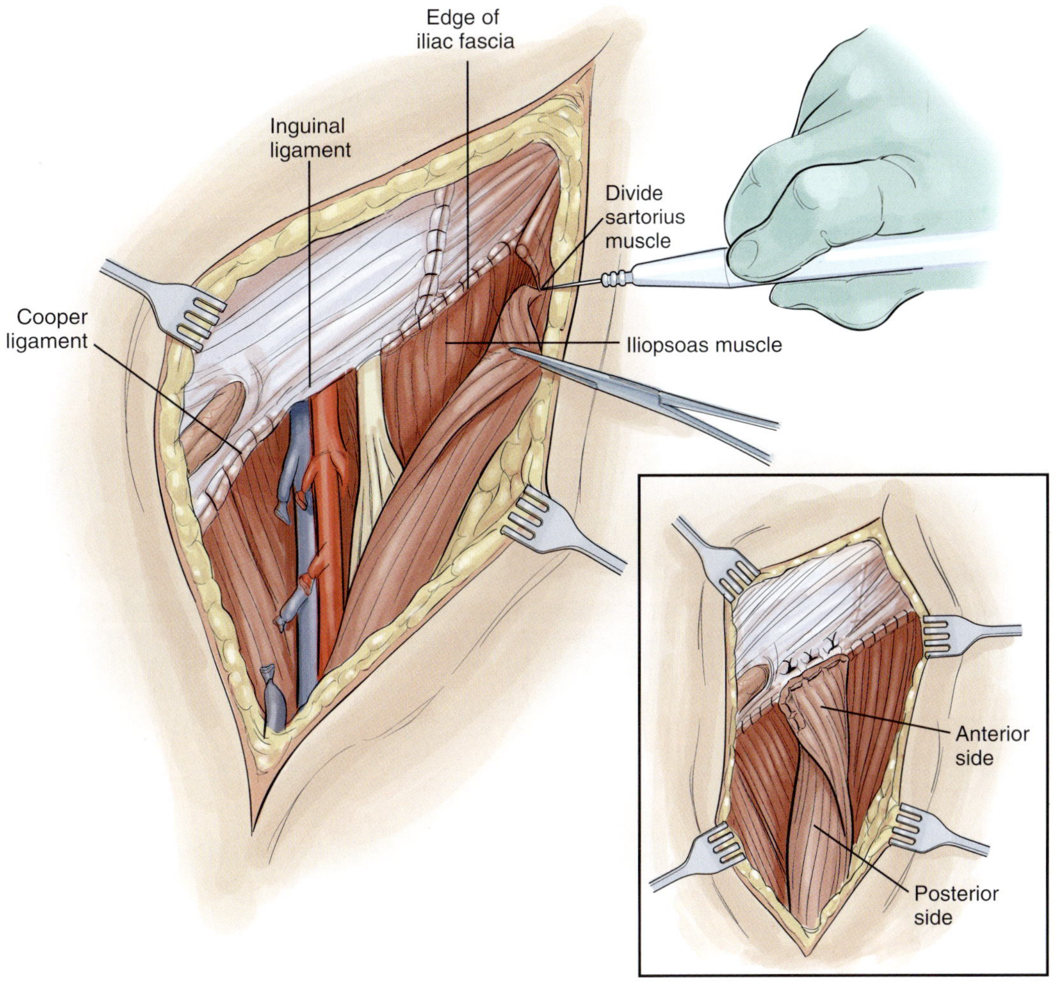

Figure 61-7.

of the adductor and vastus muscle groups (see Fig. 61-7, *inset*). The goal of the sartorius muscle transposition and rotation is to ensure optimal coverage of the femoral vessels and nerve and circulation of the proximal part of the sartorius muscle. Care must be taken to ensure that the muscle is rotated to lie over the femoral vessels without undue tension. Transposition of the sartorius muscle prevents exposure of the femoral vessels in case of wound breakdown. Occasionally the saphenous vein may be preserved as well as the sartorius muscle.

- Two low-vacuum drains are placed, one medial and one lateral, brought out through two separate stab wounds cranial to the incision, and secured with a nonabsorbable suture (Fig. 61-8). The drain should not have contact with the femoral artery and vein. Suction drainage of the pelvis is not required.
- The skin edges are examined for viability. In case of marginal circulation of the skin, the skin edges should be trimmed. The subcutaneous tissue is closed with noncontinuous, intracutaneous 2-0 absorbable sutures. The skin is closed with interrupted sutures or skin staples (see Fig. 61-8). A dry gauze is placed on the wound as dressing.

III. ALTERNATIVE TECHNICAL APPROACHES (PRO/CON) AND PEARLS

- A transplant incision is an alternative operative approach (see Fig. 61-1). The external oblique muscle is split from the iliac superior spine to the rectus sheath, and the internal oblique and transversus abdominis muscles are divided. In this case, the inferior epigastric artery and vein are ligated when indicated. The removal of the iliac nodes and obturator nodes is no different from the previously described procedure. However, the technique may leave gross residual disease behind the band of the Poupart ligament and the adjacent aponeurosis, therefore affecting the in-continuity of the dissection specimen. An abdominal-inguinal incision is an approach for the surgeon dealing with large lymph node masses in the iliac and obturator area. The incision consists of a lower midline incision from the umbilicus to the pubic symphysis, continuing transversely through the anterior rectus sheath just above the pubic crest to the midinguinal region and vertically to the femoral triangle (see Fig. 61-1).
- The peritoneal cavity is entered, and the iliac and obturator nodes are removed. If indicated, the dissection can be extended to the paraaortic and caval nodes.
- The abdominal wound is closed is standard fashion, the abdominal-inguinal part with interrupted absorbable sutures between the rectus sheath and the pubic crest. The remaining part of the superficial groin dissection is as previously described.

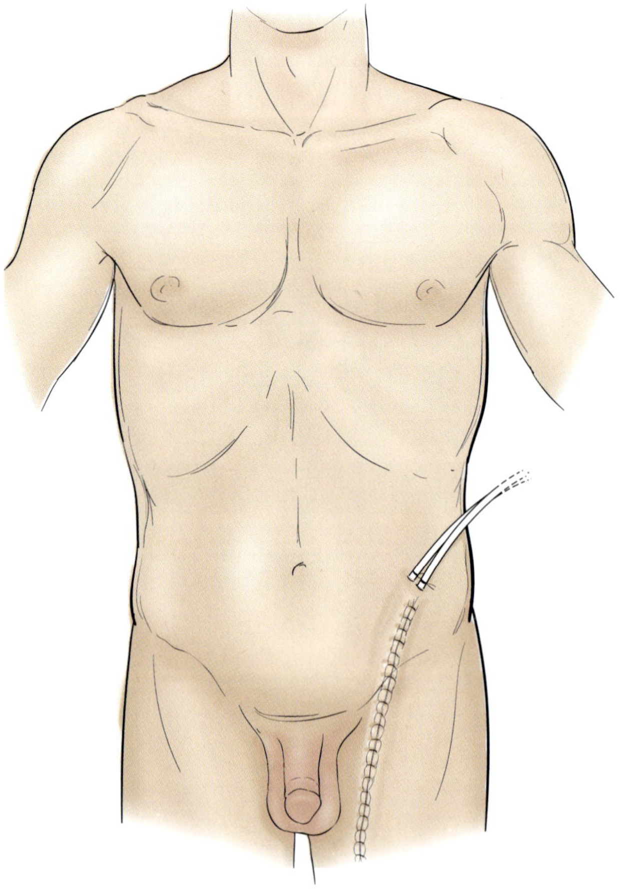

Figure 61-8.

IV. SPECIAL POSTOPERATIVE CARE

- The Foley catheter can be removed after 2 or 3 days or when the patient is fully mobilized.
- Hemorrhage is a potential immediate postoperative complication. Under general anesthesia, the wound should be opened and the hematoma evacuated.
- The patient should have 5 days of bed rest with the hip in and knee in maximal flexion to reduce tension on the wound and facilitate wound healing. Thrombosis prophylaxis with subcutaneous heparin is advised.
- Groin dissections are often complicated by wound-healing disturbances, such as wound necrosis and/or infection. The risk of infection is increased in completed groin dissections after a previous SLNB procedure. Therefore, these patients receive perioperative antibiotics. Wound necrosis is more often seen after oblique incisions than after vertical incisions or S-shaped incisions with excision of a skin ellipse. Wound healing disturbances are encountered significantly more often in patients with a high body mass index.
- On the first postoperative day, the wound dressing is removed and the wound inspected. The drain output is recorded, and the patient is instructed in how to care for both drains. Handling a low-vacuum drain is easily learned and allows discharge in a few days. If the seroma production is less than 10 mL, the drain(s) should be removed. Low-vacuum closed-suction drainage has a low risk for infection. Early removal may lead to lymphorrhea or lymphocele, impaired wound healing, and aspiration, which increases risk for infection.
- The patient is partially mobilized with a custom-made stocking and limited ambulation on the sixth postoperative day. The patient is instructed to keep the affected leg elevated when not ambulating. The patient is fully mobilized when the suction drainage is removed and primary wound healing is achieved. The patient should use the custom-fitted elastic pressure stocking at a pressure gradient of 20 to 30 mm Hg for 6 months to limit lymphedema. The stocking probably enhances the development of collateral lymphatic circulation. If after 6 months no severe lymphedema exists, the stocking may be discontinued. Elevation of the leg at night also reduces lymphedema.
- Infection in the groin incision should be avoided and treated aggressively. Infection in the groin causes fibrosis and secondary lymphedema. When lymphedema progresses, the extremity is more prone to infection.

SUGGESTED READINGS

Burmeister BH, Henderson MA, Ainslie J, et al: Adjuvant radiotherapy versus observation alone for patients at risk of lymph-node field relapse after therapeutic lymphadenectomy for melanoma: a randomised trial, *Lancet Oncol* 13:589–597, 2012.

de Vries M, Hoekstra HJ, Hoekstra-Weebers JE: Quality of life after axillary or groin sentinel lymph node biopsy, with or without completion lymph node dissection, in patients with cutaneous melanoma, *Ann Surg Oncol* 16:2840–2847, 2009.

Wevers KP, Bastiaannet E, Poos HP, et al: Therapeutic lymph node dissection in melanoma: different prognosis for different macrometastasis sites? *Ann Surg Oncol* 2012. [Epub ahead of print]

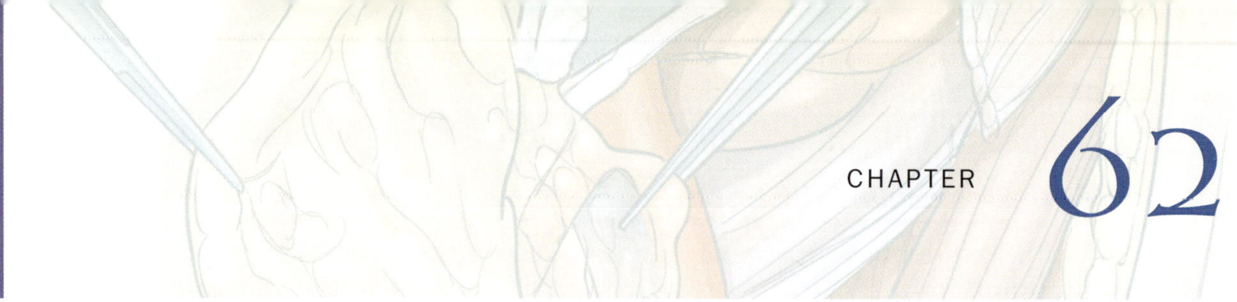

CHAPTER 62

Popliteal Lymph Node Dissection

Eliad Karin, MD, and Schlomo Schneebaum, MD

I. SPECIAL PREOPERATIVE PREPARATION

- There are two indications for popliteal node dissection: a histologically positive sentinel node in the popliteal fossa or clinical evidence of metastatic disease in this area.
- The reported prevalence of popliteal basin drainage from malignant melanoma of the distal lower extremity (in the knee or distal to the knee) ranges from 1% to 20%, depending on whether lymphoscintigraphy is used alone or combined with blue dye and a handheld gamma probe to detect the sentinel node.
- All patients with malignant melanoma that is 1 mm or more in thickness, less than 1 mm and Clark level IV or higher, or with ulceration and regression should undergo lymphoscintigraphy. A search for popliteal basin drainage of the primary distal lower extremity malignant melanoma is mandatory, and a 10-minute acquisition should be performed on every node field that can drain the site. In addition to the standard anteroposterior and oblique views of the popliteal region, a lateral view of the popliteal region with the patient standing and the knee joint flexed is performed.
- Whenever lymphoscintigraphy indicates that the popliteal basin is the draining site of the primary distal lower limb malignant melanoma, a sentinel lymph node biopsy should be done.
- It is our practice to use the combined approach of blue dye and a handheld gamma probe for the detection of the sentinel lymph node.
- It is our practice to perform the following procedures in one operation: wide local excision *and* sentinel lymph node biopsy. If the primary lesion is in the posterior distal lower extremity in proximity to the popliteal region, it is important to plan the operation so that the lines of incision will not interfere with the possibility of performing popliteal lymph node dissection.
- When planning the incision for popliteal sentinel lymph node biopsy, it is important to keep in mind the possible need to extend the incision in case the sentinel lymph node is involved. Therefore the incision should be in line with the future line of incision for popliteal lymph node dissection.
- All patients with malignant melanoma 1 mm or more in thickness are evaluated preoperatively with chest radiography, computed tomography (CT) of the abdomen, chest or positron emission tomography–CT, and CT or magnetic resonance imaging of the brain.

II. OPERATIVE TECHNIQUE

Position

- The patient is placed in a prone position. The affected lower extremity is prepped and draped circumferentially from the region of the upper thigh downward. The entire lower extremity should not be constricted by the draping so it can be moved during the procedure. The knee should be slightly flexed; we use a silicone pad under the distal shin for this purpose.

Incision

- A Z-plasty incision is made over the flexor crease (Fig. 62-1). This incision will allow optimal exposure and will heal with decreased danger of deforming knee joint contracture. If this is done after a sentinel lymph node biopsy, the incision will include the previous scar. The width and length of the Z are judged by the caliber of the lower thigh, usually with an interior angle of 100 to 120 degrees. The Z-line incision starts superiorly at the lower posterior lateral thigh and then continues downward obliquely to the upper medial part of the popliteal fossa. The Z incision then runs obliquely at 100 to 120 degrees to the popliteal fossa from upper medial to lower lateral, then at 100 to 120 degrees the incision continues obliquely downward to the upper medial shin.

Main Dissection

- The cutaneous Z-plasty incision continues downward through the subcutaneous tissue, and lateral and medial flaps are raised while traction is maintained with skin hooks.
- The lesser saphenous vein and the terminal branches of the small cutaneous nerve of the posterior femoral cutaneous nerve are exposed at the posterior deep fascia.
- The lesser saphenous vein must be ligated and divided.
- A vertical incision is made through the deep fascia. This should be done with care so as not to damage nerves below the fascia (Fig. 62-2).
- The medial sural nerve should be retracted. Sometimes it may have to be divided (this will cause cutaneous anesthesia) to allow better access to deeper structures.

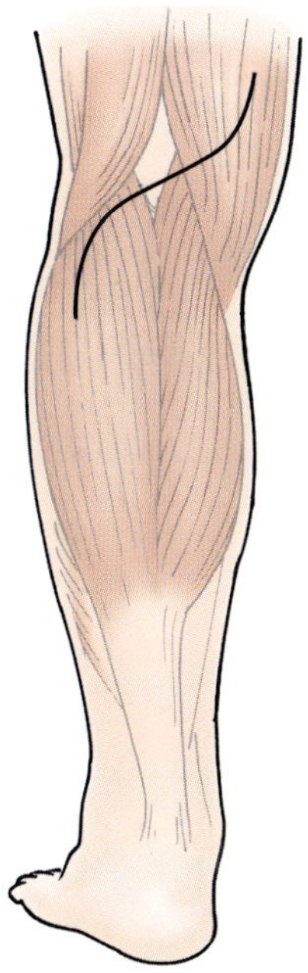

Figure 62-1.

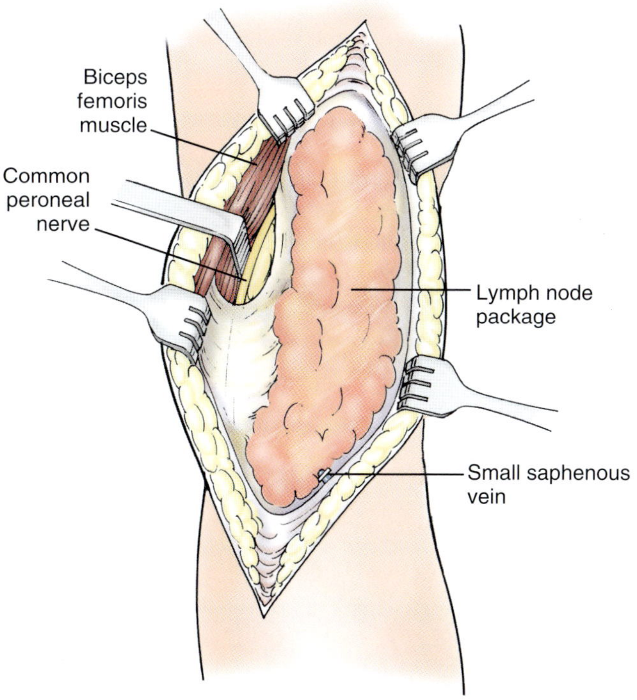

Figure 62-2.

- The tibial nerve is the most superficial midline structure that is exposed. It should be retracted laterally and gently with a vessel loop (Fig. 62-3).
- The peroneal nerve courses along the biceps femoris tendon and then turns further laterally toward the fibula. The nerve should be retracted gently with a vessel loop.
- The superior extent of dissection is bounded by the intersection of the biceps femoris and semimembranosus muscles. Inferiorly, the two heads of the gastrocnemius muscle can be further retracted to enhance distal exposure.
- A meticulous dissection is performed using diathermy and small hemoclips to remove the fat pad overlying and around the popliteal vessels (Fig. 62-4). This fat pad may contain up to seven lymph nodes. The popliteal vessels are unsheathed. The popliteal artery is slightly medial and deeper to the vein. The popliteal vein has variable small tributaries below the level of the lesser saphenous vein branch, which the surgeon should avoid.
- One lymph node is frequently located anterior to the popliteal artery and posterior to the knee joint and should be dissected.
- The popliteal space should be evaluated and palpated to ensure that all lymphatic tissue has been excised.

Closure

- Meticulous hemostasis is performed.
- The deep fascia is reapproximated with a running 2-0 absorbable suture.
- A closed suction drain remains in the subcutaneous space above the fascia, brought out through a separate incision, and secured with a 3-0 nonabsorbable monofilament suture.
- The wound edges are approximated with interrupted absorbable 2-0 subcutaneous sutures, and the skin is closed by staples (Fig. 62-5).

III. ALTERNATIVE TECHNICAL APPROACHES (PRO/CON) AND PEARLS

- An alternative skin incision can be done as a long sigmoid shape with the horizontal portion across the posterior crease of the knee.
- The medial approach to the popliteal fossa has the patient lying in a supine position. This is commonly practiced by vascular surgeons, requires extensive dissection, and is not appropriate for popliteal lymph node dissection.

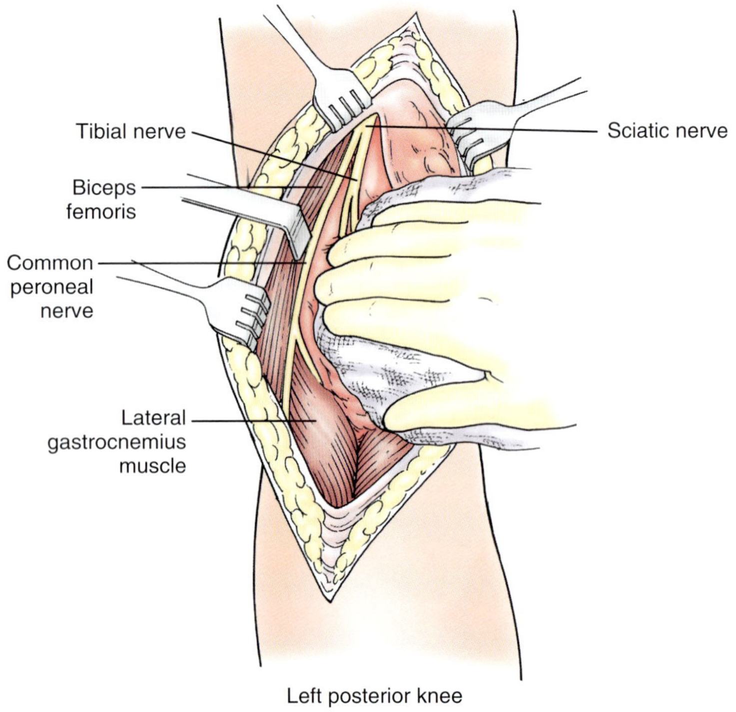

Figure 62-3.

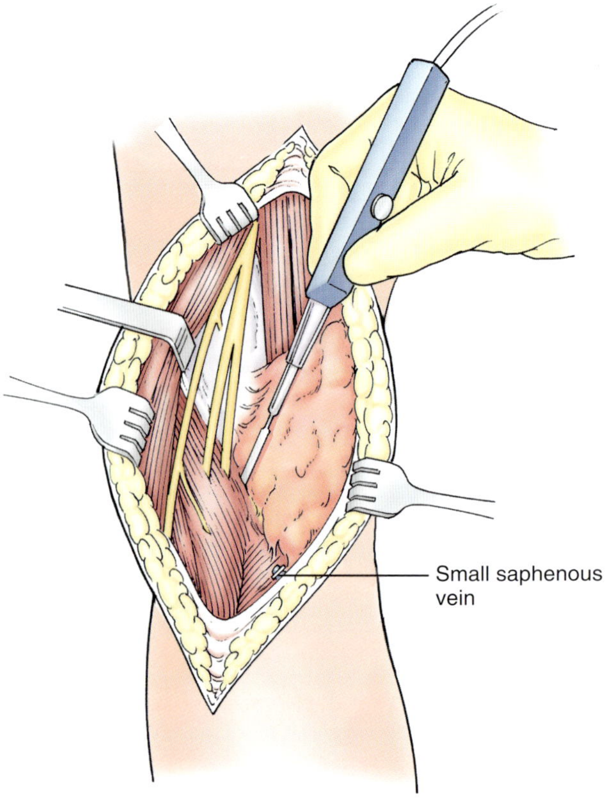

Figure 62-4.

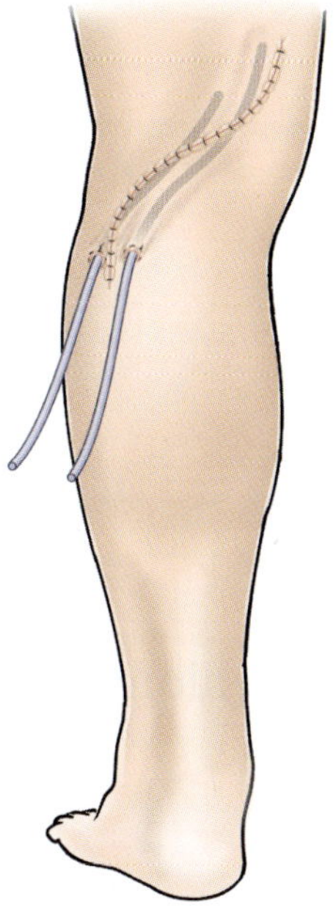

Figure 62-5.

IV. SPECIAL POSTOPERATIVE CARE

- The patient requires complete bed rest and extremity elevation for the first 2 days.
- Specific intraoperative complications of popliteal lymph node dissection are nerve injury and popliteal vascular injury. An injured medial sural nerve will cause cutaneous anesthesia over the lateral and posterior third of the leg, the lateral aspect of the foot and heel, and the lateral portion of the ankle. Injury to the peroneal nerve results in significant disability. There is a loss of capacity to lift the foot and move the toes (dorsiflexion), as well as a loss of the ability to evert the foot. The patient finds it difficult to walk and, when attempting to do so, drags the foot on the ground when bringing it forward. The patient senses a loss of control of the foot. Injury to the tibial nerve can cause weakness or paralysis of plantar flexion and adduction of the foot and toes. Sensory deficits may be seen in distribution of sural, lateral plantar, and calcaneal nerves.
- The specific immediate postoperative complications that may be encountered with popliteal lymph node dissection are hematoma, wound infection, wound disruption, neuropathic pain, deep vein thrombosis, and leg edema.
- The patient is treated with a subcutaneous injection once a day of low–molecular-weight heparin for prophylaxis of deep venous thrombosis.
- Physiotherapy for passive knee movement and instructions for active knee movement are given after postoperative day 3.
- Skin staples are left for 2 weeks or longer if necessary to avoid wound disruption.

SUGGESTED READINGS

Karakousis CP: The technique of popliteal node dissection, *Surg Gynecol Obstet* 151:420–423, 1980.
Sholar A, Martin RC 2nd, McMasters KM: Popliteal lymph node dissection, *Ann Surg Oncol* 12:189–193, 2005.
Thompson JF, Hunt JA, Culijac G, et al: Popliteal lymph node metastasis from primary cutaneous melanoma, *Eur J Surg Oncol* 26:172–176, 2000.

CHAPTER 63

Radical Axillary Dissection

Schlomo Schneebaum, MD, and Eliad Karin, MD

I. SPECIAL PREOPERATIVE PREPARATION

- The rationale of preoperative evaluation is to properly stage the patient, define the extent of involvement, confirm the diagnosis, and prepare the surgeon for unusual surgery.
- The most common indication for radical axillary lymph node dissection is melanoma with involvement of the lymph nodes.
- There are several scenarios where such an operation is indicated:
  - ▲ Positive sentinel lymph node (SLN) where the operation can be done in some instances after a frozen section in the same operation, or in a second setting if the diagnosis is by paraffin section or immunohistochemistry.
  - ▲ Following a suspicious node on physical examination verified by fine-needle aspiration in a known melanoma patient.
  - ▲ Tru-cut biopsy in cases of axillary adenopathy of unknown origin.
- In the case of a staged operation, positron emission tomography–computed tomography (PET-CT) is usually recommended to stage the patient and exclude disseminated disease.
- Axillary ultrasonography is indicated if a suspicious lymph node is identified by palpation or by PET-CT, to verify diagnosis. There is no need for ultrasonography if the diagnosis of involved SLN was done by pathology.
- Magnetic resonance imaging is indicated only in cases of grossly involved lymph nodes (lymph nodes sticking together). Involvement of blood vessels may occur, and therefore extensive surgery might be necessary.
- For assessment of correct stage, CT of the brain or magnetic resonance imaging should be done, because PET-CT is not sensitive enough to detect brain metastasis.
- There is no place for open biopsy of a lymph node suspicious for melanoma.
- The most important feature of this operation is the completeness of the dissection, including level III (lymph nodes medial to the pectoralis minor muscle). It is tragic when a patient has a recurrence in the apical axillary node because this node should have been excised in the original operation. A limited axillary dissection (level I+II axillary lymph node dissection, as for breast cancer) has no place in the management of melanoma.
- It should be remembered that a metastatic node may be present at the perimeter of a traditional axillary dissection. Lymph nodes that might be overlooked are usually along the posterior axillary line and lower chest wall, as well as along the long thoracic nerve.

II. OPERATIVE TECHNIQUE

Position

- Surgery is done under general anesthesia, with intravenous access placed in the contralateral arm.
- The patient is placed in the supine position with the ipsilateral arm placed on an arm support. We usually place a folded sheet under the scapula so that the latissimus dorsi muscle is off the operating table. The sheet is placed under the silicon mattress in the operating room.

- The chest, shoulder, and arm to the forearm are prepped. Because the technique we use requires mobilization of the arm during surgery, we drape the arm with a towel (half sheet) that is then draped with stockinet up to the elbow so the arm can be manipulated during surgery (Fig. 63-1).

Incision

- A transverse incision is made in the end of the hairline beginning at the anterior axillary line and continuing to the posterior axillary line. In the case of a previous SLN biopsy incision, an elliptical incision is placed to include the previous incision and the drain stab-wound incision (Fig. 63-2).

Main Dissection

- After the incision skin flaps are elevated, we use Allis clamps to hold the skin. Skin hooks or rake retractors can be used as well. The superior flap is raised first. The clamps are held in tension. We usually use the cutting mode of the diathermy for the first 5 mm to delineate the flap thickness, and then we use the diathermy at 45 volts in the desiccate mode.

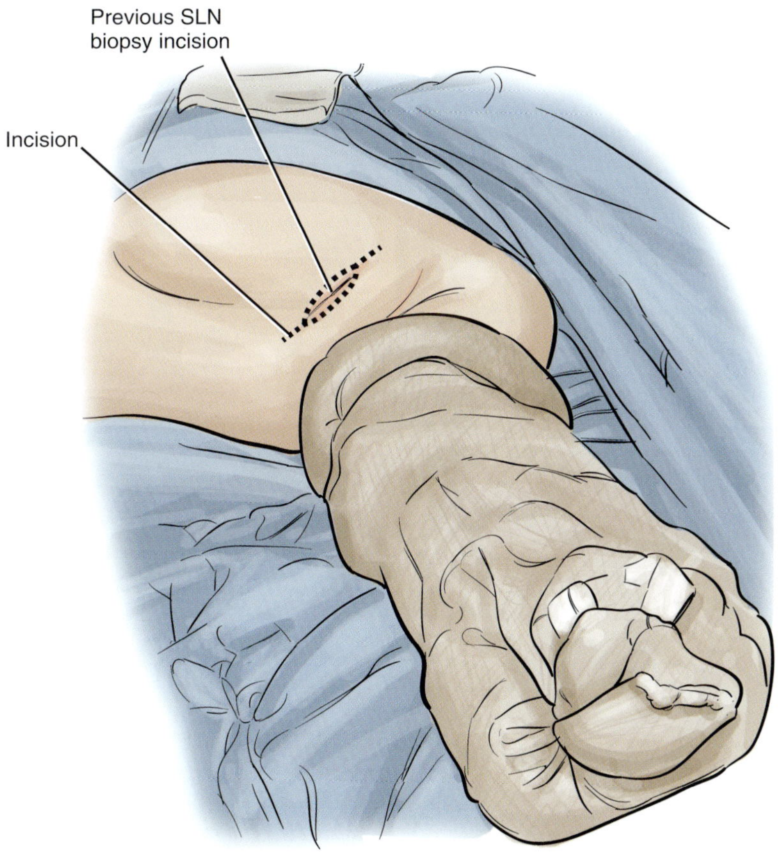

Figure 63-1. *SLN,* Sentinel lymph node.

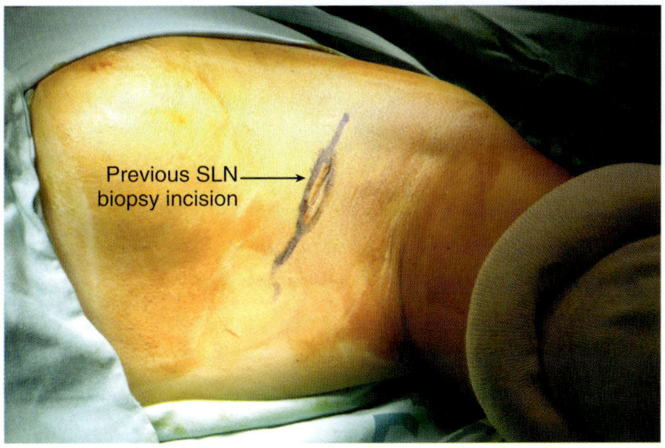

Figure 63-2. *SLN,* Sentinel lymph node.

- The flaps are raised with uniform thickness with the surgeon's nondominant hand used to apply countertraction on the soft tissue until we reach the pectoralis major fascia. We then raise the inferior flaps until we reach a point lateral to the latissimus dorsi muscle (Fig. 63-3, *A* and *B*, and Fig. 63-4).
- The superior margin of the dissection is above the pectoralis muscle fascia, near its insertion into the humerus. We continue the dissection of the fascia above and under the pectoralis major. The dissection continues to the pectoralis minor and then to the serratus muscle. The fatty and lymphatic tissue overlying the pectoralis major muscle anteriorly is dissected in a subfascial plane over the leading edge of the muscle and then on its underlying surface until the pectoralis minor (Fig. 63-5). The pectoralis major is elevated, and dissection continues along the anterior surface of the pectoralis minor muscle. At this point it is important to identify the medial pectoral nerve as it emerges through or just medial to the pectoralis minor muscle (damaging it can cause pectoralis major atrophy). We then continue to the coracobrachialis muscle and the serratus anterior muscle.
- We go cephalad to the fat pad above the axillary vein and begin to dissect it. The tissue is held with a Babcock clamp and retracted slightly (Fig. 63-6). This dissection can be done with a knife or with the assistant's help: while the surgeon uses a dissection clamp, the assistant puts hemoclips on minor blood vessels and uses the diathermy. The tissue can be swept with the blunt end of the knife handle as well.
- At this point we dissect the upper axillary lymph nodes. We use the approach of abducting the arm over the chest and retracting the pectoralis muscle in an upward direction (Fig. 63-7). This opens level III and enables dissection of all fatty tissue including the lymph nodes. It is important to be aware that

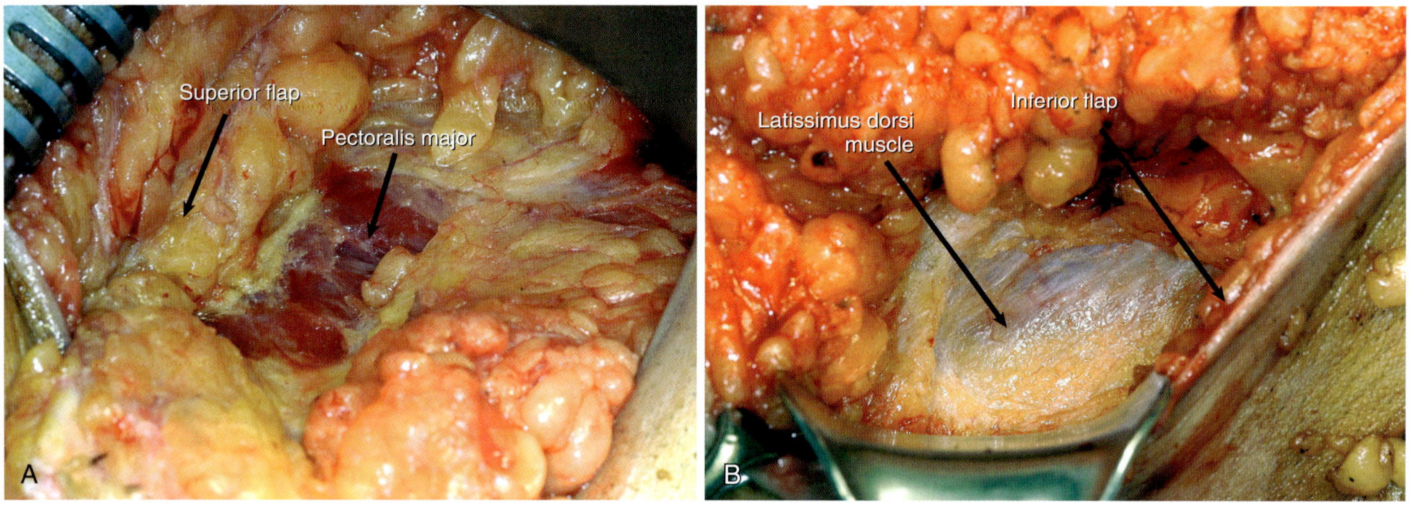

Figure 63-3.

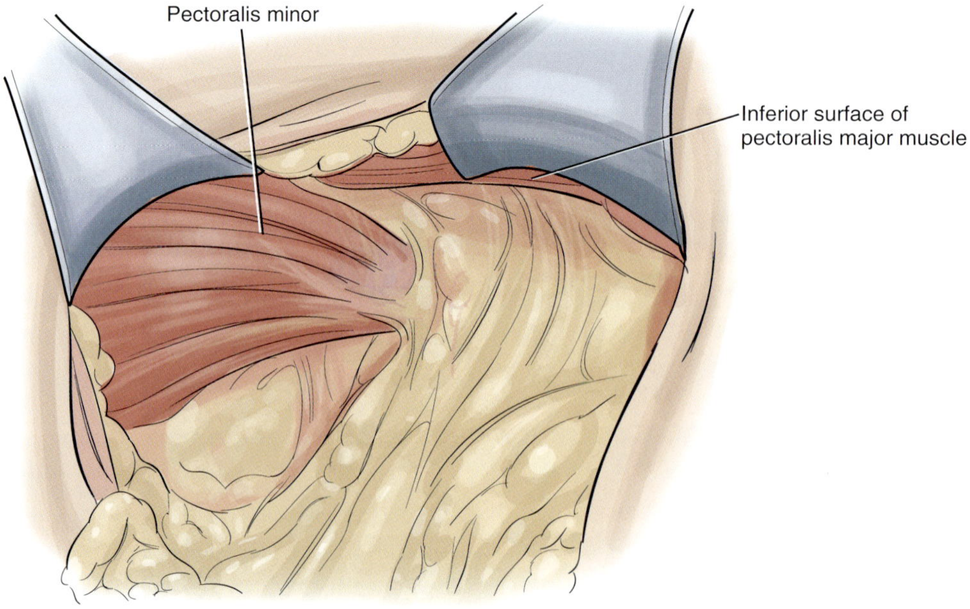

Figure 63-4.

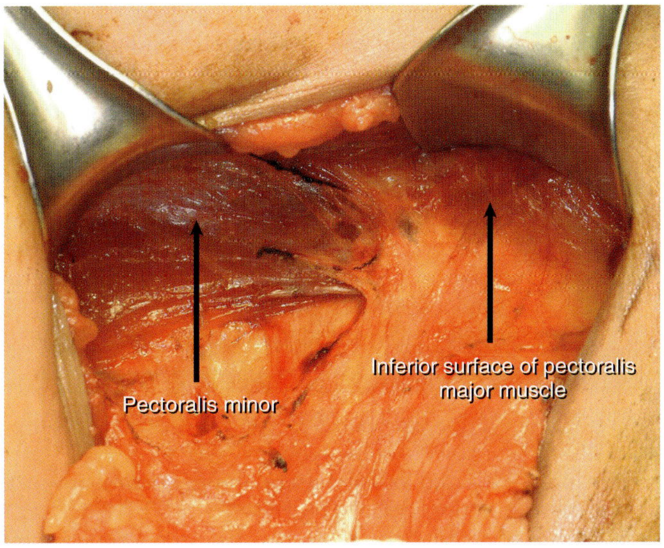

Figure 63-5.

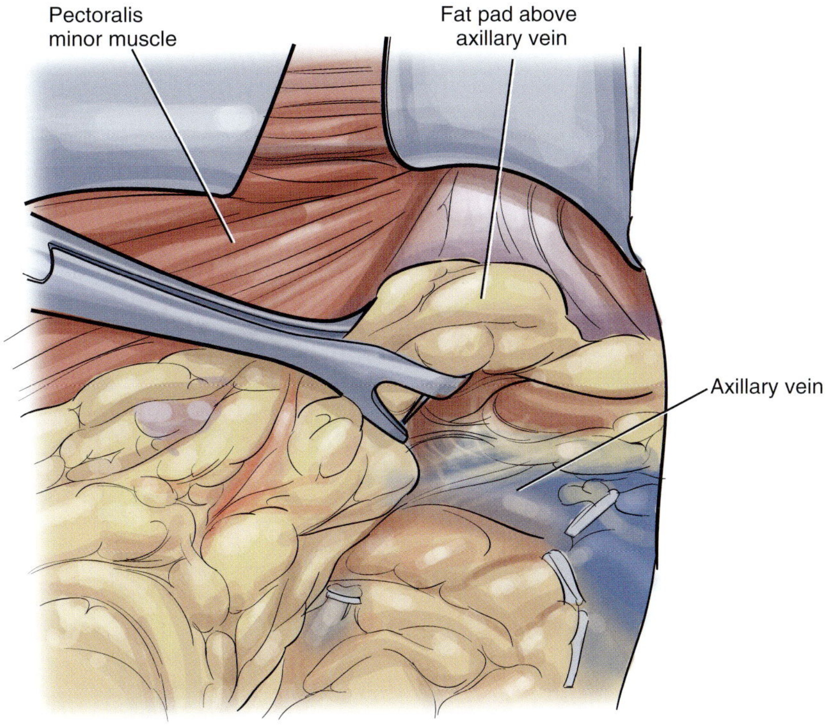

Figure 63-6.

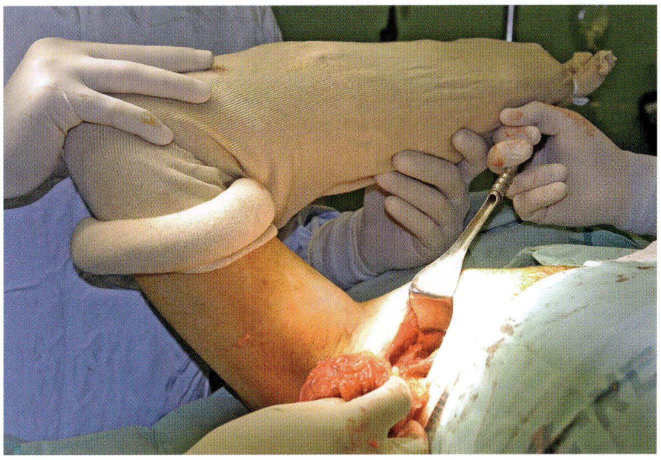

Figure 63-7.

the maneuver changes the spatial anatomy and brings the axillary vein very near to the surgeon. The dissection is done with small hemoclips for the small blood vessels (Fig. 63-8).

- The patient's arm has been brought over the chest in extreme abduction and internal rotation. The first assistant holds or steadies the arm while the second assistant sharply retracts the pectoralis muscle upward with a large retractor. This maneuver opens the axilla and greatly facilitates the dissection.
- An alternative approach is the Patey procedure to incorporate the pectoralis minor muscle as part of a dissection or taking down the pectoralis muscle at the insertion of the humerus. The advantage of this approach is that no intraoperative mobilization is needed and no alteration of the spatial anatomy.
- At the Sydney Melanoma Unit, the pectoral head of the pectoralis major muscle is detached at its insertion from the humerus and part of the pectoralis major is folded interiorly, toward the opposite side, as if opening a book. In a similar approach published elsewhere, the level III nodes are dissected freely by entering the clavicopectoral groove and retracting the clavicular and sternal heads of the pectoral muscle.
- The level III nodes are dissected freely from the axillary vein, the Halsted ligament, and other surrounding tissues. The nodes are dissected until they are positioned medially to the pectoralis minor.
- We then continue to dissect the lower axillary nodes. The fatty and lymphatic tissue is dissected downward over the brachial plexus and axillary artery and beginning at the coracoid process until the axillary vein is exposed on its anterior surface (Fig. 63-9).
- Starting at the apex of the axilla, all fatty and lymphatic tissue anterior and inferior to the axillary vein is now divided using a Babcock clamp to slightly retract the tissue. The first assistant applies hemoclips while the surgeon cuts the small branches of the axillary vein coursing the specimen.

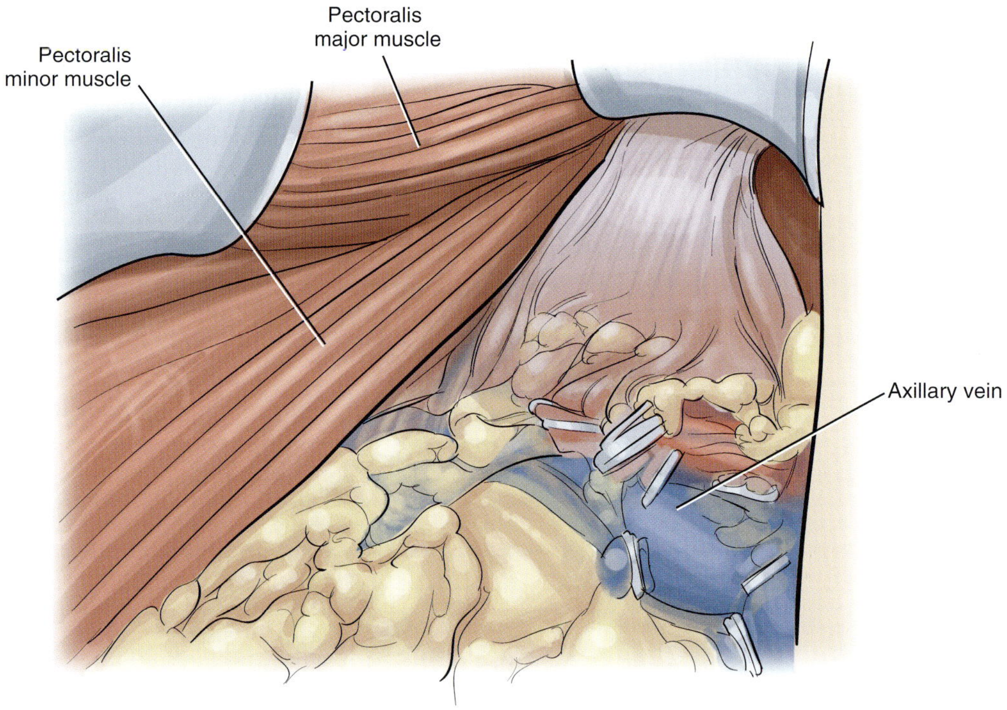

Figure 63-8.

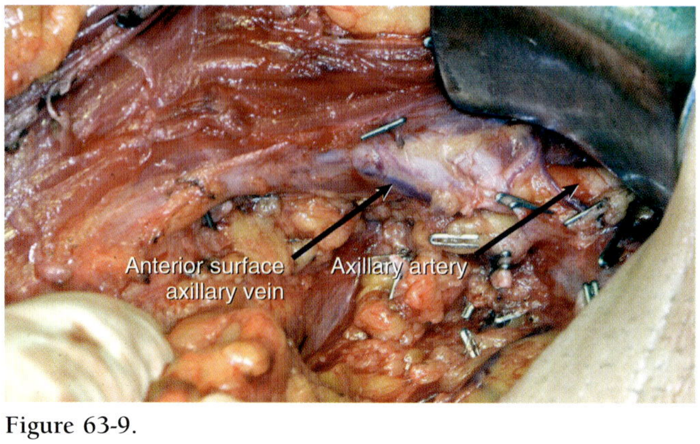

Figure 63-9.

- Another approach is to apply hemostats and ligate the blood vessels. We found this to be a disadvantage because too much manipulation may avulse the clamped branches. After the axillary vein is completely freed, dissection is continued with the diathermy. We first identify the long thoracic nerve and continue to dissect in a medial-to-lateral direction along the chest wall until the thoracodorsal vessels and nerve are identified. We usually identify them earlier when dissecting the axillary vein (Fig. 63-10, *A* and *B*). We then proceed to strip the fatty tissue from the subscapularis muscle, with the axillary vein being

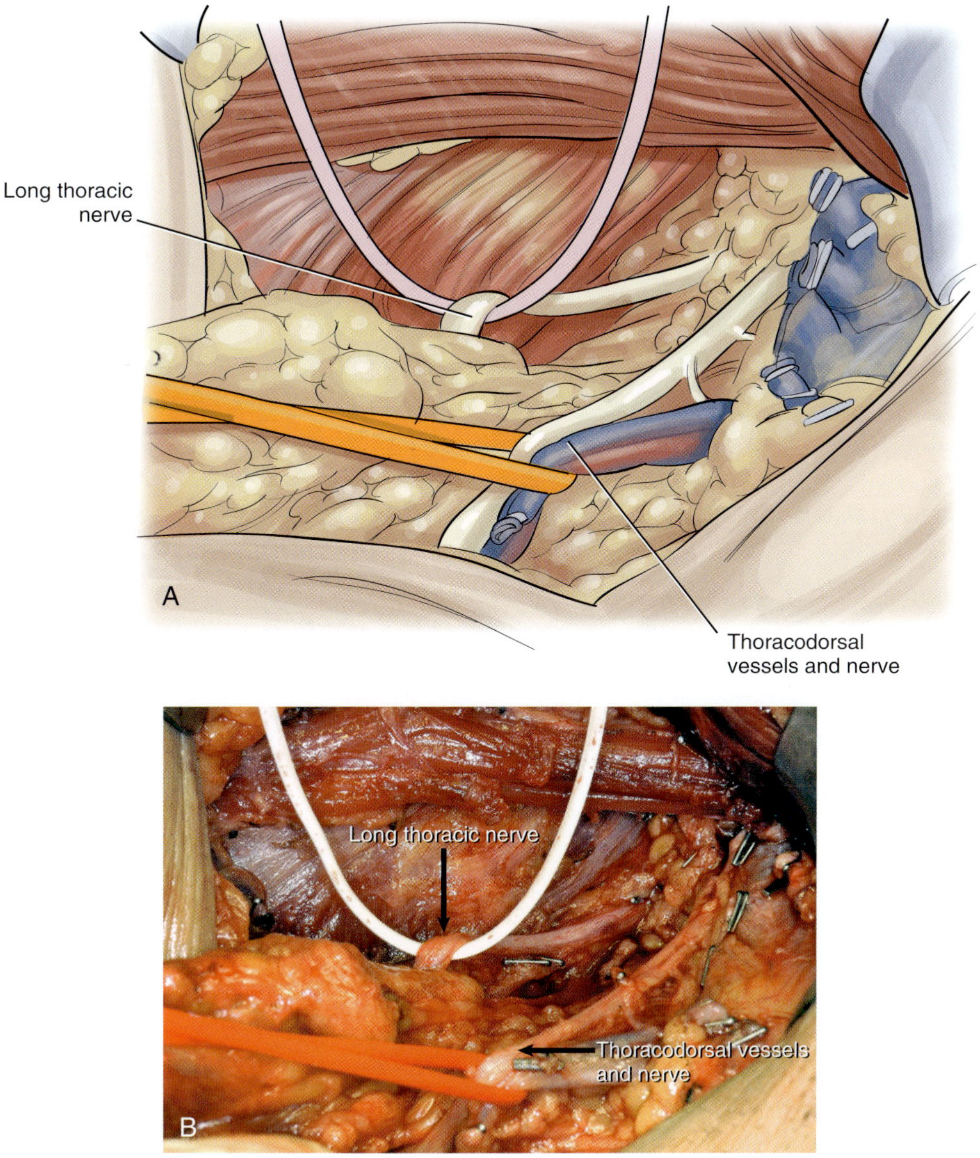

Figure 63-10.

the upper border. The fatty tissue is then removed along the latissimus dorsi to its lateral border (Fig. 63-11).

- The intercostobrachial nerve is identified as it comes from the chest wall and courses directly into the specimen, which is why it must be sacrificed. It is important to identify the nerves mentioned previously before its resection.
- The wound is irrigated with saline, and hemostasis is maintained. We usually repeat the elevation maneuver to ascertain that hemostasis is complete. A 12- or 14-Fr Hemovac drain is placed and brought out through a separate stab-wound incision.

Closure

- Closure is done with several inverted subcuticular Vicryl 3-0 sutures (or other synthetic absorbable suture), and skin staples are applied to the skin. They should remain in place 10 to 14 days. The drain is connected to a closed system (Fig. 63-12).

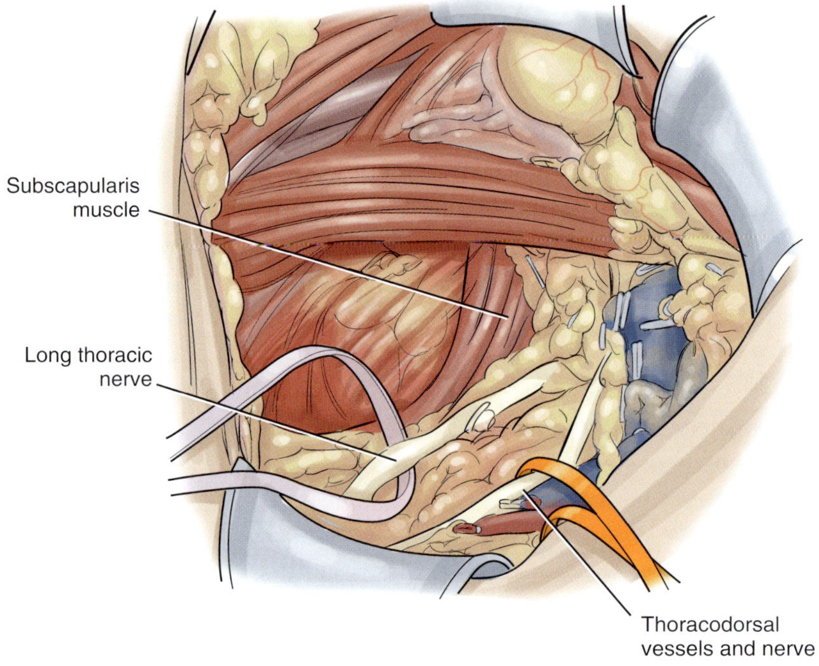

Figure 63-11.

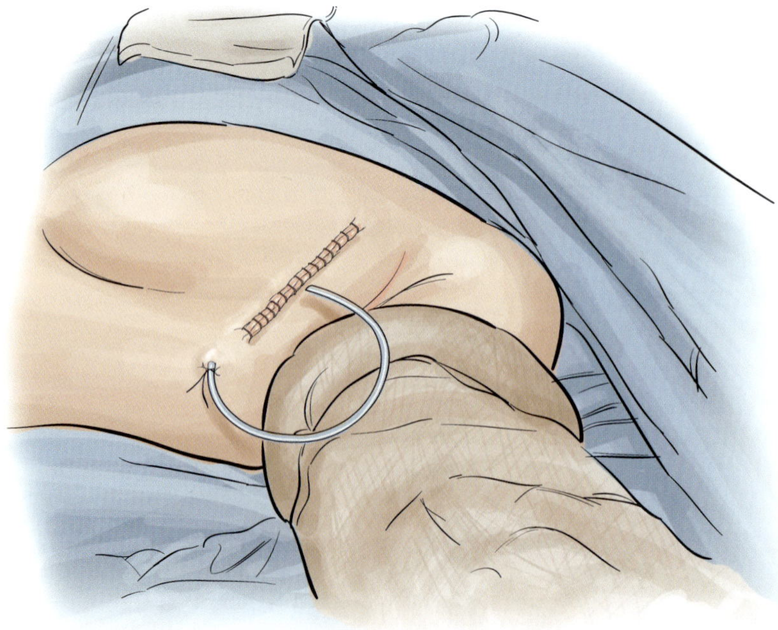

Figure 63-12.

III. ALTERNATIVE TECHNICAL APPROACHES (PRO/CON) AND PEARLS

- If the chosen approach includes detachment from the humerus, care must be taken at the conclusion of the operation. The head of the pectoralis major muscle is repaired either by attaching the tendon of the sternal head of that muscle to the humeral stump of the muscle, or alternatively by performing an intact insertion of the clavicular head as close as possible to the bicipital groove of the humerus.
- In case of involvement of the blood vessels, the vein can be ligated, but the artery should be bypassed. We place an extraanatomic bypass before resection. After removal of the specimen, an anatomic graft is placed.

IV. SPECIAL POSTOPERATIVE CARE

- The drain placed on a closed system is evacuated once daily; drainage continues until drainage is less than 40 mL, or on postoperative day 8 the drain is removed because it might be a cause of infection. If there is a collection of serum, drainage with needle aspiration under sterile conditions is done as an outpatient procedure.
- We do not limit the patient's movements. We encourage gradual physical therapy after postoperative day 3, starting with full range of motion and, after a week, exercises such as standing next to the wall and abducting the arm against it, slowly climbing with the arm on the wall. Pulley exercises are done after a week.
- We do not usually recommend an arm stocking, but if the patient had surgery on the arm such as wide excision, we recommend elevating the arm on a pillow in bed (at night).
- The patient is instructed that blood pressure measurements and blood drawing should be done in the contralateral arm. If the patient experiences a laceration or a cut, a disinfectant such as iodine should be applied, and if redness appears, a physician should be contacted.

Complications

- Specific immediate postoperative complications include seroma formation, infection, hematoma, pain, and altered sensation in the inner upper arm.
- Specific delayed complications that might be encountered are lymphedema, pain in the inner arm, and functional deficit.

Follow-Up

- At our center, if melanoma is found in the fatty tissue (extralymphatic), radiation treatment is offered. Follow-up consists of a physical exam every 3 months the first year, every 4 months the second and third years, and every 6 months the fourth and fifth years. PET-CT together with brain CT or total body CT is done on a yearly basis.

SUGGESTED READINGS

Balch CM, Urist MM, Maddox WA, et al: Management of regional metastatic melanoma. In Balch CM, Milton GW, editors: *Cutaneous melanoma: clinical management and treatment results worldwide*, Philadelphia, 1985, JB Lippincott, pp 93–113.

Karakousis CP: Surgical procedures and lymphedema of the upper and lower extremity, *J Surg Oncol* 93:87–91, 2006.

Meyer T, Merkel S, Gohl J, et al: Lymph node dissection for clinically evident lymph node metastasis of malignant melanoma, *Eur J Surg Oncol* 28:424–430, 2002.

CHAPTER 64

Composite Axillary and Supraclavicular Lymph Node Dissection

Theo Wobbes, MD, PhD, and Harald J.J. Hoekstra, MD, PhD

I. SPECIAL PREOPERATIVE PREPARATION

- Axillary lymph node dissection is a common staging procedure in surgical oncology. The most important indication is proven lymph node metastases in breast cancer and melanoma patients. In most patients of either group, a positive sentinel lymph node biopsy will lead to a complete axillary lymph node dissection. Selection for either sentinel lymph node biopsy or immediate axillary dissection is important.
- In breast cancer patients, ultrasonography of the axilla and fine-needle aspiration cytology of enlarged lymph nodes is of great value in avoiding a sentinel lymph node biopsy and planning immediately for axillary dissection. In selected cases, clinically negative axillary ultrasonography and fine-needle aspiration cytology may lead to omitting sentinel lymph node biopsy as the first step.
- In melanoma patients, a palpable lymph node should always be investigated cytologically. In extensive axillary lymph node involvement, a computed tomography scan should be performed to establish if there is continuity with lower cervical lymph nodes (levels IV and VB).
- The significance of enhanced magnetic resonance imaging using ultrasmall superparamagnetic iron oxide in the evaluation of axillary lymph node metastases in patients with breast cancer remains to be defined.
- Currently, fluorodeoxyglucose positron emission tomography (PET) is not sufficiently sensitive to replace histologic surgical staging of the axilla in patients who have breast cancer or melanoma. Gross lymph node involvement may be displayed by this diagnostic modality. Patients who have clinical stage III melanoma should be staged by fluorodeoxyglucose PET to select for a curative or palliative axillary and/or supraclavicular lymph node dissection. Patients with extensive nodal involvement should also be locally staged to prepare for the extent of the surgical procedure.

II. OPERATIVE TECHNIQUE

Position

- The patient is placed in a supine position with the arm of the involved axilla in 90-degree abduction on an arm board. Stretching of the brachial plexus should be avoided. Occasionally a lateral position can be chosen when the primary melanoma or in-transit metastasis is resected en bloc with an axillary dissection. The skin is prepared in a standard way extending across the midline, below the inframammary crease, in the supraclavicular region, and distally to the lower arm and, when required, the back. It is not necessary to drape the arm free to allow full movement, although some surgeons prefer that preparation.

Incision

- The choice of incision is dependent on the type of operation to be performed. In the case of a modified radical mastectomy, access to the axilla has already been made with the mastectomy.
- In the case of a breast-conserving operation, the incision can be performed in continuity with the lumpectomy if the tumor is located in the upper-outer quadrant of the breast. Otherwise a separate

transverse incision should be made along natural skin creases just below the hairline (see Fig. 63-1). The incision starts at the lateral margin of the pectoralis muscle and ends at the anterior margin of the latissimus dorsi muscle. Others prefer an incision along the lateral margin of the pectoralis muscle. Alternatively, an incision can be made along the deltopectoral groove and then extended laterally toward the pectoralis major border and posteriorly to the latissimus dorsi (Fig. 64-1). In the case of melanoma, particularly in muscular males, a more generous incision should be made to obtain good access for performing a complete dissection. Care should be taken to incise the full thickness of the dermis to the fascia that covers the axillary contents. Thin flaps can result in skin retraction and influence shoulder function and cosmetic outcome.

Main Dissection

- After incision of the skin, cranial and caudal flaps are prepared, extending in the dorsal direction to locate the lateral margin of the latissimus dorsi muscle and in the anterior direction to identify the pectoralis major muscle. In the case of a modified radical mastectomy, the dissection is in continuity with the ablation.
- Once the latissimus dorsi muscle is found, this muscle is further developed in the cranial direction. The cranial part of the lateral margin of the latissimus dorsi muscle is important because immediately above the transition to the tendinous part, the axillary vein can be found (Figs. 64-2 and 64-3).

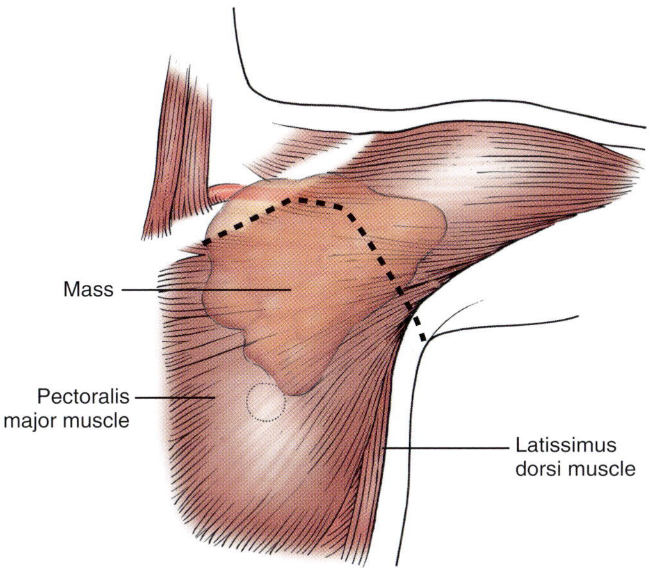

Figure 64-1.

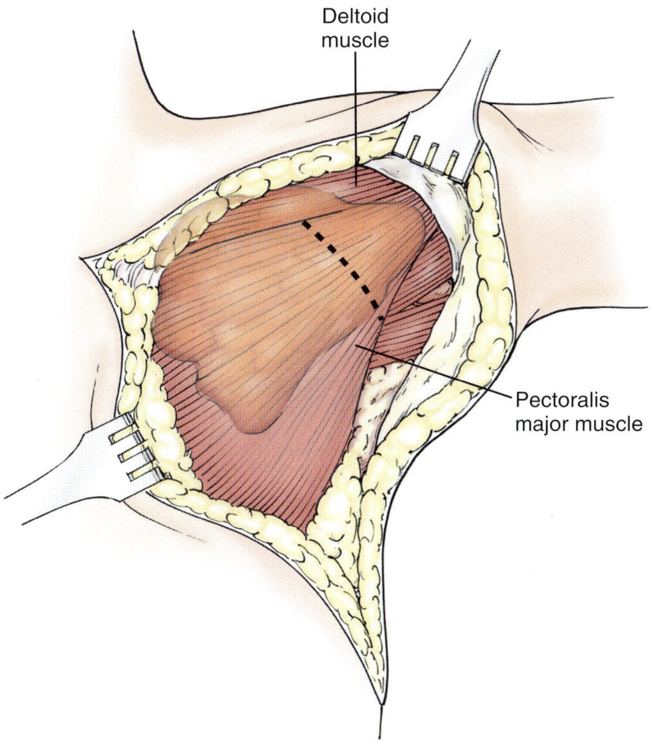

Figure 64-2.

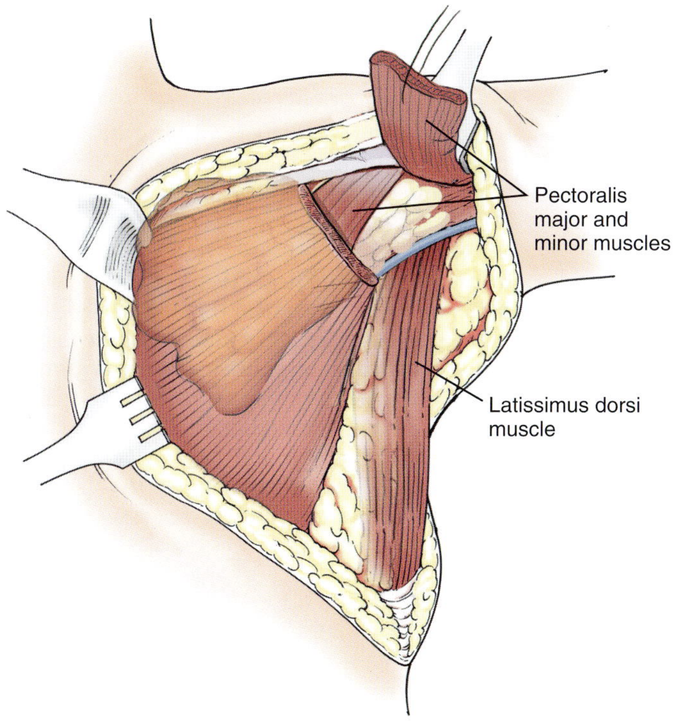

Figure 64-3.

- In a modified radical mastectomy, the axillary dissection starts generally when the lateral margin of the pectoralis major muscle is reached. In a breast-conserving procedure, it is also advisable to start the dissection medially. The muscle is dissected in the cranial direction to the top of the axilla and in the caudal direction to the thoracic wall. It is important to save the medial pectoral nerve as well as the medial pectoral vessels to prevent atrophy of the lateral part of the muscle. The structure is easily found on the undersurface of the muscle near the cranial end of the dissection. By retracting the muscle, the underlying structures can be seen and saved. Between the major and minor pectoralis muscle, the so-called Rotter lymph nodes are located. If there are lymph nodes, these are removed, sparing the intermuscular vessels.
- Subsequently, the lateral border of the pectoralis minor muscle is developed. With a retractor under the muscle, the axillary vein is presented almost automatically, and the adipose tissue and lymph nodes caudal to it can easily be removed (see Figs. 63-3 and 63-4). The region dorsal to this muscle is called level II of the axilla, whereas the fat and lymph nodes medial to the muscle are level III. Although there is a tendency to refrain from level III dissection in cases of breast cancer, a complete dissection should be performed in overt axillary lymph node involvement and in instances of melanoma and squamous cell carcinoma. To obtain better access to the level II and III region, it is advisable to remove the pectoralis minor muscle (the Patey procedure). The muscle attached to the coracoid process can easily be mobilized with the index finger just caudal to the tendinous insertion and subsequently transected just caudal to it. By retracting the muscle laterally, the connections to the thoracic wall can be mobilized and kept in continuity with the axillary dissection specimen. The so-called top axillary lymph nodes (level III) should be marked or sent separately to the pathologist.
- If the medial dissection is completed, the next step is identifying the axillary vein at the lateral side of the operating field. It should be noted that there are many variations in the anatomy of the axilla: abnormal axillary veins, abnormal muscles and tendons, and abnormal locations of the thoracodorsal nerve.
- Laterally, the axillary vein is found most easily from the point where the latissimus dorsi muscle becomes tendinous (white). The vein is unroofed over its full length, starting distally and going medially. To prevent damage to lymph vessels, the vein should not be stripped at the superior side. Then the fatty tissue can easily be detached bluntly in the caudal direction. Branching veins and large lymph vessels can be ligated or clipped and divided. Laterally and just below the vein, the intercostobrachial nerve is encountered, which should be saved to avoid numbness of the medial side of the upper arm. The nerve runs almost parallel to the vein.
- Of the axillary contents, two more structures should be saved: the thoracodorsal neurovascular bundle and the long thoracic nerve. If one is dissecting the axilla systematically from lateral to medial or medial to lateral, these structures are not difficult to find. The thoracodorsal neurovascular bundle supplying the latissimus dorsi muscle is identified below (dorsal to) a generally large vein, the anterior thoracic vein, that branches about 2 cm from the point at which the vein dissection begins (see Fig. 63-10). The thoracodorsal vessels are accompanied by the thoracodorsal nerve, which cranially is primarily located more medial to the vessels. Gentle compression with a forceps giving rise to contraction of the latissimus dorsi muscle confirms the structure. More distally, the nerve joins the vessels, coming together in the muscle. The next step is identifying the long thoracic nerve (Bell nerve) that adheres to the chest wall and runs in the craniocaudal direction to the serratus muscle (see Fig. 63-10). By retracting the axillary content in the lateral direction and dissecting the tissue from cranial to caudal parallel to the thoracic wall, the nerve is always found high in the axilla. The nerve should be left medial to the dissection plane. Subsequently, the axillary contents are dissected from the serratus anterior muscle, taking care not to violate the nerve more distally.
- The last step is the development of the thoracodorsal neurovascular bundle. Some branching vessels from the main stem should be carefully clipped. After the specimen is removed, it is labeled for the pathologist. The axillary levels in particular should be marked.

Supraclavicular Dissection

- It should be mentioned that in selected patients with melanoma, it also might be important to remove the supraaxillary lymph nodes, particularly if there is axillary metastatic involvement extending to the supraaxillary lymph nodes (levels IV and VB) (Fig. 64-4). This can be performed in continuity with the axillary dissection or through a separate supraclavicular incision. In cases of minor lymph node involvement, an extended axillary lymph node dissection will suffice. The fat pad above the level of the axillary vessels and the brachial plexus is mobilized and dissected away from these structures to the level of the axillary vein so that it can be removed in continuity with the remaining specimen.
- If there is clear continuity of extensive lymph node involvement of the lower (supraclavicular) neck basin (IV and VB) and the axillary basin, a separate supraclavicular incision should be made in the skin creases parallel to the clavicle. This incision can also be made in continuity with the axillary incision (see Fig. 64-1). After transection of the platysma, the medial border of the sternocleidomastoid muscle is developed in the cranial direction and retracted laterally and upward to expose the supraclavicular fossa. The dilemma involves the decision to keep the cervical specimen in continuity with the axillary specimen or to divide it, because keeping the continuity is technically a difficult procedure.

To perform a in-continuity resection, the middle third of the clavicle is removed (see Fig. 64-4). The level IV and VB cervical lymph nodes should be dissected, starting medially and working in the lateral direction. The cranial margin of the supraaxillary basin is the lower border of the omohyoid muscle. The floor is formed by the prevertebral fascia overlying the phrenic nerve and brachial plexus (see Chapter 1 or 2). The phrenic nerve passes over the scalenus anterior muscle from lateral to medial and lies behind the prevertebral fascia, which should not be opened to avoid severing this nerve (Fig. 64-5). After opening the sheath, the carotid artery is dissected downward as far as the subclavian artery. The same is done for the internal jugular vein to where it enters the subclavian vein (Fig. 64-6) (see Chapter 1 or 2). There are only theoretical reasons to keep continuity.

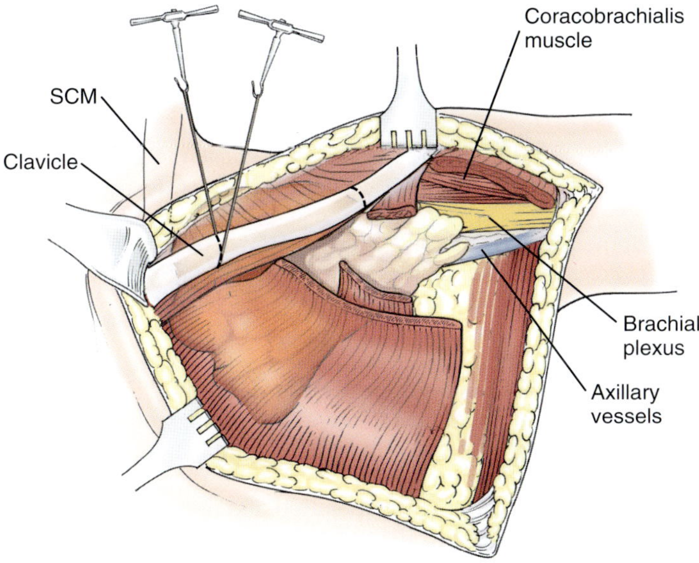

Figure 64-4. *SCM,* Sternocleidomastoid.

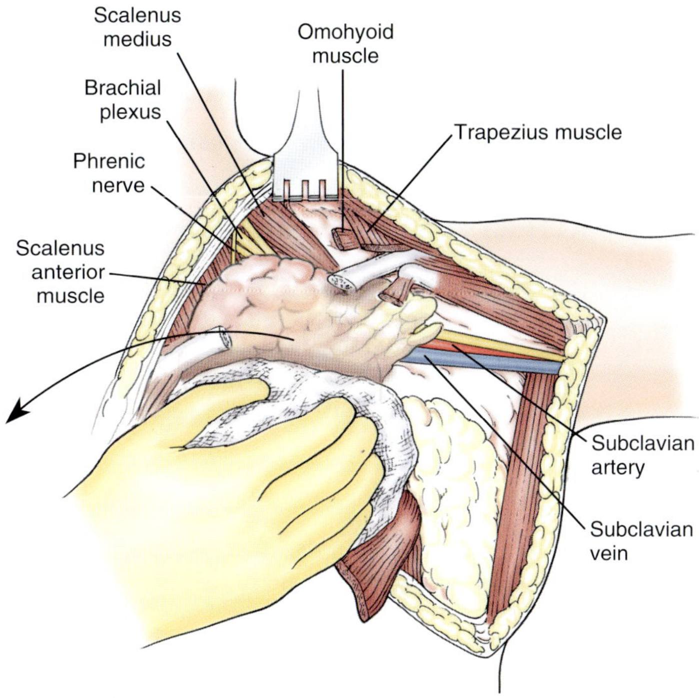

Figure 64-5.

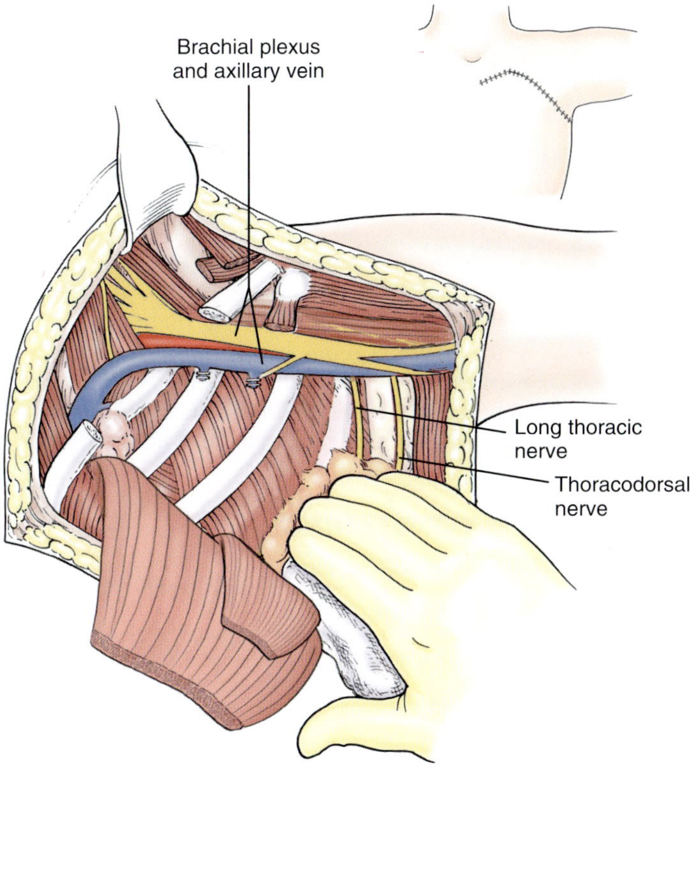

Figure 64-6.

- The fat and lymph nodes can be easily dissected from the subclavian vein by smooth upward traction. The dissection should end at the anterior border of the trapezius muscle. To gain access to this region, the posterior border of the sternocleidomastoid muscle should also be developed in the cranial direction. The external jugular vein that crosses the muscle is divided. Care should be taken not to damage the branches of the spinal accessory nerve entering the trapezius muscle at that level. Also, the transverse cervical artery that lies on the deep cervical fascia should not be severed.
- The thoracic duct, particularly at the left side, should be identified and carefully ligated.

Closure

- The wound is irrigated with warm saline solution, and meticulous hemostasis is performed. One or two low-vacuum drains are placed, brought out through separate stab wounds inferior to the incision, and secured with nonabsorbable sutures. The drains should not have contact with the axillary or jugular vein.
- The dermis is approximated with 2-0 absorbable suture, and the skin is closed with a running absorbable monofilament intracutaneous stitch. A dry gauze dressing is placed on the wound.

III. ALTERNATIVE TECHNICAL APPROACHES (PRO/CON) AND PEARLS

- Sometimes modifications of axillary lymph node dissection are indicated for patients who have melanoma or squamous cell carcinoma, and in the worst-case scenario, an axillary dissection may end as a forequarter amputation.
- When skin in the axillary region is involved, resection of the involved part is indicated. With extensive nodal involvement, resection of muscles such as the pectoralis, serratus anterior, or latissimus dorsi can be required. When the axillary vein is involved, the vein should be sacrificed.
- The axillary vessels and brachial plexus should always be covered with vital structures, and when that is impossible, reconstruction by plastic surgery or even free-tissue transfer is necessary. Therefore, before any surgical procedure, these patients should be appropriately staged locally and distantly.
- In patients with breast cancer, the sentinel lymph node procedure now leads to adequate staging and prognostic information. The question is whether limited axillary dissection in case of lymph node involvement (level I dissection) gives sufficient information for further treatment. At present, there is reason to conclude that axillary dissection in breast cancer patients is a staging operation and does not influence eventual survival. The only reason to do an extended (level II and III) dissection is to achieve local control in overt axillary involvement. It should be realized that this type of dissection, particularly in combination with radiotherapy, will lead to an increased risk of lymphedema.

IV. SPECIAL POSTOPERATIVE CARE

- The specific immediate postoperative complication that may be encountered is hemorrhage. The wound should be opened under general anesthesia and the hematoma evacuated.
- On the first postoperative day, the dressing is removed. The drain output is recorded, and the patient is instructed in how to care for the drains. Handling a low-vacuum drain is easily learned and allows hospital discharge in a few days. If the seroma production is less than 30 mL per day, the drain should be removed. There is no consensus on how long a vacuum drain should be kept in place in case of persisting seroma production. This should be handled according to departmental rules.
- From postoperative day 1, the patient should be instructed to do range-of-motion exercises help normalize shoulder function as soon as possible. The extent of the surgical procedure should be taken into account with respect to the rehabilitation.
- Late complications include lymphedema, with an incidence of 10% to 20% depending on the extent of the operation and whether it is combined with radiation. It also should be realized that more than half of patients have long-lasting complaints of the shoulder, the arm, and the scar (restricted shoulder movements, edema, pain, and numbness).

SUGGESTED READINGS

Khatri VP, Espinosa MH: Constant landmark for simplified identification of the long thoracic nerve during mastectomy, *J Surg Oncol* 64:82–83, 1997.

Kutiyanawala MA, Stotter A, Windle R: Anatomical variants during axillary dissection, *Br J Surg* 85:393–394, 1998.

Mack LA, McKinnon JG: Controversies in the management of metastatic melanoma to regional lymphatic basins, *J Surg Oncol* 86:189–199, 2004.

SECTION X

Radical Amputations

CHAPTER 65

Forequarter Amputation

Jeffrey M. Gauvin, MD, MSc, and Vijay P. Khatri, MBChB, FACS

I. SPECIAL PREOPERATIVE PREPARATION

- Preoperative radiographic imaging studies provide valuable information that aids in the diagnosis, defines the local extent of the tumor, stages the disease, and helps plan the incisional biopsy.
- Ultrasonography is particularly helpful for performing image-guided core biopsies to establish a diagnosis of soft tissue sarcoma but can also be valuable intraoperatively, as discussed later.
- Magnetic resonance remains the preferred modality for soft-tissue sarcoma, because it provides multiplanar images with improved spatial orientation. It also has the advantages of providing concurrent magnetic resonance angiography and venography, allowing delineation of tumor to adjacent vascular structures. Gadolinium contrast allows differentiation from benign tumors. Dynamic postcontrast images also help to differentiate tumor from tumor-associated edema. Preoperative imaging studies in patients who require forequarter amputation usually demonstrate malignant tumors invading the capsule of the shoulder joint and involvement of the neurovascular bundle within the axilla.
- For low-grade sarcomas, chest radiography is performed to exclude lung metastases, whereas computed tomography of the chest should be considered for patients with high-grade tumors or those larger than 5 cm.
- Office-based core needle biopsy is the first step to establish histologic diagnosis and can be performed under ultrasound guidance to avoid sampling necrotic or cystic areas, and importantly to avoid displaced neurovascular bundles.
- If core biopsy is nondiagnostic, a well-planned incisional biopsy should be performed. It is vital that placement and alignment of the incision allow it to be excised en bloc during the definitive resection.
- Patients will benefit from preoperative evaluation by orthotics to provide counseling for prosthetics, because forequarter amputation is a debilitating procedure.

II. OPERATIVE TECHNIQUE

Position

- After induction of general anesthesia and intubation, a Foley catheter is placed, and the patient is placed in a full lateral position secured with a bean bag. A roll is placed under the axilla to prevent injury to the brachial plexus. The affected upper extremity, chest, and anterior chest, as well as the back to the midline, are prepared and draped. The entire upper extremity should be draped free to allow it to be moved during the operation.

Incision

- The incision begins medially at the sternoclavicular joint, extends laterally along the clavicle, and then curves downward toward the axilla, proceeding toward the posterior axillary line. The superior part of the elliptical incision also begins at the sternoclavicular joint and travels along the clavicle, then runs over the supraclavicular region posteriorly toward the acromion and curves along the posterior axillary line to join the anterior incision. Hence, this represents a modified elliptical incision (Fig. 65-1).

Main Dissection

- Once the skin is incised, the dissection is carried downward to the level of the deep fascia. We prefer to begin the anterior dissection first. Standing anterior to the patient, the surgeon creates an anterior flap to expose the pectoralis major muscle. Next, the pectoralis major muscle is divided to expose the pectoralis minor muscle (Fig. 65-2). The clavicular head of the sternocleidomastoid muscle is severed from the clavicle. The periosteum of the clavicle is then marked with electrocautery, and the clavicle is divided with a Gigli saw near the medial third (Fig. 65-3). Alternatively, the clavicle can be disarticulated from the sternoclavicular joint, which is tougher, and the surgeon needs to avoid injury to the underlying vascular structures. When dividing the posterior capsule of the sternoclavicular joint, particular care is necessary to avoid injury to the underlying innominate vein. To allow the lateral retraction of the clavicular head along with the ipsilateral arm, the remaining attachment of the clavicle in the region of the sternoclavicular joint must be divided along with the subclavius muscle.

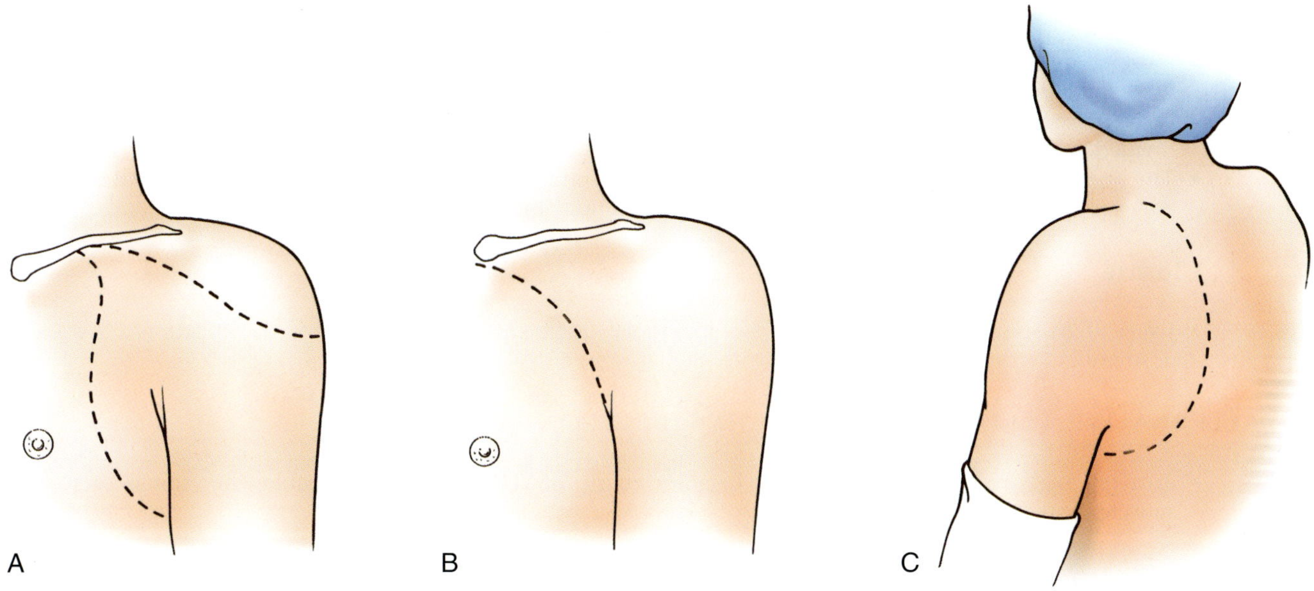

Figure 65-1.

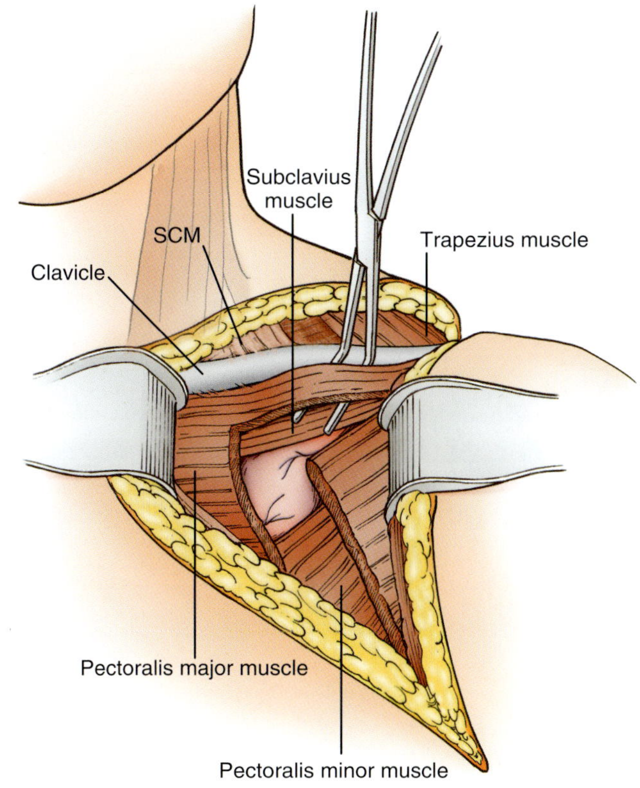

Figure 65-2. *SCM,* Sternocleidomastoid.

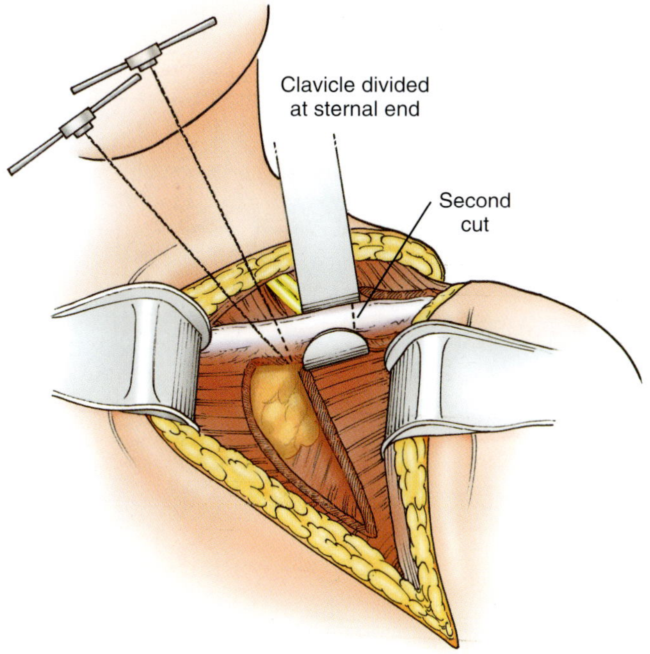

Figure 65-3.

- The subclavian vein is then isolated with a vessel loop. The external jugular vein draining into the subclavian vein is isolated, divided, and ligated with 2-0 silk suture. Dissection continues deep along the lateral border of the scalenus anterior muscle, where the subclavian artery is dissected and isolated with a vessel loop. The subclavian artery is transected and suture ligated (Fig. 65-4). Alternatively, transection can be achieved with a 2.5 linear endovascular stapler. Next, the subclavian vein is divided and suture ligated, or a 2.0 linear endovascular stapler can be used. All that remains are the trunks of the brachial plexus, which are exposed and divided sharply with a scalpel or Metzenbaum scissors (see Fig. 65-4). Bleeding from the small vessels around the nerves can be controlled with bipolar electrocautery. This essentially completes the vital anterior dissection and leaves only division of the rest of the muscular components to complete the forequarter amputation.
- The surgeon now stands posterior to the patient, completes the posterior skin incision, and deepens it downward to the fascia. A posterior flap is created to expose the broad muscle attachments of the trapezius and the latissimus dorsi muscles. The trapezius is then divided so it extends toward the medial aspect of the spinous process of the scapula. The lower aspect of the latissimus dorsi may need to be divided to expose the most inferior tip of the scapula. Once accomplished, the remaining muscles just medial to the posterior border of the scapula are exposed. Thus the levator scapulae and rhomboid muscles are divided next (Fig. 65-5). The suprascapular vessels and the transverse cervical vessels are then encountered. These are isolated, divided, and ligated with 2-0 silk suture. Moving farther in the caudal direction, the latissimus dorsi is completely transected. Finally, the serratus anterior muscle is divided at its origin on the chest wall, completing the entire resection.
- The operative area is then copiously irrigated, and 10-mm Jackson Pratt drains are placed beneath the anterior and posterior flap and secured with 3-0 monofilament suture.

Closure

- Excess flap should be trimmed and the superficial fascia then approximated with interrupted 2-0 absorbable suture. The skin is closed with staples, and a dry dressing is applied (Fig. 65-6).

III. ALTERNATIVE TECHNICAL APPROACHES (PRO/CON) AND PEARLS

- To avoid excessive blood loss, use of the LigaSure energy device can be quite valuable when transecting muscle tissue.

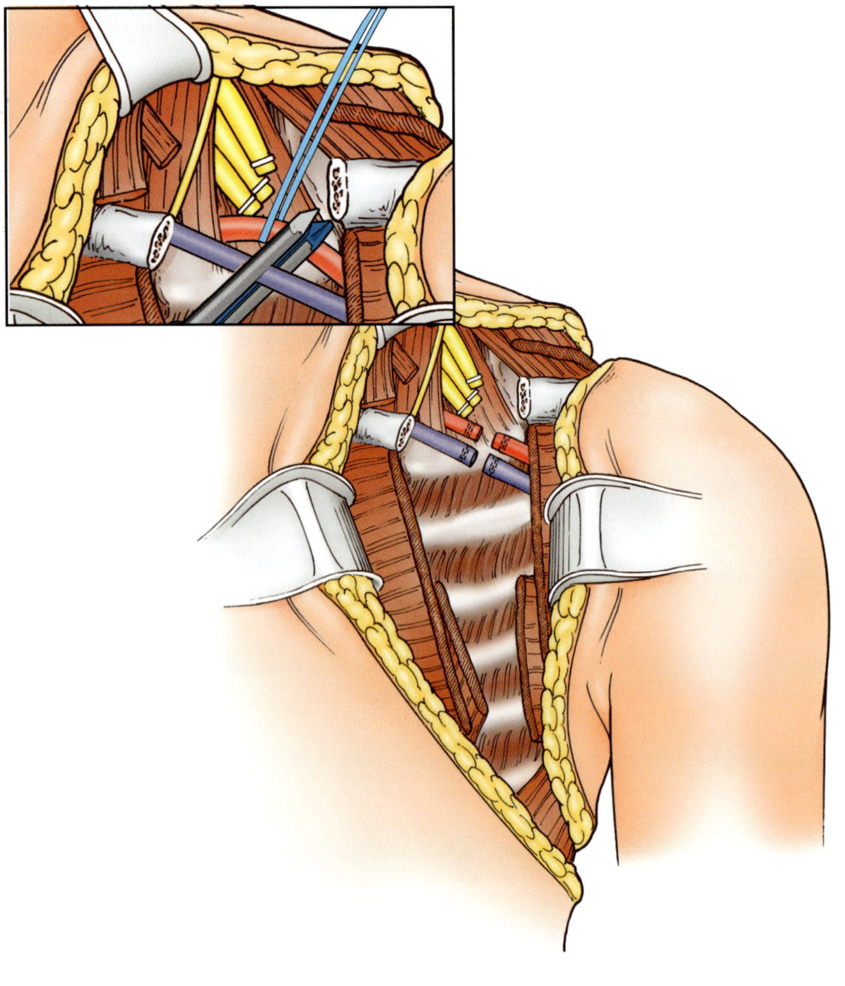

Figure 65-4.

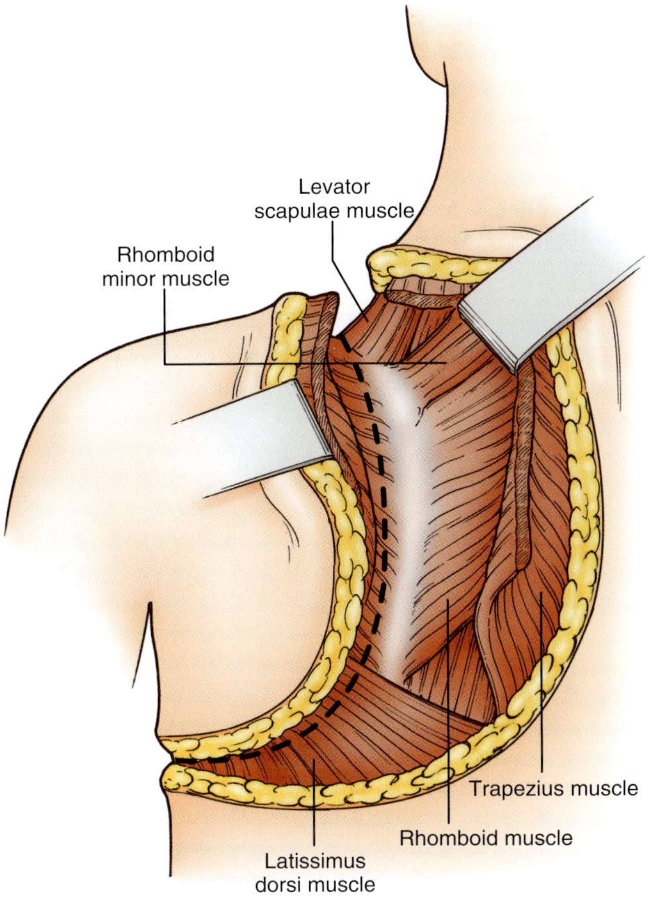

Figure 65-5.

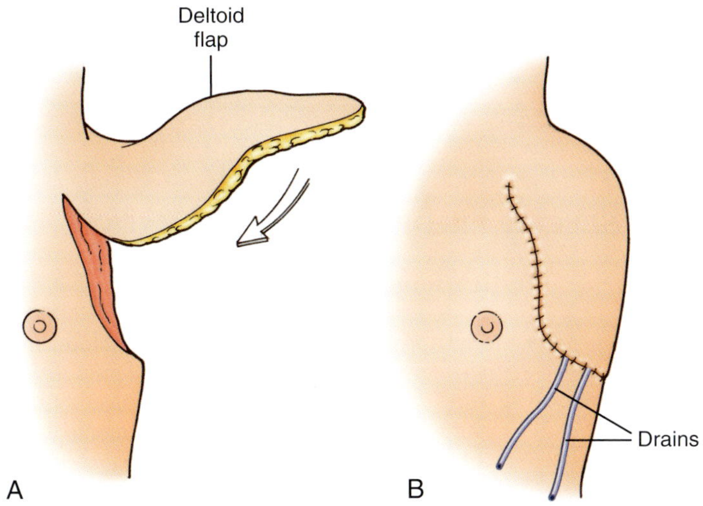

Figure 65-6.

- An alternative approach is to begin with the posterior dissection. First, all the muscles are divided; then the sternoclavicular joint is dislocated, which leaves the neurovascular bundle to be addressed last.
- Dislocating the sternoclavicular joint is difficult, so alternatively the clavicle can be transected with a Gigli saw at the medial third and the surface smoothed with a rasp.

IV. POSTOPERATIVE CARE

- Because pain can be considerable, a preoperative consultation with the pain team to place either a local block or a pain catheter may be necessary. Patient-controlled analgesia may also be needed.
- Patients are best monitored in the surgical intensive care unit for at least 24 hours or until stable, particularly as pain control can be difficult. Because there is no third-space fluid loss, all patients, even those with compromised cardiac or pulmonary function, can be managed with judicious fluid administration.
- The key to postoperative care is rehabilitation, as the patient now must learn to depend on only one arm and hand. The physical rehabilitation team is thus a crucial component of postoperative care.
- Prophylaxis against deep vein thrombosis is generally unnecessary, and we usually do not recommend it following extensive soft-tissue resection because of the likelihood of surgical-site hematoma.
- If a rather large flap had to be created and there is concern for its viability, then to prevent pressure necrosis, the patient must not lie on that side. Sometimes it may be necessary to provide the patient with a KinAir bed that will also help prevent undue pressure on the flap. This is particularly important if the patient had received prior radiation therapy, which impairs healing. In these situations we also leave the sutures or staples in place longer than normal.
- Early ambulation with assistance is recommended to avoid pulmonary complications.

SUGGESTED READINGS

Ferrario T, Palmer P, Karakousis CP: Technique of forequarter (interscapulothoracic) amputation, *Clin Orthop Relat Res* 423:191–195, 2004.

Rickelt J, Hoekstra H, van Coevorden F, et al: Forequarter amputation for malignancy, *Br J Surg* 96:792–798, 2009.

Volpe CM, Peterson S, Doerr RJ, Karakousis CP: Forequarter amputation with fasciocutaneous deltoid flap reconstruction for malignant tumors of the upper extremity, *Ann Surg Oncol* 4:298–302, 1997.

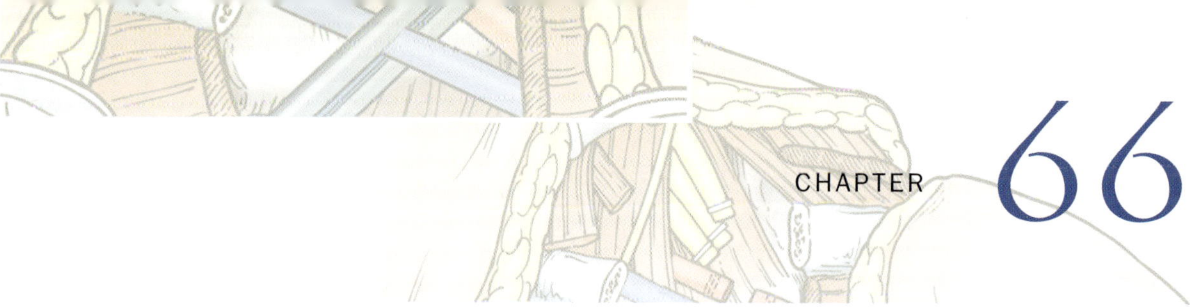

CHAPTER 66

Hip Disarticulation

Mario Mercuri, MD, and Costantino Errani, MD, PhD

I. SPECIAL PREOPERATIVE PREPARATION

Indications

- Indications for hip disarticulation include malignant tumors (of bone or soft tissues) located in the thigh, femoral diaphysis, or distal femur that are not adequately manageable by local resection. This is especially a result of tumoral involvement of the neurovascular bundle, but also owing to extremely extended tumors; extensive involvement of vessels, nerves, and bone; recurrent tumors; skin and soft tissues altered by previous surgery or radiation; pathologic fracture; infection; or a poorly functional limb caused by neurovascular impairment. Usually the association of several of these conditions is an indication for ablative surgery.
- The histotype and grade of the tumor, sensitivity to adjuvant chemotherapy and radiotherapy, age, general conditions, life expectancy, and other individual factors have a bearing on the indication.

II. OPERATIVE TECHNIQUE

Position

- The patient is placed in supine position with support under the scapula of the affected side. The entire limb is included in the sterile field, with the whole buttock, the iliac crest, and the pubic symphysis.

Incision

- The incision starts from the anterior-superior iliac spine and continues in an anterior racket shape medially inferior to the inguinal ligament to reach a point 5 cm distal to the origin of the adductor muscles (Fig. 66-1).

Main Dissection

- After dissection of the subcutis, superficial epigastric and external pudendal vessels must be ligated and divided to avoid bleeding.
- If enlarged lymph nodes are present, those proximal to the ligature are excised; those distal will be removed en bloc with the specimen.
- An incision is made just below the inguinal ligament. The femoral vessels (first the artery, then the vein) are exposed, clumped, doubly ligated, and divided; the proximal vascular stump is transfixed and ligated. The femoral nerve is also divided at this level (Fig. 66-2).

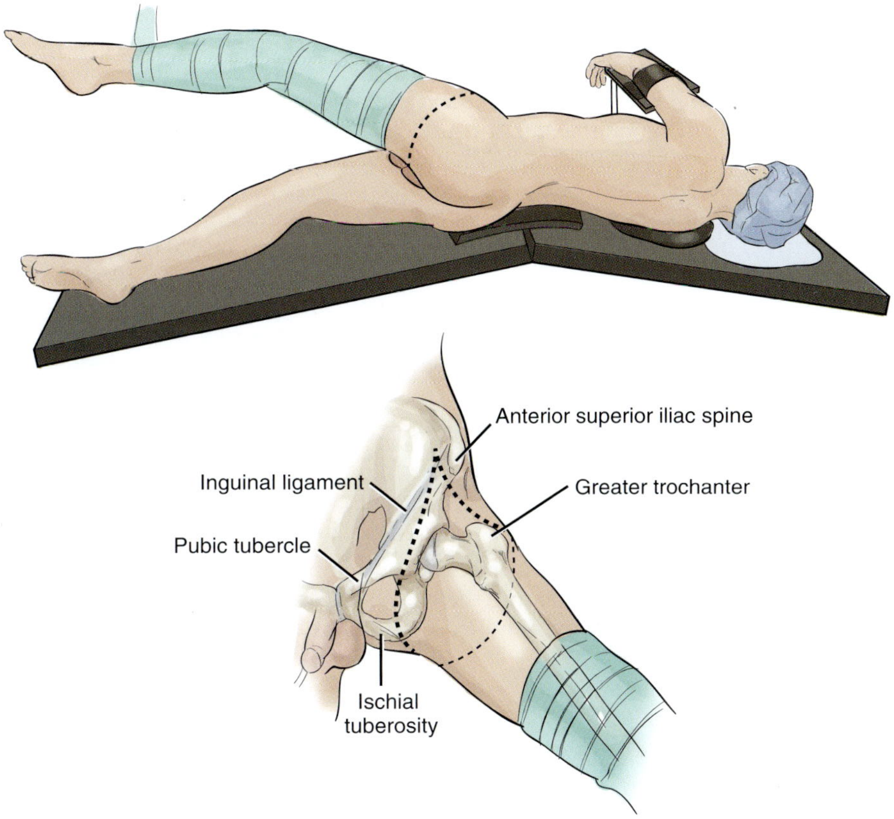

Figure 66-1.

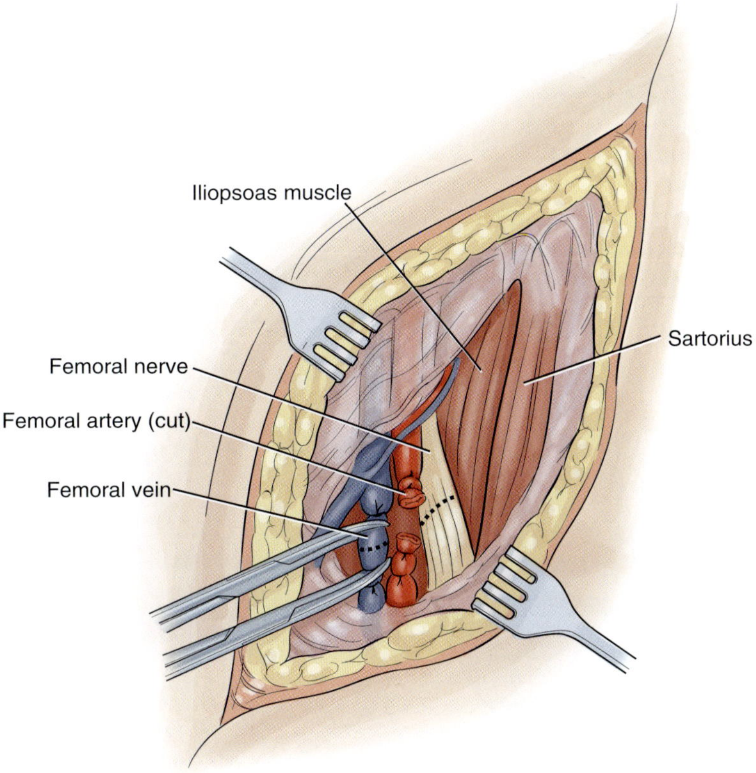

Figure 66-2.

- The muscles anterior to the hip joint (the sartorius and the rectus femoralis) are transversely divided two finger breadths below their origin and distally reflected (Fig. 66-3).
- With the hip in full abduction, flexion, and external rotation (gynecologic position), the iliopsoas is divided at its insertion to the lesser trochanter and proximally reflected (care should be taken to ligate and divide the vessels passing on the anterior surface of the iliopsoas). With the hip in the same position, the pectineus muscle is divided at its origin from the horizontal pubic ramus, followed by the adductor muscles from lateral to medial (Fig. 66-4).
- Care must be taken at this point to ligate and divide the obturator vessels and nerve, because of the risk of retraction into the pelvis of one proximal stump, which would then be impossible to reach (Fig. 66-5).
- The incision continues posteriorly from medial to lateral, with the hip fully flexed and abducted. The flexor muscles are dissected from their origin on the ischial tuberosity.
- The patient is rolled into a lateral position. The racket incision is completed posterolaterally, starting just distal to the anterosuperior iliac spine, descending in front of the greater trochanter, curving posteriorly four finger breadths distally to the tip of the trochanter, and finally transversely and posteriorly, contouring the thigh two finger breadths distally and parallel to the gluteal crease and connecting with the medial incision.
- The fascia is incised in the same line as the skin. The plane underneath the gluteus maximus is entered and completely opened, dividing the tendon of the gluteus maximus from the femur and transecting the distal fibers of the muscle. The gluteus medius and minimus muscles are divided at their insertion to the greater trochanter, internally rotating the hip, as are the short external rotators of the hip (the piriformis, gemellus, obturator internus and externus, and quadratus femoris).

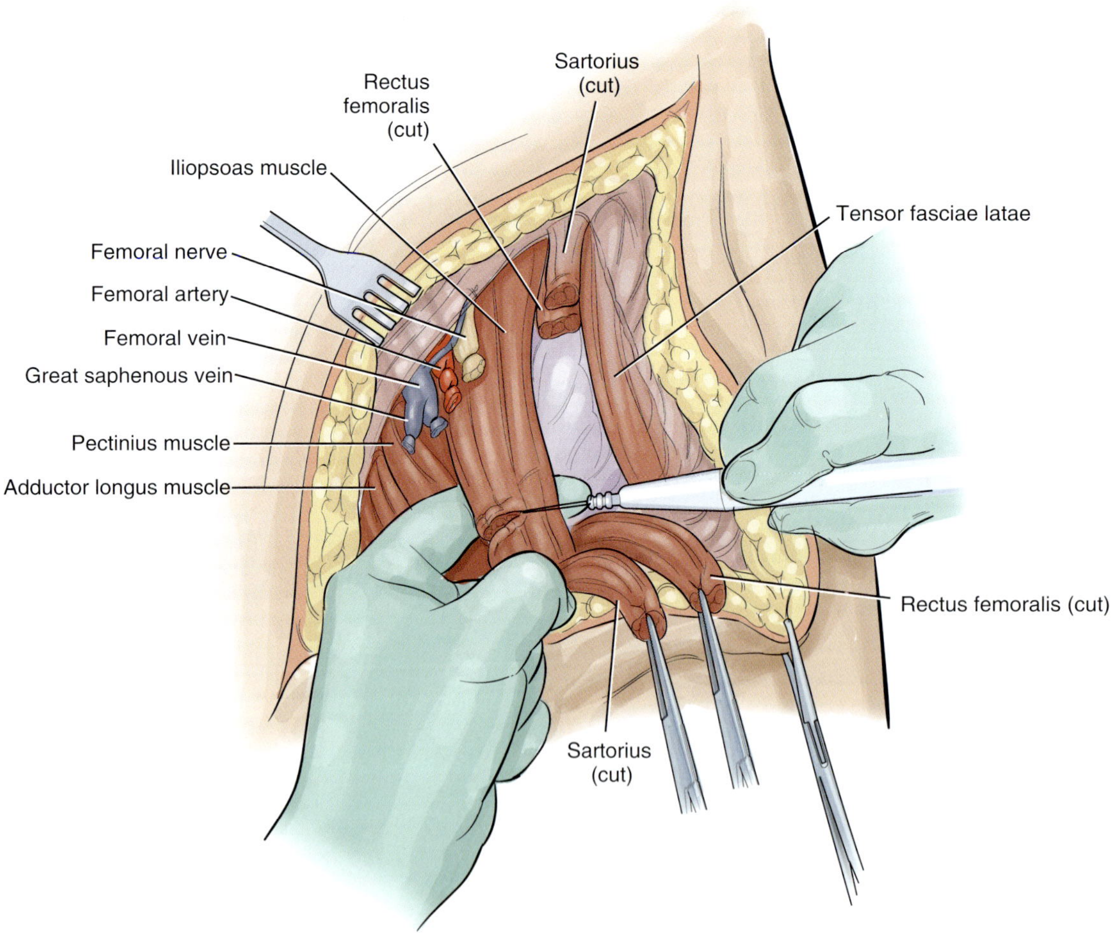

Figure 66-3.

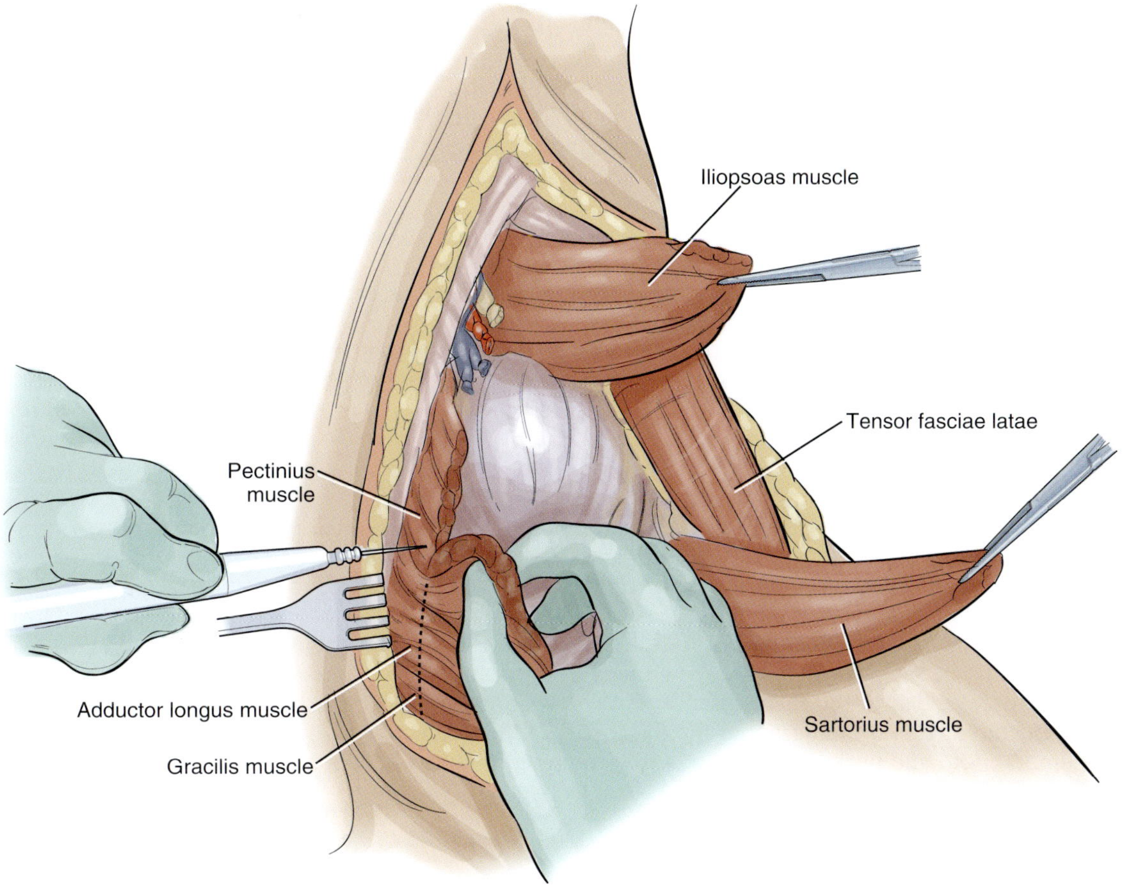

Figure 66-4.

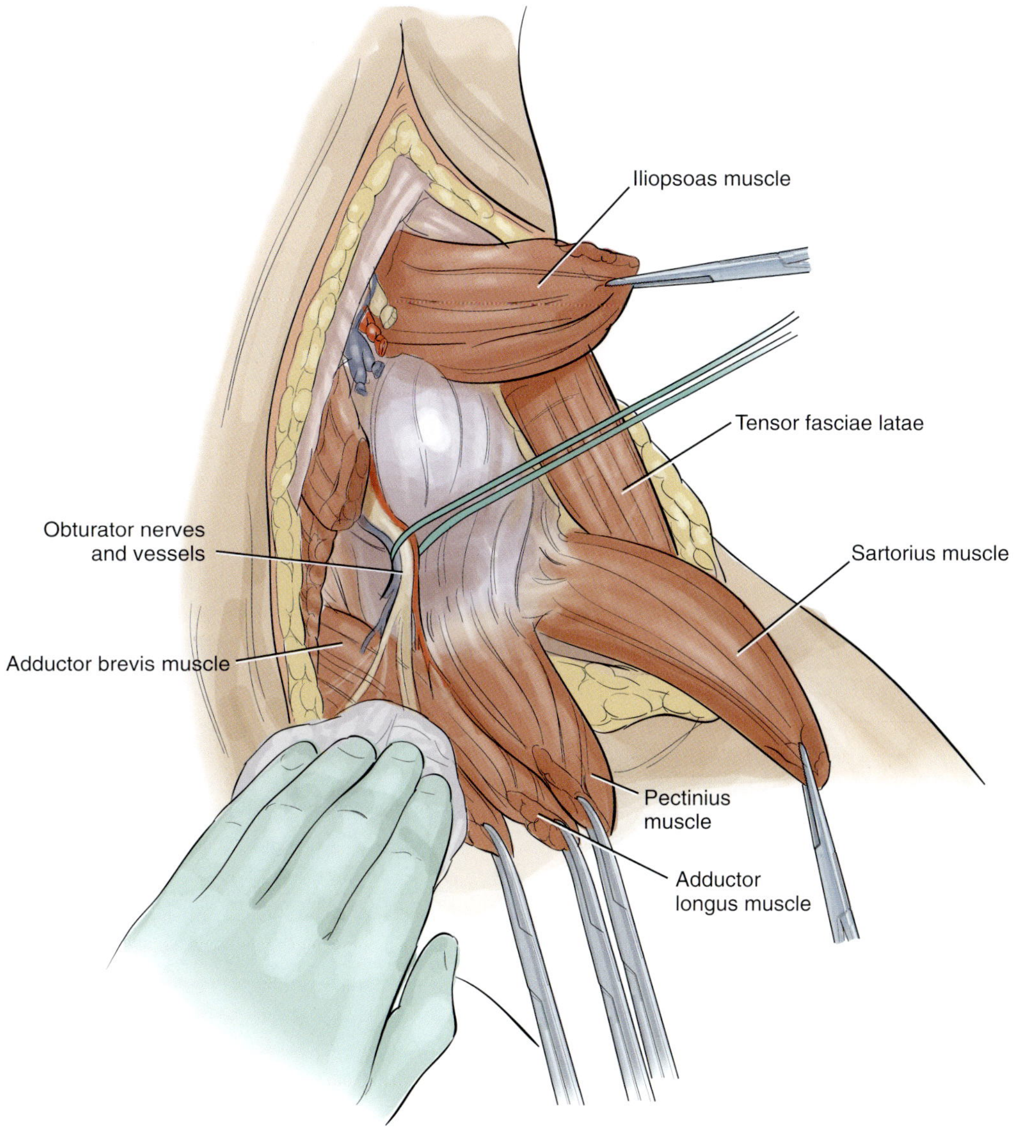

Figure 66-5.

- The hip joint capsule is incised anteriorly and posteriorly, the ligamentum teres is transected, and the hip is luxated (Fig. 66-6).
- The sciatic nerve is dissected free, ligated, and transected. Infiltrating the nerve with local anesthetic just before this procedure may reduce postoperative neurologic pain (Fig. 66-7).
- Hemostasis is secured and must be continued until the blood pressure is at least 100 mm Hg.

Closure

- For wound closure, the flaps are approximated by suturing the obturator externus and the sartorius to the gluteus medius muscle over the acetabulum.
- One suction drain is placed underneath the gluteal fascia. The fascia is then sutured to the inguinal ligament and pubic ramus (Fig. 66-8).

III. ALTERNATIVE TECHNICAL APPROACHES (PRO/CON) AND PEARLS

- When planning this procedure, the direction and position of the incision required to obtain cover flaps must be taken into account. If this type of incision passes close to the tumor, the procedure would in fact be nearly equal to a marginal resection, and it could be followed by local recurrence. These problems usually occur in tumors near the limb girdles.
- Hip disarticulation may be performed with atypical myocutaneous flaps. For example, an amputation for skeletal or soft tissue sarcomas involving the gluteus maximus may be obtained with an anteromedial skin and muscular flap of the thigh, used to cover the entire gluteal region removed up to the iliac crest. The femoral vessels are ligated at the distal part of the thigh.
- When the femoral head and neck are involved by the tumor, a modified hemipelvectomy is required. This means that the posterior portion of the ilium is not resected.

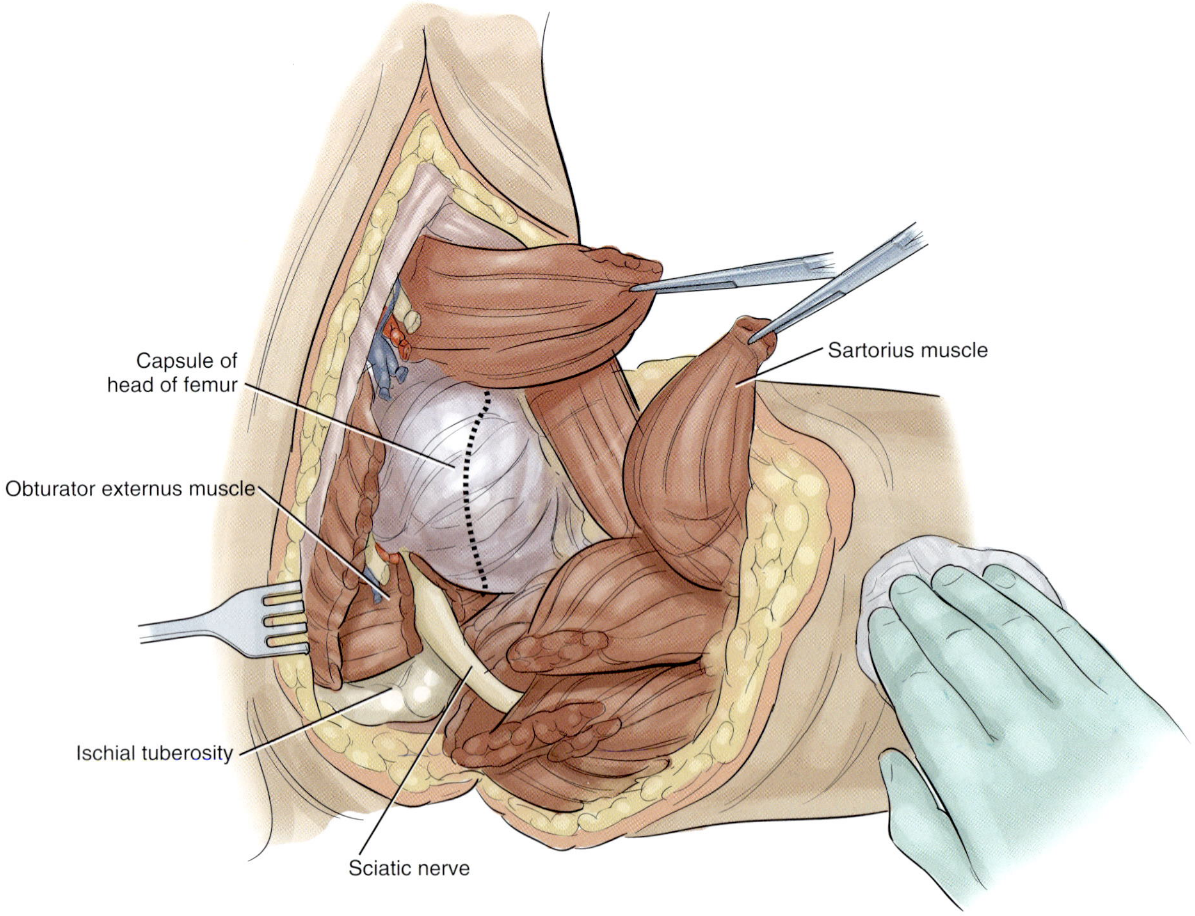

Figure 66-6.

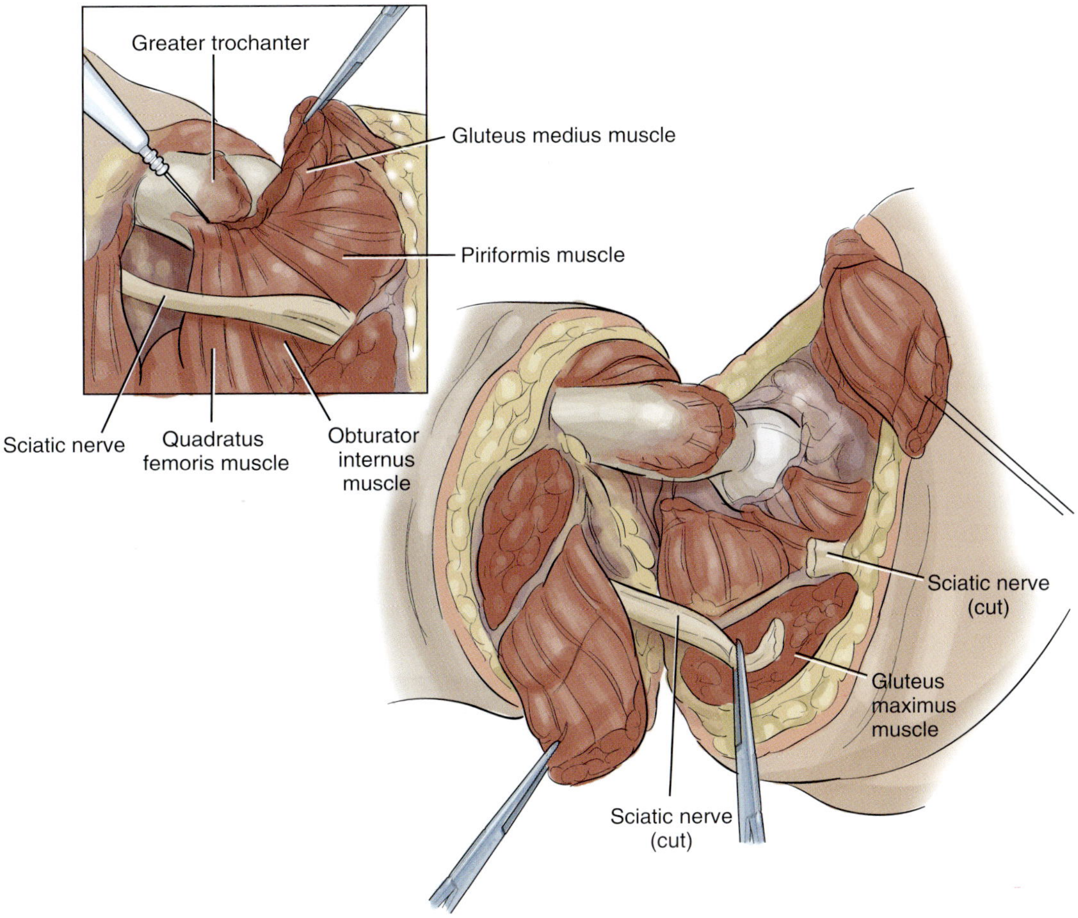

Figure 66-7.

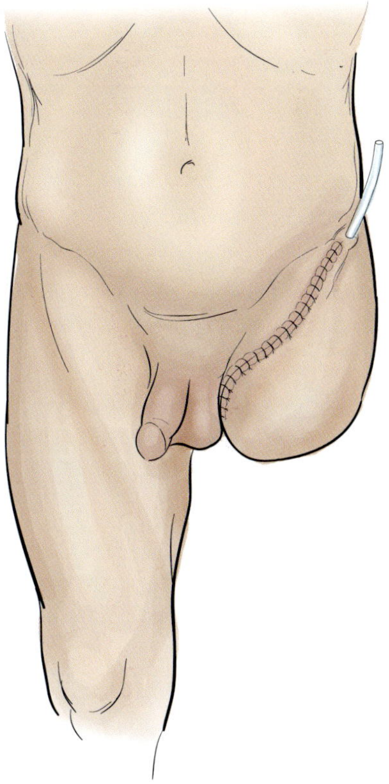

Figure 66-8.

IV. SPECIAL POSTOPERATIVE CARE

- A gently compressive dressing is applied with a spica configuration.
- The patient is encouraged to get out of bed during postoperative day 1 and no later than postoperative day 3.
- The drain is removed when its output is below 30 mL for 24 hours, usually within 3 days.
- Staples should be left for 3 weeks to avoid wound disruption.
- A hip disarticulation prosthesis for ambulation or cosmetic purposes can be obtained within a few weeks after surgery.
- With intensive physical rehabilitation, patients may become ambulatory with a cane at approximately 6 months.

SUGGESTED READINGS

Malawer MM, Sugarbaker PH, editors: *Musculoskeletal cancer surgery: treatment of sarcomas and allied diseases*, Dordrecht, The Netherlands, 2001, Kluwer Academic.

Simon MA, Springfield D, editors: *Surgery for bone and soft-tissue tumors*, Philadelphia, 1997, Lippincott-Raven.

Wakelin SJ, Oliver CW, Kaufmann MH: Hip disarticulation—the evolution of a surgical technique, *Injury* 35:299–308, 2004.

SECTION XI

Endocrine Surgery

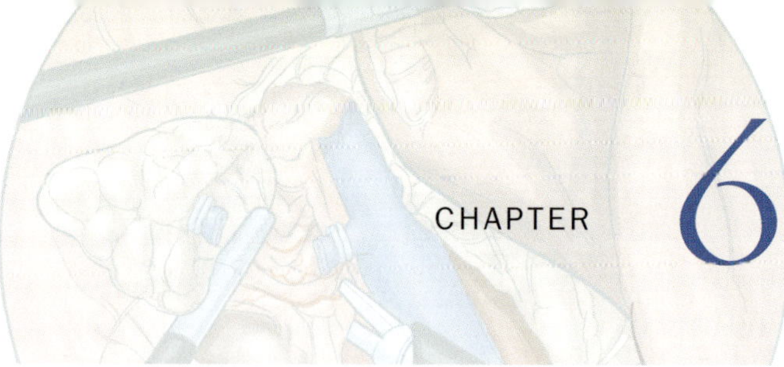

CHAPTER 67

Total Thyroidectomy with Central Neck Dissection

Rebecca S. Sippel, MD, FACS, and Orlo H. Clark, MD, FACS

I. SPECIAL PREOPERATIVE PREPARATION

- *Fine-needle aspiration:* Fine-needle aspiration is part of the standard evaluation of a thyroid nodule. It is 95% accurate in identifying malignancy and should be performed on virtually all patients preoperatively to facilitate operative planning.
- *Neck ultrasound:* Ultrasound is an essential part of the preoperative evaluation of a patient with thyroid cancer. Ultrasound can be used to identify other nodules within the thyroid that may affect the decision to perform a lobectomy versus a total thyroidectomy. Figure 67-1 shows a small heterogeneous thyroid nodule with suspicious microcalcifications. In addition, ultrasound can be used to identify neck lymphadenopathy, which can then be addressed at the time of the initial operation (Fig. 67-2).
- *Laboratory evaluation (thyroid function tests and tumor markers):* All patients should be euthyroid before undergoing surgical intervention. In the absence of symptoms, a thyroid-stimulating hormone level alone is an adequate workup of thyroid function. For patients with a suspicion of medullary thyroid cancer, serum calcitonin and carcinoembryonic antigen levels should be obtained. Serum thyroglobulin can also be a useful adjunct in patients with well-differentiated thyroid cancer.
- *Direct laryngoscopy:* Patients who have had any preoperative change in voice or hoarseness or previous neck surgery should undergo a direct laryngoscopy to confirm vocal cord function.
- *Additional workup:* A chest radiograph should be performed in all patients with thyroid cancer. If there is concern about tracheal or esophageal invasion, endoscopy or bronchoscopy should be performed. Other staging, including a radioactive iodine scan, can be performed postoperatively.

II. OPERATIVE TECHNIQUE

Position

- The patient is positioned in a supine position with the arms tucked at the sides. The base of the neck and the upper to middle back are elevated using a rolled blanket placed longitudinally between the scapulae or a bean bag that is elevated at the midpoint of the upper back. The neck is extended and the head supported with a donut pillow or foam head support. The head must be well supported to prevent posterior neck pain. The bed is placed in 20 to 30 degrees of reverse Trendelenburg position (Fig. 67-3).

Incision

- The incision is placed approximately 1 cm inferior to the cricoid cartilage, using a natural skin crease whenever possible. Placing the incision 1 cm below the cricoid cartilage puts the incision directly over the isthmus of the thyroid, allowing excellent exposure of the superior pole vessels (Fig. 67-4).
- The incision is centered using the sternal notch and chin as guidelines to the midline. The midline and length of the incision should be marked in each direction with a sterile marking pen. The incision itself is marked using a 2-0 silk tie placed in a skin crease and pressed against the neck.

- The incision length varies depending on the size of the thyroid, the site of the cricoid cartilage, the body mass index of the patient, the location of the skin crease, and how far the patient is able to extend his or her neck. A straightforward thyroidectomy and central neck dissection can be performed safely by an experienced surgeon through an appropriately placed 4-cm incision. Heavy patients with large goiters or nodules, patients who cannot extend the neck, or those who have a low cricoid cartilage require larger incisions.
- The incision should be executed sharply through the platysma. Countertraction on the skin with a sterile sponge prevents back-bleeding. Cautery on the subcutaneous bleeding sites should be limited to prevent thermal injury.

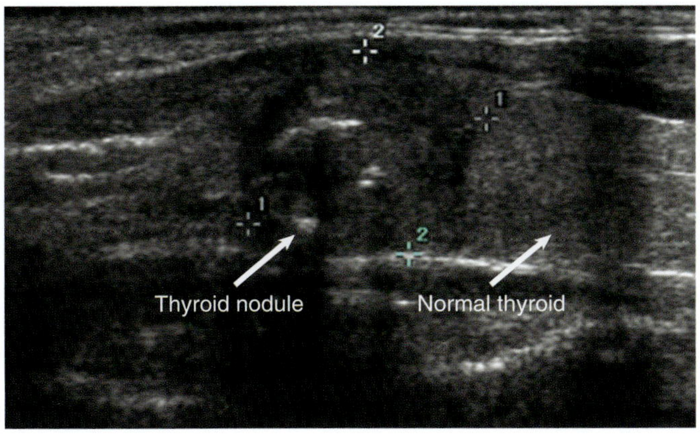

Figure 67-1.

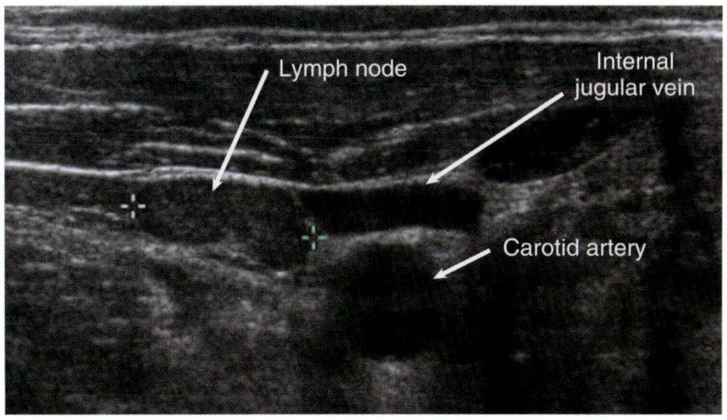

Figure 67-2.

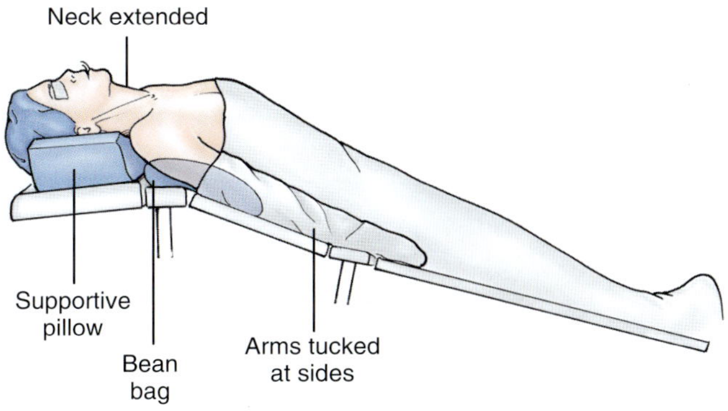

Figure 67-3.

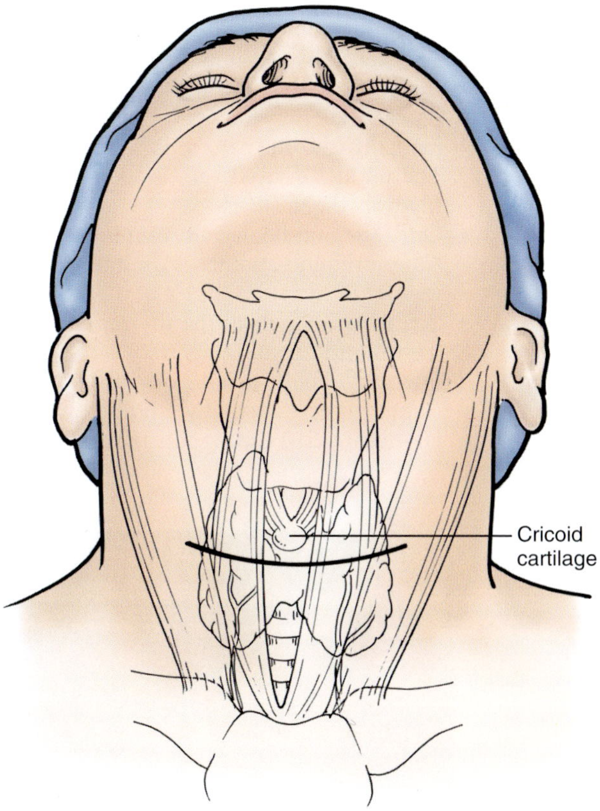

Figure 67-4.

- Five straight Kelly clamps are placed on the dermis to facilitate mobilization of the subplatysmal planes (Fig. 67-5, *A* and *B*). The dermis is retracted anteriorly and superiorly. Lateral retraction can be added using an Army-Navy retractor. Dissection is performed either sharply or with cautery in the semilunar plane immediately anterior to the anterior jugular veins and posterior to the platysma. The dissection is carried out superiorly to the notch in the thyroid cartilage and inferiorly to the suprasternal notch. The lateral dissection is completed with blunt dissection.

Main Dissection

Thyroidectomy

- The superficial cervical fascia is identified and divided using electrocautery at the midline between the strap muscles. The midline is most easily identified superiorly at the thyroid cartilage or inferiorly above the suprasternal notch (Fig. 67-6). Identification of the midline is facilitated by three points of lateral retraction.
- To facilitate exposure, the more superficial sternohyoid muscle is bluntly separated from the underlying sternothyroid muscle. This dissection is extended laterally until the ansa cervicalis is identified on the medial aspect of the internal jugular vein. This is repeated on both sides.
- Before performing our lateral dissection, we identify the isthmus and mobilize it superiorly and inferiorly just anterior to the trachea. We look for delphian lymph nodes at the level of the cricoid cartilage and remove these nodes en bloc with the specimen. If a lobectomy is to be performed, the isthmus is divided at this point. If a total thyroidectomy is planned, our preference is to remove the gland in one piece. Occasionally a gland is very large, and dividing the isthmus earlier can facilitate the lateral dissection.
- During the medial dissection, cephalad to the isthmus, we look for a pyramidal lobe, which is present in up to 80% of patients. The pyramidal lobe is dissected circumferentially and is retracted inferiorly using a right-angle clamp. The edges of the pyramidal lobe are carefully dissected from the surrounding tissues using electrocautery, and the superior end is divided once it thins out to a fibrous band, usually at the level of the thyroid cartilage.
- The lateral dissection should start on the side of the suspected tumor. The advantage of this approach is that if problems are encountered with the recurrent laryngeal nerve or parathyroid gland, a less than total thyroidectomy can be performed on the opposite side to avoid the potentially disastrous complication of bilateral vocal cord paralysis or hypoparathyroidism. Occasionally, with a very extensive or invasive tumor, it may facilitate the exposure to begin with the more straightforward side first.
- The sternothyroid muscle is then dissected free of the thyroid gland using a combination of blunt and sharp dissection. Any muscle adhering to the tumor should be removed en bloc. The dissection should proceed laterally until the middle thyroid vein is identified. The thyroid is retracted anteriorly and medially, and the carotid is retracted laterally, putting the middle thyroid vein on tension (Fig. 67-7). The middle thyroid vein is then divided to allow better exposure of the superior pole and posterior thyroid (Fig. 67-8).
- Once the middle thyroid vein is divided, a peanut dissector is used to retract the thyroid medially and superiorly, and another is used to gently push away the lateral attachments, exposing the superior pole vessels.
- The superior pole of the thyroid is then dissected free medially, between the cricothyroid muscle and the thyroid capsule (Fig. 67-9). The thyroid is grasped with a forceps and gently retracted laterally and inferiorly. The superior pole vessels are carefully skeletonized, then double-clamped with a right-angle clamp (directed laterally) and tied with 2-0 silk ties. Care must be taken to avoid injury to the external laryngeal nerve during this part of the dissection (Fig. 67-10). To prevent injury, the vessels should be

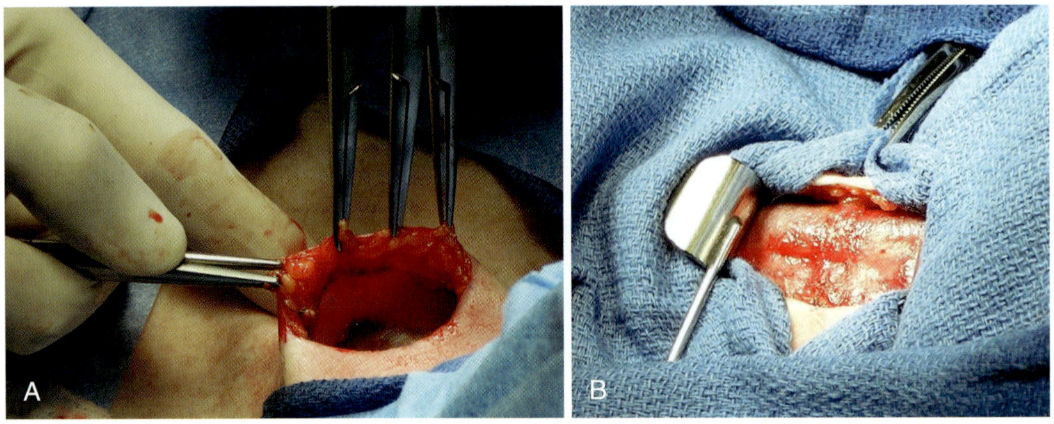

Figure 67-5.

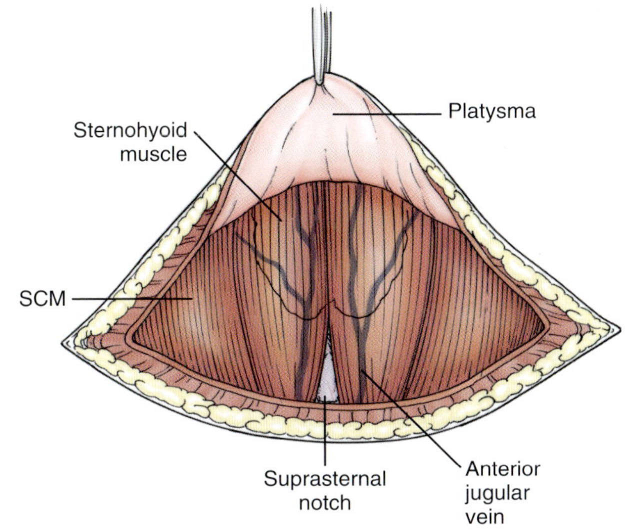

Figure 67-6. *SCM,* Sternocleidomastoid.

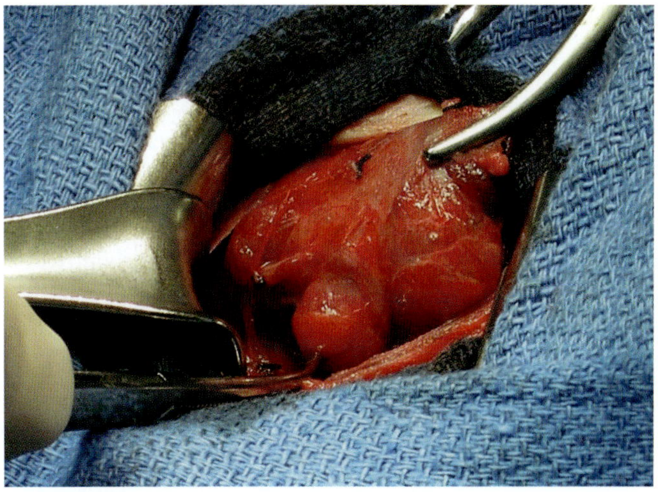

Figure 67-7.

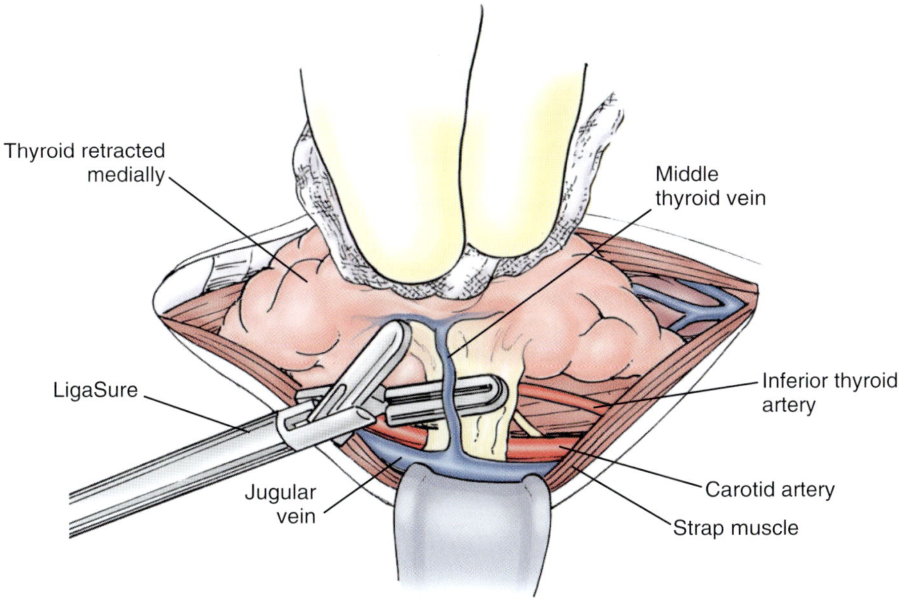

Figure 67-8.

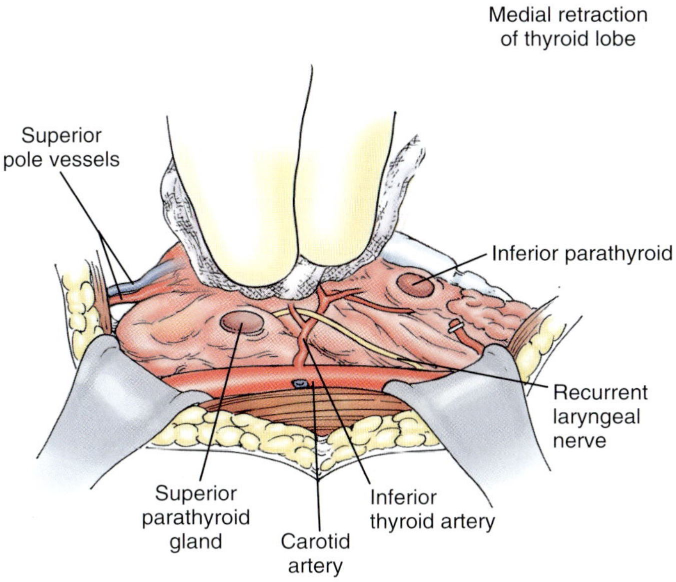

Figure 67-9.

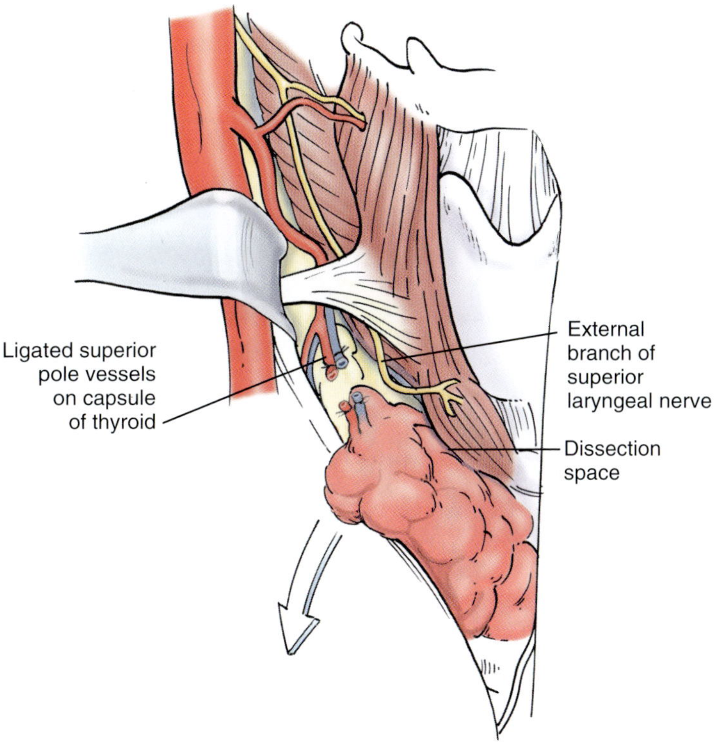

Figure 67-10.

divided immediately on the thyroid capsule, the dissection should always proceed from medial to lateral, and the medial dissection should not disrupt the cricothyroid muscle fibers.

- Once the superior pole is taken, the upper parathyroid can often be seen. The upper parathyroid lies posterior to the recurrent laryngeal nerve at or above the level of the cricoid cartilage. The parathyroid gland is gently separated from the thyroid gland, leaving as much of a vascular pedicle as possible. Clips can be used to separate the parathyroid from the thyroid to minimize disruption of its delicate blood supply and to mark the parathyroid gland.
- During every thyroid operation, it is essential to understand the anatomy of the recurrent laryngeal nerve and not to divide any lateral structures until it is clearly identified. The recurrent laryngeal nerves run in the tracheoesophageal groove and enter the cricothyroid muscle at the level of the cricoid cartilage. The right nerve takes a slightly oblique course, and the left nerve run slightly more posterior. The nerve can often be identified by the small vascular plexus that is alongside. Lateral retraction on the carotid artery and medial and anterior retraction on the thyroid gland put the inferior thyroid artery under tension, which can facilitate the identification of the recurrent laryngeal nerve (Fig. 67-11). The nerve can be identified through careful dissection of the tissue along the lateral aspect of the mid–thyroid gland, staying in the direction of the nerve.
- Once the recurrent laryngeal nerve is clearly identified, the inferior pole vessels can safely be divided using 2-0 silk ties. Care should be taken to avoid injuring the inferior parathyroid gland, which is usually located anterior to the recurrent laryngeal nerve on the posterior lateral surface of the thyroid gland or in the thyrothymic ligament.
- For the lateral dissection, the recurrent laryngeal nerve is identified at or just caudal to where it enters the larynx posterior to the cricothyroid muscle (Fig. 67-12). Dissection is performed anterior to the nerve to avoid injuring any medial branches. The ligament of Berry is divided sharply. Often a small artery and vein are present in this ligament near the recurrent laryngeal nerve. If bleeding is encountered during this dissection, gentle pressure should be applied. No structures should be clamped unless the nerve can clearly be seen and is separated from the bleeding site.
- Occasionally, either the esophagus or the trachea is invaded by tumor. If there is minimal tracheal invasion, the tumor can be shaved off of the trachea without a formal resection. If the invasion is confined, a small segment of trachea is removed and the area used for a tracheostomy, or repaired and covered with a muscle flap. If needed, up to 5 cm of trachea can be resected and reanastomosed after sufficient mobilization. If the esophagus is invaded, the muscular wall of the esophagus can be resected with the tumor provided the inner esophageal layer is left intact.
- Once the ligament of Berry is divided, there are filmy attachments between the trachea and the thyroid that can be safely divided using either electrocautery or sharp dissection.
- For a total thyroidectomy, this procedure is repeated on the opposite side.

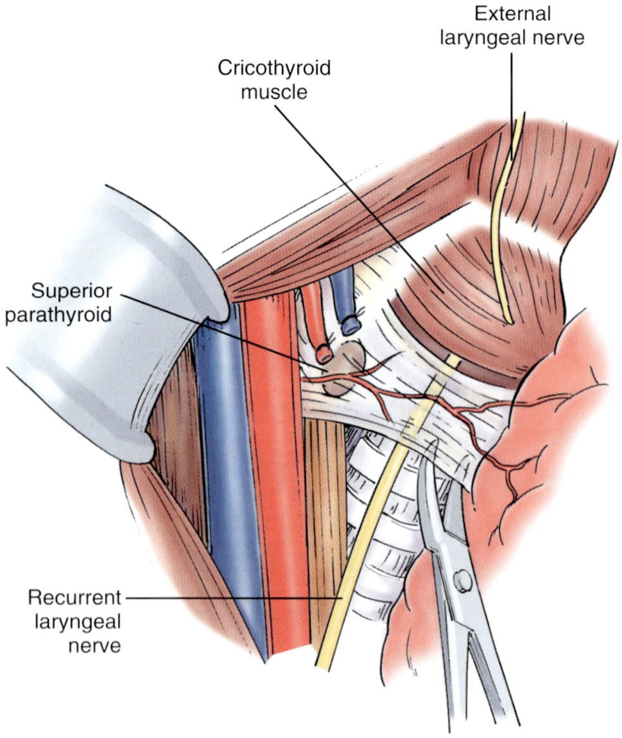

Figure 67-11.

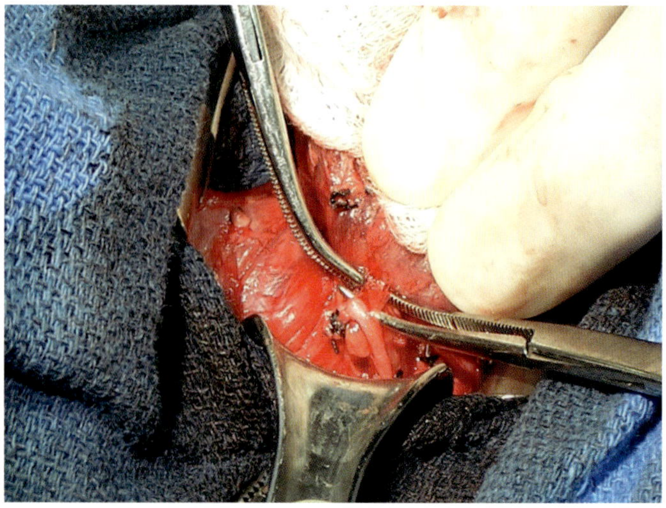

Figure 67-12.

Central Neck Dissection

- A formal central neck (level VI) dissection is typically performed after the thyroidectomy is complete. The perithyroidal and delphian lymph nodes, which are part of the level VI nodes, should already have been removed with the thyroid gland. The remaining central neck nodes are contained in the fibrofatty tissue located below the level of the cricoid cartilage between the carotid artery and the trachea. The nodes are found both anterior and posterior to the recurrent laryngeal nerve (Fig. 67-13).
- The recurrent laryngeal nerve is identified near its distal insertion into the cricothyroid muscle and is carefully dissected from the surrounding tissues proximally to the level of the clavicle. All of the fibrofatty tissue anterior to the nerve is dissected en bloc. Every attempt is made to identify the inferior parathyroid gland, which is contained within this anterior fibrofatty tissue, and to dissect it from the surrounding tissues while preserving its blood supply. If the lower parathyroid cannot be preserved in situ, a biopsy should be performed to confirm that it is parathyroid tissue and then reimplanted into the sternocleidomastoid muscle. Additional nodal tissue located posterior to the recurrent laryngeal nerve can be removed separately.

Closure

- The strap muscles are reapproximated in two separate layers using interrupted 4-0 Dexon sutures. Next, the platysma is closed using interrupted 4-0 Dexon sutures. For the final skin closure, we prefer to use surgical clips, which provide excellent cosmesis, hemostasis, and skin approximation. The surgical clips are removed the following morning and replaced with Steri-Strips. The Steri-Strips should remain for 10 to 14 days to keep tension off of the wound, minimizing scarring.

III. ALTERNATIVE TECHNICAL APPROACHES (PRO/CON) AND PEARLS

- To allow identification of both the recurrent laryngeal nerve and the normal parathyroid glands, bleeding should be kept to a minimum. If bleeding is encountered, gentle pressure should be applied. Avoid clamping any vessel unless the bleeding source is clearly identified and it is well away from the recurrent laryngeal nerve.
- Several devices are available to facilitate the division of the perithyroidal tissues, including the Harmonic Scalpel (Ethicon Endo-Surgery, Cincinnati) and the LigaSure (Valleylab, Boulder, Colo.). Care must be taken when using these instruments to avoid thermal injury to the recurrent laryngeal nerve.
- Variations in the anatomy of the recurrent laryngeal nerve are not uncommon. Either recurrent laryngeal nerve can branch before entering the larynx, although this occurs more frequently on the left side of the nerve. When branching occurs, the motor fibers usually run in the most medial branches.

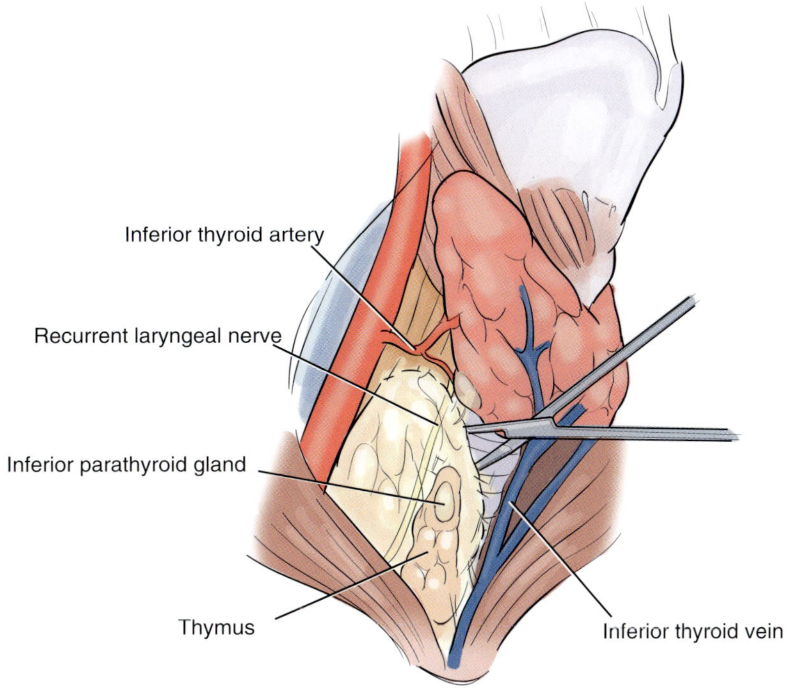

Figure 67-13.

Nonrecurrent laryngeal nerves occur in 0.5% of patients. These occur on the right side of the nerve, and the nerve can originate from either a superior or a lateral direction.

- If a parathyroid gland is devascularized or removed, a biopsy should be performed to confirm that it is parathyroid tissue and then it should be reimplanted. The parathyroid gland should be kept in physiologic saline on ice until it is ready to be reimplanted. The parathyroid gland should be cut into 1-mm cubes and be transplanted into several pockets within the sternocleidomastoid. If there is extensive lymphadenopathy or if postoperative external beam radiation therapy is to be used, the parathyroid can be autotransplanted in the forearm.

IV. SPECIAL POSTOPERATIVE CARE

- Postoperatively, the patient should be kept in a low Fowler position with the head of the bed elevated at least 10 to 20 degrees for 12 hours.
- Serum calcium levels should be measured 4 hours postoperatively and again the following morning. We treat the patient with oral calcium supplements if symptoms of hypocalcemia appear or if serum calcium falls below 7.5 mg/dL. We also check serum phosphorus the first day after surgery. An elevated serum phosphorus (above 4.5 mg/dL) in conjunction with hypocalcemia should raise concern for the possibility of hypoparathyroidism.
- Patients who have had a total thyroidectomy should be discharged home with a prescription for thyroid hormone. Patients with nonmedullary thyroid cancer should be given enough thyroid hormone to suppress their thyroid-stimulating hormone to less than 0.1 mInternational Units per mL (we use 80% of the patient's body weight in pounds as an estimation of the starting dose in mcg per day). Once the final pathology results are received in 7 to 10 days, a decision can be made whether to stop the medication before treatment with radioactive iodine.

Potential Complications after Thyroidectomy

- Unilateral injury to the recurrent laryngeal nerve manifests as hoarseness in the postoperative period. This can be either transient or permanent. Bilateral recurrent laryngeal nerve injury results in vocal cord medialization, which can cause inspiratory stridor and require emergent reintubation.
- Hypocalcemia can occur in the postoperative period because of parathyroid gland removal, injury, or devascularization. The nadir in postoperative calcium often does not occur until 48 to 72 hours after surgery. Symptoms of hypocalcemia range from mild paresthesias to tetany. Mild symptoms are treated with oral calcium replacement; more profound hypocalcemia should be treated initially with a combination of oral and intravenous calcium replacement followed by oral calcitriol (0.25 mcg twice daily).
- Neck hematoma after thyroidectomy is rare (approximately 1 in 300 patients) but is unpredictable and can be life threatening because of airway compromise. The most common presentation is increased neck pressure with difficulty breathing or swallowing. This can be associated with a change in voice, neck swelling, or the need to sit up. Most bleeding occurs within the first few hours after surgery, and virtually all within 24 hours. An unrecognized neck hematoma may have life-threatening consequences, and there should be a low threshold for immediate reexploration in these patients.
- Injury to the external branch of the superior laryngeal nerve can occur during dissection of the superior pole vessels. Injury to this nerve is associated with alterations in voice projection and pitch.
- Infection is rare after thyroidectomy, so we do not routinely recommend preoperative antibiotic prophylaxis.
- Seroma formation is common, especially after an extensive lymph node dissection. Most seromas will resorb spontaneously and do not require aspiration.

SUGGESTED READINGS

Grodski S, Cornford L, Sywak M, et al: Routine level VI lymph node dissection for papillary thyroid cancer: surgical technique, *ANZ J Surg* 77:203–208, 2007.

Kebebew E, Duh QY, Clark OH: Total thyroidectomy or thyroid lobectomy in patients with low-risk differentiated thyroid cancer: surgical decision analysis of a controversy using a mathematical model, *World J Surg* 24:1295–1302, 2000.

Lindquist S: Thyroidectomy. In Clark OH, Duh QY, Kebebew E, editors: *Textbook of endocrine surgery*, ed 2, Philadelphia, 2005, WB Saunders, 2005, pp 188–194.

CHAPTER 68

Revision Parathyroidectomy

Dina M. Elaraj, MD, FACS, and Quan-Yang Duh, MD, FACS

I. SPECIAL PREOPERATIVE PREPARATION

- When evaluating a patient with apparent persistent or recurrent hyperparathyroidism (HPT) after parathyroidectomy, the first step is to reconfirm the diagnosis. Once the diagnosis has been confirmed, prior localization studies, operative notes, and pathology reports should be reviewed to get a clear idea of what has previously been done. It is essential to consider the causes of persistent or recurrent HPT to help guide the preoperative workup and approach to reoperation.
- Persistent HPT is defined by persistent hypercalcemia diagnosed within 6 months after parathyroidectomy. The most common cause is a parathyroid adenoma in a descended upper gland that was missed in the initial lower gland parathyroidectomy. Other causes for a missed parathyroid adenoma relate to supernumerary parathyroid glands or those in ectopic sites (Fig. 68-1). Other causes of persistent HPT include failure to identify or remove all adenomatous or hyperplastic parathyroid tissue at the initial operation, parathyromatosis, or residual or metastatic parathyroid carcinoma.

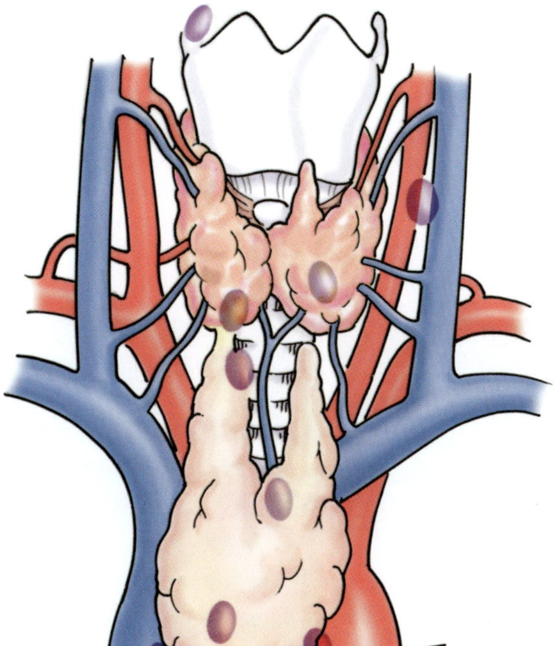

Figure 68-1.

- Recurrent HPT (defined as hypercalcemia that develops more than 6 months after curative parathyroidectomy) develops in approximately 1% of patients with sporadic primary HPT and in one third of patients with familial primary HPT. These patients have a second adenoma or multigland hyperplasia. In patients with multigland hyperplasia, the recurrent HPT is due to regrowth of a hyperplastic gland or remnant left during initial subtotal parathyroidectomy, or regrowth of autotransplanted parathyroid tissue done at the time of initial total parathyroidectomy. As in persistent HPT, other causes of recurrent HPT include parathyromatosis or residual or metastatic parathyroid carcinoma.
- Localization studies are essential in the preoperative planning for revision parathyroidectomy, as the plan should be to do a focused rather than a general exploration. We recommend two concordant studies before proceeding with reoperation. Radionuclide scanning with 99m-technetium sestamibi and ultrasound of the neck are our two preferred initial imaging studies (Fig. 68-2, *A* and *B*). If these studies are negative or discordant, we then proceed to magnetic resonance imaging (MRI) of the neck and mediastinum, which has better sensitivity than computed tomography. Invasive tests such as selective venous sampling for parathyroid hormone (PTH) or selective transarterial angiography may also be needed.
- Sestamibi scanning provides both functional and anatomic information. It can be combined with single-photon emission computed tomography, which generates a three-dimensional image of radiotracer uptake. Be aware of causes of false-positive (sarcoid, carcinoid, or thyroid nodules, both benign and malignant) and false-negative scans (small parathyroid glands, multiple adenomas or parathyroid hyperplasia, or conditions such as Hashimoto thyroiditis or multiple thyroid nodules that cause delayed washout from the thyroid).
- Ultrasound provides anatomic information such as location, size, and depth. Its major limitation is its inability to detect glands in the mediastinum, the tracheoesophageal groove, or some other ectopic locations. If a potential abnormal parathyroid gland is seen on ultrasound, one can do a fine-needle aspiration of the lesion and send the aspirate for PTH and cytology to confirm the diagnosis. Figure 68-2 illustrates the complementary information obtained from sestamibi scan and ultrasound in the case of an intrathyroidal parathyroid adenoma.
- MRI scan of the neck and mediastinum provides anatomic information for potential abnormal parathyroid glands located in both usual and ectopic sites. These glands are usually isointense on T1-weighted images, hyperintense on T2-weighted images, and enhanced with gadolinium. Figure 68-3 illustrates the complementary information obtained from sestamibi scan and MRI in the case of a parathyroid adenoma located in the tracheoesophageal groove.
- Selective venous sampling is an invasive test during which catheters are placed in veins in the neck and mediastinum that drain regions where one or more abnormal parathyroid glands might be located. PTH is measured, and the highest concentration of PTH suggests the location of the abnormal parathyroid gland(s). This test can only lateralize the location of a parathyroid tumor, and a caveat when interpreting these results is that PTH values tend to increase in veins going back toward the heart.
- All patients should have direct laryngoscopy to assess vocal cord function before any reoperation.

II. OPERATIVE TECHNIQUE

Position

- The patient is positioned supine, with the arms tucked at the sides and the neck extended. We use a bean bag covered by a gel pad as a shoulder roll to position the neck in extension. The patient's neck is prepped from chin to clavicles (or to the xiphoid if a sternotomy is planned) and draped in a diamond configuration.

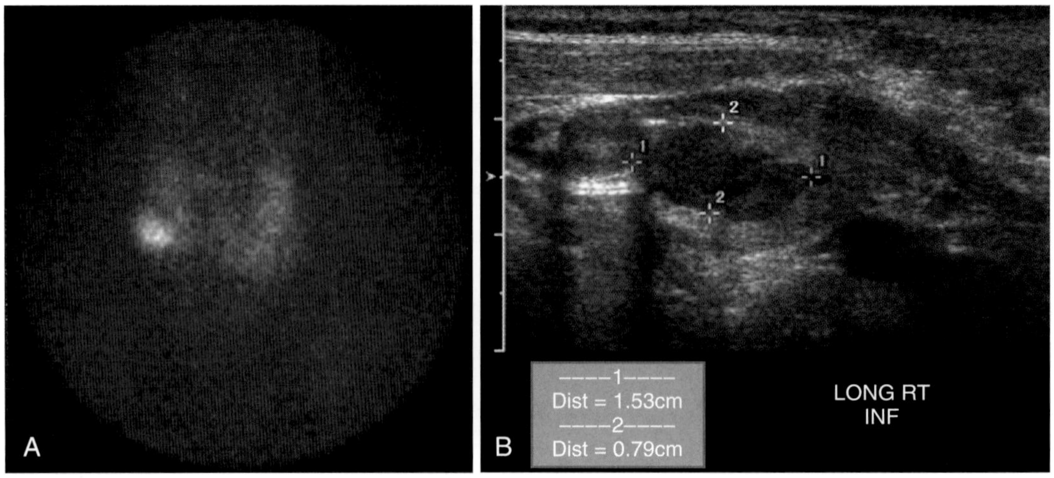

Figure 68-2. Sestamibi scan (**A**) and ultrasound (longitudinal view) (**B**) of a patient with a right lower intrathyroidal parathyroid adenoma.

Incision

- In the great majority of cases, the patient's previous skin incision can be used (Fig. 68-4). If a new incision is needed, we try to make it in a skin crease close to the location of the abnormal parathyroid gland identified on the preoperative imaging studies. If the abnormal gland is seen on ultrasound, a preincision intraoperative ultrasound is useful in deciding the exact location of the incision. A spring retractor or small handheld retractors are used to hold the incision open.

Main Dissection

- The dissection depends on the location of the abnormal parathyroid gland(s).
- In the case of an overlooked parathyroid adenoma located in the tracheoesophageal groove, a lateral approach is recommended to avoid scar tissue from the previous operation. This approach is also excellent for an ectopic gland located in the carotid sheath.
  - ▲ Develop a dissection plane along the anterior border of the sternocleidomastoid muscle. Retract this muscle laterally, and the strap muscles medially (Fig. 68-5). The ansa cervicalis, which runs along

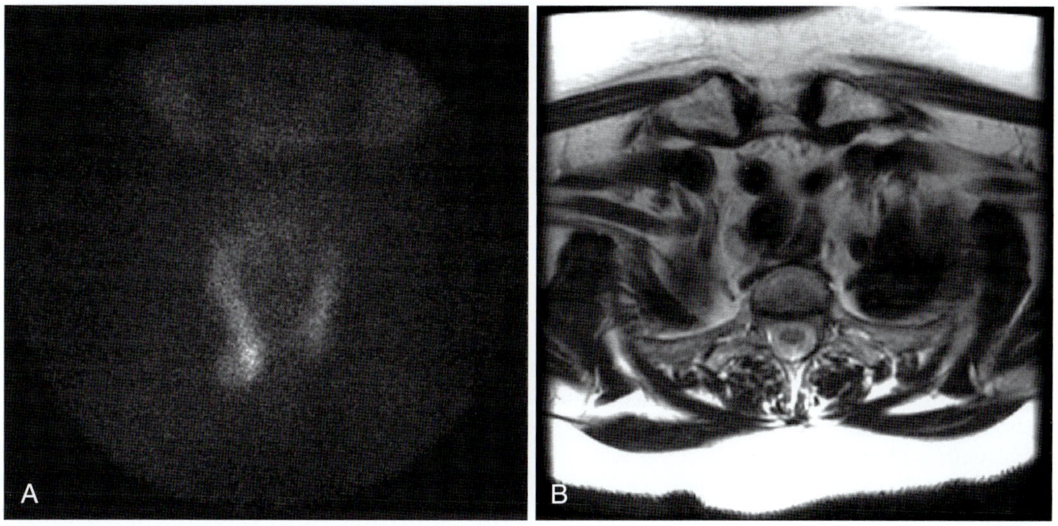

Figure 68-3. Sestamibi scan (**A**) and T2-weighted magnetic resonance imaging scan (**B**) of a patient with a parathyroid adenoma located in the right tracheoesophageal groove.

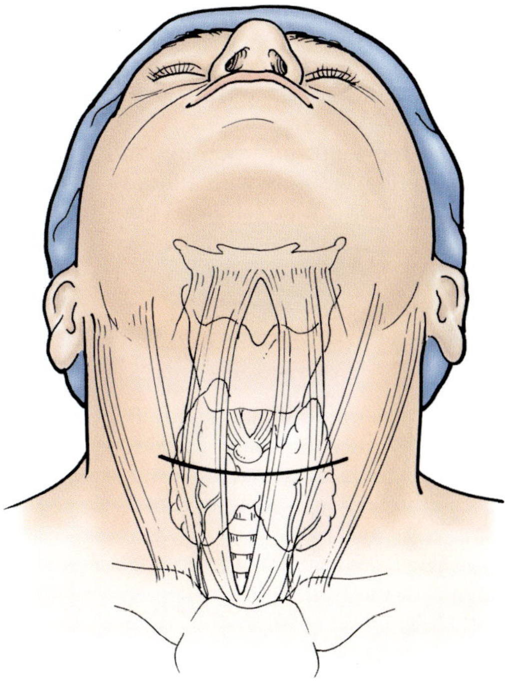

Figure 68-4.

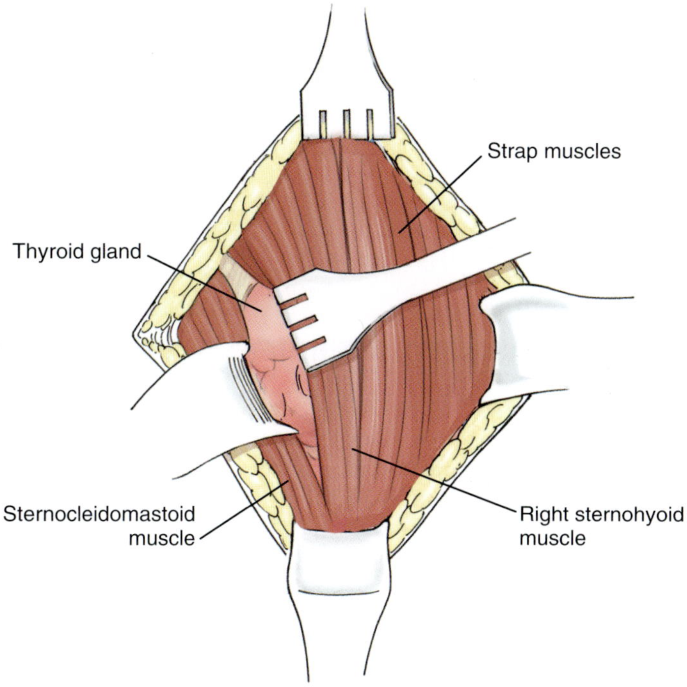

Figure 68-5.

the lateral aspect of the sternothyroid muscle, is retracted medially with the strap muscles. The omohyoid muscle, which originates from the upper border of the scapula and runs obliquely to insert on the hyoid bone, is sometimes encountered and can be retracted medially or laterally, depending on its location with respect to the incision.

- ▲ As the dissection proceeds more deeply, retract the internal jugular vein and carotid artery laterally, and the strap muscles and the thyroid gland anteromedially. A vein retractor or Kittner is useful to retract the thyroid up and outward. Be aware when doing this dissection that the incision may be deeper than originally thought.
- ▲ Look for a descended upper parathyroid gland in the tracheoesophageal groove, posterior to the recurrent laryngeal nerve (Fig. 68-6).
- ▲ Use a combination of sharp and gentle blunt dissection to free the parathyroid gland from the surrounding tissues. Be careful when using cautery near the recurrent laryngeal nerve. The gland usually has one vascular pedicle that can be clamped and ligated with a 3-0 silk tie.

- In the case of a missed lower gland located either in a normal position or in the thymus, an anterior approach is usually recommended (Fig. 68-7). It is usually possible to resect ectopic anterior mediastinal glands located in the thymus via this approach, though a median sternotomy may be necessary.
  - ▲ Create subplatysmal flaps superiorly to the level of the cricoid cartilage and inferiorly to the sternal notch. Separate the strap muscles vertically in the midline and retract them laterally (see Fig. 68-7). It is usually not necessary to divide the strap muscles, but if you need more exposure, the sternothyroid muscle can be transected at its insertion (cephalad) with minimal consequences.
  - ▲ Identify the lower pole of the thyroid gland and look for a lower gland in this area, anterior to the recurrent laryngeal nerve (Fig. 68-8). Excise the gland as described previously, using a combination of sharp and gentle blunt dissection.
  - ▲ To do a transcervical thymectomy, identify the thyrothymic ligament located in the region of the lower pole of the thyroid gland, near the trachea. This can be distinguished from other fat in the neck by its surrounding fascial layer.
    - ▲ Circumferentially dissect the thyrothymic ligament, then clamp it with two clamps and transect it. Leave the clamp on and use it like a handle to pull thymic tissue out of the mediastinum with a gentle twisting/rocking motion (Fig. 68-9). Use a combination of sharp and blunt dissection to separate the thymus from its surrounding attachments.
    - ▲ As you pull more thymus cephalad out of the mediastinum, place successively caudal clamps on the tissue to help pull it up without breaking it. Vessels and lymphatics on the surface of the thymus can be clipped or tied as the main part of the thymus is retracted cephalad. When the dissection has reached its limit, transect the thymus and ligate the tissue in the caudalmost clamp with 2-0 or 3-0 silk.
    - ▲ Open the specimen longitudinally to confirm that a parathyroid gland has been resected.

Closure

- Closure depends on the incision used.
- If a lateral-approach dissection was done, suture the sternocleidomastoid muscle to the strap muscles with interrupted 4-0 absorbable braided suture. If an anterior-approach dissection was done, suture first the sternothyroid, then the sternohyoid muscles in the same way. It is sometimes not possible to suture these muscle layers separately. Then close the platysma layer using the same interrupted 4-0 absorbable braided sutures.
- The skin may be closed in a number of ways—clips that are removed the following morning and replaced with adhesive wound closure strips, or a 4-0 monofilament subcuticular suture with adhesive wound closure strips or a liquid skin adhesive. If absorbable suture is used, it can be left in; if nonabsorbable suture is used, it can be removed the following morning.
- No drains are placed.

III. ALTERNATIVE TECHNICAL APPROACHES (PRO/CON) AND PEARLS

- Alternative technical approaches depend on the location of the abnormal parathyroid gland. For example, resection of an intrathyroidal parathyroid tumor may require thyroid lobectomy. Resection of a mediastinal parathyroid gland may require median sternotomy. Some can be removed via a minimally invasive thoracoscopic or mediastinoscopic approach. Those located in the aortopulmonary window require a thoracic approach.
- Exposure of an upper parathyroid gland sometimes requires taking down the superior-pole thyroid vessels.
- Meticulous hemostasis is essential to avoid blood staining of the tissues in the neck.
- Intraoperative PTH testing is a useful adjunct to confirm resection of hypercellular parathyroid tissue. If this technique is not available in your hospital, frozen section analysis should be used.
- Consider cryopreservation of parathyroid tissue if several parathyroid glands have been removed at previous operation(s).

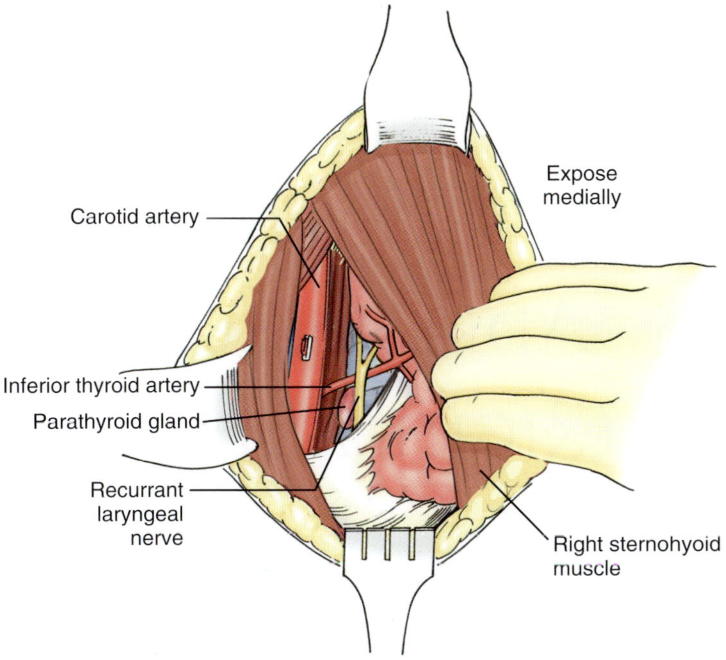

Figure 68-6.

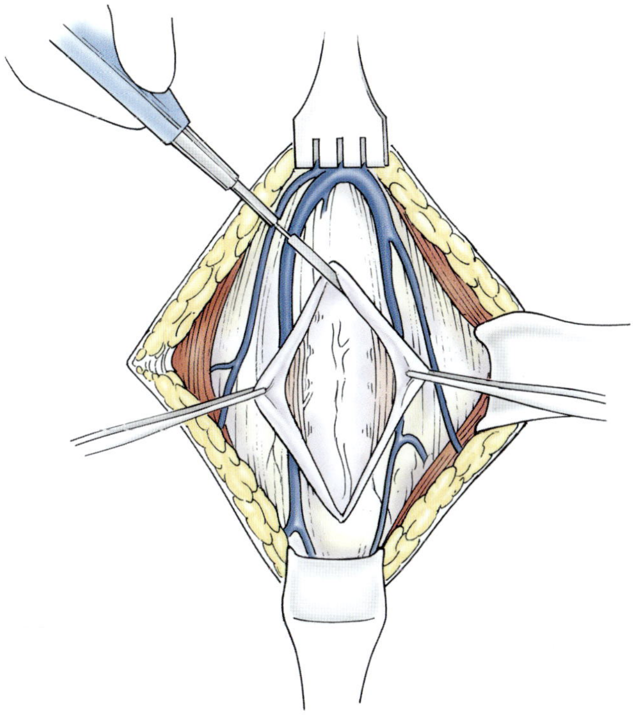

Figure 68-7.

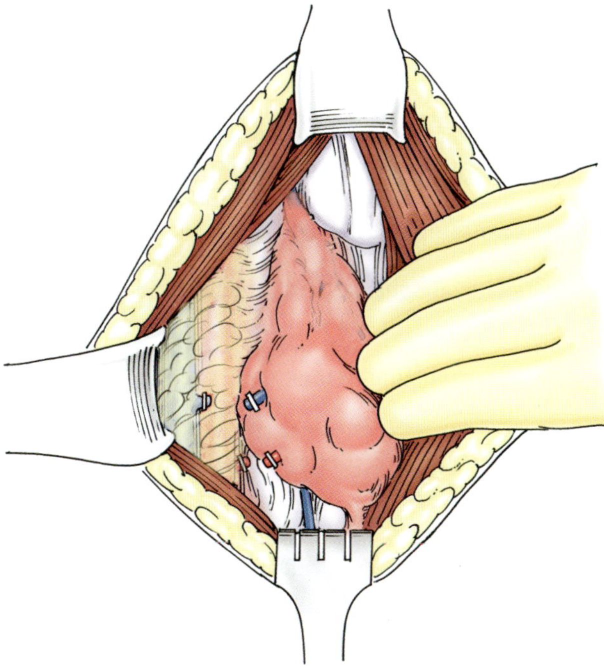

Figure 68-8.

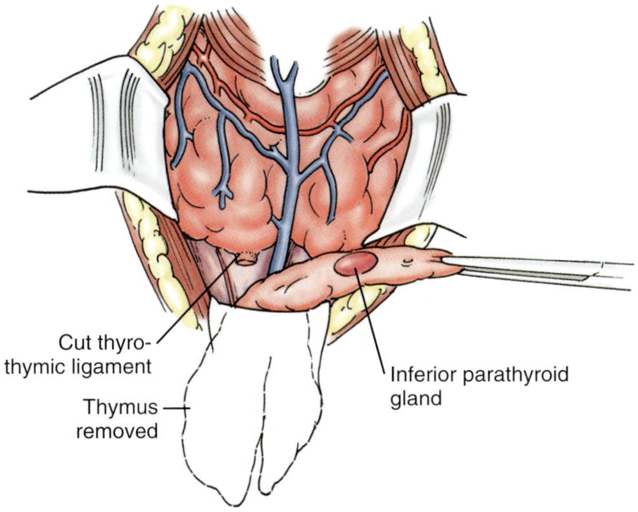

Figure 68-9.

IV. SPECIAL POSTOPERATIVE CARE

- Patients should be monitored for the development of a neck hematoma by measuring neck circumference. Neck hematoma mandates a return trip to the operating room for reexploration.
- Check serum calcium 5 hours postoperatively and the following morning. Hypocalcemia can usually be treated with supplemental oral calcium (2 to 4 g every 4 to 6 hours); the need for intravenous calcium administration is rare. Oral calcitriol (0.25 to 0.5 mcg once or twice daily) should be added if the serum calcium is less than 7.5 mg/dL.

SUGGESTED READINGS

Caron NR, Sturgeon C, Clark OH: Persistent and recurrent hyperparathyroidism, *Curr Treat Options Oncol* 5:335–345, 2004.

Gaz RD: Revision parathyroid surgery. In Randolph G, editor: *Surgery of the thyroid and parathyroid glands*, Philadelphia, 2003, Saunders.

Sturgeon C, Caron N, Duh QY: Reoperative parathyroid surgery. In Oertli D, Udelsman R, editors: *Surgery of the thyroid and parathyroid glands*, New York, 2007, Springer.

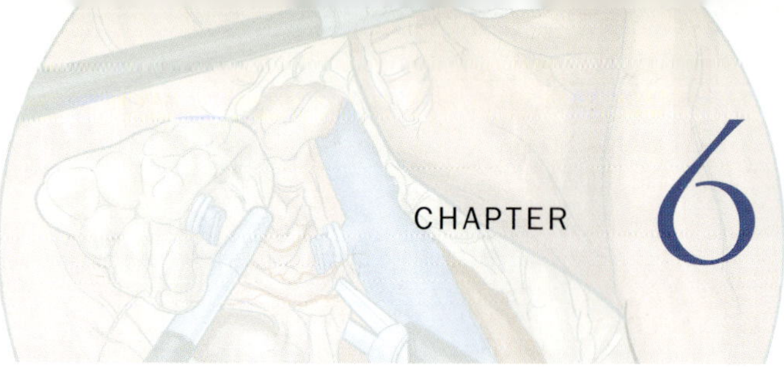

CHAPTER 69

Laparoscopic Adrenalectomy (Right and Left)

Demetrius E.M. Litwin, MD, MBA, and Mitchell A. Cahan, MD, FACS

I. SPECIAL PREOPERATIVE PREPARATION

- Either computed tomography or magnetic resonance imaging is essential in planning for surgery.
- Plasma aldosterone concentration, plasma renin activity, and serum potassium levels are mandatory if primary aldosteronism is in the differential diagnosis. Adrenal vein sampling is necessary if bilateral disease is suspected or if the lesion is unclear.
- A 24-hour urine collection for measurement of total or fractionated metanephrines and catecholamines is indicated if pheochromocytoma is suspected.
- A 24-hour urine cortisol-free analysis, low-dose dexamethasone suppression test, and basal adrenocorticotropic hormone levels are obtained to rule out corticotropin-producing lesions.

II. OPERATIVE TECHNIQUE

RIGHT ADRENALECTOMY

Position

- The approach is lateral decubitus transperitoneal, with the table bent to open the costal pelvic space. Figure 69-1 illustrates patient position for right adrenalectomy with trocar placement.

Trocar Placement

- As seen in Figure 69-1, four subcostal ports (5-12 mm) are used, one for the 30- to 45-degree laparoscope and two working ports. A fourth 5-mm port is mandatory on the right side and sometimes required on the left; it is used for retraction.

Main Dissection

- The right adrenal gland must be uncovered by mobilizing the triangular ligament and opening the bare area of the liver. As shown in Figure 69-2, this dissection is continued to the level of the vena cava, and the liver is progressively brought toward the midline.
- At this point, a flank port is placed to allow for the introduction of a grasping instrument, which then grasps two Litwin sponges and folds them to create a sponge stick that holds the right lobe up and away from the underlying adrenal gland.

- The gland is inspected, and the dissection begins at the most obvious interface between the adrenal gland and retroperitoneal fat. Often this is along the superior surface or the superior medial surface, but it can be any part of the gland. In almost all instances, one can usually identify a difference in texture and color of the gland as compared to the surrounding fat.
- Generally, the dissection of the interface is performed with the L-hook or the Harmonic scalpel. To start the plane, I prefer the L-hook, but once I achieve elevation of the gland, I prefer the Harmonic scalpel. Vessels can be adequately handled by either the L-hook or the Harmonic scalpel. Occasionally, in extremely vascular tumors, the L-hook will not achieve adequate hemostasis.
- Once the dissection of the adrenal gland has started, that aspect of the adrenal gland can be elevated and the retroperitoneal attachments progressively divided, which begins to give mobility to the gland. This mobility allows the gland some degree of movement away from the vena cava, and it is at this point that the medial dissection is performed.
- The medial dissection must be performed with very fine movements and with care to take only small pieces of tissue and vessels individually, usually with the L-hook. Otherwise, these very friable vessels will cause oozing, which will make subsequent dissection quite difficult because of the resultant poor visualization. If oozing occurs, simply pack the area with a laparoscopic sponge (e.g., Litwin sponge) and dissect elsewhere until visualization is restored. The oozing invariably stops.
- This medial dissection is usually performed from caudad to cephalad until the adrenal vein is approached. It is often useful to also do the medial dissection above the vein and the superior aspect of the gland to provide adequate mobility, which will give some length to the adrenal vein.

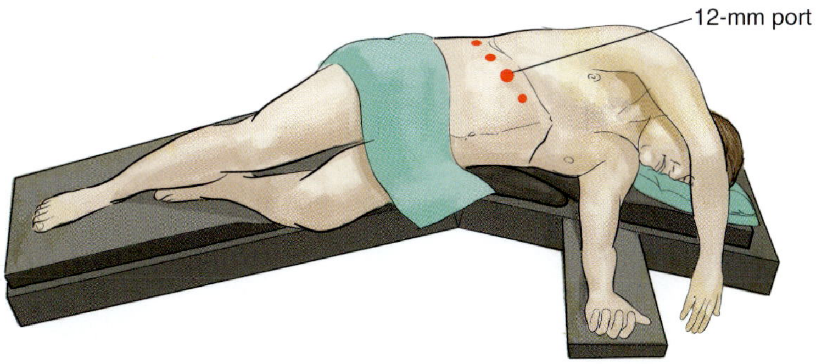

Figure 69-1.

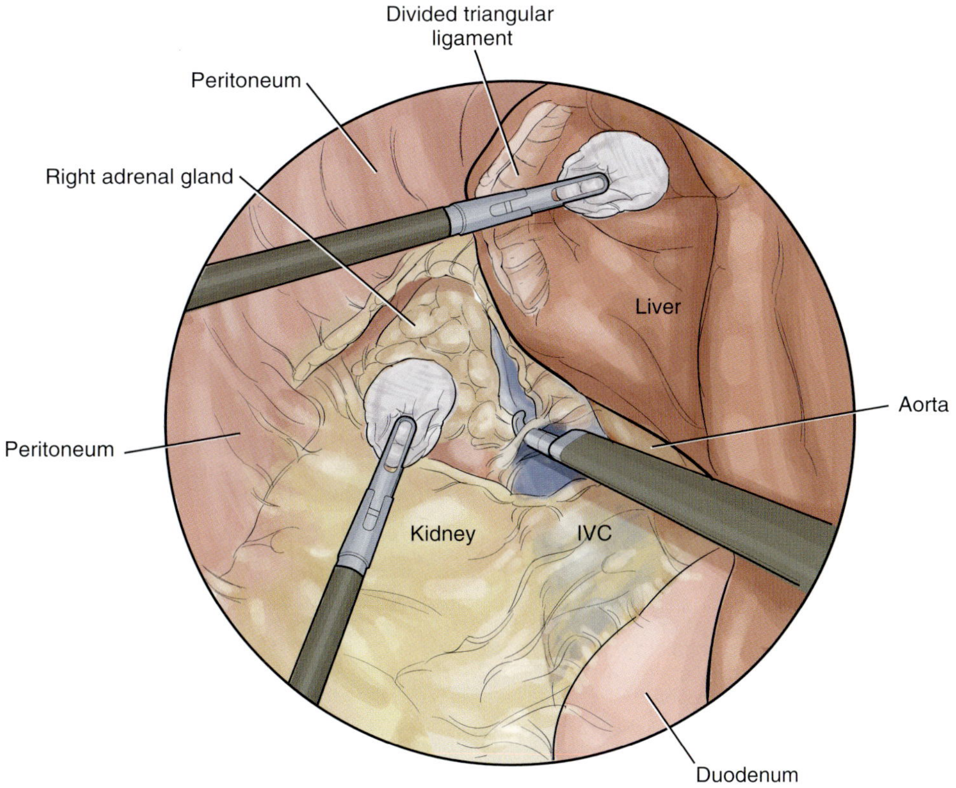

Figure 69-2. *IVC,* Inferior vena cava.

- Once adequate length is achieved, the adrenal vein can be either clipped or divided or else stapled and divided (Fig. 69-3). If the stapler is used, the 2-mm staples (gray cartridge) should be employed for hemostasis. If using clips, it is wise to use two clips on the vena cava side and one on the adrenal side. However, two properly placed clips, with a cut between that results in a margin on both sides, are better than three clumsily placed clips on a short vein. Rarely there are two adrenal veins. Occasionally the adrenal vein goes into a hepatic vein, not the vena cava. One must be vigilant because of these anatomic variations.
- Once the adrenal vein is divided, the gland can be pushed laterally as depicted in Figure 69-4, allowing for further separation from the vena cava.
- Once this medial separation from the vena cava has occurred, elevation of the vein allows for fairly rapid division of remaining attachments, including posterior retroperitoneal attachments, with a Harmonic scalpel as depicted in Figure 69-4. One must always be careful at this stage to recognize where the adrenal gland is located in relation to the fat. If one charges into the adrenal vein with the Harmonic scalpel, significant oozing can ensue.

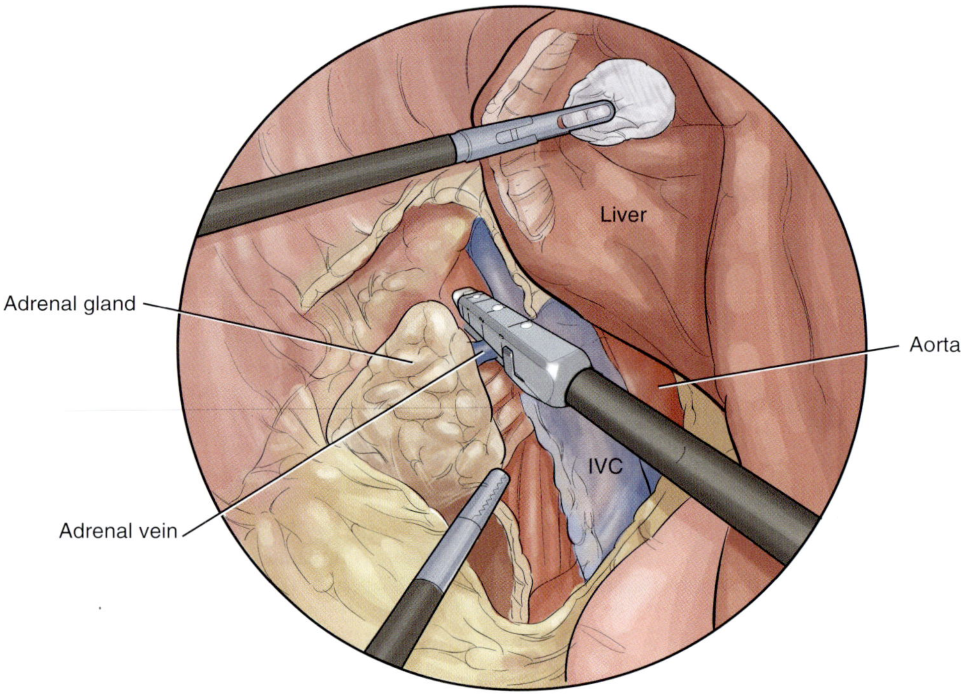

Figure 69-3. *IVC,* Inferior vena cava.

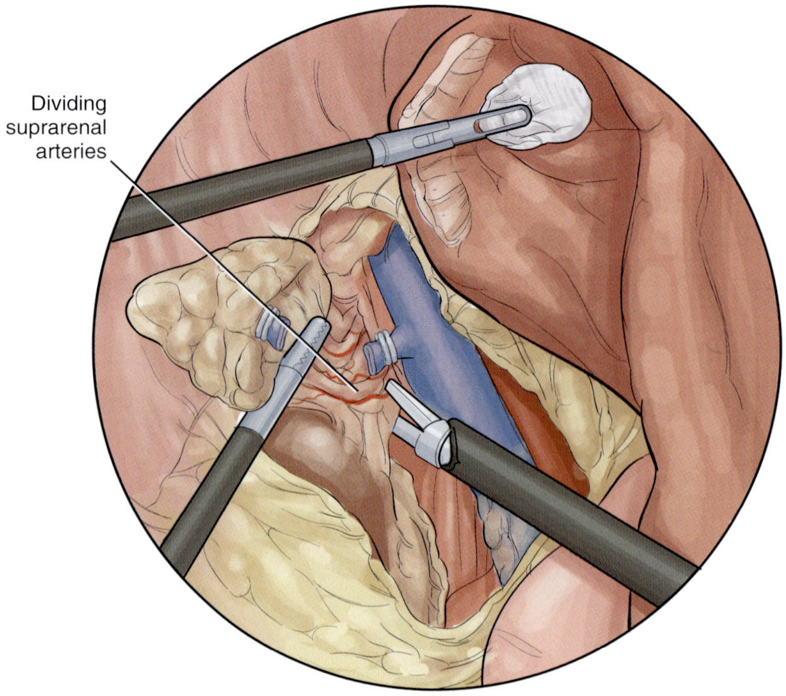

Figure 69-4.

- With the gland elevated, care must be taken to push the gland anteriorly to gain separation from the underlying kidney. Occasionally an upper-pole arterial branch to the kidney will come very close to the adrenal gland and is at risk if one does not stay close to the gland.

Closure

- Once the gland is completely detached, hemostasis is ensured. I often place Surgicel in the base.
- The gland is then placed in a bag and extracted, usually after morcellation. The fascia of the longer port sites is closed.

LEFT ADRENALECTOMY

Position and Trocar Placement

- Figure 69-5 illustrates patient positioning and trocar placement for this operation. The approach is very similar to that for right adrenalectomy, except that the spleen must be mobilized toward the midline, which will draw the tail of pancreas and the splenic vessels with it to uncover the adrenal gland. Often, but not always, the hepatic flexure of the colon must be brought down to uncover the lower portion of the adrenal gland and the kidney. The development of the plane behind the spleen is much more subtle than on the right side, and one must take great care to stay between the Gerota fascia and the pancreas and spleen.

Main Dissection

- The plane is first entered by dividing the peritoneum 0.5 cm from the spleen (Fig. 69-6).
- Using the peritoneum as a handle, the spleen is brought forward, and the peritoneum behind the spleen divided up to the level of diaphragm.

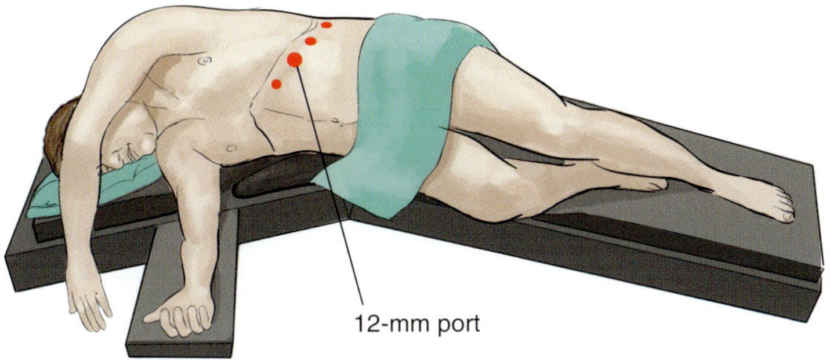

Figure 69-5.

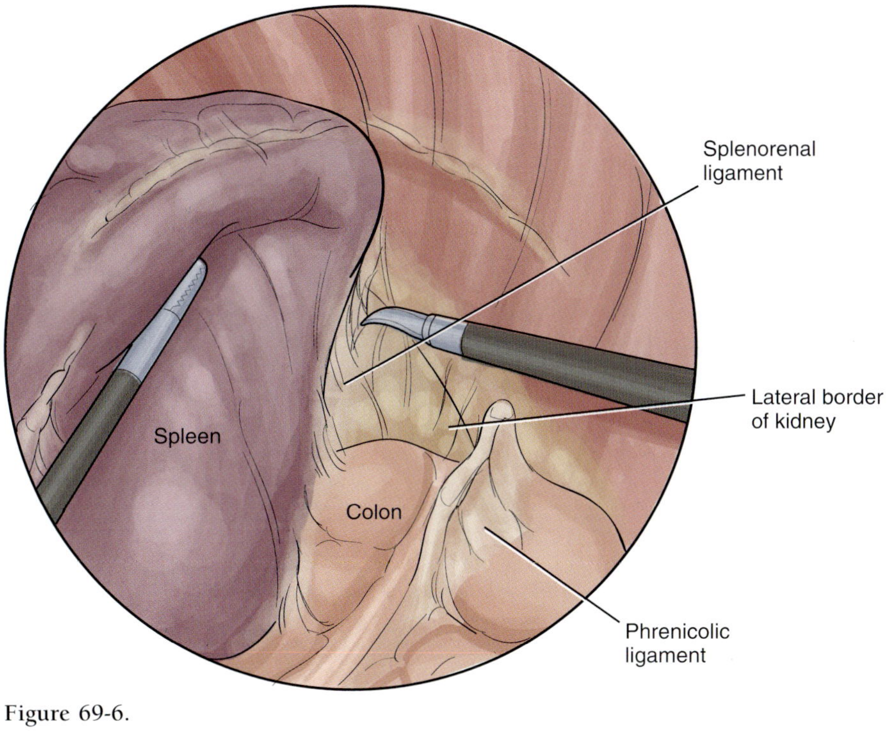

Figure 69-6.

- Blunt retraction of the spleen can be employed using the same sponge technique used for the liver. However, as the spleen falls forward and the dissection plane is developed between the spleen, the pancreas, splenic vessels, and the underlying kidney and adrenal gland, no retraction is required, as shown in Figure 69-7. This dissection must be continued until the left crus of the diaphragm is identified. Usually no additional retraction is required. One must be careful not to enter the stomach, which occasionally creeps in at the most cephalad aspect of the dissection.
- Once the adrenal gland is uncovered, occasionally the transverse colon and lateral peritoneal reflection of the descending colon also need to be mobilized, to uncover the most inferior aspect of this dissection. It is mandatory to stay in the correct plane.
- Once the gland is uncovered, the strategy deployed is similar to that for the right side. Usually one aspect of the adrenal gland can be visualized so one can clearly see the demarcation between the canary-yellow adrenal gland and the underlying retroperitoneal fat.
- Once this plane is developed, elevation of the gland from the retroperitoneum allows the gland to be easily distinguished from the retroperitoneal fat. Elevation and movement of the gland allows clear visualization of the gland edge.
- The dissection progresses around the most caudal part of the gland, and as it sweeps around to the inferior medial portion, the adrenal vein will be found.
- Conversely, as represented in Figure 69-8, if one begins to separate the left adrenal from its attachments medially and superiorly by sequentially taking small phrenic branches, then a fairly large phrenic vein will be identified. This always present phrenic vein can be followed to the adrenal vein. Remember that the adrenal vein always has a phrenic branch and an adrenal branch, which meet to create a common trunk that drains into the renal vein.
- Once there is sufficient elevation of that inferior portion of the gland and the adrenal vein is identified and encircled, it can be handled in exactly the same way as the vein on the opposite side. The phrenic vein can also be sacrificed, if this is easier.
- Once the vein is divided, more elevation of the gland can occur, and the edge of the gland usually is more evident. Division of the inferior and other attachments is usually best executed with a Harmonic scalpel.

Closure

- Once the gland is detached, Surgicel is placed at the base, and the gland is placed in a bag and extracted as on the opposite side. The fascia of the larger ports is closed.

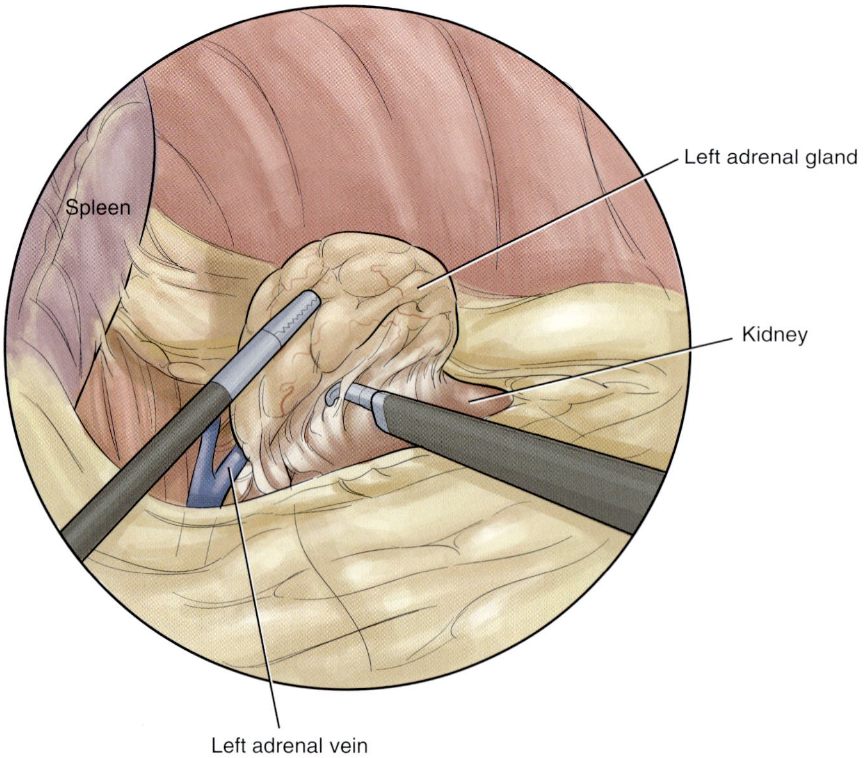

Figure 69-7.

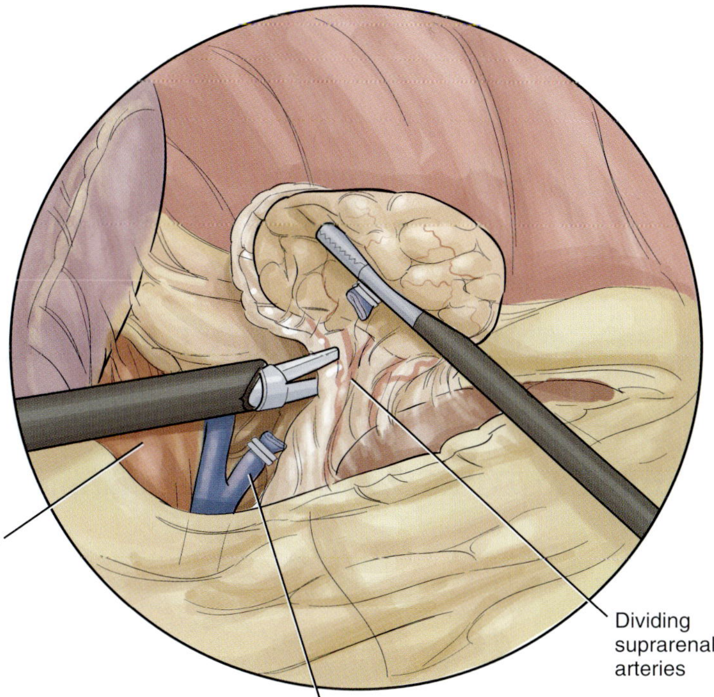

Figure 69-8.

III. ALTERNATIVE TECHNICAL APPROACHES (PRO/CON) AND PEARLS

- *Right:* Place a fourth 5-mm port in the right upper quadrant to retract the liver. Mobilize the right hepatic lobe for access to the vena cava and adrenal vein by taking down the triangular ligament to the diaphragm. Open the retroperitoneum in a longitudinal fashion medial to the adrenal gland and next to the lateral edge of the liver, until the vena cava is seen.
- *Left:* An extra port placed below the tip of the 12th rib allows for retraction of the adrenal gland or ipsilateral kidney. Mobilize the splenic flexure to visualize the splenorenal ligament. Open the retroperitoneal plane anterior to the Gerota fascia to the diaphragm, which will allow for medial rotation of the spleen and the pancreatic tail. Incise the Gerota fascia over the superior pole of the left kidney to access the adrenal gland.
- Use a vascular stapler for unusually large adrenal veins.
- On either side, if the gland cannot be clearly identified, open the Gerota fascia to expose the upper pole of the kidney, and then clear the entire pocket to tissue cephalad to the upper pole.

IV. SPECIAL POSTOPERATIVE CARE

- The patient is allowed clear liquids on the night of surgery, with advancement of diet upon return of bowel function.
- Standard intravenous postoperative narcotic regimens are used for management of pain, with transition to oral pain medications.
- The patient is discharged on postoperative day 1 to 3 after tolerating a regular diet, with follow-up in clinic within 10 days to 2 weeks after surgery.

SUGGESTED READINGS

Haveran LA, Novitsky YW, Czerniach DR, et al: Benefits of laparoscopic adrenalectomy: a 10-year single institution experience, *Surg Laparosc Endosc Percutan Tech* 16:217–221, 2006.

Novitsky YW, Czerniach DR, Kercher KW, et al: Feasibility of laparoscopic adrenalectomy for large adrenal masses, *Surg Laparosc Endosc Percutan Tech* 13:106–110, 2003.

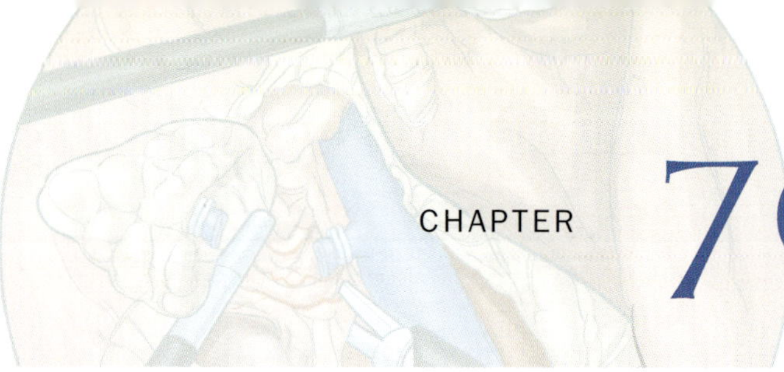

CHAPTER 70

Minimally Invasive Parathyroidectomy

Leigh Delbridge, MD, FRCS, FACS, and Catharina Ihre Lundgren, MD, PhD

I. SPECIAL PREOPERATIVE PREPARATION

- Surgery is the only available cure for primary hyperparathyroidism. Until recent decades, open four-gland parathyroid exploration via a conventional cervicotomy was the standard of care, providing a success rate of 95% to 98% in experienced hands with minimal complications. However, advances in parathyroid localization techniques have allowed alternative approaches, namely focused exploration of only the abnormal parathyroid gland with subsequent removal.
- Such procedures, performed via a small incision (by convention less than 3.0 cm in length), are now known as minimally invasive parathyroidectomy (MIP). By definition, MIP does not include the extra-thyroidal approaches (e.g., axillary or chest wall), requiring as they do an extensive dissection simply to avoid a cervical incision, nor does it include focused unilateral parathyroid exploration via a standard full-length cervicotomy. Currently described techniques for MIP include the full endoscopic approach with gas insufflation, the video-assisted approach, and the direct focused miniincision approach using either a central or lateral incision. These procedures can be performed under local or general anesthesia within an ambulatory setting and, in experienced hands, have a cure rate equivalent to open four-gland parathyroid exploration. This has been a major factor underpinning the American Association of Clinical Endocrinologists' recommendation that parathyroidectomy now be offered to all patients with a diagnosis of primary hyperparathyroidism unless contraindications to a surgical procedure exist.
- The key to the success of MIP is confident preoperative localization. An initial technetium-99m sestamibi scan should be performed (Fig. 70-1). Patients with confident localization with a single site of uptake should then have a focused ultrasound (Fig. 70-2) to define the anatomic features and precise location of the parathyroid adenoma and to assist with incision placement. Concordant localization is associated with a 98% cure on removal of the enlarged parathyroid gland. Patients with primary hyperparathyroidism with failure to localize on sestamibi scan should be offered a standard open four-gland exploration. Patients with positive sestamibi scan but negative ultrasound may still be offered MIP with a raised awareness of the possible need for conversion. Some authors have published data with MIP based on ultrasound alone; however, MIP should not be attempted in the absence of any form of positive localization.
- The technique of MIP is based on a precise understanding of the anatomy and embryology of normal and pathologic parathyroid glands. The parathyroid glands originate from the third and fourth pharyngeal pouches and are of endodermal origin. The superior parathyroids develop from the fourth pharyngeal cleft and are relatively constant in their location, being found within a 1-cm radius of the intersection of the inferior thyroid artery and the recurrent laryngeal nerve, commonly just on the superior surface of the tubercle of Zuckerkandl. Abnormal superior parathyroid glands generally lie posterior-superior to the recurrent laryngeal nerve and may descend along the tracheoesophageal groove into the posterior-superior mediastinum. The inferior parathyroid glands develop from the third pharyngeal cleft and descend along with the developing thymus. Their location is inconstant compared with the superior gland's neck. Abnormal inferior parathyroid glands are mostly found in a plane anterior-inferior to the recurrent laryngeal nerve and may descend into the anterior mediastinum, lying within the thymus. An undescended inferior parathyroid gland may be located in the carotid sheath.

II. OPERATIVE TECHNIQUE

- The technique described here is the lateral direct-focused miniincision technique. Our unit commenced MIP using a video-assisted technique, then progressed to a central miniincision technique before using the lateral technique, which significantly facilitates anatomic exposure of the parathyroid glands, especially those in a superior or posterior location.

Position

- The procedure is performed under general anesthesia or controlled regional anesthesia. The patient is positioned supine with the neck held in extension. The surgeon uses an operating headlight to provide illumination of the narrow operative field.

Incision

- The site of the incision depends on the localization to the superior or inferior position (Fig. 70-3). On-table surgeon-performed ultrasound greatly facilitates incision placement. If this is not available, the incision can be sited based on the preoperative ultrasound information using the cricoid as the most constant landmark in the neck, corresponding as it does to the upper border of the thyroid

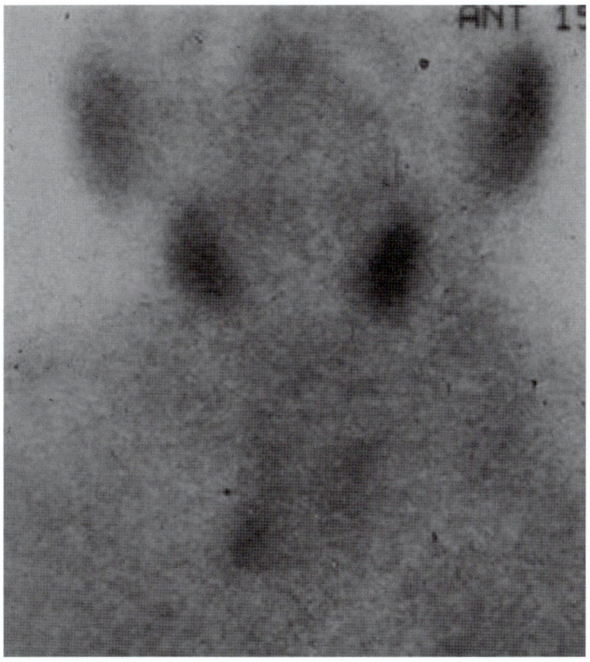

Figure 70-1.

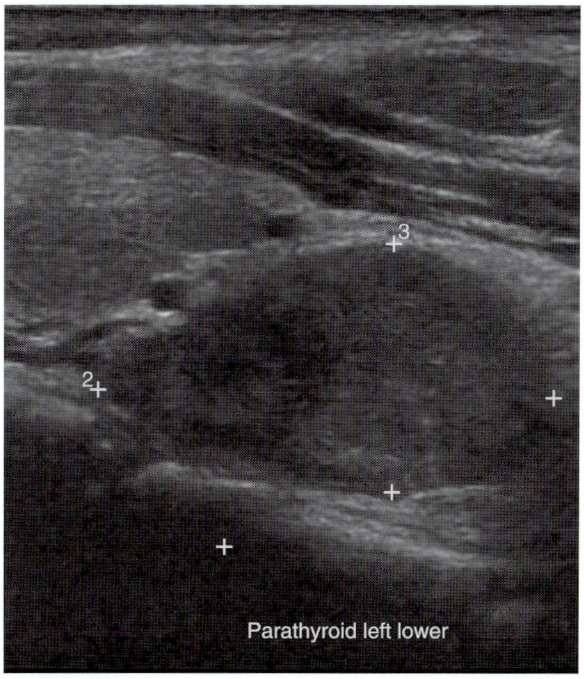

Figure 70-2.

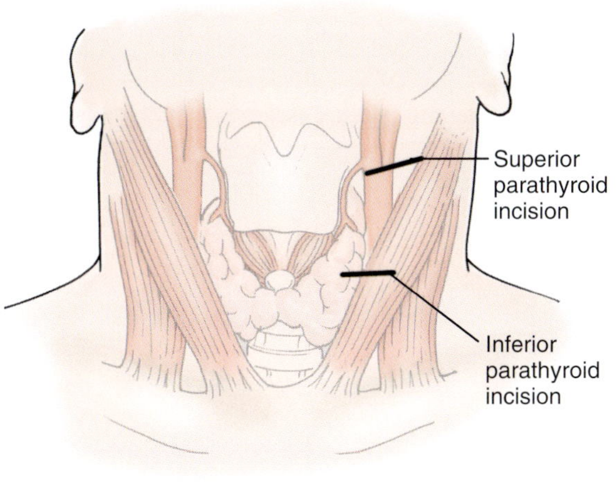

Figure 70-3.

isthmus. The incision is then marked, overlying the medial border of the sternomastoid muscle at a level corresponding precisely to the anatomic site of the localized abnormal parathyroid gland. The incision should be 2.0 to 2.5 cm long—that is, long enough to allow finger dissection of the tissue planes, providing visualization of the adenoma.

Main Dissection

- After an incision through the skin and platysma is made, the subplatysmal space is developed using a combination of blunt finger dissection and electrocautery, with any vessels encountered being divided (Fig. 70-4). The medial margin of the sternocleidomastoid muscle is defined and overlying fascia divided with electrocautery (Fig. 70-5). The sternocleidomastoid muscle is retracted laterally to expose the lateral margin of the sternothyroid muscle. The space between the two is then entered and the sternothyroid retracted medially, exposing the middle thyroid vein and omohyoid muscle, either of which may require division to expose the parathyroid-bearing area. With further blunt finger dissection, the ansa cervicalis can be visualized and preserved, and further dissection then opens the entire space down to the prevertebral fascia. Medial retraction of the thyroid gland and lateral retraction of the internal jugular vein then provide rapid visualization of more than 90% of the parathyroid-containing area in the neck.

Inferior Parathyroid Adenomas

- The thyroid lobe is retracted superiorly, and the recurrent laryngeal nerve should be identified in the tracheoesophageal groove (Fig. 70-6). Medial dissection anterior to the nerve in the region of the lower pole of the thyroid gland and thyrothymic ligament will generally demonstrate the enlarged parathyroid gland, which can be gently elevated and removed. Inferior glands often have multiple venous tributaries passing directly into the thyroid substance, and all need to be individually ligated. Occasionally part of the lower pole of the thyroid will need to be removed along with the parathyroid adenoma to avoid rupture of the capsule. Likewise, inferior glands often lie within the thymus, which can also be readily removed through the same incision (Fig. 70-7) by gentle retraction. Even intrathymic parathyroid glands located in the upper anterior mediastinum can be delivered through a cervical approach using this technique.

Superior Parathyroid Adenomas

- The thyroid lobe is elevated medially and attention directed to the prevertebral fascia. The recurrent laryngeal nerve (Figs. 70-8, 70-9, and 70-10) is then identified in relation to the inferior thyroid artery. This artery may need to be divided, especially for large adenomas, which may lay directly posterior. It is important to appreciate that the recurrent laryngeal nerve is often closely applied to such superior adenomas, indenting the anterior surface of the gland, and thus is readily injured if not identified early. Commonly, the superior adenoma will be located in the tracheoesophageal groove and can then be gently elevated on what is usually a solitary vascular pedicle (Fig. 70-11), which can then be divided between clips. The key to safe and successful delivery without capsule rupture is dissection

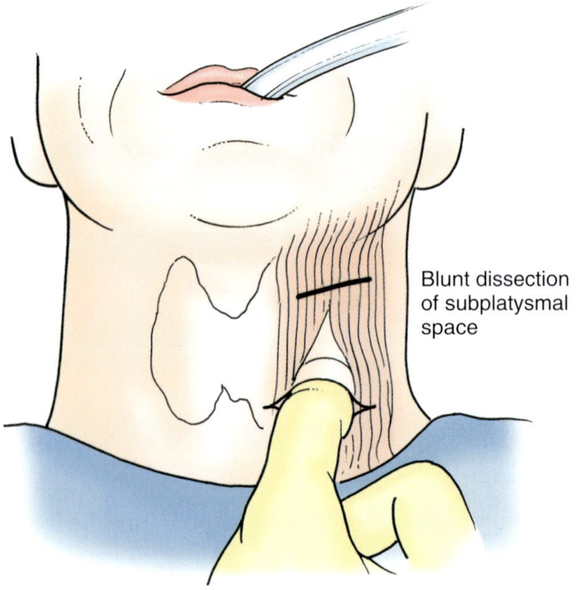

Figure 70-4.

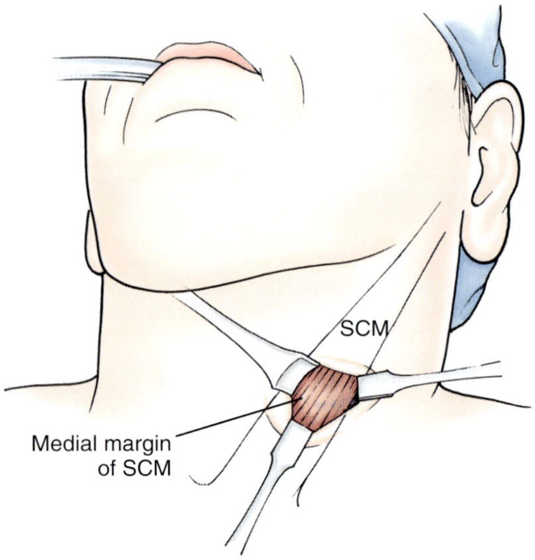

Figure 70-5. *SCM,* Sternocleidomastoid.

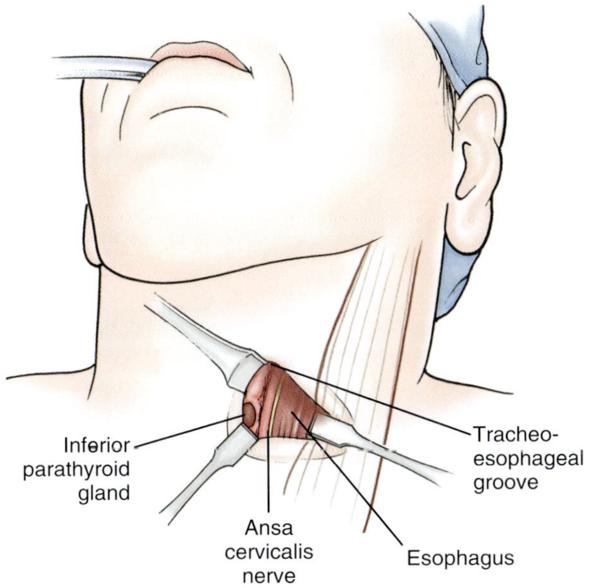

Figure 70-6.

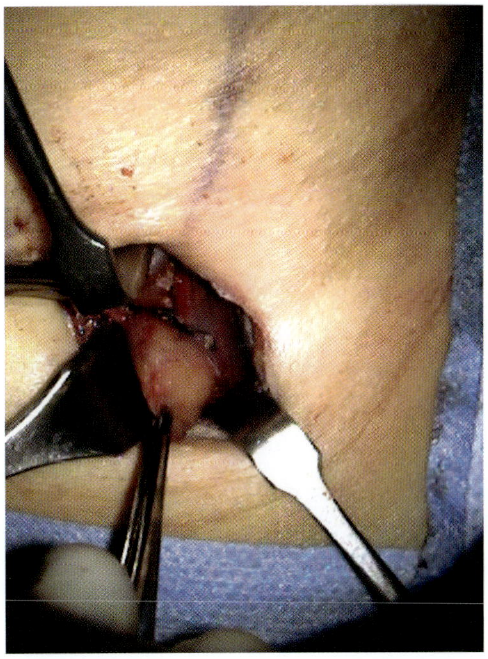

Figure 70-7.

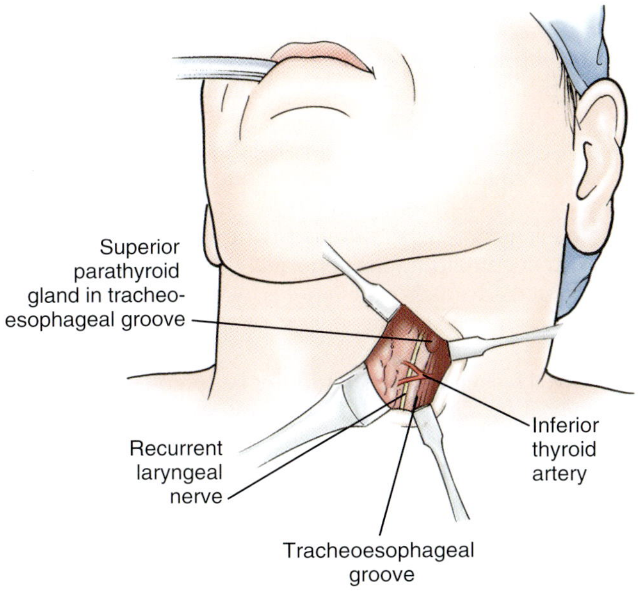

Figure 70-8.

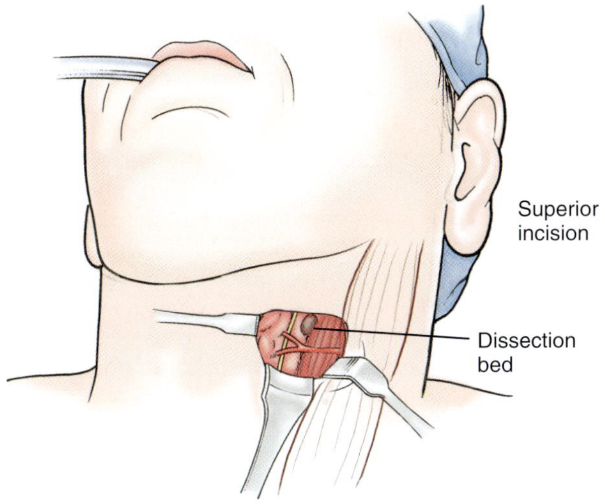

Figure 70-9.

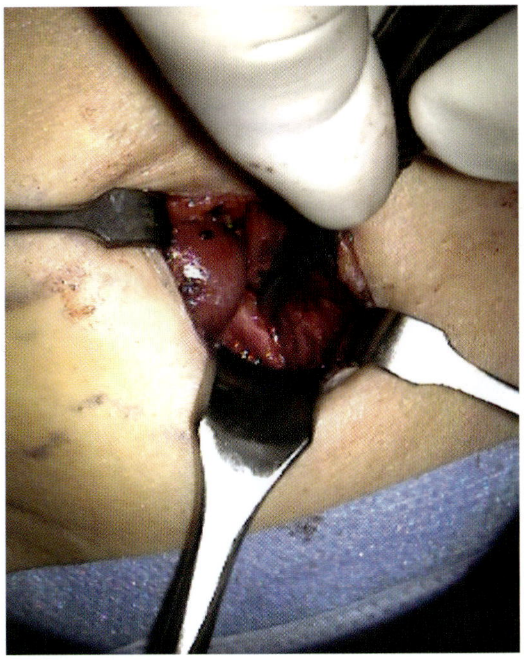

Figure 70-10.

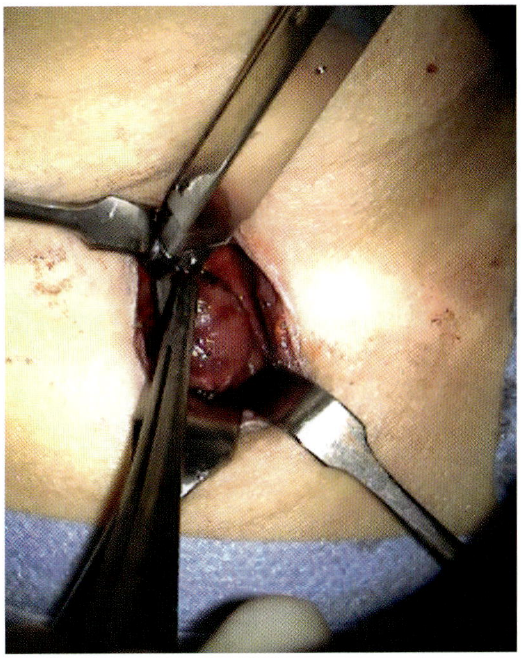

Figure 70-11.

posterolaterally in the avascular plane that surrounds such adenomas, progressively mobilizing the gland toward the pedicle, which is located superomedially. A gland that has descended along the esophagus into the posterior superior mediastinum can also be delivered by gentle finger dissection. Failure to locate an adenoma in the expected anatomic site as indicated by preoperative localization can occur, usually due to the discovery of alternative pathology such as a follicular adenoma of the thyroid. Under those circumstances, conversion to an open four-gland exploration through a standard cervicotomy should be undertaken under the same anesthetic.

Closure

- Once the tumor is removed and hemostasis is achieved, the skin incision is closed using subcuticular absorbable sutures. Any slight stretching of the incision (with subsequent extension of its length) can be reversed by using minimal plication with the subcuticular sutures, restoring the final incision length to less than 3.0 cm. A parathyroid hormone (PTH) level is measured before and after surgery to facilitate informed same-day discharge of the patient. There are no special postoperative requirements.

III. ALTERNATIVE TECHNICAL APPROACHES (PRO/CON) AND PEARLS

- *Endoscopic MIP:* This procedure is performed using one central and several lateral ports with gas insufflation. The stated advantages are excellent visualization of the anatomy; however, the technique is time consuming, is difficult to learn, and requires significant use of consumables.
- *Video-assisted MIP:* This procedure is performed via a small suprasternal incision, with finger dissection of the operative space, insertion of an endoscope to provide lighting, and specially designed dissectors to facilitate removal. The stated advantages are improved lighting and visualization of the anatomy. However, the technique is not conceptually different from the direct focused central miniincision technique and requires multiple trained assistants.
- *Direct focused central miniincision technique*: This is the most commonly performed technique, because it is based on the same operative approach as the traditional open procedure, simply through a smaller incision. A small central incision 2 cm above the sternal notch is made, the strap muscles are separated in the midline, and a focused exploration of the relevant quadrant containing the abnormal parathyroid gland is undertaken using standard surgical techniques. The stated advantages are familiarity of surgical technique and ability to explore both sides of the neck should the need arise. Access to superior or posterior adenomas, however, is clearly limited.
- *Open four-gland parathyroid exploration via standard cervicotomy:* This technique should not be forgotten as an alternative, because a patient with negative or equivocal localization should be offered open exploration. Attempts to undertake MIP in every patient with primary hyperparathyroidism will inevitably lead to failure.
- *MIP guided by intraoperative PTH measurement:* Some authors consider intraoperative PTH assay an essential prerequisite for performing any focused or minimally invasive parathyroid procedure. It involves blood sample collection preoperatively and 5 and 10 minutes after the ligation or division of the parathyroid vascular pedicle. If PTH levels are used as a guide to cure, the operation is terminated if the levels fall to less than 50% of the preoperative levels at 10 minutes. If not, an open neck exploration is performed to look for a second adenoma or multigland hyperplasia. However, the PTH seems to be inaccurate precisely in patients with multigland disease. Also, a false-negative result leads to unnecessary conversion. Numerous recent studies have demonstrated that, in appropriately selected patients, MIP can be performed without intraoperative PTH measurement with equivalent success rates.
- *Radio-guided MIP:* Introduced initially to improve localization and ensure adequate removal of tissue, this technique has largely been abandoned by most major units as providing no additional benefit.

IV. SPECIAL POSTOPERATIVE CARE

- The tape (Steri-Strip Skin Closures, 3M, Minneapolis) should not be removed for the first 2 weeks. Then it can be replaced by a Micropore tape, which can be changed every few days for 3 months, giving the best cosmetic results. No further postoperative care is usually needed.

SUGGESTED READINGS

Agarwal G, Barraclough BH, Reeve TS, Delbridge LW: Minimally invasive parathyroidectomy using the "focused" lateral approach. II. Surgical technique, *ANZ J Surg* 72:147–151, 2002.

Delbridge L: Minimally invasive parathyroidectomy: the Australian experience, *Asian J Surg* 26:76–81, 2003.

Pang T, Stålberg P, Sidhu S, et al: Minimally invasive parathyroidectomy using the lateral focused mini-incision technique without intraoperative parathyroid hormone monitoring, *Br J Surg* 94:315–319, 2007.

CHAPTER 71

Videothoracoscopic Thymectomy

Calvin S.H. Ng, BSc(Hon), MBBS(Hon)(Lond), MD(Res), FRCSEd(CTh),
and Anthony P.C. Yim, MD, FRCS, FACS

I. SPECIAL PREOPERATIVE PREPARATION

- For young patients with generalized myasthenia gravis (MG), it is now generally accepted that thymectomy should be offered. However, uncertainties remain over the role of thymectomy for patients with purely ocular symptom and those with late onset of disease.
- Between 30% and 70% of patients with initial ocular symptoms will eventually develop generalized myasthenia. Based on these statistics, we advised some of our young patients to undergo surgery even though their presentation was purely ocular (Figs. 71-1 and 71-2).
- Although some patients with purely ocular symptoms improve following thymectomy, patients should understand that the rationale for surgery is not based on symptomatic improvement, but rather on the expectation of halting progression of the disease.
- It is vital that thoracic surgeons work closely with neurologists and anesthetists to achieve optimal results.
- MG causes weakness of voluntary muscles, including those involved in respiration, so that a patient is at risk of developing postoperative respiratory failure. If bulbar palsy is present, the patient may also develop aspiration pneumonia.
- Medical treatment is associated with its own complication. Anticholinesterase treatment increases vagal tone, enhances oral secretion, and potentiates laryngeal spasm. Prolonged steroid use can result in electrolyte imbalance and increase susceptibility to infections.

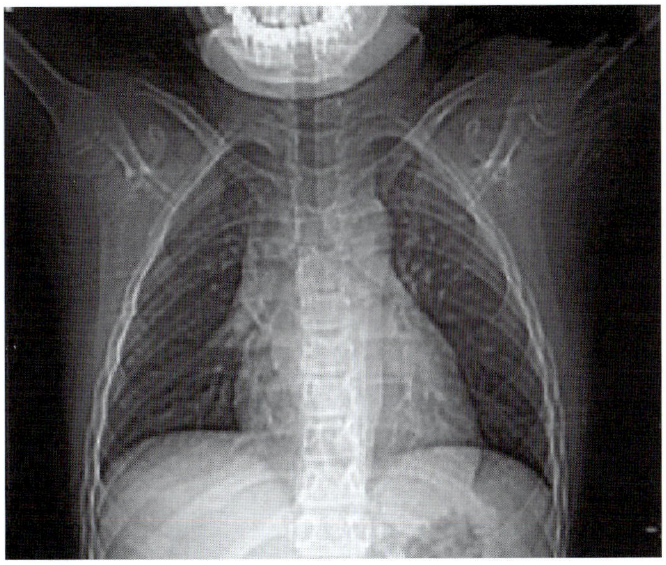

Figure 71-1. Large mediastinal mass on chest radiograph.

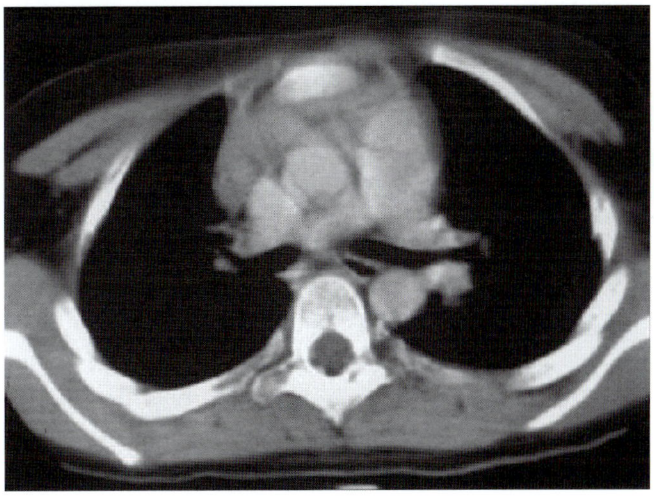

Figure 71-2. Computed tomography showing thymic hypertrophy.

- Before elective surgery, it is important that the distribution and severity of muscle weakness are carefully assessed. Respiratory function and nutritional status should also be documented and medical treatment optimized. Patients with severe weakness may require preoperative plasmapheresis, together with steroid and anticholinesterase therapy.
- Admission to the intensive care unit for ventilatory support is indicated for patients who are already in respiratory failure, but it is not necessary to wait until the patient is extubated before surgery can proceed.
- Intravenous immunoglobulin is an alternative to plasmapheresis, but there is no clear evidence that one is better. The patient should be warned of the possibility of postoperative mechanical ventilation.
- The operation is usually arranged as the first case on the elective list. Premedication is prescribed as needed, but respiratory depressant drugs are avoided. "Stress" doses of steroids may be required.
- General anesthesia involves selective one-lung ventilation to the left lung with a left-sided double-lumen endobronchial tube.
- Patients are induced with 2 mg/kg of propofol and 2 mcg/kg of fentanyl, and intubation can usually be achieved without muscle relaxants. Pretreatment of the tracheobronchial tree with local anesthetics can also facilitate intubation. Proper positioning of the endobronchial tube is confirmed with the use of the fiberoptic bronchoscope after intubation and reconfirmed after patient positioning.
- It is generally held that a body weight of at least 30 to 35 kg is necessary for the patient's airway to accommodate the smallest double-lumen device (28 Fr). This size limitation essentially precludes the use of these devices for children younger than approximately 8 years of age. Other techniques to achieve one-lung ventilation such as placement of a bronchial blocker or intentional intubation of a main stem bronchus with an endotracheal tube should be used.
- Hypoxemia during one-lung ventilation is usually caused by shunting of blood. In the case of hypoxemia, the position of the double-lumen endobronchial tube and hemodynamic stability should be confirmed. A low level of continuous positive airway pressure applied to the collapsed right lung may improve saturation. Applying positive end-expiratory pressure to the ventilated lung can also raise oxygen saturation during one-lung ventilation.
- Anesthesia is maintained with isoflurane (1% to 2%), 60% nitrous oxide in oxygen, and a single bolus of 0.1 mg/kg of morphine. Ventilation is controlled to achieve normocarbia. Patients with MG are usually more susceptible to the neuromuscular blocking effect of volatile anesthetics so that nondepolarizing muscle relaxants are usually not required.
- Patients with MG are usually also very sensitive to nondepolarizing muscle relaxants. If muscle relaxation is necessary during the course of anesthesia, a reduced dose of an intermediate-acting nondepolarizing muscle relaxant should be used, followed by a carefully titrated intravenous infusion. Monitoring neuromuscular transmission is mandatory to adjust the dosage of muscle relaxant used and to ensure complete reversal of neuromuscular blockade after the surgery.
- Electrocardiogram, invasive blood pressure, pulse oximetry, end-tidal carbon dioxide, airway pressure, ventilatory volume, inspired oxygen, and neuromuscular transmission are continuously monitored.
- There are relatively few contraindications to video-assisted thoracoscopic surgery (VATS). In addition to the general contraindications such as severe coagulopathy, specific ones include pleural symphysis and patients with severe underlying lung disease or poor lung function who are unable to tolerate the selective one-lung ventilation during general anesthesia.
- Prior operation in the ipsilateral chest should not be regarded as a contraindication. Adhesions can usually be reduced using a combination of sharp and blunt dissection under videoscopic vision.
- Contraindications to the VATS approach for resection include thymic malignancy and any evidence of invasion of the normal tissue plane. In addition, we are careful in restricting the VATS technique to small, completely encapsulated thymomas (Masaoka stage I). Clinical judgment is of paramount importance in thymic surgery, and any sign of tissue plane invasion mandates conversion to an open dissection.

II. OPERATIVE TECHNIQUE

Position

- Under general anesthesia with selective one-lung ventilation, the patient is positioned in the full left lateral decubitus position for the approach to the anterior mediastinum from the right (Fig. 71-3). Some surgeons prefer to place the patient in a 45-degree lateral decubitus position to allow for greater posterior displacement of the lung.
- The operating table is flexed to 30 degrees with the fulcrum just inferior to the level of the nipples, to open the upper intercostal spaces for thoracoscope insertion and instrumentation.
- The team of the principal surgeon, an assistant, a scrub nurse, and the anesthesiologist remain in the same positions during the whole procedure. The operating room setup consists of the anesthetic unit, videothoracoscopy unit (video monitor, image printer, recorder, and light source), video monitor for the scrub nurse to follow the surgery, electrocautery, and instrument trolley (see Fig. 71-3).

- Mostly conventional instruments are used, such as sponge-holding forceps (for retraction), dental pledget mounted on a curved clamp (for dissection), and right-angled clamp (for dissection of vascular branches).
- We advocate the use of conventional thoracic instruments such as the sponge-holding forceps whenever possible because they are less expensive and are more familiar to the surgeon. However, a few dedicated endoscopic instruments should be available to aid surgery, including endoscissors for incising the mediastinal pleura, endograsper, and endoclip applier for vascular hemostasis (Endoclip, Autosuture, United States Surgical, Norwalk, Conn.).

Incision

- The chest is the most suitable body cavity for the minimal-access approach, because once the lung is collapsed (with selective one-lung ventilation), there is plenty of room for instrument maneuvering. The use of carbon dioxide insufflation, and hence valved ports, is therefore unnecessary. In fact, there is evidence that thoracic carbon dioxide insufflation during VATS has an adverse effect on the patient's hemodynamics compared with selective one-lung ventilation.
- The use of costal or sternal hooks for anterior chest wall lifting during VATS thymectomy may increase the operative space. However, we have never found it necessary in our practice.
- Strategies to minimize chest wall trauma, avoid intercostal nerve compression, and hence minimize postoperative pain include: (1) avoiding the use of trocar ports by introducing instruments directly through the wound, (2) avoiding torquing of the thoracoscope by visualizing with an angled lens (30-degree scope), (3) using smaller telescopes (5 mm) when clinically allowed, and (4) delivering specimens through the anterior port because the anterior intercostal spaces are wider.
- Under general anesthesia, selective one-lung ventilation should be confirmed with the anesthesiologist before port incision.

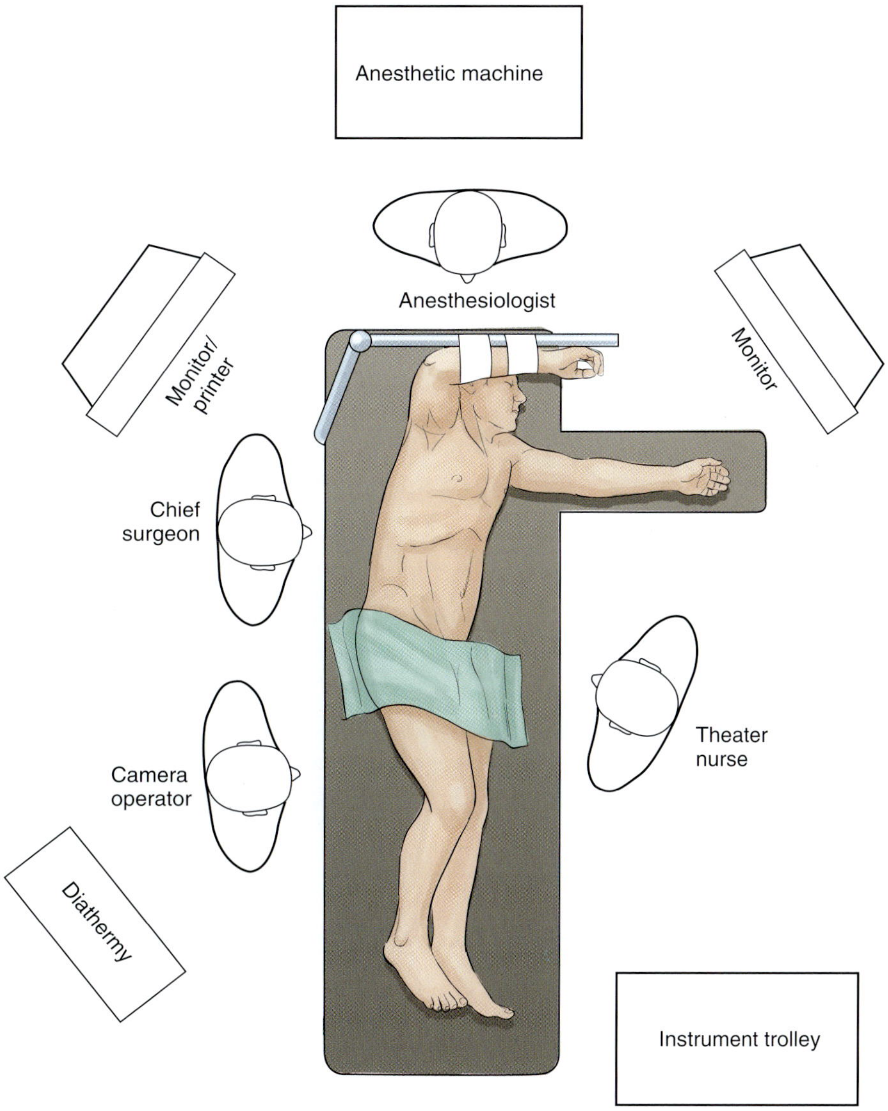

Figure 71-3.

- We advocate a right-sided approach and a three-port technique for the procedure. The thoracoscope port incision should be in front of the tip of the scapula along the posterior axillary line for the insertion of the 10-mm port and 0-degree (or 30-degree) telescope. The second and third 5-mm instrument ports should be inserted by open technique under direct thoracoscopic vision at the third intercostal space midaxillary line and the sixth intercostal space anterior axillary line (Figs. 71-4 and 71-5). Additional ports may be made for lung retraction as necessary.
- In young female patients, the instrument ports should be strategically placed over the submammary fold for cosmetic considerations.

Main Dissection

- The body of the gland is related anteriorly to the sternum and the upper four costal cartilages; posteriorly to the pericardium, ascending aorta, brachiocephalic veins, and superior vena cava; and laterally to the mediastinal pleura. Its fibrous capsule blends in with the pretracheal fascia (Fig. 71-6).
- The entire hemithorax is carefully examined with particular attention to the mediastinum. Blunt instruments such as sponge-holding forceps may be used to help collapse the lung and for manipulation to complete the exploration. The major structural landmarks should be identified, including the superior vena cava, brachiocephalic vein, and right phrenic nerve.
- It is of paramount importance that the right phrenic nerve be carefully preserved throughout the dissection, because phrenic nerve palsy represents a major complication for patients with MG. Pleural adhesions may be present and require adhesiolysis to facilitate complete lung collapse and achieve a good operating field.
- First, the right inferior horn of the thymus is identified, draping over the pericardium. The mediastinal pleura over the free edge of the right inferior thymic horn is then sharply incised anterior to the phrenic nerve (Fig. 71-7). The thymus can then be lifted and bluntly dissected off the underlying pericardium, extending on to the aorta in a cephalad manner until the left brachiocephalic vein is exposed. We have found it useful to apply deliberate and gentle traction on the thymus to allow blunt dissection using a pledget.
- The thymic venous tributaries (usually two or three) draining posteriorly into the left brachiocephalic vein can then be identified, clipped, and divided. It is important to obtain vascular control before further manipulating the thymus. Rarely, conversion to a small lateral thoracotomy for control of bleeding from a branch of the brachiocephalic vein is needed. Dissection is then carried behind the sternum.

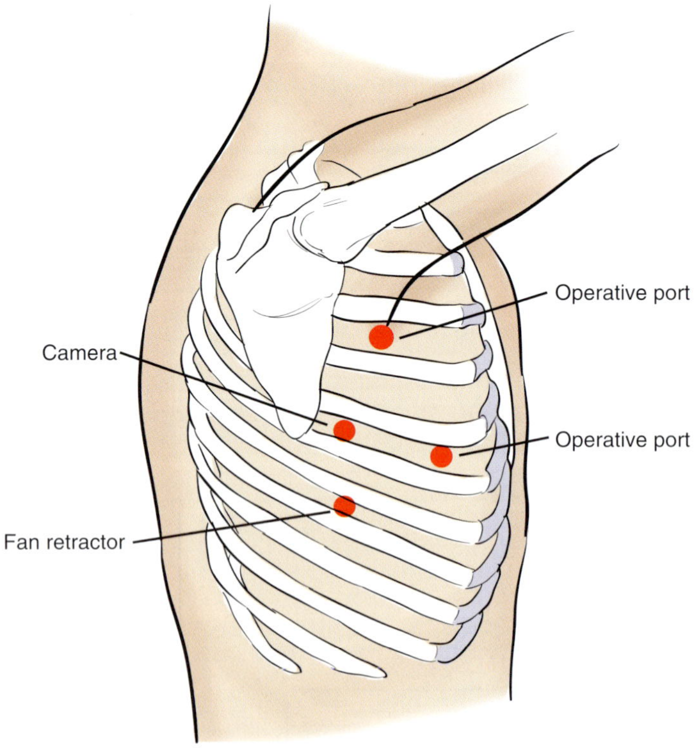

Figure 71-4.

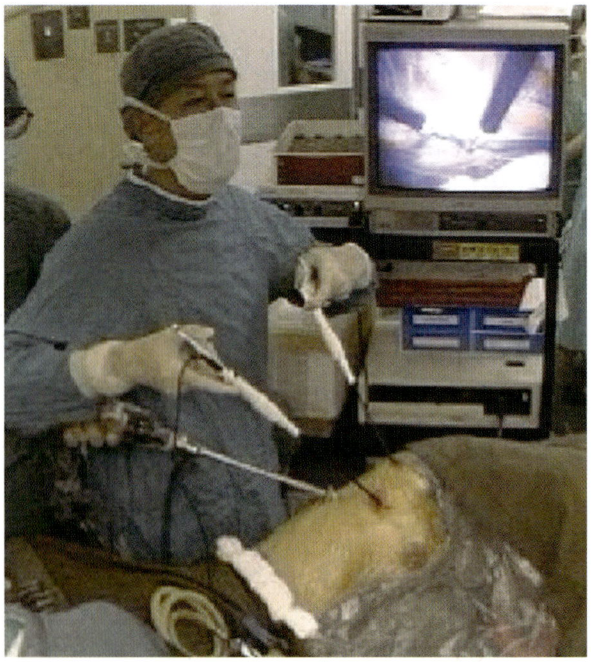

Figure 71-5.

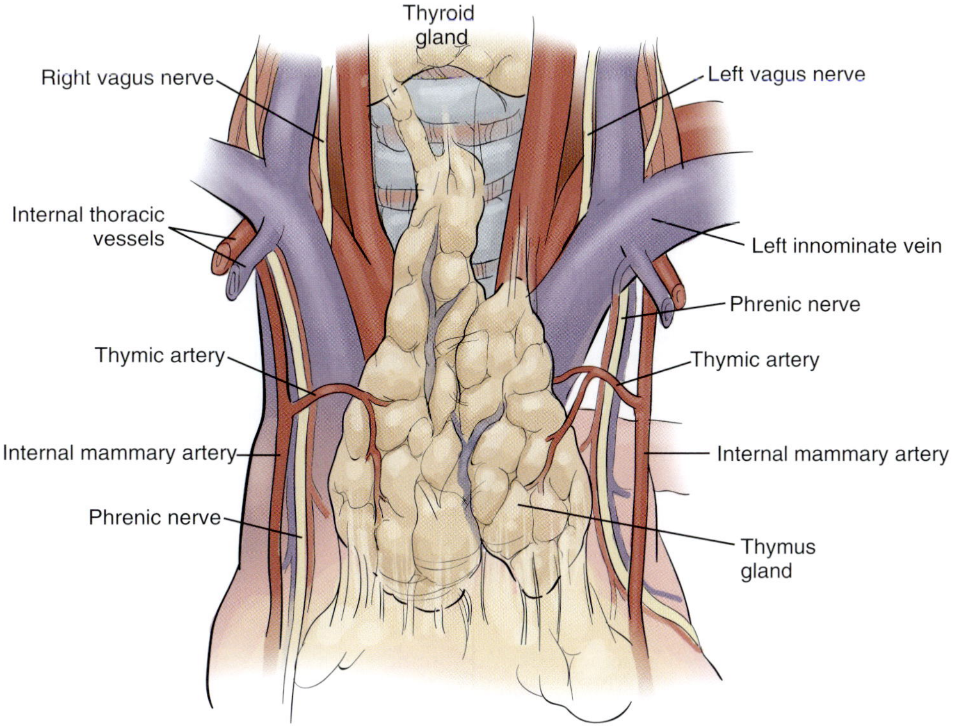

Figure 71-6.

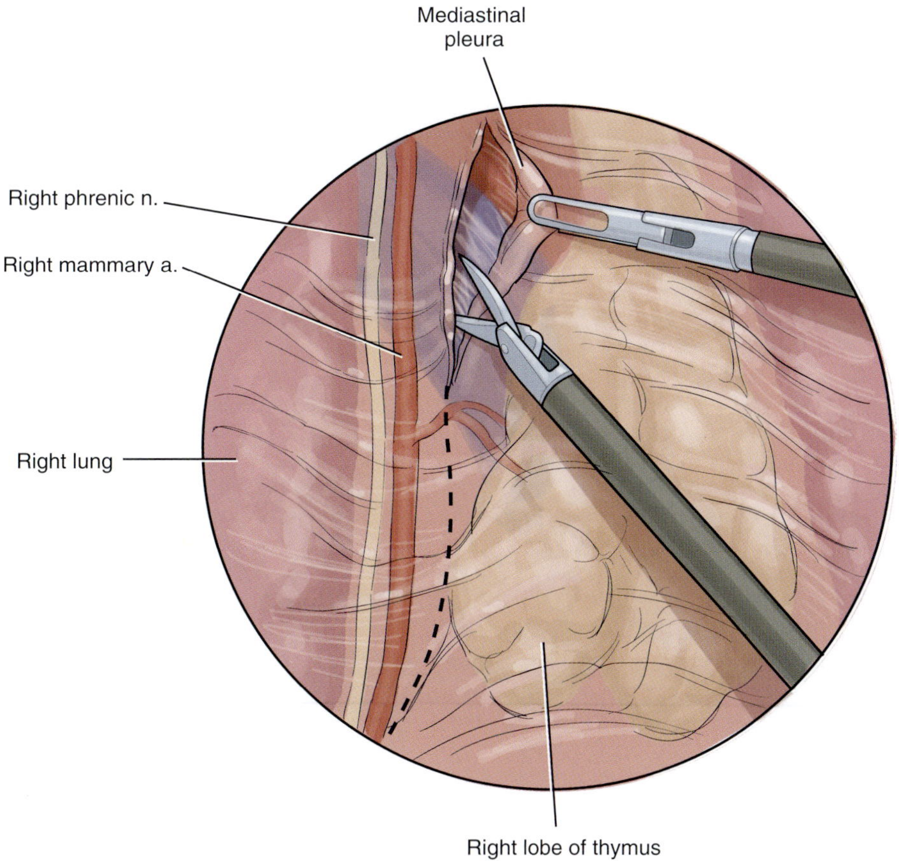

Figure 71-7.

With gentle traction on the thymus using a sponge-holding forceps, the left inferior horn can be identified and dissected up to the thymic isthmus (Fig. 71-8).

- Dissection of the superior horns is perhaps the most difficult part of the operation. The superior horns often extend into the neck, lying deep to the sternothyroid muscle. The right internal mammary vein is divided in most cases to facilitate exposure. With gentle and deliberate inferior traction on the thymus, the superior horns can be carefully dissected free from their fascial attachments, mainly using blunt dissection with the aid of mounted pledgets. The positions of the thoracoscope and inferior instrument port may be exchanged to allow better reach toward the superior parts of the thymus, particularly when conventional instruments are used.
- In a small child with a bulky hyperplastic thymus and relatively small thoracic cavity, we have found it useful to retract part of the gland out of an anteriorly placed wound, which creates more room for the instruments to facilitate further dissection.
- It is noteworthy that the left superior horn may occasionally pass behind, instead of in front, of the brachiocephalic vein, and this anatomic variation must be looked for. We have encountered it in one case; thoracoscopic dissection was successfully accomplished (Fig. 71-9).
- The thymus, as a free specimen, can then be removed in a plastic bag (Endocatch, Autosuture; or sterilized plastic "sandwich bag") through the most anterior port, because the intercostal space is wider anteriorly. After thymectomy, the anterior mediastinal soft tissue including the pericardial fat is separately removed. The specimen should be inspected for completeness of resection (Fig. 71-10).

Closure

- The thymic bed is inspected for hemostasis and completeness of resection. The brachiocephalic veins should have been skeletonized, and the junction to form the superior vena cava clearly visualized (Fig. 71-11).
- The insertion of a tube thoracostomy is optional. The lung is then reinflated under direct vision. Layered closure of the stab wounds with absorbable sutures completes the operation.

III. ALTERNATIVE TECHNICAL APPROACHES (PRO/CON) AND PEARLS

- The most commonly adopted surgical approach to thymectomy is via a median sternotomy. Other open thymectomy techniques include the transcervical, the combined median sternotomy with transcervical incision (T-incision), and partial sternotomy (involving either the upper or lower sternum).
- The thoracoscopic approach to thymectomy was first reported in 1993. Subsequently, several variants have evolved, including VATS (unilateral) thymectomy and the bilateral thoracoscopic approach combined with a cervical incision (video-assisted thoracoscopic extended thymectomy). More recently, endoscopic robot-assisted thymectomy has also been reported with good immediate results.
- There have been no randomized controlled trials of thymectomy in the treatment of MG. Therefore no consensus exists with regard to the optimum surgical approach. Furthermore, patient heterogeneity,

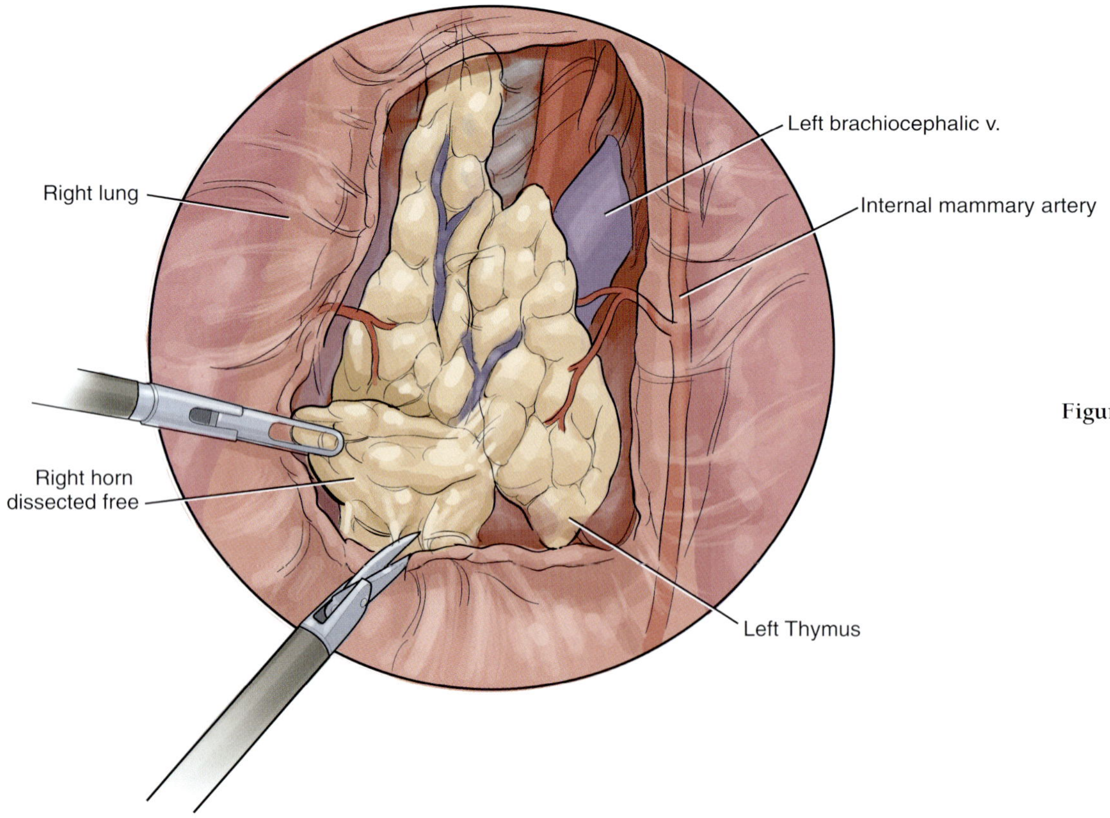

Figure 71-8.

the fluctuating nature of the disease, and different classification systems and practice guidelines make interpretation of outcomes following thymectomy difficult.

- Regardless of technique, it is generally agreed that thymectomy for MG should be complete. One group has advocated "maximal" thymectomy involving a combination of median sternotomy with cervical incision to achieve en bloc thymectomy and anterior mediastinal exenteration, which includes mediastinal pleura from the level of the thoracic inlet to the diaphragm, pericardial fat pad, and all the mediastinal fat. However, despite this radical approach, when compared with sternotomy alone or the transcervical approaches, results in terms of clinical improvement did not seem to be significantly different. In addition, a detailed autopsy study identified ectopic thymic tissue in areas (such as the retrocavinal fat) that are not accessible via a median sternotomy.
- Although it may seem intuitive to remove as much mediastinal soft tissue as possible to avoid leaving behind ectopic thymus, these remnants have never been conclusively shown to be clinically relevant, and even the most radical surgical approach does not result in a remission rate greater than 40%. Furthermore, the majority of ectopic thymus tissue is actually microscopic and may even be missed by radical thymectomy.
- The VATS approach is similar to the transcervical approach in that both are associated with minimal chest wall trauma, low postoperative morbidity, shorter hospital stay, and, perhaps more importantly, improved patient acceptance for surgery earlier in the disease compared with the transsternal approach. Only rarely is conversion from VATS to sternotomy required (2.6% to 5.5%). However, VATS has

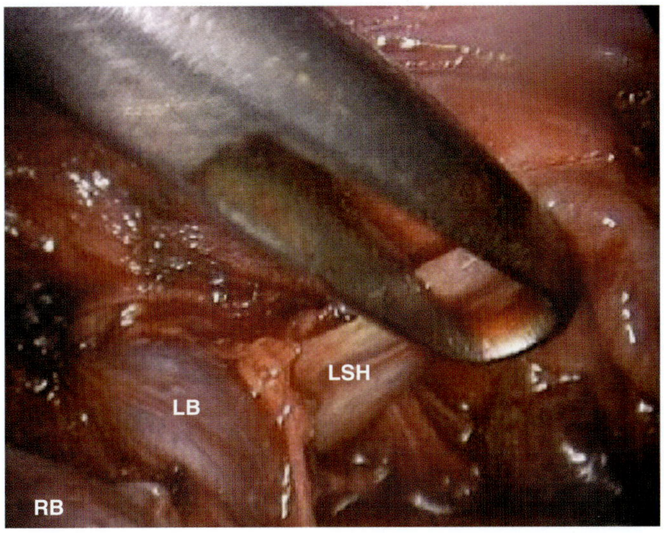

Figure 71-9. Dissection of left superior horn behind the left brachiocephalic vein. *LB,* Left brachiocephalic vein; *LSH,* left superior horn; *RB,* right brachiocephalic vein.

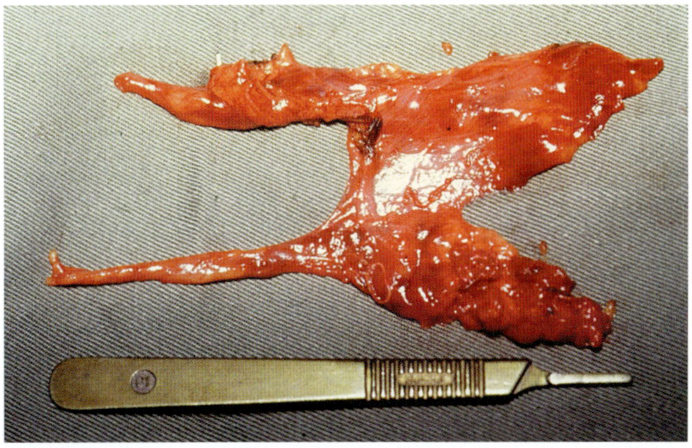

Figure 71-10.

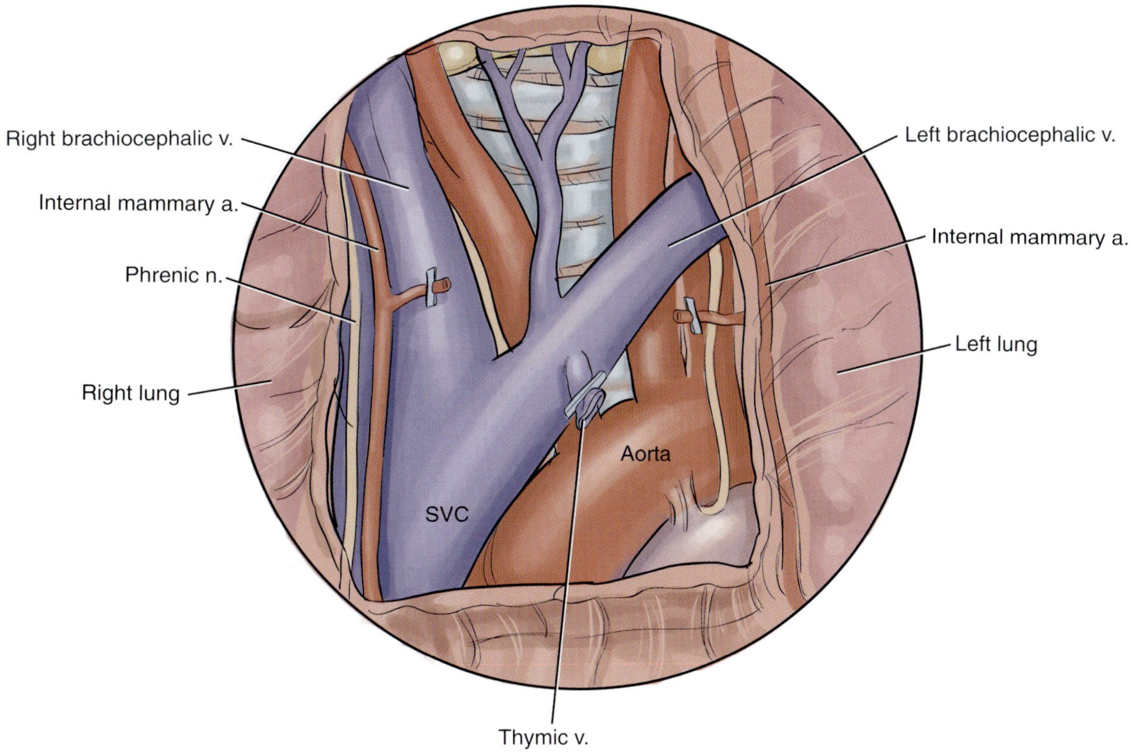

Figure 71-11. *SVC,* Superior vena cava.

additional advantages over the conventional transcervical approach: visualization is much better, and there is no crowding of instruments through a single access site. The thymus, being largely an anterior mediastinal structure, can be more directly approached through the chest than the neck.

- VATS may be a helpful approach for completion thymectomy in patients with refractory MG who have already undergone resection by prior transcervical or transsternal approach, with the potential advantage of avoiding previously dissected tissue planes and facilitating the search for residual thymic tissue. Interestingly, it has been shown that in patients who did not benefit initially from a transcervical or transsternal approach, VATS completion thymectomy can be performed to remove residual thymic tissue, resulting in improvement of symptoms.
- The cosmetic appearance of the surgical scars is seldom used to argue for a particular surgical approach. However, thymectomy may be a notable exception: the majority of patients are young and female, so the superior cosmetic appearance of VATS should be considered.
- Pulmonary function is significantly better preserved in the immediate postoperative period followed by a faster recovery after VATS when compared with the median sternotomy approach to thymectomy for MG. Such an advantage can contribute to earlier extubation and potential reduction in the incidence of postoperative pulmonary infections.
- We have shown that in our institution, patients who underwent thoracoscopic thymectomy had significantly less analgesic requirement and shorter hospital stays compared with a historical group who underwent transsternal thymectomy.
- There is controversy regarding whether the thymus should be approached from the left or right for VATS thymectomy. A left-sided approach with the use of pneumomediastinum to facilitate dissection has been advocated. From the left, it is argued, the dissection maneuvers are safer because the superior vena cava lies out of the surgical field, thus reducing risk of accidental injury. In addition, the removal of perithymic fatty tissue around the left pericardiophrenic angle and aortopulmonary window can be performed more readily from the left.
- We advocate the right-sided approach. First, the superior vena cava, easily identified from the right, provides a clear landmark for further dissection of the innominate veins. Second, the confluence of the two innominate veins to form the superior vena cava is an area most difficult to dissect well. This could be more easily accomplished from the right. Third, from the ergonomic standpoint, it is easier for right-handed surgeons performing VATS to start at the inferior poles and work cephalad from the right side. Furthermore, it allows greater maneuverability of instruments in the wider right pleural cavity, particularly in patients with cardiomegaly.
- There are two technical considerations regarding thymectomy in the prepubertal population. First, the thymus is relatively large compared to the body weight. Second, the chest is relatively small, and therefore the space for instrument maneuvering is less. Attention has to be given to achieving selective one-lung ventilation and to using finer instruments (5-mm external diameter or less).

IV. SPECIAL POSTOPERATIVE CARE

- Early extubation should be encouraged following surgery. The patient can resume full diet when fully awake from the general anesthesia, unless impaired by bulbar weakness from MG.
- A postoperative sitting chest radiograph is taken to detect pneumothorax, hemothorax, and any significant atelectasis. Postoperative chest physiotherapy and incentive spirometry should be provided and encouraged. Regular checks on oxygen saturation and bedside spirometry should be performed in the early postoperative period to give warning of respiratory muscle weakness.
- Postoperatively, patients should resume their preoperative medications for the control of MG. Pain can usually be adequately controlled by standard oral analgesics.
- Tube thoracostomy can be removed on day 1 after confirming no air leak or bleeding.
- Potential postoperative complications include acute respiratory failure, prolonged mechanical ventilation, wound infection, hypocalcemia, pneumothorax, surgical emphysema, intercostal neuralgia, and phrenic nerve palsy.
- In our experience with a median follow-up of 69 months (range 12 to 139 months), 92% of patients experienced some improvement. Our series showed complete stable remission (CSR) in 22.2% of patients, which is comparable to many other studies with CSR ranges of 14% to 41%. In addition, MM2 improvement was found in 25% and MM3 improvement in 44.4% of patients according to the MGFA postintervention status classification. The status in 5.5% of patients remained unchanged, and 2.7% died of MG.
- The number of patients experiencing postoperative CSR increased tentatively at 13 months following surgery, and then rose sharply at 117 months to 75% at 10 years follow-up.

SUGGESTED READINGS

Manlulu A, Lee TW, Wan I, et al: Video-assisted thoracic surgery thymectomy for nonthymomatous myasthenia gravis, *Chest* 128:3454–3460, 2005.

Savcenko M, Wendt GK, Prince SL, Mack MJ: Video-assisted thymectomy for myasthenia gravis: an update of a single institution experience, *Eur J Cardiothorac Surg* 22:978–983, 2002.

Tomulescu V, Ion V, Kosa A, et al: Thoracoscopic thymectomy mid-term results, *Ann Thorac Surg* 82:1003–1007, 2006.

SECTION XII

Urology

CHAPTER 72

Radical Nephrectomy with Inferior Vena Cava Tumor Thrombectomy

Gaetano Ciancio, MD, MBA, FACS, and Mark S. Soloway, MD*

I. SPECIAL PREOPERATIVE PREPARATION

- Renal cell carcinoma (RCC) infrequently extends into the inferior vena cava (IVC), and surgical extirpation is the only potential cure. How to achieve this has provoked considerable debate regarding optimal incisions, intraoperative techniques, complications, and outcomes.
- The level of the thrombus is localized with the initial computed tomography scan (Fig. 72-1) and is confirmed in some patients with magnetic resonance imaging (Fig. 72-2). Cardiac, renal, and respiratory status is evaluated preoperatively. The cranial extent of the tumor thrombus is partly defined as follows: (1) level I tumors are those extending less than 2 cm above the renal vein; (2) level II are infrahepatic; (3) level III are retrohepatic; and (4) level IV are those extending above the diaphragm into the right atrium. For a level III thrombus, we used our own modified definition.
- *Definition of level III thrombus:* Our experience suggests that a level III thrombus should be further subdivided depending on (1) the need for dissection and exposure of the major hepatic veins in addition to the IVC and (2) the degree of vascular control of the IVC required to extract this thrombus. We define as IIIa (intrahepatic) a thrombus extending into the retrohepatic vena cava but ending below the origins of the major hepatic veins; as IIIb (hepatic) a thrombus reaching the ostia of the major hepatic veins, or even extending into them; as IIIc (infradiaphragmatic) a thrombus extending above the major hepatic veins but below the diaphragm; and as IIId (suprahepatic, supradiaphragmatic) a thrombus extending into the intrapericardial vena cava but not into the right heart.
- All are managed by a transabdominal approach without bypass maneuvers, except for patients with a level IV tumor thrombus that is adherent to the atrial wall.
- Transesophageal echocardiography (TEE) is used for all the tumor thrombi that are above the infrahepatic vena cava. TEE is helpful in delineating the cranial extent of the thrombus and in monitoring embolic event. For level I or level II tumor thrombus, TEE was not used. TEE is definitely useful for RCC with levels IIIc, IIId, and IV (Fig. 72-3).

II. OPERATIVE TECHNIQUE

Position

- The patient is prepped supine with both arms abducted 90 degrees to the body. The axillary and femoral areas are prepped into the operative field in case venovenous bypass is deemed necessary.

Incision

- A triradiate incision is made commencing approximately two finger breadths below the right costal margin, extending out laterally to the midaxillary line. This is extended below the left costal margin as far as necessary, and vertically in the midline up beside the xiphoid process (Fig. 72-4).
- A Rochard self-retaining retractor (Fig. 72-5, *A*) is placed elevating the costal margins and splaying them laterally toward the axillae. This flattens the diaphragm, enabling easier liver mobilization and providing access to the retrohepatic space (see Fig. 72-5, *B*).

---

*The authors are grateful for the illustration expertise of Claudia Gutierrez.

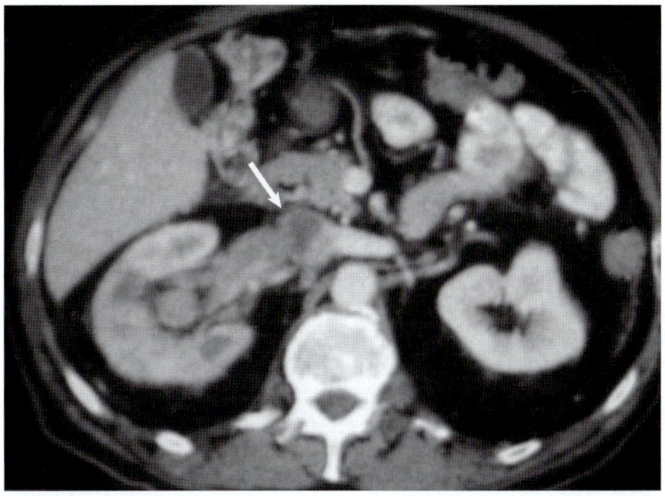

Figure 72-1. Abdominal computed tomography scan demonstrating a right renal mass with tumor thrombus extending into the right renal vein and inferior vena cava (*arrow*).

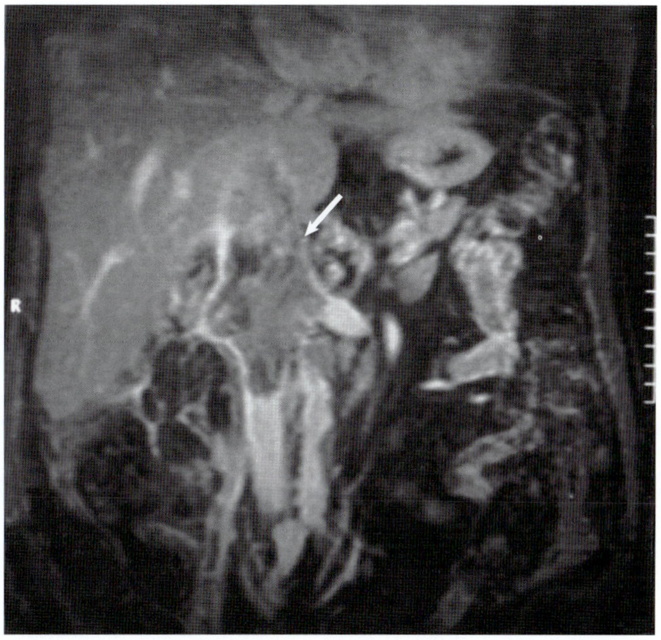

Figure 72-2. Magnetic resonance imaging demonstrating right kidney tumor and level IIIC (infradiaphragmatic) thrombus in the inferior vena cava (*arrow*).

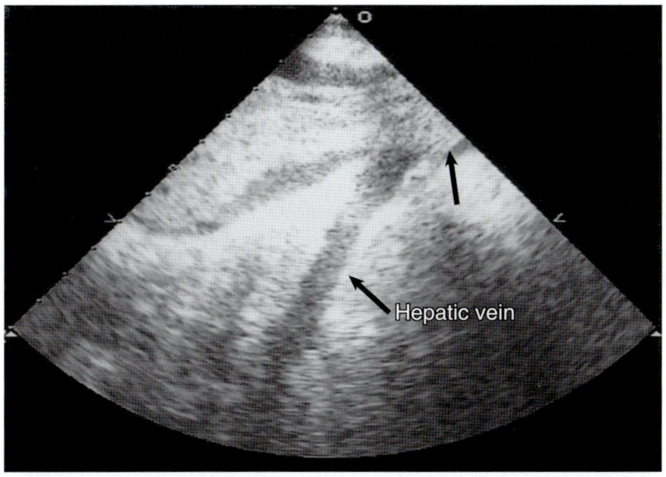

Figure 72-3. **Intraoperative transesophageal echocardiographic imaging of level IV (atrial) thrombus (*arrows*).** The *right arrow* shows the right hepatic vein obstructed by the tumor thrombus.

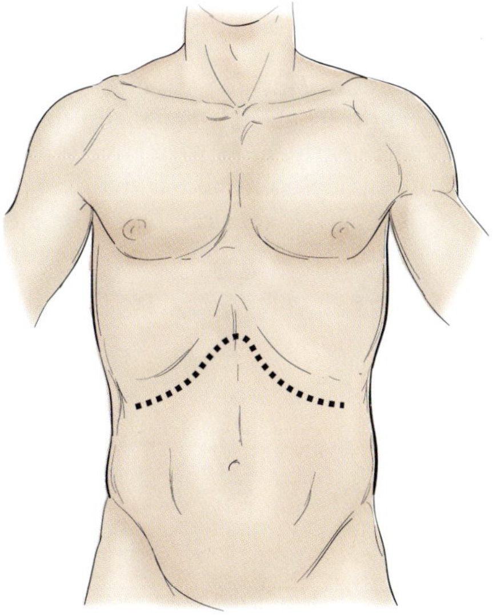

Figure 72-4.

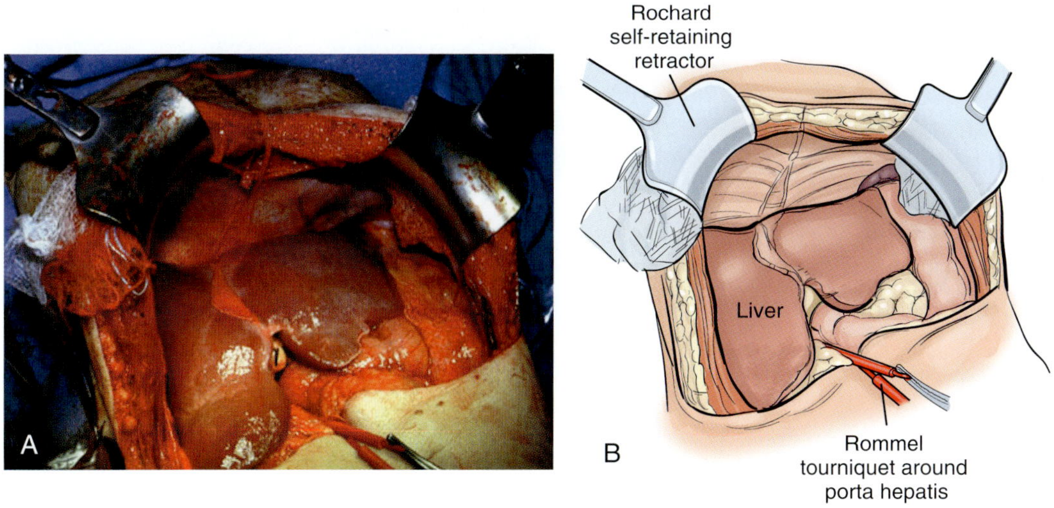

Figure 72-5.

Main Dissection

- Adequate exposure of the retrohepatic vena cava is the key to successful removal of the thrombus. To achieve this through an abdominal incision, it is imperative that the liver be well mobilized, and for a level IIIb IIIc, IIId, or IV thrombus, the major hepatic veins must also be visualized. In addition to mobilizing the liver off the vena cava, a plane between the IVC and the posterior abdominal wall is important because it permits circumferential vascular control of the vena cava.
- We do not preoperatively embolize our patients, but do pursue early ligation of the renal artery. The kidney mobilization begins laterally and proceeds posterior to the kidney, paying special attention to the perirenal collateral circulation. This posterior approach encounters fewer venous collaterals than approaching anteriorly. The kidney is mobilized medially until the renal artery is identified and ligated. The collateral circulation almost immediately decompresses, making the rest of the dissection easier and less bloody. Attention is then directed to control of the vena cava and tumor thrombus.
- *Level I:* RCC with a level I tumor thrombus can be resected with minimal IVC dissection (Fig. 72-6). The tumor can be "milked" back into the renal vein and a vascular clamp applied (Fig. 72-7). A cavotomy is performed, and the tumor is extracted. It is prudent to establish control of the left renal vein as well as the proximal and distal IVC in case of vascular invasion necessitating partial vena caval resection.
- *Level II:* Complete IVC obstruction may be present with this type of tumor thrombus extension (Fig. 72-8). As in level I, the IVC is dissected proximally and distally, including the left renal vein. For better proximal control, the liver may need to be dissected off the IVC. This maneuver is described in detail later for levels III and IV tumor extension. Once vascular control is achieved, the IVC can be clamped partially or totally (Fig. 72-9). The cava is opened along its anterolateral aspect, and the tumor thrombus is removed. If the IVC has been completely clamped, the vascular clamps can be repositioned to allow blood return from the distal IVC and the opposite renal vein. A Pringle maneuver is never needed for this level of tumor.
- *Level III:* Liver mobilization begins with division of the ligamentum teres and taking down the falciform ligament superiorly until the suprahepatic IVC is visualized entering the diaphragm. The left triangular ligament is then incised to meet the previous incision in the falciform ligament. Mobilization continues by incising the visceral peritoneum below the inferior edge of the right lobe. This area may have numerous collaterals, and thus it is advisable to ligate and divide all the tissue in this plane. The liver is gently and progressively rotated to the left, tenting the right superior coronary ligament. Incising this ligament allows the liver to be further rotated toward the midline, gradually exposing the retrohepatic vena cava. Once the direct branches from the caudate lobe to the IVC are ligated, the retrohepatic IVC is completely exposed, and any further dissection depends on where the thrombus ends

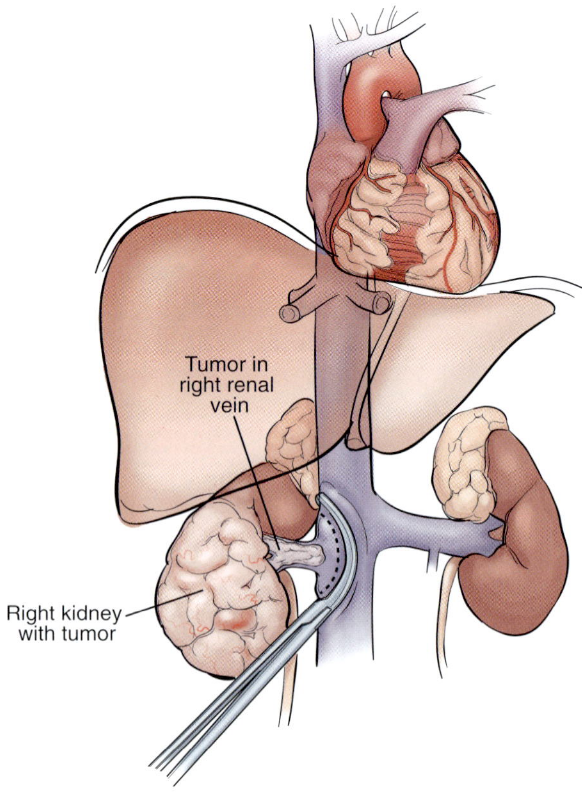

Figure 72-6.

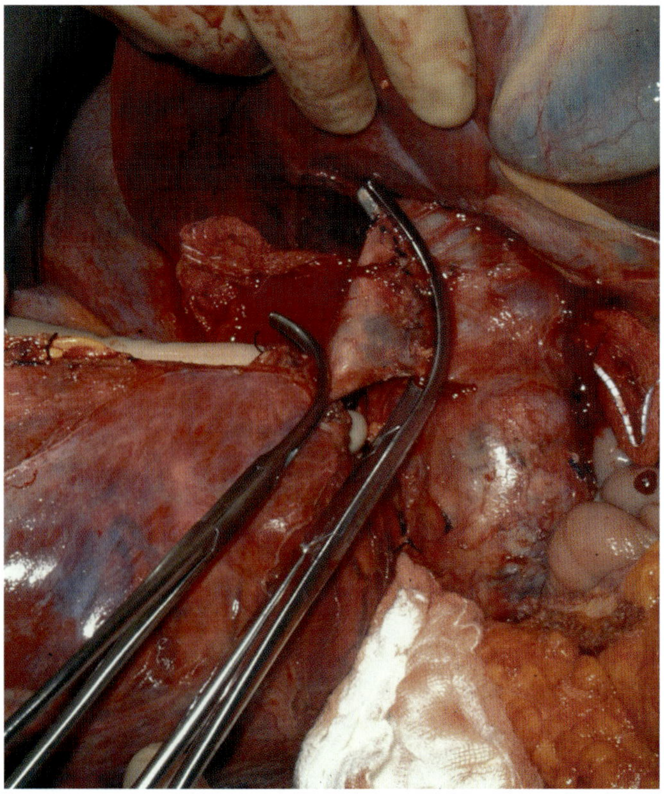

Figure 72-7.

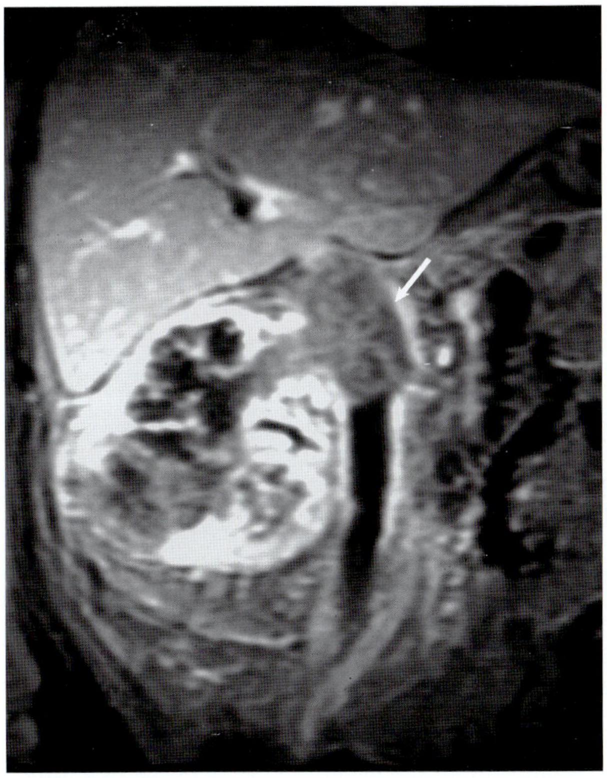

Figure 72-8. Magnetic resonance imaging demonstrating right kidney tumor and level II tumor thrombus with complete obstruction of the inferior vena cava (*white arrow*).

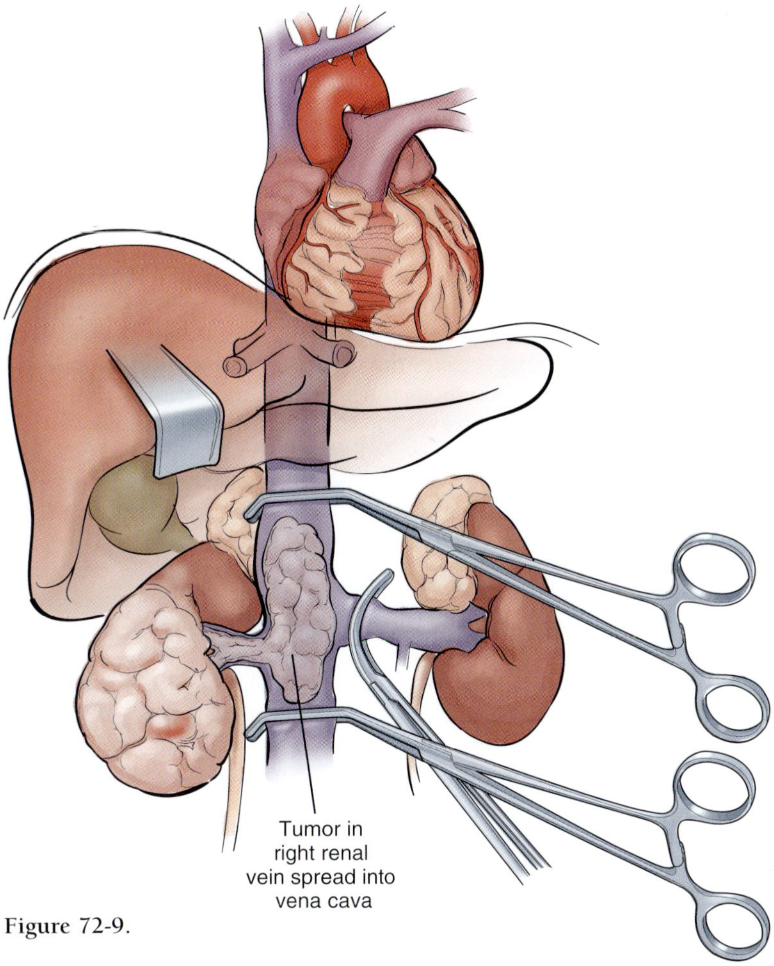

Figure 72-9.

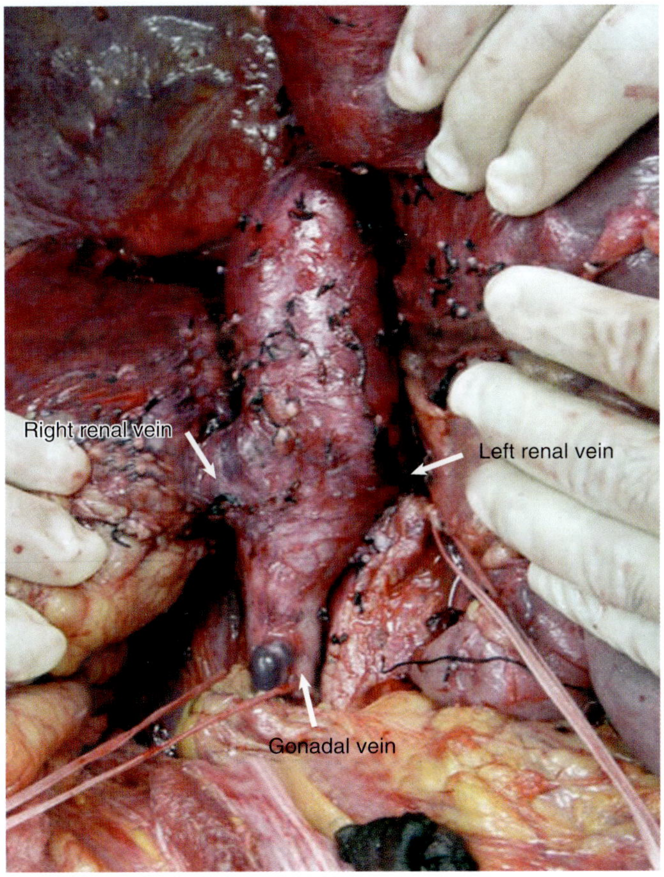

Figure 72-10.

(Fig. 72-10). In the case of a left-sided renal tumor with complete obstruction of the IVC, the right adrenal vein is ligated. In the case of partial obstruction of the IVC, the right adrenal vein is temporarily clamped during the resection of the tumor thrombus.

- *Level IIIa:* The preceding dissection is adequate for the proper placement of vascular clamps cranial to the thrombus and below the hepatic veins. After appropriate vascular isolation of the IVC is achieved, the thrombus is extracted and the IVC is closed.
- *Level IIIb:* Additional dissection is warranted because the major hepatic veins need to be visualized completely. The liver is further dissected off the IVC until it lies in a "piggyback" fashion, attached to the IVC only by the major hepatic veins. In addition, a plane is created between the IVC and the posterior abdominal wall to separate the IVC from it. This entails careful ligation of the lumbar veins that usually tether it posteriorly. It is important to appreciate the technical difficulty of this maneuver: one is essentially trying to mobilize an IVC with little or no intraluminal blood flow but many collaterals. Small tributaries can become engorged to look like lumbar vessels, and they need to be identified and ligated. Sometimes there can be an adventitial reaction that obliterates natural planes of dissection between the IVC and the posterior abdominal wall. The advantage in creating this plane is to facilitate circumferential vascular control of the IVC. This becomes particularly important if the thrombus is adherent to the caval wall, necessitating excision and graft placement. The additional mobility of the IVC also allows rotation of the liver under the IVC, enabling visualization of the hepatic ostia end-on for any potential extension of thrombus. Vascular isolation of the IVC is then achieved superior and inferior to the thrombus, as well as on the contralateral renal vein. It is advantageous to isolate the major hepatic veins to prevent blood loss from the liver. A useful technique, which we have applied routinely, is to milk the thrombus down below the level of the major hepatic veins, and then apply a vascular clamp just below the major hepatic veins. This serves a dual function. First, it allows the liver to drain into the IVC, avoiding hypotension from decreased venous return. This is especially important in older patients who may not tolerate low blood pressures. Second, by not clamping the major hepatic veins, liver congestion and postoperative hepatic dysfunction are avoided. Caution is warranted while milking the tumor down, particularly when the thrombus is adherent to the wall of the IVC. In such cases it may be safer to use venovenous bypass.
- *Level IIIc:* Thrombus at this level requires the same detailed dissection as for level IIIb. In addition, the IVC has to be dissected free from the posterior abdominal wall up to the hiatus in the diaphragm. This is where a circumferential tourniquet is placed for cranial control of the IVC. The major hepatic veins are in direct view, and the surgeon has the choice of gaining control of them by vascular isolation or with the Pringle maneuver. We routinely use the technique of milking the thrombus down the IVC to below the level of the major hepatic veins, and then clamping the IVC at that level. This maneuver also helps in patients who have Budd-Chiari syndrome. Once the thrombus is milked below the level of the major hepatic veins, the resultant decompression of the congested liver is immediate and entirely intravascular.
- *Level IIId:* At this level, there are a few adjuncts that can be quite useful. Intraoperative TEE is helpful in delineating the cranial extent of the thrombus. The diaphragm is cut in the midline anterior to the IVC. The pericardium is then opened, and the supradiaphragmatic, intrapericardial IVC is approached (Fig. 72-11, *A* and *B*). The principle is much the same as in treating level IIIb or IIIc thrombi—that is, attempts are made to milk down the thrombus into the intraabdominal IVC, below the major hepatic veins (Fig. 72-12). The advantage of freeing the IVC from the posterior abdominal wall is realized at this point. If the IVC were tethered posteriorly, any attempts to milk down the thrombus might exert traction on the wall, resulting in a tear and massive hemorrhage. Moreover, the milking-down process is facilitated by having the surgeon's fingers wrap around the IVC circumferentially (Fig. 72-13, *A*, *B*, and *C*), thereby avoiding the serious complication of tumor embolization. Vascular isolation of the IVC is then achieved at this level, and the thrombus is extracted after cavotomy.

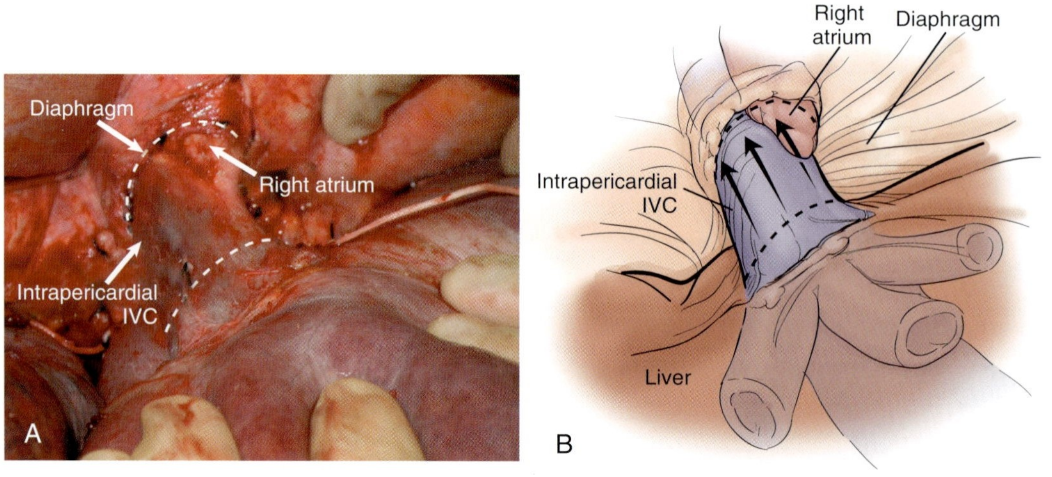

Figure 72-11. *IVC,* Inferior vena cava.

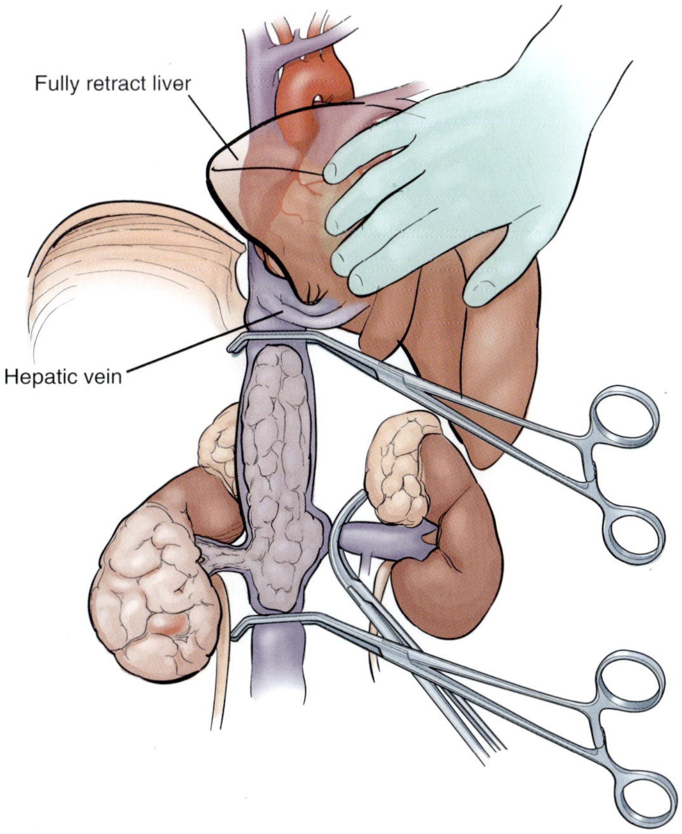

Figure 72-12.

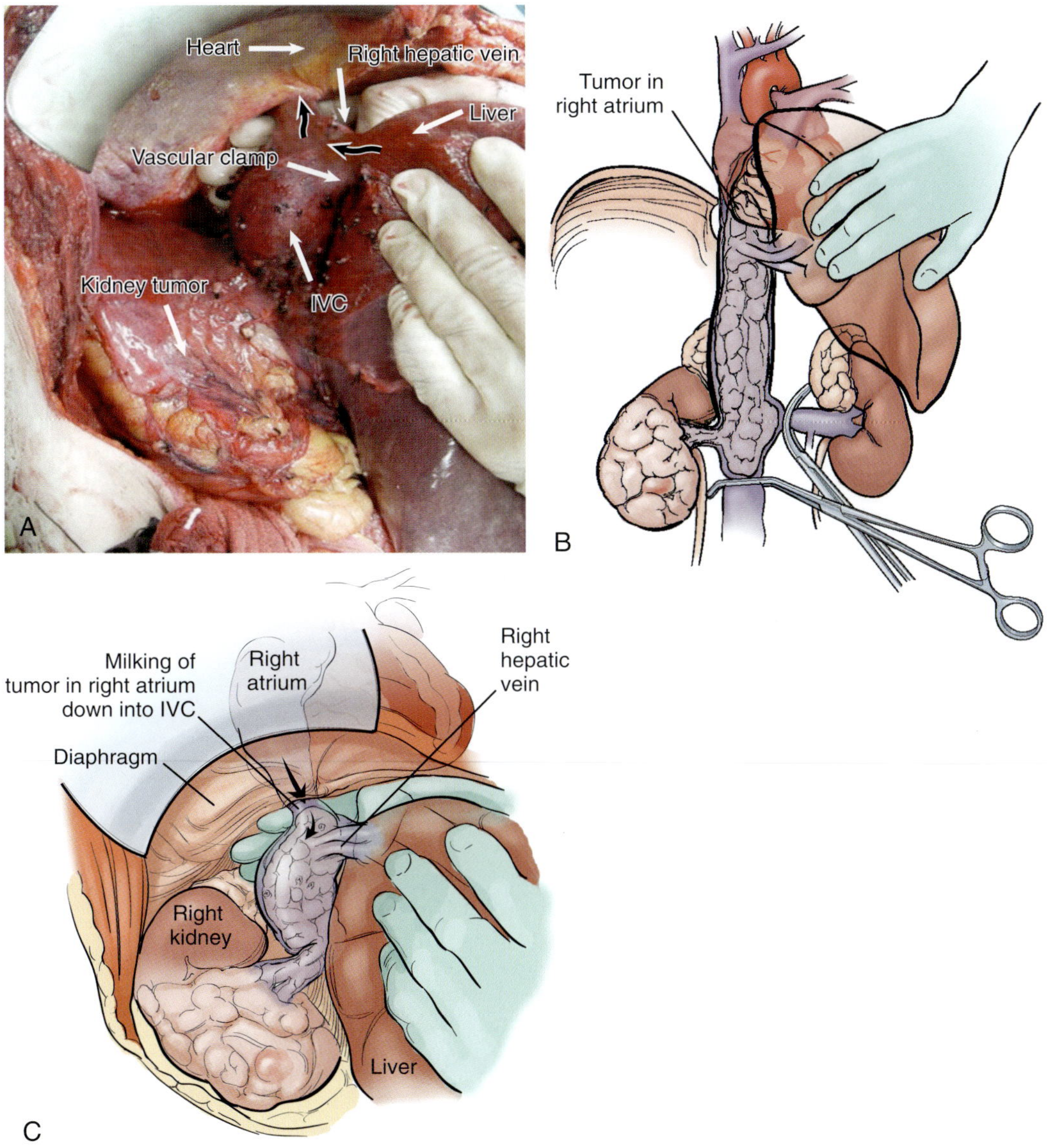

Figure 72-13. *IVC,* Inferior vena cava.

- **Level IV**: The central tendon of the diaphragm is dissected until the supradiaphragmatic, intrapericardial IVC is identified. This dissection is performed circumferentially so that the intrapericardial IVC can be encircled at its confluence with the right atrium. The right atrium is gently pulled beneath the diaphragm (Fig. 72-14). The Pringle maneuver is then performed to temporarily occlude the vascular inflow to the liver. It is recommended to wait before applying the other vascular clamps; this will allow the liver to decompress. The vascular clamps are placed in the following order: (1) the infrarenal vena cava and the left or right vein are controlled; (2) then a Satinsky clamp is placed across the right atrium under TEE monitoring. For a left side tumor, the right adrenal vein is also clamped. The IVC is incised from the diaphragm to the renals, and the tumor is sharply dissected off the atrial wall. The three hepatic veins can be directly visualized, their orifices inspected, and tumor removed if it is invading them. Following removal of the tumor thrombus and closure of the upper cava, the clamp is repositioned below the hepatic veins, the Pringle is released, and normal liver blood flow is reestablished. The remaining open IVC below the hepatic veins is oversewn. This approach can avoid sternotomy and cardiopulmonary bypass (CPB) with deep hypothermic circulatory arrest.

III. ALTERNATIVE TECHNICAL APPROACHES (PRO/CON) AND PEARLS

- CPB may be required in patients with a bulky intraatrial thrombus. However, those with a minimal, nonadherent atrial thrombus or level III tumor extension may not require CPB.
- Thoracoabdominal incision or median sternotomy provides adequate exposure and vascular control, and this also facilitates the use of CPB if needed. Although these approaches can occasionally be useful, postoperative coagulopathy and neurologic sequelae from CPB and deep hypothermic circulatory arrest can occur.
- Usually the tumor is not adherent to the wall of the IVC and can be extracted without damaging or resecting the IVC. In situations where this is not possible, the IVC can be resected en bloc with tumor (Fig. 72-15) and the proximal IVC is sutured (Fig. 72-16).
- The single most important indication for a venovenous bypass is if the patient does not tolerate cross-clamping of the IVC. Other indications include adventitial reaction around the IVC that hampers circumferential dissection, or when the vena cava requires resection and placement of a graft.
- We believe that our approach can be reproduced safely by a urologist with the help of a general, vascular, or transplant surgeon, as long as the urologist has a basic knowledge of the anatomy of the region and can appreciate the potential risks associated with different parts of the operation.
- This technique allows for removal of tumor adherent to the IVC in a bloodless field. The IVC is sutured, and an IVC graft is not needed (Fig. 72-17, *A* and *B*).
- If there is an injury to a major hepatic vein early in the surgery, CPB should be instituted.

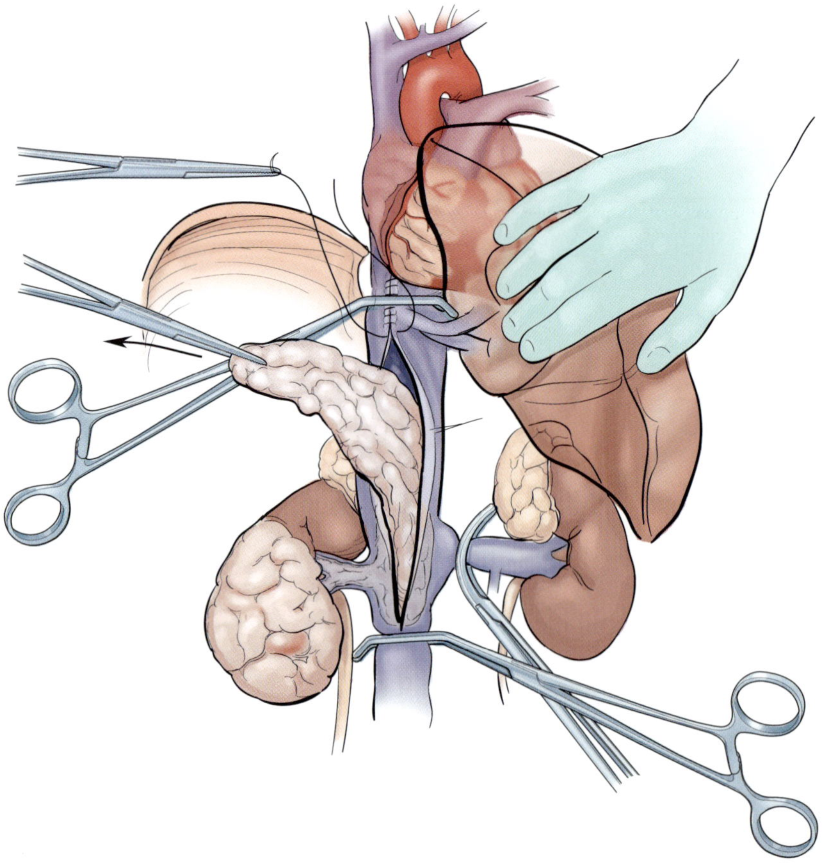

Figure 72-14.

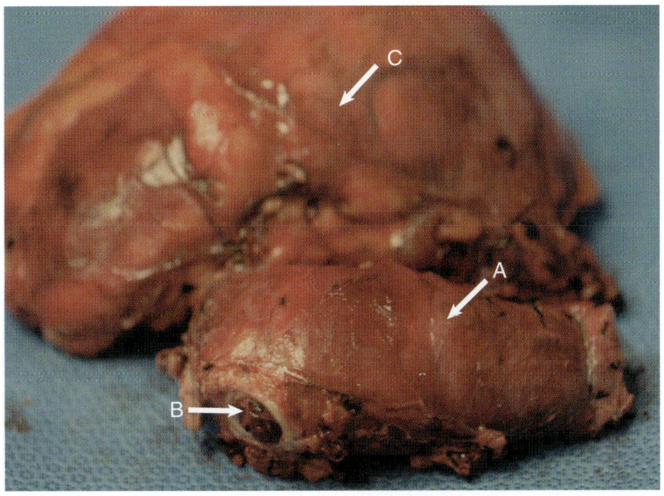

Figure 72-15. Surgical specimen includes en bloc resection of the inferior vena cava (*A*), tumor thrombus (*B*), and kidney tumor (*C*).

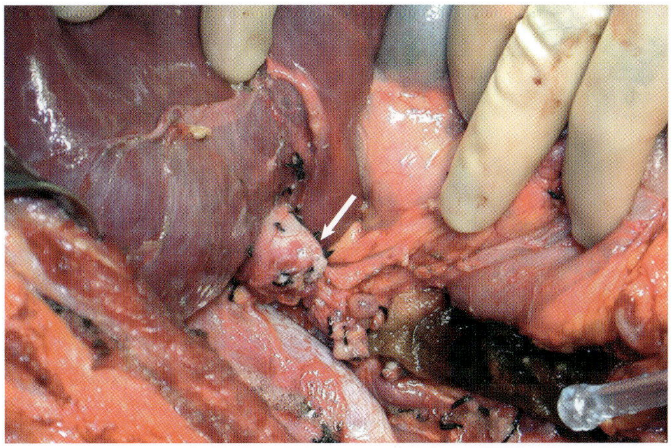

Figure 72-16. The proximal inferior vena cava below the liver was sutured (*arrow*) after en bloc resection of the renal tumor, inferior vena cava, and tumor thrombus. There was no need for inferior vena cava reconstruction.

Figure 72-17.

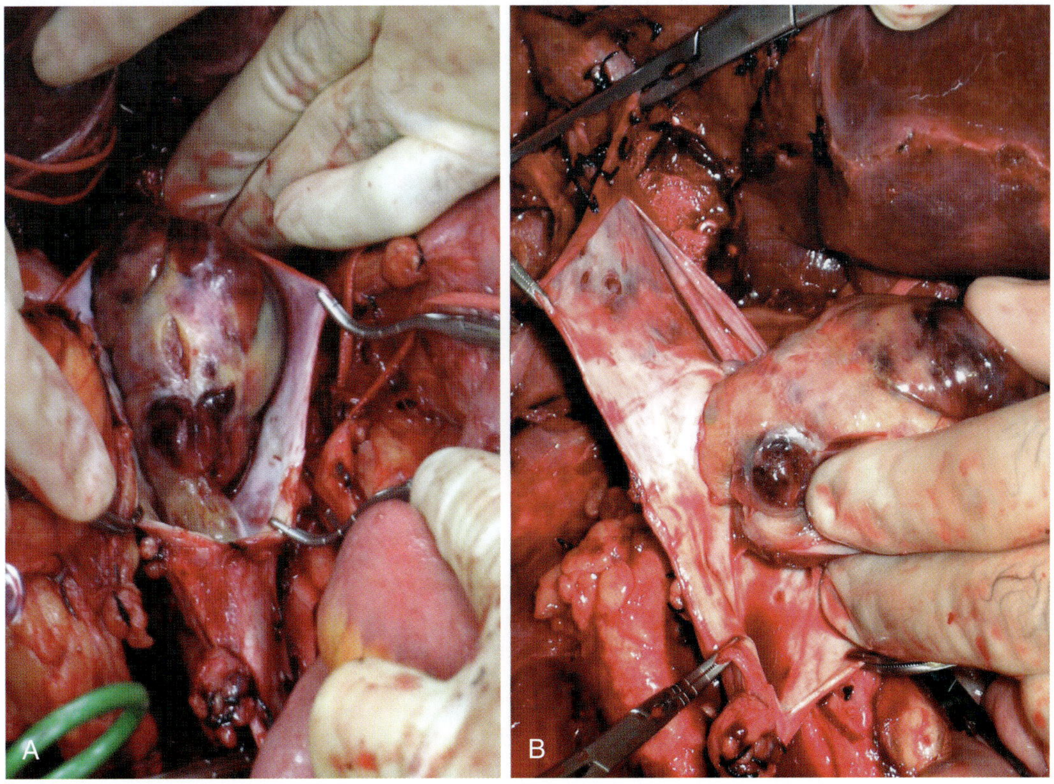

IV. SPECIAL POSTOPERATIVE CARE

- The main intraoperative goal is to prevent pulmonary embolism of the tumor thrombus. CPB should be available.
- The immediate postoperative complication is bleeding. Careful hemostasis is the key before closing the abdominal wall.
- Intravenous heparin is not needed to avoid thrombosis of the vena cava. In situations where the intima of the vena cava is stripped (see Fig. 72-17, *B*), low–molecular-weight dextran is administered for 2 days followed by daily aspirin (325 mg) orally.

SUGGESTED READINGS

Ciancio G, Hawke C, Soloway M: The use of liver transplant techniques to aid in the surgical management of urological tumors, *J Urol* 164:665–672, 2000.

Ciancio G, Soloway M: Resection of the abdominal inferior vena cava for complicated renal cell carcinoma with tumor thrombus, *BJU Int* 92:488–489, 2003.

Ciancio G, Vaidya A, Savoie M, et al: Management of renal cell carcinoma with level III thrombus in the inferior vena cava, *J Urol* 168:1374–1377, 2002.

CHAPTER 73

Radical Cystectomy

John P. Stein, MD, FACS, and Donald G. Skinner, MD, FACS

I. SPECIAL PREOPERATIVE PREPARATION

- Clinical staging for patients requiring cystectomy for bladder cancer should evaluate the retroperitoneum and pelvis along with common metastatic sites including the lungs, liver, and bones. A chest radiograph, liver function tests, and serum alkaline phosphatase should be obtained routinely. A computed tomography (CT) scan of the chest is obtained when pulmonary metastases are suspected by history or because of an abnormal chest radiograph. A CT scan of the abdomen and pelvis is routinely performed to evaluate the pelvis and retroperitoneum for any significant lymphadenopathy or local contiguous spread.
- All patients receive a mechanical and antibacterial bowel preparation the day before surgery. Intravenous hydration must be considered in these patients to prevent dehydration on arrival in the operating room. In addition, all patients should be evaluated and counseled by the enterostomal therapy nurse before surgery. A clear liquid diet may be consumed until midnight, at which time the patient takes nothing by mouth. A standard modified Nichols bowel prep is initiated the morning of admission: 120 mL of Neoloid orally at 9:00 AM; 1 g of neomycin orally at 10:00 AM, 11:00 AM, 12:00 PM, 1:00 PM, 4:00 PM, 8:00 PM, and 12:00 AM; and 1 g of erythromycin base orally at 12:00 PM, 4:00 PM, 8:00 PM, and 12:00 AM.
- Preoperative evaluation and counseling by the enterostomal therapy nurse is a critical component of the care of all patients undergoing cystectomy and urinary diversion. Patients determined to be appropriate candidates for orthotopic reconstruction are instructed in how to catheterize per urethra should it be necessary postoperatively. All patients are site marked for a cutaneous stoma, instructed in the care of a cutaneous diversion (continent or incontinent form), and instructed in proper catheterization techniques should medical, technical or oncologic factors preclude orthotopic reconstruction. The ideal cutaneous stoma site is determined only after the patient is examined in the supine, sitting, and standing positions. Proper stoma site selection is important to patient acceptance and to the technical success of lower urinary tract reconstruction should a cutaneous form of diversion be necessary. Incontinent stoma sites are best located higher on the abdominal wall, whereas stoma sites for continent diversions can be positioned lower on the abdomen (hidden below the belt line) because they do not require an external collecting device.

II. OPERATIVE TECHNIQUE

Position

- The patient is placed in the hyperextended supine position with the superior iliac crest located at the fulcrum of the operating table (Fig. 73-1, *A*). The legs are slightly abducted so that the heels are positioned near the corners of the foot of the table. In women considering orthotopic diversion, the modified frog leg or lithotomy position is employed, allowing access to the vagina. Care should be taken to ensure that all pressure points are well padded. Reverse Trendelenburg position levels the abdomen parallel with the floor and helps to keep the small bowel contents in the epigastrium. In the female patient, the vagina is also fully prepped. After the patient is draped, a 20-Fr Foley catheter is placed in the bladder and left to gravity drainage. A right-handed surgeon stands at the patient's left side.

Incision

- A vertical midline incision is made extending from the pubic symphysis to the cephalad aspect of the epigastrium (see Fig. 73-1, *B*). The incision should proceed lateral to the umbilicus on the contralateral side of the marked cutaneous stoma site. When the umbilicus is being considered as the site for a catheterizable stoma, the incision should be directed 2 to 3 cm lateral to the umbilicus at this location. The anterior rectus fascia is incised, the rectus muscles retracted laterally, and the posterior rectus sheath and peritoneum entered in the superior aspect of the incision. As the peritoneum and posterior fascia are incised inferiorly at the level of the umbilicus, the urachal remnant (median umbilical ligament) is identified, circumscribed, and removed en bloc with the cystectomy specimen (Fig. 73-2). This maneuver prevents early entry into a high-riding bladder and ensures complete removal of all bladder remnant tissue.

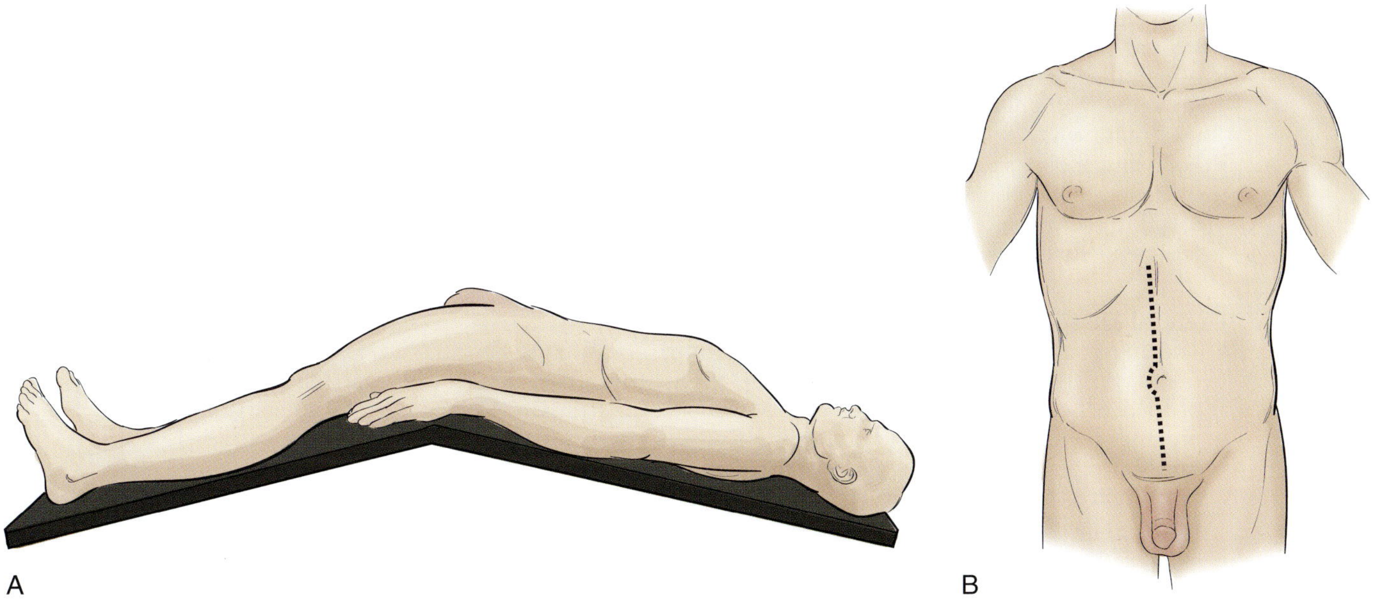

Figure 73-1.

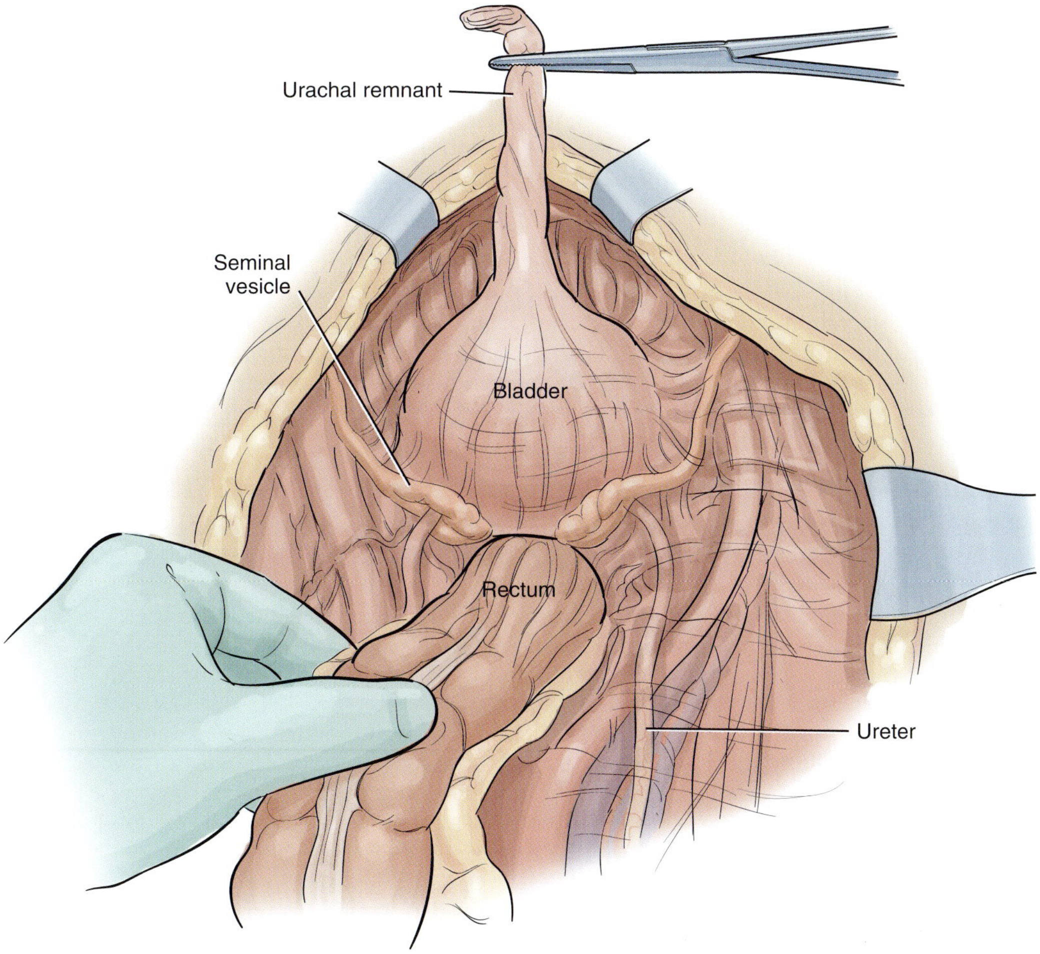

Figure 73-2.

Main Dissection

Bowel Mobilization

- The bowel is mobilized beginning with the ascending colon. A large right-angle Richardson retractor elevates the right abdominal wall. The cecum and ascending colon are reflected medially to allow incision of the lateral peritoneal reflection along the avascular/white line of Toldt. The mesentery to the small bowel is then mobilized off its retroperitoneal attachments cephalad (toward the ligament of Treitz) until the retroperitoneal portion of the duodenum is exposed. This mobilization facilitates a tension-free urethroenteric anastomosis if orthotopic diversion is performed. Conceptually, the mobilized mesentery forms an inverted right triangle: the base formed by the third and fourth portions of the duodenum, the right edge represented by the white line of Toldt along the ascending colon, the left edge represented by the medial portion of the sigmoid and descending colonic mesentery, and the apex represented by the ileocecal region (Fig. 73-3).
- The left colon and sigmoid mesentery are then mobilized to the region of the lower pole of the left kidney by incising the peritoneum lateral to the colon along the avascular/white line of Toldt. The sigmoid mesentery is then elevated off the sacrum, iliac vessels, and distal aorta in a cephalad direction up to the origin of the inferior mesenteric artery (IMA) (see Fig. 73-3). This maneuver provides a wide mesenteric window through which the left ureter will pass without angulation or tension.
- Following mobilization of the bowel, a self-retaining retractor is placed. The right colon and small intestine are carefully packed into the epigastrium with three moist lap pads, followed by a moistened towel rolled to the width of the abdomen. The descending and sigmoid colon are not packed and remain as free as possible, providing the mobility required for the ureteral and pelvic lymph node dissection.

Ureteral Dissection

- The ureters are most easily identified in the retroperitoneum just cephalad to the common iliac vessels. They are carefully dissected into the deep pelvis (several centimeters beyond the iliac vessels) and divided between two large hemoclips. A section of the proximal cut ureteral segment (distal to the proximal hemoclip) is sent for frozen section analysis to ensure the absence of carcinoma in situ or overt tumor. The ureter is then slightly mobilized in a cephalad direction and tucked under the rolled towel to prevent inadvertent injury. The rich vascular supply emanating laterally from the gonadal vessels should remain intact and undisturbed. These attachments are an important blood supply to the ureter and ensure an adequate vascular supply for the ureteroenteric anastomosis at the time of diversion. In women, the infundibulopelvic ligaments are ligated and divided at the level of the common iliac vessels.
- Leaving the proximal hemoclip on the divided ureter during the exenteration allows for hydrostatic ureteral dilation and facilitates the ureteroenteric anastomosis.

Lower Retroperitoneal and Pelvic-Iliac Lymphadenectomy

- For a combined lower retroperitoneal and pelvic-iliac lymphadenectomy, the lymph node dissection is initiated at the IMA (superior limits of dissection) and extends laterally over the inferior vena cava to the genitofemoral nerve, representing the lateral limits of dissection. Distally, the lymph node dissection extends to the lymph node of Cloquet medially (on the Cooper ligament) and the circumflex iliac vein laterally.
- The cephalad portion (at the level of the IMA) of the lymphatics is ligated with hemoclips to prevent lymphatic leak, whereas the caudal (specimen) side is ligated only when a blood vessel is encountered.
- All fibroareolar and lymphatic tissues are dissected caudally off the aorta, the vena cava, and then the common iliac vessels over the sacral promontory into the deep pelvis. The initial dissection along the common iliac vessels is performed over the arteries, skeletonizing them. As the common iliac veins are dissected medially, care is taken to control small arterial and venous branches coursing along the anterior surface of the sacrum. Electrocautery is helpful at this location and allows the adherent fibroareolar tissue to be swept off the sacral promontory down into the deep pelvis with the use of a small gauze sponge.
- Once the proximal portion of the lymph node dissection is completed, a finger is passed from the proximal aspect of dissection under the pelvic peritoneum (anterior to the iliac vessels), distally toward the femoral canal. The opposite hand can be used to strip the peritoneum from the undersurface of the transversalis fascia and connect with the proximal dissection from above. This maneuver elevates the peritoneum and defines the lateral limit of peritoneum to be incised and removed with the specimen. In men, the peritoneum is divided medial to the spermatic vessels; in women, lateral to the infundibulopelvic ligament. The only structure encountered is the vas deferens in the male or round ligament in the female; these structures are clipped and divided.
- A large right-angled rake retractor (e.g., Israel) is used to elevate the lower abdominal wall, including the spermatic cord or remnant of the round ligament, to provide distal exposure in the area of the femoral canal. Tension on the retractor is directed vertically toward the ceiling, with care taken to avoid injury to the inferior epigastric vessels. The distal limits of the dissection are then identified: the circumflex iliac vein crossing anterior to the external iliac artery distally, the genitofemoral nerve laterally, and the Cooper ligament medially.

- The lymphatics draining the ipsilateral leg, particularly medial to the external iliac vein, are carefully clipped and divided to prevent lymphatic leakage. This includes the lymph node of Cloquet, which represents the distal limit of the lymphatic dissection at this location.
- The distal external iliac artery and vein are then circumferentially dissected and skeletonized, with care taken to ligate an accessory obturator vein (present in 40% of patients) originating from the inferomedial aspect of the external iliac vein. Following completion of the distal limits of dissection, the proximal and distal dissections are joined. The proximal external iliac artery and vein are skeletonized circumferentially to the origin of the hypogastric artery (Fig. 73-4).
- At this point, the lymphatic tissue surrounding the iliac vessels is composed of a medial and lateral component attached only at the base within the obturator fossa. The lateral lymphatic compartment (freed medially from the vessels and laterally from the psoas) is bluntly swept into the obturator fossa

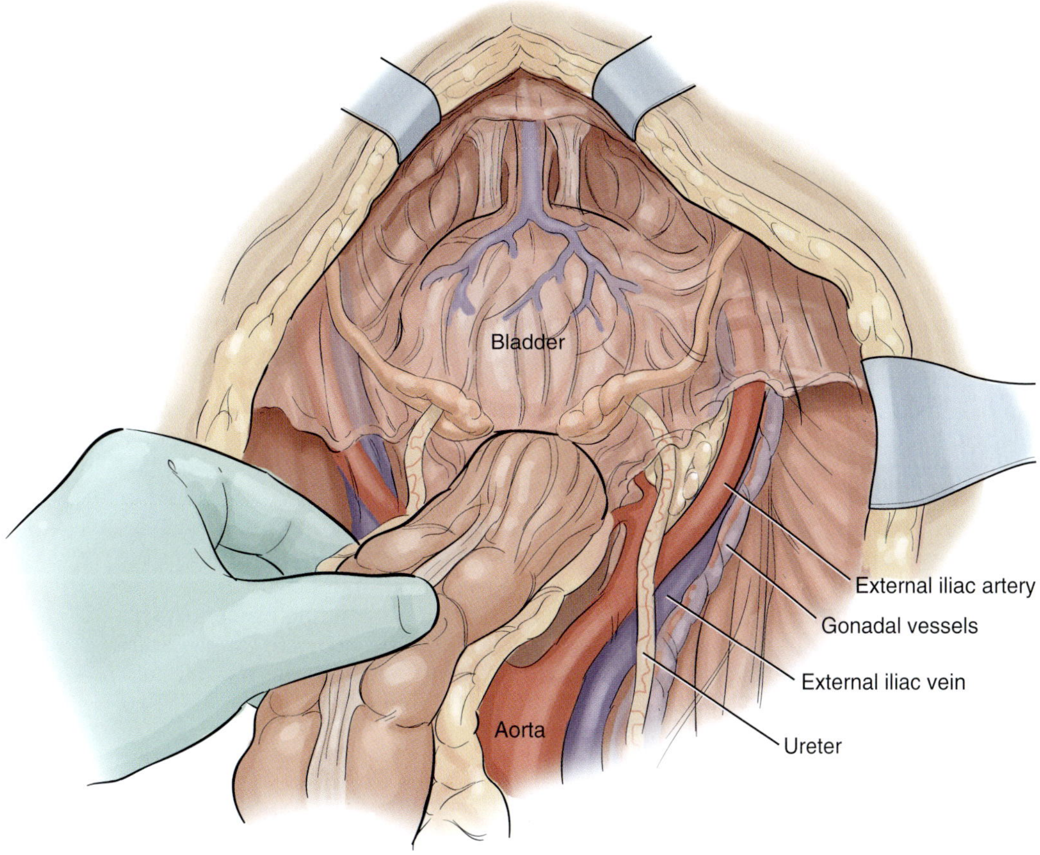

Figure 73-3.

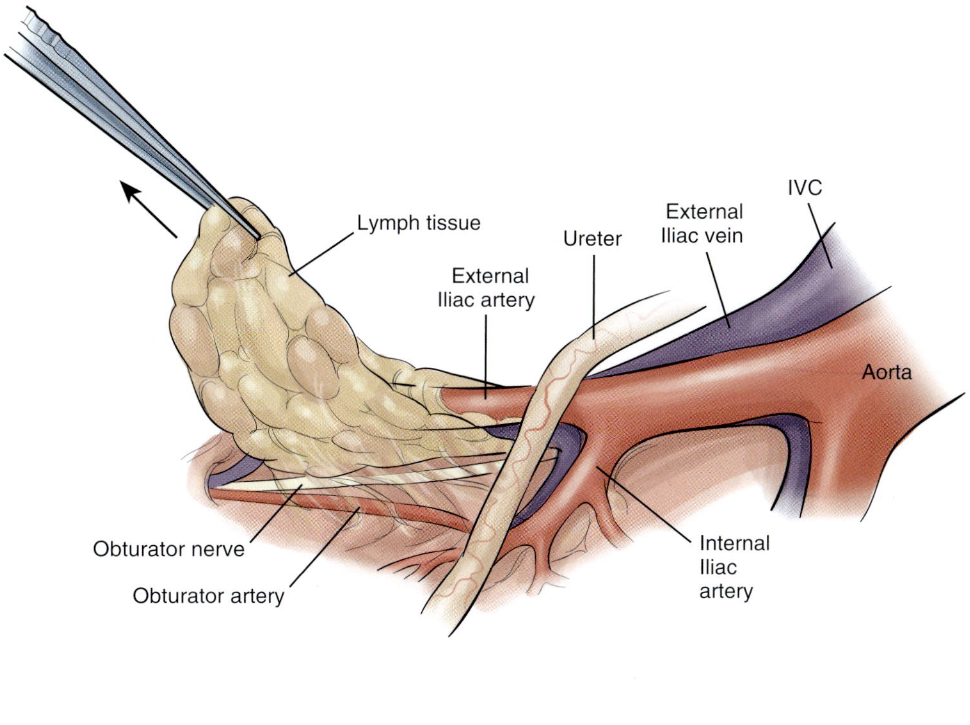

Figure 73-4. *IVC,* Inferior vena cava.

by retracting the iliac vessels medially and passing a small gauze sponge lateral to the vessels along the psoas and pelvic sidewall (see Fig. 73-4).

- This sponge should be passed anterior and distal to the hypogastric vein, directed caudally into the obturator fossa. The external iliac vessels are then elevated and retracted laterally, and the gauze sponge is carefully withdrawn from the obturator fossa with gentle traction using the left hand.
- This maneuver effectively sweeps all lymphatic tissue into the obturator fossa and facilitates identification of the obturator nerve deep to the external iliac vein. The obturator nerve is best identified proximally and carefully dissected free from all lymphatics. The obturator nerve is then retracted laterally along with the iliac vessels.
- At this point, the obturator artery and vein should be carefully entrapped between the index finger (medial to the obturator nerve) laterally and the middle finger medially with the left hand. This isolates the obturator vessels exiting the obturator canal along the pelvic floor, which are then carefully clipped and divided, taking care to stay medial to the obturator nerve.
- The obturator lymph node packet is then swept medially toward the sidewall of the bladder, ligating small tributary vessels and lymphatics from the pelvic sidewall. The nodal packet will be removed.

Ligation of the Lateral Vascular Pedicle to the Bladder

- Following dissection of the obturator fossa and dividing the obturator vessels, the lateral vascular pedicle to the bladder is isolated and divided. Developing this plane isolates the lateral vascular pedicle to the bladder, a critical maneuver in performing a safe cystectomy with proper vascular control. Isolation of the lateral vascular pedicle is performed with the left hand. The bladder is retracted toward the pelvis, placing traction and isolating the anterior branches of the hypogastric artery. The left index finger is passed medial to the hypogastric artery, posterior to the anterior visceral branches, and lateral to the previously transected ureter. The index finger is directed caudally toward the endopelvic fascia, parallel to the sweep of the sacrum. This maneuver defines the two major vascular pedicles to the anterior pelvic organs: the lateral pedicle—anterior to the index finger, composed of the visceral branches of the anterior hypogastric vessel; and the posterior pedicle—posterior to the index finger, composed of the visceral branches between the bladder and rectum.
- With the lateral pedicle entrapped between the left index and middle fingers, firm traction is applied vertically and caudally. The largest and most consistent anterior branch to the bladder, the superior vesical artery, is usually isolated and individually ligated and divided easily. Alternatively, these pedicles can be divided with endovascular linear staplers (Fig. 73-5). The remaining anterior branches of the lateral pedicle are then isolated and divided between hemoclips down to the endopelvic fascia, or as far as is technically possible. With blunt dissection, the index finger of the left hand helps identify this lateral pedicle and protects the rectum as it is pushed medially. Right-angle hemoclip appliers are ideally suited for proper placement of the clips. The endopelvic fascia just lateral to the prostate may then be incised, which helps identify the distal limit of the lateral pedicle.

Ligation of the Posterior Pedicle to the Bladder

- Following division of the lateral pedicles, the bladder specimen is retracted anteriorly, exposing the cul-de-sac (pouch of Douglas). The surgeon elevates the bladder with a small gauze sponge under the left hand, while the assistant retracts on the peritoneum of the rectosigmoid colon cephalad. This provides excellent exposure to the recess of the cul-de-sac and places the peritoneal reflection on traction, facilitating the proper division. The peritoneum lateral to the rectum is incised, and the incision is extended anteriorly and medially across the cul-de-sac to join the incision on the contralateral side. The peritoneal incision in the cul-de-sac must be made slightly on the rectal side rather than the bladder side.
- Employing a posterior sweeping motion of the fingers, the rectum can be carefully swept off of the Denonvilliers fascia (with the seminal vesicles, prostate, and bladder anteriorly in men) and off of the posterior vaginal wall in women. This sweeping motion, when extended laterally, helps to thin and develop the posterior pedicles, which appear like a collar emanating from the lateral aspect of the rectum.
- Once the posterior pedicles have been defined, they are clipped and divided to the endopelvic fascia in the male patient. The endopelvic fascia is then incised adjacent to the prostate, medial to the levator ani muscles (if not done previously), to facilitate the apical dissection.
- In the female patient, the posterior pedicles including the cardinal ligaments are divided 4 to 5 cm beyond the cervix. With cephalad pressure on a previously placed vaginal sponge stick, the apex of the vagina can be identified and incised posteriorly just distal to the cervix. The vagina is then circumscribed anteriorly with the cervix attached to the cystectomy specimen. If concern exists regarding an adequate surgical margin at the posterior or base of the bladder, then the anterior vaginal wall should be removed en bloc with the bladder specimen, subsequently requiring vaginal reconstruction if sexual function is desired.
- The anterior vaginal wall is then sharply dissected off the posterior bladder down to the region of the bladder neck (vesicourethral junction), which is identified by palpating the Foley catheter balloon. At this point, the specimen remains attached only at the apex in men and at the vesicourethral junction in women.

Anterior Apical Dissection in the Male Patient

- Once the cystectomy specimen is completely freed posteriorly, attention is then directed anteriorly to the pelvic floor and urethra. All fibroareolar connections between the anterior bladder wall, prostate, and undersurface of the pubic symphysis are divided. The endopelvic fascia is incised adjacent to the prostate, and the levator muscles are carefully swept off the lateral and apical portions of the prostate. The superficial dorsal vein is identified, ligated, and divided.
- The puboprostatic ligaments are identified and only slightly divided just beneath the pubis, lateral to the dorsal venous complex that courses between these ligaments. Care should be taken to avoid any extensive dissection in this region along the pelvic floor. The puboprostatic ligaments need only be incised enough to allow for a proper apical dissection of the prostate.
- Several methods can be performed to control the dorsal venous plexus. We prefer to gather the dorsal venous complex at the apex of the prostate with a long Allis clamp (Fig. 73-6). This may help better

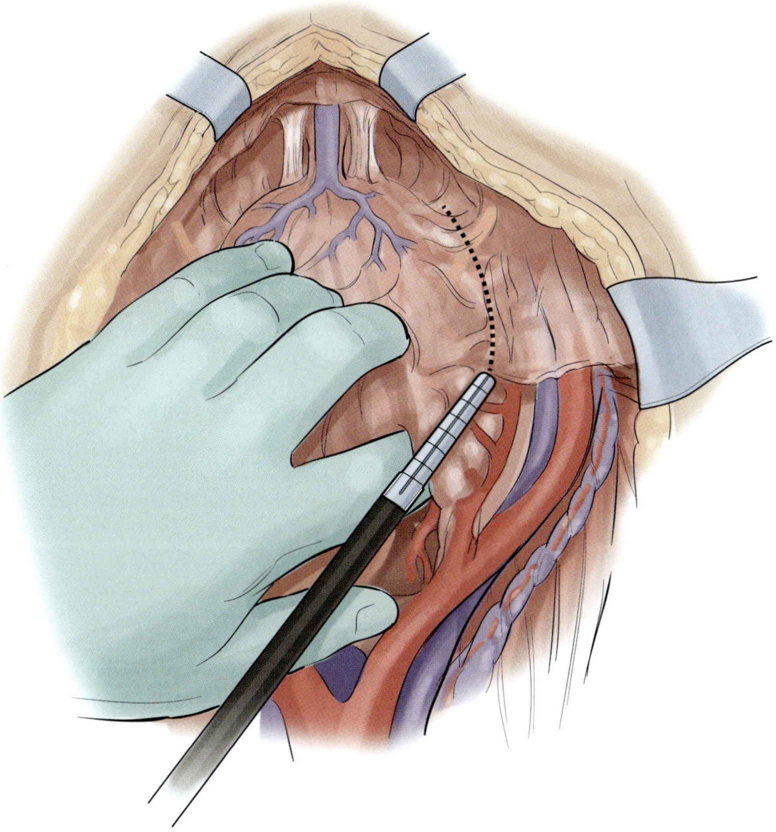

Figure 73-5.

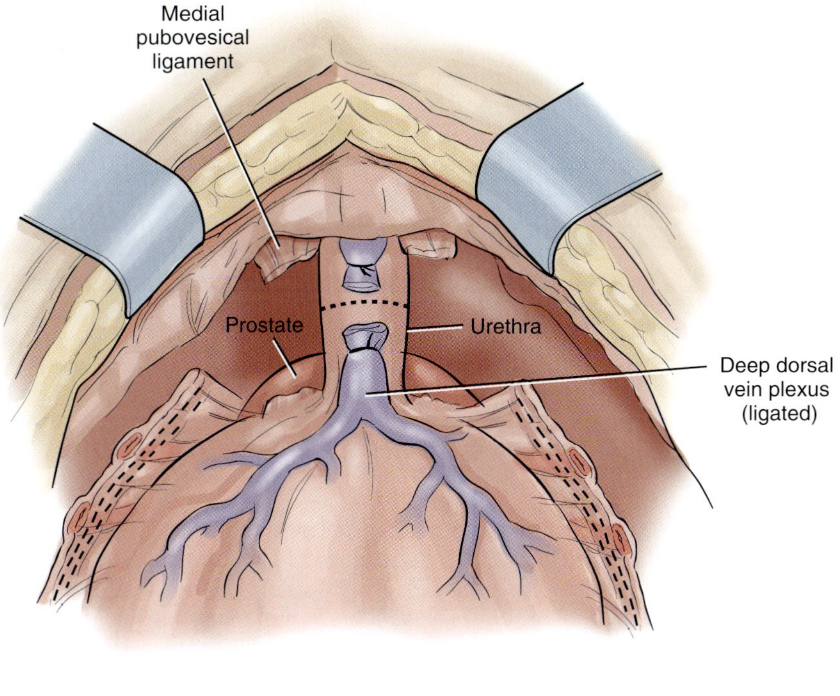

Figure 73-6.

define the plane between the dorsal venous complex and the anterior urethra. A figure-of-eight 2-0 absorbable suture can then be carefully placed under direct vision anterior to the urethra (distal to the apex of the prostate) around the gathered venous complex. This suture is best placed with the surgeon facing the head of the table and holding the needle driver perpendicular to the patient. The suture is then tagged with a hemostat.

- After the complex has been ligated, it can be sharply divided with excellent exposure to the anterior surface of the urethra. Once the venous complex has been severed, the suture can be used to further secure the complex. The suture is then used to suspend the venous complex anteriorly to the periosteum to help reestablish anterior fixation of the dorsal venous complex and puboprostatic ligaments, which may enhance continence recovery.
- The urethra is then incised 270 degrees just beyond the apex of the prostate (see Fig. 73-6). Six 2-0 polyglycolic acid sutures are placed in the anterior urethra, carefully incorporating only the mucosa and submucosa of the striated urethral sphincter muscle anteriorly. Following this, two posterior urethral sutures are placed. The posterior urethra can then be divided and the specimen removed after dividing the Foley catheter between clamps to prevent spillage of any bladder contents.
- If a patient is considering an orthotopic diversion, frozen section analysis of the distal urethral margin of the cystectomy specimen is then performed to exclude tumor involvement.

Anterior Dissection in the Female

- When developing the posterior pedicles in women, the posterior vagina is incised at the apex just distal to the cervix. This incision is continued anteriorly along the lateral and anterior vaginal wall, forming a circumferential incision. The anterolateral vaginal wall is then grasped with curved Kocher clamps.
- Careful dissection of the proper plane will prevent entry into the posterior bladder and also reduce the amount of bleeding in this vascular area. Development of this posterior plane and vascular pedicle is best performed sharply and continued just distal to the vesicourethral junction. Palpation of the Foley catheter balloon assists in identifying this region. This dissection effectively maintains a functional vagina.
- In the case of a deeply invasive posterior bladder tumor in a woman, with concern for an adequate surgical margin, the anterior vaginal wall should be removed en bloc with the cystectomy specimen. After dividing the posterior vaginal apex, the lateral vaginal wall subsequently serves as the posterior pedicle and is divided distally. This leaves the anterior vaginal wall attached to the posterior bladder specimen.
- The Foley catheter balloon again facilitates identification of the vesicourethral junction. The surgical plane between the vesicourethral junction and the anterior vaginal wall is then developed distally at this location. A 1-cm length of proximal urethra is mobilized while the remaining distal urethra is left intact with the anterior vaginal wall.
- Vaginal reconstruction by a clamshell (horizontal) or side-to-side (vertical) technique is required. Other means of vaginal reconstruction may include a rectus myocutaneous flap, a detubularized cylinder of ileum, a peritoneal flap, or an omental flap.
- When the posterior dissection is completed (taking care to dissect just distal to the vesicourethral junction), a Satinsky vascular clamp is placed across the bladder neck. The Satinsky vascular clamp placed across the catheter at the bladder neck prevents any tumor spill from the bladder. With gentle traction, the proximal urethra is completely divided anteriorly, distal to the bladder neck and clamp. A total of 10 to 12 sutures are placed.
- The vaginal cuff may be closed in two layers with absorbable sutures. The vaginal cuff is then anchored via a colposacropexy using a strut of Marlex mesh to the sacral promontory. This fixates the vagina without angulation or undue tension.
- In the final parts of the operation, a well-vascularized omental pedicle graft is placed between the reconstructed vagina and neobladder and secured to the levator ani muscles to separate the suture lines and prevent fistulization.
- Following removal of the cystectomy specimen, the pelvis is irrigated with warm sterile water. The presacral nodal tissue previously swept off the common iliac vessels and sacral promontory into the deep pelvis is collected and sent separately for pathologic evaluation. Nodal tissue in the presciatic notch bilaterally, anterior to the sciatic nerve, is also sent for histologic analysis.
- Hemostasis is obtained, and the pelvis is packed with a lap pad while attention is directed to the urinary diversion.
- After the cystectomy is completed, the urinary diversion is performed accordingly (Fig. 73-7).

Closure

- The pelvis is drained for urine or lymph leak with a 1-inch Penrose drain for 3 weeks, and a large suction Hemovac drain is placed for the evacuation of blood for 24 hours.
- A gastrostomy tube with an 18-Fr Foley catheter is routinely placed using a modified Stamm technique, which incorporates a small portion of omentum (near the greater curvature of the stomach) interposed between the stomach and the abdominal wall.

III. ALTERNATIVE TECHNICAL APPROACHES (PRO/CON) AND PEARLS

- An understanding of the fascial layers is critical for the appropriate dissection of the posterior plane and pedicle to the bladder. The anterior and posterior peritoneal reflections converge in the cul-de-sac to form the Denonvilliers fascia, which extends caudally to the urogenital diaphragm. This anatomic boundary in the male separates the prostate and seminal vesicles anteriorly from the rectum posteriorly. The plane between the prostate and seminal vesicles and the anterior sheath of the Denonvilliers will not develop easily. However, the plane between the rectum and the posterior sheath of Denonvilliers (the Denonvilliers space) should develop easily with blunt and sharp dissection. Therefore, the peritoneal incision in the cul-de-sac must be made slightly on the rectal side rather than the bladder side. This allows proper and safe entry and development of the Denonvilliers space between the anterior rectal wall and the posterior sheath of the Denonvilliers fascia. Care should be taken as one develops this posterior plane more caudally, because the anterior rectal fibers reflect anteriorly, often are adherent to the specimen, and can be difficult to bluntly dissect. In this region, just cephalad (proximal) to the urogenital diaphragm, sharp dissection may be required to dissect the anterior rectal fibers off the apex of the prostate to prevent rectal injury at this location.
- There are several situations that may impede the proper development of this posterior plane. Most commonly, when the incision in the cul-de-sac is made too far anteriorly, proper entry into the Denonvilliers space is prevented. Improper entry can occur in between the two layers of the Denonvilliers fascia, or even anterior to this, making the posterior dissection difficult and increasing the risk of rectal injury. Furthermore, posterior tumor infiltration or previous high-dose pelvic irradiation can obliterate this plane, making the posterior dissection difficult. To prevent injury to the rectum in these situations, sharp dissection should be performed under direct vision. It is important to avoid blunt dissection with the finger in areas where normal tissue planes have been obliterated by previous surgery or radiation. Sharp dissection under direct vision will dramatically reduce the potential for rectal injury.
- Several methods can be used to control the dorsal venous plexus. One may carefully pass an angled clamp beneath the dorsal venous complex, anterior to the urethra. The venous complex can then be ligated with an absorbable suture and divided close to the apex of the prostate. If any bleeding occurs from the transected venous complex, it can be oversewn with an absorbable suture.
- Approximately 80% of all patients undergoing cystectomy for transitional cell carcinoma of the bladder are appropriate candidates for an orthotopic neobladder substitute. From an oncologic perspective,

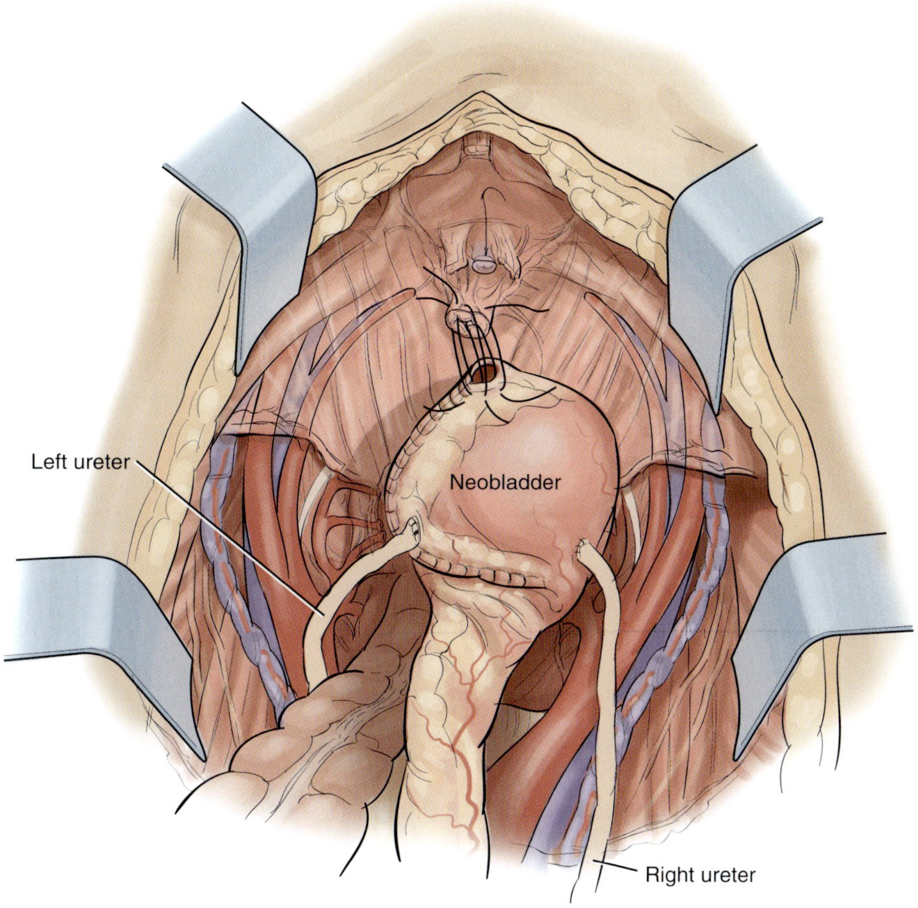

Figure 73-7.

only those patients found to have a positive margin at the proximal urethra (distal to the apex of the prostate in men and just distal to the bladder neck in women) on intraoperative frozen section are absolutely excluded from orthotopic reconstruction. Contraindications to orthotopic urinary diversion include the presence of tumor within the urethra or extending to the urethral margin, as determined by frozen section analysis of the distal surgical margin at the time of cystectomy; compromised renal function (creatinine greater than 2.5 ng/mL); or the presence of inflammatory bowel disease. Even in patients with locally advanced disease, orthotopic diversion can be employed without concern over subsequent tumor-related reservoir complications.

- If the frozen section demonstrates tumor, a cutaneous diversion should be performed as discussed preoperatively.

IV. SPECIAL POSTOPERATIVE CARE

- Patients are best monitored in the surgical intensive care unit for at least 24 hours or until stable. Careful attention to fluid management is imperative, because third-space fluid loss in these patients can be tremendous and deceiving. Patients with compromised cardiac or pulmonary function may require invasive cardiac monitoring with a pulmonary artery catheter placed before surgery to precisely ascertain the cardiac response to fluid shifts. A combination of crystalloid and colloid fluid replacement is given on the night of surgery and converted to crystalloid on postoperative day 1.
- Prophylaxis against stress ulcer is initiated with a histamine receptor (H_2) blocker. Intravenous broad-spectrum antibiotics are continued in all patients and subsequently converted to oral antibiotics as the diet progresses.
- Prophylaxis against deep vein thrombosis is important in patients undergoing extensive pelvic operations for malignancies. The anticoagulation is initiated in the recovery room with 10 mg of sodium warfarin via a nasogastric or the gastrostomy tube. The daily dose is adjusted to maintain a prothrombin time in the range of 18 to 22 seconds. If the prothrombin time exceeds 22 to 25 seconds, 2.5 mg of vitamin K is administered intramuscularly to prevent possible bleeding.
- Pain control by a patient-controlled analgesic system provides comfort and enhances deep breathing and early ambulation.
- The gastrostomy tube is generally removed on postoperative day 7, or later if bowel function is delayed. Management of the catheter and drain is specific to the form of urinary diversion. Some patients may develop a prolonged ileus or some other complication that delays the quick return of oral intake. In such circumstances, it is wise to institute total parenteral nutrition earlier rather than later, or the patient may become farther behind nutritionally.
- Most early complications (85%) following radical cystectomy are unrelated to the urinary diversion and can be managed conservatively. The most common early, diversion-unrelated complication after radical cystectomy is dehydration, whereas the most common early, diversion-related complication is urinary leakage.
- Although we have found that preoperative treatment with chemotherapy and/or radiation therapy does not increase perioperative morbidity or mortality, neoadjuvant treatment strategies have not been routinely employed in our patients before radical cystectomy for invasive bladder cancer.
- Preoperative radiation therapy is considered only in those patients with a history of previous partial cystectomy or those who experienced extravesical tumor spill at the time of endoscopic management of the primary bladder tumor.
- Although there has been recent interest in the application of neoadjuvant chemotherapy in patients with muscle-invasive bladder cancer, its routine administration is clearly a debatable issue. We are strong advocates of postoperative adjuvant chemotherapy when the administration is given to high-risk patients, based on accurate pathologic evaluation of the primary bladder tumor and regional lymph nodes.
- Proper patient selection and strict attention to perioperative details, along with a dedicated and meticulous surgical approach, are all critical to minimizing the morbidity and mortality of surgery and ensuring the best clinical outcomes in patients following radical cystectomy.

SUGGESTED READINGS

Stein JP, Ginsberg DA, Skinner DG: Indications and technique of the orthotopic neobladder in women, *Urol Clin North Am* 29:725–734, 2002.

Stein JP, Quek MD, Skinner DG: Contemporary surgical techniques for continent urinary diversion: continence and potency preservation. In Libertino JA, Zinman LN, editors: *Atlas of the urologic clinics of North America*, Philadelphia, 2001, WB Saunders, pp 147–173.

Stein JP, Skinner DG: Orthotopic bladder replacement. In Walsh PC, Retik AB, Vaughan ED, Wein AJ, editors: *Campbell's urology*, ed 8, Philadelphia, 2002, WB Saunders, pp 3835–3864.

CHAPTER 74

Laparoscopic Retroperitoneal Lymph Node Dissection for Low-Stage Nonseminomatous Testis Cancer

Philip Fransen, MD, and Guenter Janetschek, MD

I. SPECIAL PREOPERATIVE PREPARATION

Clinical Stage I—Nonseminomatous Testis Cancer

- Imaging should include computed tomography of the abdomen and the chest.
- All tumor markers (α-fetoprotein, β-human chorionic gonadotropin, and lactate dehydrogenase) should be normalized for surgery.
- Indication for surgery depends further on risk factors and local treatment protocols:
  - ▲ *High-risk factors:* Vascular invasion, pT2 to pT4
  - ▲ *Low-risk factors:* No vascular invasion, pT1

Stage II—After Chemotherapy

- At this stage, surgery is indicated in any of the following cases:
  - ▲ Residual mass after chemotherapy
  - ▲ Tumor markers returned to normal levels
  - ▲ Initial tumor size up to 5 cm (stage IIA and stage IIB); in stage IIC (more than 5 cm), an individual decision has to be made according to tumor size, localization, and the experience of the surgeon.
- Bilateral spread of the disease is a relative contraindication for laparoscopy.

Preoperative Measures

- On preoperative day 1, oral mechanical bowel preparation, including clear fluid diet and laxatives, is performed.
- Low-dose systemic antibiotic coverage is provided on the day of surgery.
- Typing and cross-matching are performed for two units of blood.
- Special attention should be paid to the patient who has undergone preoperative chemotherapy with bleomycin, because pulmonary toxicity may ensue after oxygen administration during anesthesia. In such cases, a preoperative consultation with the anesthetist and pulmonary function tests may be required.

Equipment

- Three-chip video camera, high-quality video equipment
- 30-degree laparoscope
- AESOP robot, used to hold and guide the laparoscope; it has the advantage of providing stable video images even in lengthy procedures.
- An insufflator with a high flow rate prevents the pneumoperitoneum from collapsing.
- Four trocars, 10/11 mm; one or two of these can be replaced by a 5-mm trocar if desired.
- Reusable scissors with monopolar cautery
- Bipolar dissector, used for dissection and hemostasis
- Ultrasonic scalpel is useful for hemostatic dissection of lymphatic tissue but is dangerous for the fine dissection of the vessels.
- Suction device: 5 mm, one row of holes at the tip only
- Right-angle dissector for dissection of vessels
- Clips for the ligation of vessels: We have replaced the metallic clips with Hem-o-lok clips because the latter do not slide off transected vessels. However, metallic clips may be required when there is a risk of injury to delicate structures by the sharp tip of the Hem-o-lok clip.
- A small surgical sponge held with a 5-mm traumatic grasper is used for retraction. This tool is also very helpful in applying pressure to stop sudden bleeding. In this situation it replaces the finger of the surgeon, which would stop the bleeding during open surgery. A fan retractor is helpful to retract the liver. Retraction of the bowel is seldom necessary.

II. OPERATIVE TECHNIQUE

Position

- For retroperitoneal lymph node dissection (RPLND) to the right side, the patient is placed on the operating table with the right side elevated 45 degrees upward so that by rotating the table the patient can be brought into a supine or lateral decubitus position without repositioning. In addition, the table is slightly flexed at the umbilicus. If necessary, the Trendelenburg or anti-Trendelenburg position is used (Fig. 74-1).
- For left-sided dissection, an identical mirror-image positioning is used.

Trocar Placement

- A Veress needle is used for the initial stab incision at the umbilicus to create the pneumoperitoneum. The first trocar (10/11 mm) for the laparoscope is placed at the site of the umbilicus (see Fig. 74-1).
- Two secondary 10/11-mm trocars for the surgeon are placed at the lateral edge of the rectus muscle approximately 8 cm above and below the umbilicus.
- The fourth trocar (10/11 mm or 5 mm) is positioned in the anterior axillary line to facilitate retraction.
- The position of trocars does not differ for the right and left side.
- A fifth trocar might be necessary in the case of a large liver.

Templates

- Templates have been described that include the primary landing sites of lymph node metastases for patients diagnosed with nonseminomatous germ cell tumor clinical stage I.
- We have showed that the primary landing sites of lymph node metastases are exclusively ventral to the lumbar vessels. Therefore, for a diagnostic RPLND, there is no need to transect the lumbar vessels and remove the tissue behind the vena cava and aorta.

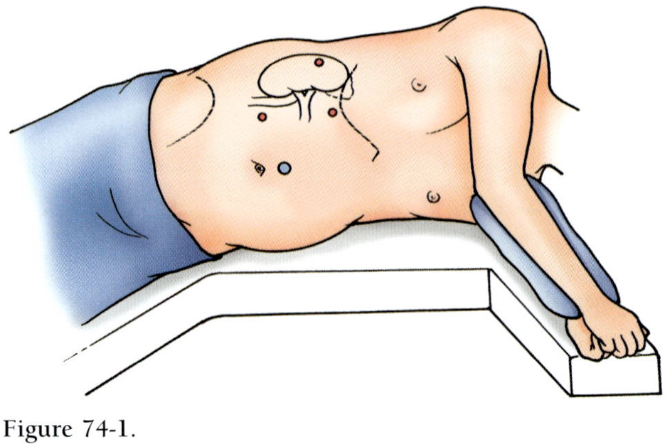

Figure 74-1.

- The right template (Fig. 74-2, *A*) includes the interaortocaval lymph nodes, preaortic tissue between the left renal vein and the inferior mesenteric artery, precaval tissue, and all the tissues lateral to the vena cava and the right common iliac artery; the lateral border of dissection is the ureter.
- The left template (see Fig. 74-2, *B*) includes preaortic tissue between the left renal vein and the inferior mesenteric artery, all the tissue lateral to the aorta and the left common iliac artery, and the interaortocaval lymph nodes; the lymphatic tissue ventral to the aorta below the inferior mesenteric artery is preserved. The lateral border of dissection is the ureter.

Main Dissection

Right Side (Figs. 74-3 and 74-4)

- The peritoneum is incised along the line of Toldt from the cecum to the right colic flexure. Cephalic dissection is carried out parallel to the transverse colon and lateral to the duodenum along the vena cava upward to the hepatoduodenal ligament, whereas the caudal dissection is continued along the spermatic vessels down to the internal inguinal ring. In the next step, the colon, duodenum, and head of the pancreas are reflected medially until the anterior surface of the vena cava, aorta, and opening of the left renal vein are completely exposed.
- This first step, exposure of the retroperitoneum, differs completely from open surgery. In contrast, RPLND is more or less the same procedure.
- The spermatic vein is dissected free along its entire course and excised. The spermatic artery is clipped and transected at its crossing over the vena cava, whereas the spermatic artery origin will be approached later.

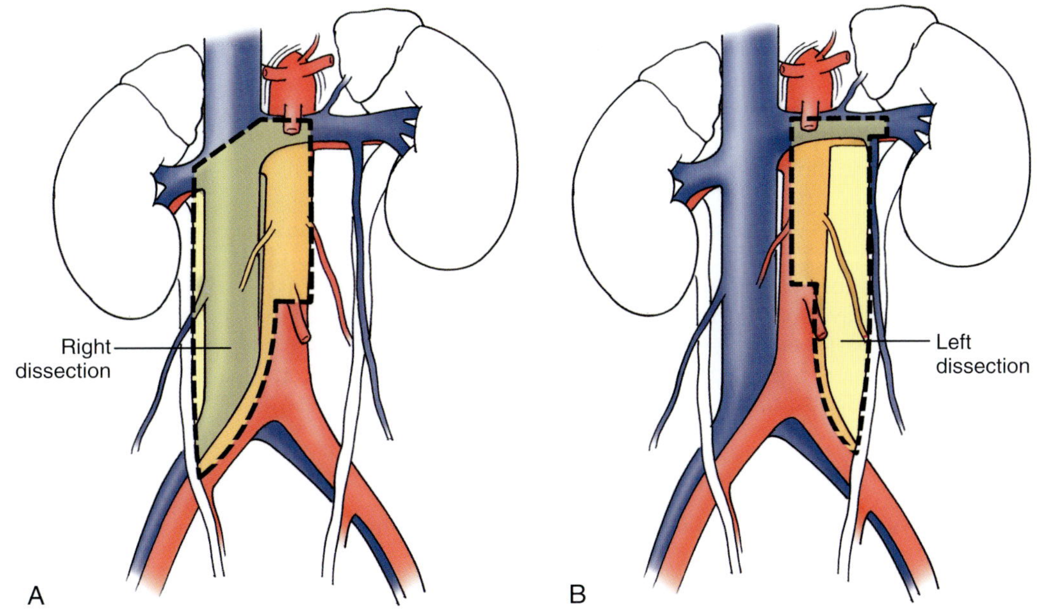

Figure 74-2.

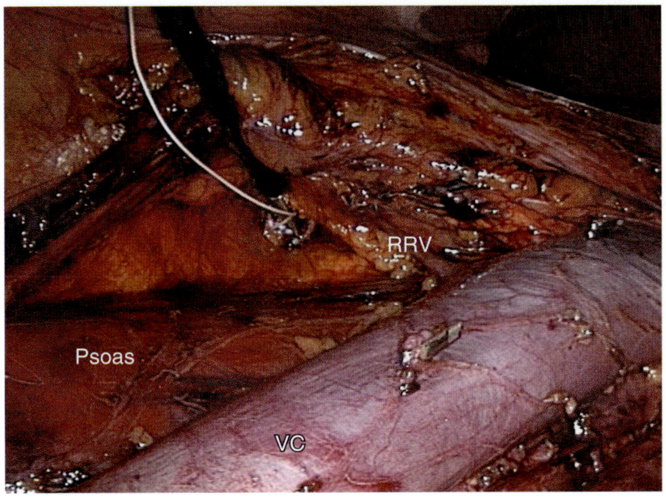

Figure 74-3. *RRV,* Right renal vein.

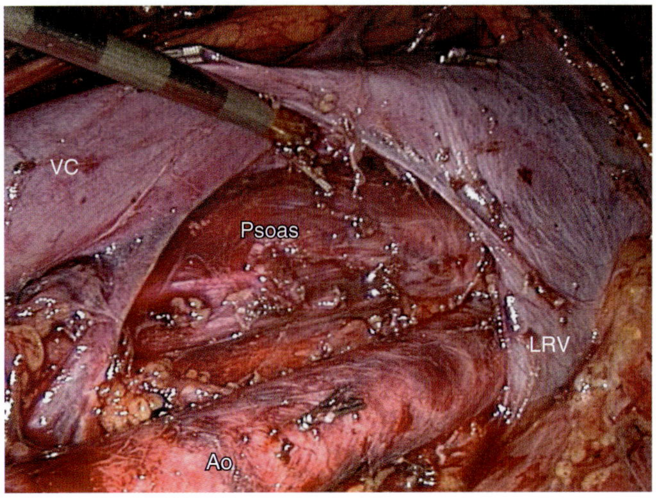

Figure 74-4. *LRV,* Left renal vein; *VC,* vena cava.

- Excision of the lymphatic tissue around the great vessels is performed in a split-and-roll technique as described by Donohue.
- Cranial to caudal, the lymphatic tissue overlying the vena cava is split open, then the lateral and anterior surfaces of the vena cava are dissected free. Both renal veins are then dissected free. Lymphatic tissue overlying the right common iliac artery is incised, and the dissection is continued from caudal to cranial upward to the origin of the inferior mesenteric artery (Fig. 74-5). Cranial to the inferior mesenteric artery, dissection is continued upward along the left margin to the aorta, completely freeing the ventral surface of the aorta. The spermatic artery is then clipped at its origin.
- Cranial to caudal, the interaortocaval space is then dissected, starting from the lower edge of the right renal artery down to the lumbar vessels, and the lymphatic tissue is removed step by step. The right renal vein and artery lateral to the vena cava delineate the cranial border of the dissection, whereas the caudal border is the point where the ureter crosses the iliac vessels (Figs. 74-6 and 74-7). The lymphatic tissue is clipped distally; then the dissection is continued cephalad until the lymphatic package is freed. The lumbar veins are exposed, but they are transected only in exceptional cases (Figs. 74-8 and 74-9). Lymph nodes lateral to the vena cava and medial to the ureter are dissected free. The nodal package can then be removed within a specimen retrieval bag. The colon and duodenum are returned to their anatomic positions and secured with one suture laterally, which is tied extracorporeally.

Left Side

- The peritoneum is incised along the line of Toldt, starting from the left colonic flexure down to the pelvic brim and distally along the spermatic vein to the internal inguinal ring. The splenocolic ligament is transected, and the colon is dissected until the anterior surface of the aorta is exposed. In the next step, the spermatic vein is dissected along its entire course and excised. The ureter is then identified laterally and separated from the lymphatic tissue, taking care to preserve its blood supply. That step facilitates dissection of the left renal vein until it is freed completely (Fig. 74-10).
- Dissection of the lymphatic template is started caudally at the crossing of the ureter with the common iliac vessels, by splitting the lymphatic tissue over the anterior surface of the left common iliac artery in a cranial direction along the lateral border of the aorta, circumventing the inferior mesenteric artery on the left side and preserving it (see Fig. 74-6). Cranial to the inferior mesenteric artery, dissection is continued along the anterior and medial surfaces of the aorta up to the left renal vein, and during this dissection, the origin of the spermatic artery is clipped and transected. Next to that, the lateral surface of the aorta is dissected down to the origin of the lumbar arteries (see Fig. 74-10; Fig. 74-11). To gain access to the left renal artery, the lumbar vein draining in to the left renal vein must be transected. Other lumbar vessels are dissected free from the lymphatic tissue to the point at which they disappear in the layer between the spine and psoas muscle, and then the sympathetic chain lateral to that point can be identified (Fig. 74-12). When the nodal package is completely freed, it can be retrieved in a laparoscopic retrieval bag. The colon is then secured in its anatomic position with an extracorporeally tied suture.

Closure

- To prevent lymphocele formation, the peritoneal incision is not closed.
- No drain is placed to prevent lymphocele formation.
- At the 10/11-mm ports, the peritoneum and fascia are closed.
- The skin is closed by a skin stapler.
- Dressings to 5 cm are used to cover the wounds.

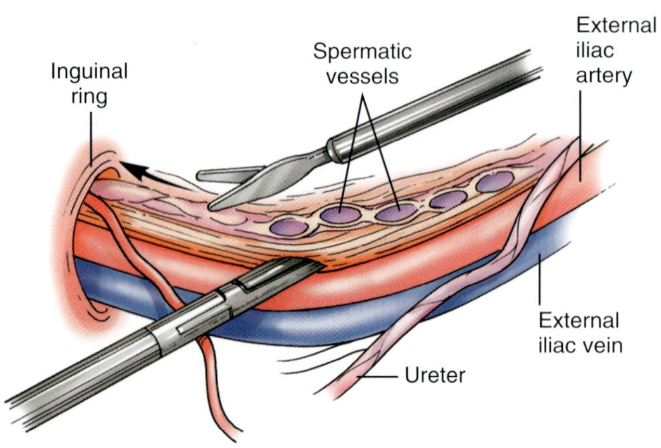

Figure 74-5.

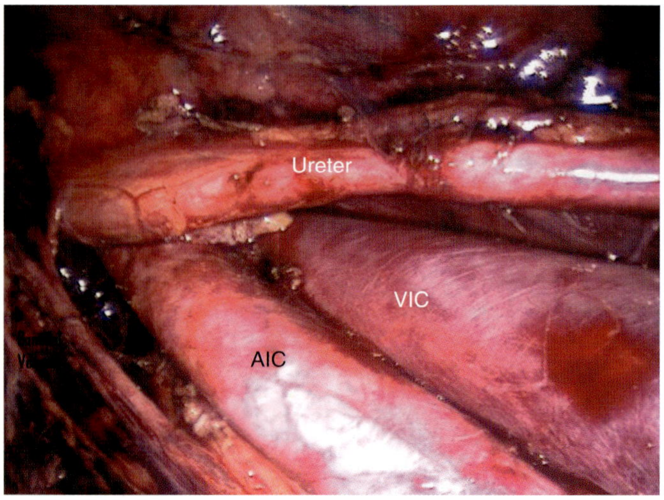

Figure 74-6. *AIC,* Common iliac artery; *VIC,* common iliac vein.

III. ALTERNATIVE TECHNICAL APPROACHES (PRO/CON) AND PEARLS

- At present there is no consensus about the optimal treatment for clinical low-stage nonseminomatous germ cell tumors. After orchiectomy, the treatment options are surveillance, chemotherapy, or RPLND, followed by surveillance or chemotherapy.
- The best treatment option should combine maximal safety and cure together with minimal morbidity for the patient.

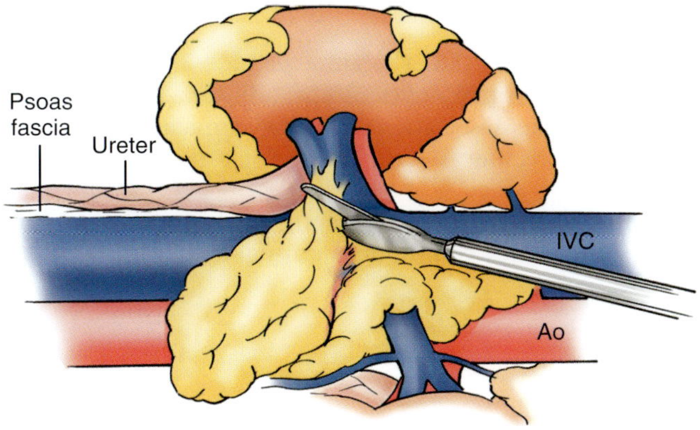

Figure 74-7. *Ao,* Aorta; *IVC,* inferior vena cava.

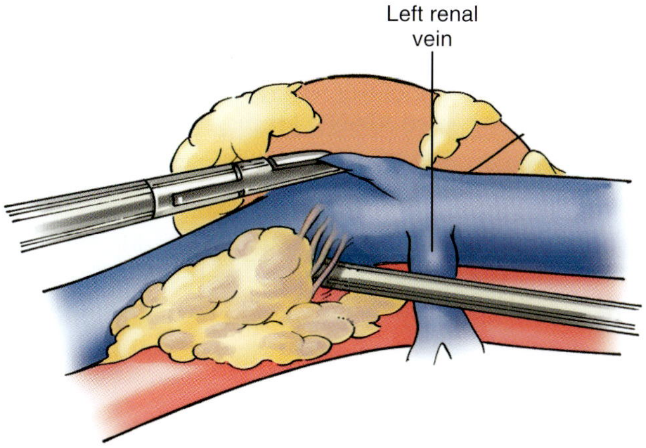

Figure 74-8.

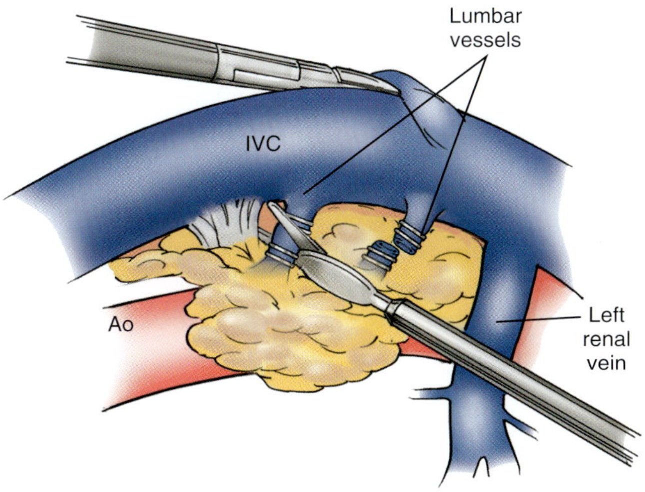

Figure 74-9. *Ao,* Aorta; *IVC,* inferior vena cava.

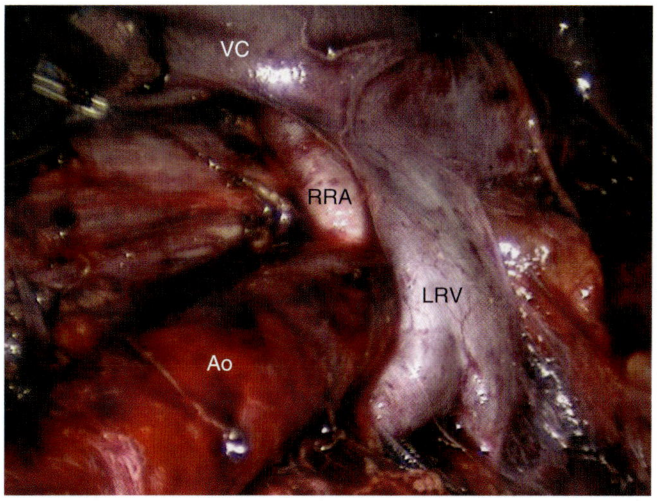

Figure 74-10. *Ao,* Aorta; *LRV,* left renal vein; *RRA,* right renal artery; *RRV,* right renal vein; *VC,* vena cava.

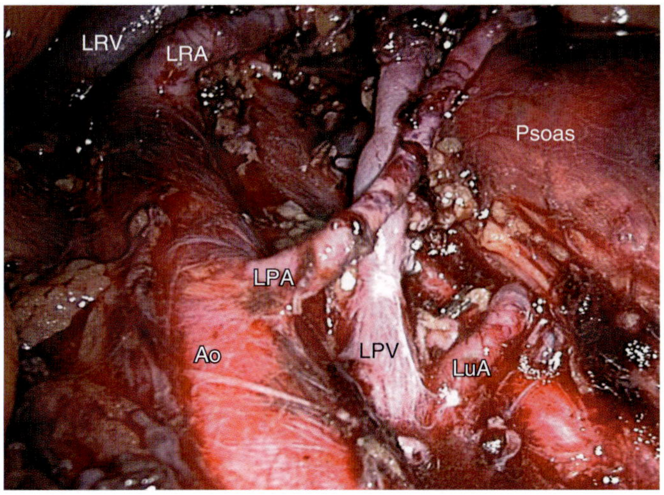

Figure 74-11. *Ao,* Aorta; *LPA,* left pulmonary artery; *LPV,* left pulmonary vein; *LRA,* left renal artery; *LRV,* left renal vein; *LUA,* left uterine artery.

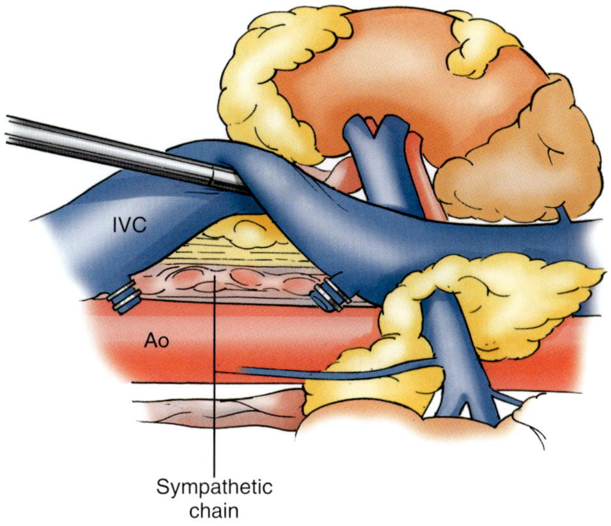

Figure 74-12. *Ao,* Aorta; *IVC,* inferior vena cava.

- In Europe there is a greater tendency for surveillance or chemotherapy, whereas in North America there is a greater propensity for surgery.
- When surveillance protocols are used, the literature reports a clinical relapse rate as high as 30%. As a consequence, chemotherapy must be offered to patients in a later stage of the disease. Because of patient noncompliance or the lack of sensitivity of current diagnostic imaging studies (computed tomography, magnetic resonance imaging, positron emission tomography), there is a greater probability that second-line treatment modalities will fail. The dose of chemotherapy will also be higher in this setting, and the toxicity of chemotherapy increases exponentially relative to the dosage.
- Giving chemotherapy with bleomycin, etoposide, and platinum to every patient as an adjuvant therapy will induce overtreatment and subjects the patient to both acute and long-term toxicity (pulmonary fibrosis or secondary malignancies).
- Use of RPLND in a therapeutic setting yields high relapse rates, up to 50%. Therefore we have always used RPLND for diagnostic purposes only, and all patients with positive nodes receive adjuvant chemotherapy. This approach is strongly recommended by the European Association of Urology guidelines, and most U.S. patients also receive adjuvant chemotherapy for clinical stage I/pathologic stage II tumors.
- Diagnostic and therapeutic RPLND differ in template, which therefore has to be clearly defined.
- The template of diagnostic RPLND has the advantage that it does not compromise normal antegrade ejaculation.

Pearls

- Especially in laparoscopic RPLND, exposure of the complete retroperitoneum and the great vessels is of utmost importance. This is achieved through wide mobilization of the colon on either side, allowing free access to the retroperitoneum with no need to retract the bowel later during the procedure. While mobilizing the left colon for exposure, the surgeon should take care not to enter the plane behind the kidney, thus reclining it and making further dissection almost impossible.
- To avoid iatrogenic organ injury, the surgeon should maintain clear dissection borders by remaining on the vessels at all time during dissection. The use of clips on the resected margins of lymphatic tissue should help minimize lymphocele formation.
- While splitting the tissue overlying the aorta in the cranial direction, the surgeon should be alert to the presence of the left renal vein, as this structure could be inadvertently injured. Similarly, accessory arteries to the kidney may be encountered during the dissection between the aorta and the kidney; severing them may result in troublesome bleeding and loss of renal function (see Fig. 74-11).
- Hemostasis is probably the most frequent problem encountered by the surgeon during laparoscopic RPLND. Generally, the best solution for hemostasis is prevention, using appropriate preoperative imaging to discover aberrant vessels (see Fig. 74-11) and good surgical technique with excellent exposure.
- If bleeding is still encountered, the following may prove very helpful:
  - Compression with suction or sponge replaces the finger of the surgeon in open surgery.
  - In the case of venous bleeding, the pneumoperitoneum can be raised to 20 mm Hg for a short period.
  - Supplementary support can be given.
  - Exposure can be improved.
  - Blood flow should be controlled with upstream clamps.
  - The surgeon should not hesitate to add an extra trocar to manage the situation, as this may make the difference between a laparoscopic procedure and a conversion.
  - Use 7-cm sutures prepared with a Lapra-Ty or a Hem-o-lok clip to avoid time-consuming knotting.
  - A conversion kit should always be readily at hand.

IV. SPECIAL POSTOPERATIVE CARE

- Postoperative medication is limited to standard analgesia and subcutaneous thromboprophylaxis.
- Oral intake is resumed on postoperative day 1, and early mobilization is encouraged.
- If chylous ascites occurs despite the preventive measures described earlier, a low-fat diet can be recommended until the problem is solved.
- The urinary catheter is removed on postoperative day 1 if urinary output is adequate.

SUGGESTED READINGS

Albqami N, Janetschek G: Laparoscopic retroperitoneal lymph-node dissection in the management of clinical stage I and II testicular cancer, *J Endourol* 19:683–692, 2005.

Holtl L, Peschel R, Knapp R, et al: Primary lymphatic metastatic spread in testicular cancers occurs ventral to the lumbar vessels, *Urology* 59:114–118, 2002.

Steiner H, Peschel R, Janetschek G, et al: Long-term results of laparoscopic retroperitoneal lymph node dissection: a single-center 10-year experience, *Urology* 63:550–555, 2004.

CHAPTER 75

Laparoscopic Nephrectomy

H. Christoph Klingler, MD, FEBU, and Michael Marberger, MD, FRCS

I. SPECIAL PREOPERATIVE PREPARATION

- Renal ultrasonography is highly recommended as a first-step investigation, particularly to investigate localization of tumor site and size. Although renal ultrasonography may be diagnostic as to whether lesions are cystic or solid, it may not rule out or prove malignancy. In addition, structure and anatomy of left and right renal units should be investigated, to clarify if a radical removal of one kidney seems possible. However, even with Doppler power mode or contrast enhancement, renal function may not be reliably investigated. Consequently, renal ultrasonography must be regarded as an additional tool, but not as the primary investigation.
- Renal diagnostic workup is best performed by renal helical contrast-enhanced computed tomography (CT) scan, provided renal function is normal. CT scan is highly diagnostic for renal cell cancer, particular when contrast enhancement of the tumor is possible, but ruling out small benign lesions may be difficult (see the discussion of renal biopsy). Renal anatomy, lymphatic status, and function of both renal units can be tested simultaneously. In selected cases an intravenous pyelogram may add to the diagnostic capabilities, particularly when upper urinary tract transitional-cell cancer must be ruled out. This, however, can be replaced by four-phase contrast CT including a urographic phase. Contrast-enhanced magnetic resonance imaging (Fig. 75-1) is an excellent alternative, particularly when renal function is impaired (serum creatinine greater than 2.0 mg/dL) but will not routinely add to diagnostic capabilities. Magnetic resonance or CT angiography is another recommended tool in cases where

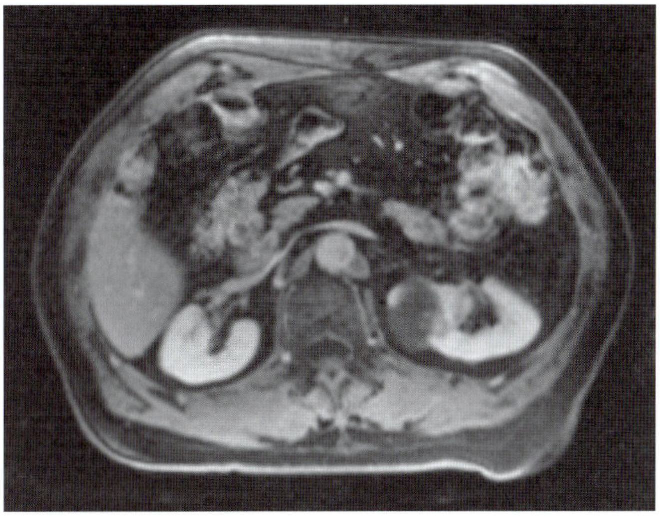

Figure 75-1. A 5-cm left renal tumor on magnetic resonance imaging T1 flash.

vascular pathology is present or may be expected (Fig. 75-2). Renal isotope scan is recommended only in selected cases, particularly when preterminal renal insufficiency may call for nephron-sparing surgery rather than complete nephrectomy.

- If there is any suspicion of upper urinary tract transitional-cell cancer, cystoscopy with retrograde ureteropyelography and selective urine cytology may be performed under general anesthesia before radical nephrectomy. In the case of upper urinary-tract cancer that has been proved by positive cytologic or radiologic findings, we proceed with a modified laparoscopic nephroureterectomy. This combines laparoscopic radical nephrectomy (as indicated later) with open excision of the distal ureter including the bladder cuff, leaving the entire specimen intact. It leaves the patient with the advantages of minimally invasive surgery.
- Accumulating results in the literature demonstrate that core needle biopsy of solid renal lesions should be considered more frequently. This, however, applies more to solid tumors smaller than 4 cm. However, larger masses that may potentially be resectable should be considered for CT-guided biopsy, because benign or less aggressive malignant tumors may be an argument for nephron-sparing surgery in selected cases.
- There is no specific preoperative patient care for laparoscopic radical nephrectomy. Bowel enema and low–molecular-weight heparin the night before surgery are highly recommended, and the patient should be well hydrated. Compression stockings are placed on the patient's legs before surgery. A broad-spectrum antibiotic is administered intravenously 2 hours before surgery and continued through postoperative day 3. After introduction of general anesthesia, a nasogastric tube and an indwelling bladder catheter are inserted to decompress both stomach and bladder. An external warming system (Bair Hugger, Arizant Healthcare, Eden Prairie, Minn.) is draped around the patient.

Choice of Access

- Commonly, urologists favor transperitoneal access because of its resemblance to open transperitoneal access. Likewise, surgical working space is wider and landmarks are more easily accessible throughout the entire procedure. This, however, has changed because of increased experience with retroperitoneal laparoscopic surgery. Today, both surgical techniques must be readily available and should be chosen according to patients' needs. There are only a few contraindications for laparoscopic transperitoneal surgery, but previous extensive abdominal surgery, septic renal disease, or morbid obesity may be reasons to choose a retroperitoneal technique. Even severe cardiopulmonary comorbidity favors retroperitoneal access, because there may be less gas absorption during retroperitoneoscopy, provided the peritoneal cavity remains intact. From the surgical standpoint, there are few differences between radical and simple nephrectomy. Differences exist in conjunction with oncologic principles rather than in the surgical techniques, and benign pathology may be an argument for a retroperitoneal nephrectomy to minimize operative trauma.

Oncologic Principles

- There have been concerns that the principles of surgery for renal cancer may be compromised by laparoscopic procedures in general. However, all surgical steps are similar to the open ablative techniques. In particular, early vascular control (see Figs. 75-7 and 75-8) gives early oncologic control and also prevents hemorrhage. Likewise, a no-touch surgical technique must be maintained by leaving the Gerota fascia intact, thus primarily preventing potential tumor cell spillage. In addition, intact organ retrieval in a cell-tight organ bag via a muscle-splitting incision in the lower abdomen (Fig. 75-3) significantly decreases the risk of drop or port-site metastasis compared with that for manual or electric organ morcellation. Thus far, reported local recurrences, intraperitoneal drop, or port-site metastases have been found predominantly in patients in whom these principles were not followed. Consequently, laparoscopic surgery has proven to be oncologically effective when these principles are strictly followed.

II. OPERATIVE TECHNIQUE

Position

Transperitoneal Access

- The patient is placed in a slightly overstretched 45-degree lateral decubitus position (Fig. 75-4). Special care must be taken to pad all positional pressure points and to secure the patient to the table, preferably with cushions and tapes, to allow safe intraoperative rotation of the table when needed during surgery.
- The surgeon faces the patient's face. The assistant stands on the opposite side of the table, and the scrub nurse at the surgeon's side by the patient's legs.

Retroperitoneal Access

- The patient is placed in a slightly overstretched 90-degree lateral flank position (Fig. 75-5).
- The surgeon faces the patient's back. The assistant stands on the opposite side of the table, and the scrub nurse at the surgeon's side by the patient's legs.

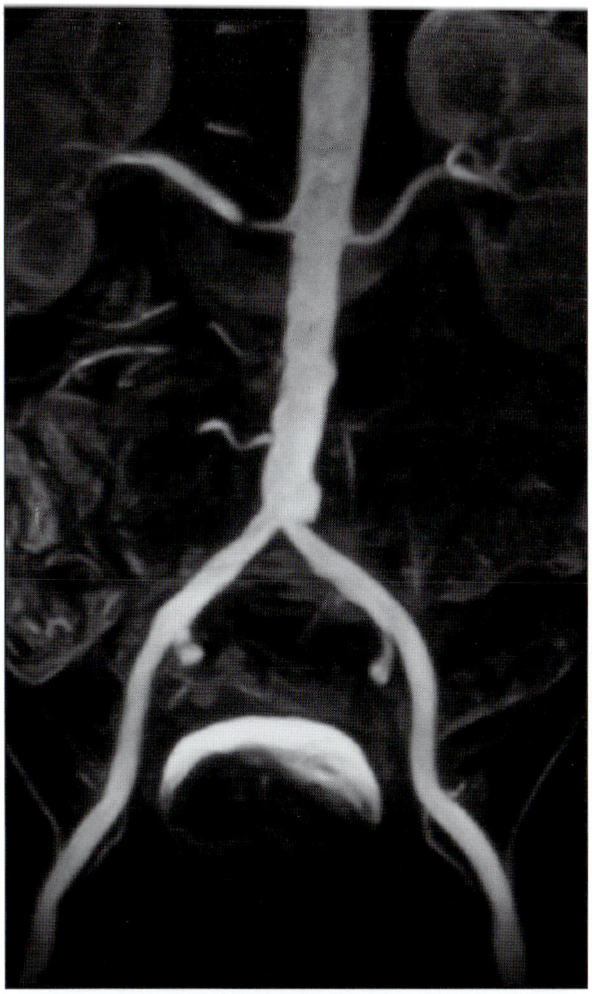

Figure 75-2. Magnetic resonance angiogram in the same patient demonstrating right renal artery stenosis.

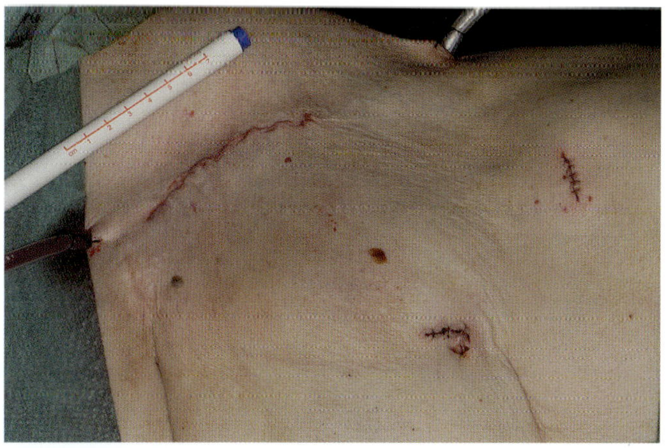

Figure 75-3. Postoperative site after successful radical transperitoneal laparoscopic nephrectomy. Specimen retrieval was performed via the lower abdominal incision.

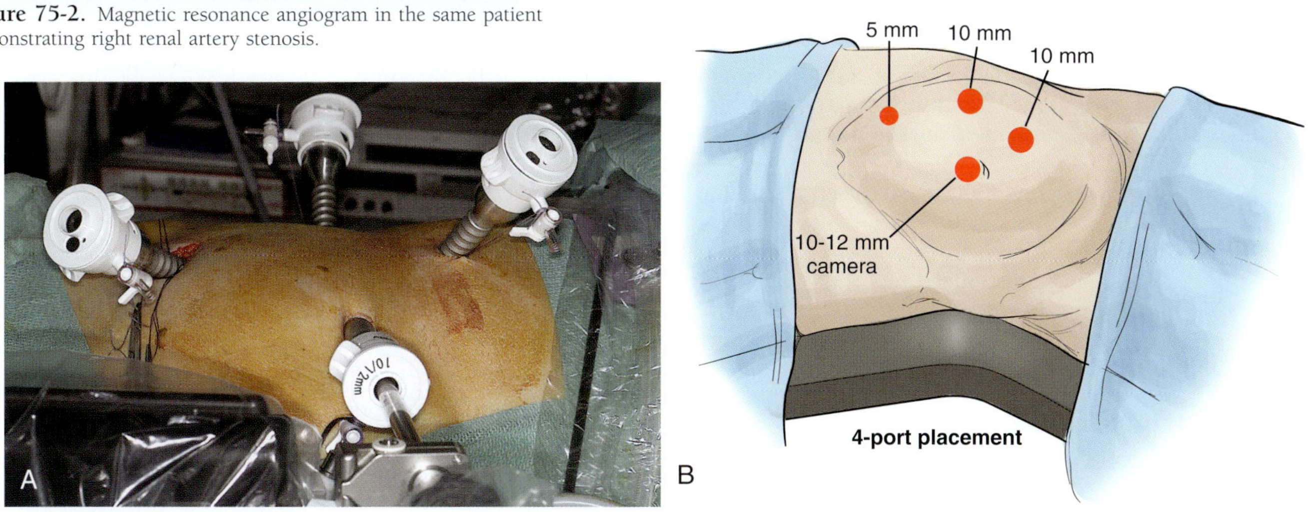

Figure 75-4.

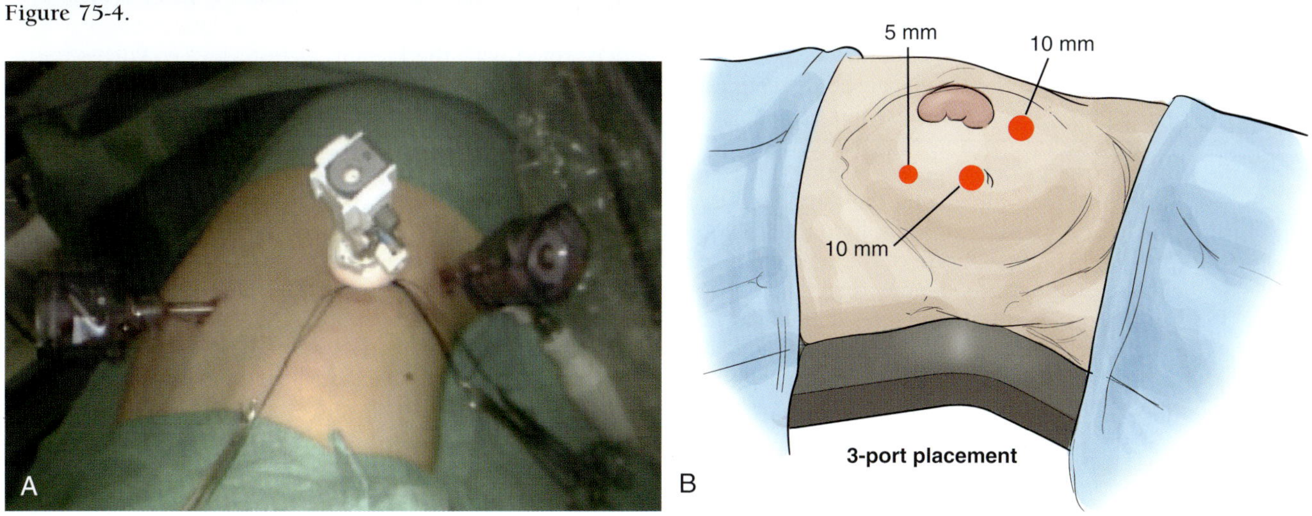

Figure 75-5.

Incision

Transperitoneal Access

- To create a pneumoperitoneum, either a Veress needle is set blindly at the umbilicus, or, in the case of previous surgery or in children, an open 3-cm minilaparotomy (Hasson technique) is used. Commonly, the Hasson technique is regarded as safer for gaining access for the first port.
- Intraabdominal pressure is maintained at a maximum of 12 to 14 mm Hg in adults.
- For the standard transperitoneal technique, a four-port approach (see Fig. 75-4, *A* and *B*) is used. The 10/12-mm trocar for the laparoscope is placed at the umbilicus, and two trocars for the surgeon are placed at the lateral edge of the rectus muscle, one in the subcostal area and one in the lower abdomen. At least the port in the lower abdomen must be a 12-mm port to allow introduction of the 12-mm vascular endoscopic stapler for control of the renal vein when needed. This port is also used for organ retrieval after nephrectomy (see Fig. 75-3). With the use of modern 5-mm ultrasonic and bipolar hemostatic dissection instruments or clips, the standard subcostal upper port is 5 mm, but a 12-mm port may be necessary when difficulties with control of large renal vessels occur. The lateral 10/12-mm port for the assistant is placed at the midaxillary line; this port is used for placing the drainage tube at the end of surgery.
- Fixation of the ports by sutures is helpful, particularly when instruments must be changed repeatedly during dissection.
- In laparoscopic transperitoneal surgery, a voice-controlled robotic arm (AESOP, Computer Motion, Goleta, Calif.) for camera guidance may be helpful, giving a video image without tremor and leaving both surgeons hands-free for the intervention. In addition, only one assistant is needed to assist and to serve as a backup in case of complications (see Fig. 75-4, *A*).

Retroperitoneal Access

- To gain the initial retroperitoneal access, the Hasson technique is used as discussed earlier.
- A 3- to 5-cm muscle-splitting incision is made at the midaxillary line between the iliac crest and the tip of the 12th rib. This port is later used for intact organ retrieval and must therefore be carefully planned. The retroperitoneal cavity is enlarged, first digitally and then with a balloon distention device (balloon catheter or blunt-tipped balloon port, Tyco, Norwalk, Conn.), creating a space outside the Gerota fascia and the lateral abdominal wall by insufflating about 800 to 1000 mL of normal saline air into the balloon (Fig. 75-6). Preferably, a so-called 12-mm Hasson trocar (blunt-tip Hasson port, Ethicon, Cincinnati; balloon port, Tyco) is used to seal this port site, preventing gas leakage. Before this, two more 12-mm ports may be placed under digital control at the lateral abdominal wall and in the lower abdomen. Intraabdominal pressure is maintained at a maximum of 10 to 12 mm Hg in adults.
- Another 5-mm port can be used after final dissection of the retroperitoneal cavity, but this port is optional.
- In retroperitoneoscopy, the voice-controlled robotic arm is of less help, because the position of the camera may be changed repeatedly during dissection, and this can be done more quickly by the assistant. Mounting of the robotic arm may even not allow camera maneuvers at extreme positions. Therefore, we no longer use the robotic camera arm in retroperitoneal nephrectomy.

Main Dissection

- For laparoscopic dissection and cutting, monopolar scissors (Richard Wolf, Knittlingen, Germany) and bipolar forceps (Ethicon) can be used. Alternatively, the Harmonic scalpel (Harmonic ACE, Ethicon) or bipolar dissectors (LigaSure, Valleylab, Boulder, Colo.) may be used, but for pure ablative surgery these are expensive tools. Blunt dissection can be performed with the Elefant suction device (Porges, Paris) because the tissue can be dissected bluntly and simultaneously cleared of fat and liquids. For retraction, grasping forceps and flexible endoscopic retractors can be used. The latter are particularly helpful in retroperitoneal nephrectomy because of the limited working space.
- On the right side, surgery is begun with incision of the peritoneum at the Toldt line, freeing the cecum pole, and then mobilizing the ascending colon up to the hepatic flexure. The peritoneal lining below the liver is incised transversely to the lateral abdominal wall. This creates an access to the supraadrenal area and the dorsal side of the renal pedicle. Thereafter the duodenum is mobilized according to the Kocher technique, gaining direct access to the vena cava and the renal vein. The ureter is best approached at its crossing above the iliac vessel running right below the gonadal veins, which may be easily identified, are on the right side, and are usually not resected. Further dissection of both structures is continued cranially to the lower renal pole, leaving the Gerota fascia intact. By lifting the lower renal pole, access to the renal pedicle can be obtained, and after the renal artery and vein are cleared from surrounding lymphatic tissue, both are secured with clips (Hem-o-lok, Weck, Durham, N.C.; Figs. 75-7 and 75-8) and divided using scissors or the endostapler (Ethicon or Tyco), starting with the artery. Care must be taken not to overlook any additional upper pole artery; otherwise, back-flow bleeding

may occur. Thereafter, a decision must be made as to whether the adrenal gland must be resected. If so, all relevant vessels are clipped next to the vena cava. Special care must be taken to clip the subhepatic region, because there are usually additional vessels located there. Otherwise the dissection of the upper pole is performed by using bipolar dissection, but the use of the Harmonic scalpel (Harmonic ACE) or a bipolar dissector (LigaSure) may ease mobilization of the upper renal pole. Finally, the kidney is fully mobilized from the psoas muscle, which can be done bluntly, and the lateral border of the kidney is released, preferably with monopolar cutting. The ureter is clipped and dissected, and the entire organ is enclosed in a cell-tight organ retrieval bag.

- If necessary, a staging lymphadenectomy may now be performed, including hilar and ventral caval lymph nodes, retrieved within a small cell-tight organ bag (Rüsch, Kernen, Germany) via the lower 12-mm port and sent for frozen section. As a last step, the port in the lower abdomen is enlarged to a 7- to 10-cm incision (depending on the overall size of the specimen). The intact specimen (Fig. 75-9) is then removed within the cell-tight organ bag and sent for frozen section to prove negative margins.
- Radical nephrectomy on the left side varies significantly at some steps. Because the kidney is covered completely by the descending colon and the splenic flexure, dissection is more tedious and time

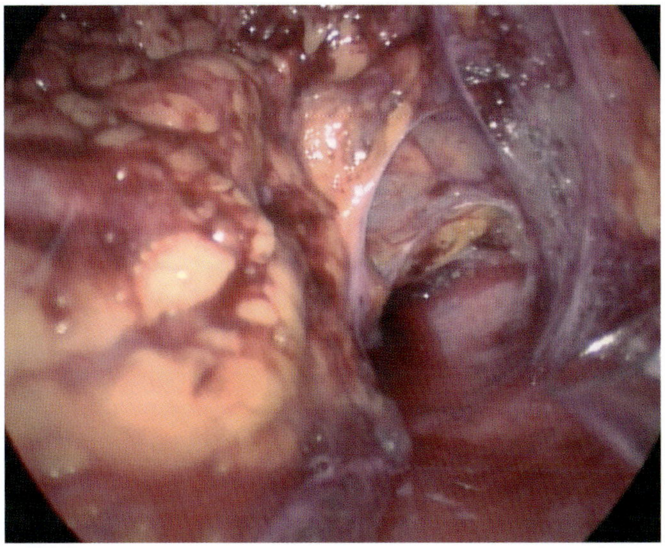

Figure 75-6.

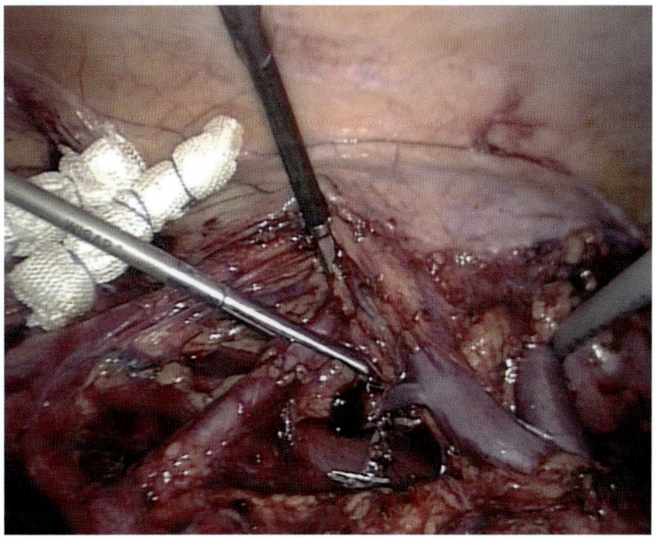

Figure 75-7.

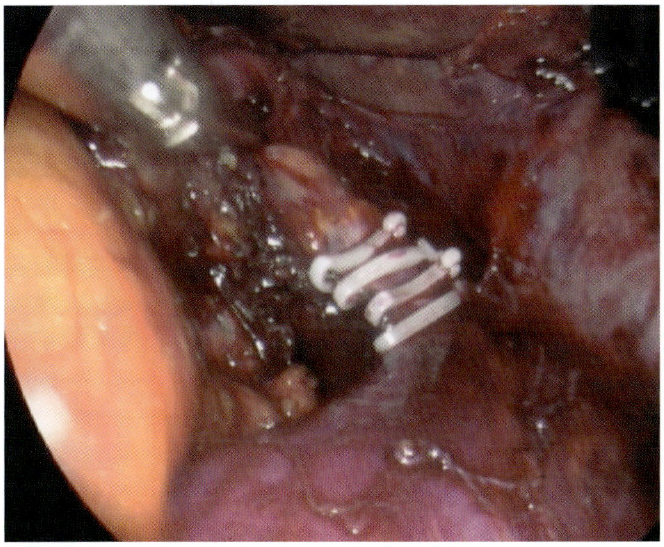

Figure 75-8.

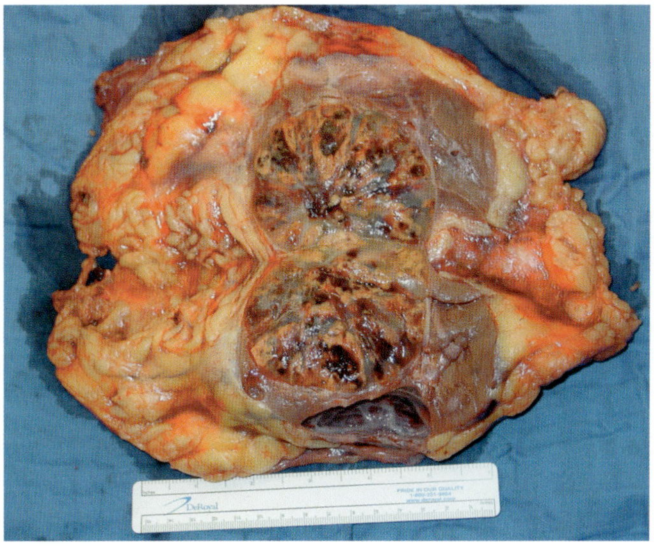

Figure 75-9.

consuming (Fig. 75-10). The splenic flexure must be completely dissected to achieve access to the retroperitoneal cavity (Fig. 75-11). If a simple nephrectomy is to be performed for a benign condition, the Gerota fascia is incised (Fig. 75-12), whereas for radical nephrectomy, the Gerota fascia is left intact. Dissection of the ureter and gonadal veins is similar to that for the right side, but the gonadal veins should be resected and removed with the specimen (Fig. 75-13). A number of lumbar veins that open

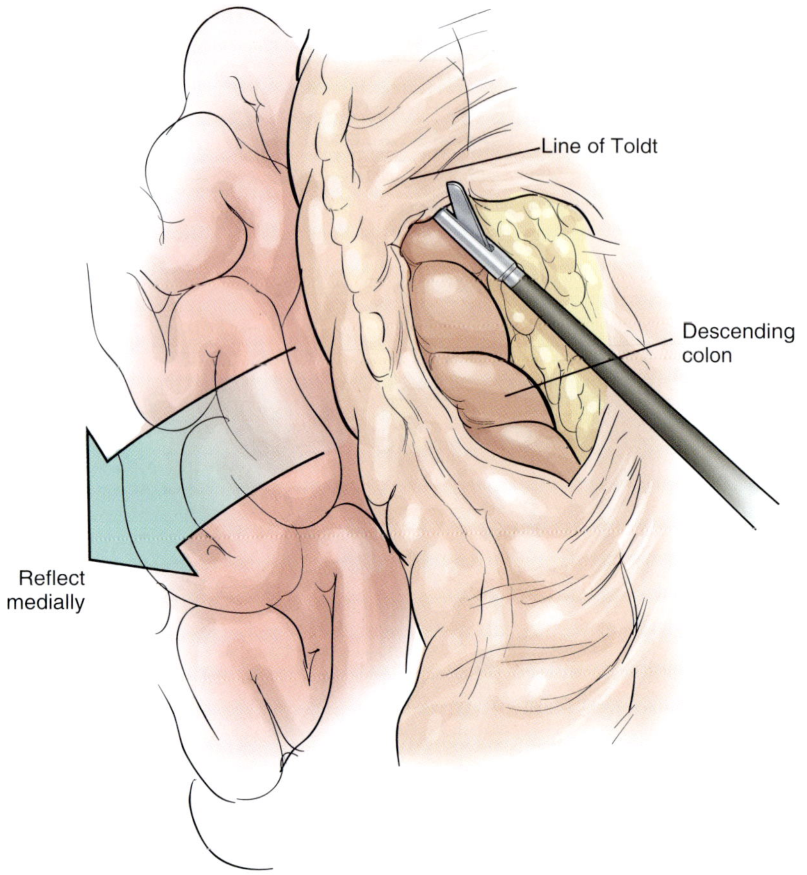

Figure 75-10.

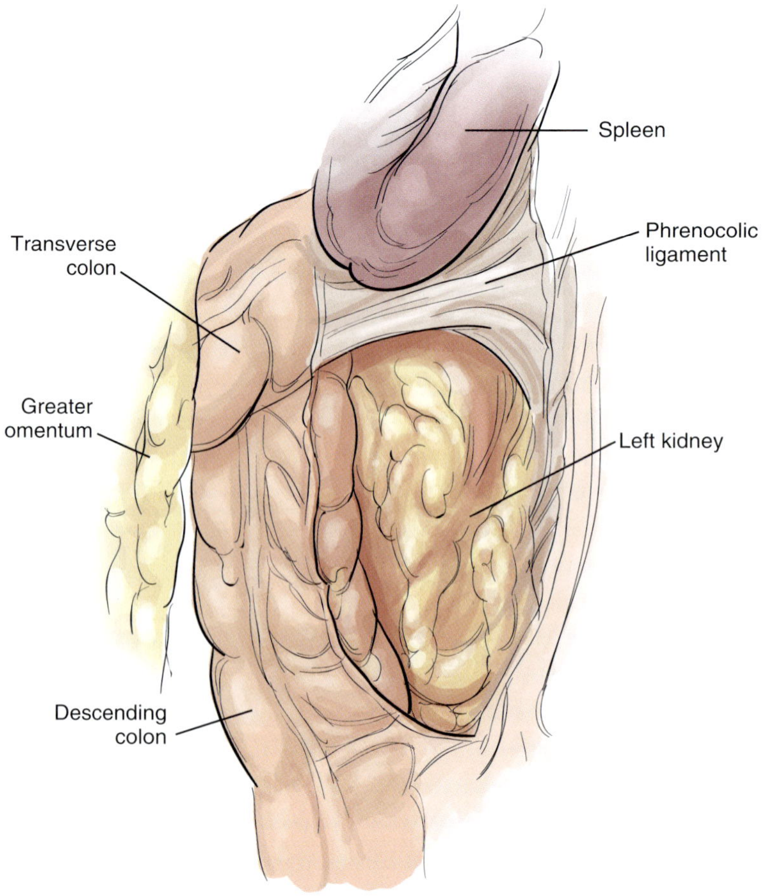

Figure 75-11.

into the renal veins make dissection of the renal pedicle more cumbersome. The ureter is then divided between clips (Fig. 75-14). The renal vein must be transected either distally or peripherally to the opening of the adrenal vein, depending on whether the adrenal gland is to be resected. If necessary, hilar and ventral aortic lymph nodes may be removed, with the psoas muscle serving as the lateral and the iliac vessels as the caudal boundary. All other surgical steps are similar to the technique

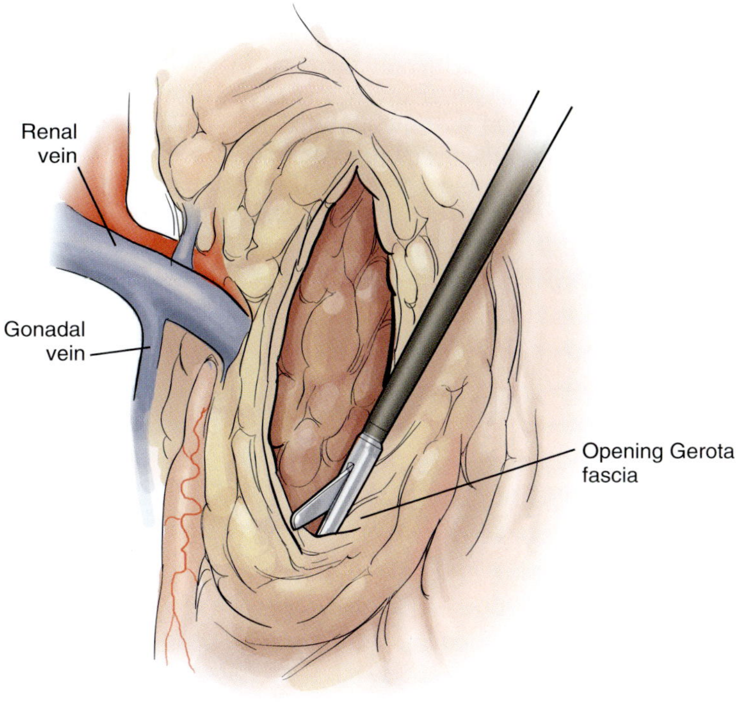

Figure 75-12.

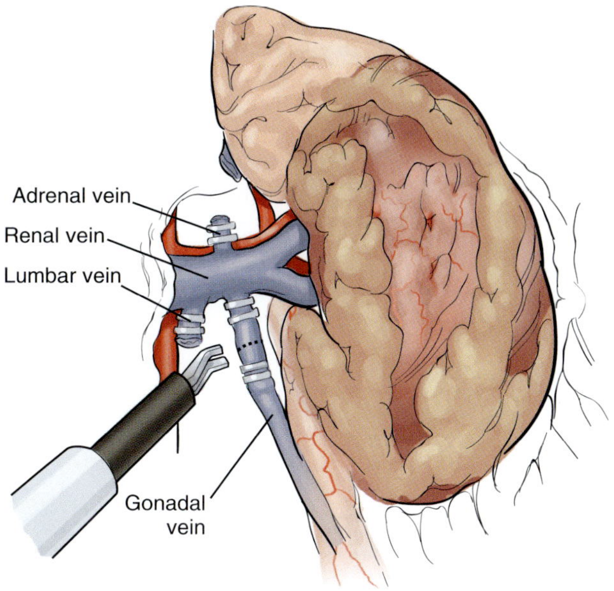

Figure 75-13.

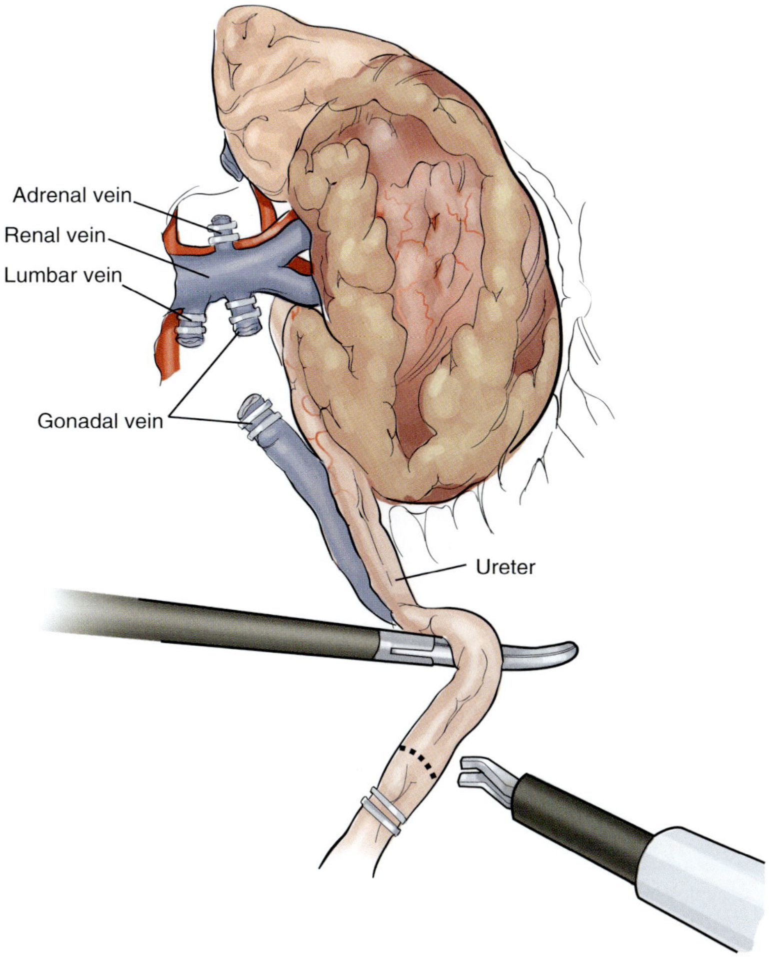

Figure 75-14.

described for right-sided radical nephrectomy: namely, the left renal artery is isolated and can be transected with a linear endovascular stapler (Fig. 75-15).

Special Considerations for Retroperitoneoscopy

- The psoas muscle and the lateral abdominal wall are the primary landmarks with retroperitoneal nephrectomy (see Fig. 75-6). Starting at the lower renal pole and with the help of an endoscopic retracting fan, the entire kidney is mobilized anterolaterally, and the lateral and posterior aspect of the kidney up to the upper pole is dissected, mainly bluntly. The Gerota fascia is incised at the area of the renal pedicle, parallel and next to the psoas muscle. The next step is to identify the renal artery, which may be dissected after it is secured with clips or the endostapler. Alternatively, the Gerota fascia is incised at the lower anterior renal pole, and the peritoneal lining of the anterior renal aspect may be easily dissected. In addition, the ureter can be found more easily at the lower pole, guiding the surgeon to the renal pelvis. Now the renal vessels may be safely identified (Fig. 75-16), and unless this was done primarily, the renal artery and then the renal vein are secured with clips or the endostapler and dissected. By dissection of the upper renal pole, the adrenal gland may be resected simultaneously or left behind. Finally, the ureter is secured with clips and dissected, and the specimen is wrapped in a cell-tight organ retrieval bag.

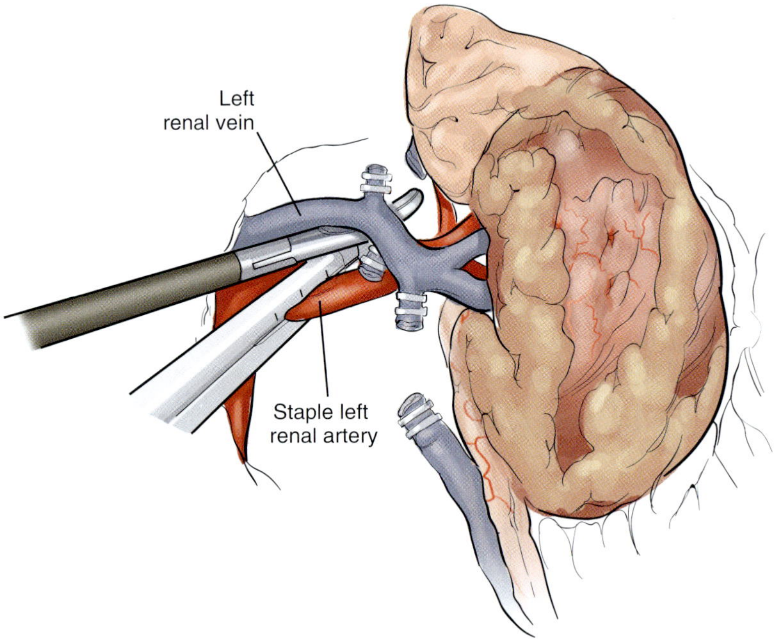

Figure 75-15.

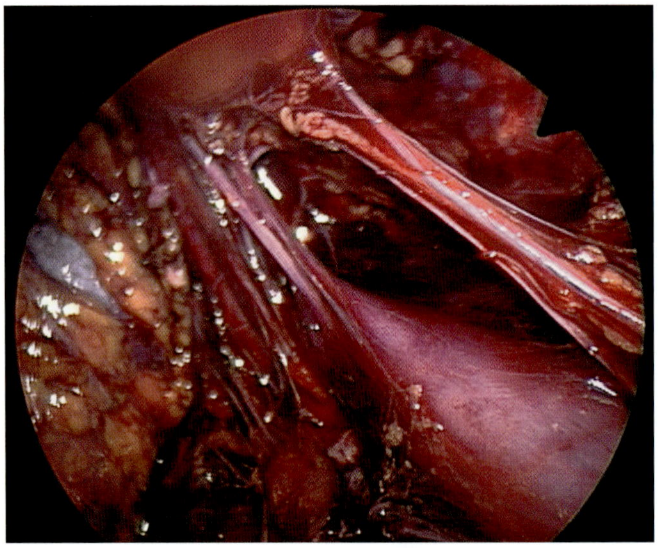

Figure 75-16. Retroperitoneal nephrectomy with renal pedicle in a child. Ureter at *right*, renal vein at *center*, and renal artery at *left*.

- Staging lymphadenectomy of hilar lymph nodes as indicated in the transperitoneal technique is feasible; however, dissection of a larger template is difficult with retroperitoneal access. In rare cases in which a radical lymphadenectomy is imminent, a transperitoneal technique is therefore the better technical approach. The middle port is then enlarged to 7 to 10 cm, and the specimen is removed intact for frozen section to prove negative margins.

Closure

- The 7- to 10-cm incision is closed in layers with Vicryl size 0 running sutures. Laparoscopic instruments are brought into the operative cavity and the operative site checked for hemorrhage. Intraabdominal pressure should be lowered to 8 to 10 mm Hg. A 21-Fr drainage tube is placed via the lateral port and fixed to the skin with a nonabsorbable suture. The 12-mm ports are routinely closed with Vicryl size 0 endostitches under laparoscopic visual control. The 5-mm ports are checked for local bleeding during removal under laparoscopic vision but are not routinely closed as described earlier. The skin is sutured with absorbable Monocryl 4-0 sutures, but skin staples may be used as well.

III. ALTERNATIVE TECHNICAL APPROACHES (PRO/CON) AND PEARLS

Alternative Approaches

- Hand-assisted laparoscopic radical nephrectomy is an alternative technique combining laparoscopic and open surgery. By the aid of a special access sheath, the surgeon places one hand into the abdominal cavity, making it possible to dissect and hold the renal specimen during laparoscopic dissection. In addition, the hand access port is used at the end of surgery to remove the specimen. For a right-handed surgeon, however, a right radical nephrectomy is difficult to perform, because the dominant hand is in the peritoneal cavity and the surgeon must perform difficult surgical steps with the left hand. The other surgical steps are quite similar to transperitoneal radical nephrectomy as indicated earlier. The only proven advantage of this technique is in patients undergoing live-donor nephrectomy, because ischemia time may be reduced significantly compared to laparoscopic donor nephrectomy.

Pearls

- Modern reusable instruments are more cost effective, but disposables should be available as backup instruments and must be used when infectious diseases (human immunodeficiency virus, hepatitis) are present. Before surgery, all instruments must be checked carefully for any defect; otherwise, significant hemorrhage can occur. Instruments transmitting current should preferably be disposable, but high-quality reusable bipolar dissectors and scissors with disposable blades are available (Richard Wolf).
- After dissection of all renal arteries, continuous urine production must be carefully monitored to check for contralateral urine production. This is of particular importance when multiple vessels are present and dissection is cumbersome. If the contralateral renal artery is accidentally ligated, this may be noticed in time, and immediate reanastomosis of the artery might save the renal unit.

IV. SPECIAL POSTOPERATIVE CARE

- The most common complication after laparoscopic nephrectomy is hemorrhage. Therefore, postoperative red blood cell count and pressure monitoring are mandatory. Fluid production via the drainage tube must also be checked continuously. On postoperative day 1, mobilization of the patient is enforced, the indwelling catheter is removed, and a combination of oral and intravenous fluids are given. On postoperative day 2, wound drainage is removed and bowel function is stimulated. On postoperative day 3, regular alimentation is scheduled. For postoperative pain relief, nonsteroidal analgesics (diclofenac, tramadol) are given intravenously twice daily on the postoperative days 1 and 2 and thereafter orally on demand only.

SUGGESTED READINGS

Allan JDD, Tolley DA, Kaouk JH, et al: Laparoscopic radical nephrectomy, *Eur Urol* 40:17–23, 2001.

Klingler HC, Lodde M, Pycha A, et al: Modified laparoscopic nephroureterectomy for treatment of upper urinary tract transitional cell cancer is not associated with an increased risk of tumour recurrence, *Eur Urol* 44:442–447, 2003.

Nambirajan T, Jeschke S, Al-Zahrani H, et al: Prospective, randomized controlled study: transperitoneal laparoscopic versus retroperitoneoscopic radical nephrectomy, *Urology* 64:919–924, 2004.

SECTION XIII

Gynecology

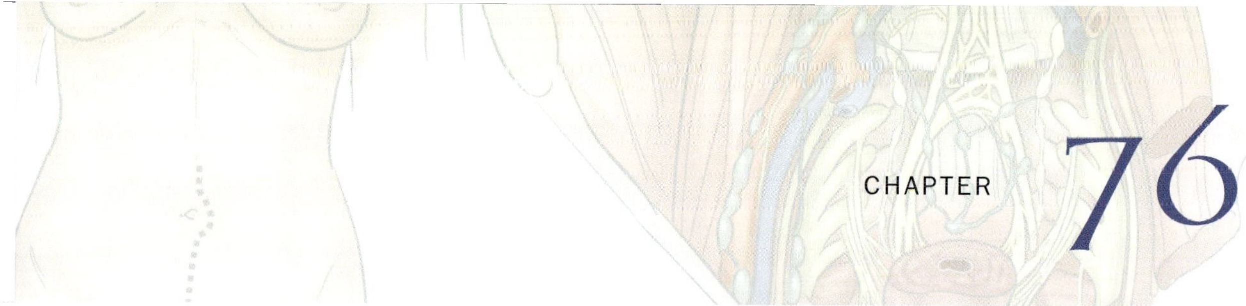

CHAPTER 76

Nerve-Sparing Radical Abdominal Hysterectomy with Regional Lymphadenectomy

Francesco Raspagliesi, MD, and Antonino Ditto, MD

I. SPECIAL PREOPERATIVE PREPARATION

- According to the International Federation of Gynecology and Obstetrics (FIGO), cervical cancer must be staged clinically. However, pretreatment radiologic imaging provides valuable information that aids in diagnosis, defines the local extent of the tumor, and helps in staging of the disease. Plain radiographs are of limited value.
- Ultrasonography is also of limited value. Computed tomography scan (Fig. 76-1) and positron emission tomography scan can be used in the evaluation of lymph node status. The current imaging modality of choice is magnetic resonance imaging (MRI). Understanding the normal anatomy, especially on axial images, allows the surgeon to decipher the abnormal MRI, particularly parametrial status and involved lymph node groups.
- MRI is the preferred imaging modality for cervical cancer, as it can provide multiplanar images with better spatial orientation (Fig. 76-2). Concurrent dynamic postcontrast images can also be obtained that delineate the relationship of the tumor to adjacent paracervical tissue. Behavior of the primary tumor following administration of gadolinium contrast allows differentiation from scar tissue due to neoadjuvant treatment. Dynamic postcontrast images may also help differentiate viable tumor from tumor-associated edema.
- For cervical cancer, chest radiography is performed to look for lung metastases. Computed tomography of the chest should be considered for patients with suspicious images on chest radiography.
- To establish histologic diagnosis, office-based cervical biopsy is appropriate. Its yield can be further enhanced by use of colposcopy in the IA stages, or examination under anesthesia in locally advanced cases. The biopsy provides enough tissue to establish a histologic diagnosis, depth of invasion, and tumor grade.
- If a biopsy reveals nondiagnostic material, then a conization biopsy can be performed on an outpatient basis with local anesthesia, ideally as part of a well-planned treatment strategy.

II. OPERATIVE TECHNIQUE

Position

- The patient is placed in the supine position.

Incision

- A linear median incision is outlined from the umbilicus to the pubic area (Fig. 76-3, *A*). The incision is sometimes oriented longitudinally over the umbilicus to facilitate resection of the lymph nodes of the common iliac region.

Main Dissection

- Once the skin is incised, a Bookwalter retractor is used to maintain retraction of the abdominal wall.
- The principle of the nerve-sparing radical abdominal hysterectomy technique is to resect the uterine support ligaments based on a rational approach that minimizes damage to the pelvic autonomic innervations without compromising oncologic radicality. The Piver-Rutledge class III radical hysterectomy (RH) with pelvic lymph node dissection (PLD) has been modified to spare the nerves at the level of the landmarks referred to later (Fig. 76-3, *B*). These modifications are covered on the following page.

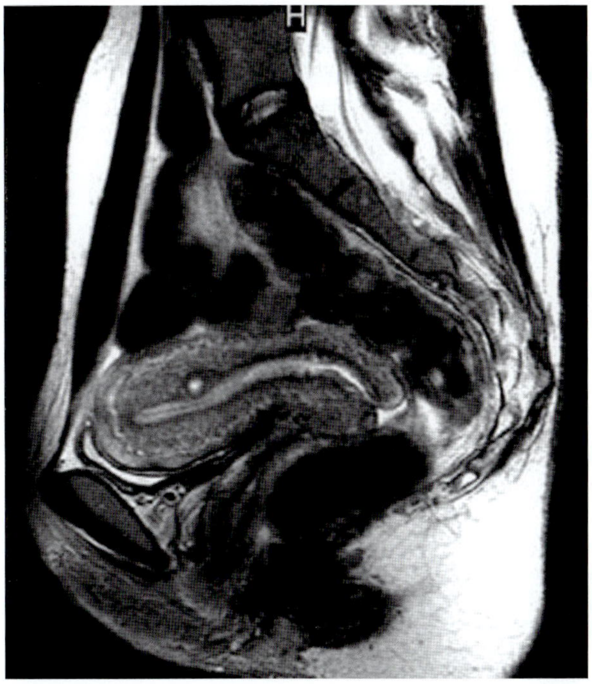

Figure 76-1. Longitudinal cross-sectional image illustrating the normal anatomy of the uterine cervix.

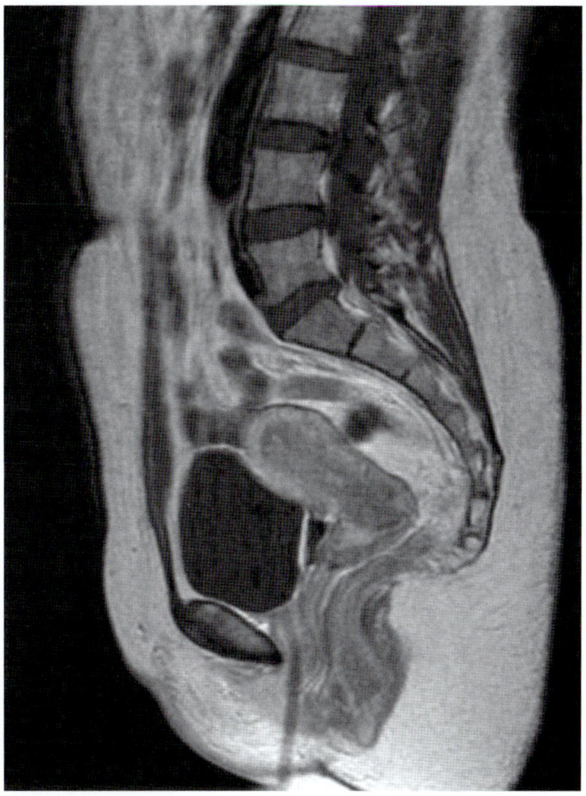

Figure 76-2. Longitudinal cross-sectional magnetic resonance images of a cervical cancer.

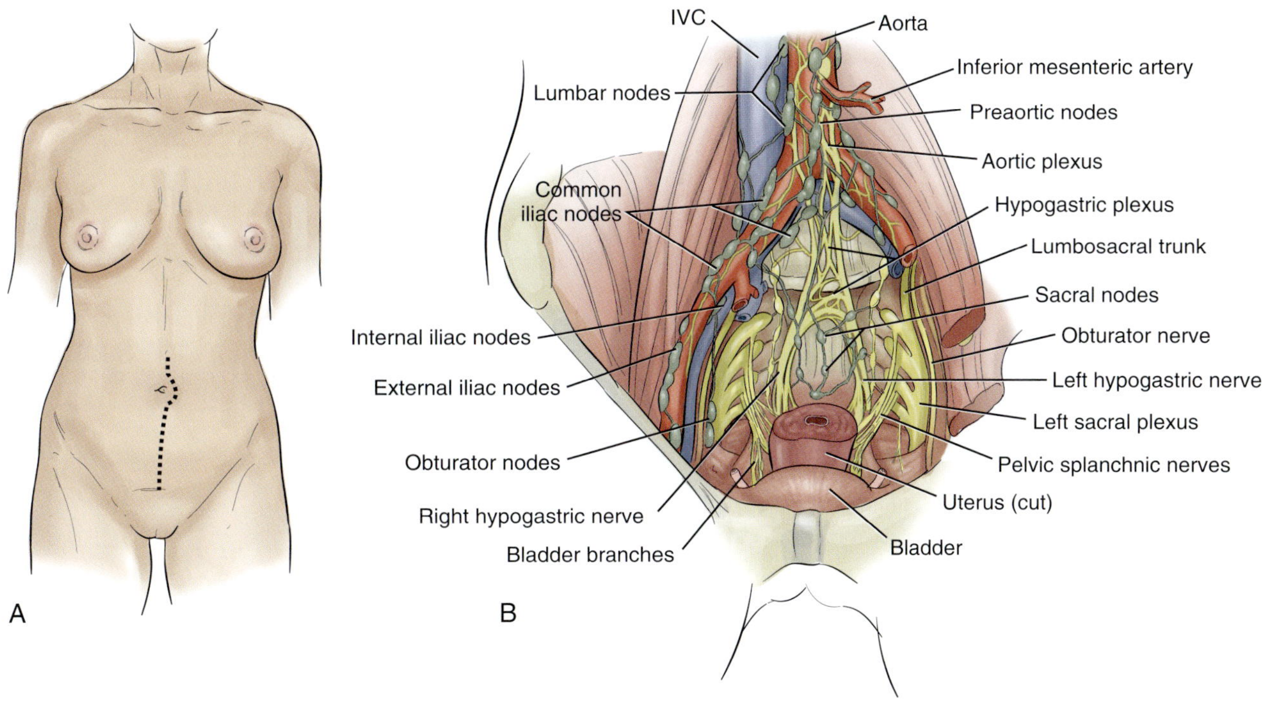

Figure 76-3. *IVC*, Inferior vena cava.

- *Preserving the sympathetic nerves during pelvic lymphadenectomy.* After preparation of the pararectal and paravesical spaces, dissection begins at the origin of the external iliac vessels and continues caudally along the medial border of the psoas muscle. The lower limit of external iliac lymphadenectomy is represented by the deep inferior epigastric vessels. The lateral boundaries of dissection are superficially delineated by the fascia covering the psoas muscle and deeply by the fascia covering the internal obturator and levator ani muscles. The medial margin of the lymphadenectomy is represented by a plane that is parallel to the umbilical artery and is delineated by the umbilicopubic fascia, the bladder, and the rectum. The clearing of the obturator fossa begins with mobilization of the obturator nodes, which are completely dissected after the identification of the upper face of the obturator nerve.
- During the first step of PLD, the sympathetic fibers running over the aorta are identified. The superior hypogastric plexus and medium hypogastric plexus are detached from the aortic bifurcation, presacral nodes, and left common iliac nodes (Fig. 76-4). The dissection continues cranially to detach the fibers from the paraaortic lymph nodes up to the point where the inferior mesenteric artery emerges. Then, the dissection continues caudally down to the origin of the two hypogastric nerves (Fig. 76-5). The uterosacral ligaments (USLs) are divided into lateral and medial layers by blunt dissection, as described by Trimbos and colleagues. As outlined, the lateral layer of the USL contains nerve fibers and the medial layer is fibrous.
- *Preserving the hypogastric nerve and the proximal part of the inferior hypogastric plexus (IHP).* The hypogastric nerve and the initial part of the IHP are situated in the lateral part of the USL. During dissection of the USL and rectal pillars and after incision of the peritoneum of the Douglas pouch, the prerectal space is developed by blunt dissection (Fig. 76-6). The USLs between the prerectal and the pararectal

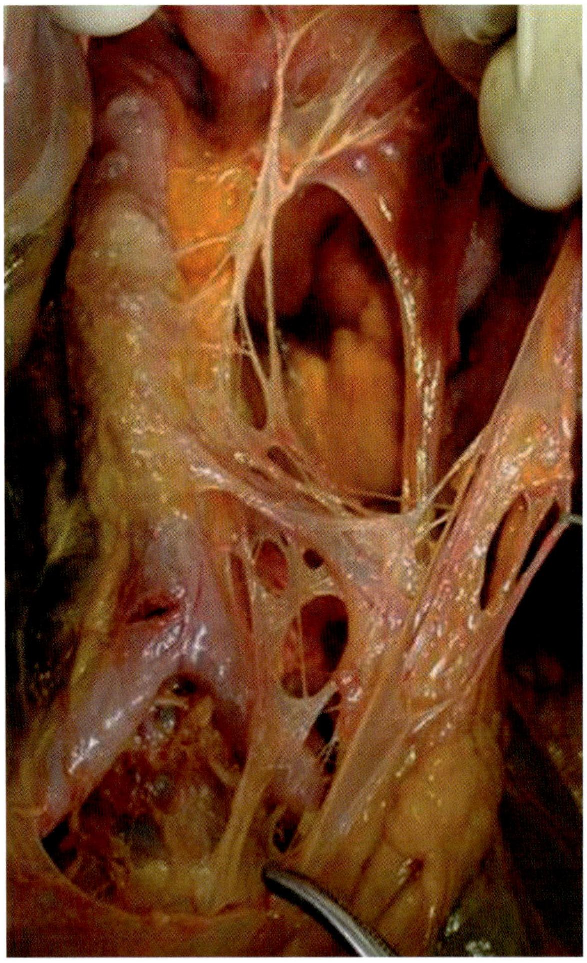

Figure 76-4.

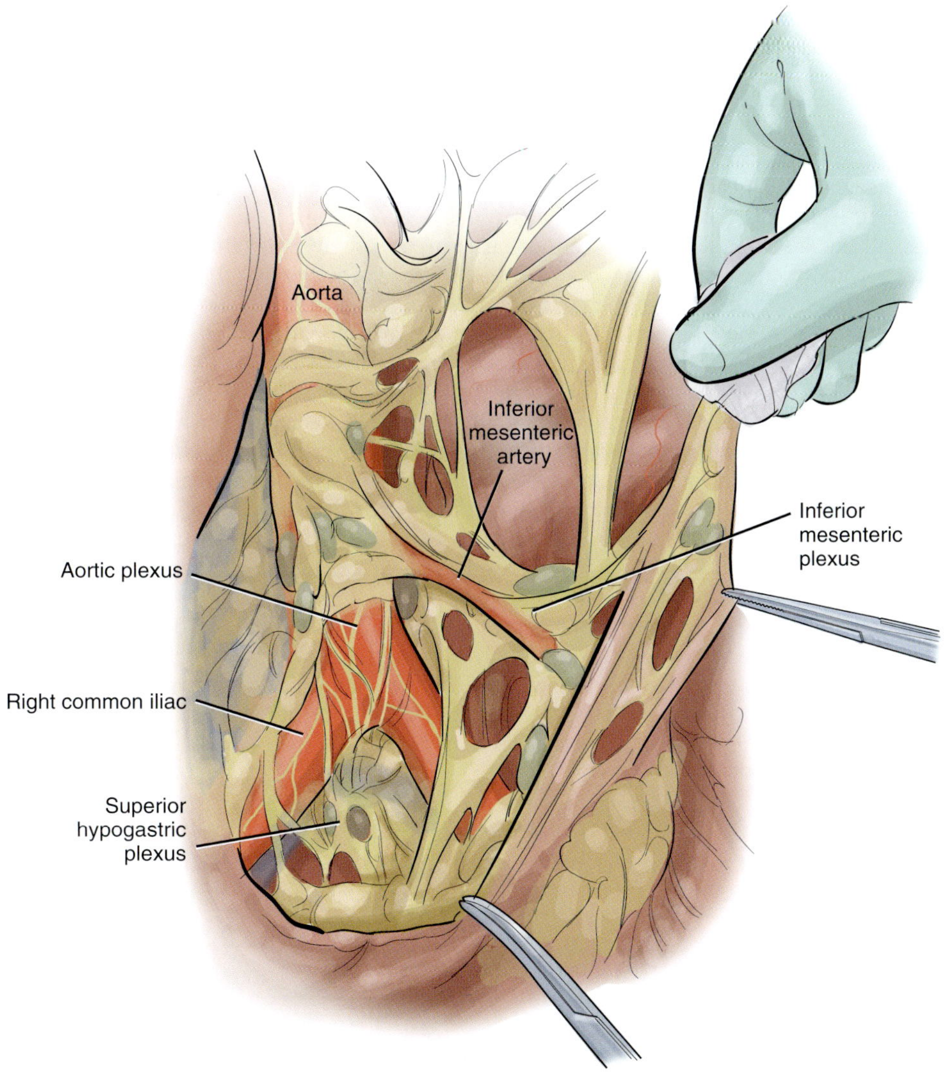

Figure 76-5.

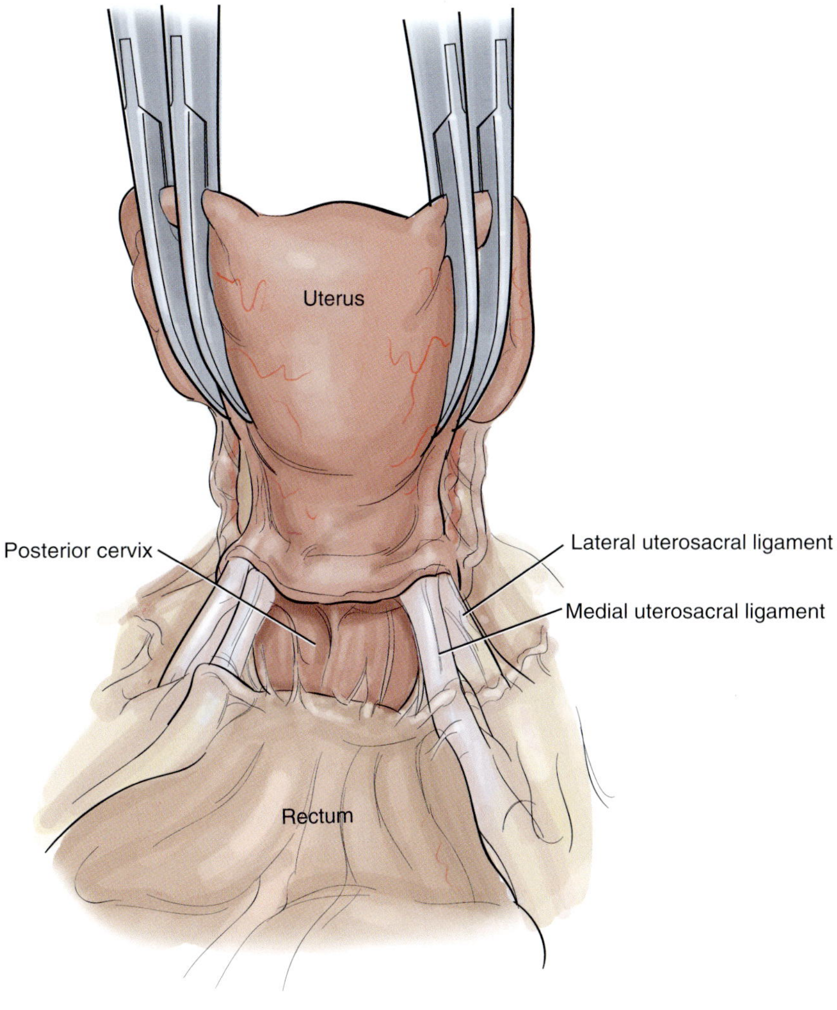

Figure 76-6.

spaces are identified. The medial USLs are separated from the lateral nerve fibers (Fig. 76-7). The medial ligaments are resected, whereas the lateral parts are saved. This maneuver preserves the terminal part of the hypogastric nerve and the cranial part of the IHP (see Fig. 76-5).

- *Preserving the pelvic splanchnic nerves and middle part of the IHP.* The cardinal ligaments (CLs) are dissected and cut close to the pelvic wall with the assistance of a hemoclip, according to the technique of Burghardt and co-workers. All the vascular structures (venous, arterial, and lymphatic) that constitute the CL are isolated. After isolation, these structures are clamped with hemoclips. All the vessels are cut, and the loose connective tissue attached to the pelvic sidewall is removed radically along with the CL. Unfortunately, during this step some fibers of the first group of parasympathetic fibers that run along the dorsomedial section of the CL are inevitably sacrificed.
- The caudal part of the IHP runs along the lateral vaginal wall (Fig. 76-8). The ureter tunnel is developed in the usual fashion, and the anterior part of the vesicovaginal ligament (VVL) is cut. After further dissection of the ureter, the fibers in the lateral vaginal wall are first identified, and then the posterior part of the VVL is cut. To clarify the anatomy of the vesicouterine ligament, it can be meticulously separated under magnification (2.5×) during Okabayashi RH. A precise network of blood vessels in the vesicouterine ligament is identified. Knowledge and meticulous dissection of this anatomy creates a safe RH and reduces blood loss during the operation. This anatomic knowledge aids in performing the nerve-sparing technique during RH.
- *Preserving the distal part of the IHP.* After dissecting the VVL, nerve fibers (bladder branches) located along the lateral vaginal wall are identified, and the CL from the paracolpium is resected, detaching it from the vaginal fornix. The CLs are pulled up, maintaining slight tension to uncover the fibers that extend from the IHP to the base of the bladder (Fig. 76-9). The nerve fibers along the vaginal fornix for about 2 cm are gently moved down. Nerve fibers from the IHP run beside the lateral wall of the

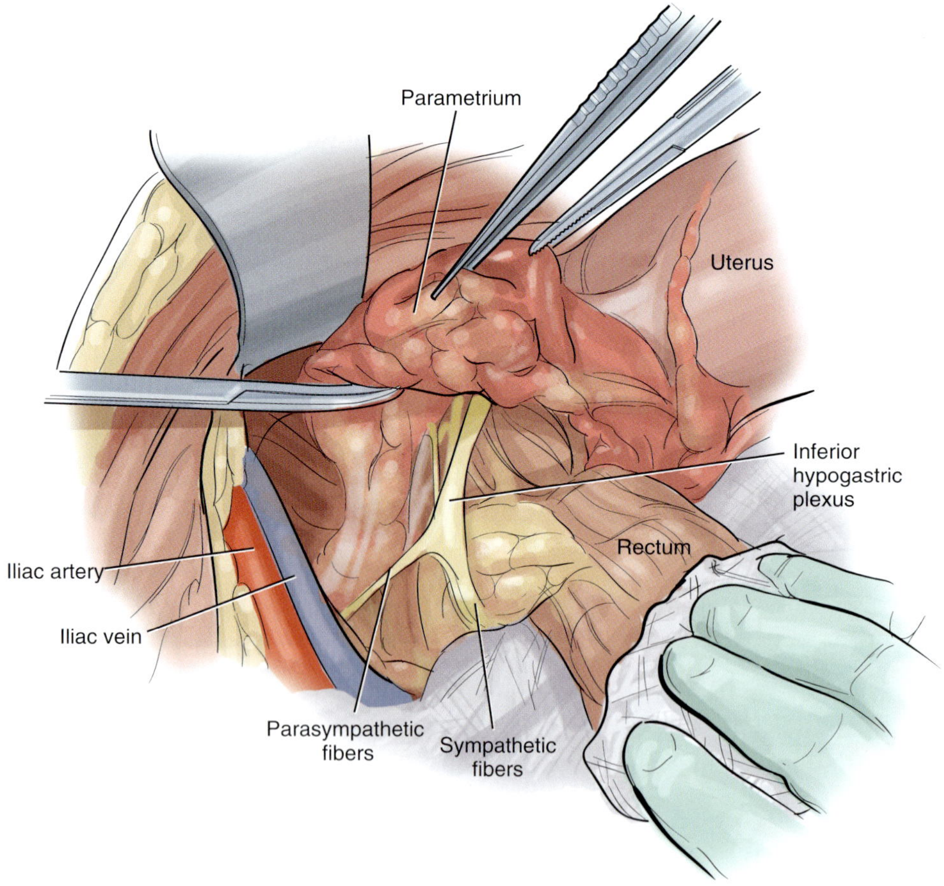

Figure 76-7.

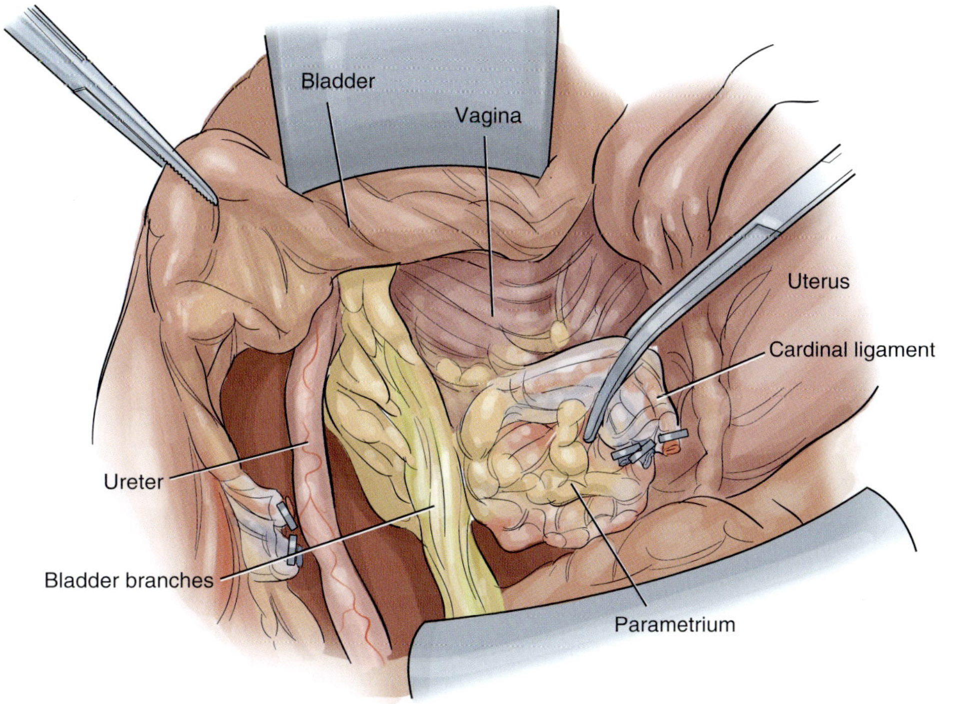

Figure 76-8.

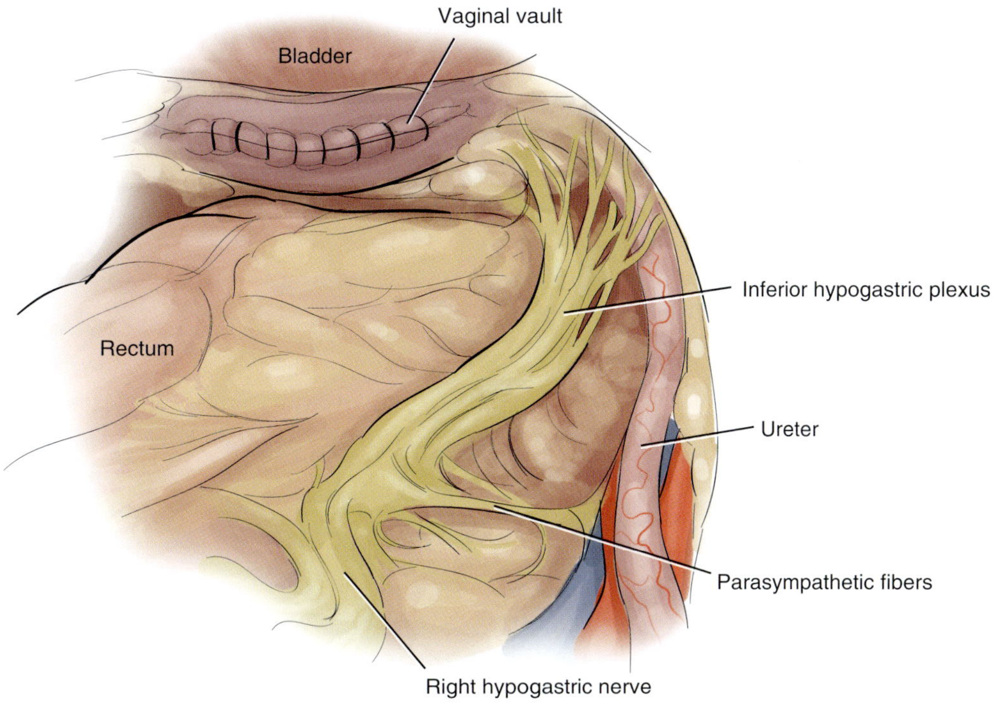

Figure 76-9.

vagina to the bladder, and these are preserved during this step in surgery, restricting the level of colpectomy to 2 cm below the cervix instead of resecting the cranial half of the vagina (Fig. 76-10). After this step, the pelvic plexus is completely identifiable.

Closure

- After hemostasis is obtained, one drain is placed in the Douglas pouch and secured with 3-0 nonabsorbable monofilament suture.
- The fascia of the rectus abdominis muscle is closed with a 1-0 absorbable monofilament suture.
- The dermis is then carefully approximated with 2-0 absorbable suture, and the skin is closed with staples.

III. ALTERNATIVE TECHNICAL APPROACHES (PRO/CON) AND PEARLS

- There is a growing body of data on nerve-sparing RH in cervical cancer. However, to date there is no consensus regarding the area of the uterine support ligaments to which a nerve-sparing approach should be directed, in part because of fragmentary knowledge of pelvic and urogenital neuroanatomy.
- Hockel and associates studied the topographic anatomy of the parametrial tissue with high-resolution MRI and by dissection of fresh human cadavers. The perispinous adipose tissue contains the pelvic plexus, the pelvic splanchnic nerves, small blood vessels, and lymphatic tissue. They performed a liposuction-assisted nerve-sparing abdominal RH technique. Hockel stated that nerve-sparing removal of perispinous adipose tissue by liposuction is a feasible addition to wide en bloc parametrectomy in anatomically defined planes.
- Possover and colleagues have investigated the parasympathetic innervations of the bladder in the CL in patients undergoing laparoscopically assisted class III radical vaginal hysterectomy. During laparoscopic dissection of the CL, the middle rectal artery is identified as a landmark separating the vascular from the neural part of the CL. The CL is completely freed of all lymphatic and fat tissue by blunt dissection, and all vessels of the vascular part are identified, recognizing the border between the last vessels of the vascular part of the CL and the first branches of the pelvic splanchnic nerves. Thereafter,

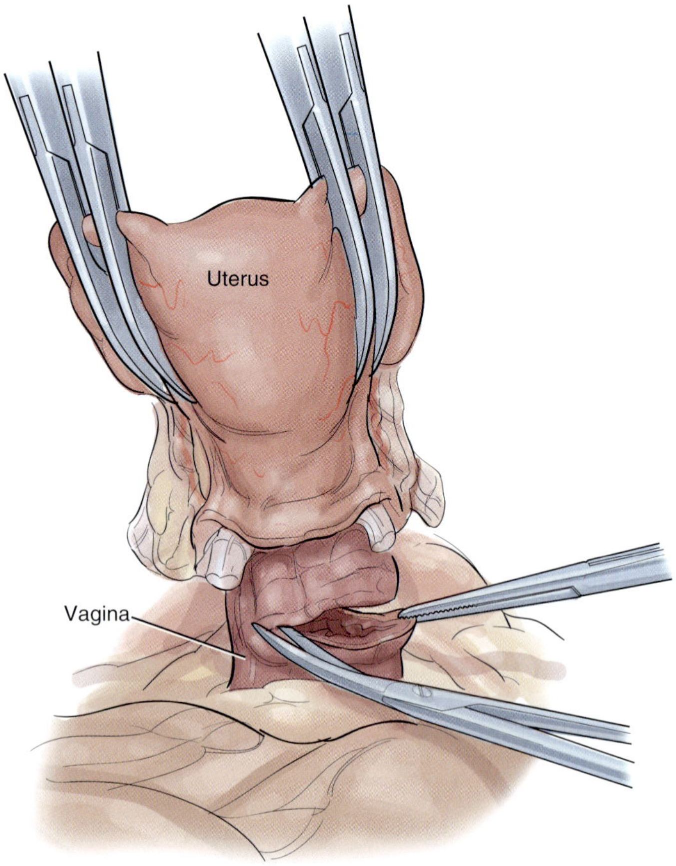

Figure 76-10.

the neural part of the CL is freed of fat and lymphatic tissue anteriorly. After bipolar coagulation, the vascular part of the CL is divided as laterally as possible at the pelvic sidewall, including the middle rectal vessels. The pelvic splanchnic nerves are completely exposed and preserved. Then, the operation is completed transvaginally.

- Trimbos and co-workers introduced elements of the Japanese nerve-sparing techniques and carried out a feasibility study. The following surgical steps help prevent surgical damage to the pelvic autonomic nerves during RH and are performed in sequence during the course of the operation. The sacrouterine dissection plane separates the medial ligamentous tissue (USL) and the lateral nerve fibers. The USL can then be safely clamped, cut, and ligated without damaging the hypogastric nerve or proximal part of the IHP. Dividing the parametrium unites the paravesical and pararectal spaces. In a frontal section through the parametrium, two separate parts can be distinguished: an upper part containing vascular structures, fat, and loose connective tissue; and a lower part that feels tight on palpation and contains denser connective tissue and the nerve fibers of the middle part of the IHP. To avoid the IHP, the dissection follows the shape of the bow of a ship from a lateroventral to a mediodorsal position.
- Surgeons variously use an ultrasonic surgical aspirator, liposuction, laparoscopy, and sharp or blunt dissection to clear the ligament from the nerves. These different approaches hamper the wide application of the method, which in turn could represent an obstacle to the conduction of randomized controlled studies.

IV. SPECIAL POSTOPERATIVE CARE

- Preventive intraoperative ureteral stenting positioned with cystoscopy can be used to minimize the likelihood of ureteral fistulas.
- Specific intraoperative complications that may be encountered with nerve-sparing RH plus PLD are obturator nerve injury, injury to superficial genitofemoral nerves, and injury to pelvic vessels.
- Specific immediate postoperative complications that may be encountered with nerve-sparing RH plus PLD are infection, wound disruption, hematoma, pelvic bleeding, neuropathic pain, deep vein thrombosis, neurogenic bladder, and intestinal slow-transit constipation.
- Specific delayed complications that might be encountered with nerve-sparing radical abdominal hysterectomy plus PLD are lymphedema, lymph cyst, ureteral fistulas, neurogenic bladder, and slow-transit constipation.
- Subcutaneous heparin injection as prophylaxis for deep vein thrombosis should be used the day before the procedure and continued for 30 days. Early ambulation is advisable. Brief preoperative antibiotic prophylaxis is also advisable.
- Staples should be left for at least 7 days to avoid wound disruption that might delay postoperative radiation therapy.

SUGGESTED READINGS

Possover M, Stober S, Plaul K, Schneider A: Identification and preservation of the motoric innervation of the bladder in radical hysterectomy type III, *Gynecol Oncol* 79:154–157, 2000.

Raspagliesi F, Ditto A, Fontanelli R, et al: Nerve-sparing radical hysterectomy: a surgical technique for preserving the autonomic hypogastric nerve, *Gynecol Oncol* 93:307–314, 2004.

Trimbos JB, Maas CP, Deruiter MC, et al: A nerve-sparing radical hysterectomy: guidelines and feasibility in Western patients, *Int J Gynecol Cancer* 11:180–186, 2001.

CHAPTER 77

Radical Vulvectomy with Groin Dissection

Francesco Raspagliesi, MD, and Francesco Hanozet, MD

I. SPECIAL PREOPERATIVE PREPARATION

- A biopsy should be performed when any lesion of the vulva is discovered.
- For squamous cell carcinoma of the vulva that's been confirmed with a biopsy, the resectability of the lesion should be assessed. If the lesion involves the upper urethra or anus or cannot be completely resected because of fixation to the pelvic bone, neoadjuvant radiation and chemotherapy should be considered before surgical intervention. This type of therapy can allow future resection with preservation of the urethral or rectal sphincter in most cases.
- Imaging studies other than routine chest radiographs have not been helpful in the evaluation of women with vulvar carcinoma, except to evaluate specific symptoms or nodal enlargement.
- A computed tomography scan may be useful to help evaluate nodal spread in the pelvis in women with evidence of groin node metastasis, but the sensitivity of such scans for detection of pelvic lymphadenopathy is approximately 30%. Because of the low sensitivity of imaging in detecting pelvic-node metastases, some authors have suggested laparoscopic assessment of the pelvic lymph nodes as an alternative (Figs. 77-1 and 77-2).
- Positron emission tomography (PET) scanning holds some promise in improving the sensitivity of detecting small nodal metastases. However, no report documents the sensitivity or specificity of PET scan findings in persons with vulvar carcinoma.

II. OPERATIVE TECHNIQUE: GROIN

Position

- The patient is placed supine with the thighs wide apart at approximately 45 degrees, slightly externally rotated to better expose the adductor longus muscle by placing it in a horizontal position to the plane of the Scarpa triangle, and lowered approximately 10 to 15 degrees with respect to the plane of the operating table. The knees can be extended or flexed.

Incision

- The groin incision is performed using an elliptical incision parallel to and approximately 1 cm below the inguinal ligament from the anterosuperior iliac spine to the pubic tubercle (Fig. 77-3, *A* and *B*).

Main Dissection

- Once the skin is incised, the inguinal ligament flap is developed by undermining the superficial fascia, kept on traction, for approximately 2 cm above the inguinal ligament, to reach the aponeurosis of the external oblique muscle. During this procedure, the superficial epigastric vessels are encountered, secured by diathermy or ligature, and sectioned. The dissection is extended medially to reach the pubic

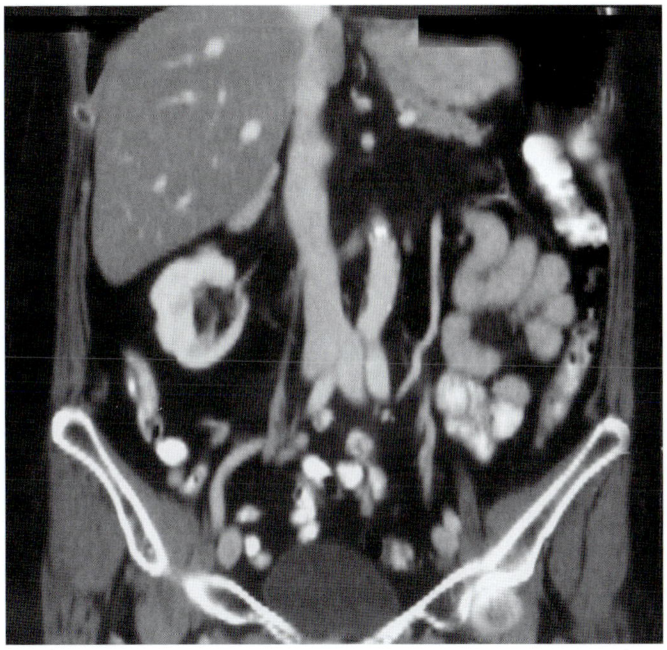

Figure 77-1. Sagittal cross-sectional computed tomography image illustrating inguinal and pelvic adenopathy.

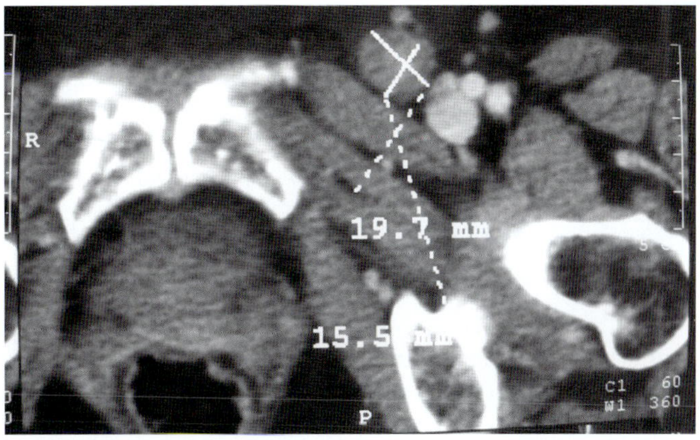

Figure 77-2. Axial cross-sectional computed tomography image illustrating inguinal and pelvic adenopathy.

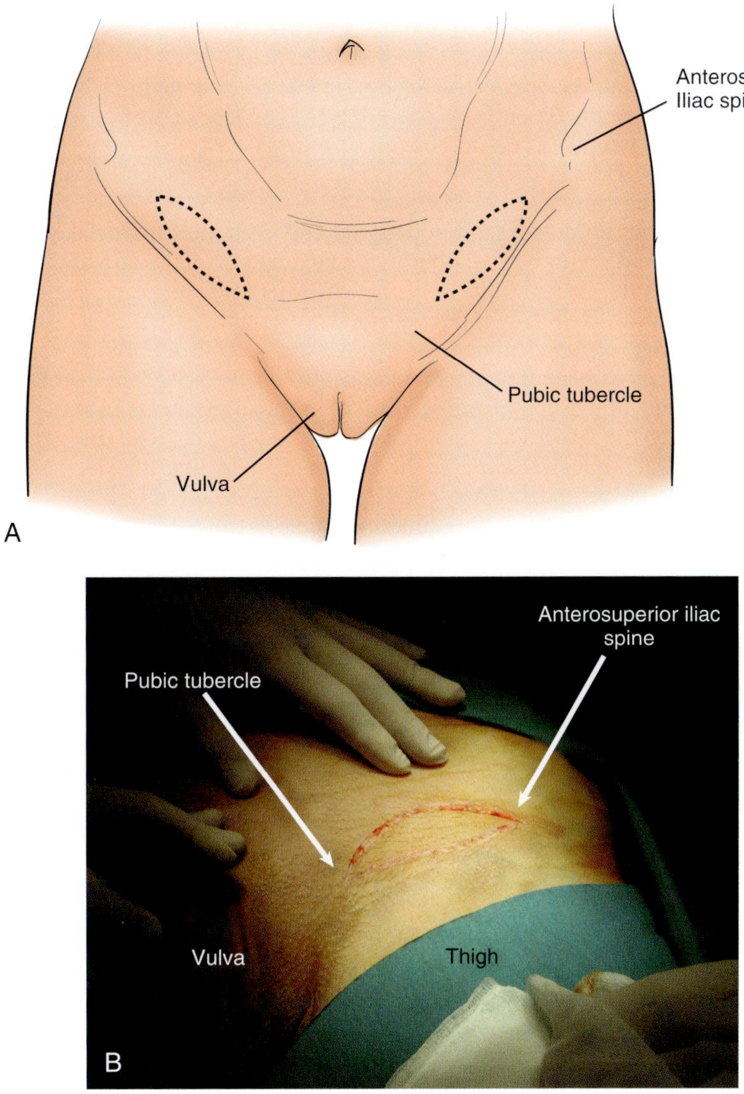

Figure 77-3.

tubercle, encountering the round ligament, and then laterally in the direction of the anterosuperior iliac spine, stopping when the superficial circumflex iliac vessels are encountered. These vessels represent the surgical landmark for stopping the lateral extent of the inguinal dissection. At this point, through a combination of blunt and sharp dissection, approximately 2 cm above the inguinal ligament, the fatty and fibrous tissue containing the superficial inguinal nodes is detached from the external oblique muscle aponeurosis to the plane where the inguinal ligament encounters the femoral fascia (Figs. 77-4 and 77-5, *A*).

- The lateral flap of the Scarpa triangle is developed along the medial border of the sartorius muscle fascia, which must be preserved; it marks the lateral boundary of the dissection. The deep dissection should not be carried too far laterally, identifying the medial portion of the sartorius muscle fascia and avoiding important bleeding. Moving medially, attention must be paid to the dissection of the tissue above the portion of the femoral fascia, from the medial border of the sartorius muscle to the lateral border of the fossa ovalis. Dissection then moves medially and downward to the apex of the Scarpa triangle. Using sharp and blunt dissection, it is easy to detach the lateral portion of the tissue containing the saphenous vein and the superficial femoral nodes overlying the femoral fascia (see Fig. 77-5).
- The medial flap of the Scarpa triangle is developed along the lateral border of the adductor longus muscle fascia, which must be preserved and marks the medial boundary of the dissection. Care must be taken not to carry the dissection too far medially. The deep dissection is continued to identify the lateral portion of the adductor longus muscle fascia. Moving laterally and downward, using sharp and blunt dissection, the great saphenous vein is suddenly encountered and can be detached from the underlying femoral fascia with the surrounding superficial femoral lymph nodes (Fig. 77-6).
- The apex of the Scarpa triangle is developed using blunt dissection with a small gauze swab, taking advantage of the natural plane of cleavage to create a tunnel between the femoral fascia and the tissue containing the saphenous veins. By placing the forefinger in the tunnel and slightly upward, and grasping, it is easy to dissect the block of tissue and avoid damage to the femoral fascia. The great and accessory saphenous veins are isolated and preserved. The block of adipose tissue containing the nodes surrounding the great saphenous vein is then separated from the vein, moving toward the inferior margin of the fossa ovalis.
- The medial angle of the Scarpa triangle is developed, moving cranially to the pubic tubercle, along the adductor longus fascia, via blunt dissection with a small gauze swab, taking advantage of the natural plane of cleavage. To facilitate the surgical dissection, a tunnel is created close to the pubic tubercle, between the adductor longus fascia and the overlying tissue. The dissection can then start from the pubic tubercle to free all lymphatic tissue above the femoral fascia, moving laterally to the medial border of the fossa ovalis. During this procedure, the superficial pudendal vessels are isolated and secured by diathermy or ligature.
- The lateral angle of the Scarpa triangle is developed, moving from the superficial circumflex iliac vessels (which are now isolated and secured by diathermy or ligature) medially and slightly downward along the inguinal ligament and the cranial portion of the sartorius fascia to reach the upper portion of the lateral border of the fossa ovalis, freeing the lymph nodes along the superficial circumflex iliac vessels. Care must be taken during this dissection because there are several perforating vessels, which may be exposed and secured to avoid bleeding and retraction of these vessels under the femoral fascia.
- The surgical development of the fossa ovalis consists in grasping and elevating the entire block of adipose tissue containing the superficial inguinofemoral nodes such that the portion of the femoral vein within the fossa ovalis is better exposed. It is now easy to free the deep femoral nodes, lying medially to the femoral vein, through careful scissors dissection, moving from the inferior border of the falciform ligament to the level of the inguinal ligament. During this procedure, the medial aspect of the lamina cribrosa is removed, and the lateral aspect covering the femoral artery is left intact. At

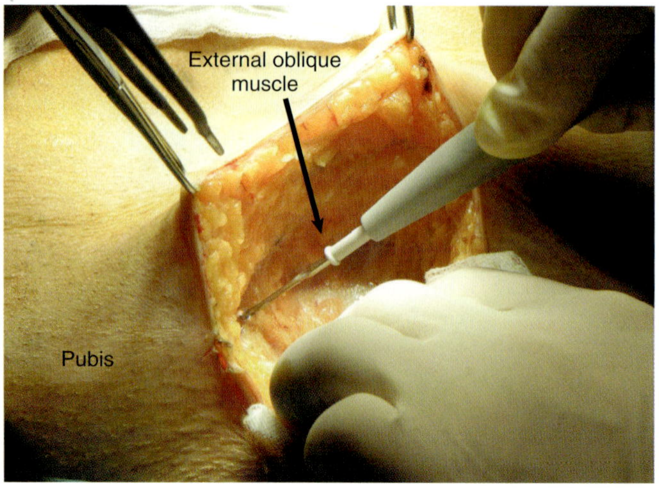

Figure 77-4.

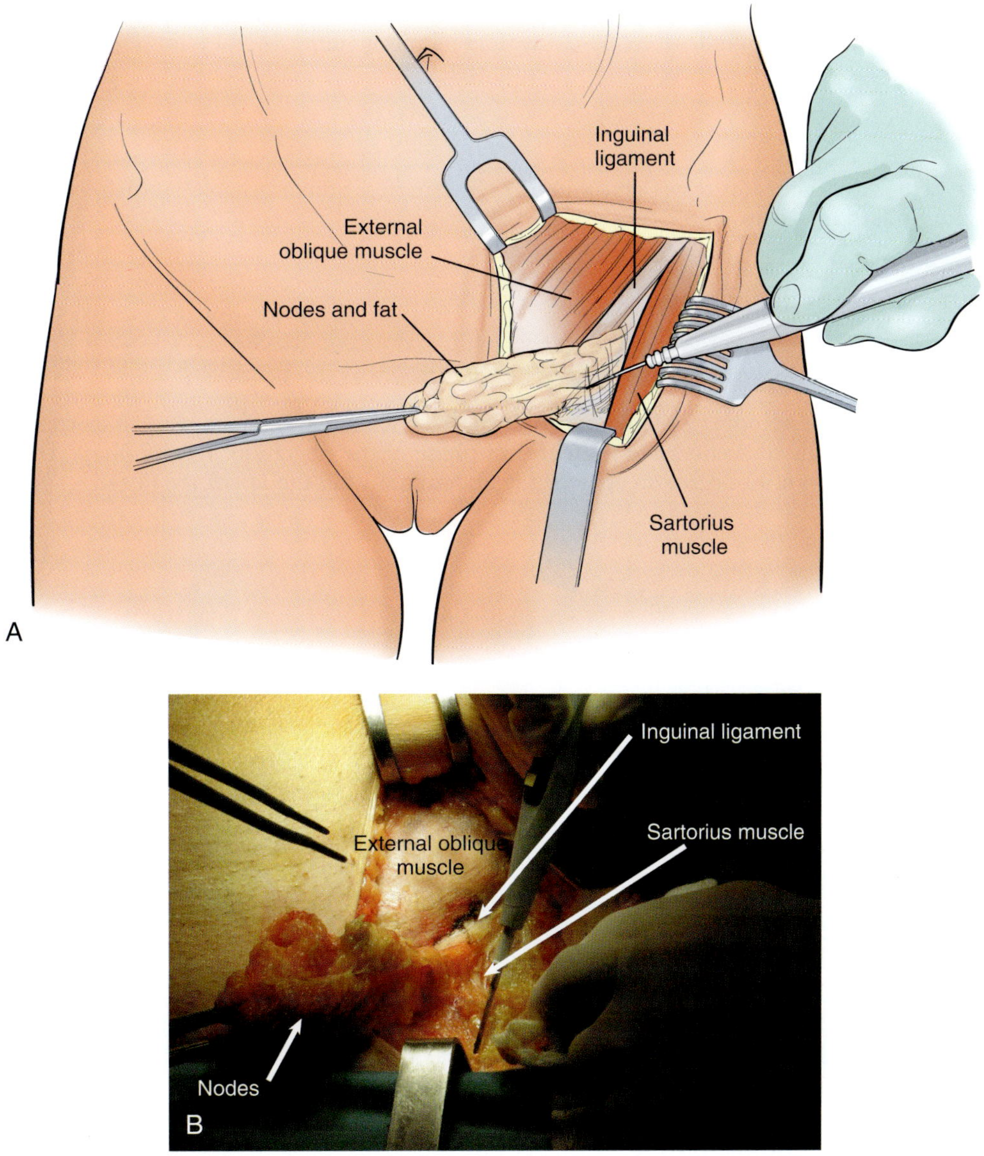

Figure 77-5.

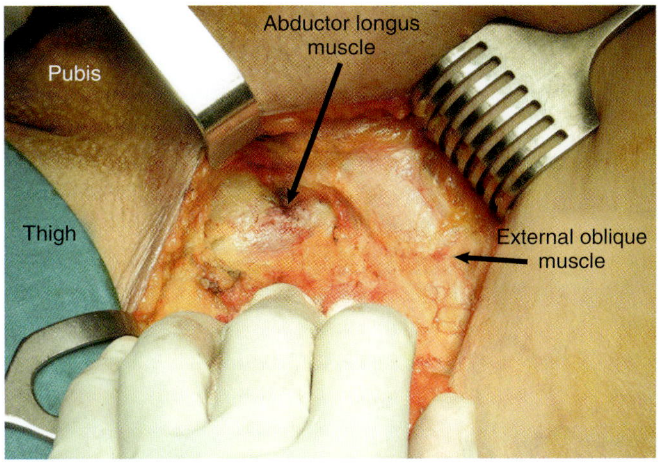

Figure 77-6.

this point, the entrance of the great saphenous vein into the femoral vein is exposed. It is now possible to remove en bloc the bundle of tissue containing all the inguinofemoral lymph nodes (Fig. 77-7).

Closure

- After hemostasis, the skin edges are united by interrupted nonabsorbable sutures, such as Prolene. Suction drains are left in place.

III. OPERATIVE TECHNIQUE: VULVA

Position

- Surgery for vulvar carcinoma is often performed with the woman's legs in adjustable stirrups to facilitate both the groin node dissection and the perineal phase of the operation. In this phase, the thighs are abducted and form a 90-degree angle with the abdominal wall; the knees are flexed.

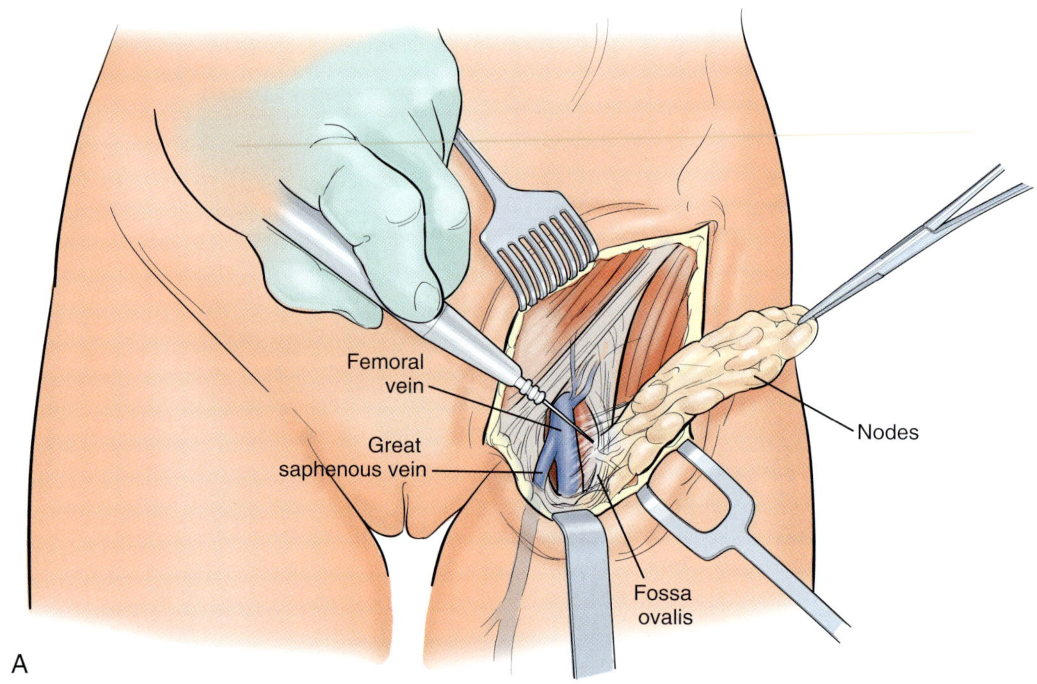

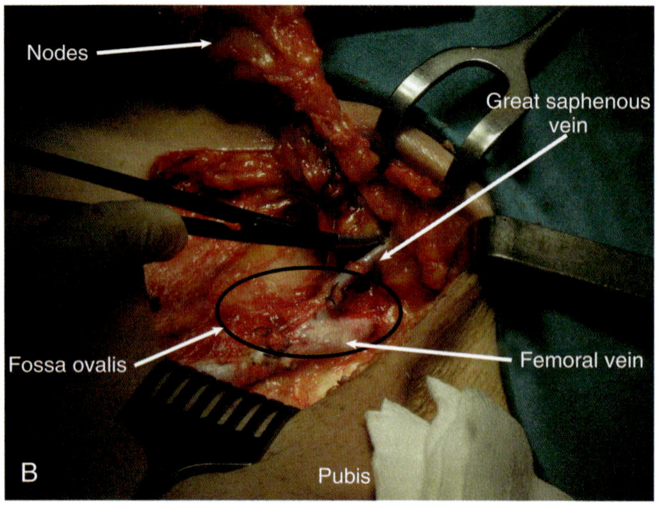

Figure 77-7.

Incision

- The radical vulvectomy incisions are placed according to the location and size of the primary tumor. The surgeon should attempt to obtain a 2-cm margin of normal tissue around the tumor in all directions. However, a 1-cm margin is reasonable around the urethral meatus, clitoris, and anus, to preserve the structures and their function (Fig. 77-8).

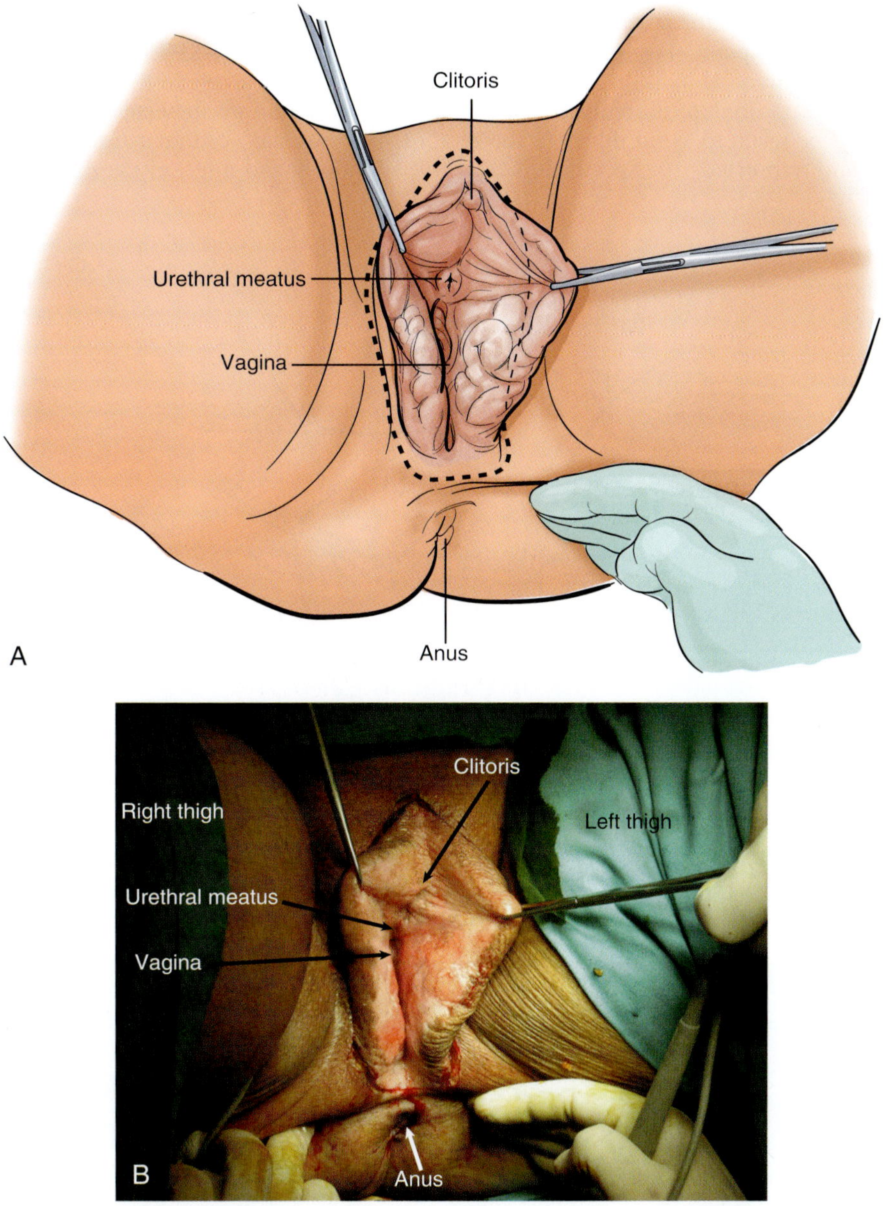

Figure 77-8.

Main Dissection

- The labiocrural incisions are carried through the fatty tissue bilaterally; extension through the tissue is necessary to the level of the deep fascia of the urogenital diaphragm bilaterally, and this is usually performed with electrocautery (Fig. 77-9). Care should be taken to identify the internal pudendal vessels; these can be individually clamped, transected, and ligated. Inferiorly, the perineal body and posterior vulvar tissue are dissected from the anus.
- Superiorly, the specimen is dissected off the pubic periosteum; the dissection is continued in this manner inferiorly. The lateral portions of this part of the procedure are also taken deeply until the adductor fascia is encountered.
- The dissection of the superior portion of the vulva continues medially and laterally to expose the pubic periosteum and adductor fascia bilaterally. The base of the clitoris is identified, clamped, transected, and ligated at this point (Fig. 77-10). The dissection is completed and joined medially by making a transvestibular mucosal incision above the urethra.
- Inferiorly, the portions of the vulvar tissue along the perineum are dissected upward to the vagina; care should be taken to avoid injury to the rectum. The vascular vestibular tissue along the vagina is clamped and transected. The specimen is now free superiorly and inferiorly, and removal of the vulva is complete.

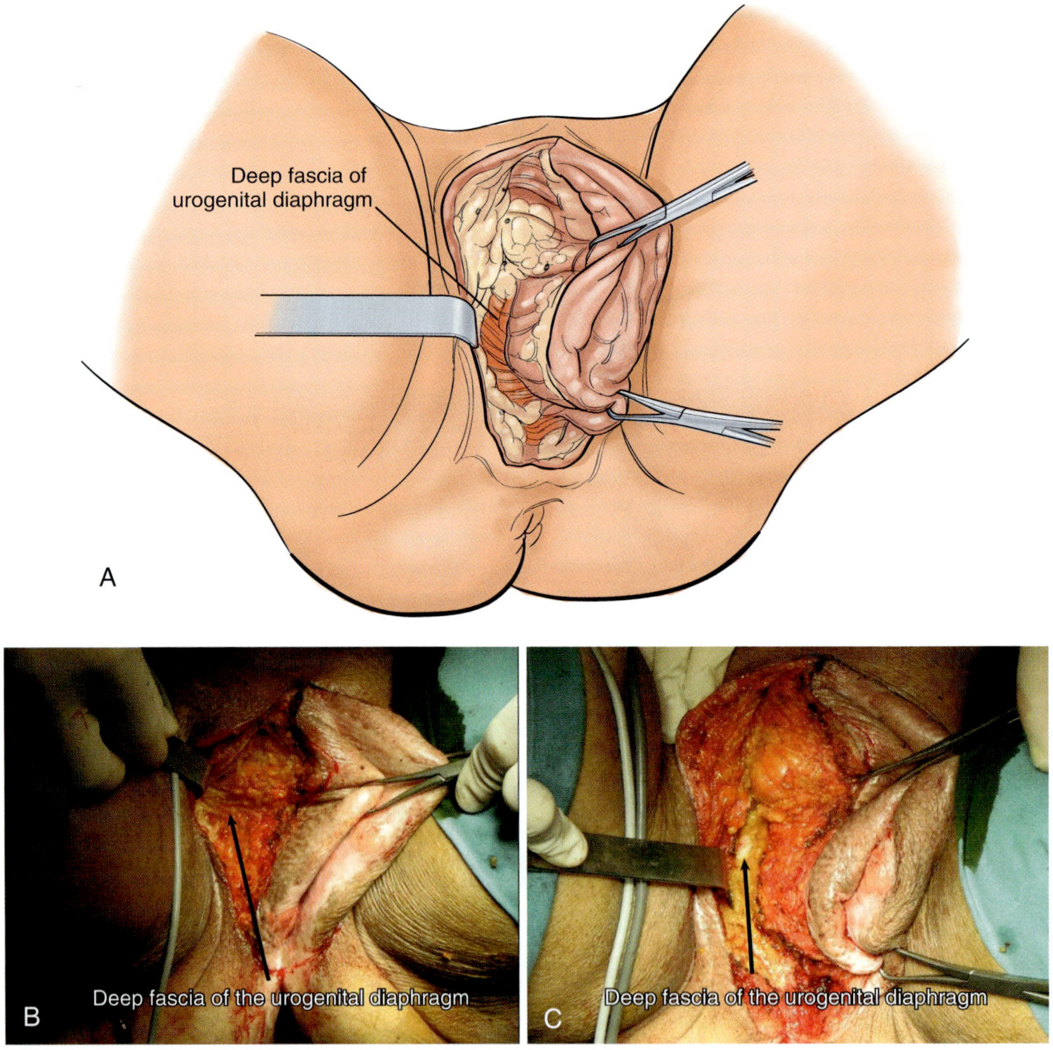

Figure 77-9.

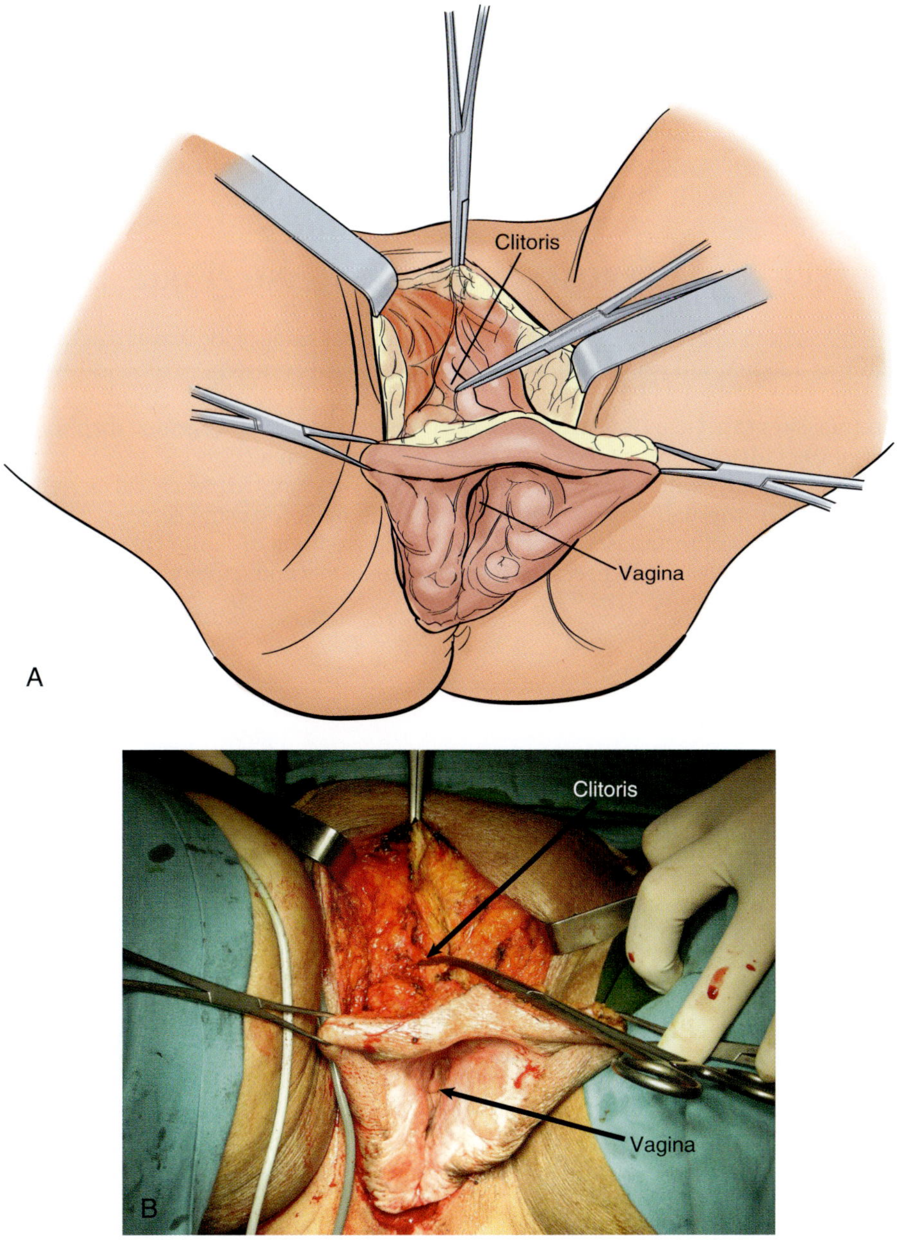

Figure 77-10.

Closure

- The edges of the wound and the perineum are closed with vertical mattress sutures. The urethra should be secured on a straight course without tension. The vaginal edges should be everted over the perineum and anus (Fig. 77-11). In some instances, such as when a large defect is present or the patient has had prior radiation, a primary tension-free closure is not possible; it may be necessary to use a myocutaneous flap to provide healthy tissue with adequate blood supply.

IV. ALTERNATIVE TECHNICAL APPROACHES (PRO/CON) AND PEARLS

- Great effort has been devoted to decreasing the morbidity of surgery for vulvar carcinoma. A less radical approach was adopted following the discovery that the local recurrence risk was low when the pathologic margin around the primary lesion was 8 mm. Taking into account shrinkage during tissue fixation, this translates to a 1-cm clinical margin. Deep dissection to the urogenital diaphragm is performed, but most of the vulva can be spared if the primary lesion is small.
- A decrease in morbidity without compromising survival was reported when vulvar and inguinal surgeries were performed through separate incisions. The rationale for using separate incisions is based on the mechanism of nodal metastases, which arise from the emboli of tumor cells. In comparative studies of en bloc vulvectomy/lymphadenectomy versus separate-incision surgery, the use of separate incisions

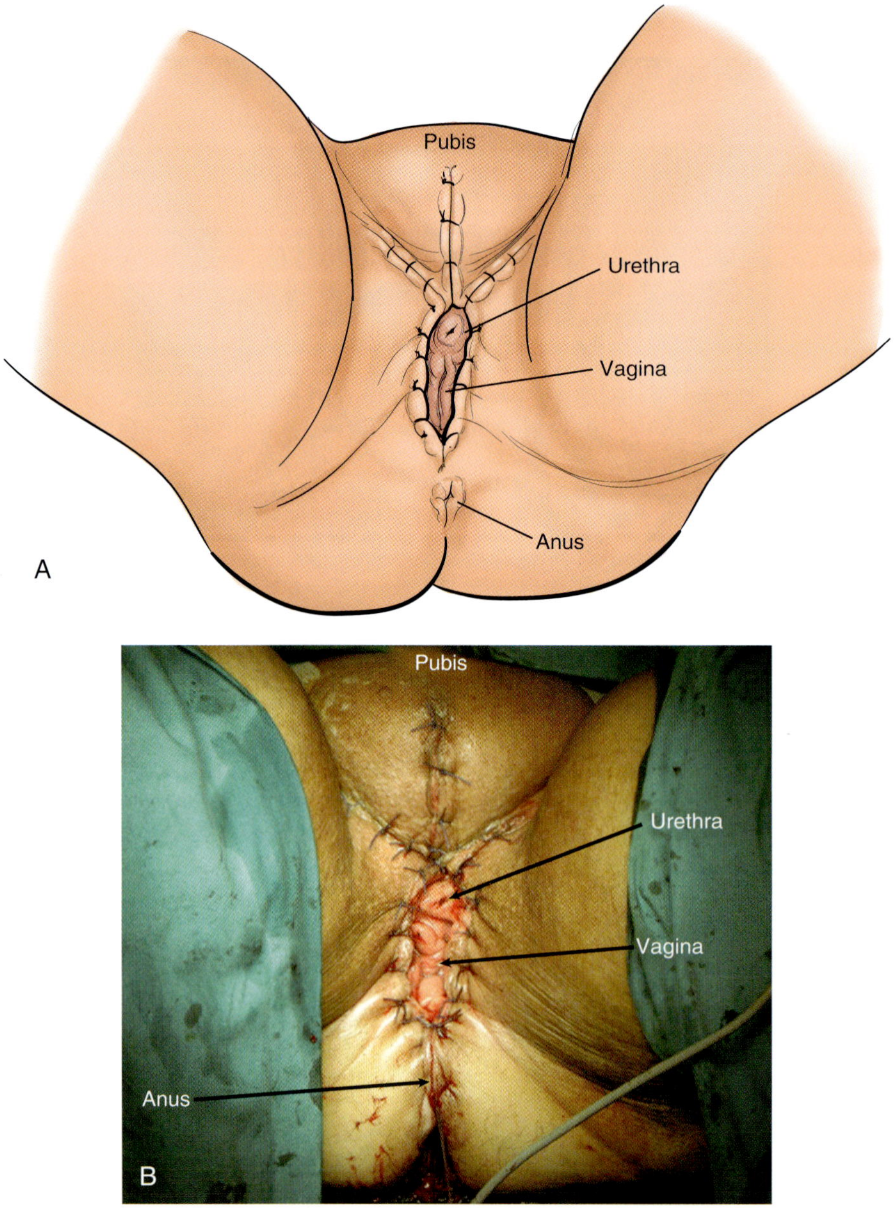

Figure 77-11.

resulted in less morbidity than was seen with en bloc resection. Nonetheless, some reports of skin bridge metastasis may favor the use of en bloc resection in cases of bulky metastatic nodes.

- Concerning inguinofemoral management, the standard procedure for lymph node dissection consists of the removal of all superficial inguinal nodes and the femoral nodes medial to the femoral vein. This procedure does not require removal of the fascia lata and great saphenous vein. In fact, preservation of these structures decreases postoperative morbidity. Nonetheless, in cases of bulky nodal disease, the removal of the fascia lata and great saphenous vein is necessary, and en bloc incision is a legitimate procedure.
- In lateralized tumors, lymph node metastases are generally ipsilateral, and isolated contralateral metastases are rare. Tumors with a medial margin 0.1 cm from the midline structures are lateralized lesions; all other tumors are medial. Lateralized tumors can be treated with unilateral lymphadenectomy if there is no pathologic involvement of ipsilateral nodes. Therefore, adequate treatment may require an additional procedure if the diagnosis of nodal metastasis is made postoperatively.
- Sentinel lymph node biopsy is a promising technique. The main problem is that, although the first reports demonstrated a high accuracy, further studies reported false-negative cases. Because it yields a poor outcome, groin relapse after a negative sentinel lymph node biopsy is of concern and suggests that long-term follow-up data are required before lymphatic mapping and sentinel lymph node biopsy alone can be considered standard treatment for patients with squamous cell carcinoma.

V. SPECIAL POSTOPERATIVE CARE

- After surgery, frequent sitz baths are recommended. Patients should dry the vulva completely after each sitz bath. A Foley catheter may be needed for a prolonged period after surgery around the urethra. Heparin should be used in all women to prevent postoperative venous thrombosis. Drains should be placed at the time of lymphadenectomy because of the flow through the groin lymphatics. These drains should be left in place until drainage is approximately 25 mL or less per day. In many cases, this may take more than 2 weeks.
- Lymphocyst formation is noted in 7% to 19% of patients after groin lymphadenectomy. Lymphocysts usually manifest as an asymptomatic mass in the groin. Multiple aspirations are often required.
- Cellulitis and lymphangitis can occur after groin node dissection. The incidence rate of cellulitis requiring antibiotics ranges from 20% to 40%. The etiologic agent is most often a streptococcal species, and treatment with penicillin is adequate. If drains are still in place, first-generation cephalosporins may be more appropriate to cover *Staphylococcus aureus*.
- Chronic lymphedema has been reported in 10% to 20% of women after groin node dissection. This problem is more common if radiation is required. Preserving the saphenous vein decreases the incidence of this problem. If edema does develop, the use of compression stockings, massage therapy, and limb wraps can help control the accumulation of fluid.

SUGGESTED READINGS

Marsden DE, Hacker NF: Contemporary management of primary carcinoma of the vulva, *Surg Clin North Am* 81:799–813, 2001.
Micheletti L, Bogliatto F, Massobrio M: Groin lymphadenectomy with preservation of femoral fascia: total inguinofemoral node dissection for treatment of vulvar carcinoma, *World J Surg* 29:1268–1276, 2005.
Rouzier R, Haddad B, Atallah D, et al: Surgery for vulvar cancer, *Clin Obstet Gynecol* 48:869–878, 2005.

CHAPTER 78

SURGICAL MANAGEMENT OF OVARIAN CANCER

Pedro T. Ramirez, MD, and David M. Gershenson, MD

I. SPECIAL PREOPERATIVE PREPARATION

Demographics and Staging

- Ovarian cancer is the third most common gynecologic malignancy in the United States. Approximately 22,280 women were expected to be diagnosed with the disease in 2012, and nearly 15,500 women were predicted to die of it during the same time period.

Preoperative Evaluation

- The high mortality rate is due primarily to the fact that the majority of patients present with advanced-stage disease (Table 78-1).
- Approximately 80% of ovarian malignancies are epithelial in origin. The remaining cell types include germ cell tumors and sex cord–stromal tumors. The International Federation of Gynecology and Obstetrics (FIGO) staging criteria for ovarian cancer are outlined in Table 78-2.
- The surgical approach to patients with a presumptive diagnosis of ovarian cancer differs depending on whether the patient presents with an isolated adnexal mass with ultrasonographic and serologic findings suggestive of ovarian cancer or with gross evidence of upper abdominal disease.
- It is important to emphasize that any patient suspected of having an ovarian malignancy should be referred to a gynecologic oncologist. Previous studies have shown that patients with early-stage disease who are operated on by a gynecologic oncologist are more likely to undergo comprehensive staging, which allows for the more accurate selection of patients requiring adjuvant therapy. In addition, patients with advanced disease who are operated on by gynecologic oncologists are more likely to receive optimal cytoreductive surgery leading to improved median and overall 5-year survival.

Early-Stage Disease

- The routine evaluation of a patient with ovarian cancer varies according to the patient's initial presentation. The diagnosis of early-stage ovarian cancer is often the result of an incidental finding, because most patients are asymptomatic. Generally, an adnexal mass is detected as part of a routine pelvic examination.

TABLE 78-1 Approximate Stage Distribution by Category of Ovarian Malignancy

	Percentage of Ovarian Malignancies		
STAGE	EPITHELIAL	GERM CELL	SEX CORD–STROMAL
I	15-25	50-70	85-100
II	15-20	5-15	0-5
III	40-50	25-35	0-10
IV	10-20	2-5	0-2

Modified from Gershenson DM, Wharton JT: Surgery for ovarian cancer. In: Gershenson DM, DeCherney AH, Curry SL, Brubaker L, editors: *Operative Gynecology*, Philadelphia, 2001, WB Saunders, p 690-712.

- Fortunately, most adnexal masses in premenopausal women are not malignant—ovarian cancer represents fewer than 5% of all adnexal masses in this age group. Typically, in this setting, the patient will undergo pelvic ultrasonography to define the characteristics of the adnexal mass.
- Findings on ultrasound such as irregular borders, solid components, papillary projections, thick septations, and bilateral tumors are suggestive of malignancy. If these findings are noted, patients generally undergo computed tomography (CT) evaluation of the abdomen and pelvis to rule out metastatic spread of disease. Pulmonary metastases are rare in the setting of early-stage ovarian cancer, but all patients routinely undergo chest radiographic evaluation before surgery to rule out pulmonary disease or pleural effusions.
- In addition to the imaging studies discussed, a serum CA-125 test should be ordered to provide additional information on the level of suspicion of malignancy. CA-125 levels are elevated in approximately 50% of patients with early-stage ovarian cancer. Values that exceed 35 units/mL are considered abnormal.

Advanced-Stage Disease

- Unfortunately, the majority of patients with ovarian cancer present with advanced-stage disease. The typical symptoms described by patients with advanced ovarian cancer include abdominal swelling, pain, dyspepsia, urinary frequency, and weight changes (Fig. 78-1). Generally, on pelvic examination, palpation reveals evidence of enlarged adnexal masses that are fixed, solid, and irregular in shape. In such cases, ultrasonography offers little or no useful information; instead, the patient should undergo CT of the abdomen and pelvis. This is an important study because it helps identify patients who are ideal candidates for surgical exploration and tumor cytoreduction versus patients who are ideal candidates for neoadjuvant chemotherapy.

TABLE 78-2 FIGO Staging for Primary Carcinoma of the Ovary

STAGE	DESCRIPTION
I	Limited to the ovaries.
IA	Limited to one ovary. Capsule intact. No ascites.
IB	Limited to both ovaries. Capsule intact. No ascites.
IC	Stage IA or IB but with tumor on surface or capsule rupture or with ascites.
II	Growth to one or both ovaries with pelvic extension.
IIA	Extension to the uterus and/or tubes.
IIB	Extension to other pelvic tissue.
IIC	Stage IIA or IIB but with tumor on surface of one or both ovaries or capsule rupture or with ascites.
III	Tumor involving one or both ovaries but with peritoneal implants outside of the pelvis and/or positive retroperitoneal or inguinal nodes or with superficial liver metastases.
IIIA	Tumor grossly limited to the pelvis but with microscopic extension outside of the pelvis.
IIIB	Tumor in one or both ovaries with peritoneal implants outside of the pelvis <2 cm.
IIIC	Abdominal implants >2 cm in diameter and/or positive retroperitoneal or inguinal nodes.
IV	Distant metastases to the liver parenchyma. Positive pleural effusion for metastatic disease.

FIGO, International Federation of Gynecology and Obstetrics.

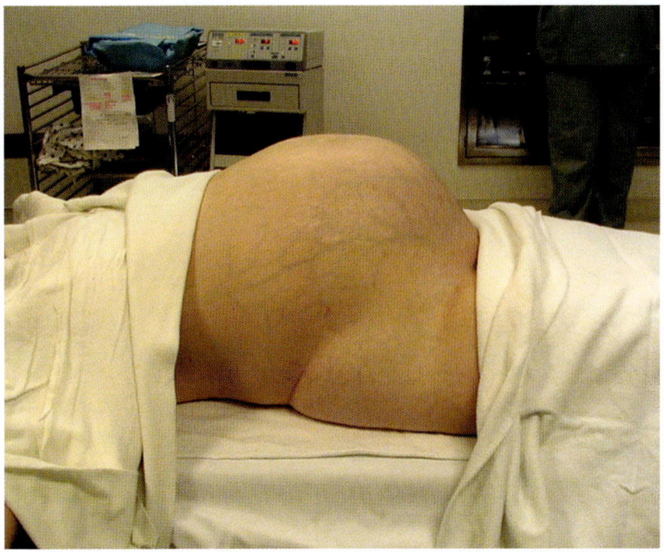

Figure 78-1. Typical presentation of a patient with advanced ovarian cancer. Abdominal examination is consistent with an extensive amount of ascites and carcinomatosis.

- Patients who are not considered surgical candidates are those with evidence of intraparenchymal liver disease, disease in the lesser sac invading retroperitoneal tissue, extensive mesenteric lymphadenopathy, and/or suprarenal lymphadenopathy (Fig. 78-2). These patients will generally undergo treatment in the form of neoadjuvant chemotherapy followed by interval tumor reductive surgery.
- Patients should also undergo either a chest radiograph or CT to rule out the possibility of either large pleural effusions or metastatic disease (Fig. 78-3). Patients with lung metastases are often considered to have inoperable disease and are treated with neoadjuvant chemotherapy.

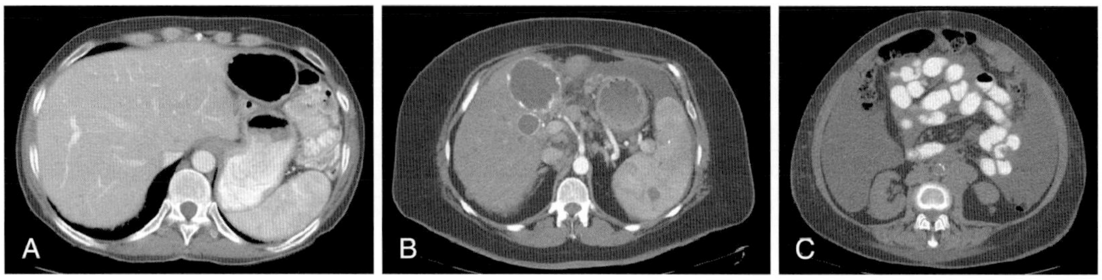

Figure 78-2. **A**, Normal computed tomography scan of the upper abdomen. **B**, Multiple liver and splenic metastases. **C**, Extensive para-aortic lymphadenopathy.

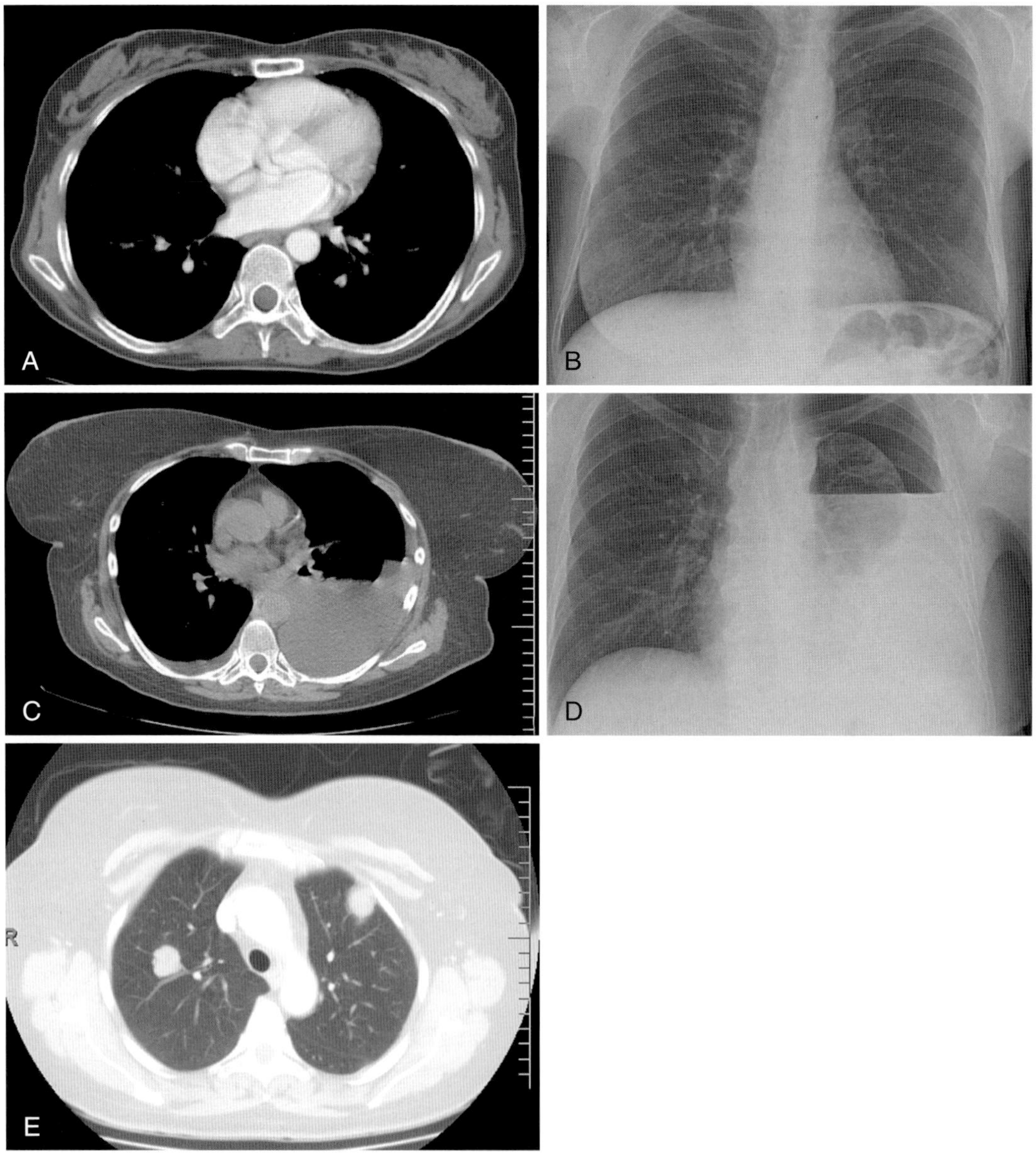

Figure 78-3. **A**, Normal computed tomography (CT) scan of the chest. **B**, Normal chest radiograph. **C**, Unilateral pleural effusion on CT scan. **D**, Bilateral pulmonary effusions with evidence of a complete pneumothorax on the left side. **E**, Bilateral pulmonary metastases.

- A serum CA-125 test should always be performed before surgery, as this will serve as an indicator of response to therapy in the postoperative period. Serum CA-125 levels are elevated in approximately 80% of patients with advanced-stage disease.
- Barium studies of the gastrointestinal tract are not routinely obtained unless indicated by symptoms such as rectal bleeding or bowel obstruction. A recent normal mammogram should always be verified because occasionally primary breast cancer with metastases to the abdomen and pelvis can mimic advanced ovarian cancer. Ovarian cancer rarely metastasizes to the brain or to bone, and brain magnetic resonance imaging or bone scans are therefore unnecessary unless indicated by the patient's symptoms.

II. OPERATIVE TECHNIQUE: EARLY-STAGE DISEASE

- In patients with suspected early-stage ovarian cancer, surgical staging is traditionally performed via a laparotomy; however, recently there is increasing evidence that a laparoscopic or robotic-assisted, minimally invasive approach is safe and feasible.

Position

- In our institution, patients are placed in the dorsal lithotomy position in preparation for surgical staging. All patients receive prophylactic antibiotics before surgery, and we routinely use lower-extremity compression devices to prevent or decrease the risk of thromboembolic events.

Incision

- For laparotomy procedures, a midline vertical incision is performed so that in the event of the diagnosis of a malignancy, the surgeon will have adequate access to the upper abdomen to perform the indicated staging biopsies. A Bookwalter or Thompson retractor is typically used to expose the abdomen and pelvis.

Main Dissection

- The procedure begins with a thorough evaluation of the pelvis and the upper abdomen. After this is completed, pelvic and abdominal washings are obtained and sent for cytologic evaluation. At this point, attention is placed on removing the affected ovary.
- The patient's age plays a large role in determining the surgical approach. In young women who want to remain fertile, it is acceptable to perform a unilateral salpingo-oophorectomy to remove the affected ovary, which is sent for frozen-section evaluation.
- The salpingo-oophorectomy is performed by making an incision along the peritoneum lateral to the infundibulopelvic ligament and mobilizing the ovary and fallopian tube medially to expose the ureter. Once this has been performed, the infundibulopelvic ligament is clamped and transected. The salpingo-oophorectomy is completed by transecting the utero-ovarian ligament.
- Care should be taken not to rupture the capsule of the ovarian neoplasm. If a malignancy is confirmed by frozen-section evaluation, one may opt for removal of the contralateral ovary and uterus if the patient is not interested in future fertility. However, in a nulliparous patient, one may consider leaving the uterus and contralateral ovary in situ if these appear normal.
- It is imperative that details of the procedure and the intended approaches and various intraoperative options be discussed with the patient during preoperative counseling and while obtaining informed consent.
- If there is no other evidence of disease, the surgeon should perform pelvic and para-aortic lymphadenectomy or lymph node sampling. We routinely advocate removal of lymphatic tissue in the pelvis from the common iliac vessels proximally to the circumflex iliac vein distally. Lymphatic tissue is also removed from the obturator space. The obturator lymph nodes are removed by separating the lymphatic bundle from the external iliac vein superiorly and then from the obturator nerve inferiorly. The proximal resection extends to the bifurcation of the external and internal iliac vessels. This is generally performed bilaterally. For the para-aortic dissection, our margin extends from the renal vessels proximally to the aortic bifurcation distally.
- After the lymphadenectomy is completed, we then perform an omentectomy or omental biopsy. The omentum is fanned out, and its attachments to the transverse colon are identified. An avascular plane between the transverse colon and the omentum is opened with electrocautery. Only the posterior leaf of the omentum should be incised. An avascular plane between the omentum and the underlying transverse mesocolon is developed to the level of the lesser sac, which is posterior to the stomach wall. The gastroepiploic and short gastric vessels are isolated by electrocautery. These vessels are transected.

The omentectomy is performed from the hepatic flexure to the splenic flexure of the transverse colon. Once the omentectomy is completed, biopsies are obtained from the bilateral paracolic gutters and peritoneal surfaces of the pelvis and along the bilateral diaphragmatic surfaces.

Closure

- Before closure, we routinely perform one last thorough inspection of the abdominal and pelvic cavity to ensure that there is no evidence of residual disease. The abdomen and pelvis are irrigated before closure of the abdominal wall. We routinely place an adhesion barrier material such as Seprafilm (Genzyme, Cambridge, Mass.) over the bowel before fascial closure.

III. OPERATIVE TECHNIQUE: ADVANCED-STAGE DISEASE

Position

- In patients with advanced ovarian cancer (Fig. 78-4), our routine approach is to place the patient in a dorsal lithotomy position. This allows the surgeon to have access to the pelvis in the event that a digital examination of the vagina or the rectum is required during the surgery to help identify the surgical planes.
- All patients receive prophylactic antibiotics before surgery, and prophylactic measures similar to those described for patients with early-stage disease are taken to prevent thromboembolic events.

Incision

- A generous midline vertical incision should be performed to gain access to and excellent exposure of the upper abdomen. The incision may need to be extended superiorly to the level of the xiphoid process in cases where the patient has disease involving the upper abdomen or diaphragm (Figs. 78-5 and 78-6). Retractors similar to those described previously are used. Once the abdomen is exposed, the surgeon should remove all ascites encountered and send them for cytologic evaluation.

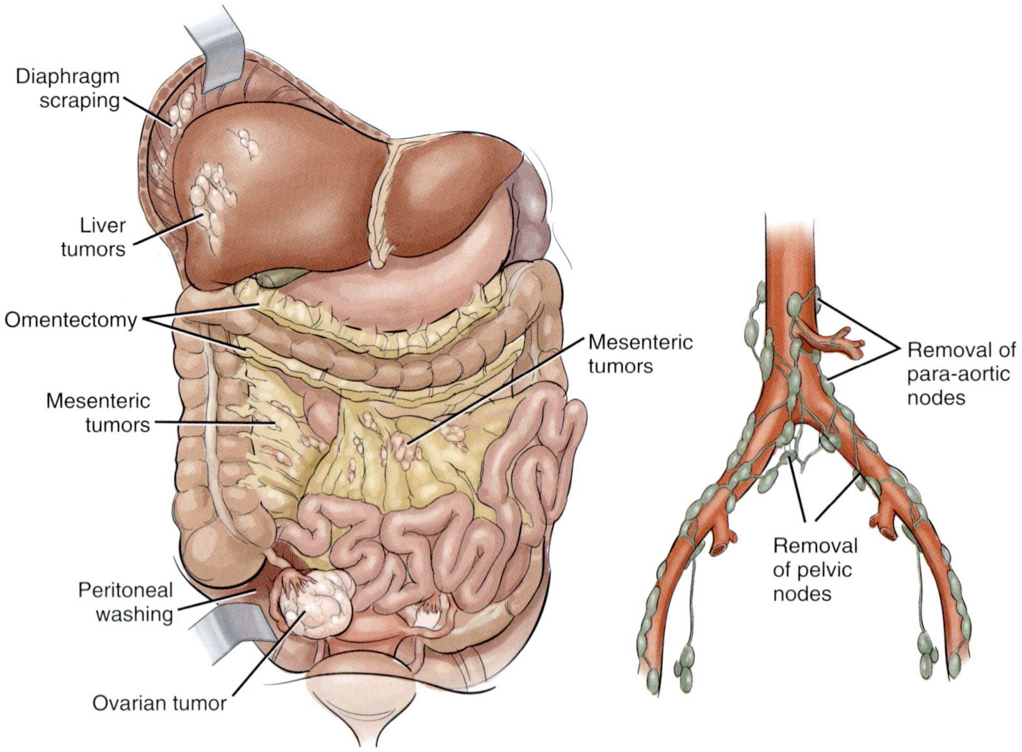

Figure 78-4.

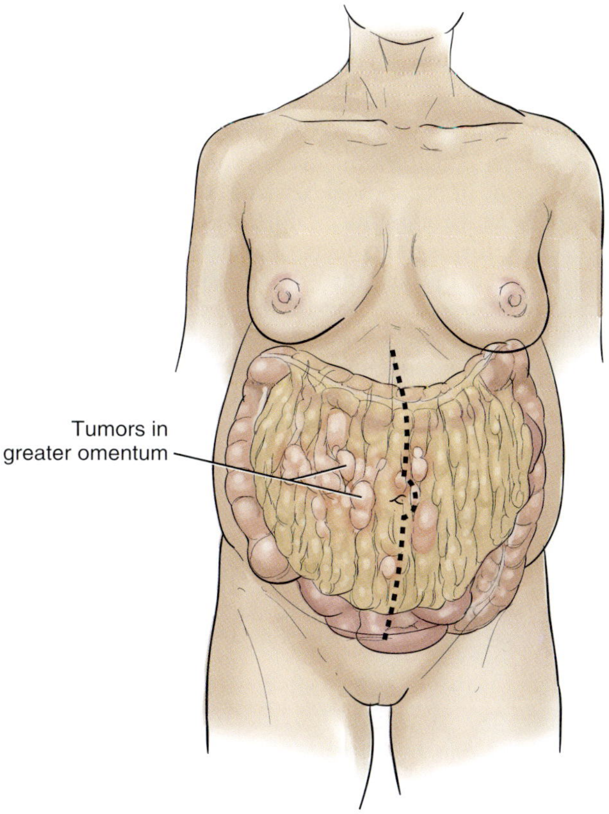

Figure 78-5.

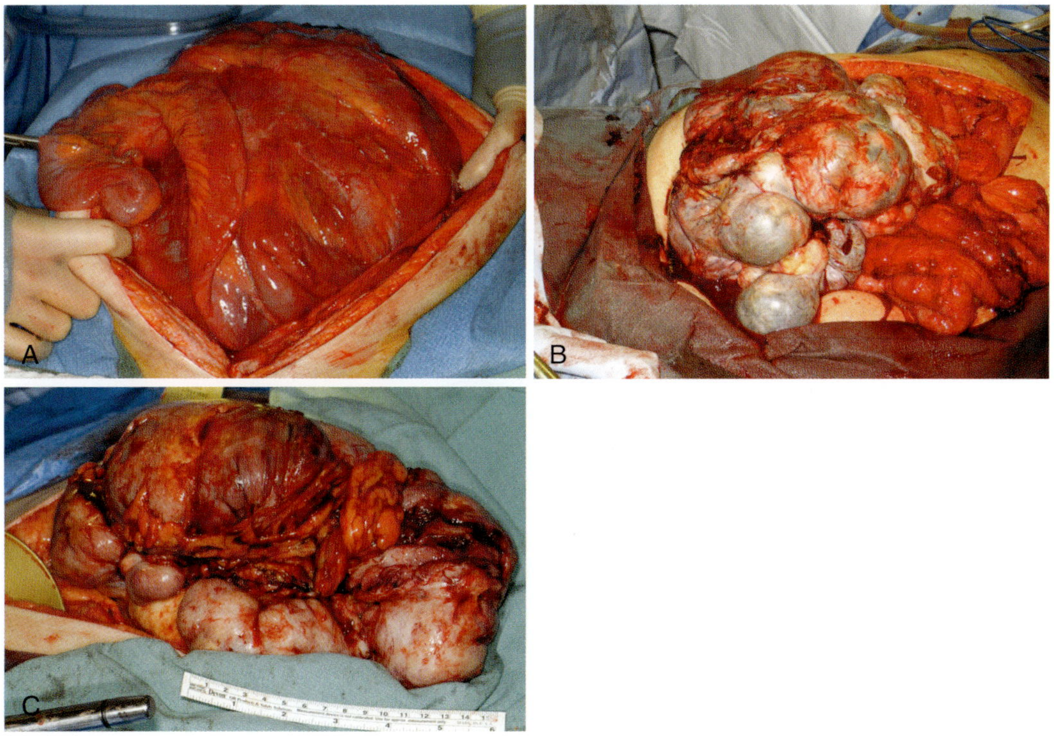

Figure 78-6. **A** through **C**, Midline vertical incision performed to remove large ovarian tumor involving the mesentery of the small bowel.

Main Dissection

- Tumor resection begins with a total abdominal hysterectomy and bilateral salpingo-oophorectomy (Fig. 78-7). If the primary ovarian disease is densely adherent to the distal sigmoid colon or to sections of the small bowel, a partial resection of the bowel will be required. Ideally, the surgeon should attempt to perform a primary anastomosis of the remaining bowel to avoid the undesirable effects of an ostomy.
- Attention is then focused on the upper abdomen, where a complete omentectomy should be performed. Care should be taken not to cause any injury to the lower pole of the spleen at the splenic flexure of the transverse colon, because this is often a site of disease.
- If there is evidence of enlarged (greater than 1 cm) retroperitoneal lymph nodes, these should be removed by making an incision on the peritoneum immediately overlying the aorta and vena cava (Fig. 78-8). This incision should be performed from the level of the mid–right common iliac vessels distally to the level of the reflection of the duodenum over the aorta and vena cava (Fig. 78-9). However, it is important to recognize that no evidence in the literature supports routine lymphadenectomy in the setting of advanced ovarian cancer in patients with normal-size lymph nodes.

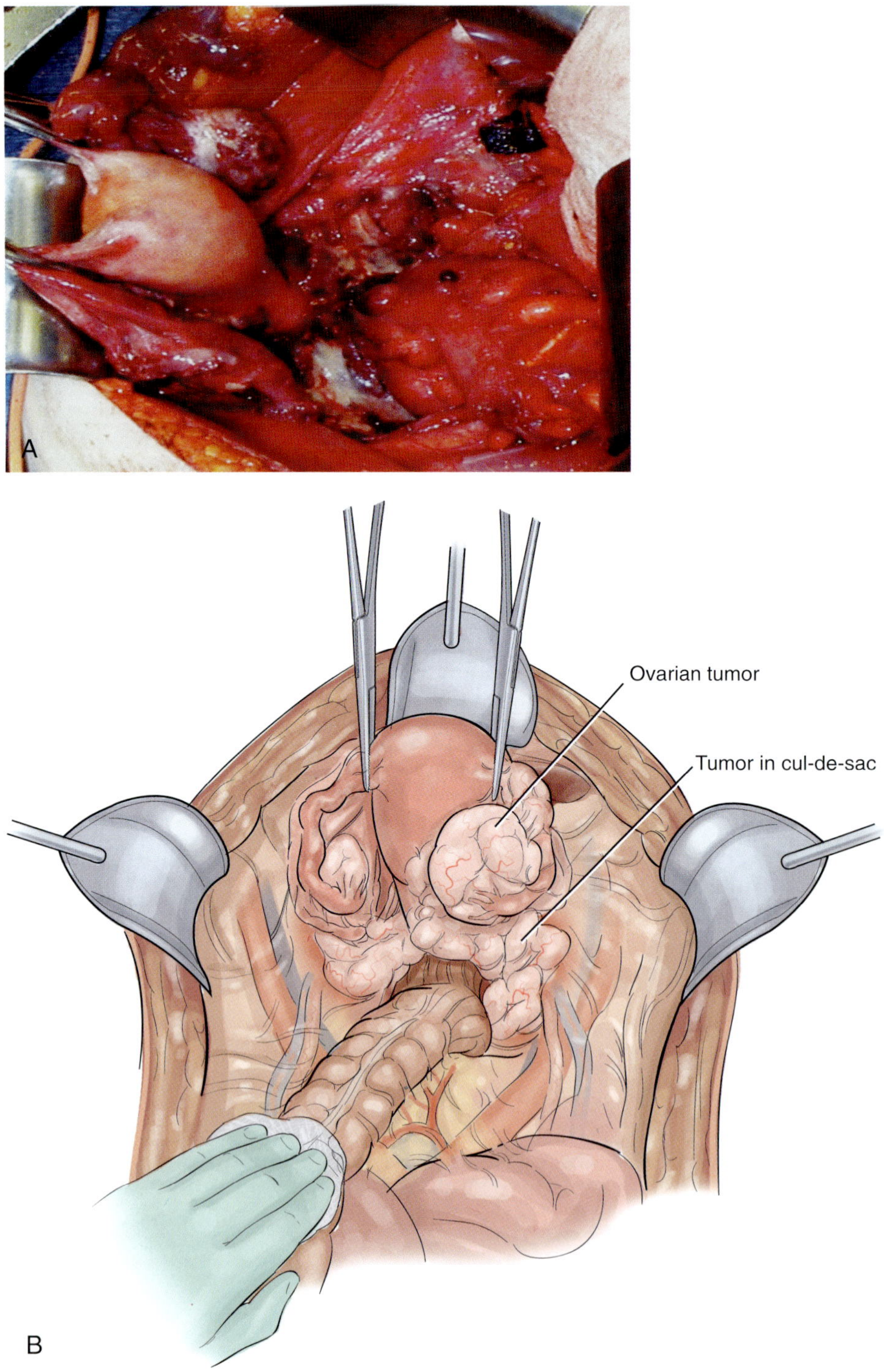

Figure 78-7. A and B, Total abdominal hysterectomy and bilateral salpingo-oophorectomy during advanced ovarian cancer tumor reductive surgery.

- Occasionally, patients will require diaphragmatic peritoneal resection. To achieve adequate access to the diaphragm, it is important that the midline incision be extended to the level of the xiphoid process. The liver must be mobilized by transecting the entire falciform ligament and the coronary and triangular ligaments. The peritoneum overlying the diaphragm can then be removed using either Metzenbaum scissors or electrocautery. A recent study evaluated the therapeutic value of diaphragmatic surgery in advanced ovarian cancer. The results showed that surgical procedures to treat diaphragmatic disease increase the rate of complete and optimal debulking and correlate with improved survival.

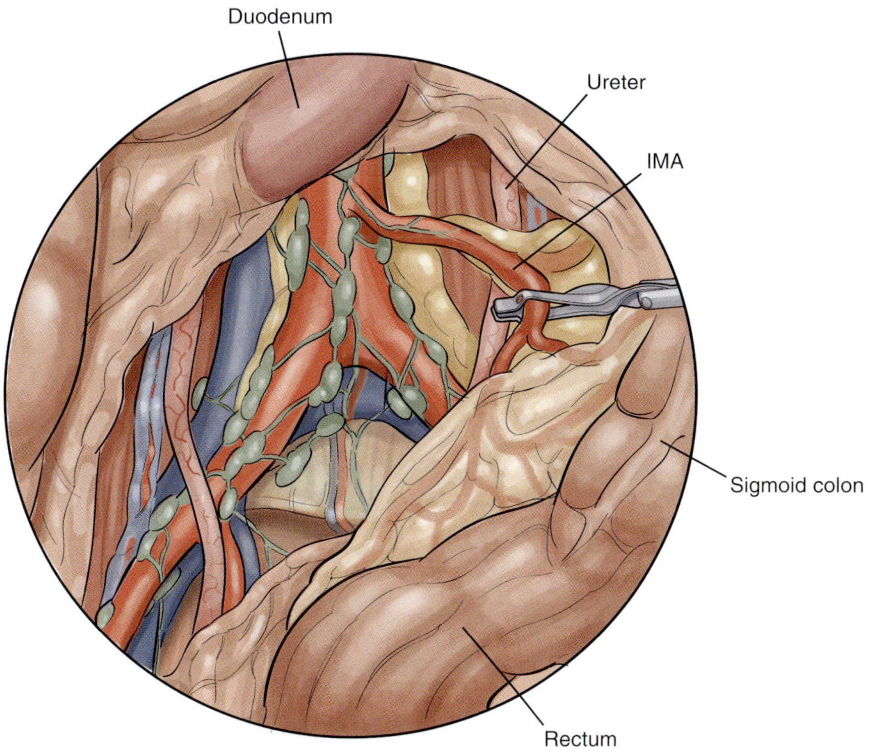

Figure 78-8. Retroperitoneal para-aortic lymph node dissection. *IMA,* Inferior mesenteric artery.

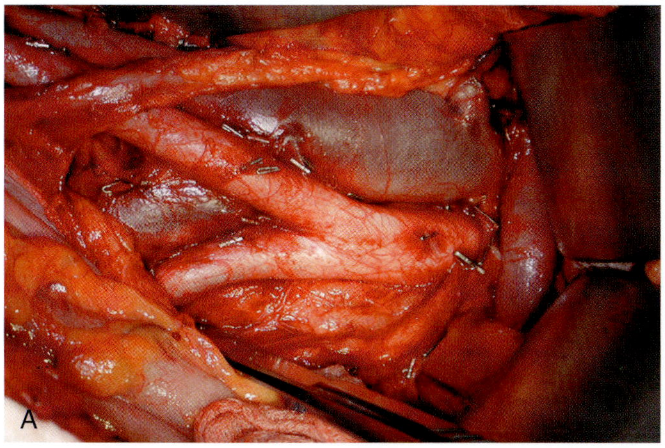

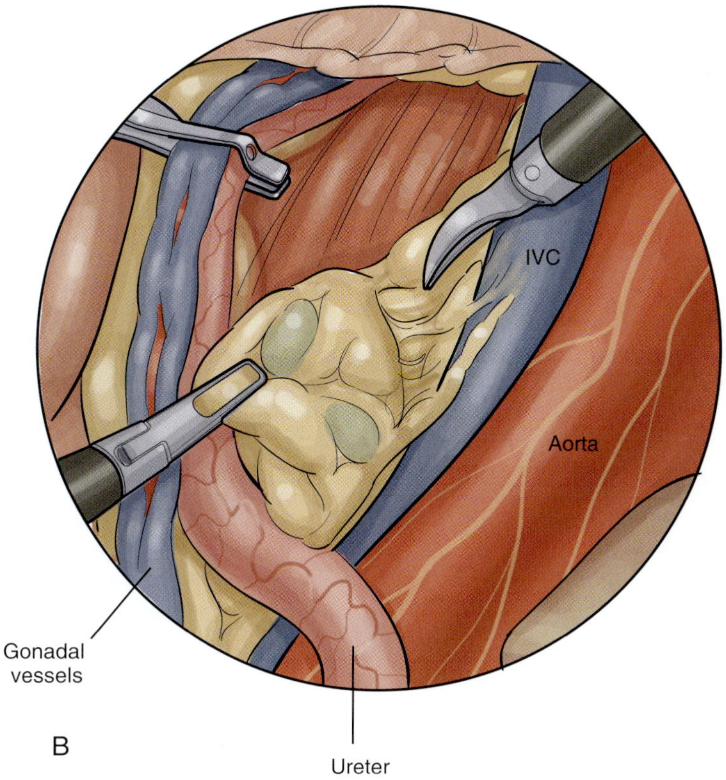

Figure 78-9. A and B, Complete para-aortic lymphadenectomy in a patient with enlarged para-aortic lymph nodes in advanced ovarian cancer. *IVC,* Inferior vena cava.

- Splenectomy is another procedure that is performed in approximately 8% of patients with advanced ovarian cancer undergoing surgical cytoreduction (Fig. 78-10). When the spleen is removed, the majority of patients have involvement of the hilum, but one can also see capsular and parenchymal involvement. In addition to direct involvement of the spleen with metastatic ovarian cancer, other indications for splenectomy in this setting are to accomplish resection of the omentum as an en bloc specimen or intractable bleeding from a traction injury.
- The usual steps for performing a splenectomy include entry into the lesser sac by transecting the short gastric vessels and then transection of the ligamentous attachments such as the splenocolic, splenophrenic, splenorenal, and gastrosplenic ligaments. Finally, once the major vessels have been identified at the hilum, we recommend transection of the splenic artery and vein using a vascular stapler or a clamping technique followed by placement of size 0 silk sutures to secure the vascular pedicle. It should be emphasized that routine drainage of this site postoperatively is not necessary unless there is suspicion of trauma to the pancreatic tail.
- One should make every effort to remove tumor that involves the small or large bowel to achieve optimal cytoreduction. This may often require bowel resection with reanastomosis or placement of a diverting colostomy if an anastomosis is not feasible.

Closure

- An adhesion barrier material is placed over the bowel before fascial closure. Closure of the incision is typically performed using size 0 polydioxanone continuous sutures. The subcutaneous tissue is thoroughly irrigated, and the skin is closed using staples.

IV. ALTERNATIVE TECHNICAL APPROACHES (PRO/CON) AND PEARLS

- In patients with presumed early-stage ovarian cancer, one can also consider surgical staging through a minimally invasive approach. The patient is placed in the dorsal lithotomy position, and a uterine manipulator is placed in the uterus to ensure adequate uterine mobilization during the procedure.
- Our approach is to use a four-port technique (Fig. 78-11). The initial entry port is at the umbilicus, and this is placed under direct visualization using Xcel bladeless trocars (Ethicon Endo-Surgery, Cincinnati). Three additional trocars are then placed: one each at the right and left lower quadrants and a third at the midline suprapubically. The steps of the procedure are exactly the same as those used in the laparotomy approach.
- The benefits of a minimally invasive approach include a shorter hospital stay, faster return of bowel function, less pain, and a much earlier return to normal daily activities. Among the disadvantages of

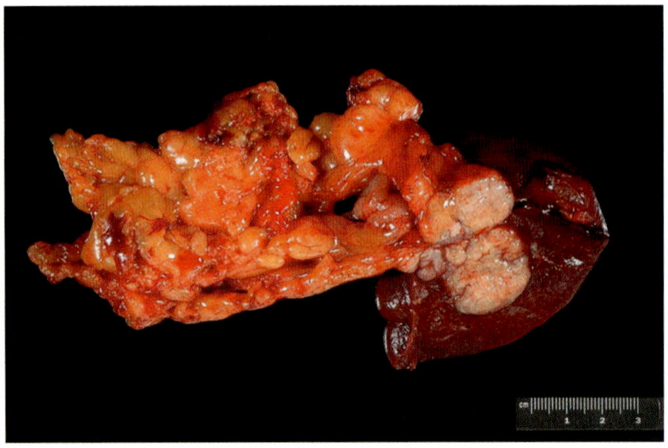

Figure 78-10. Surgical specimen after splenectomy for metastatic disease to the hilum of the spleen.

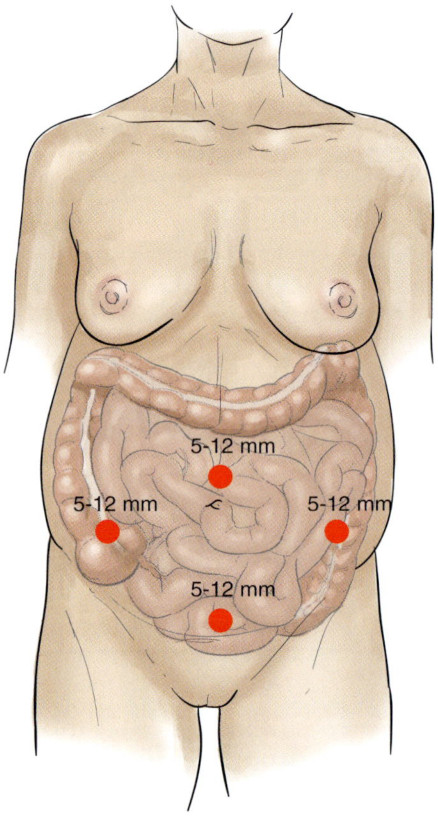

Figure 78-11.

laparoscopy are that it requires surgical expertise and is associated with a steep learning curve, particularly in the performance of pelvic and para-aortic lymphadenectomy. It can also be limiting in that if a patient has a large adnexal mass (larger than 8 to 10 cm), it would be difficult to remove it intact, thus increasing the likelihood of rupture, which would certainly be undesirable. Finally, the time in the operating room during the laparoscopic approach may be longer, and the cost associated with this technique is higher because of the sophisticated technology used.

- Laparoscopy has also been proposed in the setting of advanced ovarian cancer to determine the amount of disease and therefore assess the likelihood of tumor resection to achieve optimal cytoreduction. Although this approach appears promising, most studies published thus far have been retrospective in nature and conducted in small cohorts of patients. Laparoscopy in advanced ovarian cancer has the following potential disadvantages: it does not allow the surgeon to directly palpate the degree of tumor involvement in the abdomen or pelvis, and it does not allow for the accurate determination of the amount of retroperitoneal disease.

Pearls

Early-Stage Ovarian Cancer

- Always discuss the possibility of intraoperative diagnosis of malignancy and approach to the contralateral ovary and uterus in the setting of consideration of fertility preservation.
- When performing a laparotomy, a midline vertical incision should be used in all patients so that in the event of a diagnosis of malignancy, the surgeon will be able to extend the incision superiorly and perform an adequate staging procedure.
- When performing a laparoscopy, the surgeon must be skilled in performing not only the oophorectomy and possible hysterectomy but also pelvic and para-aortic lymphadenectomy as well as omental biopsy.

Advanced-Stage Ovarian Cancer

- A thorough evaluation of the preoperative CT scan will help the surgeon determine if the patient is an ideal candidate for surgery versus neoadjuvant chemotherapy. Patients with disease within the mesentery of the bowel, suprarenal lymph nodes, or the lesser sac extending to the porta hepatis or with multiple intraparenchymal liver metastases are rarely ideal candidates for surgical cytoreduction.
- In a patient with an extensive amount of ascites, extensive disease in the abdomen, and multiple comorbidities, it is strongly recommended that a central venous access catheter be placed before surgery, and it is wise to reserve an intensive care unit bed for the patient postoperatively.
- To eradicate small amounts of disease from the surfaces of the peritoneum, we recommend using the argon beam coagulator. This is an electrosurgical device that conducts current to tissue in a beam of inert argon gas. Another useful instrument is the Cavitron Ultrasonic Surgical Aspirator (CUSA). It combines tissue fragmentation, irrigation, and aspiration to remove tumor from the surfaces of vital structures such as the liver, spleen, or blood vessels.

V. SPECIAL POSTOPERATIVE CARE

- *Resection of pelvic tumor:* Possible complications include injury to the pelvic vascular structures, ureter, or obturator nerve. If there are extensive adhesions of the tumor to the bladder or rectum, inadvertent injury to these structures may occur, and such injuries should be repaired immediately.
- *Intestinal resection:* Complications associated with bowel resection include anastomotic leakage and subsequent abscess formation, bowel perforation, intestinal stricture, and bowel obstruction. In cases where an ostomy is performed, the patient may experience parastomal herniation or retraction, stomal stricture or prolapse, stomal bleeding, and skin erosion around the stoma.
- *Splenectomy:* Complications include hemorrhage, abscess formation, left-sided atelectasis or pneumonia, thrombocytosis and thromboembolic events, pancreatic tail injury, and stomach injuries resulting in gastric fistulas.
- *Diaphragmatic resection:* Complications include pneumothorax, hemorrhage from the phrenic arteries, infection, injury to the pericardial sac, and injury to the lung, vena cava, liver, or phrenic nerves.

SUGGESTED READINGS

American Cancer Society: Cancer facts & figures. 2007. Available at http://www.cancer.org.
Eisenhauer EL, Abu-Rustum NR, Sonoda Y, et al: The addition of extensive upper abdominal surgery to achieve optimal cytoreduction improves survival in patients with stages IIIC-IV epithelial ovarian cancer, *Gynecol Oncol* 103:1083–1090, 2006.
Leblanc E, Querleu D, Narducci F, et al: Surgical staging of early invasive epithelial ovarian tumors, *Semin Surg Oncol* 19:36–41, 2000.

SECTION XIV

Breast

CHAPTER 79

Nipple- and Areola-Sparing Mastectomy

Jean Yves Petit, MD, and Francesca De Lorenzi, MD, PhD

I. SPECIAL PREOPERATIVE PREPARATION

- Preoperative mammogram and breast ultrasound are mandatory for the diagnosis of breast cancer and provide valuable information of the local tumor extent. Despite the increasing use of breast-conserving treatment, mastectomy remains the most appropriate treatment for large or multicentric tumors, a medium-size tumor located in a very small breast, or recurrences after conservative treatment.
- Magnetic resonance imaging is a second-step investigation, generally required when the standard examinations are doubtful (Fig. 79-1).
- To establish histologic diagnosis, fine-needle aspiration and core biopsy are appropriate. The core biopsy provides enough tissue to establish a histologic diagnosis, tumor grade, and biologic characteristics.
- Nipple and areola preservation is indicated when the primary tumor is located at least 1 cm outside the areola margins, when there is no nipple retraction or bloody discharge, and when no microcalcifications are present in the retroareolar area at mammogram (Fig. 79-2).
- Preoperative drawings with the patient in the standing position are mandatory to check the symmetry with the contralateral healthy breast and mark anatomic landmarks (i.e., the bilateral level of the inframammary fold; the distance between the sternal notch and the areola; and the midline, width, height, and projection of the breast) that will guide breast-mound reconstruction (see later).

II. OPERATIVE TECHNIQUE

Position

- The patient is placed in the supine position with both arms abducted to explore the axilla. Both breasts are included in the sterile field to allow assessment of breast symmetry at the end of reconstruction. The operating table allows the patient to be raised to a sitting position during surgery.

Incision

- The skin incision for the mastectomy is usually drawn over the tumor site. An elliptical skin paddle can be removed according to the distance between the tumor and the dermis. This skin paddle does not include the areola, and the incision should stop at about 0.5 to 1 cm from the lateral border of the areola (Figs. 79-3 and 79-4). Periareolar incision is not recommended to prevent areola damage and devascularization during surgery; it is not necessary since nipple-sparing mastectomy is indicated for tumors located far from the areola.

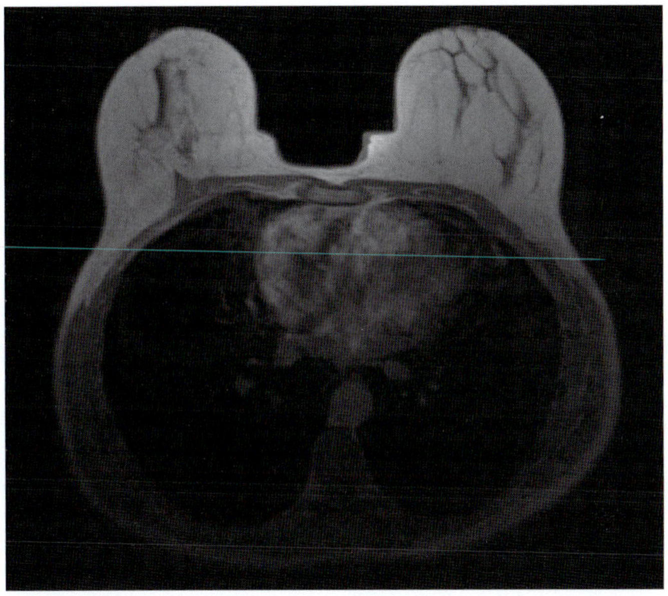

Figure 79-1.

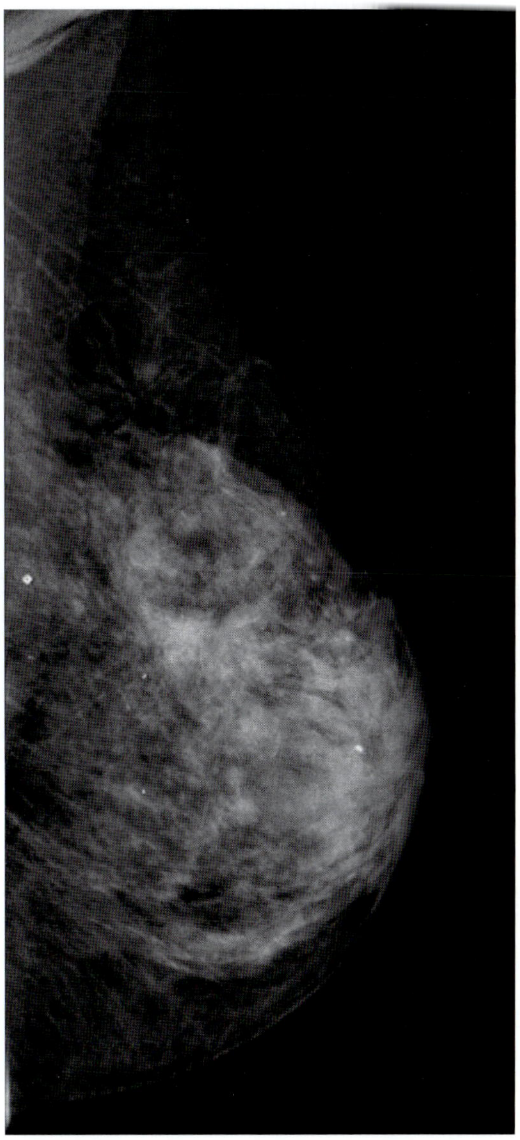

Figure 79-2.

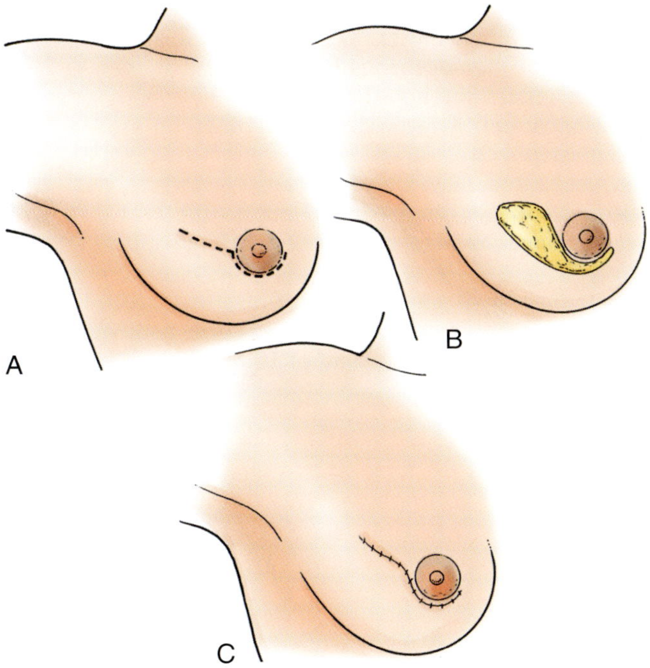

Figure 79-3.

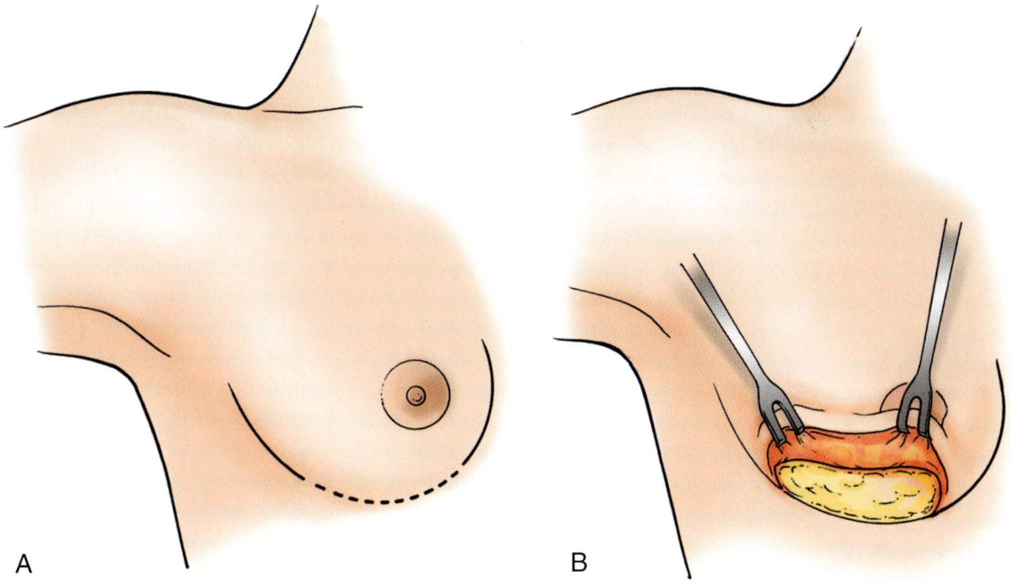

Figure 79-4.

Main Dissection

- The subcutaneous dissection can be performed with scissors to avoid any injury to the subdermal vessel network (see Figs. 79-4 and 79-5). A glandular layer 0.5 cm thick remains attached to the dermis to preserve the blood supply and the sensitivity of the nipple and areola. This glandular "patch" should extend 1 to 2 cm beyond the lateral border of the areola. Anatomically, connections between the gland and the dermis are tight only in the retroareolar area. As the dissection gradually extends laterally, the thicker subcutaneous fat makes the glandular dissection easier.
- A thin specimen is removed from the remaining retroareolar tissues for immediate frozen histologic examination. Nipple and areola preservation is possible only if the frozen-section is negative for carcinoma.
- The deep dissection of the gland over the pectoral fascia can be performed in the same way as in the classic mastectomy (Fig. 79-6). If this prepectoral dissection is performed first, the bleeding of the subcutaneous dissection is decreased by the ligature of the perforator vessels.
- As soon as the dissection is completed, the specimen is marked with sutures for pathologic examination.
- Sentinel node biopsy or complete axillary dissection is performed, depending on the individual case.

Intraoperative Electron Therapy

- To complete the surgical treatment and decrease the risk of local relapse in the tissues behind the preserved nipple and areola, intraoperative radiotherapy with electrons (ELIOT) is delivered to the nipple and areola complex (NAC).
- Two protective devices are placed between the NAC and the pectoralis muscle to minimize irradiation of the thoracic wall and to guarantee the delivery of a full and homogeneous radiation dose at the NAC site. For this purpose, we use a lead disk 5 mm thick and an aluminum disk 4 mm thick, both available in various diameters (4, 5, 6, 8, and 10 cm). Protection of the wall is guaranteed by the absorption properties and thickness of the lead and aluminum.
- The sterile collimator of the mobile linear accelerator is placed in contact with the NAC. The target of irradiation includes the remaining glandular tissue behind the NAC and corresponds to the NAC diameter and its periphery. The thickness of the target tissue is measured to choose the right irradiation energy.
- The total dose of 16 Gy is delivered to the NAC in a single fraction. According to the linear quadratic model and computing the surviving fraction of clonogenic units, a single dose of 16 Gy corresponds to a fractionated dose of about 45 Gy for early-responding tissue (tumor cells) and of 70 to 80 Gy for late-responding normal tissues (vessels, fat, nerves).
- Irradiation lasts about 2 minutes.

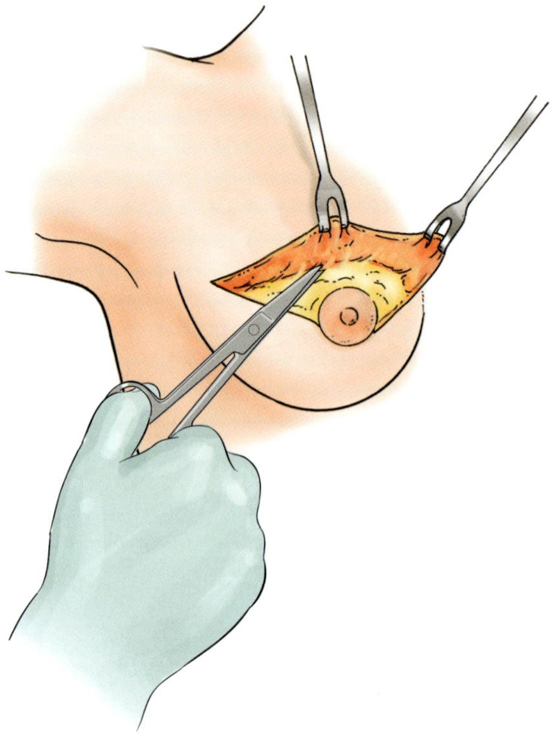

Figure 79-5.

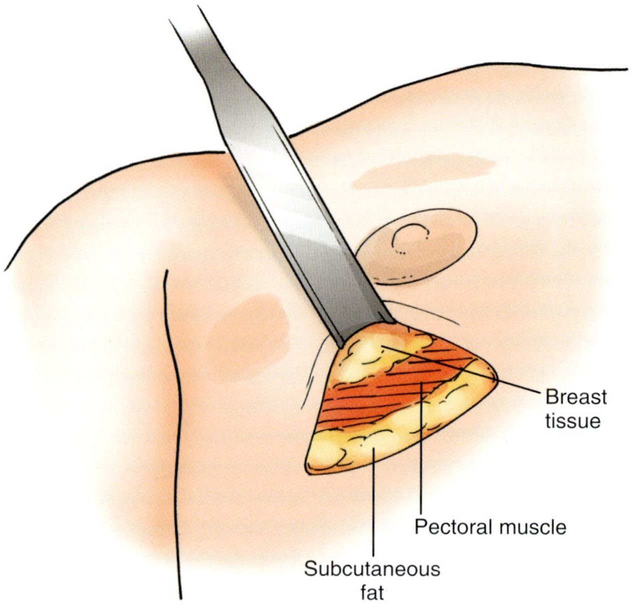

Figure 79-6.

Breast Reconstruction

- Breast reconstruction is performed immediately after irradiation with the use of implant or autologous tissues (Fig. 79-7).
- The use of a silicone gel implant is generally indicated for small to medium-size breasts with minor ptosis. The implant is placed behind the pectoralis major muscle and serratus anterior muscle (Fig. 79-8, *A* and *B*).
- In cases of a large and ptotic breast, an autologous de-epithelialized flap (transverse rectus abdominis muscle flap from the abdomen or latissimus dorsi flap) is preferred (Fig. 79-9, *A* and *B*).

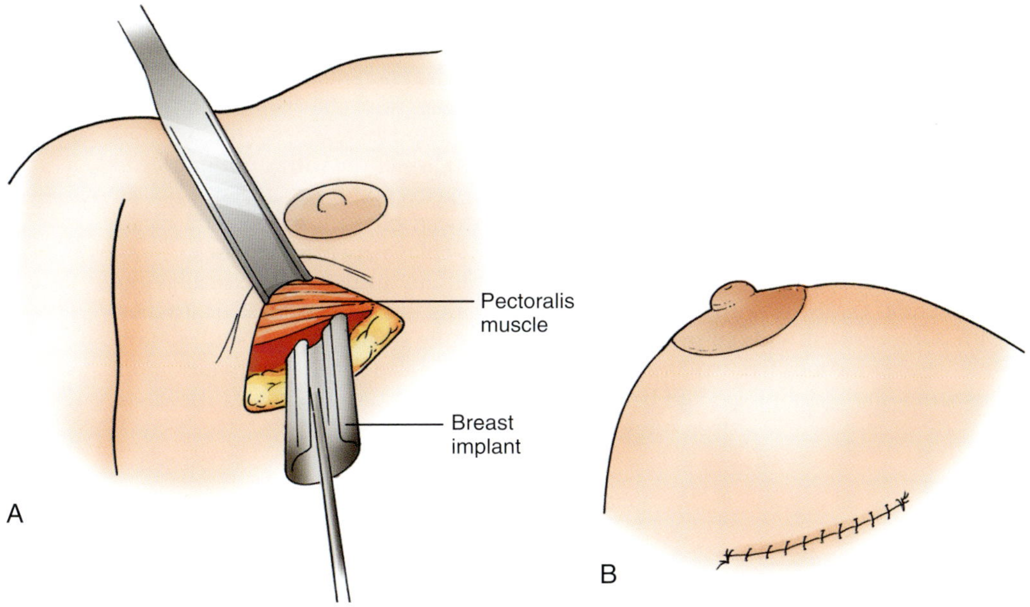

Figure 79-7.

Figure 79-8.

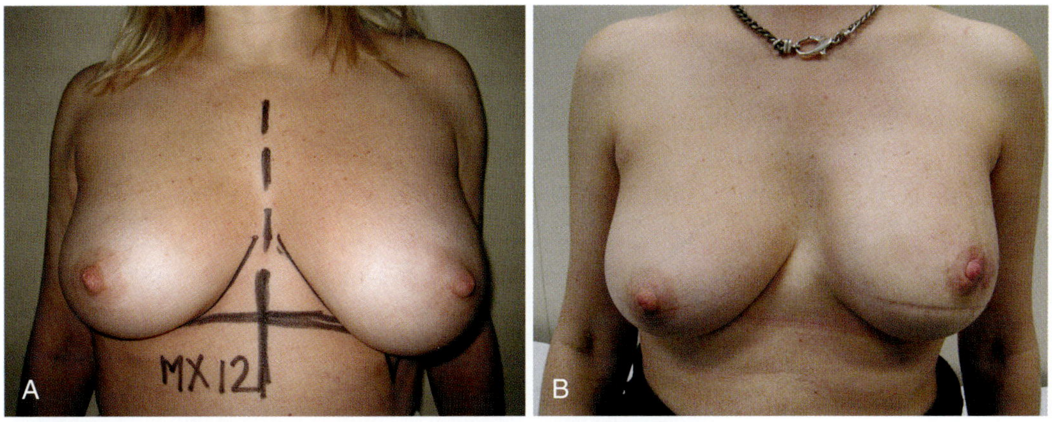

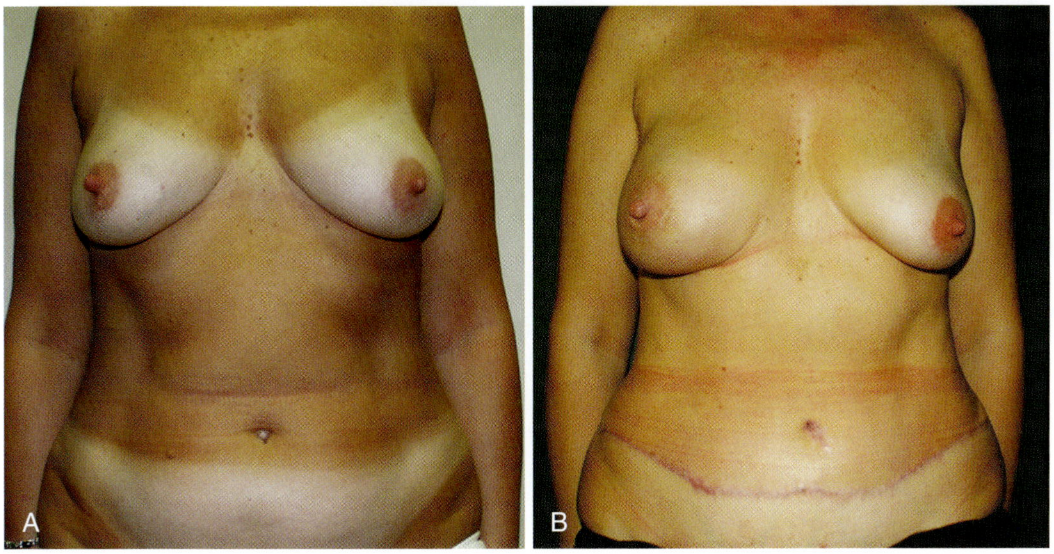

Figure 79-9.

Closure

- After hemostasis is obtained and breast reconstruction is performed, a Jackson-Pratt or Bellovac drain is placed through a separate stab incision and secured with 2-0 nonabsorbable monofilament suture. In the case of complete axillary dissection, an additional drain is positioned toward the axilla.
- The dermis is carefully approximated with 3-0 absorbable suture, and an intradermal running 4-0 absorbable suture is used for skin.

III. ALTERNATIVE TECHNICAL APPROACHES (PRO/CON) AND PEARLS

- Technically, the skin incision could be placed far from the tumor site (i.e., at the level of the inframammary fold) in cases of deeply located tumors. In these cases, there is an inherent risk of having two breast scars if a positive retroareolar specimen requires nipple and areola removal.
- If possible, the skin incision is placed below the décolleté line.
- At the beginning of our experience, we performed the subcutaneous dissection with a blunt Hegar dilator (no. 6 or 8) to reduce undesirable injuries to the subdermal plexus. With the advent of electrocautery, the subcutaneous dissection could be performed with reduced blood loss in a very clean operative field, but in these cases the risk of injuries to the dermic vascular network increases.
- Many authors perform nipple- and areola-sparing mastectomy without any intraoperative irradiation of the remaining tissues behind the NAC with apparently similar results in terms of local recurrence rate. In comparison with our technique and our series, those series include smaller tumors and tumors located farther from the areola, and positive axillary lymph nodes are considered a contraindication for nipple- and areola-sparing mastectomy with no irradiation. In addition, 10% to 15% of the cases in most of these studies are prophylactic mastectomies without breast cancer.

IV. SPECIAL POSTOPERATIVE CARE

- Prophylactic antibiotics are delivered following an ultrashort protocol (2 g second-generation Cephalosporin within 30 minutes before skin incision) or a short administration (an additional 1 g second-generation Cephalosporin after 4 hours of surgery or in case of massive bleeding, and an additional 1 g 8 hours after the second administration).
- Subcutaneous low–molecular-weight heparin injections are administered daily within 24 hours after surgery for 1 week, as with every cancer patient, to prevent vein thrombosis.
- A specific intraoperative complication is the necessity of nipple and areola removal if frozen-sections are positive for malignant cells. In these cases, of course, no irradiation is delivered.
- Specific immediate postoperative complications that may be encountered are infection, wound dehiscence, partial or total nipple and areola necrosis, and hematoma. In the case of implant breast reconstruction, wound dehiscence and/or infection may lead to implant exposure and removal even though the implant is placed behind the pectoralis major and serratus anterior muscles. In cases of flap reconstruction, spontaneous healing by second intention usually occurs.
- Partial or total nipple and areola necrosis is generally a result of poor blood supply of the NAC at the end of nipple- and areola-sparing mastectomy. Technically, an aggressive subcutaneous dissection damaging the dermal vascular network could be one of the causes. Moreover, this complication is more frequent in patients who are heavy smokers and in large and ptotic breasts because of the length of skin flaps. Skin necrosis generally requires surgical removal and skin reapproximation.
- The specific delayed complications include areola depigmentation and dislocation, radiodystrophy, loss of nipple projection, and lack of nipple and areola sensitivity. Moreover, any specific complication related to breast reconstruction technique impairs the cosmetic outcome. Areola depigmentation and nipple flattening are mainly due to poor vascularization. Skin radiodystrophy is due to irradiation and is rare; when present, it is characterized by a circular erythema and mild pigmentation corresponding to the irradiation field. It usually improves with time. Nipple and areola dislocation is due to scarring and scar contracture; it is difficult to predict and prevent.

SUGGESTED READINGS

Petit JY, Veronesi U, Orecchia R, et al: The nipple-sparing mastectomy: early results of a feasibility study of a new application of perioperative radiotherapy (ELIOT) in the treatment of breast cancer when mastectomy is indicated, *Tumori* 89:228–291, 2003.

Petit JY, Veronesi U, Orecchia R, et al: Nipple sparing mastectomy with nipple areola intraoperative radiotherapy: one thousand and one cases of a five years experience at the European Institute of Oncology of Milan (EIO), *Breast Cancer Res Treat* 117:333–338, 2009.

Petit JY, Veronesi U, Rey P, et al: Nipple-sparing mastectomy: risk of nipple-areolar recurrences in a series of 579 cases, *Breast Cancer Res Treat* 114:97–101, 2009.

CHAPTER 80

Skin-Sparing Mastectomy and Sentinel Lymph Node Biopsy

Grant W. Carlson, MD

I. SPECIAL PREOPERATIVE PREPARATION

- The procedure is useful in patients having prophylactic mastectomy and patients with stage 0 to stage II breast cancer. It used in conjunction with immediate breast reconstruction.
- Defining the location and extent of the breast cancer is essential before performing a skin-sparing mastectomy (SSM). Careful review of mammograms and pathology of excisional biopsies is necessary to prevent close or involved margins.
- Injection of radioactive colloid is performed either the day before or the morning of surgery. When used in conjunction with blue dye, radioactive colloid has the greatest sensitivity in finding axillary sentinel lymph nodes.

II. OPERATIVE TECHNIQUE

Position

- The patient is placed supine; the arms are abducted 90 degrees, supported on arm boards, and secured with gauze. This is in preparation for immediate breast reconstruction.
- Draping is performed in such a way that an assistant can stand cephalad to the operative arm. Both breasts are prepped in the operative field, with exposure from above the sternal notch to below the costal margin. The arms are exposed to the midhumerus.

Incision

- The inframammary fold is delineated preoperatively with a marking pen with the patient in the upright position. The nipple-areolar complex, skin overlying superficial cancers, and previous biopsy incisions are removed. The type of SSM has been classified by the type of incision used and the amount of skin removed (Fig. 80-1).

- A type I SSM is commonly used in prophylactic cases and for nonpalpable cancers diagnosed by needle biopsy. In patients with a small-diameter areola, a lateral extension of the incision is sometimes necessary to improve exposure to the axillary tail. A type II SSM is used when a superficial tumor or previous biopsy is in proximity to the areola. A type III SSM is used when a superficial tumor or previous incision is remote from the areola. Care must be taken to ensure the viability of the intervening skin. A type IV SSM is used in large, ptotic breasts when a reduction is planned on the opposite breast. A common problem with this technique is the occurrence of native skin flap necrosis of the most distal portions of the flap, particularly at the T junction (see Fig. 80-1).
- A separate axillary incision is made transversely behind the border of the pectoralis major muscle one finger breath below the axillary hair line.

Main Dissection

Sentinel Lymph Node Biopsy

- The sentinel lymph node biopsy is performed before mastectomy. After the patient is premedicated with steroids and antihistamines, 2 mL of blue dye is injected into the subareolar lymphatic plexus. In patients who have had prior upper outer-quadrant biopsies, an intraparenchymal injection is made in the lateral wall of the biopsy cavity.
- The axillary incision is extended through the clavipectoral fascia to expose the axillary contents. Care is taken to preserve the intercostal-brachial nerves that run transversely on the axilla.
- The dissection is begun along the lateral border of the pectoralis major muscle. Blue channels can be identified crossing over the muscle to course into the axilla. The channels are followed to the sentinel lymph nodes. In obese patients or when the blue channels are not readily apparent, the gamma probe aids this dissection. The lymphatic channels are clipped to reduce the incidence of lymphocele formation. Drains are not routinely used.
- The following lymph nodes are removed and sent to pathology for frozen-section examination:
  - ▲ Radioactive lymph nodes
  - ▲ Blue lymph nodes
  - ▲ Lymph nodes with blue channels entering them
  - ▲ Clinically suspicious lymph nodes
- Radioactive lymph nodes are removed until the lymphatic basin has a cumulative radioactive count over 10 seconds that is 10% or less of the cumulative count of the hottest sentinel lymph node.

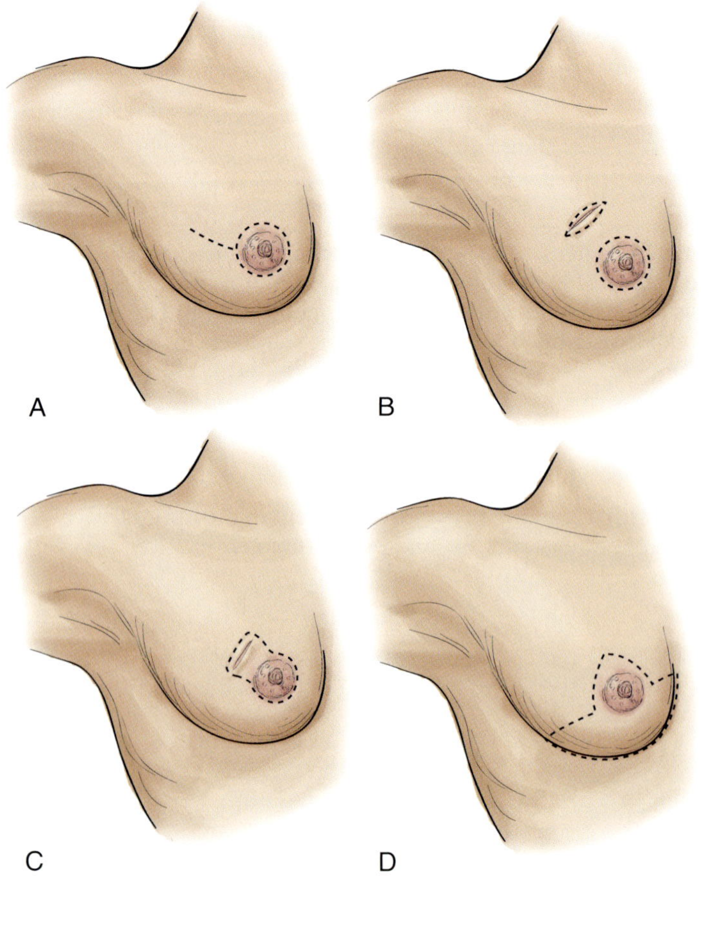

Figure 80-1. **A**, Type I skin-sparing mastectomy (SSM). **B**, Type II SSM. **C**, Type III SSM. **D**, Type IV SSM.

Skin-Sparing Mastectomy

- The skin flaps are elevated superficial to the enveloping fascia of the breast (Fig. 80-2). The skin flap thickness depends on the location on the breast and the body habitus of the patient. Breast tissue extends closer to the skin in the lower quadrants, and the subcutaneous tissue is thicker in the upper, outer quadrant of the breast. In a thin patient, skin flap thickness may be only 2 to 3 mm and may transmit light. In the obese patient, the flaps may be 5 to 10 mm in thickness.
- Electrocautery on low blended coagulation current is used for flap elevation. The majority of the blood vessels lie deep to the fascia, but perforating vessels to the skin are encountered and controlled with coagulation current. Skin retraction is performed with double-pronged skin hooks (Fig. 80-3). Because the skin opening is small, the flaps are elevated centripetally to assist in exposure.

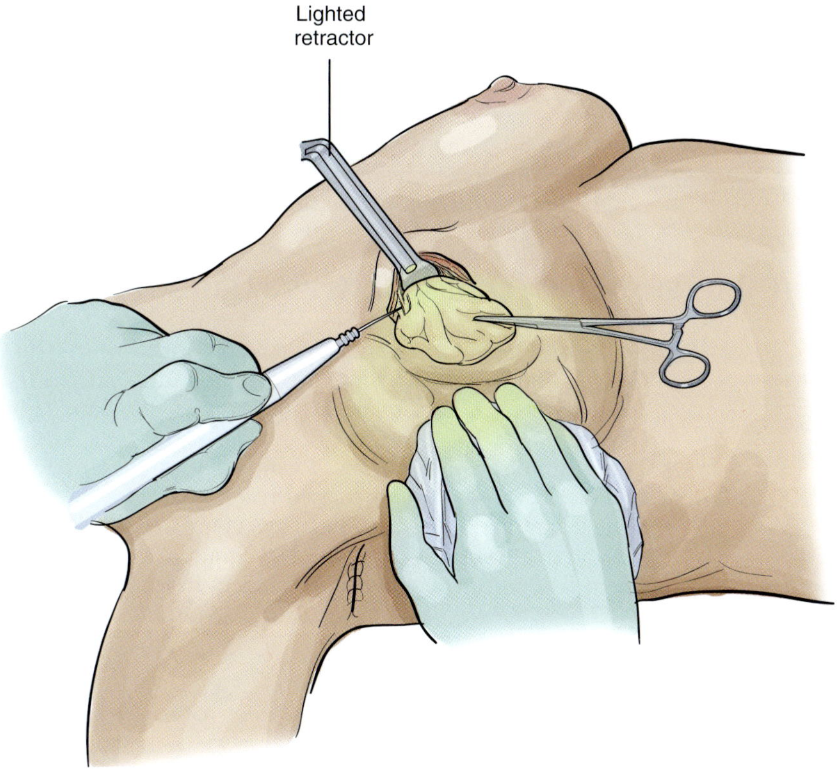

Figure 80-2.

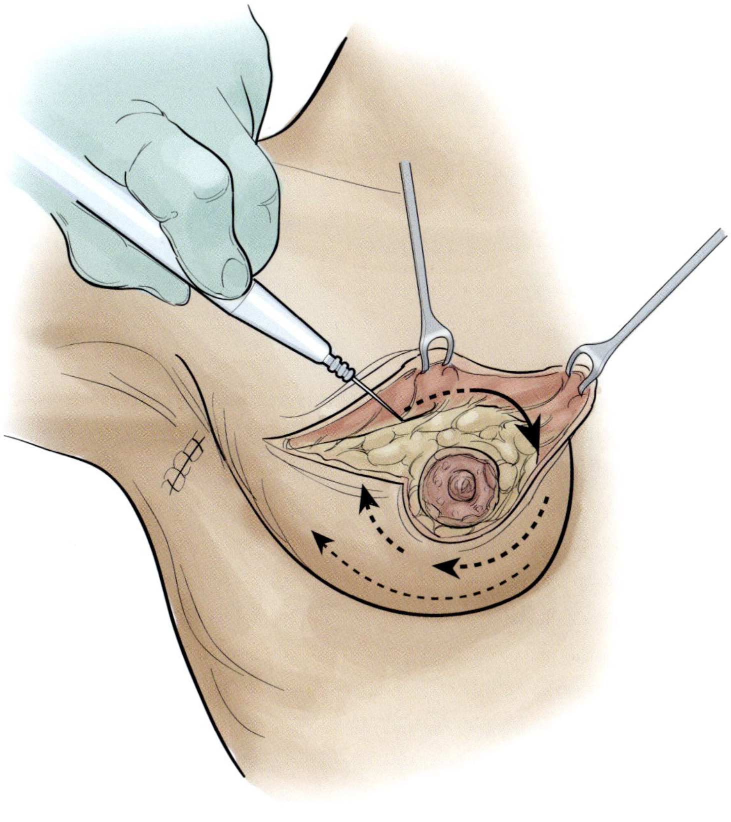

Figure 80-3.

- Superiorly, the breast falls away from the skin as the clavicle is approached. The fascia is followed down to the pectoralis major muscle. Medially, the fascia is not as defined, and the dissection ends at the border of the sternum (Fig. 80-4). Perforating vessels of the internal mammary artery are frequently encountered along the sternal border and can be controlled with electrocautery. Inferiorly, the dissection follows the superficial layer of the fascia to its junction with the deep layer. The skin is adherent to the anterior abdominal wall at this juncture. This is appreciated by observing the previous skin marking of the fold. This fascial junction occurs at the inferior edge of the pectoralis major muscle. Laterally, the dissection continues over the pectoralis muscle toward the humerus, enabling removal of the axillary tail.
- The breast is removed by elevating the fascia of the pectoralis major muscle with the specimen. This is best accomplished by dissecting parallel to the muscle fibers.

Closure

- Preservation of the skin envelope and inframammary fold facilitates breast shaping during reconstruction (Figs. 80-5 and 80-6). The abundant native skin reduces the amount of tissue transfer required. In cases of autologous reconstruction, there is less need for surgery on the contralateral breast to achieve symmetry. The periareolar incisions are relatively inconspicuous and are easily hidden by clothes.

III. ALTERNATIVE TECHNICAL APPROACHES (PRO/CON) AND PEARLS

- An SSM is technically more demanding and time consuming than a modified radical mastectomy. Careful handling of the skin flaps is required to prevent ischemic complications. Deep retractors are avoided to prevent damage to the base of the skin flaps, and low electrocautery is used for flap elevation.
- The procedure should be used cautiously in patients with a history of chest irradiation or tobacco smoking because of the increased risk of skin loss.
- Several nonrandomized studies have compared the local recurrence of breast cancer associated with SSM and conventional (non-SSM) techniques. The local recurrence rate in these studies ranged from 0% to 7%, and no significant differences in local recurrence rate between the techniques was found.

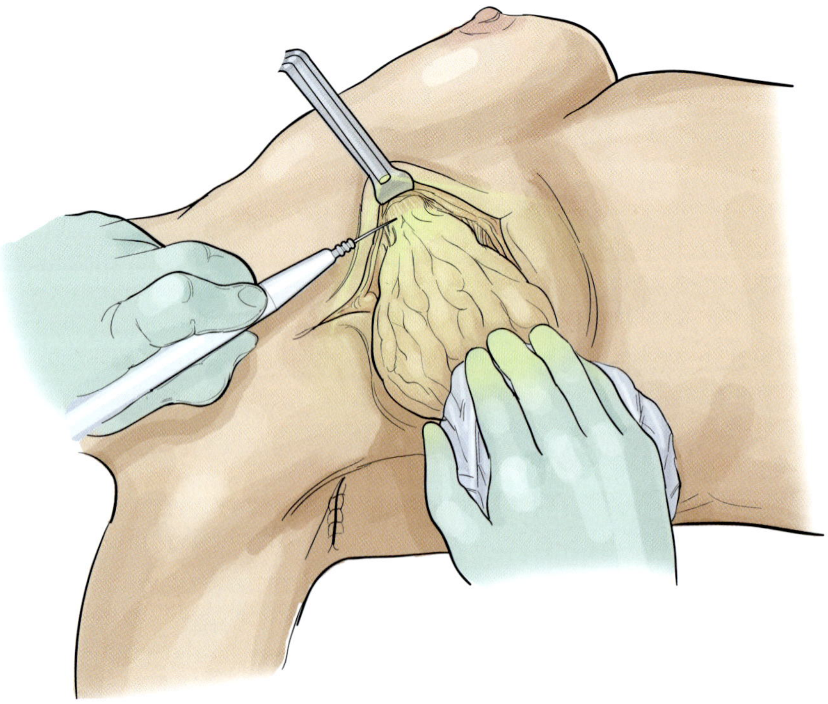

Figure 80-4.

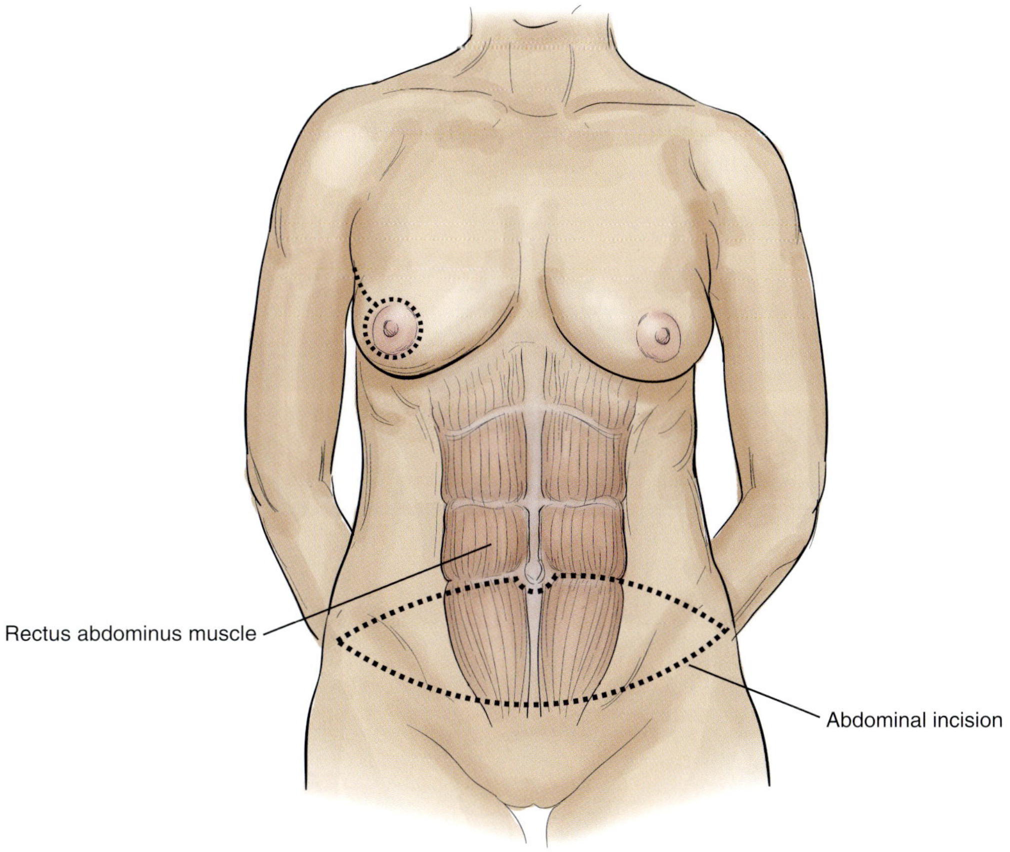

Figure 80-5.

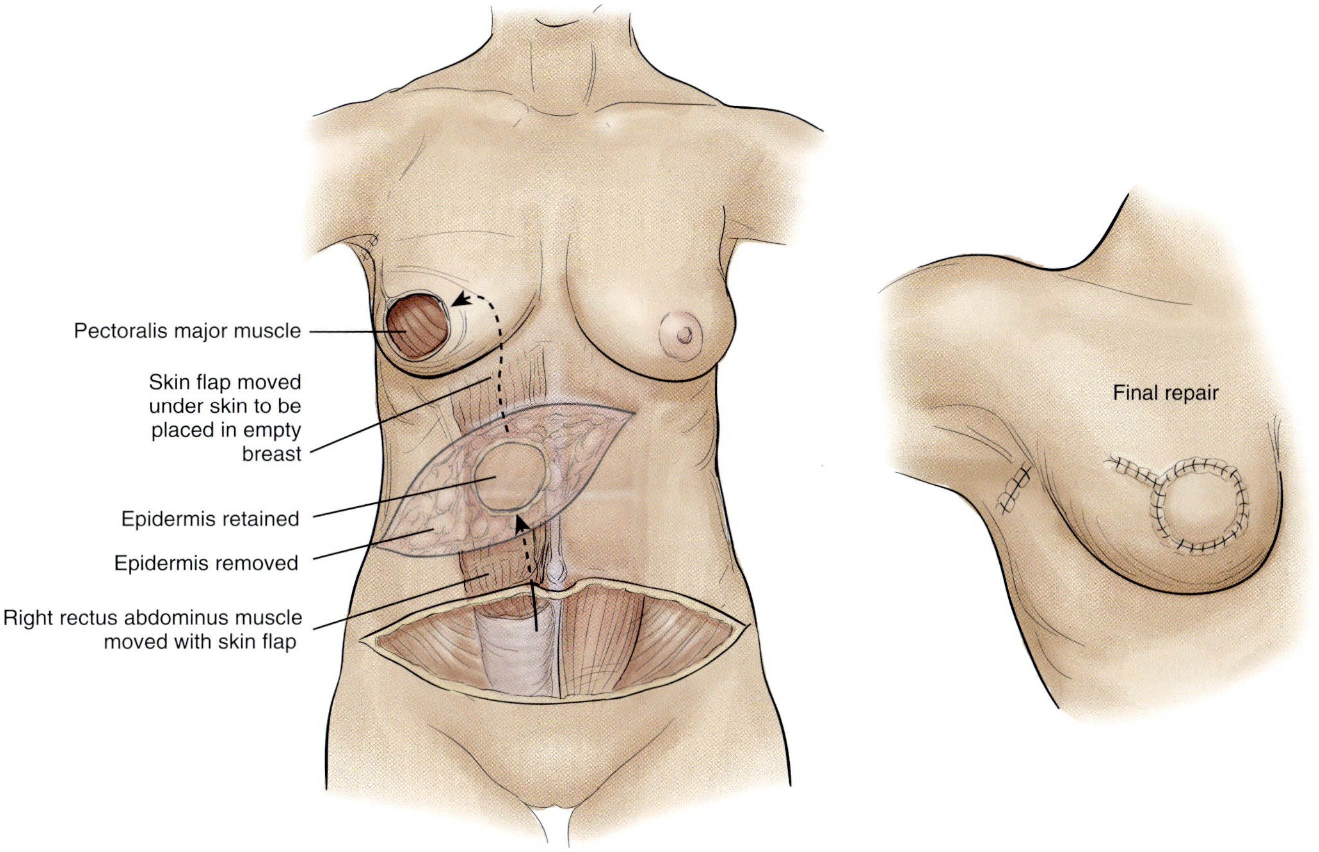

Figure 80-6.

IV. SPECIAL POSTOPERATIVE CARE

- Skin flap viability is assessed clinically, and ischemic skin is resected, especially in cases of immediate implant reconstruction where native skin necrosis could result in implant exposure. If there is a question of skin perfusion, fluorescein can be employed. The incidence of native skin flap necrosis is similar for SSM and non-SSM techniques.

SUGGESTED READINGS

Carlson GW: Tailored surgery for early breast cancer: surgical techniques. In Piccart M, Wood WC, Hung MC, et al, editors: *Breast cancer management and molecular medicine: towards tailored approaches*, New York, 2007, Springer, pp 161–182.

Carlson GW, Page A, Johnson E, et al: Local recurrence of ductal carcinoma in situ after skin sparing mastectomy, *J Am Coll Surg* 204:1074–1080, 2007.

Carlson GW, Styblo TM, Lyles R, et al: Local recurrence after skin sparing mastectomy: tumor biology or surgical conservatism? *Ann Surg Oncol* 10:108–112, 2003.

SECTION XV

Hernia

CHAPTER 81

Laparoscopic Ventral Hernia Repair

Alexander P. Nagle, MD, FACS, and Nathaniel J. Soper, MD

I. SPECIAL PREOPERATIVE PREPARATION

Patient Selection

- The technique for laparoscopic repair of abdominal wall hernias was described in 1993. The repair is based on the principles of the Rieves-Stoppa open retrorectus tension-free mesh repair. The Rieves-Stoppa repair has been shown to be superior to other open techniques in terms of recurrence. The laparoscopic approach differs in that the mesh is positioned in the intraperitoneal cavity rather than in the retrorectus plane. The laparoscopic approach has the advantages of fewer wound complications, avoidance of large soft tissue dissection, and shorter recovery. The laparoscopic approach allows for clear visualization of the abdominal wall, wide mesh coverage beyond the defect, and secure fixation to healthy abdominal wall fascia, improving chances of a successful repair. The laparoscopic approach to abdominal wall hernias has become the procedure of choice in most cases in which a prosthetic mesh is needed (Fig. 81-1). Small hernias (2 to 3 cm) are still best approached anteriorly and repaired primarily. However, in the setting of obesity, history of smoking, or prior surgical repair, even small hernias may best be approached laparoscopically using a prosthetic mesh. Nonmidline hernias are ideally suited for a laparoscopic approach. There remains debate regarding the best approach to larger abdominal wall hernias (greater than 12 to 15 cm). These can be significantly more challenging and should not be approached laparoscopically early in a surgeon's learning curve. An open repair using an underlay mesh or a separation of components should be considered for larger hernias. Clearly, in the presence of loss of abdominal domain, a laparoscopic approach should not be attempted. In the setting of contamination, such as enterocutaneous fistula or bowel resection, an open approach may be preferred. An open hernia repair is also favorable when a combined abdominoplasty or panniculectomy is indicated.

Preoperative Preparation

- Preoperative preparation begins with the operative consent. It is important to discuss the expected outcomes and to specifically address the issues of postoperative pain, seroma formation, and the risk of enterotomy. The risk of enterotomy will be greater in patients with multiple previous abdominal operations or multiple prior ventral hernia repairs, especially prior mesh repairs. In particular, previously placed polypropylene mesh should heighten the suspicion for dense adhesions. All prior operative reports should be obtained and reviewed if possible. A bowel prep is recommended in most cases to decrease the amount of contamination should an intraoperative enterotomy occur. Preoperative antibiotics (first-generation cephalosporin) are administered because a prosthetic mesh will be used. Sequential compression devices are placed on the lower extremities for deep venous thrombosis prophylaxis. A Foley catheter is typically used to decompress the bladder. In the setting of a suprapubic hernia, a three-way Foley catheter is helpful to distend the bladder and facilitate its identification and mobilization.

II. OPERATIVE TECHNIQUE

Position

- The patient is placed in the supine position with both arms tucked along the side. In large patients, if it is not possible to tuck both arms, the operating table can be moved away from the anesthetist so that the surgeon or assistant can stand cephalad to the arm boards if needed. The patient is securely strapped to the operating table to facilitate maximum tilting and lateral rotation of the table. Two video monitors are used, one on each side of the operating table. The abdomen is prepped widely to allow lateral placement of trocars. Additionally, an Ioban skin protector is used to prevent direct contact of the prosthetic mesh with the skin flora.

Trocar Placement

- The initial trocar is placed in a location away from all previous incisions and on the opposite side of the hernial defect (Fig. 81-2). A subcostal location at the anterior axillary line is often free of adhesions. The initial trocar can be placed with a Veress needle, open (Hasson) technique, or an optical viewing

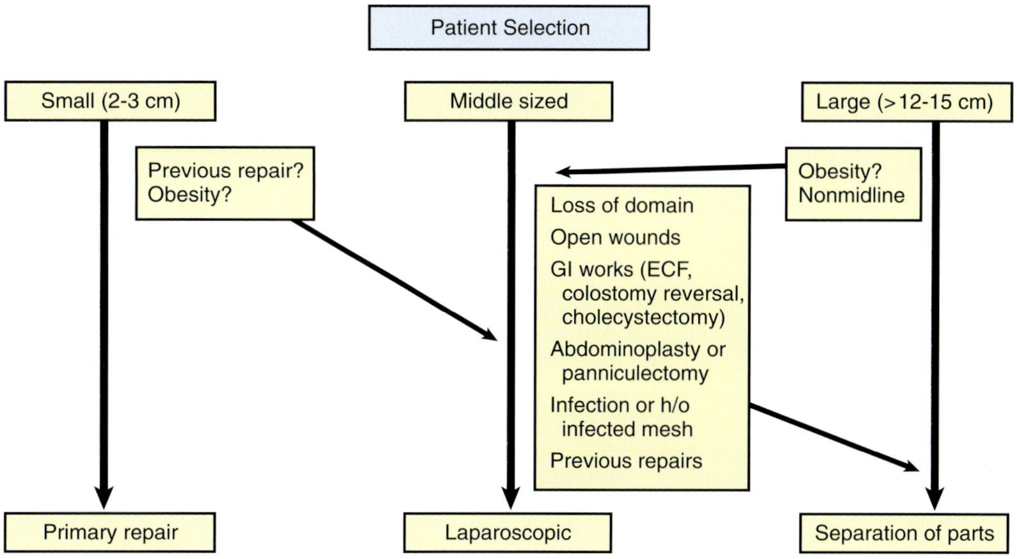

Figure 81-1. *ECF,* Enterocutaneous fistula; *GI,* gastrointestinal; *h/o,* history of.

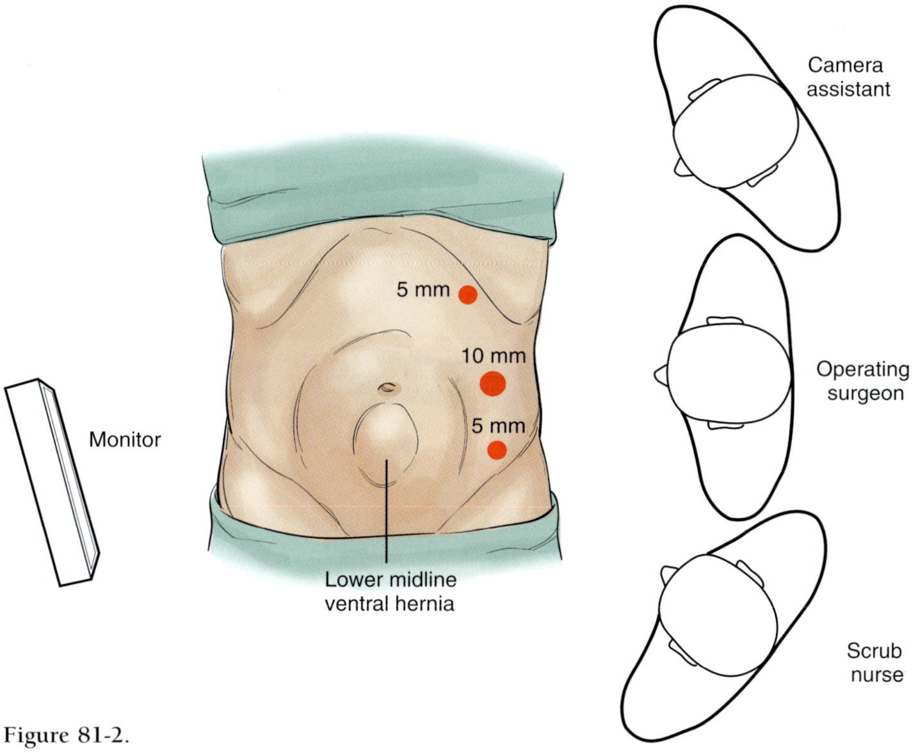

Figure 81-2.

trocar. Surgeons should use the access method with which they have the most experience and feel the most comfortable. The initial trocar can be either 5 or 10 mm, depending on the diameter of the laparoscope being used. The 5-mm laparoscope is more versatile because it can be moved to other 5- or 10-mm trocar sites. Angled laparoscopes (30 or 45 degrees) are helpful to maximize the ability to view "around corners" and to view the anterior abdominal wall.

- The additional trocars are then placed under direct laparoscopic visualization. At least one 10-mm trocar will be needed to allow insertion of the mesh into the peritoneal cavity. The density of the intraperitoneal adhesions will determine how many additional trocars are needed. In the setting of dense or numerous adhesions, typically two additional lateral trocars are needed on the same side as the initial trocar. This allows the surgeon to work inline with the camera and to perform the adhesiolysis with two hands (see Fig. 81-2). Additionally, at least one 5-mm trocar will be needed on the opposite side to accommodate mesh fixation.

Main Dissection

Adhesiolysis and Hernia Reduction

- Adhesiolysis can be the most difficult and time-consuming aspect of the operation. Not all adhesions are alike. Filmy adhesions may be taken down bluntly. Dense adhesions will require sharp dissection (Fig. 81-3). The use of energy sources, such as monopolar or bipolar cautery and ultrasound dissection, should be limited to avoid thermal tissue damage to the intestines. One difficult situation involves dense adhesions between the bowel and the anterior abdominal wall or previously placed mesh—in particular, previously placed polypropylene mesh. In this case, the plane between the bowel and the peritoneum is often obliterated, and it is necessary to dissect in the preperitoneal space. Surgeons should be flexible about trocar placement, and additional trocars should be placed as needed to accomplish the necessary adhesiolysis. A 5-mm laparoscope allows the surgeon to use different trocars to improve visualization. Direct manipulation of the intestinal wall should be avoided if possible. If necessary, the mesentery or epiploic fat should be grasped to provide countertraction. The hernia content is reduced in a hand-over-hand manner using atraumatic graspers. External manual compression will assist with safe reduction. The hernial sac is not excised, and therefore some degree of postoperative seroma formation should be expected in all cases. It may also be necessary to divide the falciform ligament should it be within 4 to 5 cm of the edge of the hernial defect. It is important to dissect all adhesions beneath the entire length of the incision. This will often identify multiple small fascial defects ("Swiss cheese") that could not be appreciated preoperatively. Once adhesiolysis is complete, the area lysed should be thoroughly inspected for possible bleeding or bowel injury. If found, these complications should be treated appropriately. Small bleeding points may be sutured or controlled with clips or with cautious application of low-wattage cautery. Serosal tears and enterotomies can be repaired laparoscopically; however, there should be a low threshold to convert to laparotomy. If there is any concern about the integrity of the bowel, we recommend a minilaparotomy to examine the bowel under direct vision.

Mesh Preparation and Insertion

- Once all the adhesions have been removed, the size of the hernial defect is measured in at least two dimensions. To ensure accuracy, measurement should be performed intraperitoneally rather than at

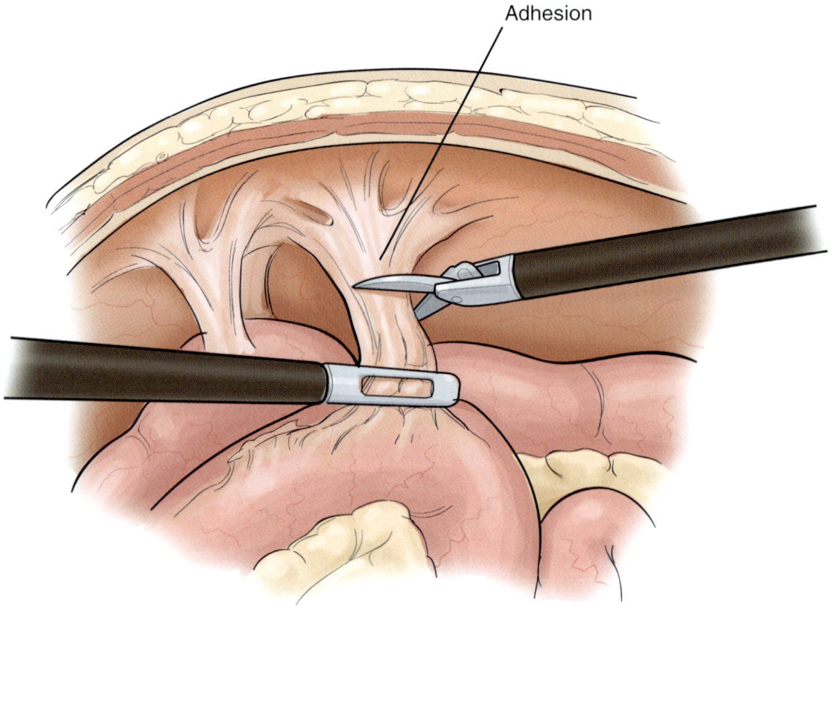

Figure 81-3.

the level of the skin. Considering the pneumoperitoneum and thickness of the abdominal wall, there can be a great discrepancy between a measurement at the surface of the skin and a measurement at the peritoneal level. We place a malleable ruler inside the peritoneal cavity to obtain an accurate measurement (Fig. 81-4). Typically, in the presence of multiple fascial defects, the maximum distance between all defects is measured, and one piece of mesh is used to cover them all. Once the fascial defect is measured, 4 to 5 cm is added in all directions to determine the appropriate size of the prosthetic mesh. In general one should err on the side of a larger mesh. The overlap distance is important for mesh ingrowth and fixation. The intraabdominal pressure will be distributed evenly across the mesh (Pascal's law); therefore the tendency will be to push the mesh up into the hernial defect. The greater the mesh overlap, the more pressure holding the mesh against the abdominal wall and the more surface area for mesh ingrowth. One must also assume some degree (up to 20%) of mesh shrinkage. It is also important to consider the type of mesh and the expected ingrowth—that is, polypropylene or polyester would be expected to have better tissue ingrowth than polytetrafluoroethylene.

- The mesh is prepared by first identifying which side (surface) of the mesh should be against the anterior abdominal wall and which side should face the peritoneal contents. The mesh is then oriented and marked appropriately (superior, inferior, right and left lateral). Four stay-sutures (U-stitches) are placed near the edge of the mesh (Fig. 81-5). The suture tails are left long to accommodate passage across the anterior abdominal wall and to allow a knot to be tied down to the fascia. We use a permanent monofilament suture. The mesh is then rolled as tightly as possible along its long axis to minimize its diameter (Fig. 81-6). The rolled mesh is then placed into the peritoneal cavity through a 10-mm trocar.

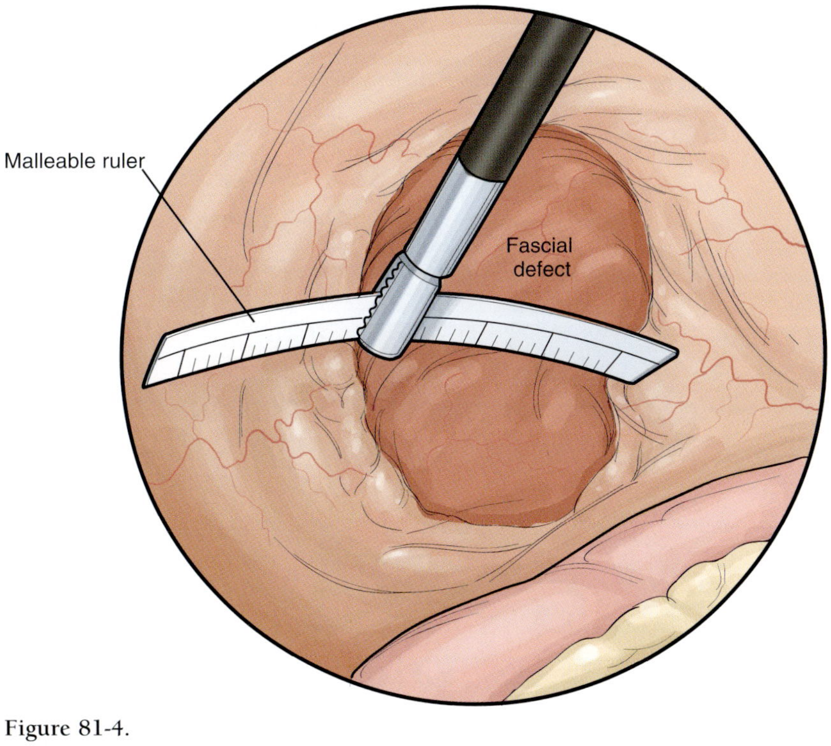

Figure 81-4.

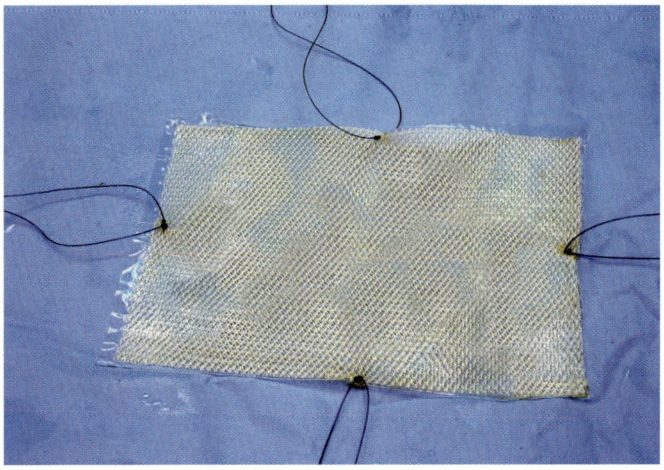

Figure 81-5.

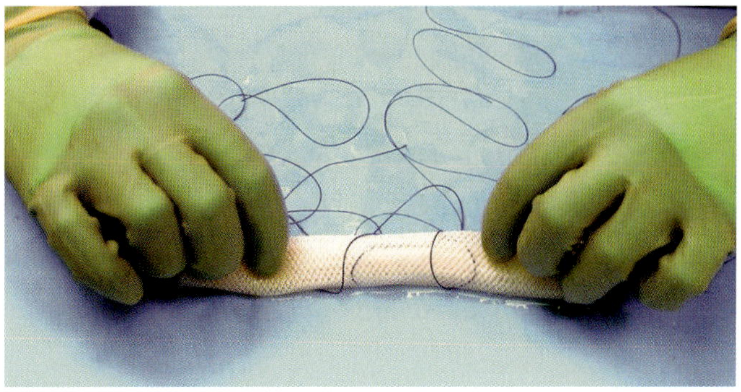

Figure 81-6.

This typically involves temporarily removing the cap from the 10-mm trocar (Fig. 81-7). It is preferable to insert the mesh through the trocar to minimize contamination of the mesh. However, for a very large mesh, it may be necessary to temporarily remove the 10-mm trocar and pass the mesh across the abdominal wall through the skin incision. Once the mesh is within the peritoneal cavity, the mesh is unrolled and oriented appropriately. Care is taken to ensure that the appropriate side (surface) of the mesh is against the abdominal wall. An angled telescope is advantageous to allow looking at the anterior abdominal wall and down at the mesh stay sutures.

Mesh Fixation

- The stay sutures are brought out across the entire abdominal wall through small incisions in the skin using a suture-passing instrument (Fig. 81-8). Both paired suture tails pass across the abdominal wall through the same skin incision, but each tail passes through a different fascial defect separated by approximately 1 cm. The sutures are not tied until all four stay sutures have been passed across the

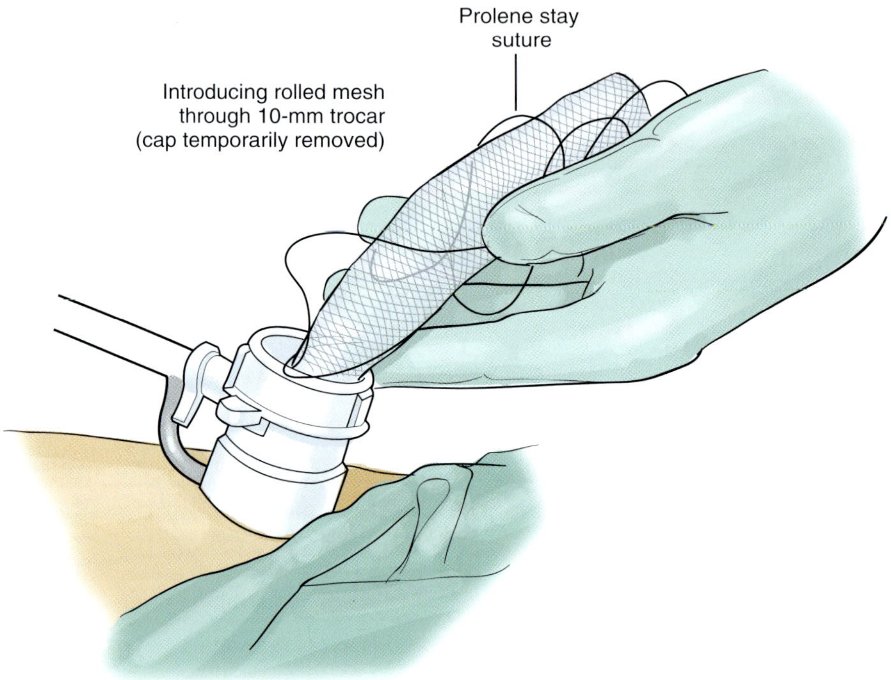

Figure 81-7.

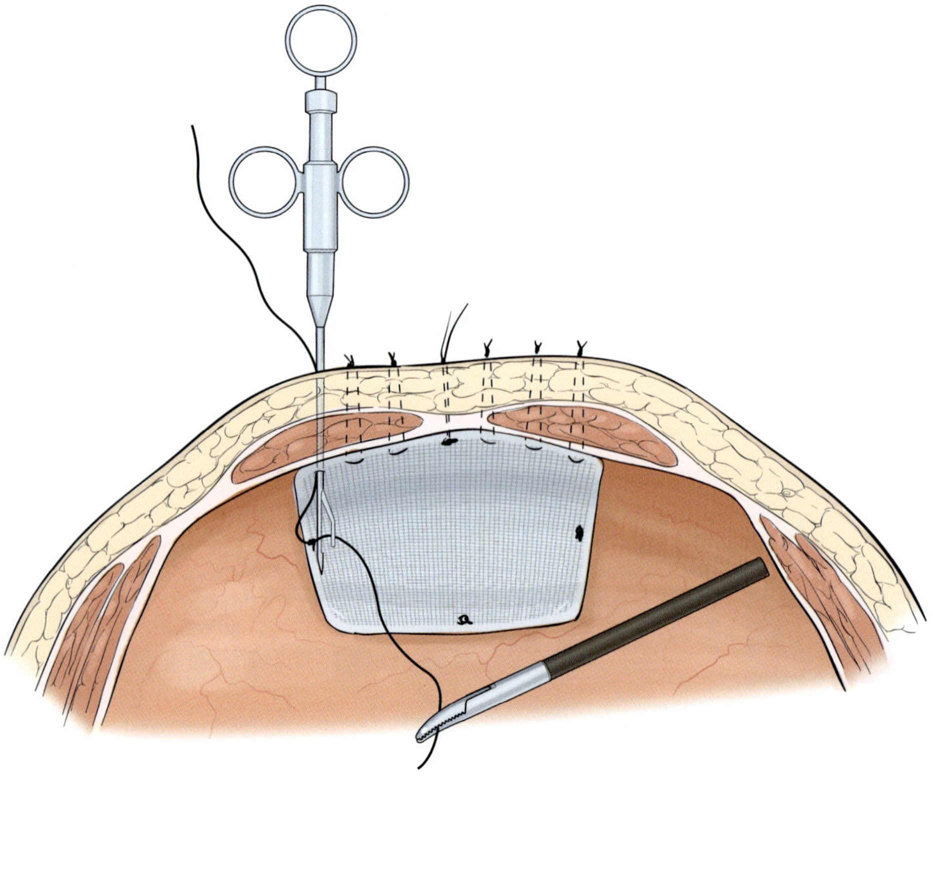

Figure 81-8.

abdominal wall and lifted to demonstrate the appropriate tautness of the mesh. If the stay suture is in an unacceptable position, it is pulled back into the abdominal cavity and repositioned so that the mesh is taut. It is important to stretch the mesh tightly so that when the pneumoperitoneum is released, the mesh does not bow into the hernial defect. Once the mesh is confirmed to be taut and in an appropriate position, the four stay sutures are tied extracorporeally downward to the fascia. To avoid puckering at this site, the skin and subcutaneous tissue can then be elevated back into place using a hemostat. The tacking device is then used to tack the mesh circumferentially (360 degrees) along its perimeter. It is important to apply strong countertraction (opposite hand) externally against the abdominal wall to ensure that the tacks are driven well into the abdominal wall (Fig. 81-9). Also, with the opposite hand on the abdominal wall, the stapler achieves a more perpendicular angle, which improves reliability. There is concern that an exposed tack can lead to bowel adhesions or even bowel injury. Most tacks penetrate only 2 to 3 millimeters into the abdominal wall, and therefore there is a theoretical concern that the entire mesh could migrate or shift along the peritoneum. The tensile strength has been shown to be 2.5 times greater when transfascial sutures are used compared to tacks. We do not recommend relying on tacks as the sole method of fixation. Although the tacks may not provide long-term fixation, they stretch the mesh taut for additional suture fixation and help to prevent internal herniation between the mesh and the abdominal wall. Using the suture-passing instrument, additional transfascial U stitches are then placed at 5-cm intervals. For larger fascial defects or in obese patients, there is more of a tendency (pressure) for the mesh to be pushed into the fascial defect, and transfascial U stitches should therefore be placed at more frequent intervals (every 2 to 3 cm) (Fig. 81-10). In the setting of multiple small defects (Swiss cheese), fewer transfascial sutures are needed. It is also important to consider the type of mesh material being used and the expected tissue ingrowth. For example, when using polytetrafluoroethylene, more transfascial sutures should be used because of poor tissue ingrowth.

Closure

- Before releasing the pneumoperitoneum, a final inspection of the underlying bowel and assessment of hemostasis should be performed. If possible, the greater omentum should be placed in the pelvis, thereby covering the small intestine and minimizing the possibility of intestinal adhesions to the mesh. It is also important to close the fascia at any 10-mm trocar site.

III. ALTERNATIVE TECHNICAL APPROACHES (PRO/CON) AND PEARLS

- Trocars should be placed far from the hernial defect to allow adequate space for adhesiolysis and mesh overlap.
- If necessary, one should not hesitate to add trocars to facilitate safe adhesiolysis.

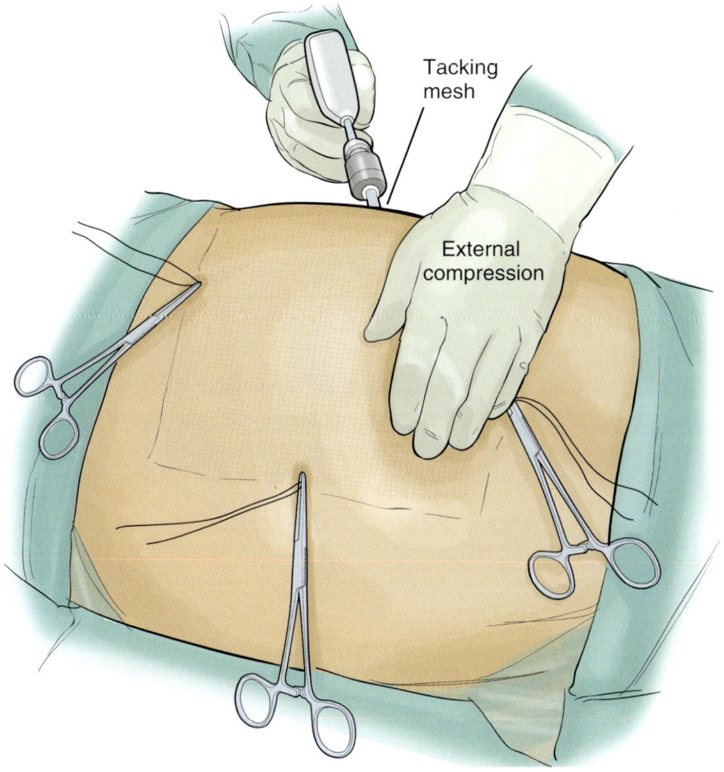

Figure 81-9.

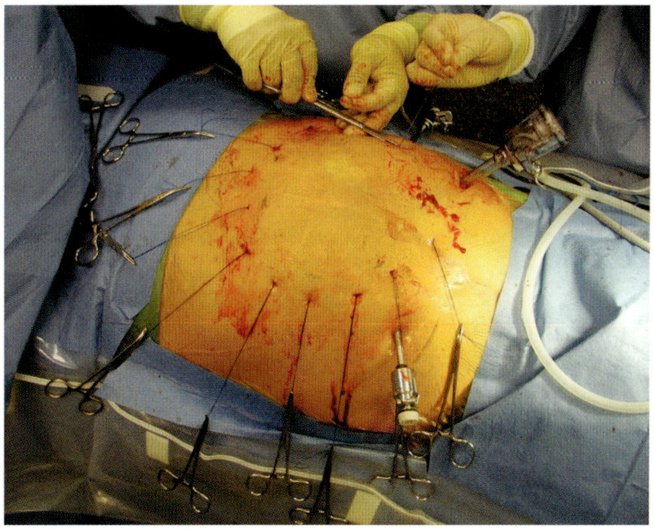

Figure 81-10.

- When selecting mesh size, it is best to err on the side of a larger mesh rather than too small.
- Transfascial sutures should be used at least every 5 cm around the perimeter of the mesh.
- An alternative technique involves closing the hernial defect primarily before placement of the mesh. Techniques have been described to close the hernial defect intracorporeally, using a transfascial suture passer, or making a small skin incision over the hernia to close the fascia via an open technique. Closing the hernial defect may minimize seroma formation and reduce the abdominal pressure pushing the mesh into the hernial sac. Restoring the rectus muscles to a more medial position may also improve body wall function.

IV. SPECIAL POSTOPERATIVE CARE

- Most patients are discharged the day after surgery. Patients have significantly more pain following laparoscopic ventral hernia repair than most other laparoscopic operations. There is significant peritoneal and muscle irritation from the transfascial sutures and tacks. Postoperative pain is controlled with scheduled intravenous ketorolac 30 mg every 6 hours while the patient is in the hospital. Oral pain medication is also initiated soon after surgery, and intravenous narcotics are used for breakthrough. However, for very large hernias, intravenous narcotics may be required for the first 24 hours postoperatively. We instruct our patients to limit their activity level for 4 weeks postoperatively.

Complications

- The surgeon should warn the patient about seroma formation, which occurs in every case because the hernial sac is not excised. Many of these seromas are not noticed by the patient, but some are visible and cause the patient to believe that the hernia has recurred or was not repaired. Most of these seromas will resolve on their own after 8 to 12 weeks. Aspiration of the seroma should be reserved for significant associated symptoms or if the seroma does not spontaneously resolve. Persistent pain at a transfascial suture site occurs in a small percentage of patients. This site can be injected with local anesthesia (several times if required) for resolution. Surgical intervention to remove the culprit suture is rarely needed. One of the most dreaded complications is an enterotomy. An enterotomy can occur intraoperatively or can be missed or present in a delayed fashion. Patient selection is important to avoid patients at high risk for dense adhesions. The possibility of an enterotomy should be addressed with the patient preoperatively, and a plan for dealing with it should be outlined. Although there may be several options (Table 81-1), the surgeon must recognize and appreciate his or her own technical limitations and should also err on the side of being conservative. Experience and good surgical judgment are invaluable.
- There are very limited data regarding the long-term recurrence rate following a laparoscopic ventral hernia repair. Even short-term outcomes can be difficult to interpret. One of the major reasons for this uncertainty has been the great variability in the technique of repair, such as the use and number of transfascial sutures, as well as the type of prosthetic mesh used. Nonetheless, most authors report a recurrence rate of around 10%. There are many potential mechanisms of recurrence (Table 81-2) following a laparoscopic ventral hernia repair.

TABLE 81-1 Intraoperative Enterotomy: Surgical Options

1. Convert to open, repair the enterotomy, and close the hernial defect primarily.
2. Convert to open, repair the enterotomy, and attempt a laparoscopic repair at a later date.
3. Laparoscopically repair the enterotomy and place mesh as planned.
   a. Only consider this option if there is minimal or no spillage of enteric content.
   b. If there is spillage of enteric content, consider a biologic mesh.
4. Laparoscopically repair the enterotomy, complete the adhesiolysis, and plan a delayed laparoscopic repair in 48 hours.

TABLE 81-2 Potential Mechanisms for Recurrence

1. Missed defect
2. Mesh contraction
3. Mesh migration
4. Fixation failure or inadequate fixation
5. Mesh failure
6. Tissue failure

SUGGESTED READINGS

Heniford BT, Park A, Ramshaw BJ, Voeller G: Laparoscopic repair of ventral hernias: nine years' experience with 850 consecutive hernias, *Ann Surg* 238:391–399, discussion 399–400, 2003.

LeBlanc KA: Laparoscopic incisional hernia repair: are transfascial sutures necessary? A review of the literature, *Surg Endosc* 21:508–513, 2007.

Pierce RA, Spitler JA, Frisella MM, et al: Pooled data analysis of laparoscopic vs. open ventral hernia repair: 14 years of patient data accrual, *Surg Endosc* 21:378–386, 2007.

CHAPTER 82

Preperitoneal Repair of Recurrent Hernia with Giant Prosthesis (Stoppa Repair)

Pierre Verhaeghe, MD, PhD, FACS, and René Stoppa, MD, PhD, FACS

I. SPECIAL PREOPERATIVE PREPARATION

- Before performing this procedure, the surgeon should be familiar with the surgical anatomy, purpose of the procedure, and preoperative preparation.

Anatomy

- Groin hernias result from a deficiency of the transversalis fascia in the weak area (Fig. 82-1) of the osteomuscular orifice—the Fruchaud myopectineal orifice—through which the femoral vessels and the spermatic cord pass. Treatment of these hernias may be unified and requires, after resection of the

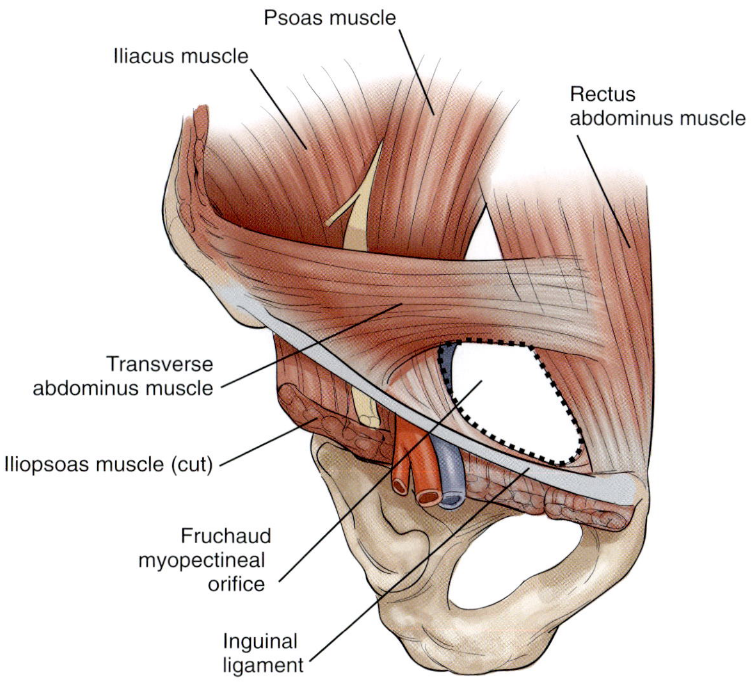

Figure 82-1.

sac, reinforcement of the transversalis fascia behind the myopectineal orifice. When one avoids the superficial inguinal nerves in the preperitoneal approach, the incidence of testicular atrophies and painful sequelae is decreased. As a side benefit, this approach preserves the mechanisms that protect the inguinal region from the effects of intraabdominal pressure (Keith's "inguinal shutter," Lytle's Hesselbach ligament sling, Ogilvie's cord lifting).

Aim of the Operative Procedure

- The central focus of our procedures is the placement of a wide sheet of nonresorbable mesh between the muscles and peritoneum. The mesh extends broadly (Fig. 82-2) beyond the internal inguinal orifice in all directions. When the peritoneal sac is replaced, intraabdominal pressure forces the prosthesis against the inner face of the abdominal wall. It quickly attaches as connective tissue develops through the mesh. With this method, the surgeon is using the forces that have created the hernia (that is, pressure of the abdominal contents) to obtain a radical repair and to prevent recurrence of the hernia. The prosthesis could be compared to a patch between an inner tube and a tire. The surgeon places a large prosthesis, extending from one anterior superior iliac spine to the opposite one, which reinforces the peritoneum, rendering it inextensible.

Physical Preparation

- The skin of the abdomen, scrotum, and perineum must be carefully disinfected because of the risk of sepsis in surgery using prostheses. If the patient has any skin diseases, the operation must be deferred until the lesions are healed. Extensive hernias require respiratory preparations and sometimes the use of progressive pneumoperitoneum (the so-called Goni Moreno technique).

Prosthesis Used

- We use Dacron or Mersilene mesh in all of our operations. It is a light, supple, elastic tissue of wide-meshed net that permits rapid infiltration by the connective tissue.

II. OPERATIVE TECHNIQUE

Position

- The patient lies in a mild Trendelenburg position. The surgeon and scrub nurse stand on the side opposite the hernia that is to be dissected first, and the assistant stands on the other side.
- General anesthesia is usually used. Spinal and especially peridural anesthesia are useful in patients at respiratory risk.

Incision

- The abdominal wall is cut strictly in the midline. The umbilical prevesical fascia is cut along its entire length, with Mayo scissors, beginning at the suprapubic space and moving cephalad (Fig. 82-3).

Main Dissection

- Dissection begins inferiorly in the Retzius space to cleave the preperitoneal and prevesical space.
- Dissection progresses laterally under the fascia covering the rectus abdominis (Fig. 82-4) and protecting the inferior epigastric vessels. The surgeon does not try to dissect the hernia first. Dissection proceeds laterally, a little higher than the internal inguinal opening, unsticking the peritoneum to expose the iliopsoas muscle and iliac vessels laterally and dorsally.

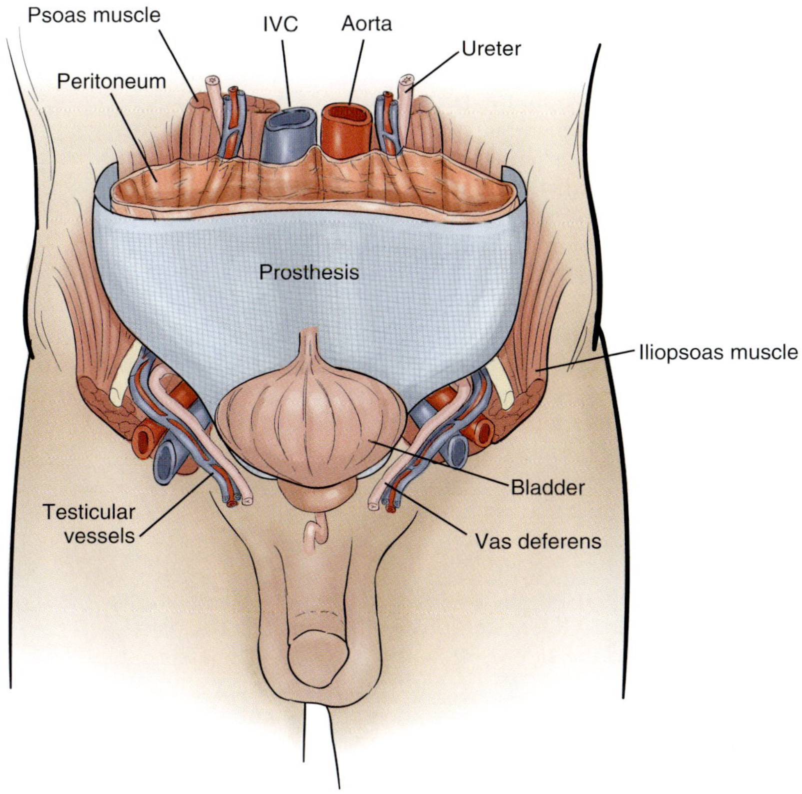

Figure 82-2. *IVC,* Inferior vena cava.

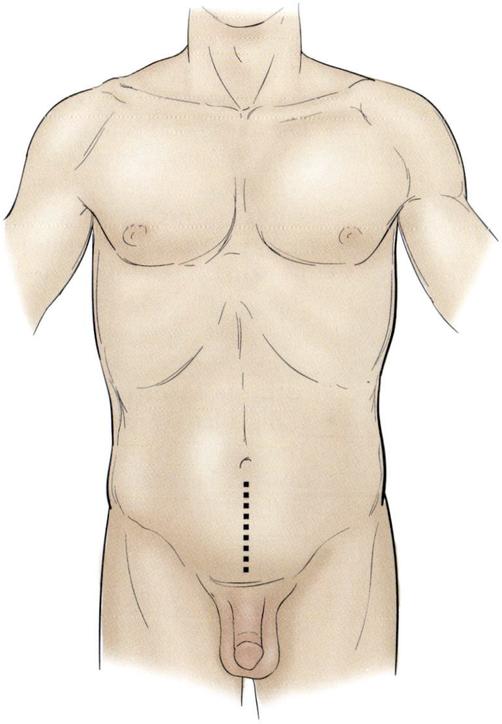

Figure 82-3.

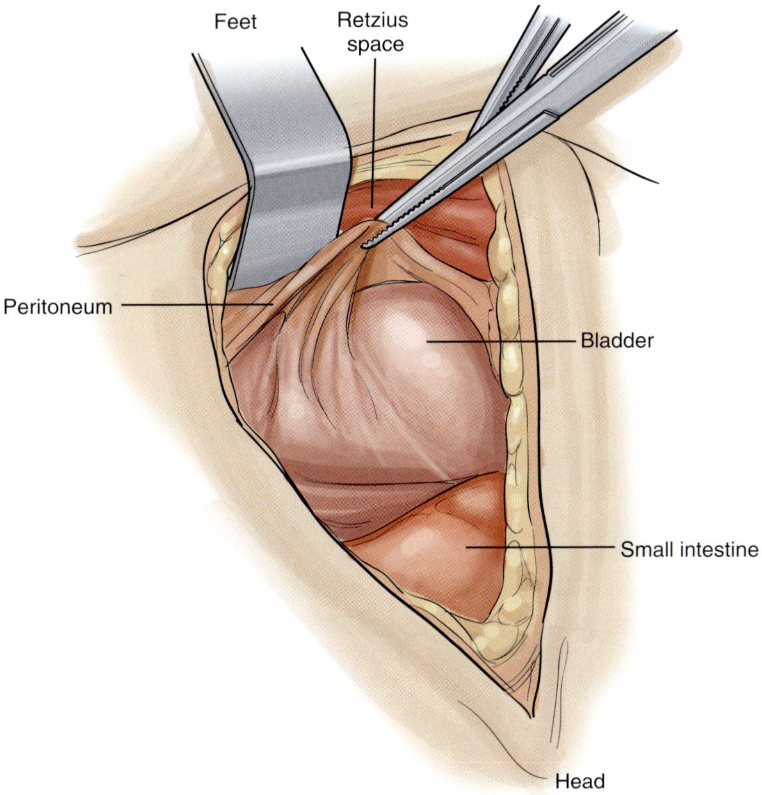

Figure 82-4.

- Using both hands, the surgeon can easily perform a circular motion (Fig. 82-5) passing anteriorly to the iliac vessels and allowing a Silastic band to encircle the spermatic cord and hernia. The cord is seized in its retroparietal course with a Silastic band, and moderate traction is applied (Fig. 82-6) so the scissors can dissociate the various elements of the cord from the peritoneal sac.
- This dissection is finished with a blunt swab. Then the peritoneal sac is found on the inner aspect and the urogenital fascia with a posterosuperior base on the outer aspect, the sides of which contain the deferent canal on the inside and the spermatic vascular pedicle on the outside. When the spermatic cord elements are released, as when the Silastic band is taken off, these elements join themselves by gravity with the posterior wall so no element can cross the preperitoneal prevesical space.
- To perform the retroparietal dissection on the opposite side, the surgeon, scrub nurse, and assistant change sides and proceed in the same manner to treat the second hernia.

Prosthesis Insertion

- Using a large prosthesis to reinforce the visceral sac renders repair of the hernial defects unnecessary. The size of the prosthesis is measured on the patient. The correct transverse dimension is equal to the distance between the anterosuperior iliac spines minus 2 cm, the height of the prosthesis being equal to the distance between the umbilicus and the pubis. The patch is chevron-shaped (Fig. 82-7), measuring on average 24 cm transversely and 16 cm vertically, with extreme values ranging from 20 to 30 cm transversely and 14 to 20 cm vertically.
- The prosthesis is easily cut with a pair of straight scissors using the no-touch technique. The patch is then grasped at all four corners and in the middle with long Rochester forceps that facilitate the placement procedure (Fig. 82-8). The patch is first placed on the side opposite the surgeon. The assistant retracts the parietal wall as the surgeon depresses the peritoneal sac with the left hand, pulling it upward; this opens the parietoperitoneal cleavage space. The prosthesis is then pushed into this space with the Rochester forceps. First, the inferior median forceps (*1* in Fig. 82-8) is placed between the pubis and bladder, followed by the inferior angle forceps (*2*), median lateral forceps (*3*), and superior angle forceps (*4*). Each is pushed as far as possible. This action unfolds the prosthesis on all points of the parietoperitoneal cleavage space and surrounds the part of the visceral sac opposite the surgeon. As each of the forceps is pushed into its correct place, the assistant immobilizes the visceral sac until the surgeon releases it with the left hand, which enables it to take its place as the valve is removed from under the parietal wall. A forceps (*5*) fixes the prosthesis to the umbilical prevesical fascia under the umbilicus (Fig. 82-9). The forceps (*4*, *3*, *2*, one after another in Fig. 82-8) used to place the prosthesis are then removed delicately at the same angle at which they were placed, passing along the inner side of the parietal wall.
- The surgeon and the assistant again change sides and perform the same procedure on the opposite side. The Dacron mesh prosthesis is fully unfolded and inserted without excessive tension to surround the visceral sac, generously overlapping the hernial defects and also protecting the median subumbilical

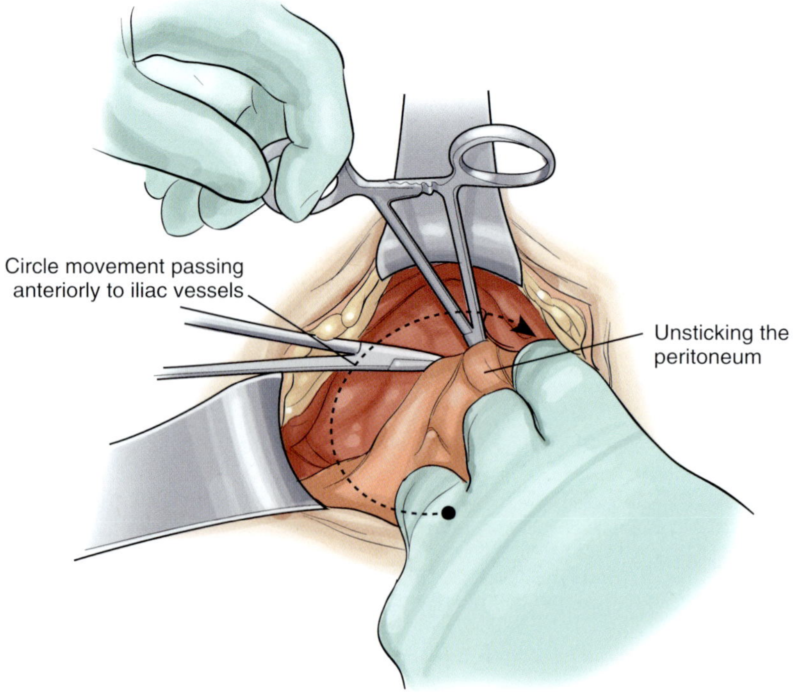

Figure 82-5.

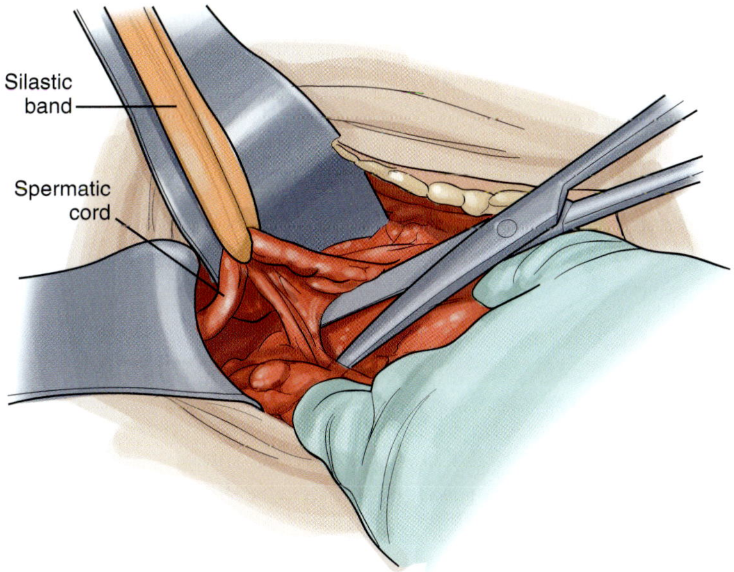

Figure 82-6.

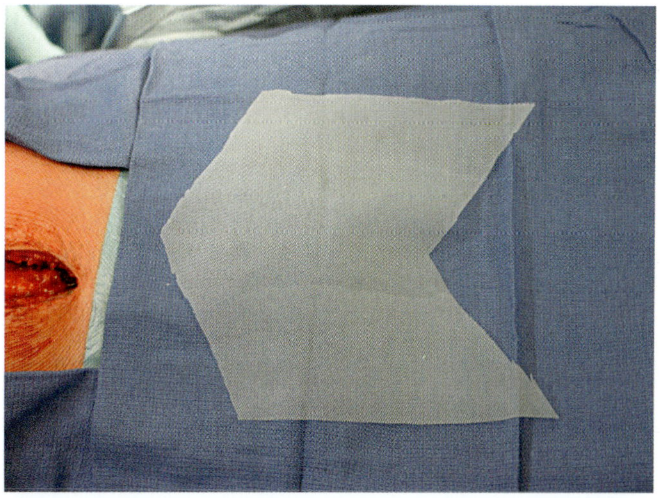

Figure 82-7. Chevron-shaped prosthesis to facilitate three-dimensional adaptation of the prosthesis in the pelvis.

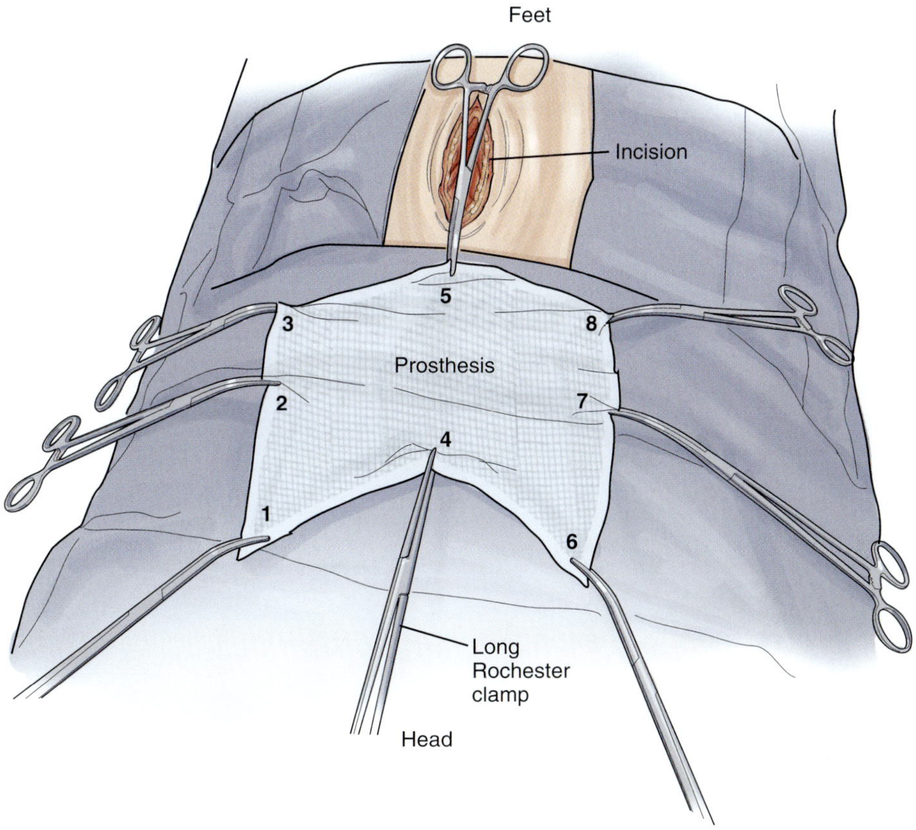

Figure 82-8. See text for explanation of numbers.

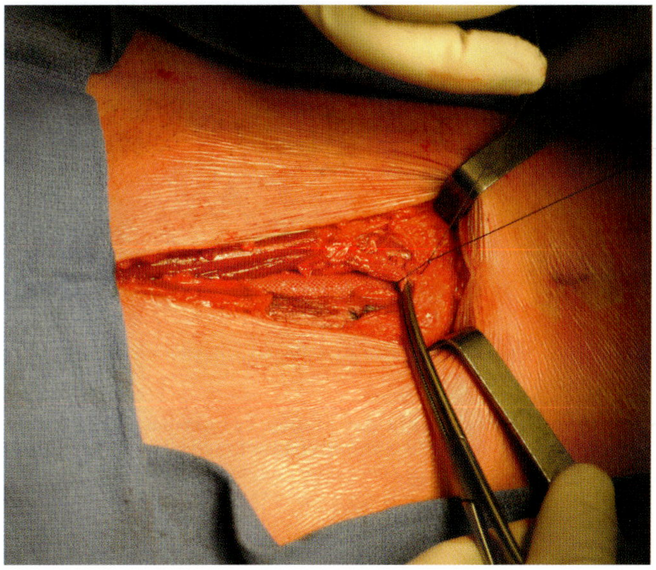

Figure 82-9. Prosthesis fixed to umbilical prevesical fascia.

incision. The inferior angle forceps (6), median lateral forceps (7), and superior angle forceps (8) are successively placed (Fig. 82-10, *A* and *B*). The middle of the superior border of the patch is then fixed with a synthetic resorbable suture to the inferior border of the Richet umbilical fascia.

Closure

- The parietal suture is made with slow-resorption synthetic suture material. The subcutaneous fat is padded with small slow-resorption synthetic material and the skin is sutured with fine subcutaneous nylon or glue. When suction drainage tubes seem necessary, they are placed in front of the prosthesis.

III. ALTERNATIVE TECHNICAL APPROACHES (PRO/CON) AND PEARLS

- A horizontal Pfannenstiel incision (Fig. 82-11) can be used for better cosmetic results. Surgeons in training are warned that the lateral side of this incision is very near the internal inguinal ring, which makes it more difficult to avoid the urogenital fascia and expose the iliopsoas muscle in the lateral and upper part of the dissection.
- In females, the lack of a spermatic cord may make the dissection easier, but the round ligament cannot be unstuck and must be cut to insert the mesh.
- A voluminous inguinoscrotal hernia can be a challenge. The first step involves surrounding the spermatic cord and hernia with a Silastic band. Expression of the scrotum can aid in reduction of the hernia. If this expression cannot be easily obtained, it is better to forego reduction and to open the sac. The inferior part of the sac (with Redon tube) will be left in the scrotum to limit the risk of testicular atrophy.
- For inguinal and suprapubic incisional hernias, the same dissection is performed, but with larger and higher dissection of the properitoneal space. The mesh must be fixed laterally to avoid early incisional hernia recurrence.

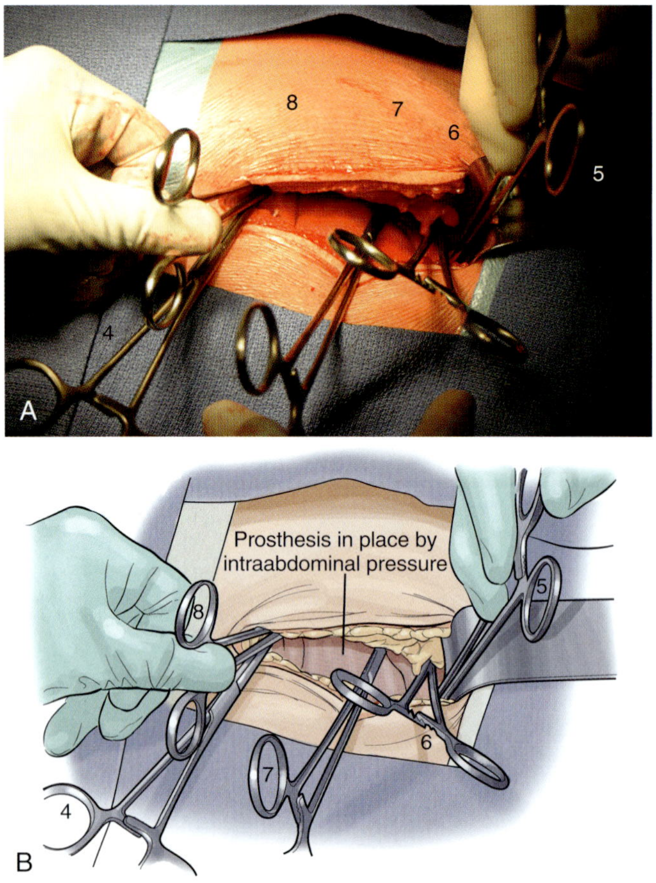

Figure 82-10. Prosthesis held in position by intraabdominal pressure against the inner face of the abdominal wall. Inferior angle forceps (6), median lateral forceps (7), superior angle forceps (8).

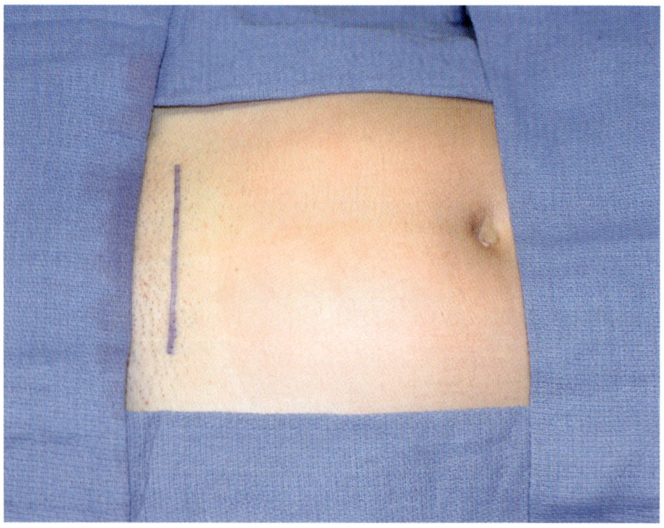

Figure 82-11.

Incidence of Primary Hernia Repair

- When no prosthesis is used, a Lichtenstein repair is performed. This intact posterior approach is typically easy to do. If adhesions of the spermatic cord, sequelae of peritoneal resection, are found, it is better to open the peritoneum near this adhesion to allow the position of the peritoneal sac to be controlled intraperitoneally. The peritoneum is then sewn with synthetic, slowly resorbable sutures.
- When a retromuscular laparoscopic prosthesis is inserted (transabdominal preperitoneal, total extraperitoneal, or intraperitoneal onlay mesh), the dissection is more difficult. The correct approach is in front of the anterior prosthesis, which is left sticking to the peritoneum. The difficulty with the spermatic cord depends on the width of the previous dissection.
- When the Stoppa repair is used, an anterior approach is taken to suture the inferior side of the previous prosthesis to the inguinal ligament (as in the Shouldice repair). In older patients, this repair can be performed under local anesthesia.

IV. SPECIAL POSTOPERATIVE CARE

- Usually, no suction drain is needed. The patient is urged to resume early unrestricted activity. Prophylactic antibiotic therapy is not routinely used. The patient is discharged from the hospital on postoperative day 2 or 3.
- The patient must be informed of the possible occurrence of a penis root ecchymosis. The color can be frightening, but the ecchymosis is harmless.
- Scrotal hematoma is a complication of voluminous inguinoscrotal hernia that is not always prevented by a suction drain.
- Testicular ischemia is more frequent after recurrent hernia repair than after primary repair. A posterior approach (Stoppa repair or laparoscopic repair) limits the risk but not completely.
- Postoperative infection is very rare if skin is carefully disinfected and if postoperative infection did not complicate the previous repair.

Conclusion

- Familiarity with this approach and with prostheses encourages surgeons to no longer distinguish between types of groin hernias (inguinal or femoral). The main appeal of this approach is the ability to place a large piece of synthetic mesh behind the weak inguinal area to tighten the wall, regardless of the damage to all layers of its structure. The preperitoneal approach is convenient for even the most difficult hernial repairs, such as those of multirecurrent, prevascular, sliding, enormous, or bilateral hernias. Its principles are valuable for all posterior prosthesis implantation by laparotomy or by a laparoscopic approach.

SUGGESTED READINGS

Forte A, Zullino A, Manfredelli S, et al: Rives technique is the gold standard for incisional hernioplasty. An institutional experience, *Ann Ital Chir* 82:313–317, 2011.

Fruchaud H: *The surgical anatomy of hernias of the groin*, Bendavid R, Cunningham P, translators. Toronto, 2006, Pandemonium Books. Originally published 1956.

Verhaeghe P, Rohr S: *Chirurgie des hernies inguinales de l'adulte*. Monographie de l'Association Française de Chirurgie. Paris, 2001, Arnette edit, p 10.

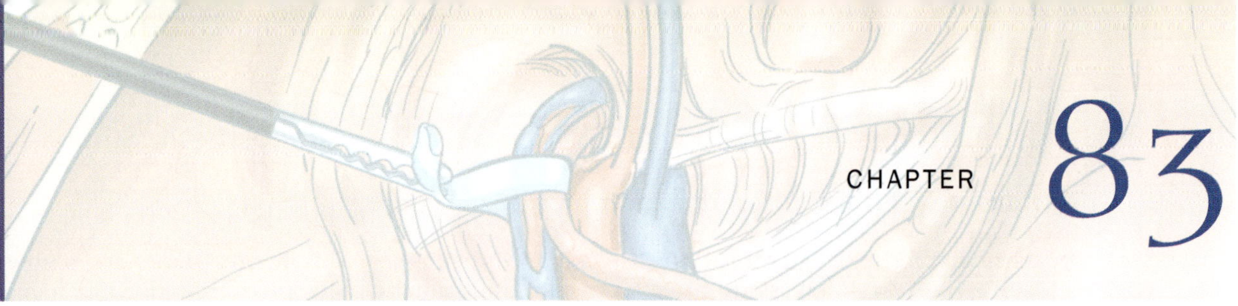

CHAPTER 83

Laparoscopic Transabdominal Preperitoneal Repair of Inguinofemoral Hernia

Alexander P. Nagle, MD, FACS, and Nathaniel J. Soper, MD

I. SPECIAL PREOPERATIVE PREPARATION

Patient Selection

- When evaluating a patient for an inguinal hernia repair, it is important to consider both the open anterior and the laparoscopic approach. This allows for selection of an operation that best fits the patient's overall condition and the particular type of hernia being treated.
- In general, patients who are not candidates for general anesthesia should have an open anterior repair. Patients who have previously undergone a retropubic prostatectomy should also undergo an open operation, because the posterior groin anatomic planes are often obliterated.
- For unilateral primary inguinal hernias, the role of laparoscopic repair remains debatable. In experienced hands, excellent results can be achieved in terms of recurrence, complications, and patient satisfaction.
- For recurrent or bilateral inguinal hernias, the advantages of a laparoscopic repair become more obvious.
- There are two different laparoscopic repair techniques, and debate continues as to whether the transabdominal preperitoneal (TAPP) or totally extraperitoneal (TEP) technique is superior. Each technique has its advantages and disadvantages.
- There are two major criticisms of the TAPP procedure. The first is the need to enter the peritoneal cavity, which increases the possibility of iatrogenic injury and adhesion formation. The second is the need to close the peritoneum over the mesh, which is time consuming and has been associated with bowel obstruction caused by herniation through gaps in the closure.
- The TEP approach requires more specialized instruments and is technically more demanding because of the limited working space.
- The surgeon should be comfortable with a TAPP repair before progressing to a TEP, because the TAPP is a potential fallback alternative in cases when the TEP proves technically impossible, such as with extensive peritoneal tears.
- There are also specific situations in which the TAPP may be preferred, such as many cases of recurrent inguinal hernia. After a primary repair that violated the preperitoneal space, especially if it involved the placement of mesh, a TAPP technique is advisable. This indication includes a prior laparoscopic repair or any of the open techniques that place mesh in the preperitoneal space. However, following a primary open (anterior) repair that did not significantly violate the preperitoneal space, the TEP approach is reasonable in the hands of an experienced surgeon.

- Large scrotal hernias are best approached with a TAPP because the increased working space facilitates reduction of the hernia. Similarly, incarcerated hernias are ideally suited for a TAPP because it allows easier inspection of the viability of the entrapped viscera and also provides a better angle for reduction (Fig. 83-1). The TAPP is also preferred in the presence of a lower abdominal incision where the preperitoneal space may be obliterated.

Anatomy

- The anatomy of the inguinofemoral region viewed via a laparoscope placed in the peritoneal cavity differs radically from the anatomy observed via an open or anterior approach. The laparoscopic surgeon needs to become familiar with the anatomic structures of this region to perform a safe and secure hernia repair. This knowledge and familiarity with the anatomy represents the most difficult aspect of the learning curve. In the TAPP technique, the anatomic landmarks are covered with peritoneum, which must first be incised and a peritoneal flap developed to expose the region adequately. The important landmarks that need to be unequivocally identified include the Cooper ligament, the epigastric vessels, the spermatic cord, and the iliac vessels (see Fig. 83-4). In addition, the laparoscopic anatomic distinctions among direct inguinal, indirect inguinal, and femoral hernias must be well understood (see Fig. 83-4). A structure that is not routinely exposed, but nonetheless must be appreciated, is the iliopubic tract, because this marks the inferior boundary for staple placement when fixing the mesh.
- The location of several nerves in the preperitoneal space is important to prevent neuralgia, which was seen early in the developmental stages of the laparoscopic approach. The genitofemoral nerves arise from the first and second lumbar nerves and course through the psoas muscle, dividing into a genital and femoral branch proximal to the internal ring. The genital branch continues along the psoas muscle and joins the spermatic cord at the internal inguinal ring. It supplies the sensory innervations to the scrotal skin and the medial thigh and motor innervations to the cremaster muscle. The femoral branch follows the psoas muscle more laterally and continues posterior to the iliopubic tract, supplying sensation to the proximal anterior thigh. The femoral nerve passes under the inguinal ligament lateral to the iliac artery and supplies sensation to the anteromedial thigh and motor fibers to the quadriceps femoris. The lateral femoral cutaneous nerve emerges from the lateral midpsoas and continues across the iliacus toward the anterior superior iliac spine, passing under the lateral portion of the iliopubic tract (approximately 2 cm lateral to the internal ring). This nerve supplies sensation to the lateral thigh.

Preoperative Preparation

- The patient should undergo appropriate testing to ensure suitability for general anesthesia. Preoperative antibiotics (first-generation cephalosporin) should be administered because a prosthetic material is to be inserted. The bladder must be decompressed, either with insertion of a Foley catheter or by having the patient void immediately before entering the operating room. Sequential compression devices are placed on the lower extremities for deep venous thrombosis prophylaxis.

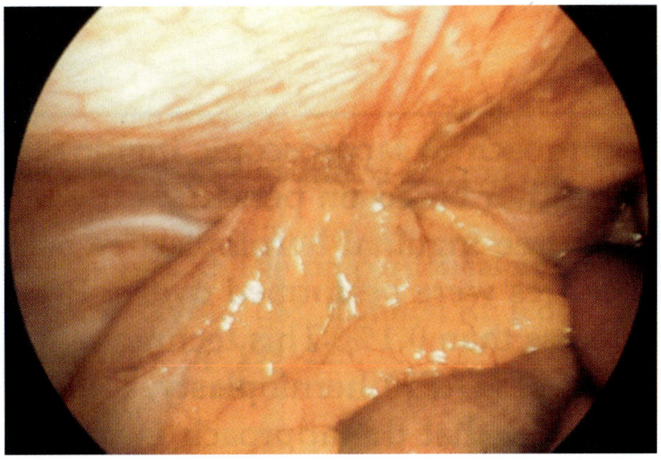

Figure 83-1. Incarcerated hernia.

II. OPERATIVE TECHNIQUE

Position

- The patient is placed in the supine position with both arms tucked along the side. The patient is securely strapped to the surgical bed to facilitate the Trendelenburg position. Two video monitors are used at the foot of the bed, one on each side of the operating table. The surgeon stands opposite the side to be repaired with the assistant (camera operator) opposite the surgeon. The abdomen is prepped and draped for laparoscopy as well as for a possible open procedure. Additionally, an Ioban skin protector is used to prevent direct contact of the prosthetic mesh with the skin.

Trocar Placement

- The initial trocar is placed in the umbilicus or in an alternative site in patients with a prior midline incision. The initial trocar can be placed with a Veress needle, open (Hasson) technique, or an optical viewing trocar. Surgeons should use the access method with which they have the most experience and feel the most comfortable. The initial trocar can be either 5 or 10 mm, depending on the diameter of the laparoscope being used. Angled laparoscopes (30 or 45 degrees) are helpful to maximize visibility. Under laparoscopic visualization, two 5-mm operating trocars are placed just lateral to the rectus muscles at the level of the umbilicus (Fig. 83-2).

Main Dissection

- After routine diagnostic surveillance laparoscopy is completed, the patient is placed in Trendelenburg position to allow the bowel to fall away from the pelvis. Adhesions are removed as necessary to ensure good visualization and access to the inguinal floor. Both inguinal regions are inspected; the internal ring and the cord structures should be immediately evident (Fig. 83-3). If an asymptomatic hernia is identified on the contralateral side, it should be repaired laparoscopically during the same anesthesia. The median umbilical ligament (obliterated urachus), medial umbilical ligaments (obliterated umbilical artery), and lateral umbilical folds (containing inferior epigastric vessels) are identified (Fig. 83-4). Commonly, the inferior epigastric vessels and the vas deferens can be seen through the intact peritoneum.
- Using sharp scissors, a peritoneal incision is made extending from the lateral edge of the medial umbilical ligament and extending toward the anterior superior iliac spine. The peritoneal incision should be

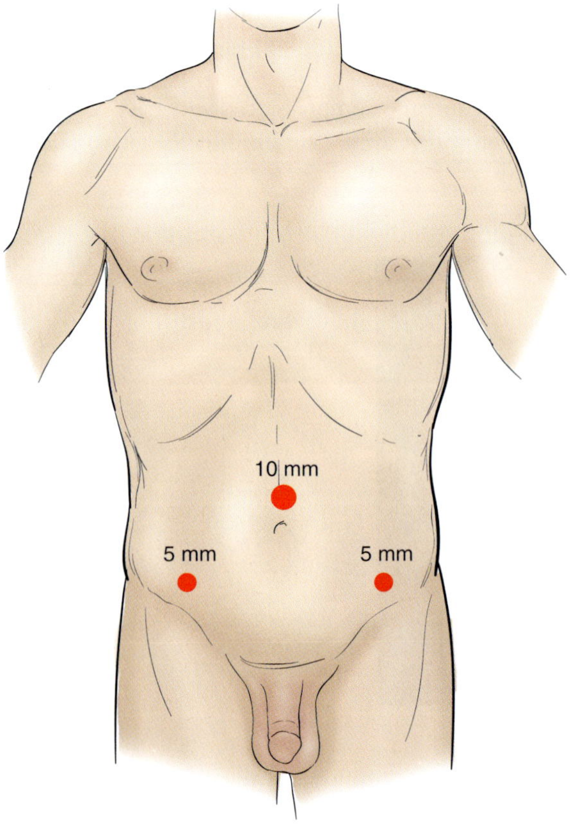

Figure 83-2.

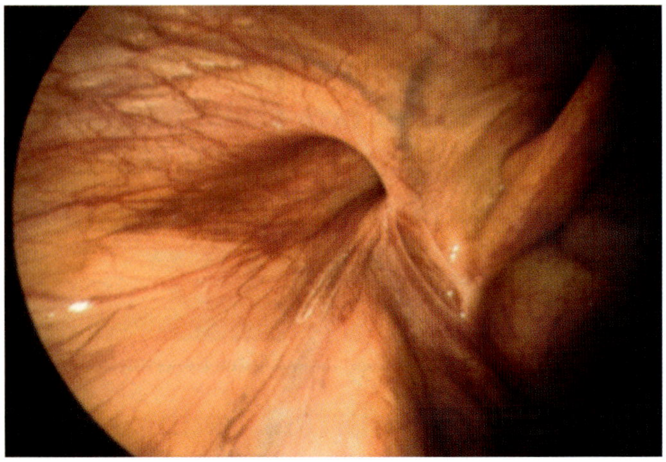

Figure 83-3. Indirect hernial defect, visualized from the peritoneal cavity.

long and made as high as possible (at least 2 to 4 cm above the defect) to maximize the exposure (Fig. 83-5). The preperitoneal space and resulting peritoneal flap are then developed using a two-handed technique with blunt-tipped instruments. The plane of dissection should be generally avascular, and therefore the need for electrocautery or sharp dissection should be minimal.

- As the peritoneal flap is being developed, the inferior epigastric vessels are exposed, and care is taken not to dissect these vessels from the anterior abdominal wall (Fig. 83-6). It is also important to maintain the integrity of the peritoneal flap to allow future coverage of the newly placed mesh. Should the

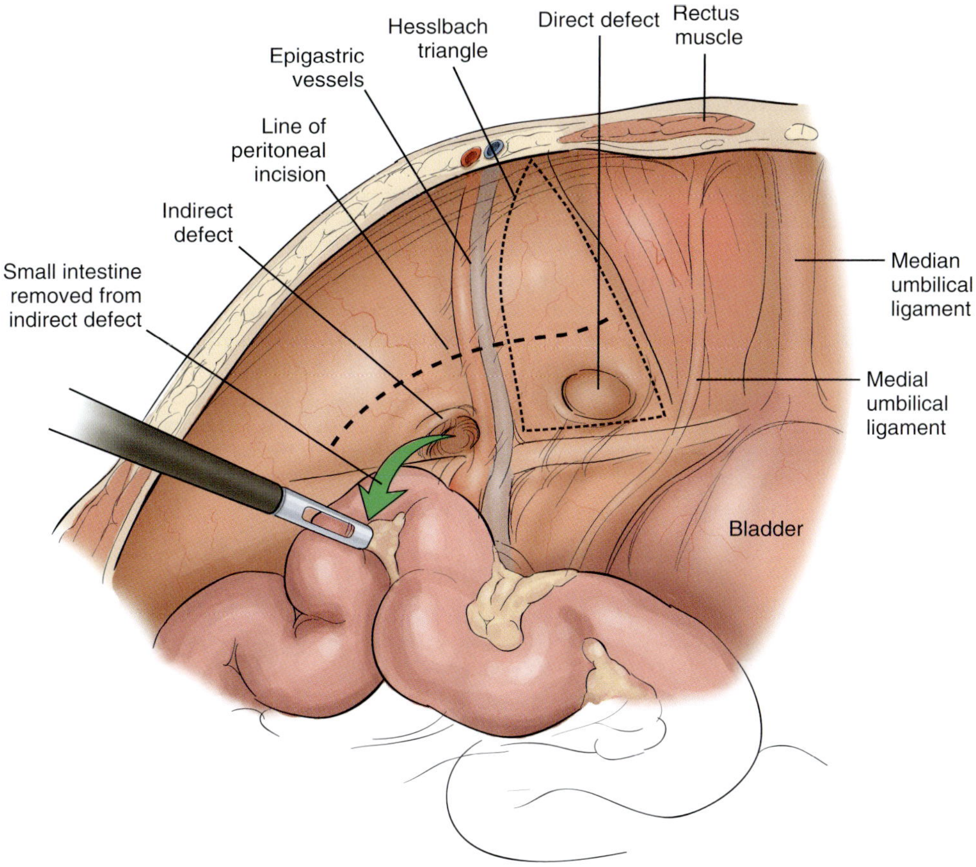

Figure 83-4.

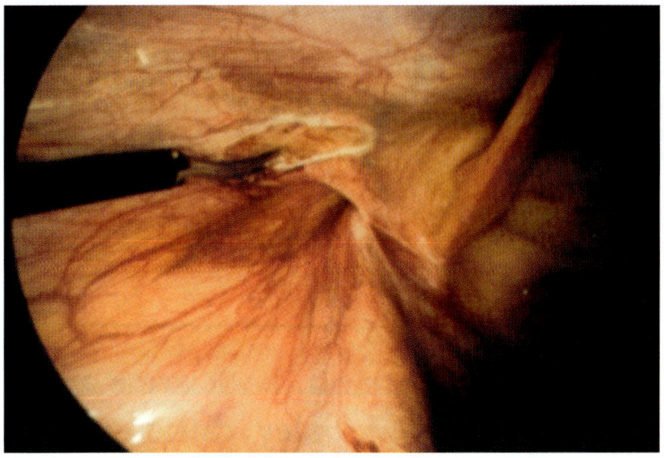

Figure 83-5. Incision of the peritoneum.

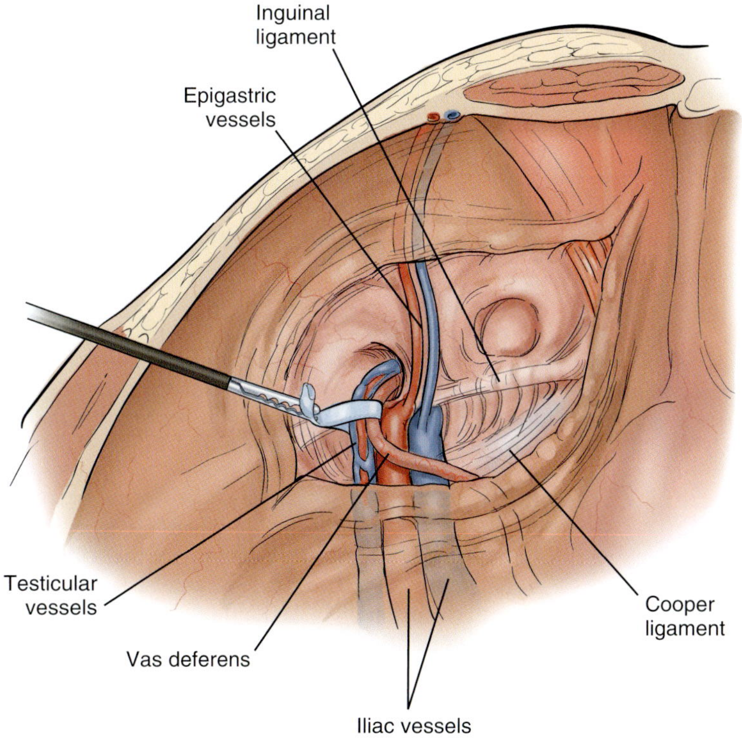

Figure 83-6.

peritoneum become significantly fragmented, polypropylene or polyester mesh should not be used because of concern for intestinal adhesions to the mesh. In this setting a composite mesh with one surface that is bioabsorbable should be used.

- The initial dissection begins at the symphysis pubis, which can usually be visualized, and progresses along the Cooper ligament, stopping just above the crossing vein and medial to the iliac vein. The iliac vessels are not dissected, but their position should be clearly identified and noted. It is important to clearly expose the Cooper ligament, because this point marks the most medial aspect of fixation (see Fig. 83-6).
- Next, attention is directed to the most lateral aspect of the preperitoneal space. This area needs to be well developed to allow the mesh to lie smoothly against the posterior wall. The dissection is then carried medially toward the internal ring and spermatic cord. The indirect space is explored for an indirect hernial sac. An indirect sac is usually located on the anterolateral side of the cord structures, as opposed to conventional surgery, where they appear anteromedial. The hernial sac should be reduced in a hand-over-hand manner to ensure the countertension essential to creating a plane between the cord and the sac. If an instrument can be manipulated to the most distal end of the hernial sac, excellent countertraction can be achieved by pulling the sac cephalad and lateral, creating a visible plane between the cord structures and the sac.
- Using blunt dissection, the indirect sac is dissected completely free of the spermatic cord. Care is taken to prevent damage to the vas deferens or the blood supply to the testicle. It is important to completely reduce the hernial sac back into the peritoneal cavity. Particular care should also be taken not to dissect lateral and inferior to the Cooper ligament, because the iliac vessels will enter the femoral canal at this site. Indirect sacs are more difficult to deal with than direct sacs, as they can adhere tenaciously to the cord structures. If the sac cannot be mobilized from the cord without undue trauma, the sac can be divided, leaving the distal sac in situ, with the understanding that a seroma will almost certainly develop in the retained distal sac. The proximal sac will need to be ligated to reestablish the integrity of the peritoneum.
- It is also important to completely reduce or remove any excessive fatty tissue (so-called lipomas of the cord). If this fat is not removed, the patient might believe that the hernia has recurred or was not repaired. Similarly, direct hernial sacs must be completely reduced and dissected free of the cord structures.

Mesh Preparation and Insertion

- In the United States, polypropylene is the most commonly used mesh, whereas in Europe, many prefer polyester. The mesh needs to be large enough (at least 10 by 15 cm) to provide adequate coverage of the direct, indirect, and femoral spaces. When determining the appropriate mesh size, it is also important to consider that most meshes will contract up to 20% secondary to tissue ingrowth with the resultant contraction. Many surgeons use a contoured or three-dimensional mesh (such as Bard 3DMax) because they feel it is easier to handle and conforms better to the preperitoneal space than a flat piece of mesh. In the end, the particular product used by a surgeon is simply a matter of personal preference.
- The mesh is rolled and then grasped with a 5-mm instrument and inserted into the peritoneal cavity via the umbilical 10-mm camera trocar (Fig. 83-7). The laparoscope is replaced, and the mesh is gently pushed into the pelvis with the scope. Using two graspers, the mesh is then unrolled and oriented appropriately over the inguinal region. When the mesh is smoothed out, it should provide adequate coverage of the indirect, direct, and femoral spaces. The medial aspect of the mesh should overlap the pubic bone and cross the midline. If the patient has bilateral hernias, the mesh from each side will overlap. The mesh can be simply laid over the cord structures, and there is no need to cut a slit for the cord.

Fixation

- Fixation is another aspect of surgery about which there is varying opinion. If a large enough mesh is used, little fixation is probably necessary, and in fact some surgeons use none. The use of a large mesh allows the intraabdominal pressure to act uniformly over a large area of normal abdominal wall, thus holding the mesh in place and preventing herniation. The avoidance of tacks has the theoretical advantage of avoiding complications such as nerve entrapment. A few surgeons have advocated the use of biologic adhesives, such as fibrin, for securing the mesh. However, most surgeons have enough concern about mesh migration that the use of fixation tacks is the rule rather than the exception. There is no minimum number of tacks that should be used to hold the mesh in place, but most surgeons try to limit the number of tacks (Fig. 83-8). We typically use three tacks to secure the mesh. Their purpose is not to give strength to the repair but to hold the mesh smoothly against the posterior abdominal wall until the mesh becomes incorporated into the wall.
- When placing tacks, the first step is to identify the landmarks. The iliopubic tract is recognized as a white fibrous band running transversely at the lower edge of the internal ring. In some patients it is

quite prominent and obvious, whereas in others it is subtle and barely visible. The location is confirmed by placing one hand on the abdominal wall and the other hand holding a laparoscopic grasper. The grasper is pressed against the abdominal wall, and the tip is felt with the opposite hand. If the surgeon cannot feel the instrument, it is below the iliopubic tract and in an area where the nerves are at risk for injury. No tacks should be inserted in the mesh or abdominal wall unless the anchoring device can be felt with opposite hand. In addition, with the opposite hand on the abdominal wall, the stapler achieves a more perpendicular angle, which improves reliability.

- The mesh is initially secured medially to the Cooper ligament. It is mandatory to feel the pubic bone when placing this anchor. The mesh should extend medially 1 to 2 cm beyond the Cooper ligament. This stabilizes the mesh and allows the surgeon to fan it out in a lateral direction, taking out any wrinkles or folds. The mesh is then secured to the anterior abdominal wall above the iliopubic tract. We recommend one tack medial to the inferior epigastric vessel and one tack lateral to the epigastric vessels. It is important to apply strong countertraction (opposite hand) externally against the abdominal wall to ensure that the tacks are driven into the abdominal wall. This also ensures that the fixation is done above the iliopubic tract.

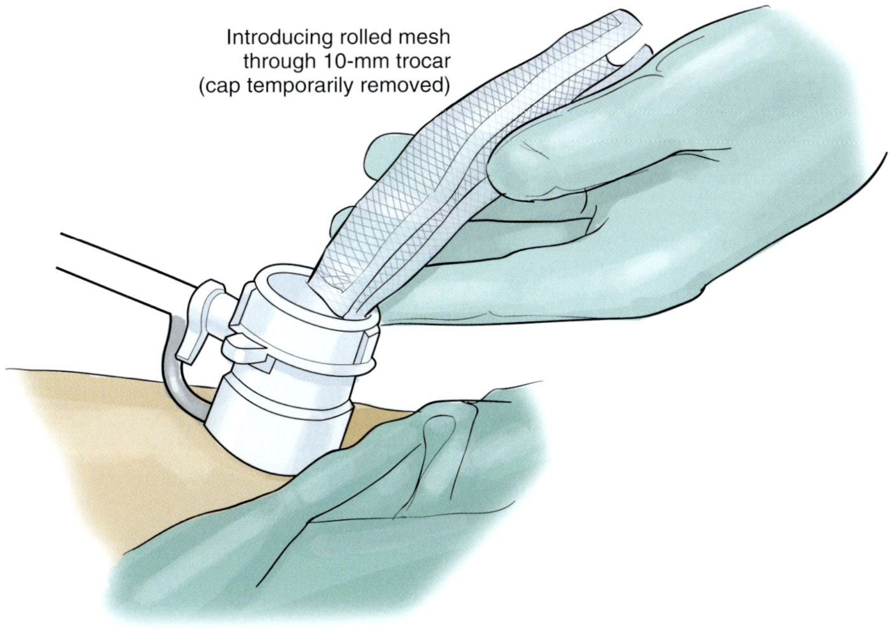

Figure 83-7.

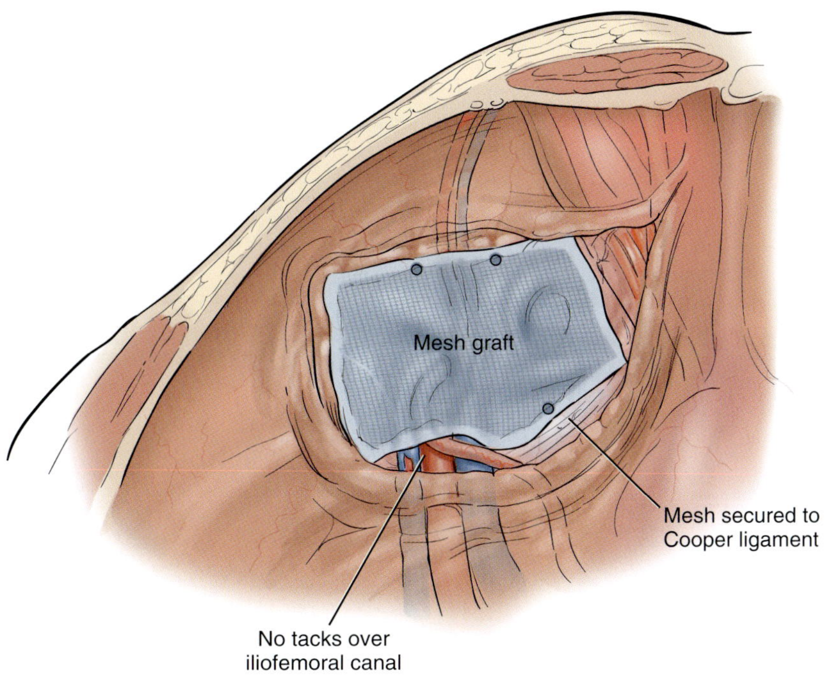

Figure 83-8.

Closure

- The peritoneal closure should be initiated on the lateral aspect of the repair. The peritoneal flap is held by a grasper and pulled over the upper peritoneal layer. It is not important that the peritoneal edges be approximated exactly. The most important issue is that the peritoneal flap must completely cover the mesh (Fig. 83-9). Tenting of the peritoneum can occur if too much tension is required to approximate the two edges. The tenting effect may leave space between the peritoneal flap and the prosthesis. There is concern that bowel might herniate into this space and result in a bowel obstruction. Running sutures, staples, or fibrin glue have been used for fixation of the peritoneal flap. Spiral tacks commonly do not work well because the peritoneum is too thin. The epigastric vessels should be meticulously visualized during the fixation of the peritoneal flap. After the mesh is fixed, the two 5-mm trocars are removed under direct vision. The fascia of the subumbilical trocar site is closed as needed.

III. ALTERNATIVE TECHNICAL APPROACHES (PRO/CON) AND PEARLS

- Fixation tacks should be used sparingly to avoid nerve entrapment; typically two or three tacks will suffice.
- The fixation tacks should never be placed below the level of the iliopubic tract.
- The peritoneal flap must be completely closed to prevent internal herniation and exposure of the mesh to the intestines.

IV. SPECIAL POSTOPERATIVE CARE

- Most patients are discharged on the day of surgery. The patient is allowed clear liquids in the immediate postoperative period and is advanced to a regular diet as tolerated. Patients are required to void before discharge. Postoperative referred shoulder and neck pain may occur transiently because of diaphragmatic irritation. Immediate postoperative pain is controlled with intravenous ketorolac 30 mg. Oral pain medication is also initiated soon after surgery, and intravenous narcotics can be used for breakthrough. The surgeon should warn the patient about bruising and scrotal swelling.
- We instruct our patients to limit their activity level for 2 weeks postoperatively. The patient may return to work as soon as the discomfort is tolerable, often within the first week. Written instructions are given to the patient and the family with detailed advice concerning signs of potential problems. Routine postoperative follow-up at 2 to 4 weeks is advised for all patients.

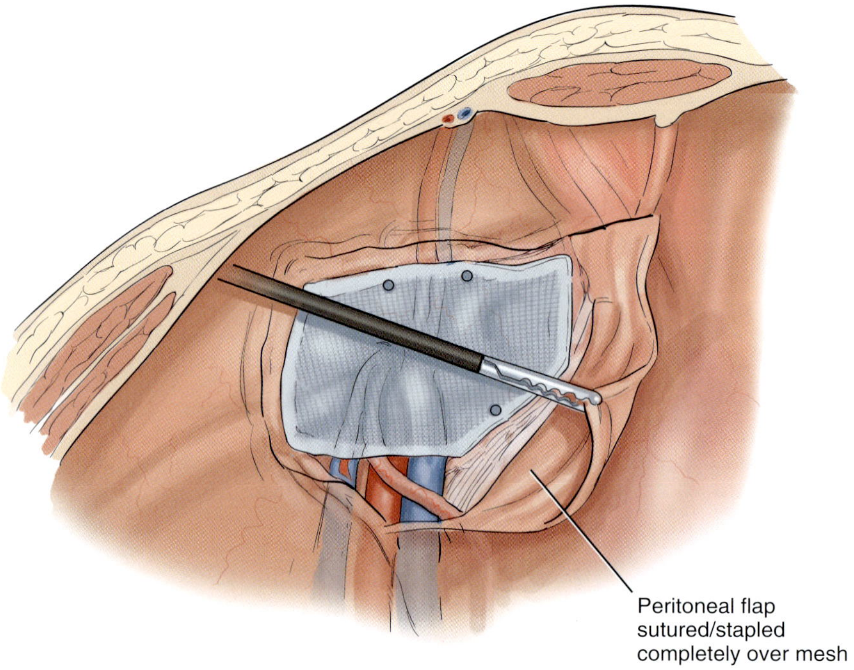

Figure 83-9.

TABLE 83-1 Potential Complications Following Laparoscopic TAPP Repair

COMPLICATIONS	STRUCTURES/ORGAN INVOLVED	CAUSES	RECOGNITION	MANAGEMENT
Vascular injuries	Inferior epigastric, spermatic, external iliac, deep circumflex iliac, obturator	Insertion of Veress needle or trocar, inexperience, anatomic variations	Bleeding during surgery, postoperative signs of shock	Ligation of all the bleeding vessels except external iliac
Urinary retention, infection, and hematuria	Bladder, ureter, and kidneys	Extensive preperitoneal dissection, urinary catheterization, bladder injury during dissection, off-center trocar insertion	During surgery, postoperative intravenous pyelography, ultrasound, CT scan	Antibiotics for urinary tract infection Surgical repair for bladder injury
Small bowel obstruction	Small bowel	Small bowel herniation into preperitoneal space, incomplete closure of peritoneal flap	Postoperative abdominal pain, nausea, and vomiting; CT scan	Surgical reduction of small bowel and complete closure of the peritoneal flap
Nerve injuries	Femoral branch of genitofemoral, lateral cutaneous nerve of the thigh, and intermediate cutaneous branch of anterior branch of the femoral nerve	Variable anatomy and inappropriate tack placement, extensive dissection below iliopubic tract	Burning pain, hyperesthesia, paresthesia, and anesthesia	Analgesia, reexploration, and removal of tack
Complications related to mesh	Bladder, small bowel, large bowel	Migration, infection, adhesions, and erosion of the mesh into intraabdominal organs	Clinical suspicion, small bowel obstruction, fistula, abscesses	Conservative or operative
Recurrence	Inguinal region	Incomplete dissection, too small a mesh, migration of the mesh, displacement of mesh by hematoma	Groin lump or pain	Repeat repair, laparoscopic or conventional
Pubic and pelvic osteitis	Pubic tubercle	Staple into the bone	Diagnosis of exclusion	Self-limiting, analgesia
Groin seroma and hematoma	Groin/testicle	Extensive dissection, inadequate hemostasis	Lump or bruising in the groin or scrotum	Self-limiting or evacuation
Wound infection	Trocar site	Usually endogenous	Pain, cellulitis, pus from the trocar site	Open skin, dressing changes, antibiotics

CT, Computed tomography; *TAPP*, transabdominal preperitoneal.

Complications

- One of the major criticisms of laparoscopic inguinal hernia repair is the steep learning curve. This is clearly reflected in the literature, as studies have consistently shown improvement in both the complication and recurrence rates with experience. Furthermore, complications after laparoscopic hernia repair tend to be more severe than after open repairs (e.g., bowel obstruction, vascular injury, or injury to the bladder or bowel). Once the surgeon is beyond the learning curve, the incidence of serious complications is extremely rare. It is important to distinguish between complications unique to the hernia repair itself and those inherent in laparoscopic surgery. Recurrence after a laparoscopic TAPP repair is rare when the operation is performed properly. Once beyond the learning curve, many authors report recurrence rates around 0.3% (Table 83-1).

SUGGESTED READINGS

Lovisetto F, Zonta S, Rota E, et al: Use of human fibrin glue versus staples for mesh fixation in laparoscopic transabdominal preperitoneal hernioplasty: a prospective, randomized study, *Ann Surg* 245:222–231, 2007.

Neumayer L, Giobbie-Hurder A, Jonasson O, et al: Open mesh versus laparoscopic mesh repair of inguinal hernia, *N Engl J Med* 350:1819–1827, 2004.

Novitsky YW, Czerniach DR, Kercher KW, et al: Advantages of laparoscopic transabdominal preperitoneal herniorrhaphy in the evaluation and management of inguinal hernias, *Am J Surg* 193:466–470, 2007.

SECTION XVI

Soft Tissue/ Bone Resection

CHAPTER 84

Anterior Thigh Tumor Resection

Fritz C. Eilber, MD, and Frederick R. Eilber, MD

I. SPECIAL PREOPERATIVE PREPARATION

- *Physical exam:* Any mass of the anterior thigh that is large, deep to the subcutaneous tissue, nonmobile, and/or firm should be considered to be a soft tissue sarcoma until proven otherwise. In the presence of any clinical features that raise the suspicion of soft tissue sarcoma, cross-sectional imaging and tissue diagnosis are critical in guiding appropriate care.
- *Imaging:* Plain radiographs and ultrasounds are of little value, and angiograms are not necessary. Cross-sectional imaging is critical, because it provides the anatomic information necessary to guide surgical resection. Cross-sectional imaging can be performed by either computed tomography (CT) or magnetic resonance imaging (MRI) and should include the appropriate intravenous contrast agent to delineate the vascular anatomy (Figs. 84-1 and 84-2).
- *CT versus MRI:* Too much emphasis is placed on this distinction, and there are very few instances in which one modality is preferred over another. Although certain soft tissue sarcomas image better with MRI and others better with CT, this choice should be driven by both the surgeon's comfort with the imaging technique and the availability and ease of obtaining the study.
- *Tissue diagnosis:* CT-guided core biopsy is the optimal method to obtain tissue diagnosis. CT guidance allows for precise tissue sampling, including targeting specific areas of concern within a tumor. Fine-needle aspiration is inadequate. Core biopsies needs to be done with large-bore needles, as this allows for adequate tissue collection for histologic diagnosis, grade, and often critical ancillary studies such as cytogenetics and electron microscopy. In the rare instance (<5%) that a CT-guided core biopsy is unable to provide an adequate histologic diagnosis, an incisional biopsy can be performed. Such a biopsy should be placed in line with the incision required for definitive surgical resection, with attention to hemostasis to avoid a hematoma. Transverse incisions in the extremity are to be avoided.
- *Staging:* Patients with high-grade thigh sarcomas should have a CT scan of the chest, as this is the most common site of metastatic disease. Staging for high-grade liposarcomas should also include a CT of the abdomen and pelvis because these lesions can metastasize to other sites. For low-grade sarcomas, the routine preoperative chest radiograph is sufficient. Positron emission tomography scans have not been validated as a screening modality and are not done in the setting of primary disease unless under a study protocol.
- *Neoadjuvant therapy:* Patients with large (≥5 cm), high-grade, deep sarcomas should be considered for protocol neoadjuvant therapy (chemotherapy, radiation therapy, and/or chemoradiation), which should only be administered at a sarcoma center or cancer center with expertise in sarcomas.

II. OPERATIVE TECHNIQUE

Position

- The patient is placed in the supine position. A Foley catheter should be placed. It is generally best to prep the entire extremity including the groin. Stockinet is placed over the foot and ankle, and the extremity is draped free to allow it to be moved during the operation. The groin and knee should be included in the field.

Incision

- A vertical incision is made over the palpable mass or over its location based on cross-sectional imaging. The incision should ellipse out the previous incisional biopsy site if present. A generous incision should be made that extends both above and below the lesion to allow for appropriate exposure (Fig. 84-3).

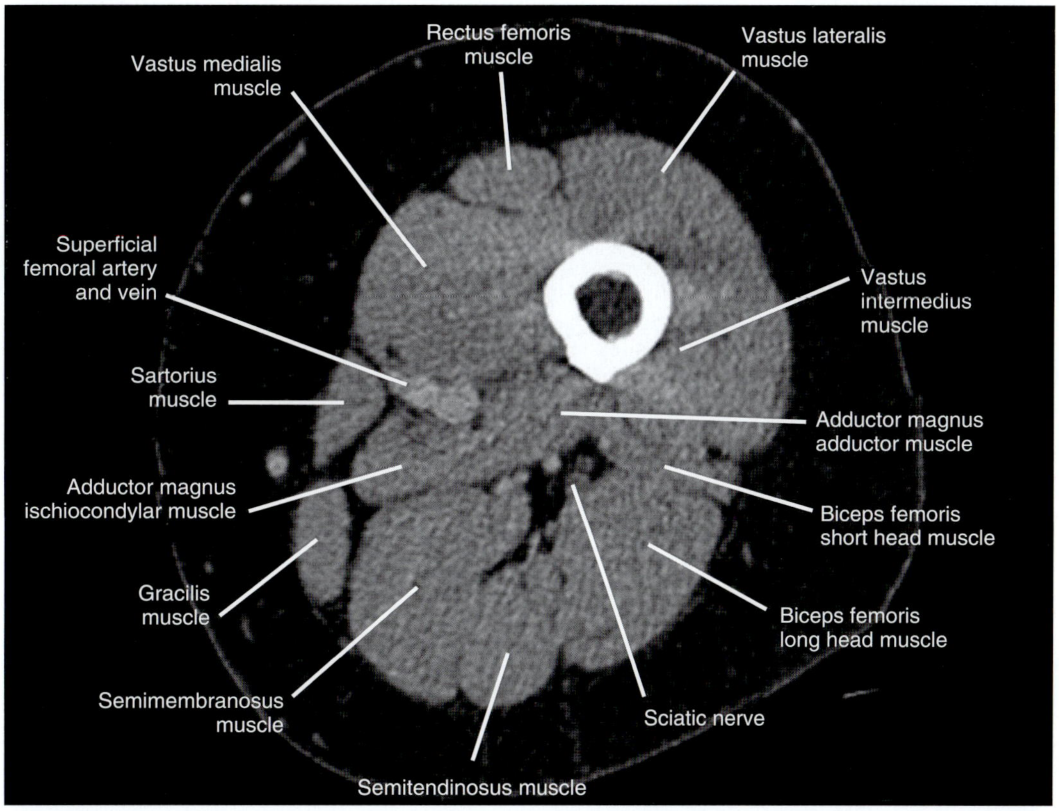

Figure 84-1. Computed tomography scan illustrating the normal anatomy of the left thigh.

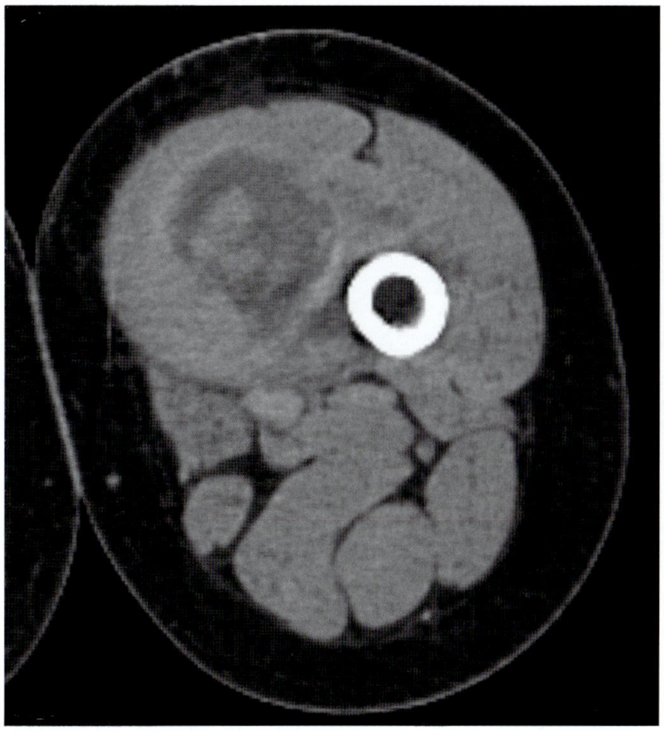

Figure 84-2. Computed tomography scan of a left anterior thigh sarcoma.

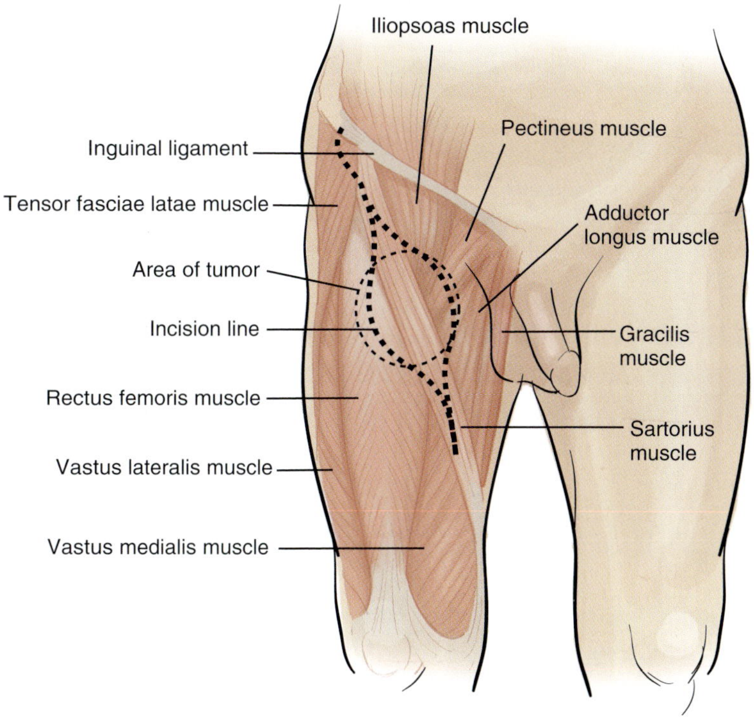

Figure 84-3.

Main Dissection

- Flaps of skin and subcutaneous fat are raised off the fascia of the anterior thigh both medially and laterally (Fig. 84-4).
- The initial aspect of any dissection is becoming anatomically oriented, as these tumors are often large and can distort normal anatomy. Because most tumors of the anterior thigh are within the general proximity of the femoral vessels, it is important to identify them before beginning the resection of the tumor. The femoral artery, vein, and nerve are easily identified proximally as they enter the anterior thigh below the inguinal ligament. More distally in the midthigh, the superficial femoral artery, vein, and saphenous nerve can be found within the adductor canal underneath the sartorius muscle (Fig. 84-5).
- En bloc resection of the tumor is the primary surgical goal, with dissection being performed through normal adjacent tissue planes. A clamp (tonsil or right angle) and Bovie cautery are used for the dissection. Vessels are ligated as necessary with 2-0 or 3-0 silk ties.
- Surgical resection should include normal soft tissue adjacent to the tumor. At a minimum, the pathologic specimen needs to be free of tumor at the resection margins, and this can be accomplished without a complete muscle group resection. There is no role for an incomplete resection or "debulking" of a soft tissue sarcoma.
- Tumors of the anterior thigh are often are close to either the superficial or deep (profunda) femoral vessels. Resection of these structures en bloc with the tumor is usually not necessary. Exposure of the vessels both proximally and distally allows meticulous dissection to be performed along their length (Fig. 84-6), and if necessary, the adventitia of the artery and vein can be removed with the tumor.

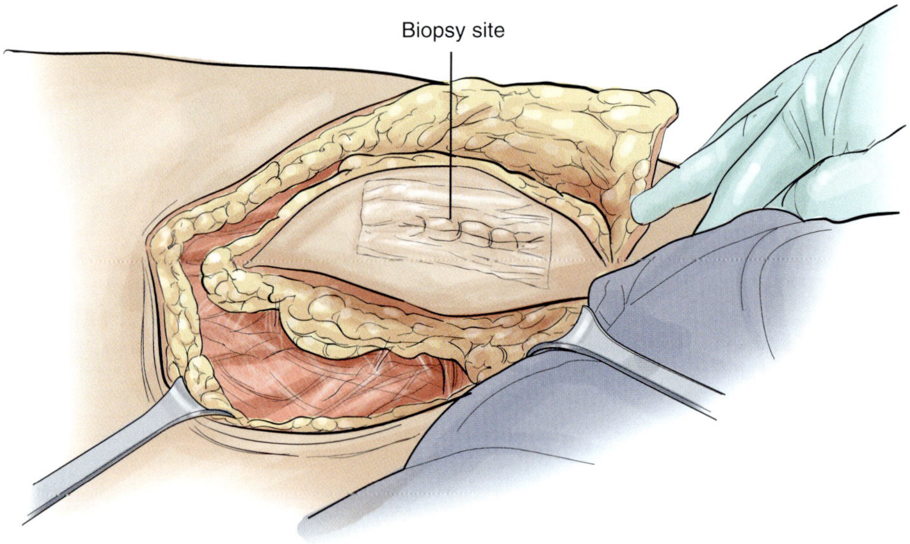

Figure 84-4.

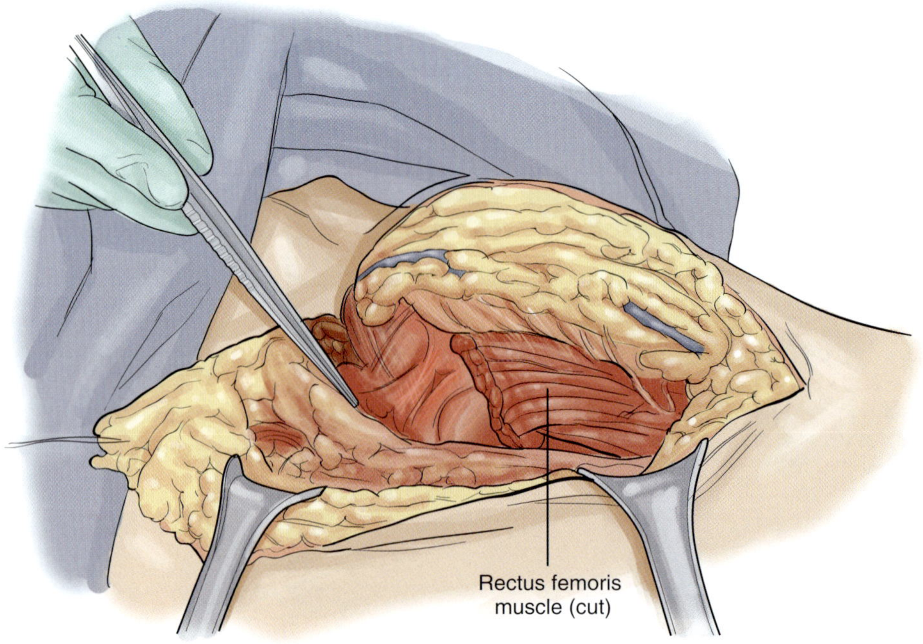

Figure 84-5.

- Resection of neurovascular structures is essentially never done for a primary low-grade tumor. If a primary high-grade tumor directly involves or arises from a neurovascular structure, then that structure should be resected en bloc with the sarcoma.
- The deep femoral artery can be resected without the need for an arterial reconstruction. Resection of the superficial femoral artery requires reconstruction with autologous vein or polytetrafluoroethylene.
- The deep femoral veins and the saphenous vein can usually be resected without causing severe extremity swelling. Resection of the superficial femoral vein puts the patient at risk for permanent, severe venous swelling of the extremity. Unlike the arteries of the thigh, the veins cannot be reconstructed with any degree of success.
- Because the femoral nerve branches to innervate the muscles of the anterior thigh just below the inguinal ligament, it is rarely directly involved by an anterior thigh tumor. Loss of motor function following resection of an anterior thigh tumor usually has more to do with the muscular resection than any neural resection or injury.
- Marking sutures are placed on the resected tumor to allow for orientation and appropriate margin assessment by the pathologist. If the tumor is close to a particular resection margin, additional tissue at that region of the resection cavity can be sent for pathologic results and an additional margin assessed. The resection bed is inspected for the integrity of the vessels, and hemostasis is achieved (Fig. 84-7).

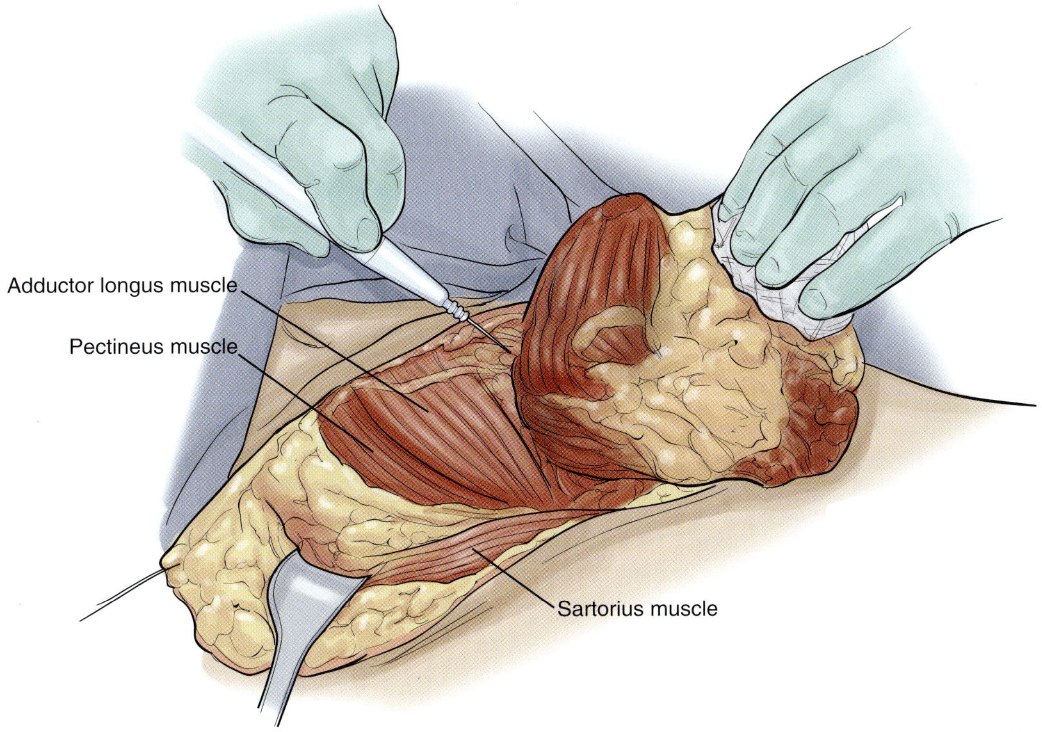

Figure 84-6.

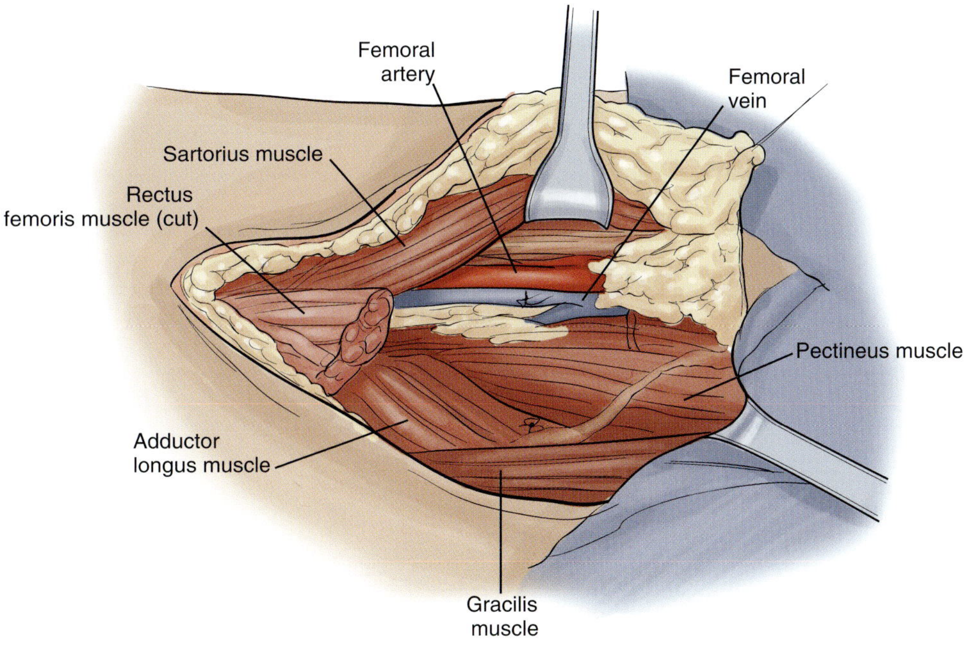

Figure 84-7.

Closure

- At least one and often two round 19-Fr Jackson-Pratt drains are placed into the resection cavity. They are brought through the skin through a separate stab incision and anchored to the skin with a stitch.
- Subcutaneous fat and skin are approximated using 2-0 Vicryl, and the skin is closed with staples. After a gauze dressing has been applied to the incision, the leg is wrapped with two 6-inch Ace wraps, and a knee immobilizer is placed.

III. ALTERNATIVE TECHNICAL APPROACHES (PRO/CON) AND PEARLS

- If an extensive vascular dissection is required, resulting in exposure of the femoral vessels, they should be covered with additional layer of tissue before the skin closure in the event the wound opens or becomes infected. Rotation of a sartorius muscular flap is the easiest way to accomplish this coverage. The sartorius is divided at its origin at the anterior superior iliac spine and rotated in a medial manner to lie over the femoral vessels. It is then anchored to the inguinal ligament and adductor fascia.
- By far the most common anterior thigh tumor is a soft-tissue sarcoma. These are rare, high-risk malignancies that are best managed by an experienced multidisciplinary team of physicians at a sarcoma center or a cancer center that has expertise in these tumors.
- A multidisciplinary team of surgeons is intermittently needed for resection of these lesions, and thorough preoperative planning is therefore critical. Complex reconstruction by plastic surgery, with either a local rotational flap or a free flap, and vascular reconstructions by vascular surgery are occasionally required.
- The development of locally recurrent disease is a morbid and potentially limb-threatening event that is associated with decreased survival. The optimal treatment of locally recurrent disease is to prevent it, which necessitates aggressive and definitive surgery in the setting of the primary disease.

IV. SPECIAL POSTOPERATIVE CARE

- While the patient is in bed, the extremity should be elevated.
- Patients should have a physical therapy evaluation on postoperative day 1 and are encouraged to perform touch-down weight bearing with the physical therapist. The Ace wrap and knee immobilizer placed while in the operating room should be continued for the first several weeks. Significant range of motion of the knee is thus limited over this time period. Patients are discharged home with either crutches or a walker depending on their strength and age.
- Patients are taught Jackson-Pratt drain care and sent home with the drains in place. The drains are not removed until the output is less than 20 mL/day. Staples are left in for at least 1 week and often up to 2 weeks if there are concerns for neoadjuvant radiation therapy or the condition of the wound.
- The most common immediate postoperative complications include infection, hematoma, and wound dehiscence or slough.
- The most common delayed complications include seroma and leg edema.

SUGGESTED READINGS

Eilber FC, Brennan MF, Eilber FR, Kattan MF: Validation of the postoperative nomogram for 12-year sarcoma specific death, *Cancer* 101:2270–2275, 2004.

Eilber FC, Rosen G, Nelson SD, et al: High grade extremity soft tissue sarcomas: factors predictive of local recurrence and its effect on morbidity and mortality, *Ann Surg* 237:218–226, 2003.

Eilber FC, Tap WD, Nelson SD, et al: Advances in chemotherapy for patients with extremity soft tissue sarcoma, *Orthop Clin North Am* 37:15–22, 2006.

CHAPTER 85

Posterior Thigh Tumor Resection

Vijay P. Khatri, MBChB, FACS

I. SPECIAL PREOPERATIVE PREPARATION

- Pretreatment radiologic imaging provides valuable information that aids in diagnosis, definition of the local extent of the tumor, planning of the biopsy, and staging of the disease. Plain radiographs are of limited value except for cases of chronic hematoma that may reveal diagnostic calcification.
- Ultrasonography is also of limited value except to guide percutaneous biopsies. The current imaging modality of choice is magnetic resonance imaging (MRI). Understanding the normal anatomy, especially on axial images, allows the surgeon to decipher abnormal MRIs, particularly the involved muscle groups. It also allows formulation of the three-dimensional approach to resection (Fig. 85-1).

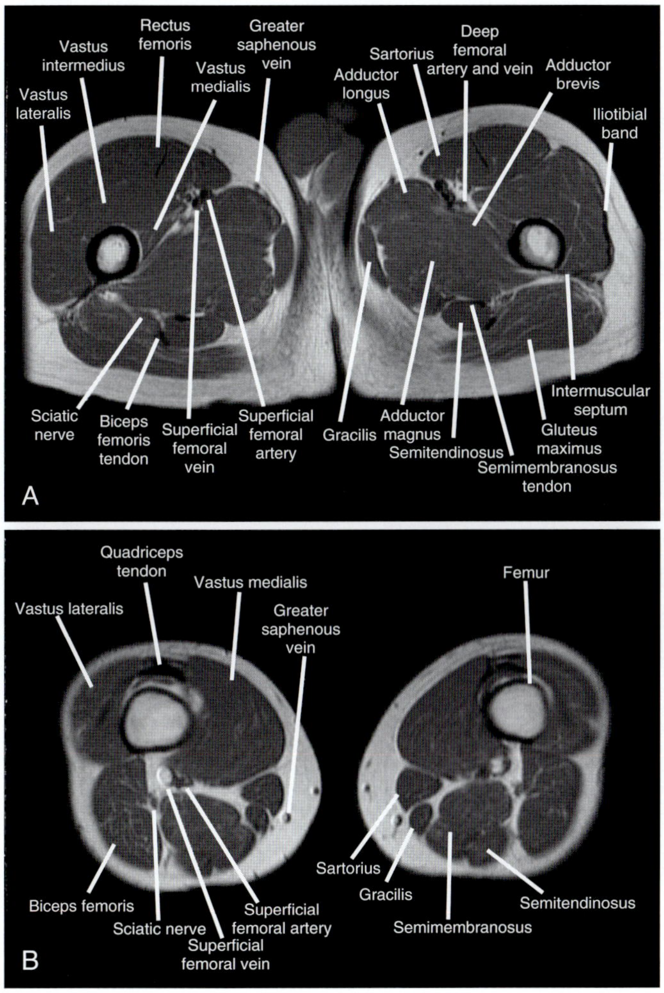

Figure 85-1. Axial cross-sectional image illustrating the normal anatomy of the proximal thigh (**A**) and the distal third of the thigh (**B**).

- MRI is the preferred imaging modality for extremity sarcoma, because it can provide multiplanar images with better spatial orientation. Also, concurrent magnetic resonance angiography can be obtained that delineates the relationship of the tumor to adjacent vascular structure. Behavior of the primary tumor following administration of gadolinium contrast allows differentiation from lipomatous benign tumors (Figs. 85-2 and 85-3). Dynamic postcontrast images may also help differentiate viable tumor in adjacent muscle from tumor-associated edema.
- For low-grade sarcomas, chest radiography is performed to look for lung metastases. Computed tomography of the chest should be considered for patients with high-grade tumors or tumors larger than 5 cm.
- To establish histologic diagnosis, office-based core needle biopsy is appropriate, as it has a diagnostic accuracy of about 95%. Its yield can be further enhanced by use of ultrasonography to avoid sampling necrotic and cystic areas, and importantly avoiding neurovascular bundles that may have been displaced superficially. The core biopsy provides enough tissue to establish a histologic diagnosis and tumor grade. For difficult cases, it allows additional diagnostic tests, such as electron microscopic examination and cytogenetic analysis. It also has an advantage over open biopsies, which can be associated with wound complications, particularly if the tumor is very large and primary closure is under tension.
- If a core biopsy reveals nondiagnostic material, an incisional biopsy can be performed but should ideally be part of a well-planned treatment strategy. When performing a biopsy, proper placement of the incision is vital: it should be performed at a site that can be excised en bloc during the definitive surgery resection. Transverse incisions in the extremities are always contraindicated.

II. OPERATIVE TECHNIQUE

Position

- The patient is placed in the prone position. The affected lower extremity is prepped and draped circumferentially from the region of the buttock downward. The entire lower extremity should be draped free to allow it to be moved during the operative procedure.

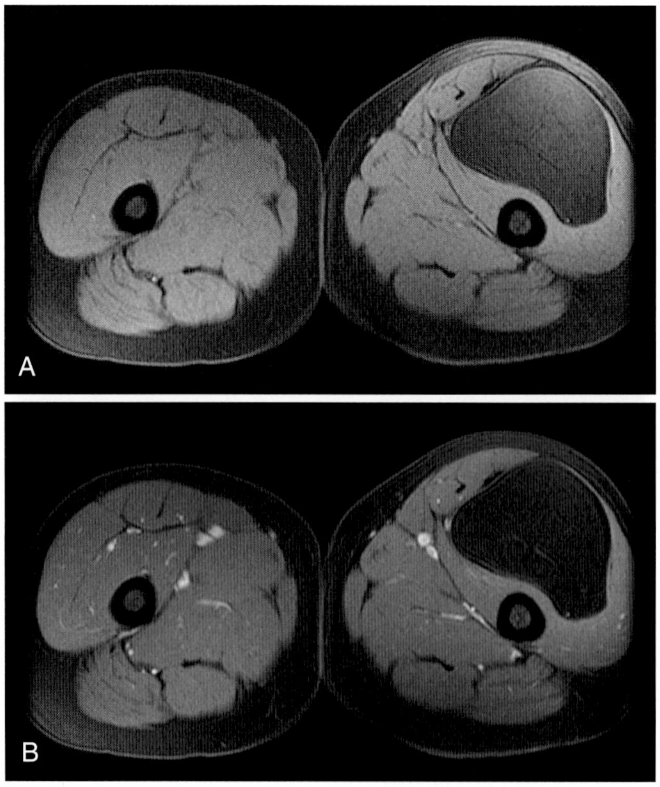

Figure 85-2. Axial cross-sectional image of a lipoma. This is an example of a benign soft tissue mass, which demonstrates lack of enhancement following administration of gadolinium. **A**, Precontrast axial image; **B**, postcontrast axial image.

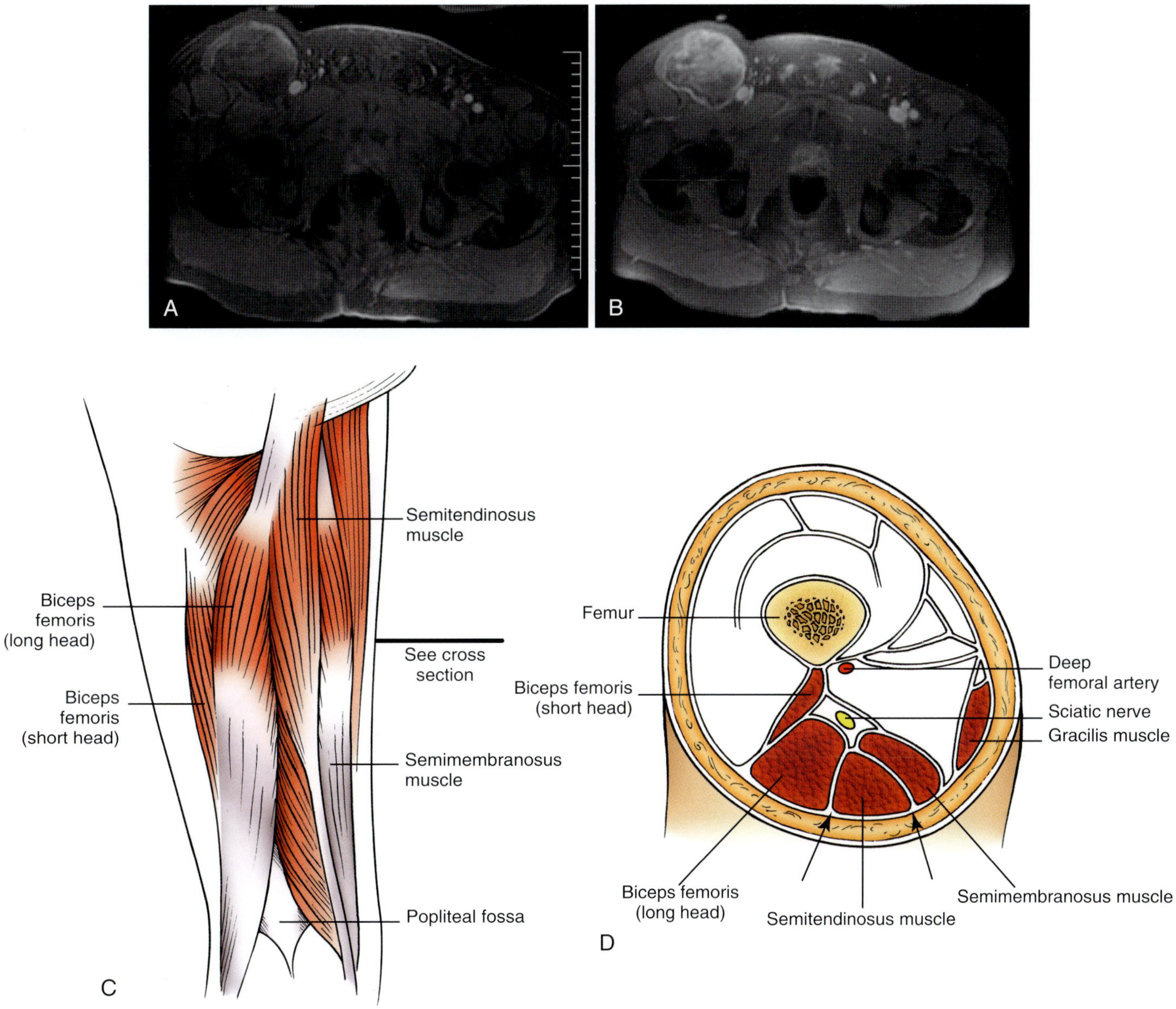

Figure 85-3. Axial cross-sectional image of a liposarcoma. Soft tissue sarcomas show enhancement following administration of gadolinium. **A,** Precontrast axial image; **B,** postcontrast axial image. Posterior (**C**) and cross-sectional (**D**) anatomic view of the thigh.

Incision

- An elliptical incision is outlined over the mass to include any previous incisional biopsy performed (Fig. 85-4). The ellipse is oriented longitudinally because this facilitates resection of the tumor and, if necessary, compartmental resection.

Main Dissection

- Once the skin is incised, medial and lateral flaps are raised and developed beyond the palpable edge of the tumor. To maintain retraction of the flaps, multiple stay sutures using 2-0 silk are placed in the dermis (Fig. 85-5). The fascia is then identified and incised circumferentially beyond the palpable border of the tumor.

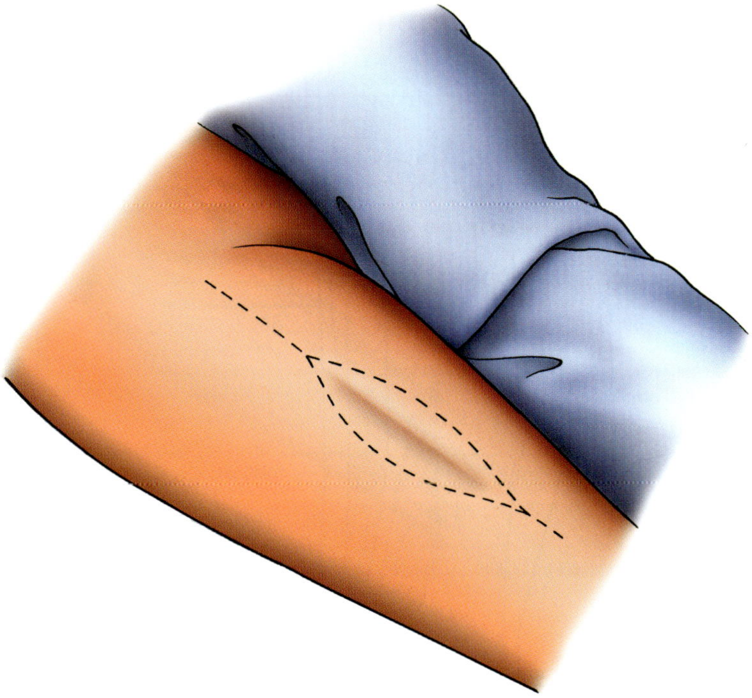

Figure 85-4.

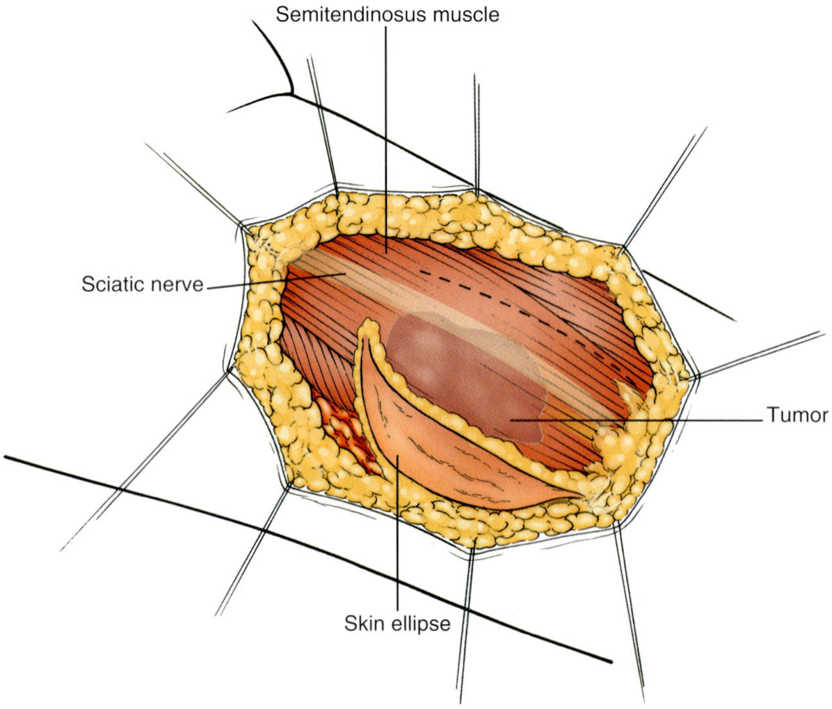

Figure 85-5.

- The long head of the biceps femoris muscle, the semimembranosus muscle, and the semitendinosus muscle are exposed. If further proximal exposure is necessary, the gluteus maximus muscle can be retracted upward or partially incised. The medial extent of the dissection is to the level of the gracilis muscle, whereas the lateral extent is to the iliotibial tract.
- The proximal aspect of the popliteal fossa is encountered, which is bordered by the biceps femoris laterally and the semimembranosus/semitendinosus tendons medially. Here the popliteal vessels are identified and vessel loops are placed. In a similar fashion, the distal portion of the sciatic nerve and its terminal branches, the tibial and common peroneal nerves, are carefully isolated, and vessel loops are placed. The critical structure in the posterior thigh is the sciatic nerve. Its proximity to the tumor should have been clearly delineated by the preoperative MRI scan.
- The sciatic nerve is identified after division of the biceps, semimembranosus, and semitendinosus muscles. Before any muscle groups are divided, it is important to expose the sciatic nerve proximally where it can be seen coursing midway between the greater trochanter and the ischial tuberosity (Fig. 85-6). The long head of the biceps femoris is retracted medially to identify the sciatic nerve. While keeping the nerve under direct view, the long head of the biceps femoris as well as the semimembranosus and semitendinosus muscles are divided with electrocautery.
- Dissection then proceeds in the caudal direction with frequent assessment of the adequacy of the deep margin. The divided hamstring muscles, along with the tumor mass, are then elevated from the underlying adductor magnus muscle. If the tumor encroaches closely on the adductor magnus, this muscle should also be resected in order to achieve adequate margins. If a portion of the adductor magnus needs to be resected, beware of the proximity of the superficial femoral vessels that lie just within the

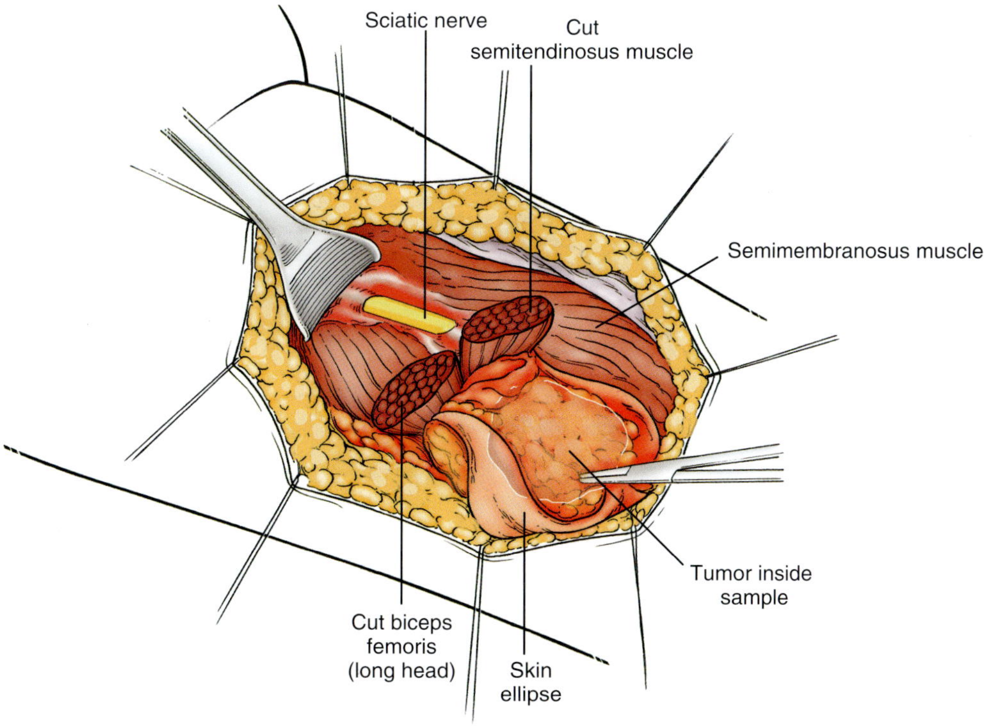

Figure 85-6.

adductor canal (Fig. 85-7, *A*). These vessels can be inadvertently injured because they are being exposed from a rather unconventional direction.

- While performing the deep dissection, if the tumor mass is felt to be in close proximity to the sciatic nerve, dissection is performed on top of the nerve just beneath the perineurium (Fig. 85-7, *B*). In this fashion, the perineurium can act as a thin layer of margin. The dissection is continued distally, and the long head of the biceps femoris is separated from the underlying short head of the biceps femoris.
- Laterally, the fascia lata is incised, exposing a portion of the vastus lateralis and the short head of the biceps femoris. Medially, the gracilis muscle can be preserved if it is uninvolved with the malignant process. Keeping the structures within the popliteal fossa under view, the long head of the bicep femoris is transected distally on the lateral side of the posterior thigh. In a similar fashion, the insertions of the semimembranosus and semitendinosus muscles are divided, thus exposing the underlying medial head of the gastrocnemius muscle.

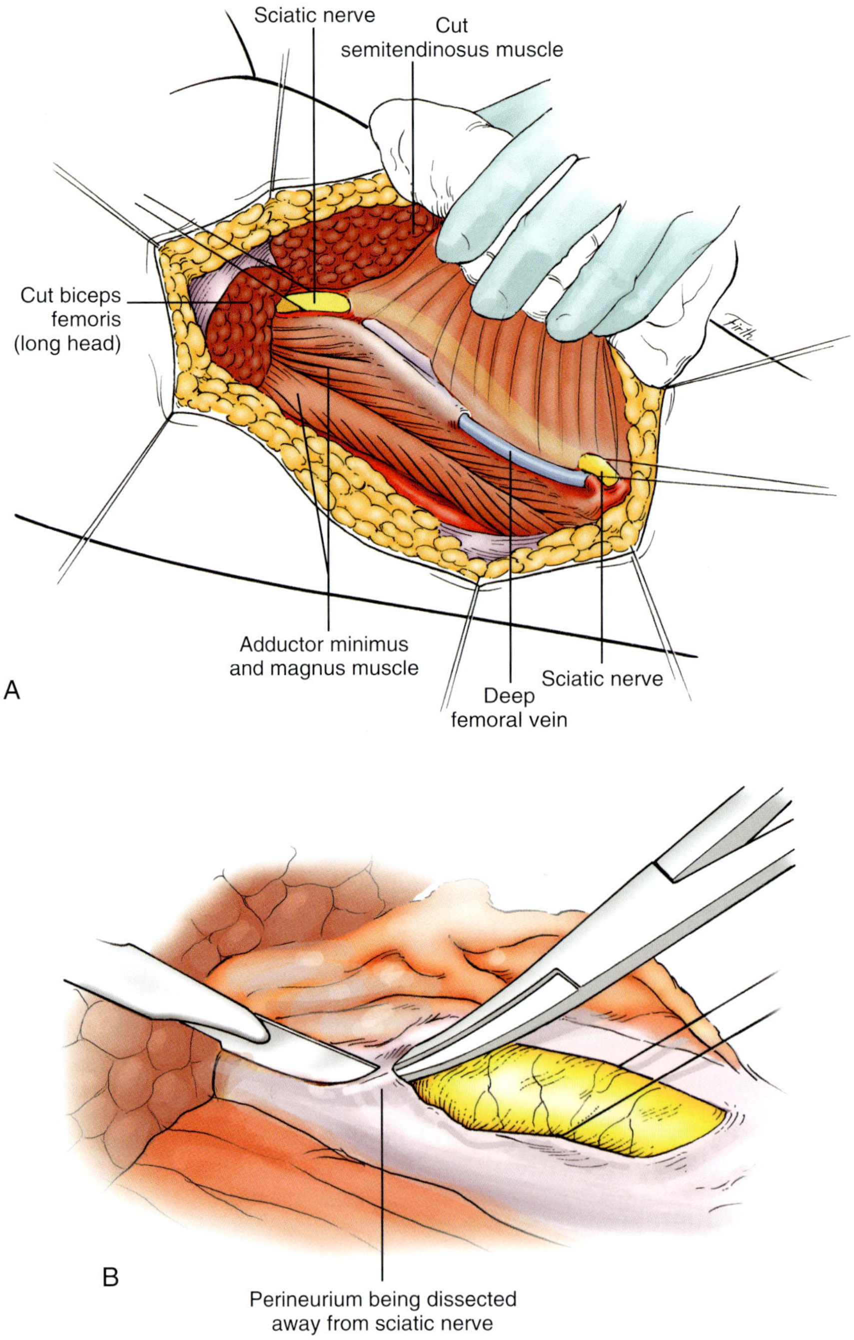

Figure 85-7.

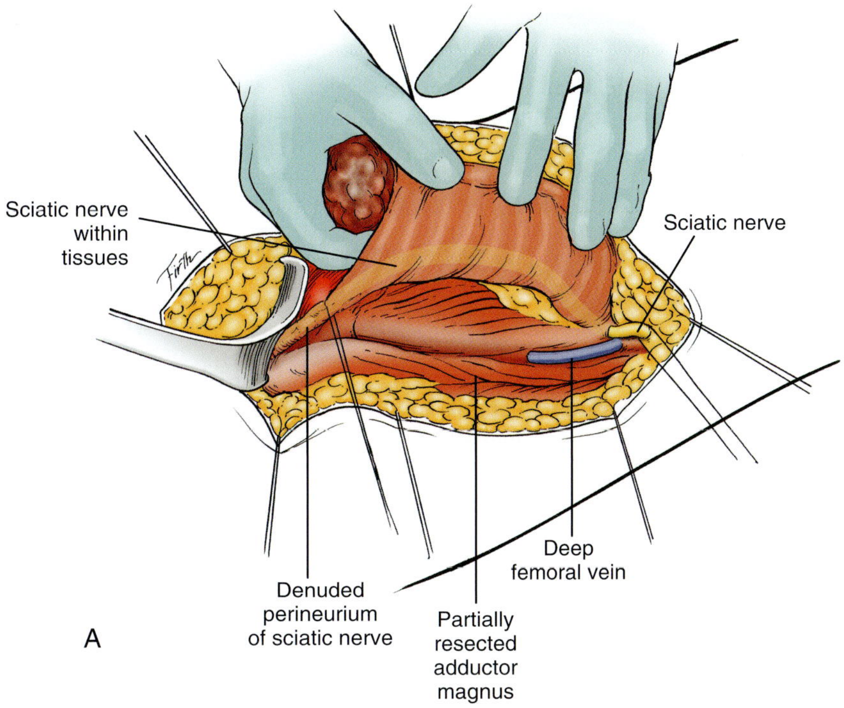
Sciatic nerve within tissues
Sciatic nerve
Deep femoral vein
Denuded perineurium of sciatic nerve
Partially resected adductor magnus
A

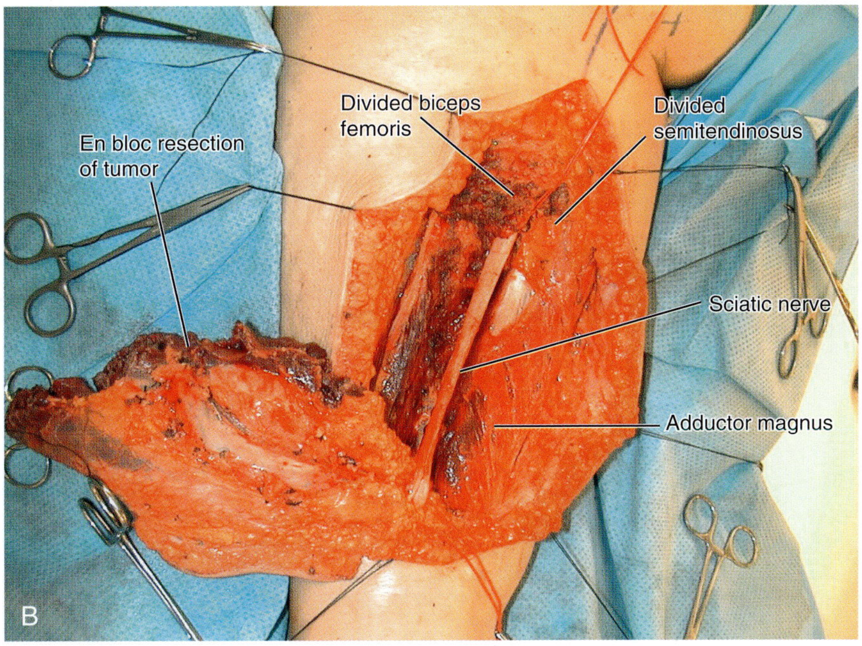
Divided biceps femoris
Divided semitendinosus
En bloc resection of tumor
Sciatic nerve
Adductor magnus
B

Figure 85-8.

- The sciatic nerve with its terminal branches is seen lying on the adductor magnus (Figs. 85-8 and 85-9). Now that the muscles of the posterior thigh have been resected, the operative bed reveals the adductor magnus, the short head of the biceps femoris, and the sciatic nerve. Inferiorly, the two heads of the gastrocnemius muscle are also visible. During the inferior dissection, particular care is taken to avoid injuring the blood vessels that supply the gastrocnemius muscle, as this muscle may be needed for reconstructive purposes, especially if primary closure of the skin is not feasible.
- The specimen has to be oriented for the pathologist (Fig. 85-10) to allow appropriate margin assessment, particularly in the region where the tumor was in close proximity to the neurovascular structures.

Closure

- After hemostasis is obtained, two Jackson-Pratt drains are placed through a separate stab incision and secured with 3-0 nonabsorbable monofilament suture.
- The dermis is then carefully approximated with 2-0 absorbable suture, and the skin is closed with staples. If a large skin ellipse has had to be resected and primary closure is not feasible, reconstruction with a local rotational flap or free flap is necessary.

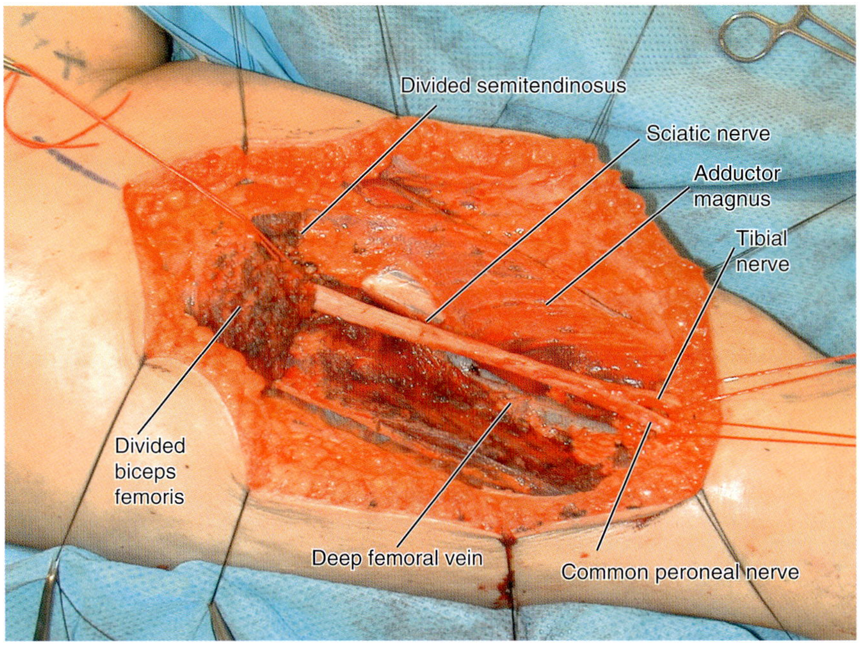

Figure 85-9.

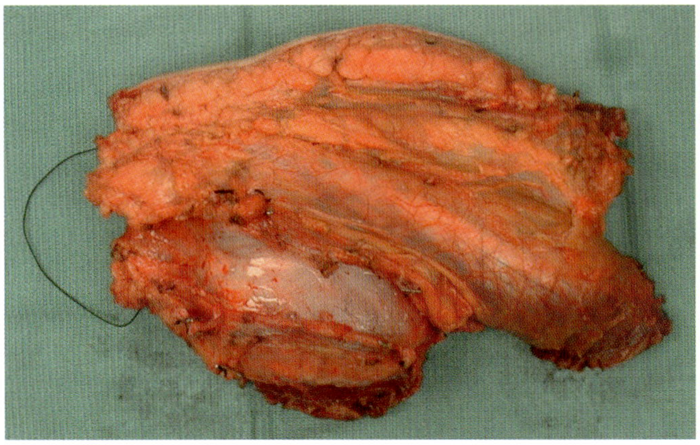

Figure 85-10.

III. ALTERNATIVE TECHNICAL APPROACHES (PRO/CON) AND PEARLS

- Technically, the many new hemostatic instruments allow division of the muscles with reduced blood loss. Unless the neurovascular bundle is encased, it can invariably be preserved because of the expansive, noninfiltrative growth characteristic of soft tissue sarcomas. In these circumstances, when dissecting along the vessels or nerves, the adventitia of the vessel or perineurium is incised, and the planes just beneath these layers are opened. Division of these filmy layers is best achieved with a sharp no. 15 blade. The layers should be left on the specimen side to serve as a margin.
- Diagnosis of the histologic subtype, such as either a leiomyosarcoma or a malignant peripheral nerve sheath tumor, usually suggests that the vessel or nerve of origin must be resected. When the vessel of tumor origin is a vein, usually it does not require reconstruction, because collateral venous drainage has often developed. In contrast, if the artery must be resected, reconstruction can be achieved with either autologous vein or polytetrafluoroethylene.
- In the event that a decision is made to treat the patient with brachytherapy, the operative area that needs to be radiated is carefully mapped in collaboration with the radiation oncologist. The brachytherapy catheters are passed through the skin at 1-cm intervals and secured in the operative bed with simple plain 3-0 chromic sutures. Exposed vessels should be covered with adjacent musculofascial tissue or an appropriate-size Alloderm.

IV. SPECIAL POSTOPERATIVE CARE

- To minimize the likelihood of edema and wound disruption, particularly in patients who have received preoperative radiation, it is important to institute complete bed rest and extremity elevation.
- Specific intraoperative complications that may be encountered with extremity sarcoma resection are sciatic nerve injury, injury to superficial femoral vessels, and tumor rupture.
- Specific immediate postoperative complications that may be encountered are infection, wound disruption, hematoma, neuropathic pain, and deep vein thrombosis.
- Specific delayed complications that may be encountered are lymphedema, recurrent sarcoma, and radiation necrosis.
- Subcutaneous heparin injection for deep vein thrombosis prophylaxis should be avoided because of the risk of operative-bed hematoma. Instead, a compression device can be placed on the contralateral extremity, though level I evidence is lacking. A similar approach is necessary if the patient has had brachytherapy catheters inserted, to avoid altering their careful intraoperative placement. Bed rest is continued for 3 to 5 days, followed by limited ambulation with the aid of a walker and instructions to avoid excessive ambulation.
- If there is any suggestion of tension on the skin closure, staples should be left for at least 2 weeks, or longer if necessary to avoid wound disruption that may delay postoperative radiation therapy. In patients who have received preoperative radiation therapy, healing may be impaired, and similar cautious postoperative care is needed to reduce wound-related morbidity.

SUGGESTED READINGS

Geisinger KR, Ward WG, Levine EA: Soft-tissue sarcoma, *N Engl J Med* 353:2303–2304, 2005.

Khatri VP, Goodnight JE: Extremity soft tissue sarcoma: controversial management issues, *Surg Oncol* 14:1–9, 2005.

Pisters PW, Leung DH, Woodruff J, et al: Analysis of prognostic factors in 1,041 patients with localized soft tissue sarcomas of the extremities, *J Clin Oncol* 14:1679–1689, 1996.

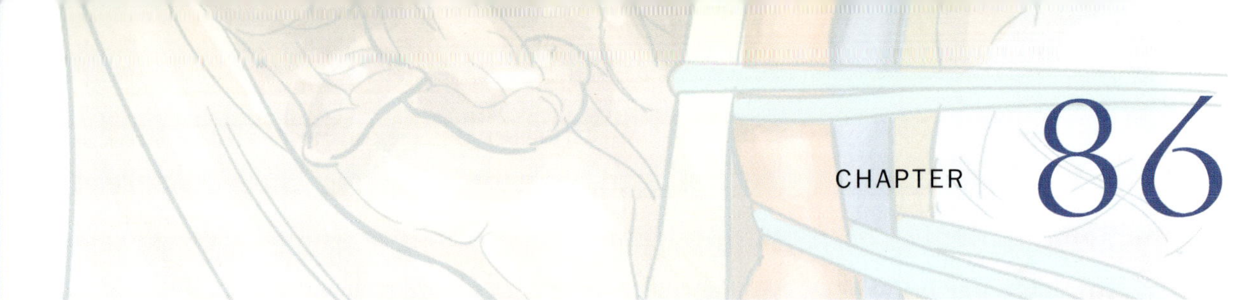

CHAPTER 86

Resection of Flexor Fossa (Axilla and Groin) Sarcoma

Fritz C. Eilber, MD, and Frederick R. Eilber, MD

I. SPECIAL PREOPERATIVE PREPARATION

- *History and physical exam:* The history and physical exam are particularly important in patients with tumors of the axilla and groin. Specific attention should be focused on a history of malignancies that metastasize to regional lymph nodes (melanoma, squamous cell carcinoma, breast cancer) or develop within the nodal tissue (lymphoma). Physical exam should look for skin lesions, masses, or surgical scars on the extremity or breast. In addition, the popliteal or epitrochlear and cervical regions should be examined for lymphadenopathy. In the absence of nodal disease, soft tissue sarcoma should be considered if the tumor is large, deep, immobile, and firm. In the presence of any of these clinical features, cross-sectional imaging and tissue diagnosis are critical in guiding appropriate care.
- *Imaging:* Cross-sectional imaging is critical because it provides the anatomic information necessary to guide surgical resection. Cross-sectional imaging can be performed by either computed tomography (CT) or magnetic resonance imaging (MRI) and should include the appropriate intravenous contrast agent to delineate the vascular anatomy (Figs. 86-1 through 86-3).
- *CT versus MRI:* Too much emphasis is placed on this distinction, and there are very few instances in which one modality is preferred over the other. Although certain soft tissue sarcomas are imaged better with MRI and others better with CT, this choice should be driven by both the surgeon's comfort with the imaging technique and the availability and ease of obtaining the study.
- *Tissue diagnosis:* CT-guided core biopsy is the optimal method of obtaining tissue diagnosis. CT guidance allows for precise tissue sampling, including targeting specific areas of concern within a tumor. Fine-needle aspiration is inadequate. Core biopsies need to be done with a large-bore needle to allow adequate tissue collection for histologic diagnosis, grade, and often critical ancillary studies such as cytogenetics and electron microscopy. In the rare instance (<5%) that a CT-guided core biopsy is unable to provide an adequate histologic diagnosis, an incisional biopsy can be performed. Such a biopsy should be placed in line with the incision required for definitive surgical resection, with attention to hemostasis to avoid a hematoma.
- *Staging:* Patients with groin sarcomas should have a CT scan of the chest, abdomen, and pelvis. CT of the pelvis is particularly important, because local extension into the pelvis is not uncommon for these tumors. Patients with axillary sarcomas should have a CT scan of the chest. Positron emission tomography scans have not been validated as a screening modality and are not done in the setting of primary disease unless under a study protocol.
- *Neoadjuvant therapy:* Patients with large (≥5cm), high-grade sarcomas of the flexor fossa (axilla or groin) should be strongly considered for protocol neoadjuvant therapy (chemotherapy, radiation therapy, and/or chemoradiation). The ability to obtain adequate margins in the flexor fossa is more limited than in the extremity. Neoadjuvant therapy often shrinks lesions in the flexor fossa, improving their resectability and margin status. Neoadjuvant therapy should be administered only according to a protocol, and at a sarcoma center or a cancer center with expertise in sarcomas.

II. OPERATIVE TECHNIQUE

Position

- The patient is placed in the supine position. A Foley catheter should be placed. It is generally best to prep the entire extremity (leg or arm). Stockinet is placed over the foot or hand, and the extremity is draped free to allow it to be moved during the operation. The prep should include the chest wall for axillary sarcomas and the lower abdomen for groin sarcomas.

Incision

- *Groin*: A curvilinear incision is initiated from the lower-lateral abdominal wall superior and medial to the anterior superior iliac spine. The incision is carried along the inguinal crease, ending medially and distally over the adductor muscles of the thigh (Fig. 86-4).

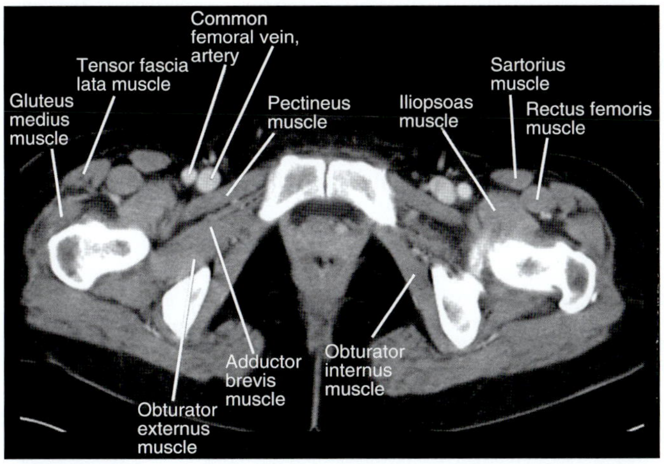

Figure 86-1. Computed tomography scan illustrating the normal anatomy of the left groin.

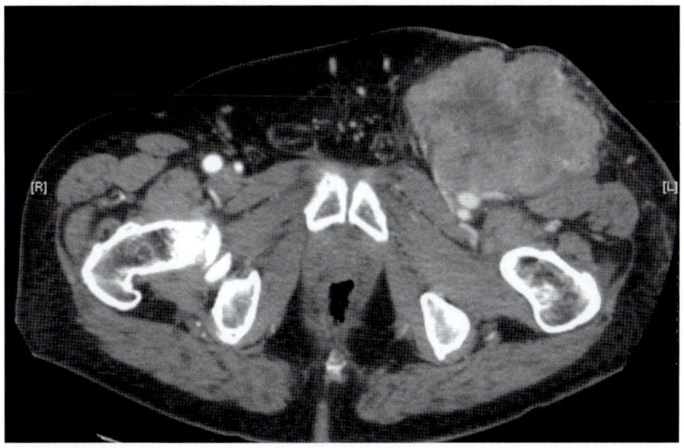

Figure 86-2. Computed tomography scan of a left groin sarcoma.

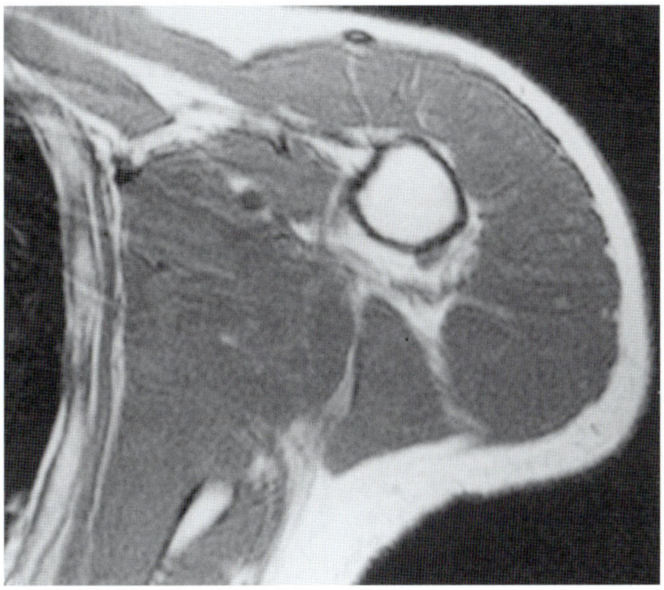

Figure 86-3. Magnetic resonance image of a left axillary sarcoma.

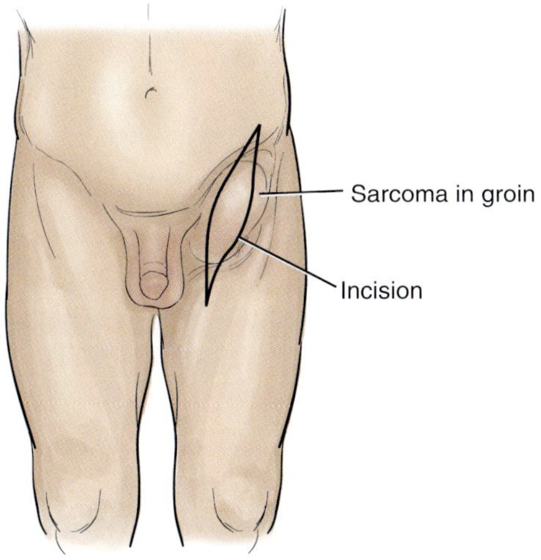

Figure 86-4.

- *Axilla*: An incision is made about two finger breadths below the axillary crease, from the lateral border of the pectoralis major muscle to the latissimus dorsi muscle (Fig. 86-5).
- The incision should ellipse out the previous incisional biopsy site if present. A generous incision should be made to allow for appropriate exposure.

Main Dissection

Axilla

- Flaps of skin and subcutaneous fat are raised superiorly and inferiorly.
- The initial aspect of the dissection is focused on becoming anatomically oriented to the lateral border of the pectoralis major muscle, the latissimus dorsi, the axillary artery and vein, and the brachial plexus. Sarcomas in the axilla are close to neurovascular structures, and it is critical to identify them before beginning resection of the tumor (Fig. 86-6).
- The thoracodorsal vessels should be identified and preserved if they are not directly involved with the tumor.
- Both the thoracodorsal and long thoracic nerve should be identified and preserved if they are not directly involved with the tumor.

Groin

- Flaps of skin and subcutaneous fat are raised superiorly, exposing the inferior aspect of the lower abdominal wall and inguinal ligament and inferiorly exposing the fascia of the anterior thigh musculature.
- The initial aspect of the dissection is focused on becoming anatomically oriented to the femoral artery, vein, and nerve. Sarcomas in the groin are close to neurovascular structures, and it is critical to identify these structures before beginning resection of the tumor (Fig. 86-7).
- Tumors of the groin may extend into the pelvis, and division of the inguinal ligament and lower abdominal wall fascia and musculature is often required for exposure.
- Attention to the inferior epigastric vessels is important because they arise from the distal iliac vessels just before the inguinal ligament.

Axilla and Groin

- En bloc resection of the tumor is the primary surgical goal, with dissection being carried out through normal adjacent tissue planes. A clamp (tonsil or right angle) and Bovie cautery are used for the dissection. Vessels are ligated as necessary with 2-0 or 3-0 silk ties.

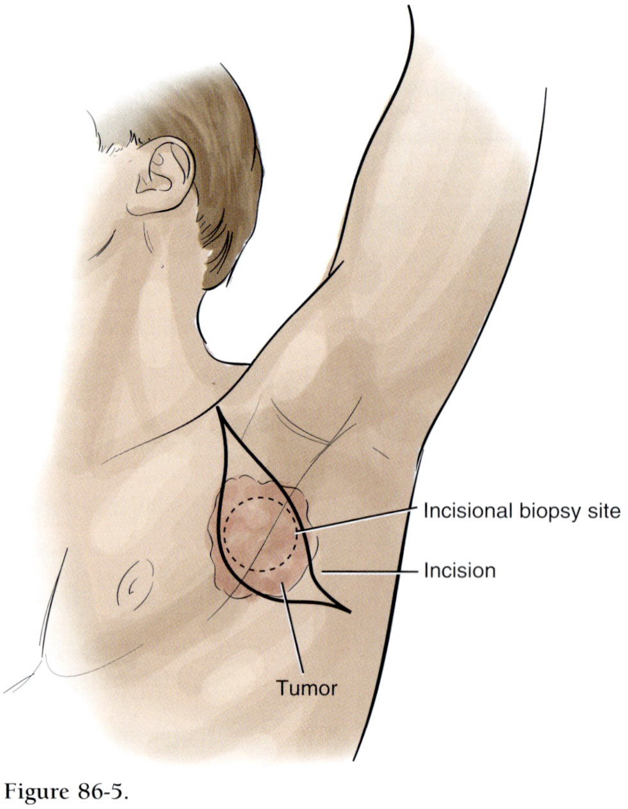

Figure 86-5.

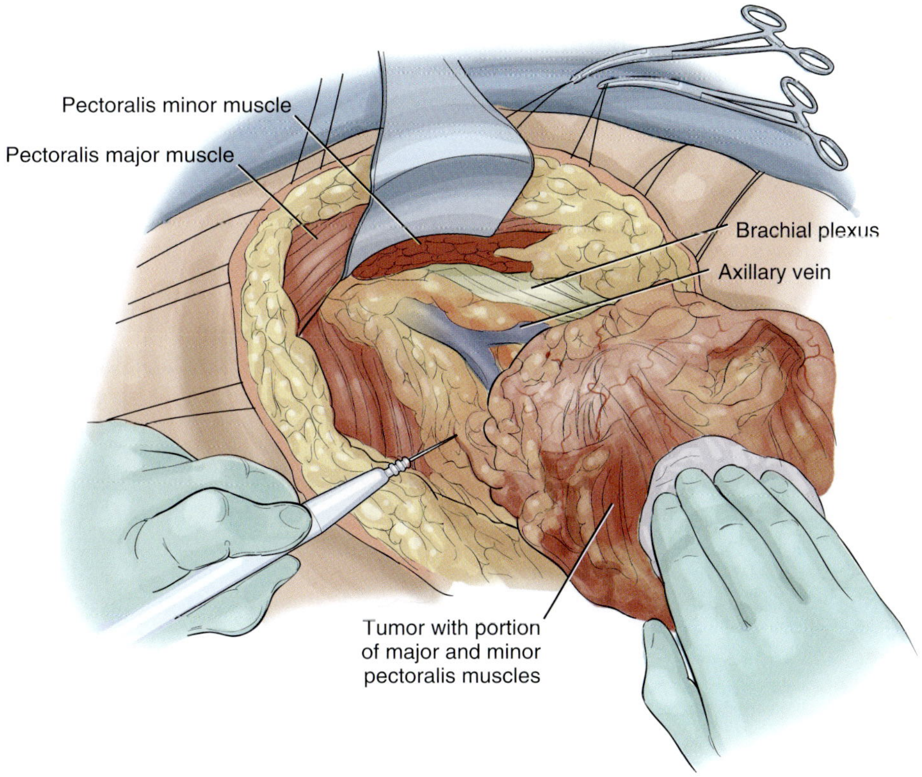

Figure 86-6.

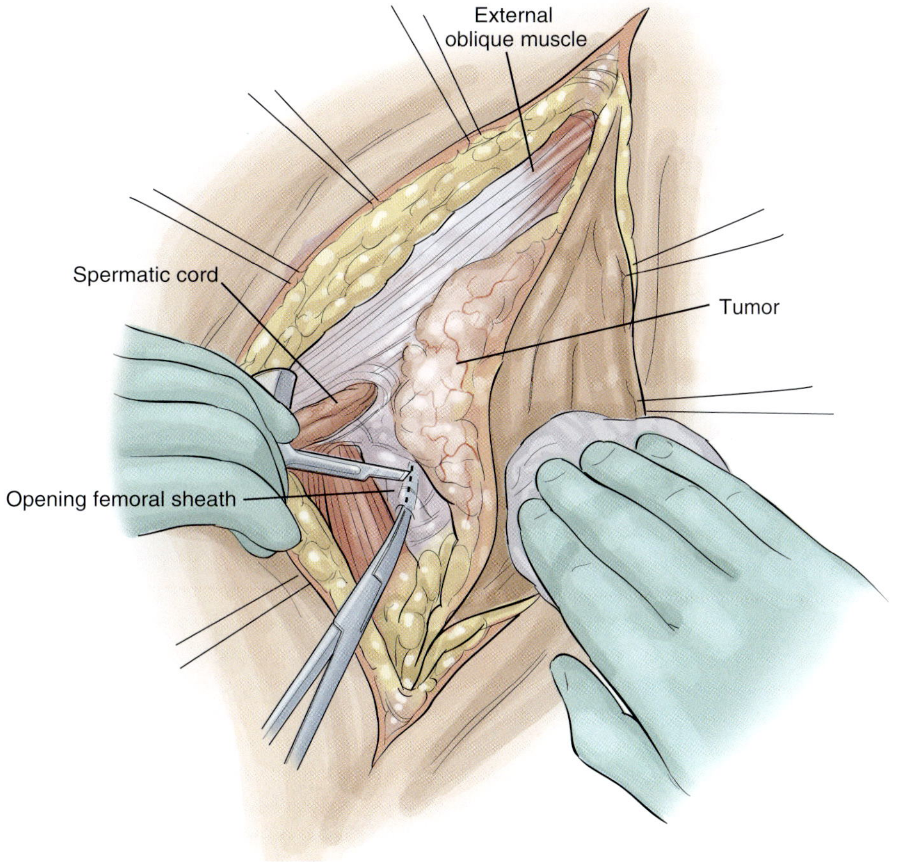

Figure 86-7.

- Surgical resection should include normal soft tissue adjacent to the tumor. At a minimum, the pathologic specimen must be free of tumor at the resection margins (see Fig. 86-6).
- Resection of the neurovascular structures en bloc with the tumor is usually not necessary unless the sarcoma arises from the vessels or nerve. Exposing the neurovascular structures both proximally and distally allows meticulous dissection to be performed along the neurovascular bundle, and if necessary, the adventitia of the artery and vein or perineurium can be removed with the tumor (Figs. 86-8 and 86-9).
- Resection of neurovascular structures is rarely done for a primary low-grade tumor. If a primary high-grade tumor directly involves or arises from a neurovascular structure, the structure requires en bloc resection with the sarcoma.
- Resection of the femoral or axillary artery requires reconstruction with autologous vein or polytetrafluoroethylene.
- Resection of the femoral or axillary vein puts the patient at risk for permanent severe venous swelling of the extremity, as these veins cannot be reconstructed with any degree of success.
- Resection of either the femoral nerve or brachial plexus results in significant functional deficits. Patients are usually able to tolerate resection of the femoral nerve to the point where the limb is still reasonably functional with a knee brace. The loss of the brachial plexus usually results in a nonfunctional extremity, and if the brachial plexus is directly involved, amputation should considered.
- Marking sutures are placed on the resected tumor to allow for appropriate margin assessment by the pathologist. If the tumor is close to a particular resection margin, additional tissue at that region of the resection cavity can be sent for pathologic results and an additional margin assessment obtained.

Closure

- At least one and often two round, 19-Fr Jackson-Pratt drains are placed into the resection cavity. They are brought through the skin through a separate stab incision and anchored to the skin with a stitch (Fig. 86-10).
- In the groin, if the femoral vessels are exposed, they should be covered with a transposed sartorius muscular flap (see Fig. 86-9, *inset*). Subcutaneous fat and skin are approximated using 2-0 Vicryl, and the skin is closed with staples. After a gauze dressing has been applied, compression is applied with two 6-inch Ace wraps around the proximal thigh and pelvis or around the chest wall.

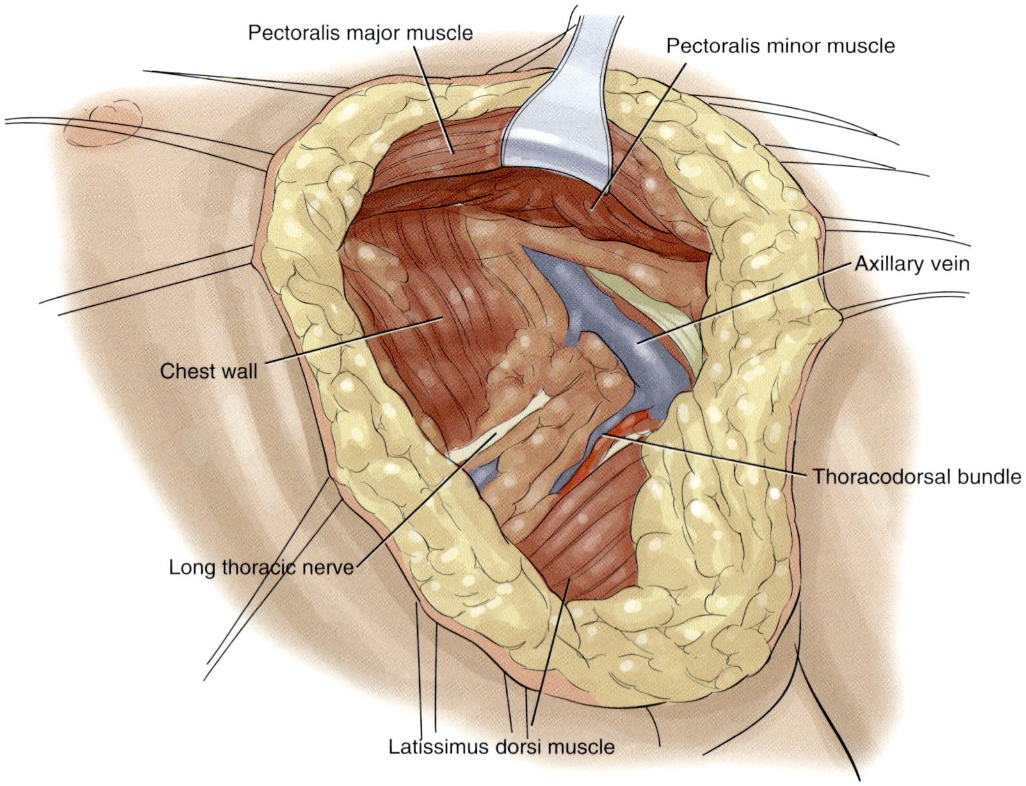

Figure 86-8.

III. ALTERNATIVE TECHNICAL APPROACHES (PRO/CON) AND PEARLS

- There is no role for either axillary or inguinal lymphadenectomy. Sarcomas rarely if ever involve or metastasize to lymph nodes. Including a lymphadenectomy with the tumor resection will significantly add to the risk of permanent extremity edema.
- Particularly in the groin, resection of a flexor fossa sarcoma results in exposure of the vessels. The femoral vessels should be covered with additional layer of tissue before the skin closure in case the

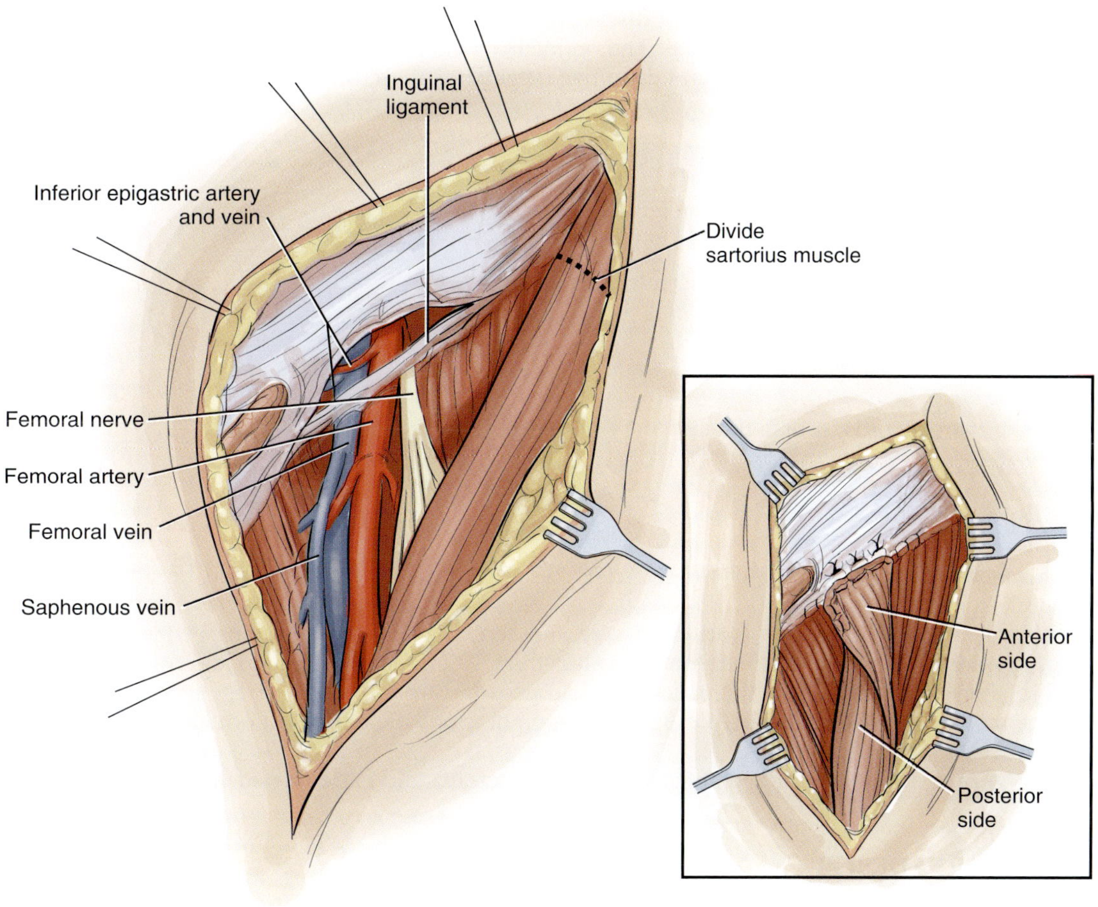

Figure 86-9.

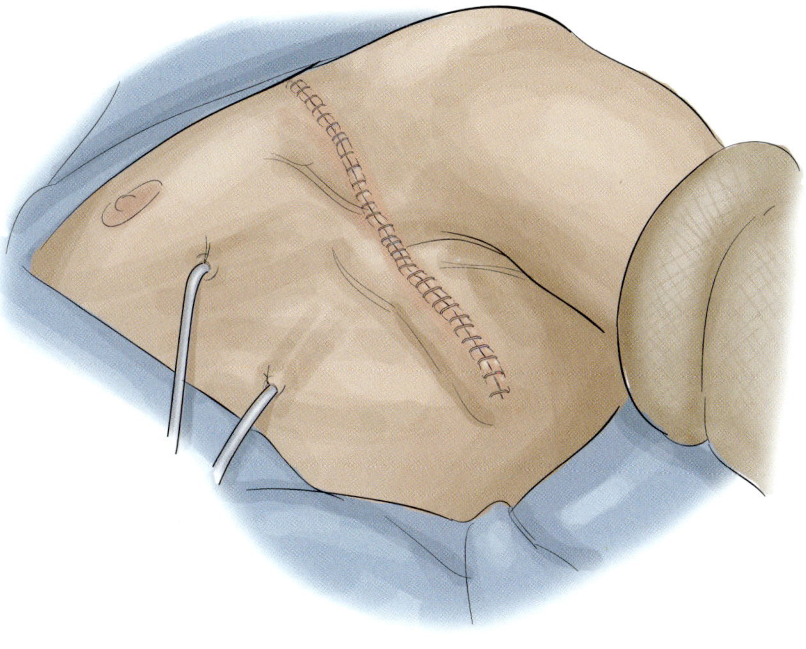

Figure 86-10.

wound opens or becomes infected. Rotation of a sartorius muscular flap is the easiest way to accomplish this coverage. The sartorius is divided at its origin at the anterior superior iliac spine and rotated 180 degrees in a medial manner to lie over the femoral vessels. It is then anchored to the inguinal ligament and adductor fascia.

- Soft tissue sarcomas are rare, high-risk malignancies that are best managed by an experienced multidisciplinary team of physicians at a sarcoma center or a cancer center that has expertise in these tumors.
- A multidisciplinary team of surgeons is often needed for resection of these lesions, and thorough preoperative planning is therefore critical. Complex reconstruction by plastic surgery with either a local rotational flap or a free flap and vascular reconstruction by vascular surgery are occasionally required.
- The development of locally recurrent disease is a morbid and potentially limb-threatening event that is associated with decreased survival. The optimal treatment of locally recurrent disease is to prevent it, which necessitates aggressive and definitive surgery in the setting of the primary disease.

IV. SPECIAL POSTOPERATIVE CARE

Axilla

- The arm of the affected side is placed in a sling.

Groin

- While the patient is in bed, the extremity should be elevated.

Axilla and Groin

- Significant range of motion of the extremity distal to the surgical site should be limited for several weeks.
- Patients are taught Jackson-Pratt drain care and sent home with the drains in place. Jackson-Pratt drains are not removed until the output is less than 20 mL/day. Staples are left in for at least 1 week and often up to 2 weeks, if the patient has had neoadjuvant radiation therapy or wound concerns.
- The most common immediate postoperative complications include infection, hematoma, and wound dehiscence or slough.
- The most common delayed complications include seroma and extremity edema.

SUGGESTED READINGS

Brooks AD, Bowne WB, Delgado R, et al: Soft tissue sarcomas of the groin: diagnosis, management, and prognosis, *J Am Coll Surg* 193:130–136, 2001.

Eilber FC, Eckardt JJ, Rosen G, et al: Large, deep, high-grade extremity sarcomas: treating tumors of the flexor fossae, *Surg Oncol* 8:211–214, 1999.

Yang RS, Lane JM, Eilber FR, et al: High grade soft tissue sarcoma of the flexor fossae. Size rather than compartmental status determine prognosis, *Cancer* 76:1398–1405, 1995.

CHAPTER 87

Scapular Resections

Mario Mercuri, MD, and Laura Campanacci, MD, PhD

I. SPECIAL PREOPERATIVE PREPARATION

Indications for Total Scapulectomy

- Indications include chondrosarcoma, Ewing sarcoma, metastases, and osteosarcoma.
- Resection of the whole scapula with its musculofascial covering may realize a radical surgical margin in the case of tumors contained in that osteomuscular compartment.

Contraindications for Total Scapulectomy

- If the tumor involves the glenohumeral joint, an extra-articular resection of scapula and humeral head (Tikhoff-Linberg) is indicated.
- If the subclavian-axillary neurovascular bundle is involved, it is necessary to resort to a forequarter amputation.

II. OPERATIVE TECHNIQUE: TOTAL SCAPULECTOMY

Position

- The patient lies on the unaffected side, to provide full access to the posterior and anterior aspects of the shoulder and the thorax. The entire upper limb, the thorax from the sternum to the spinous processes, and the base of the neck are included in the sterile field.

Incision

- A longitudinal, slightly curved incision extending from the tip of the acromion to the inferior angle of the scapula or an elliptical incision needs to be used to encompass any prior incision. The incision can be modified according to the conditions of the skin (S or T shaped; Fig. 87-1).

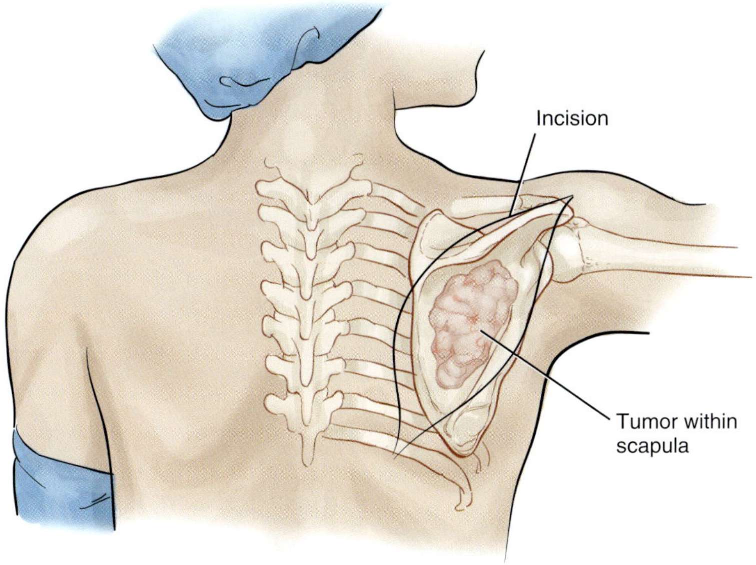

Figure 87-1.

Main Dissection

- Flaps are created beyond the confines of the palpable tumor (Fig. 87-2). Subsequently, the muscles on the medial and lateral aspect of the scapula are exposed (Fig. 87-3).
- The trapezius and deltoid insertions are detached from the spine of the scapula, the acromion, and the lateral clavicle and retracted, exposing the rotator cuff and the entire vertebral border of the scapula (Fig. 87-4).
- The latissimus dorsi is detached from the inferior angle of the scapula. This angle and the vertebral border of the scapula are pulled backward, and the rhomboids, levator scapulae, and omohyoideus are divided. On the deep (anterior) surface of the levator scapulae, the transverse cervical vessels are ligated and divided.
- When the subscapularis muscle appears to be sufficient to achieve wide margins anteriorly, the serratus anterior muscle is detached near the vertebral border of the scapula, and an easy dissection plane is bluntly developed between the subscapularis and the serratus anterior.
- If safer margins are possible toward the thoracic wall, three progressively more extended margins are feasible:
  - ▲ The serratus anterior is not detached from the scapula, but from the ribs, and is removed en bloc with the scapula.
  - ▲ In addition, a layer constituted by the periosteum of the ribs and the external intercostal muscles over an appropriate area can be included.
  - ▲ Exceptionally, if the tumor is not freely movable on the chest wall and involves the ribs, a full-thickness patch of the thoracic wall, including the pleura, should be included in the resection.
- Progressively, the teres major, teres minor, and infraspinatus muscles are divided close to their humeral insertion, and the long head of the triceps is divided at a distance from its scapular insertion. The acromioclavicular joint is opened, and the supraspinatus tendon is divided near the humerus. On the deep aspect of the supraspinatus muscle, the suprascapular vessels are ligated and divided. The glenohumeral joint capsule is circumferentially divided near the humeral head. The subscapularis tendon is divided at the anterior aspect of the joint. The intra-articular tendon of the long head of the biceps is divided near its insertion to the glenoid.
- Finally, the coracoid process is freed from its muscular insertions, and the coracoclavicular ligaments are sectioned near the clavicle. These are the last strong structures affixing the scapula. After their transection, it can be completely mobilized and removed.
- In cases of less extensive tumors, the uninvolved muscular compartments such as the subscapularis and supraspinatus can be subperiosteally detached from the scapula and preserved. Similarly, through subperiosteal exposure, the acromion can be transected at its base by a Gigli saw, the neck of the scapula osteotomized outside the articular capsule and parallel to the glenoid surface (thus allowing for better stability of the humeral head), and the coracoid process also osteotomized at its base.

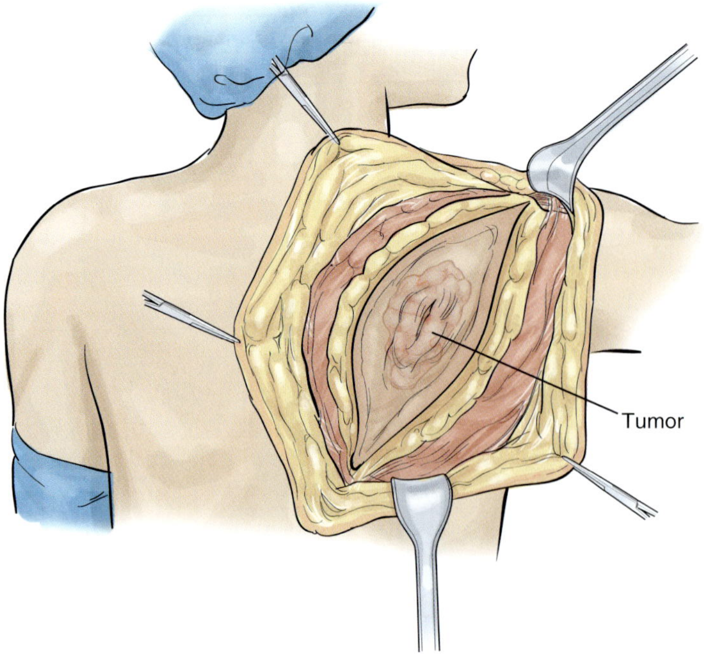

Figure 87-2.

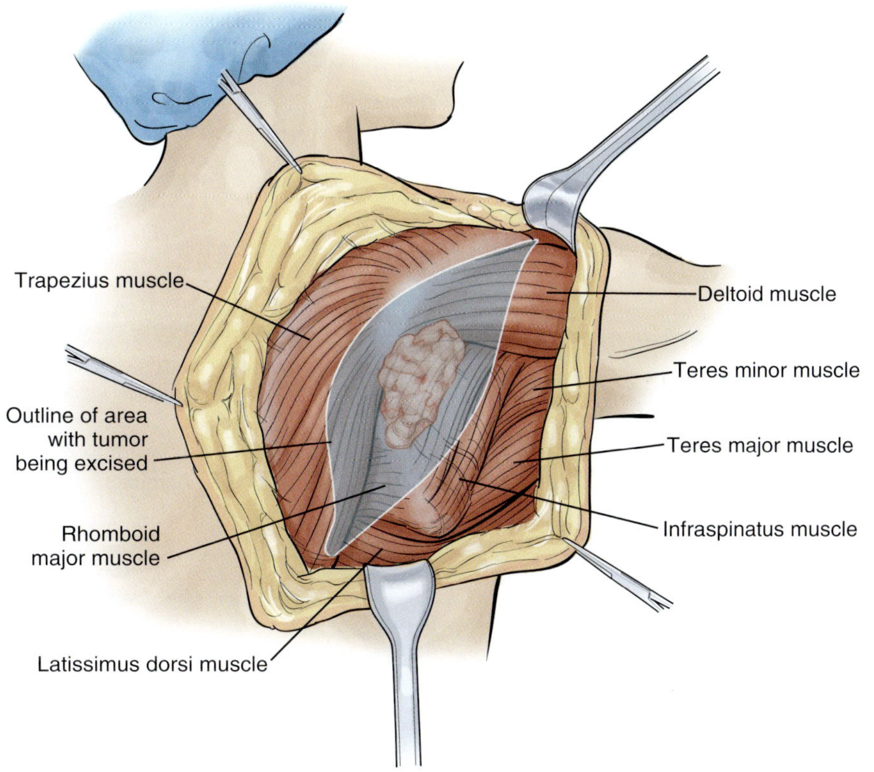

Figure 87-3.

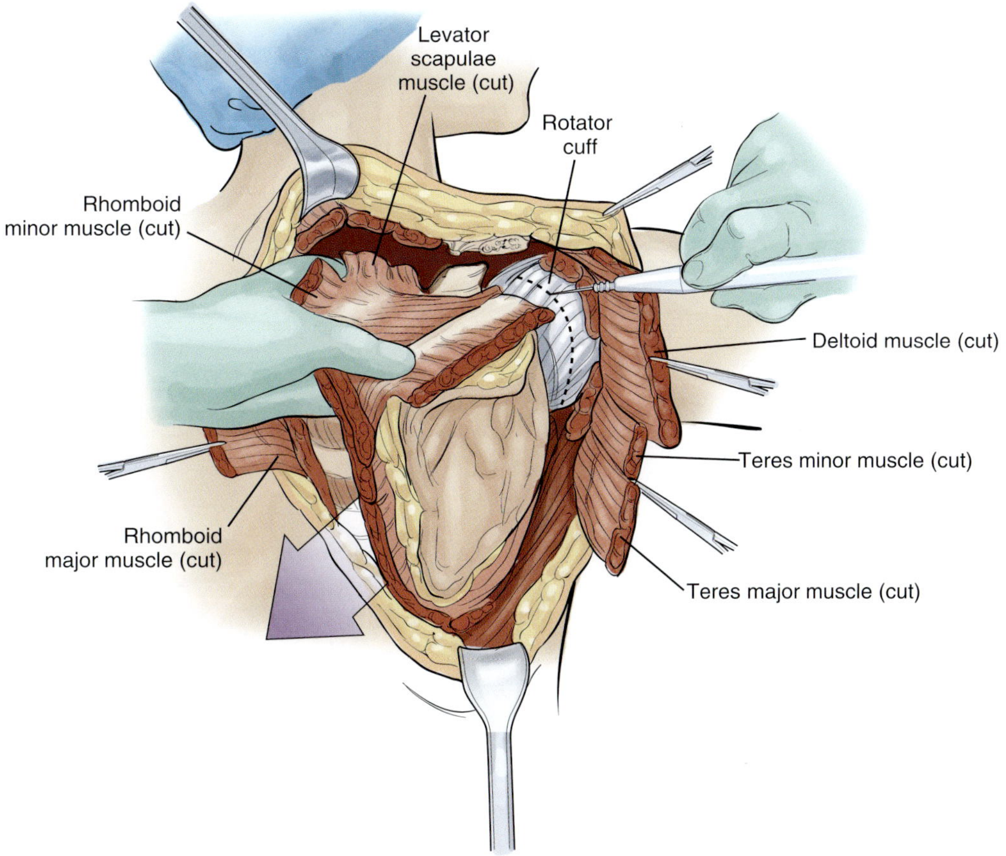

Figure 87-4.

Reconstruction

- The resected scapula does not need to be replaced. The deltoid is sutured to the trapezius. The coracoid muscles and the tendon of the long head of the biceps can be sutured to the clavicle (Fig. 87-5).

Closure

- The wound is closed and drains are inserted (Fig. 87-6).

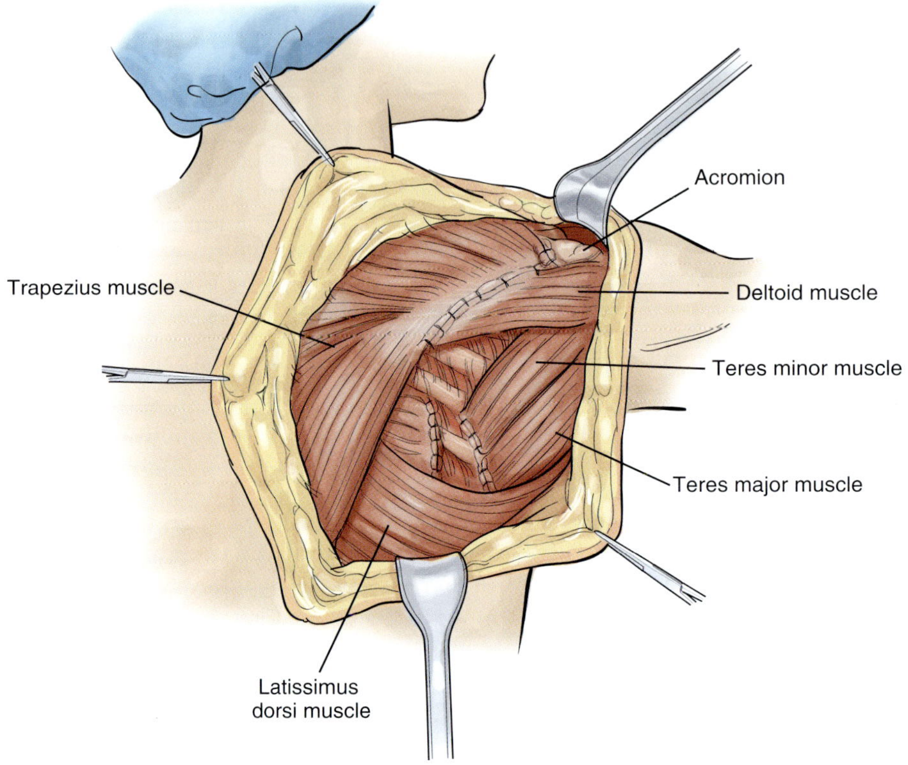

Figure 87-5.

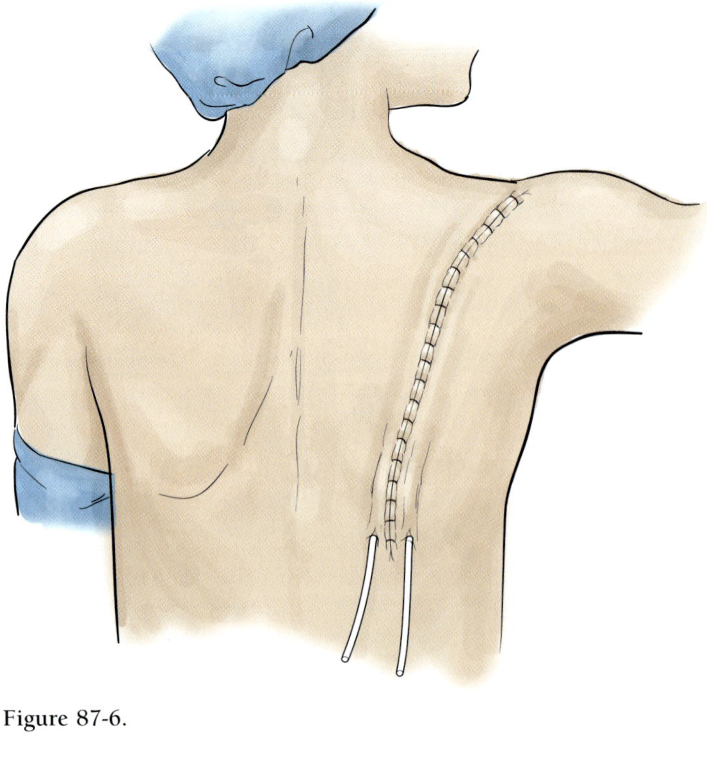

Figure 87-6.

III. ALTERNATIVE TECHNICAL APPROACHES (PRO/CON) AND PEARLS

Partial Scapulectomy

- When the tumor involves only the inferior part of the scapula, this can be osteotomized below the spine of the scapula and the scapulohumeral joint, and only the inferior body of the scapula is widely resected.
- Rarely, the resection can be limited to the glenoid, preserving the scapular body. This resection is done through the anterior approach, transecting the subscapularis at the level of the medial extent of the glenoid resection to expose the area of scapula through which the osteotomy can be performed.
- *Reconstruction:* The resected portion of the scapula does not need to be replaced. Reconstruction consists of suturing the remaining muscles to the retained portion of the scapula, and one suction drain is placed underneath the fascia.

IV. SPECIAL POSTOPERATIVE CARE

- Adequate pain control is necessary and is achieved with narcotic patient-controlled analgesia. Nonsteroidal antiinflammatory agents can be added as narcotic-sparing agents.
- The patient is encouraged to begin passive motion in the early postoperative period as soon as pain is adequately controlled.
- The patient is prescribed a comfortable arm sling and is allowed to increase activity as tolerated. In particular, the patient is encouraged to passively move the elbow, forearm, and hand to maintain normal function.
- A postoperative consultation with physical therapy and rehabilitation service is initiated to begin the rehabilitative process that will continue after discharge.

SUGGESTED READING

Bickels J, Wittig JC, Kollender Y, et al: Limb-sparing resections of the shoulder girdle, *J Am Coll Surg* 194:422–435, 2002.

Malawer MM, Sugarbaker PH: *Musculoskeletal cancer surgery: treatment of sarcomas and allied diseases*, Dordrecht, The Netherlands, 2001, Kluwer Academic.

Volpe CM, Pell M, Doerr RJ, Karakousis CP: Radical scapulectomy with limb salvage for shoulder girdle soft tissue sarcoma, *Surg Oncol* 5:43–48, 1996.

CHAPTER 88

Tikhoff-Linberg Procedure and Modifications for Shoulder Girdle Resections

Paul H. Sugarbaker, MD, FACS, FRCS, and Martin M. Malawer, MD, FACS

I. SPECIAL PREOPERATIVE PREPARATION

- The Tikhoff-Linberg resection and its modifications are limb-sparing surgical options to be considered for bony and soft tissue tumors in and around the proximal humerus and shoulder girdle. Careful selection of patients whose tumors do not involve the neurovascular bundle or chest wall is required. Portions of the scapula, clavicle, and/or proximal humerus are resected in conjunction with all muscles inserting into and originating from the involved bones. Optimal function is achieved by muscle transfer and skeletal reconstruction. A custom prosthesis is used to maintain length and stabilize the distal humerus after resection of sarcomas of the proximal humerus. Function of the hand and forearm after most shoulder girdle resections should be nearly normal; elbow flexion plus stability of the shoulder may be achieved without the need of an orthosis.

Indications

- Indications for limb-sparing procedures include high-grade and some low-grade bone and soft tissue sarcomas of the shoulder girdle.
- Selection of patients for this procedure is based on the anatomic location of the cancer and on a thorough understanding of the natural history of osteosarcomas and soft tissue sarcomas.
- Absolute contraindications include extension of tumor to involve the neurovascular bundle or to the chest wall.
- Relative contraindications may include pathologic fracture, extensive involvement of the shaft of the humerus, tumor contamination of the operative area from hematoma after biopsy, or unwise placement of the biopsy incision. Pathologic fracture through the tumor is a relative contraindication because it may result in extensive tumor-contaminated hematoma disseminating into the operative field.

Preoperative Studies

- Useful preoperative evaluations include the physical examination, computed tomography of the shoulder girdle, magnetic resonance imaging (MRI), arteriogram and venogram, and bone scan. Neurovascular involvement may be suggested by the position of the tumor at the shoulder, an abnormal neurologic examination, or absent pulses. However, these symptoms may be produced by tumor compression as well as by invasion by tumor. Computed tomography and MRI are especially useful for assessing chest wall involvement. They will also show the position of the tumor mass and suggest the amount of soft tissue extension.
- The arteriogram and venogram may be necessary to assess the interval between tumor and neurovascular structures. The bone scan and MRI are used to determine the extent of intramedullary involvement of the humerus and the site through which the humerus is to be transected. The humerus is resected to 6 cm beyond the area of technetium uptake. MRI is useful to determine intraosseous extent and skip metastases.

Classification of Shoulder Girdle Resections

- A classification system for resections of bony and soft tissue neoplasms involving the shoulder girdle has been developed. Types I through VI are classified according to the bony structures removed during surgery and their relationship to the glenohumeral joint. Types I through III and IV through VI are performed intra-articularly and extra-articularly, respectively. The major variable is the presence or absence of the major motor group, the abductor mechanism.
- In the classification system, A denotes that the shoulder abductors have been spared, and B denotes that abductor muscles are partially or completely resected. In general, the loss of any component of the abductor mechanism (rotator cuff and/or deltoid muscle) creates a similar functional disability. The abductor mechanism is almost always resected when there is extraosseous extension of a bone tumor in this area. Procedures that are type A (abductors preserved) accomplish an intracompartmental resection, type B procedures (abductors resected) an extracompartmental resection.
- In general, type I, II, and III resections are performed for benign or low-grade lesions of the proximal humerus or scapula. Types IV, V, and VI are most often used for the treatment of high-grade sarcomas of the scapula and humerus. In this system, the original Tikhoff-Linberg resection is classified as type IVB. The most common procedure for high-grade sarcomas (especially osteosarcoma of the proximal humerus) is type VB and is illustrated in this chapter.
- In summary, this proposed system considers the status of the structures removed (bone/abductor mechanism) and the type of resection performed (intracompartmental vs. extracompartmental), reflects the status of the glenohumeral joint (intra-articular vs. extra-articular), denotes the type of surgical margin achievable (marginal, wide, or radical), and indicates an increasing surgical magnitude of the resection.

Biopsy

- The biopsy site should be carefully selected. If possible, it should be through the deltoid muscle and away from the major vessels and nerves. The biopsy site should be placed so it can be widely excised by the definitive excision.

II. OPERATIVE TECHNIQUE

Position

- The patient is placed in an anterolateral position, which allows some mobility of the upper torso. The skin is prepared down to the level of the operating table, to the umbilicus, and cranially past the hairline (Fig. 88-1, *A*).

Incision

- The incision starts over the junction of the inner and middle thirds of the clavicle. It continues along the deltopectoral groove and down the arm over the medial border of the biceps muscle. The biopsy site is excised, leaving a 3-cm margin of normal skin. The posterior incision is not opened until the anterior dissection is complete (see Fig. 88-1, *A*).

Main Dissection

Exploration of the Axilla to Determine Resectability

- The skin is opened through the superficial fascia. Care is taken to preserve the deep fascia on muscles. Anteriorly, the skin flap is dissected off the pectoralis major muscle to expose its distal third, and the short head of the biceps muscle is uncovered. The pectoralis major muscle overlying the axilla is dissected free of axillary fat so that its insertion on the humerus can be visualized. This muscle is divided just proximal to its tendinous insertion on the humerus, and the portion of the muscle remaining with the patient is tagged with a suture (see Fig. 88-1, *B*). The axillary sheath is now identified and the coracoid process visualized. In order to expose the axillary sheath along its full extent, the pectoralis minor, short head of the biceps, and coracobrachialis muscles are divided at their insertion on the coracoid process. Again, all proximal muscles are tagged with a suture for their later identification and use in the reconstruction (see Fig. 88-1, *B*).
- Before exploration of the neurovascular bundle, the skin flaps are minimally developed. The patient's tumor may be found unsuitable for limb-salvage surgery, and more extensive flap dissection at this point would lead to tumor contamination of the anatomic site that would constitute flaps of a forequarter amputation.

Dissection of the Neurovascular Bundle

- Vessel loops are passed around the neurovascular bundle near the proximal and distal ends of the dissection. Medial traction on the neurovascular bundle allows visualization of the axillary nerve, posterior circumflex humeral artery, and anterior circumflex humeral artery. These three structures are ligated and then divided. If the neurovascular bundle is found to be free of any extension of the tumor, dissection for the limb-salvage procedure proceeds. The musculocutaneous nerve is isolated and carefully preserved. Although sacrifice of this nerve is occasionally required to preserve tumor-free margins of resection, its loss means lack of active elbow flexion after surgery.
- The deep fascia between the short and long heads of the biceps muscle is divided below the tumor mass to maximally separate the short and long heads of the biceps. This permits easy visualization of the musculocutaneous nerve. The radial nerve is identified at the lower border of the latissimus dorsi muscle, passing around and behind the humerus into the triceps muscle group. The profunda humerus artery that accompanies this nerve is ligated and divided. The radial nerve passes posterior to the humerus in its midportion (spiral groove). To dissect it free of the bone, a finger is passed around the humerus to bluntly move the nerve away from the bone. Similarly, the ulnar nerve is traced down the arm; the intermuscular septum is divided between biceps and triceps over the nerve to clearly visualize it (Fig. 88-2).

Division of Muscle Groups Anteriorly to Expose the Neck of the Scapula

- The short and long heads of the biceps are widely separated to expose the humerus (see Fig. 88-2). The site for the humeral osteotomy is determined, and the long head of the biceps and brachialis muscles are transected at this level. The inferior border of the latissimus dorsi muscle is identified, and a fascial incision is made that allows one to pass a finger behind the latissimus dorsi and teres major muscles several centimeters from their insertion into the humerus or scapula. The latissimus dorsi and teres major muscles are transected using electrosurgery. External rotation of the humerus exposes the subscapularis muscle, which is transected at the level of the coracoid process. Care must be taken not to enter the joint space. The portions of these muscles that are to remain with the patient are tagged for future reconstruction. By transecting these muscles, the anterior portion of the neck of the scapula has been exposed.

Posterior Incision and Lateral Skin Flap

- The surgeon now changes his or her orientation from the anterior to the posterior aspect of the patient. Rotation of the table away from the surgeon may allow for better visualization.

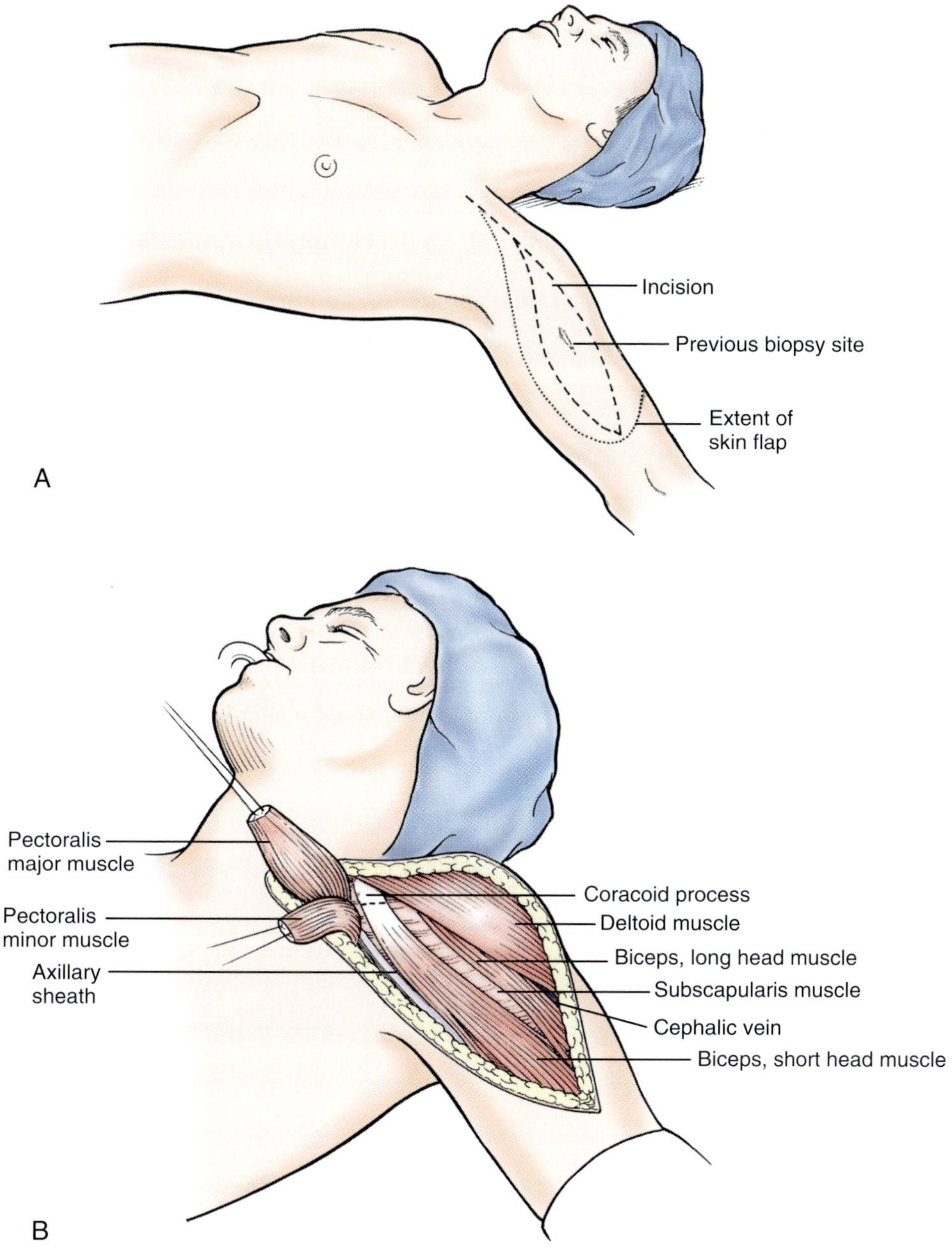

Figure 88-1.

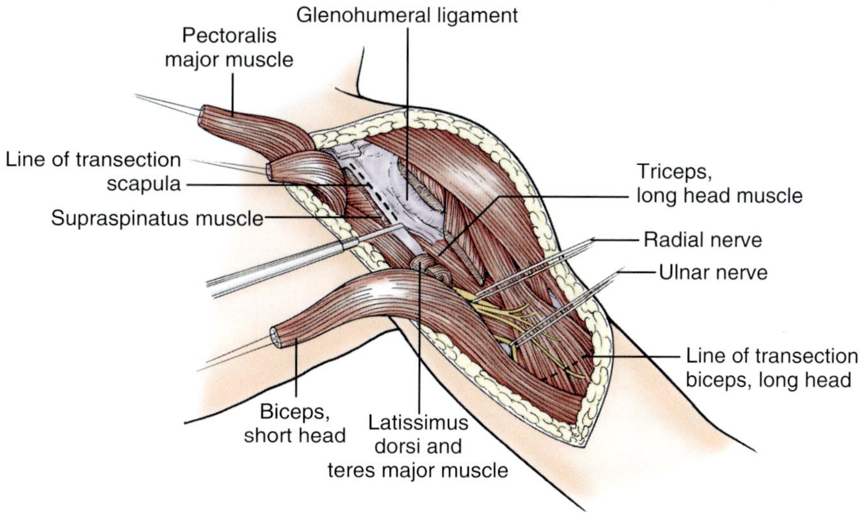

Figure 88-2.

- The posterior incision begins anteriorly over the junction of the middle and lateral thirds of the clavicle. It continues downward over the lateral third of the scapula until it passes the lower edge of this bone. A skin flap is developed by dissecting the skin and subcutaneous tissue between the anterior and posterior incisions from the underlying deltoid muscle downward to the level of the mid-humerus (Fig. 88-3). If the entire scapula is to be removed, this posterior incision is made longer to allow the skin flap to expose muscle over the entire scapula.

Division of Muscle Groups Posteriorly

- The thick fascia joining the posterior border of the deltoid muscle to the infraspinatus muscle and scapular spine is divided (see Fig. 88-3). The deltoid muscle is left intact as a covering over the tumor mass. The trapezius muscle is transected from its insertions on the scapular spine and acromion. The surgeon's index finger is passed beneath the teres minor upward to the area of the planned scapular osteotomy. The supraspinatus, infraspinatus, and teres minor muscles are transected over the neck of the scapula; this allows the plane of transection through the neck of the scapula to be exposed. All transected muscles are tagged proximally.
- While shielding the radial and ulnar nerves, the triceps muscles are transected at the level selected for the humeral osteotomy.

Clavicular, Scapular, and Humeral Osteotomies

- The clavicle is divided at the junction of its middle and inner thirds (Fig. 88-4). This is usually accomplished with a Gigli saw. The scapula is divided through its surgical neck medial to the coracoid process, also using a Gigli saw. Usually the clavicular and scapular osteotomy are performed before the humeral osteotomy.
- If the entire scapula is to be resected, the skin flap is taken back to the medial edge of the scapula. After this is accomplished, the rhomboid, levator scapuli, and trapezius muscles are divided from their insertions on the scapula. The teres major, teres minor, supraspinatus, infraspinatus, and subscapularis muscles need not be divided if a full scapula resection is to be performed.
- If the procedure is being performed for an osteosarcoma of the proximal humerus, the humerus is transected 6 cm distal to the tumor as determined by preoperative bone scan. Cryostat sections of tumor margins and touch preparations for cytologic examination of the marrow at the site of the osteotomy are obtained. The section of humerus removed is measured, and a prosthesis 4 to 6 cm shorter is selected. Some shortening of the extremity allows better soft tissue coverage.
- On removing the specimen, one should note that a generous amount of soft tissue still covers the tumor. The long and lateral heads of the triceps muscle remain on the humerus. The upper portion of the long head of the biceps and the upper portion of the brachialis muscle remain with the specimen. The entire deltoid muscle covers the tumor. The insertions of the supraspinatus, infraspinatus, pectoralis major, latissimus dorsi, teres major, teres minor, and subscapularis muscles remain covering the tumor and constitute the free margins.

Securing the Prosthesis

- If a prosthesis is to be used, 5 to 7 cm of distal humerus must be preserved. A power reamer is used to widen the medullary canal of the remaining humerus; it is reamed until it is 1 mm larger than the stem of the prosthesis. The length of the bony specimen is measured so that a prosthesis of appropriate length is used. Methyl methacrylate cement is injected into the medullary canal, and the prosthesis is positioned (Fig. 88-5). The head of the prosthesis should be oriented so that it lies anterior to the

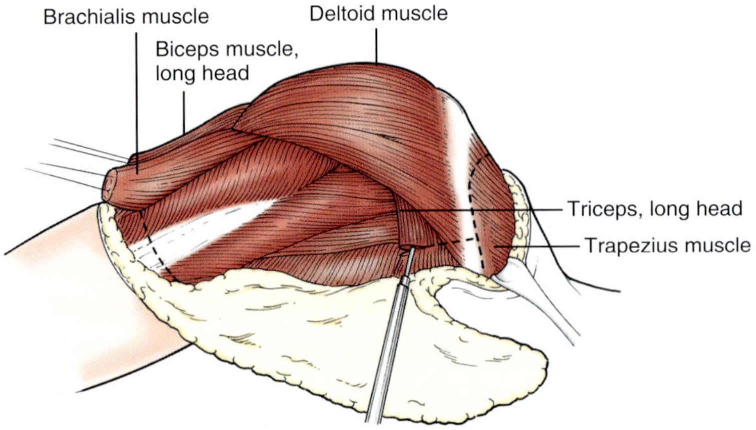

Figure 88-3.

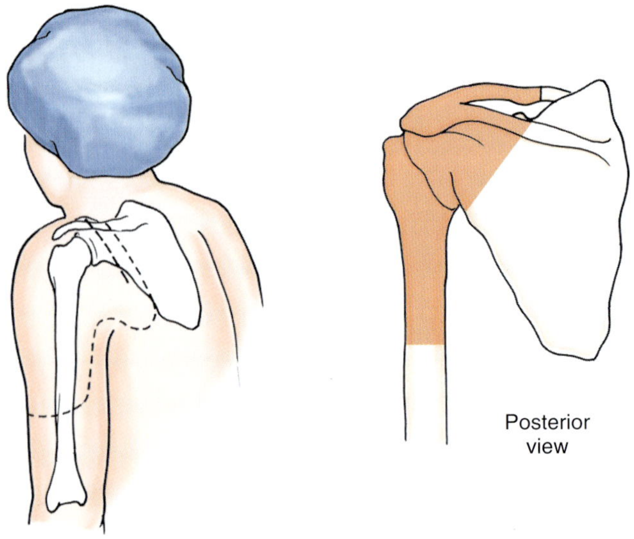

Figure 88-4.

transected portion of scapula while the arm is in neutral position. The radial nerve should be positioned anterior to the prosthesis so it does not become entrapped between muscle and prosthesis during the reconstruction. Drill holes are made through the scapula at the level of its spine. Drill holes also are made through the distal portion of the transected clavicle. The head of the prosthesis is secured by Dacron tape to the remaining portion of the scapula so that the prosthesis is suspended mediolaterally for horizontal stability. It is suspended in a craniocaudal direction by a second tape from the end of the clavicle for vertical stability. A 3-mm Dacron tape is used.

Reconstruction

- The pectoralis minor muscle is sutured to the subscapularis muscle over the neurovascular bundle to protect it from the prosthesis (Fig. 88-6). The pectoralis major muscle is closed over the prosthesis to

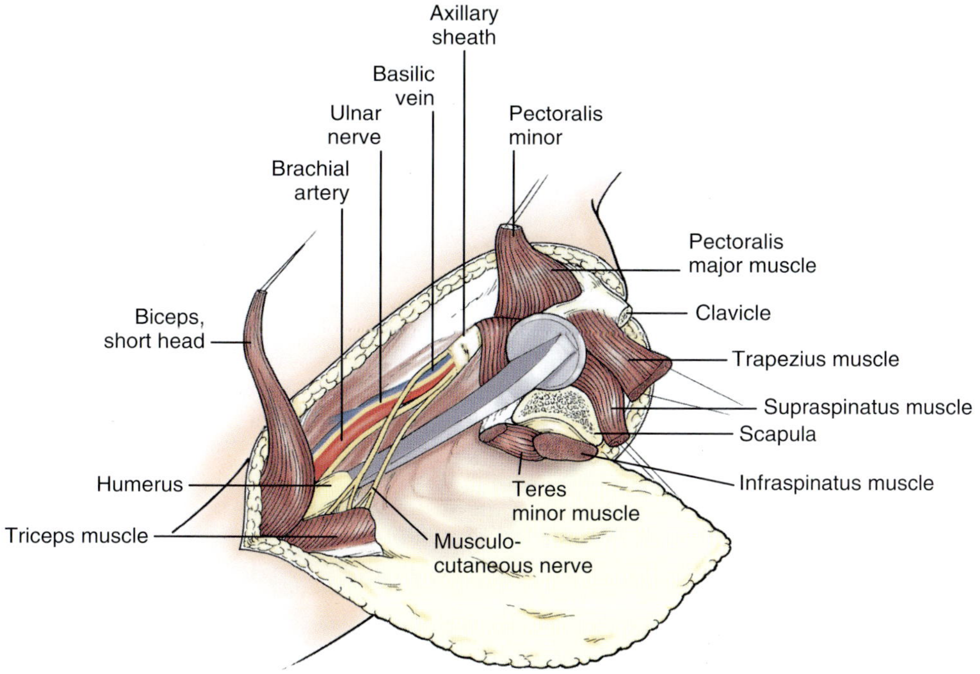

Figure 88-5.

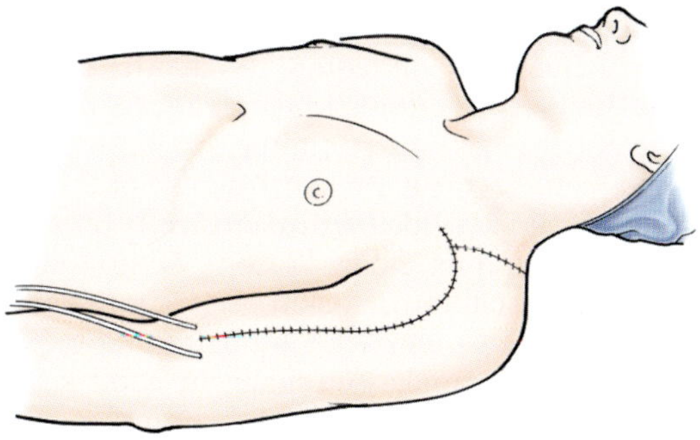

Figure 88-6.

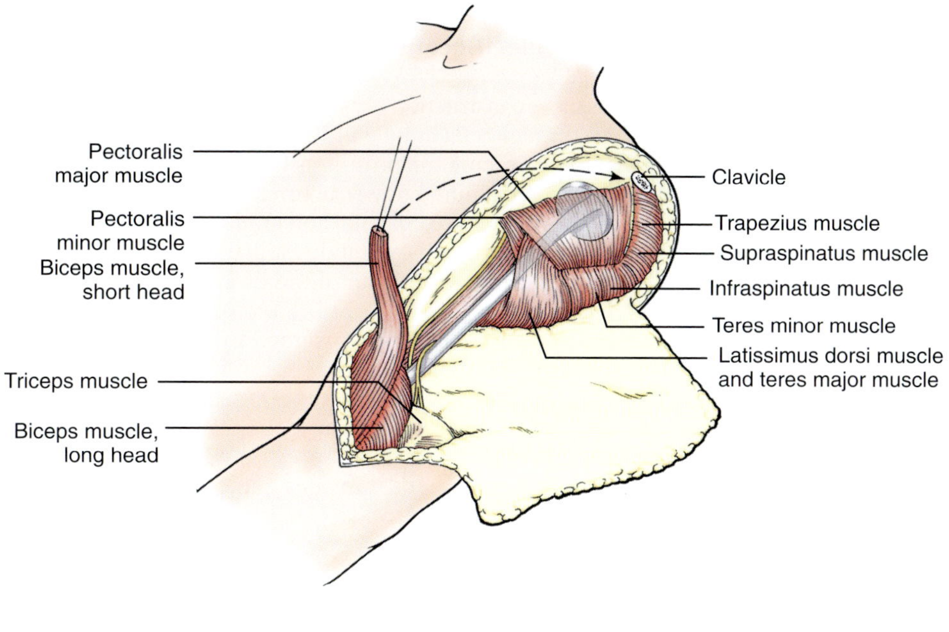

the cut edge of the scapula and secured by nonabsorbable sutures through drill holes. Next, the trapezius, supraspinatus, infraspinatus, and teres minor are secured to the superior and lateral borders of the transected pectoralis major. The teres major and latissimus dorsi muscles are secured to the inferior border of the pectoralis major muscle. The tendinous portion of the short head of the biceps is secured anteriorly under appropriate tension to the remaining clavicle. The long head of the biceps and the brachialis muscles are sutured to the short head of the biceps muscle under appropriate tension so that these two muscles can work through the short biceps tendon. The remaining triceps muscle is secured anteriorly along the lateral border of the biceps to cover the lower and lateral portion of the shaft of the prosthesis. Ideally, when the proximal and distal muscular reconstruction is complete, the prosthesis is covered in its entirety by muscle.

Closure

- Multiple suction catheter drainages are secured. The superficial fascia is closed with absorbable suture, and the skin is closed with clips (see Fig. 88-6). A sling and swathe are applied in the operating room.

III. ALTERNATIVE TECHNICAL APPROACHES (PRO/CON) AND PEARLS

Discussion

- High-grade sarcomas of the shoulder girdle have been treated traditionally by interscapulothoracic amputation. Nonablative extirpation has been rare. This chapter contains a complete description of the technique for a modified Tikhoff-Linberg procedure in patients who have sarcomas of the proximal humerus. Also, modifications of the procedure for tumors at other anatomic sites have been used. Proximal humeral lesions require resection of a greater length of humerus and adjacent soft tissues than described in the original Tikhoff-Linberg procedure.
- The technique of resection and reconstruction requires a thorough knowledge of the regional anatomy and technique of musculoskeletal reconstruction. Essential aspects of the treatment plan should be emphasized. The initial biopsy should be performed through the anterior portion of the deltoid muscle for a lesion of the proximal humerus. The deltopectoral interval should not be used, because performing a biopsy here would contaminate the deltopectoral fascia, the subscapularis, and pectoralis major muscles and would jeopardize the ability to perform an adequate resection through uninvolved tissue planes.
- For the definitive resection, the initial incision extends along the medial aspect of the biceps muscle, divides the pectoralis major, and exposes the neurovascular structures, thereby enabling the surgeon to determine resectability early in the dissection. This incision does not jeopardize construction of an anterior skin flap in patients who will require forequarter amputation.
- The length of bone resection is determined preoperatively from a bone scan and MRI. To avoid a positive margin at the site of humeral transection, the distal osteotomy is performed 6 cm distal to the area of abnormality on the scan. Segmental reconstruction of the resultant humeral defect is necessary if resection is performed distal to the deltoid tuberosity. A prosthesis is necessary to maintain length of the arm and to create a fulcrum for elbow flexion. We no longer use a Kuntscher nail because of the risk of proximal migration, instability, and skin perforation. Rather, a custom prosthesis is fixed distally with methyl methacrylate into the remaining humerus and proximally with Dacron tape to the clavicle and remaining portion of the scapula. Alternatively, good results have been reported with autograft (usually fibulas) or allograft used as spacers in obtaining an arthrodesis.

Principles of Shoulder Reconstruction

- Proximal soft tissue reconstruction is essential to cover the prosthesis and create shoulder stability. This is accomplished through a technique of "dual suspension" through static and dynamic reconstruction. Dacron tape is used to secure the prosthesis horizontally. Vertical suspension is by Dacron tape secured by drill holes in the remaining bony structures (clavicle and scapula or clavicle alone). These two sets of Dacron tapes provide for mediolateral and craniocaudad stability. This interposition prosthetic device provides a strut between the rib cage and residual humerus for static suspension. Dynamic suspension provided by transfer of the short head of the biceps muscle to the stump of the clavicle allows elbow flexion.
- Motor reconstruction and soft tissue coverage is as follows. The short head of the biceps brachii is secured to the end of the clavicle. Also, to assist in elbow flexion, the severed long head of the biceps brachii is sutured along the cut edge of its short head. Mobility at the shoulder is provided by preservation and transfer of the pectoralis major, trapezius, supraspinatus, infraspinatus, teres minor, teres major, and latissimus dorsi muscles. Use of these muscle groups offers dynamic support, assists in suspension of the prosthesis, and provides soft tissue coverage. Soft tissue coverage is essential in preventing skin problems and secondary infection.

- Preserving the musculocutaneous nerve is important. The short biceps muscle is responsible for elbow flexion postoperatively and is also used for soft tissue coverage of the prosthesis. It is the most important arm muscle remaining after resection. Flexion of the elbow is possible in patients with function of the biceps muscle. Muscle transfer also allows some flexion and extension motion at the shoulder. The pectoralis major muscle allows forward flexion of the shoulder. The trapezius and latissimus dorsi muscles cause posterior motion.
- Extra-articular, rather than intra-articular, resection of the glenohumeral joint by scapular osteotomy medial to the coracoid is recommended for proximal humeral lesions because it removes en bloc the potentially contaminated extension of the tumor. Scapular osteotomy not only removes the potential for tumor contamination of the operative field, but also permits medialization of the prosthesis and a decrease in bulk in the area to be covered.
- To minimize the incidence of transient nerve palsies, care should be taken not to place undue traction on nerves during resection. The radial nerve should pass in front of, rather than around, the prosthesis. The scapular osteotomy should be performed before the humeral osteotomy to minimize traction that may occur during manipulation of the extremity.
- On follow-up, none of our patients complained of shoulder instability or fatigue. This is attributed to our technique of prosthetic suspension and soft tissue reconstruction. In general, forward and backward shoulder flexion ranges from 30 to 45 degrees with good strength. Shoulder abduction was initially absent, but with scapulothoracic motion (because of the remaining scapula), about 30 degrees was eventually obtained. Elbow strength and motion depended on the status of the remaining biceps. This emphasizes the need for careful preservation, when possible, of musculocutaneous nerve and the short head of the biceps.
- The technique of resection and reconstruction as described in this chapter permits a curative, nonablative alternative to forequarter amputation. Despite the magnitude of resection, the surgical morbidity is minimal, and functional results are good. We recommend this procedure in carefully selected patients.

IV. SPECIAL POSTOPERATIVE CARE

- Patients undergoing shoulder girdle resection retain hand function and good elbow function, but lose shoulder function. From a rehabilitation perspective, shoulder girdle resection clearly offers an outcome superior to that for a forequarter amputation or shoulder disarticulation procedure. Further, shoulder girdle resection is less disfiguring and is associated with only minimal pain and edema. In our experience, patients' acceptance of the outcome of surgery has been good.
- The rehabilitation process begins with a patient orientation program, often showing pictures of patients who have undergone the procedure and demonstrating what one can do postoperatively and what limitations in function are likely to follow surgery. Preoperatively, a shoulder mold is fashioned, using the involved shoulder if its contours are not distorted. The cosmetic shoulder helps preserve the symmetry and appearance of the shoulder contour and can support a bra strap or heavy overcoat.
- On postoperative day 1, an arm sling is provided for support and to restrict abduction. The motion restriction should be maintained until the incision is healed; sutures are usually removed after about 2 weeks. Edema should be controlled with an elasticized glove or elastic stockinet. At the same time active, maximal head motion is begun to preserve strength and range and to help mobilize edema. Teaching the patient to be aware of proper head and neck positioning and cervical range of motion is initiated when the patient first becomes ambulatory.
- If the incision heals by first intention and after suction catheters have been removed, active and assistive elbow motion within the confines of the sling is started. At about 3 weeks, the sling is removed for passive shoulder range of motion (ROM) and pronation and supination of the wrist. The sling is used intermittently after the suture line is healed, primarily for upright activities in which arm support increases comfort. Once the arm is out of the sling, full ROM of the elbow (flexion, extension, pronation, and supination) should be performed. Passive ROM to the shoulder (flexion, abduction, external and internal rotation) and pendulum exercise should be done with the help of a family member or physical therapist.
- Normal daily activities are encouraged, but weights in excess of 20 lb should not be lifted with the arm that has undergone a Tikhoff-Linberg procedure. Pain and shoulder or arm discomforts have not been significant management problems, and control is achieved with minimal analgesia.

SUGGESTED READINGS

Malawer MM, Meller I, Dunham WK: A new surgical classification for shoulder-girdle resections: analysis of 38 cases, *Clin Orthop Rel Res* 267:33–44, 1991.

Malawer MM, Wittig J: Proximal humerus resection. The Tikhoff-Linberg procedure and its modifications. In Malawer MM, Sugarbaker PH, editors: *Musculoskeletal surgery. Treatment of sarcomas and allied diseases*, Dordrecht, The Netherlands, 2001, Kluwer Academic, pp 519–551.

Voggenreiter G, Assenmacher S, Schmit-Neuerburg KP: Tikhoff-Linberg procedure for bone and soft tissue tumors of the shoulder girdle, *Arch Surg* 134:252–257, 1999.

CHAPTER 89

Total and Subtotal Sacrectomy for En Bloc Resections of Primary Tumors of the Sacrum

Jean-Paul Wolinsky, MD, and Ziya L. Gokaslan, MD, FACS

I. SPECIAL PREOPERATIVE PREPARATION

- Primary and metastatic tumors of the sacrum are rare occurrences. Many different histologic tumor types may occur in the sacrum. Each tumor needs to be approached uniquely, and the goals of treatment need careful consideration. Treatments for sacral tumors can result in significant morbidity and should not be embarked on lightly.
- As with all tumors of the spine, the assessment should determine whether the treatment is palliative or curative, and a treatment regimen should be based on this. Most metastatic tumors to the sacrum should be treated with palliation as the goal (intralesional resection and/or adjuvant therapy). Primary tumors of the sacrum should be treated with hope of a potential cure (en bloc resection) if possible, and the functional consequences of the treatment required need to be evaluated.
- Treatment modalities for primary sacral tumors are limited. They include en bloc surgical resection and, to a lesser extent, radiation therapy (conventional, stereotactic, and proton beam irradiation) and chemotherapy. Metastatic tumors to the sacrum can most often be treated with radiation therapy and chemotherapy, as well as intralesional surgical resection if necessary.
- Clearly the pathologic evaluation of a tumor is paramount in the treatment strategy. If there is a known history of metastatic disease, the diagnosis is more easily made. If the sacral tumor is the first presentation of a tumor, then a more thorough evaluation is required. This would involve a workup for other sites of metastasis as well as the primary site (computed tomography of the chest, abdomen, and pelvis; bone scan; and positron emission tomography scanning). A biopsy should be performed of the most readily accessible lesion. Once a tissue diagnosis is made, subsequent treatment is dictated by the histology of the lesion in addition to the status of the systemic disease.
- Obtaining a tissue diagnosis is paramount in treating sacral tumors, because some primary lesions are treated predominantly by surgical excision, whereas others are amenable to treatment with radiation or chemotherapy. Sometimes a tumor appears to be one for which surgical resection is the only option, and yet after biopsy results, it becomes apparent that the tumor may be more suitable for treatment with radiation or chemotherapy. An excellent example of this similarity would be lymphomatous myeloma. In addition, care should be taken when planning a biopsy of a sacral tumor. A percutaneous transsacral biopsy is the preferable method to obtain tissue (Fig. 89-1). A ventrally located sacral tumor, although easily accessible via a transrectal or transvaginal biopsy, should be biopsied through a posterior transsacral route. A transrectal or transvaginal biopsy may seed the biopsy tract and, with certain tumors (chordoma), can result in spread to another body cavity, requiring a more extensive surgical procedure for tumor control. In addition to planning a transsacral approach, marking the skin where the percutaneous biopsy was performed is beneficial so the biopsy tract can be excised with the specimen during surgery.

- Functional considerations need to be understood when proceeding with surgery. Sacral tumors can be classified by location within the bony sacrum (area of sacrum involved) and according to what neural elements will be preserved if an en bloc resection is pursued. Unilateral preservation of an S3 nerve root, with bilateral S2 root preservation, is necessary for nearly normal bowel, bladder, and sexual function. Sacrifice of the S2 nerve roots and below will result in loss of voluntary control of the bowel and bladder and in sexual dysfunction. Loss of the L5 roots and below will result in inability to ambulate in addition to loss of bowel and bladder control and sexual function. Based on the level of neurologic preservation, a classification scheme for sacral resection has been developed: low sacral amputation (osteotomy through S2-S3, with preservation of S3 and above); midsacral amputation (osteotomy through S1-S2, with preservation of S2 and above); high-sacral amputation (osteotomy through S1, with preservation of S1 and above); total sacrectomy (will require an anterior and posterior approach, with an osteotomy through L5-S1, with sacrifice of S1 and below); and hemicorporectomy (sacrifice of at least L5 and below)—an operation beyond the scope of this chapter.

Prep

- The rectum is irrigated with saline and Betadine irrigation until the effluent is clear. This is performed in case of a rectal perforation during resection of the tumor.
- The lumbosacral region is prepped in the usual sterile fashion from the upper-lumbar region rostrally and below the rectum caudally. The lateral extent of the prep will go to the greater trochanter bilaterally.

II. OPERATIVE TECHNIQUE

- The following illustrations describe the technique for resection of primary tumors of the sacrum via an en bloc approach. The technique described highlights the steps of the operation but is an oversimplification. Successful outcome of such a large operation requires the cooperation of an experienced team—neurosurgery, plastic surgery, vascular surgery, general surgery, nurses, physical therapists, and rehabilitation physicians.
- A total sacrectomy will be performed in two stages—an anterior approach and a posterior approach. The anterior approach facilitates vascular control of the internal iliac arteries and veins, as well as the middle-sacral artery and vein. During the anterior approach, a myocutaneous rectus flap with the pedicle off of the inferior epigastric vessels can be harvested for use in closure of the second-stage posterior approach and tumor resection. Sacral tumors not requiring a total sacrectomy can be approached entirely posteriorly.
- All patients will receive a bowel prep before the operation.

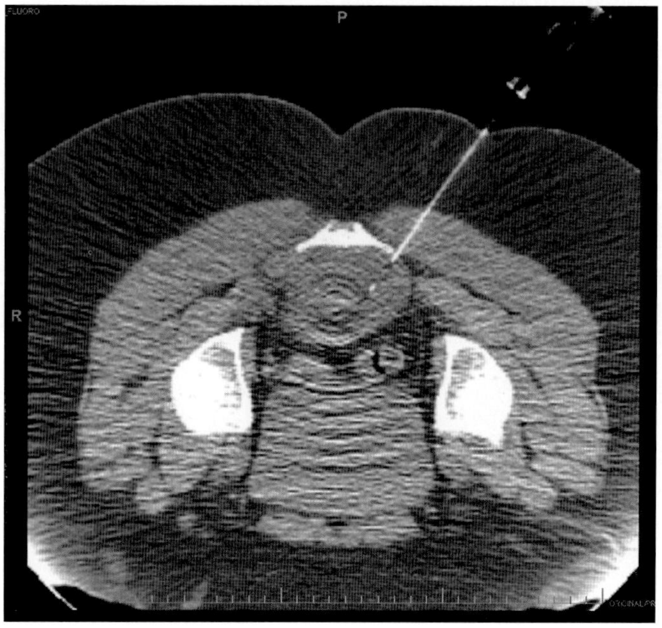

Figure 89-1.

ANTERIOR APPROACH (USED ONLY FOR TOTAL SACRECTOMY)

- The patient is positioned supine for a midline laparotomy on a standard operating table.
- A standard incision is made for a midline laparotomy, and care is taken to avoid the inferior epigastric vessels. The incision is also planned so that the plastic surgery team can harvest a myocutaneous rectus flap.
- The internal iliac arteries and veins are identified, ligated, and sectioned.
- The middle sacral artery and vein are identified, ligated, and sectioned.
- A complete L5-S1 diskectomy is performed (Fig. 89-2).
- The myocutaneous rectus flap is then harvested with the pedicles based on the inferior epigastric vessels (Fig. 89-3). The flap is placed deep into the pelvis so that it can be retrieved in the second stage and pulled through the posterior sacral defect for closure.

POSTERIOR APPROACH

Position

- The patient is positioned prone on the Andrews table.
- The head is fixed via a Mayfield head holder and, with the Mayfield sitting adapter, is suspended over the table (Fig. 89-4). This allows the head to be positioned with no pressure points on the face.

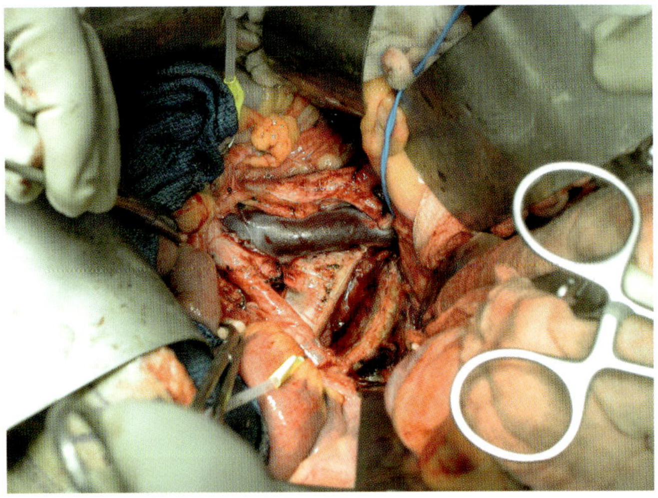

Figure 89-2.

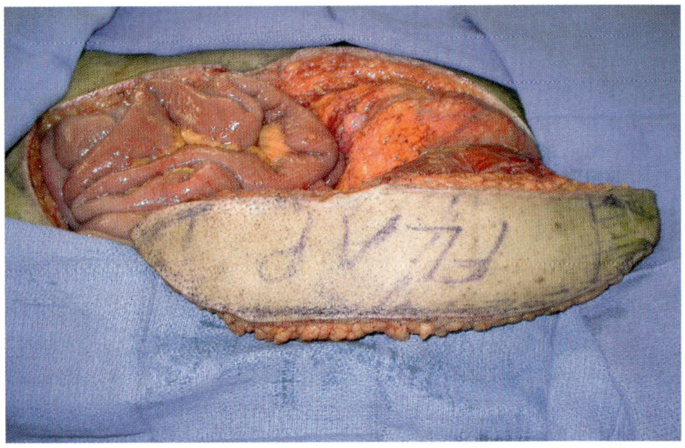

Figure 89-3.

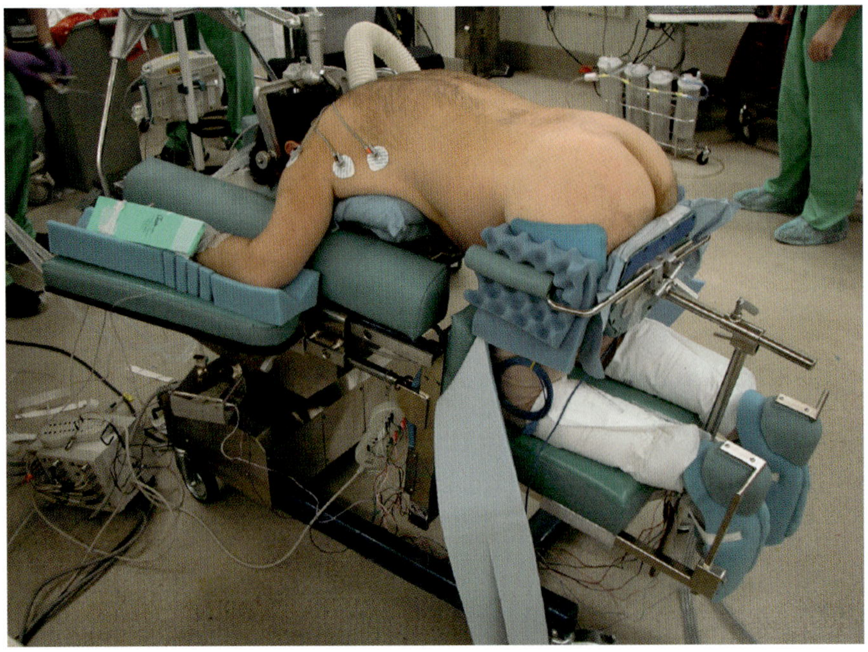

Figure 89-4.

Care must be taken not to change the position of the operative table during the operation. The table may be raised or lowered, but any tilting of the table or Trendelenburg maneuvers could result in a cervical injury if the patient were to move in the head frame.

Incision

- A midline incision is made. The initial biopsy tract is incorporated into the incision. The tract through the skin, as well as the underlying subcutaneous tissue and muscle along the tract, will be removed with the specimen. Therefore an elliptical skin incision is made around the biopsy tract (Fig. 89-5).

Main Dissection

- The incision is carried through the subcutaneous tissue and the lumbosacral fascia (Fig. 89-6). After the fascia is incised, it is elevated off the paraspinous muscles laterally. There is an avascular plane that can be followed to the iliac crest bilaterally. The fascia is elevated off of the iliac crest. A transverse incision is made in the fascia just rostral to the planned rostral extent of the tumor resection. This provides the rostral margin of the en bloc resection. The fascia is retracted laterally with a self-retaining retractor.
- Using a subperiosteal technique, the paraspinous muscles are elevated off of the spinous process, the lamina, the facets, and the transverse processes of the spine. If a total sacrectomy is planned, this exposure must encompass L3 through L5. If a subtotal sacrectomy is to be performed, then exposure of L5 is sufficient. The paraspinous muscles are then cut transversely at the same level at which the fascia was incised. Using a subperiosteal technique, the paraspinous muscles are mobilized laterally off of the ilium. The muscles can now be retracted rostrally.

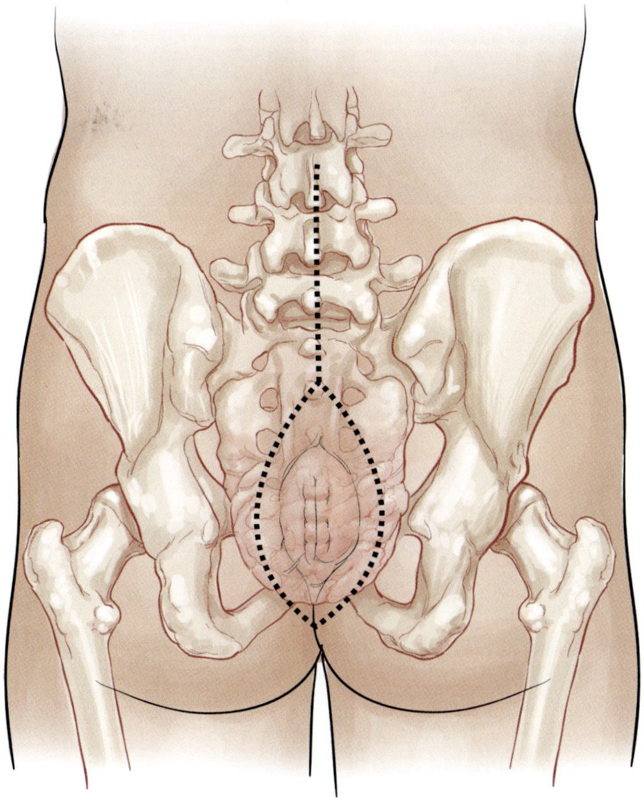

Figure 89-5.

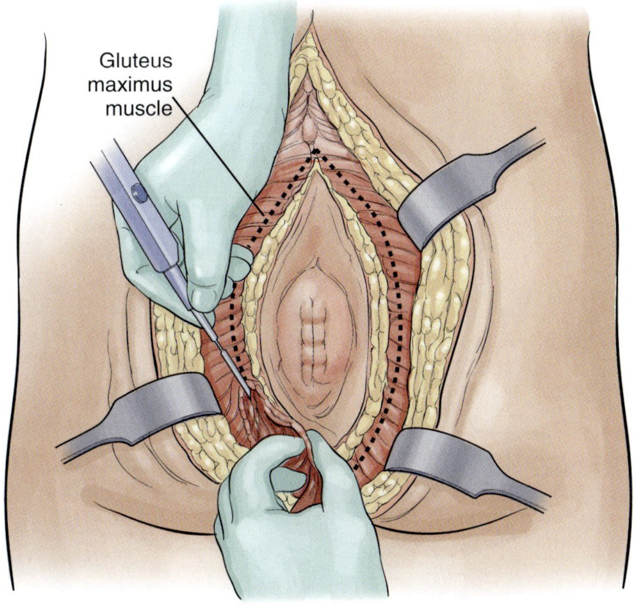

Figure 89-6.

- The gluteal muscles inserting on the lateral aspect of the ilium are elevated, allowing visualization of the sciatic notch. A self-retaining retractor is placed to maintain the exposure (Fig. 89-7, *A* and *B*).
- A laminectomy is performed at the level of the most caudal nerve root to be preserved (Fig. 89-8, *A* and *B*). After the laminectomy is complete, the nerve to be preserved is identified and followed laterally. The laminectomy is extended laterally to the dorsal foramen of the sacrum, and the dorsal root at that foramen is released. Care must be taken to release the dorsal root, because failure to do so can result in a traction injury to the motor root.
- Once the dorsal root has been released from the foramen, the lateral osteotomies are performed. The osteotomy follows a line created by the dorsal foramen proximally and the sciatic notch distally (Fig. 89-9, *A* and *B*). Using a high-speed diamond burr, an osteotomy is performed along this path. The bony cut is made until the ventral periosteum is encountered. The periosteum is cut using a Kerrison punch, after which the ventral root is visualized.
- On completion of the lateral osteotomy, attention is turned to the midline. Using size 0 silk suture, the nerve roots to be sacrificed are identified, ligated, and cut. The nerves to be preserved can then be carefully retracted rostrally. Using the high-speed diamond burr, the midline osteotomy is performed

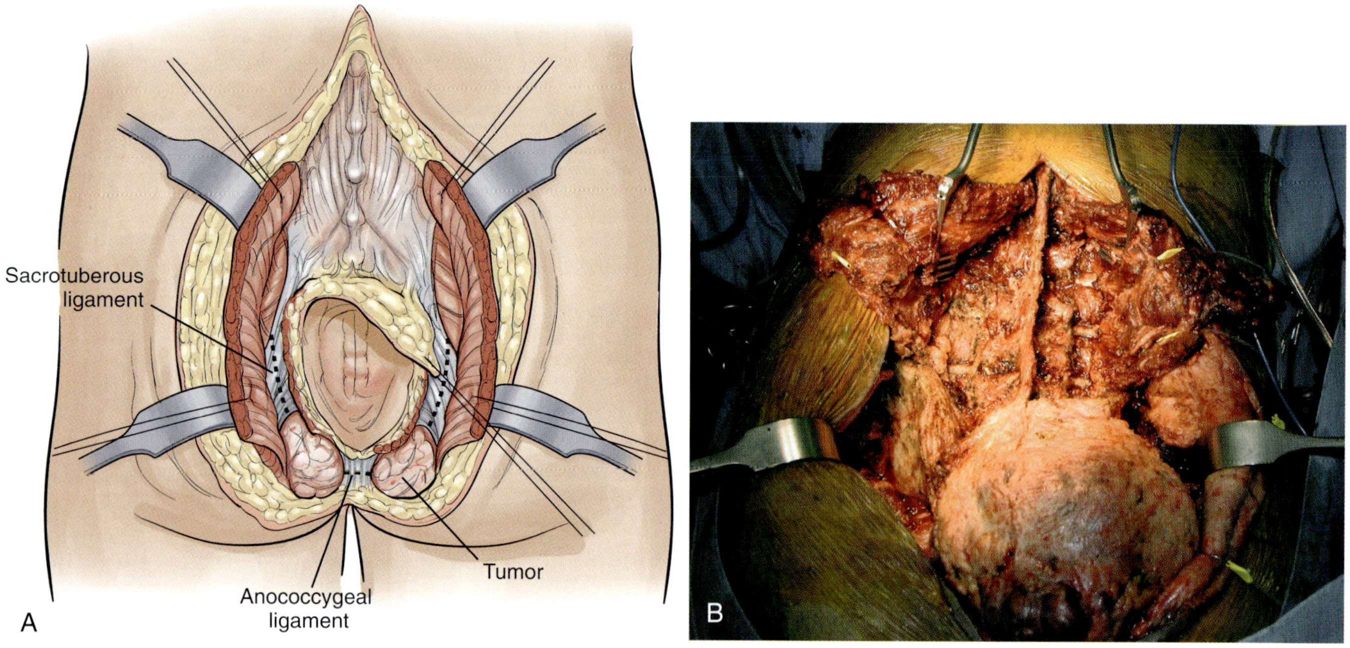

Figure 89-7.

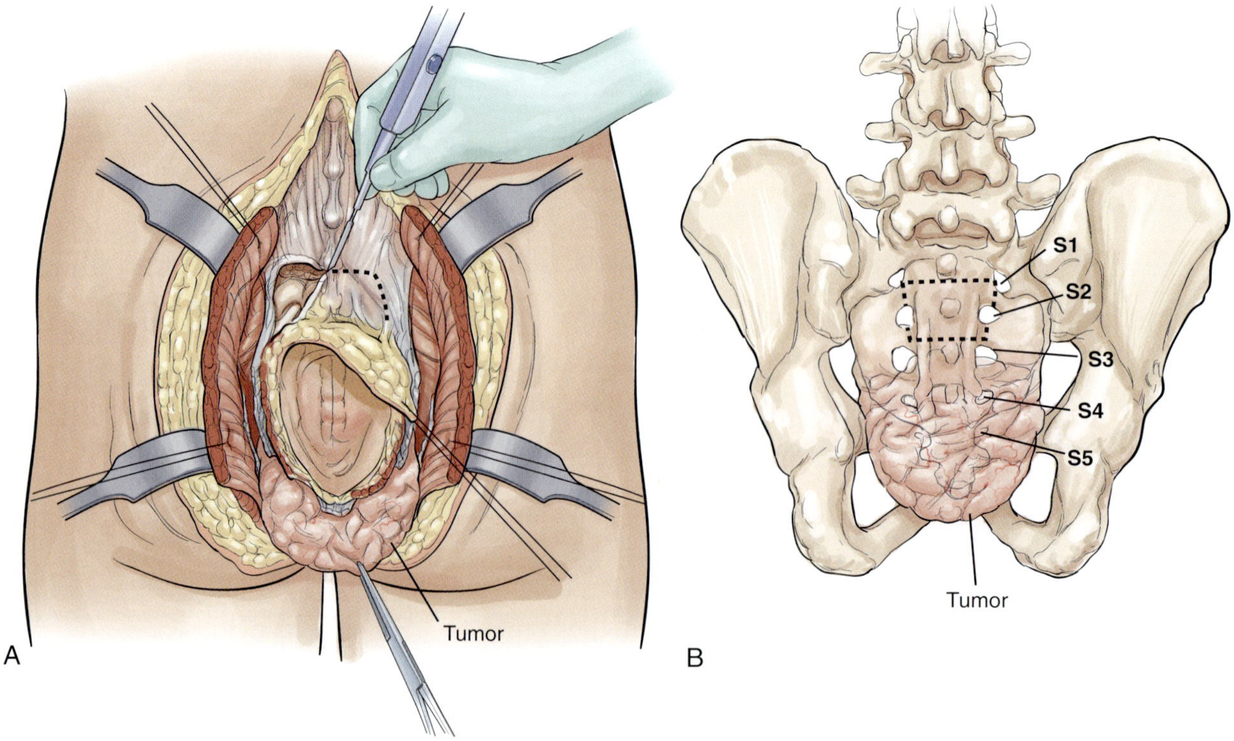

Figure 89-8.

(see Fig. 89-9), connecting the lateral osteotomies through the vertebral body (this will be the L5-S1 disk space for a total sacrectomy).

- The ligamentous and muscular attachments on the distal sacrum and coccyx must now be cut (see Fig. 89-7, *A*). The most distal nerve to be spared is identified as it joins the sciatic nerve at the sciatic notch. Care must be taken not to injure this nerve or the sciatic nerve. The muscular (gluteus muscles, piriformis muscles) and ligamentous structures (sacrotuberous ligament and sacrospinous ligament) are cut using the Bovie cautery. The sacrum is now mobile.
- The rostral aspect of the specimen is now secured with a penetrating towel clamp and gently rotated posteriorly, out of the pelvis. The mesorectum is carefully dissected off of the capsule of the tumor. Care must be taken to avoid injury to the rectum or violation of the tumor. As the tumor is delivered, the anococcygeal ligament is identified and cut. The specimen can now be delivered.

Lumbopelvic Reconstruction

- Subtotal sacrectomies do not result in lumbopelvic instability and usually do not require reconstruction. Total sacrectomies do result in significant instability, and in these instances lumbopelvic reconstruction is recommended (Fig. 89-10, *A* and *B*).

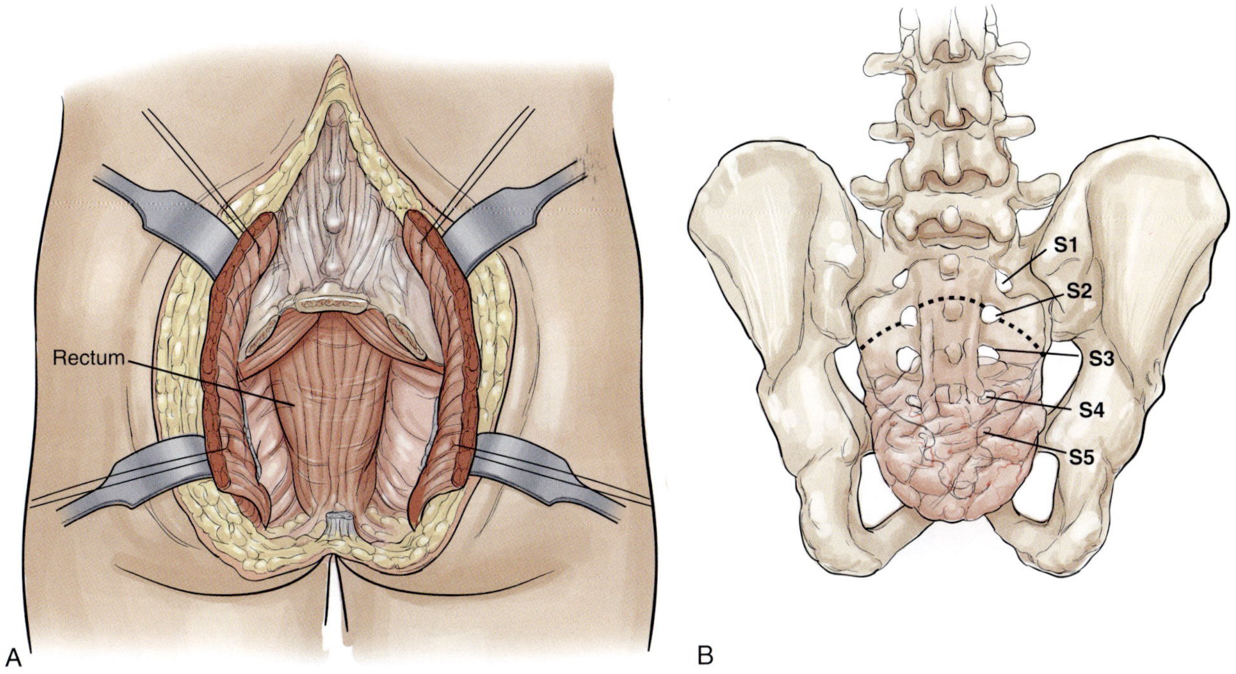

Figure 89-9.

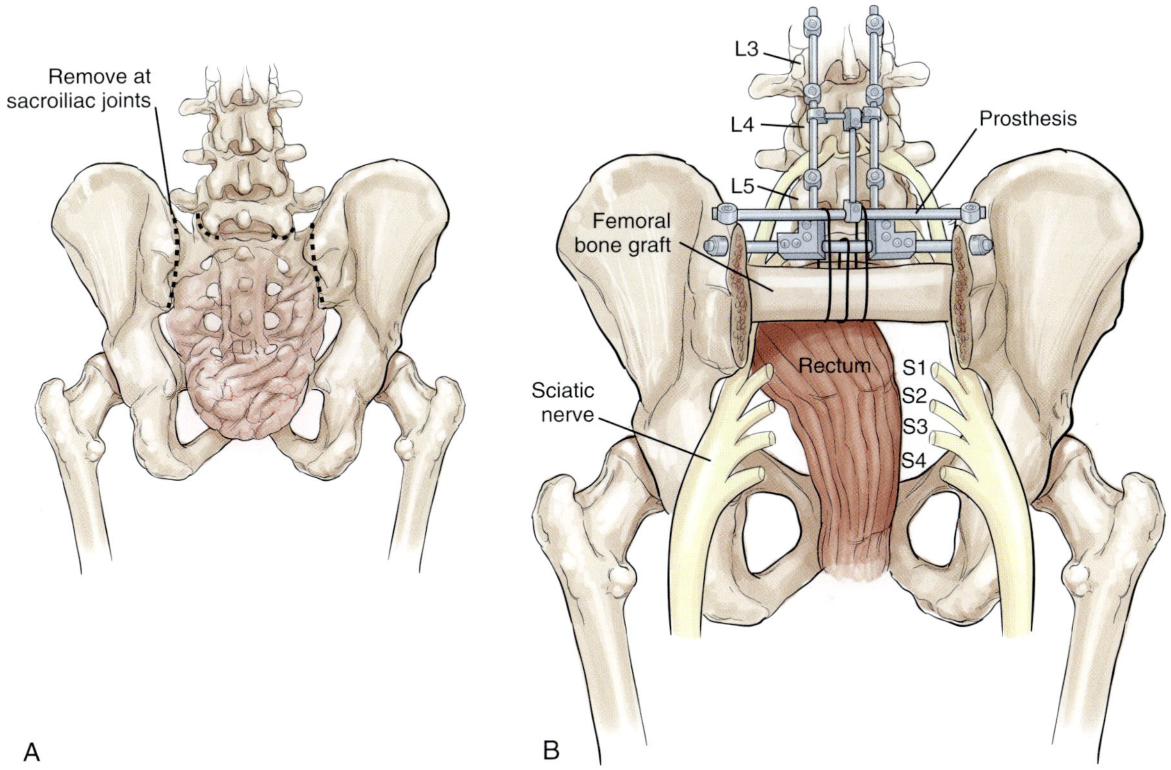

Figure 89-10.

- For reconstruction, pedicle screws are placed at L3, L4, and L5 bilaterally. Bilateral iliac screws are placed. A transiliac rod is placed. The iliac screws are linked via a contoured rod to the pedicle screws on either side. The transiliac rod is cross-linked to this construct to provide further load sharing. A femoral-shaft allograft is contoured so that it will span the remaining ilium. This allograft is secured in place via titanium cables around the allograft and transiliac rod (see Fig. 89-10). The area is decorticated, and graft is packed from the ilium to L3 along the transverse processes and facet joints to produce the arthrodesis. Postoperatively, the patient has no weight-bearing restrictions and can ambulate.

Closure

- If an anterior approach was performed, the myocutaneous rectus flap can now be identified through the sacral defect. The flap is delivered (Fig. 89-11). If adequate viable muscles remain, these are approximated, and then the skin is approximated (Fig. 89-12).
- Using a piece of Alloderm, a barrier is sewn into position to keep the rectum and pelvic contents ventral to the sacral defect. This will decrease the chance of a hernia of the rectum through the sacral

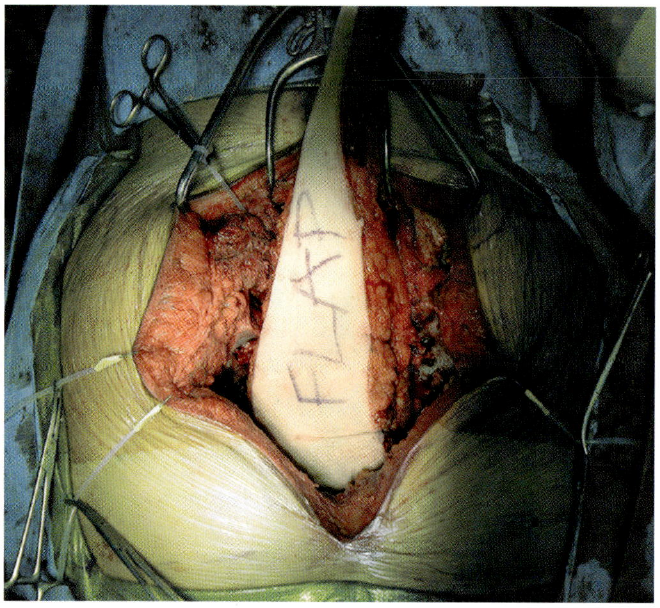

Figure 89-11.

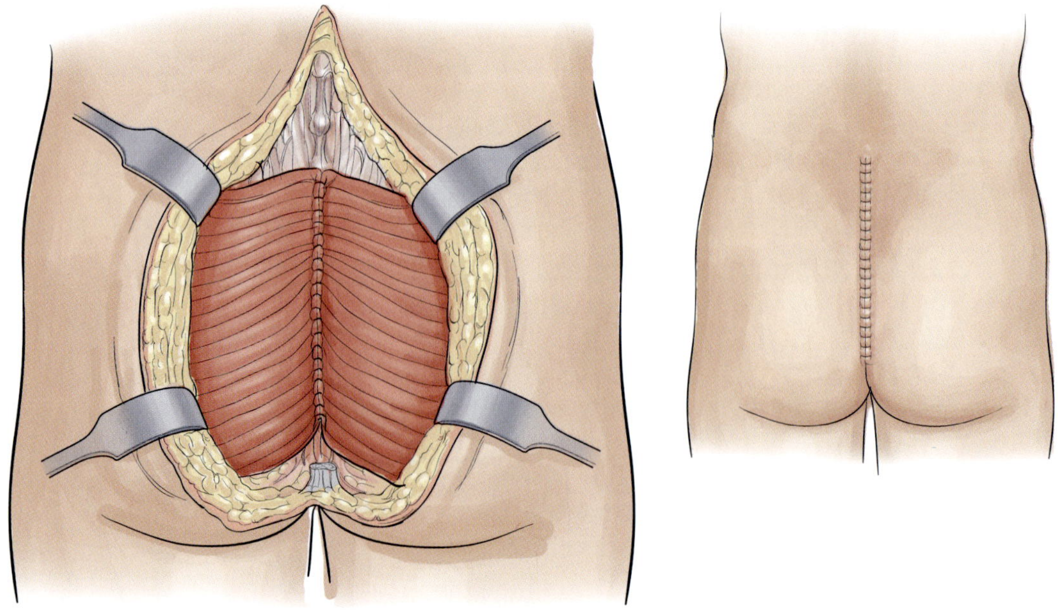
Figure 89-12.

defect and will keep the rectum ventral if postoperative radiation therapy is required. The Alloderm is sewn into the bony pelvis along the osteotomies.
- If a myocutaneous rectus flap is available, then this is used to fill the soft tissue defect. If no flap is available, then the closure is made in the usual multilayered fashion.

III. ALTERNATIVE TECHNICAL APPROACHES (PRO/CON) AND PEARLS

- The osteotomies can be performed with an osteotome, sagittal saw, Gigli saw, or high-speed drill. We prefer the high-speed diamond burr because it provides the highest degree of control and allows for hemostasis of the bony edges as the osteotomy progresses.
- If a myocutaneous rectus flap is not available (previous surgery), then an omental flap can be a good alternative.
- Subtotal sacrectomies can be performed through an entirely posterior approach. If vascular control or wound healing is a concern, then a staged combined anterior and posterior approach can be applied.
- If bowel, bladder, and sexual function are to be preserved in a subtotal sacrectomy, great care must be used to identify and preserve the pudendal nerves as they emerge from the nerve roots proximal to the sciatic nerve.

IV. SPECIAL POSTOPERATIVE CARE

- Postoperative bladder and bowel dysfunction must be appropriately managed. Patients should undergo straight catheterization to decrease the chance of urinary tract infections. Bowel incontinence can usually be controlled with a constipating diet and a bowel evacuation regimen.
- Wound infections are the major complication of sacrectomies. Careful attention to the wound post-operatively is paramount. Pressure on the wound should be avoided. To allow the wound to heal, 3 to 4 days of bed rest is recommended before mobilization.

SUGGESTED READINGS

Fourney DR, Gokaslan ZL: Current management of sacral chordoma, *Neurosurg Focus* 15:E9, 2003.

Fourney DR, Rhines LD, Hentschel SJ, et al: En bloc resection of primary sacral tumors: classification of surgical approaches and outcome, *J Neurosurg (Spine 3)* 2:111–122, 2005.

Miles WK, Chang DW, Kroll SS, et al: Reconstruction of large sacral defects following total sacrectomy, *Plast Reconstr Surg* 105:2387–2394, 2000.

CHAPTER 90

Abdominoinguinal Incision for Resection of Pelvic Tumors

Tristan D. Yan, BSc(Med), MBBS, MS, MD, PhD,
and Paul H. Sugarbaker, MD, FACS, FRCS

- Pelvic tumors with lateral fixation present difficulties in their resection, primarily because of inadequate exposure through conventional abdominal incisions. The difficulty arises with tumors in the lower part of the pelvis where the anterior abdominal wall converges with the retroperitoneal structures. In this area, the inguinal ligament spanning between the anterior superior iliac spine and the pubic tubercle provides an obstacle to unhindered exposure. A midline, paramedian, or oblique abdominal incision usually does not provide adequate exposure for safe resection of these tumors. Traditional incisions provide enough exposure for the dissection and control of the common iliac vessels proximally, below the bifurcation of the aorta, but do not afford exposure of the terminal portion of the external iliac vessels because the tumor mass hinders further visibility. Often these tumors are considered unresectable.
- Karakousis has described a solution for these problems with exposure. What is needed for the resection of these tumors is an incision that simultaneously provides an in-continuity exposure of the abdominal cavity and one or both groins so iliac and femoral vessels are exposed in one field. For this incision, both an abdominal component and an in-continuity inguinal component are needed—that is, an abdominoinguinal incision. The inguinal ligament may have to be divided to allow uninterrupted exposure and control of the iliofemoral vessels. A transverse incision connecting with the midline incision, by dividing the origin of the rectus abdominis from the pubic crest and the insertion of the inguinal ligament to the pubic tubercle, provides the necessary link that allows a single in-continuity field and optimizes exposure.
- In practice there are variations of this incision, depending on the location, size, and complexity of the pelvic sidewall tumor. The abdominoinguinal incision may function much in the same way that the thoracoabdominal incision is used for the upper quadrant of the abdomen.

I. SPECIAL PREOPERATIVE PREPARATION

- The indications for the abdominoinguinal incision are: (1) abdominal or pelvic tumors extending over the iliac vessels, (2) tumors in the iliac fossa (Fig. 90-1), (3) primary tumors possibly involving the iliac vessels or large iliac lymph node metastases, (4) tumors with fixation to the wall of the true pelvis or large obturator nodes, (5) tumors involving the pubic bone with or without extension to the pelvis or adductor group of muscles, and (6) tumors of the groin when involving the vessels or the lower abdominal wall or extending into the retroperitoneal area.
- A computed tomography scan of the abdomen and pelvis provides an assessment of the extent of the pelvic tumor (see Fig. 90-1), its relationship with the iliac vessels and femoral nerve, and whether there is invasion of the iliac bone.

II. OPERATIVE TECHNIQUE

Position

- The patient should be placed in the supine position.

Incision

Abdominal Incision

- A midline abdominal incision is made from above the umbilicus to the pubic symphysis (Fig. 90-2). The peritoneal cavity is entered and explored to assess the extent of disease. Preliminary dissection between the tumor mass and common iliac vessels may be performed. Involvement of the common iliac vessels does not necessarily mean they cannot be resected, because they can be removed en bloc with the tumor. When there is a question of involvement of the iliac vessels distally, the common iliac vessels are dissected free, and vessel loops are passed around them.

Inguinal Incision

- If the decision is made to proceed with the resection, the lower end of the midline abdominal incision is extended transversely either along the inguinal ligament (Fig. 90-3) or to the midinguinal point and then vertically, over the course of the femoral vessels, for a few centimeters.

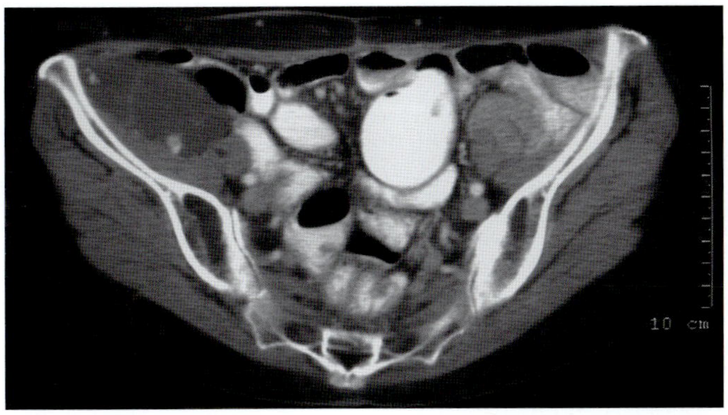

Figure 90-1. A tumor mass is situated in the right iliac fossa invading the iliacus muscle and immediately adjacent to the femoral nerve and external iliac vessels.

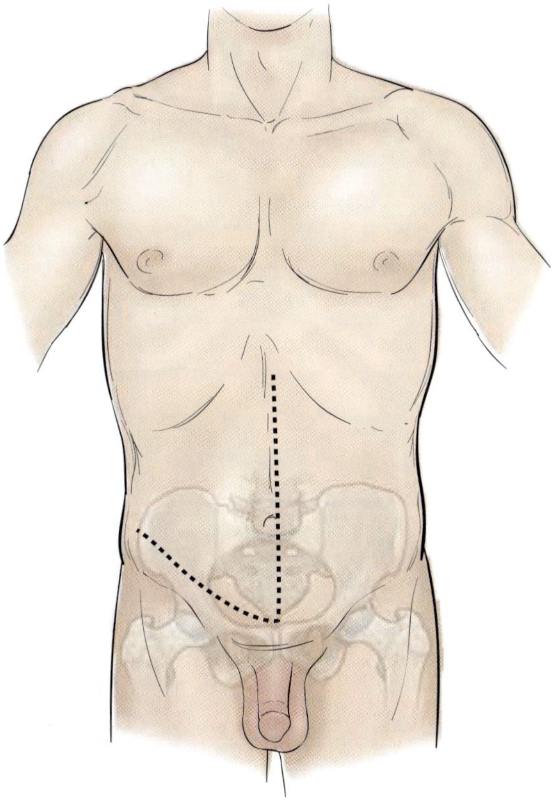

Figure 90-2. A midline abdominal incision is made from above the umbilicus to the pubic symphysis.

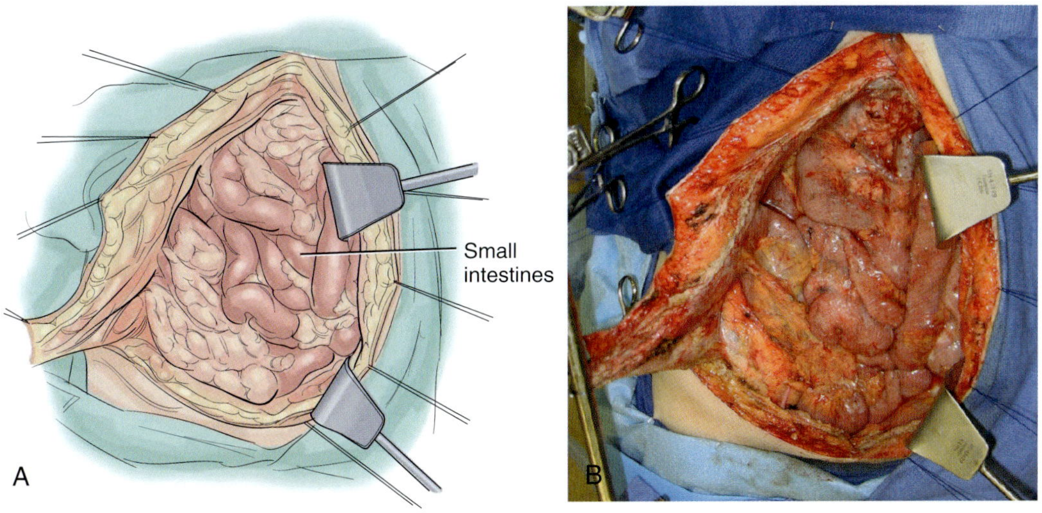

Figure 90-3. An inguinal incision is made by extending the lower end of the midline abdominal incision transversely along the inguinal ligament. The transverse portion of the incision is deepened to the surface of the anterior rectus sheath, which is divided. The rectus abdominis muscle is transected a few millimeters from its origin on the pubic crest. The dissection is viewed from the left side of the patient.

- The transverse portion of the incision is deepened to the surface of the anterior rectus sheath, which is divided, and the rectus abdominis muscle is transected a few millimeters from its origin on the pubic crest. This incision is through its tendinous portion. At the same time, the inferior deep epigastric arteries and veins are ligated and divided (Fig. 90-4).

Main Dissection

- The selection of the incision either parallel to or across the inguinal ligament is dependent on the location of the tumor. In many situations in which the tumor is large and distal and pressing against the obturator foramen (foramina) or the obturator areas, one can obtain sufficient exposure with a unilateral or bilateral use of the transverse portion of the full incision. In other words, the lower end of the midline incision is extended transversely from the pubic symphysis to the pubic tubercle, and the ipsilateral-rectus sheath and muscle are divided off the pubic crest.
- If the tumor is simply a pelvic mass extending over and obscuring the iliac vessels, the improved exposure allows the dissection of the mass off the vessels and safe ligation of any tumor-feeding branches (Fig. 90-5). For a tumor located in the iliac fossa, the incision is extended parallel to the inguinal ligament.
- The femoral nerve is located lateral to the femoral artery, immediately posterior to the continuation of the iliac fossa. Further cautious dissection along this nerve determines its relation to the tumor and whether it can be saved (Fig. 90-6). With lateral retraction and elevation of the musculocutaneous

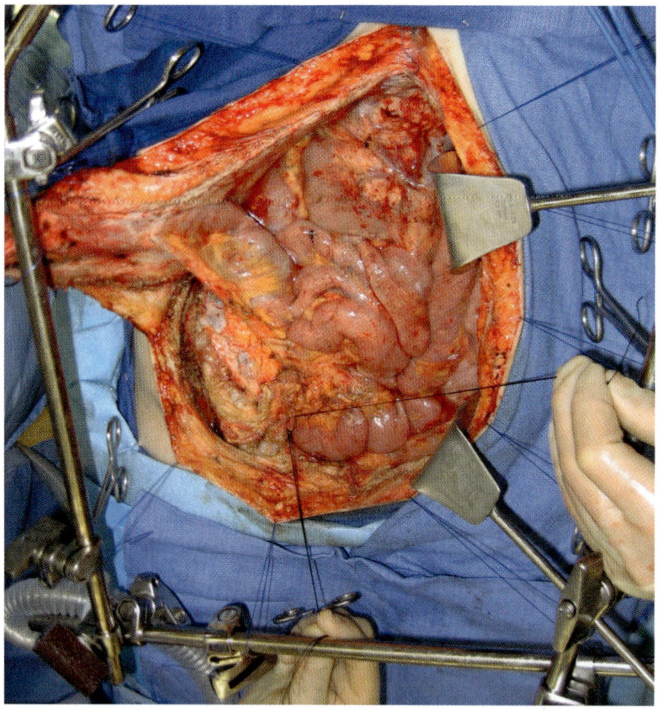

Figure 90-4. The inferior deep epigastric artery and vein are ligated in continuity, then divided.

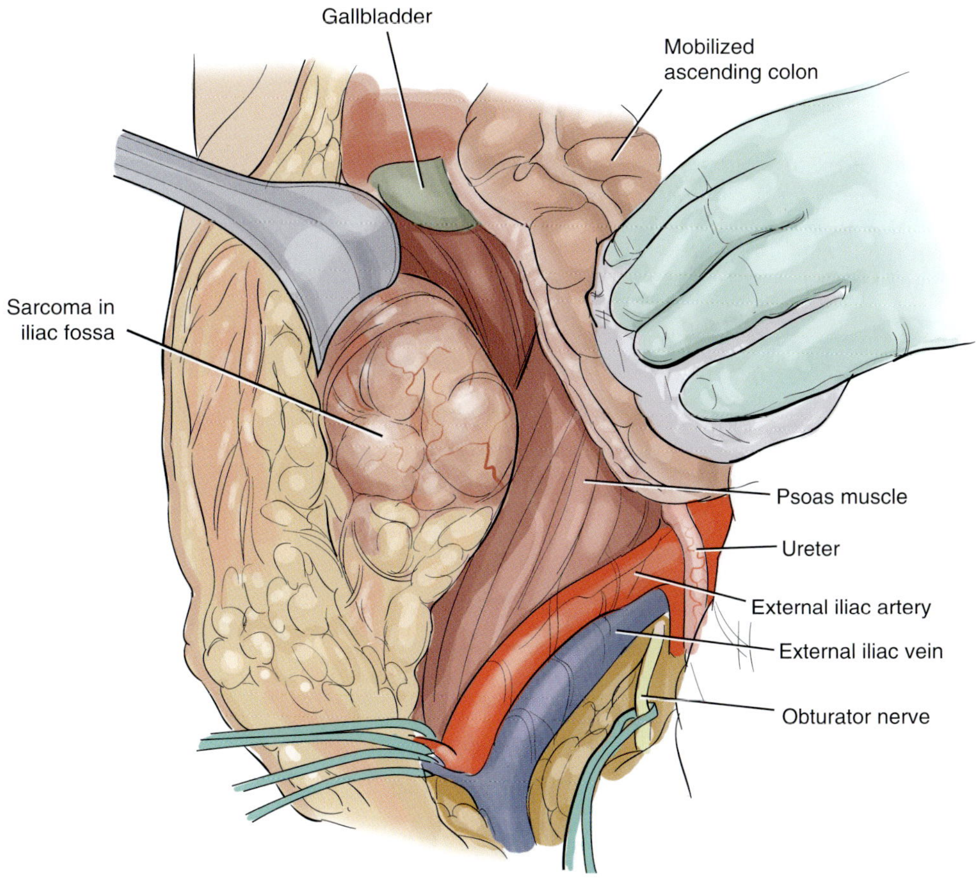

Figure 90-5.

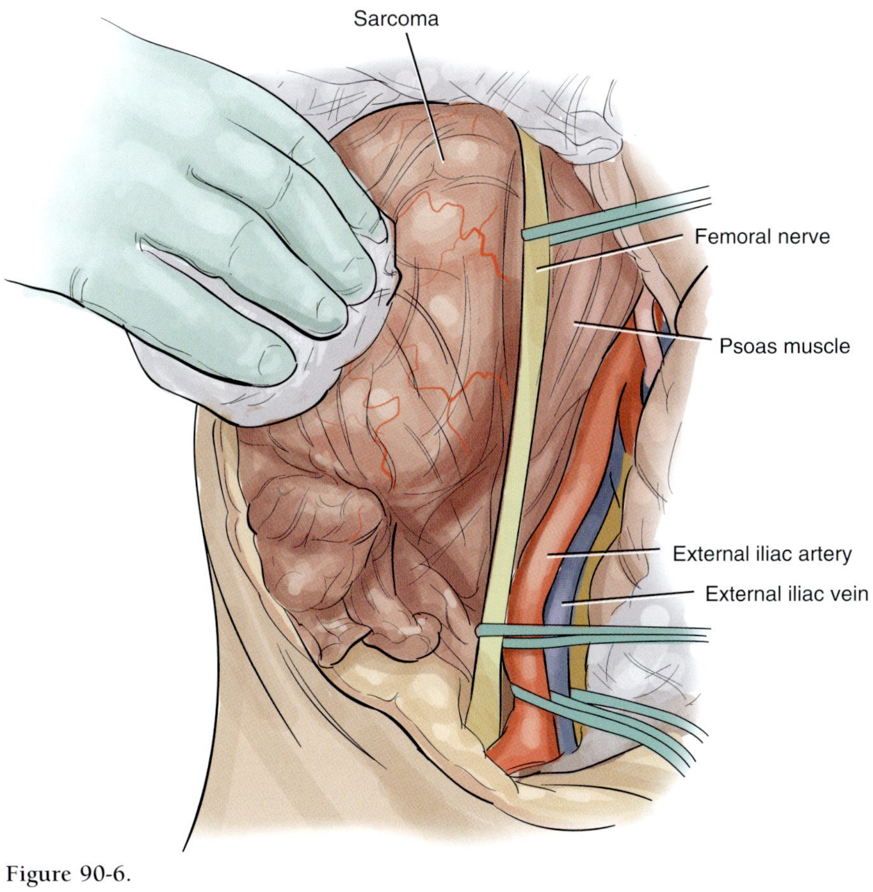

Figure 90-6.

flap, dissection of the tumor off the anterior abdominal wall is made possible. The tumor is removed en bloc with adequate surgical margin (Fig. 90-7, *A* and *B*, and Fig. 90-8).

Closure

- The closure of the abdominoinguinal incision involves approximation of the rectus sheath and muscle to their remnants on the pubic crest using nonabsorbable suture. Lateral to the vessels, the inguinal ligament is approximated to the iliac fascia and medial to the vessels to the Cooper ligament. When a defect in the fascia has been created, it may be covered with an allogeneic mesh, which also replaces the inguinal ligament (Fig. 90-9). The midline abdominal incision is closed in continuity with the

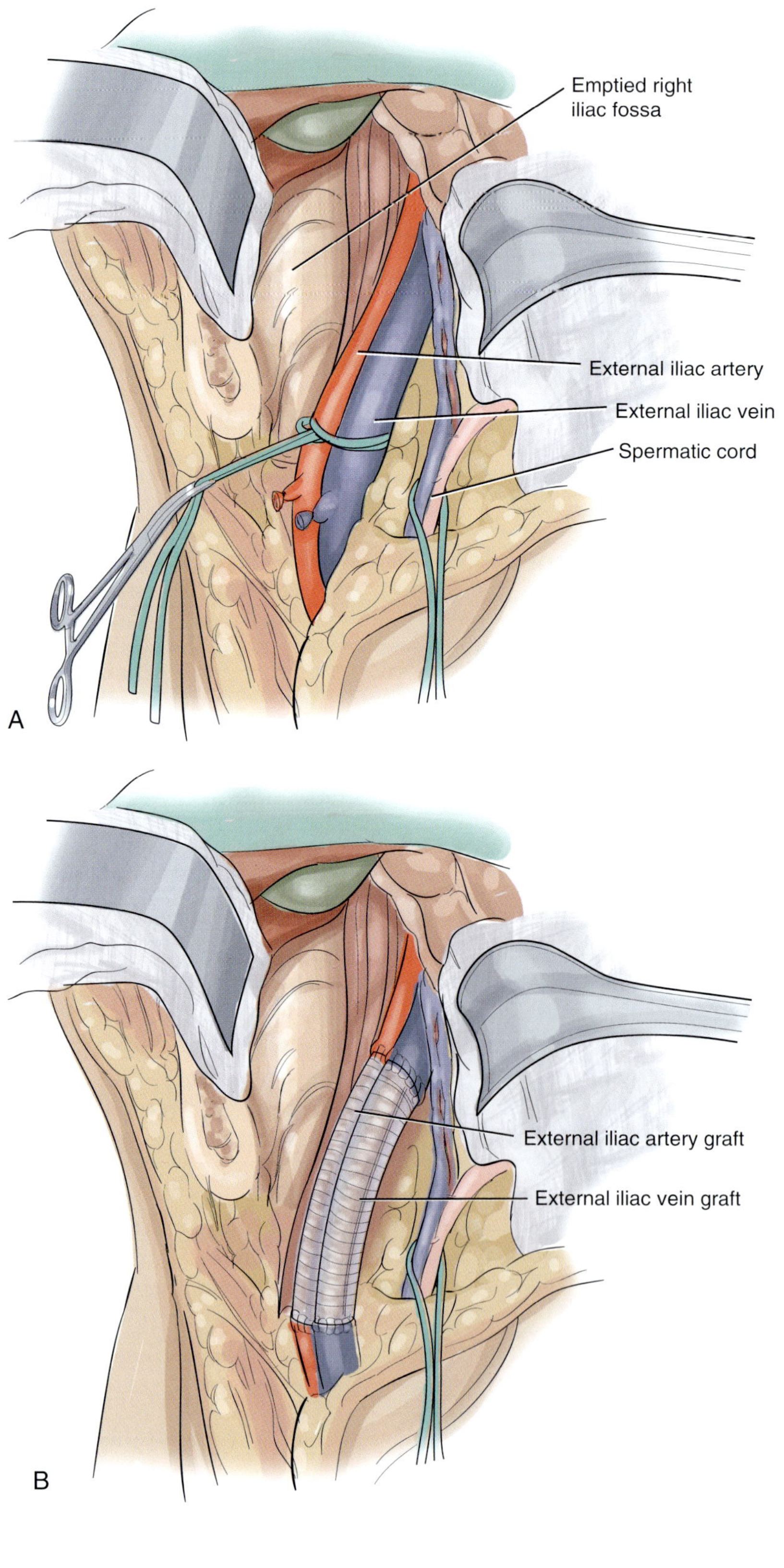

Figure 90-7.

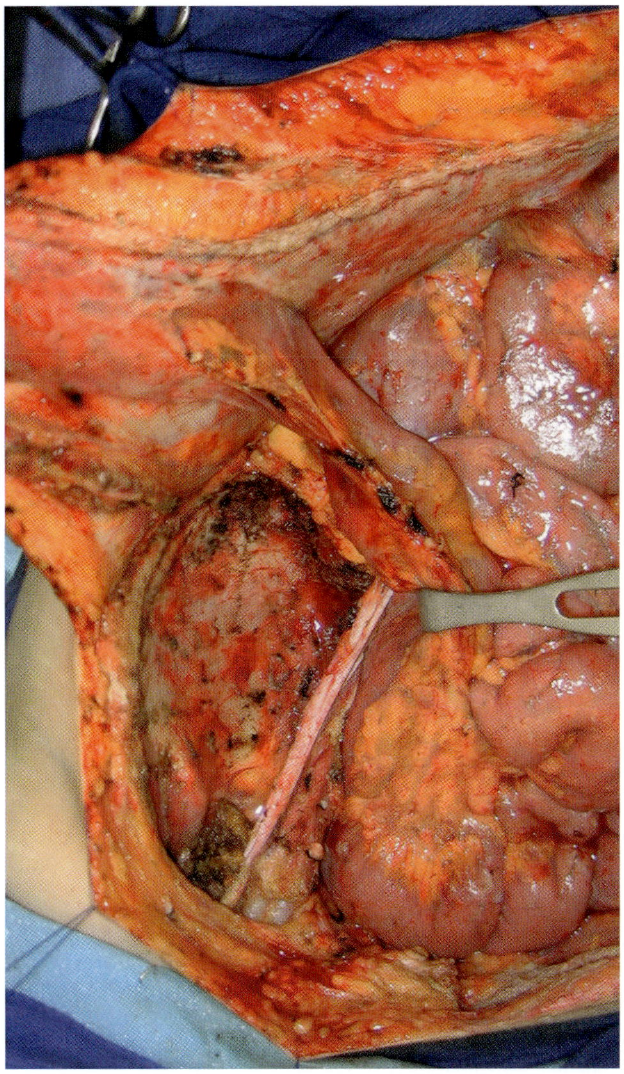

Figure 90-8. Dissection of the tumor away from the anterior abdominal wall, wing of the ilium, femoral nerve, and common and iliac artery allows en bloc resection with a minimal surgical margin.

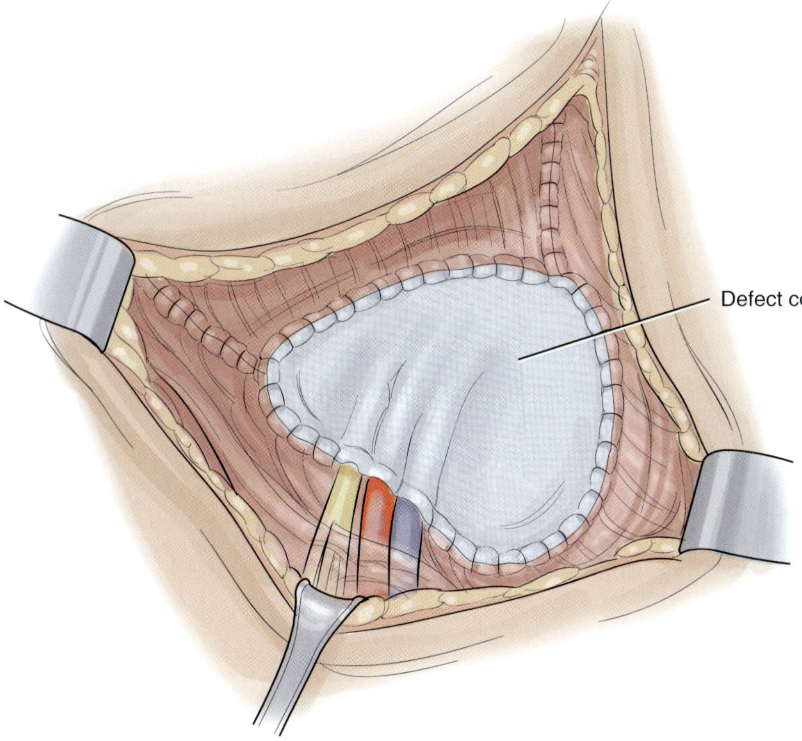

Figure 90-9.

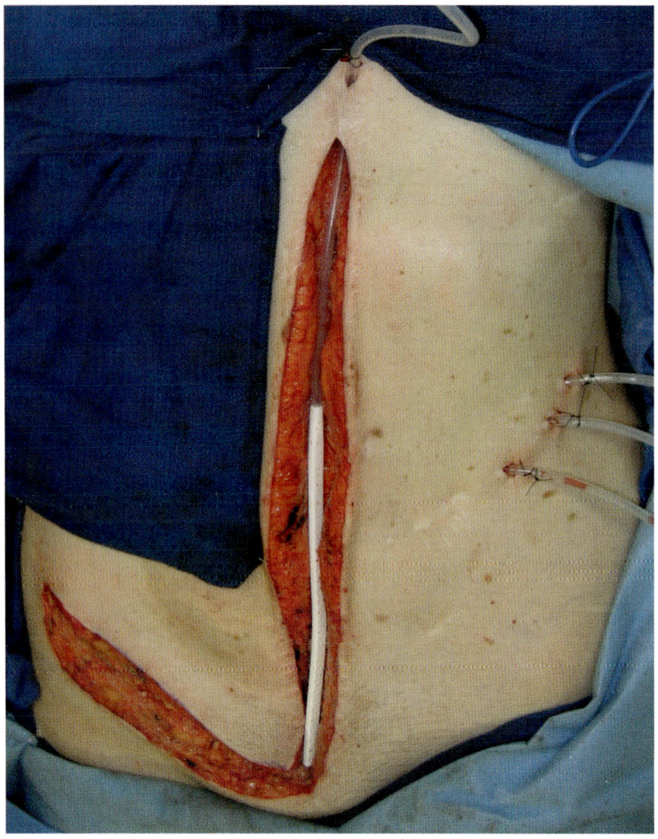

Figure 90-10. The midline abdominal incision is closed in continuity with the inguinal incision. Suction drains are placed beneath the abdominal wall and in the subcutaneous layer.

inguinal incision. A suction drain is placed in the subcutaneous layer (Fig. 90-10). The skin is closed in a routine fashion.

III. ALTERNATIVE TECHNICAL APPROACHES (PRO/CON) AND PEARLS

- The abdominoinguinal incision has been used in patients with a variety of tumors, usually soft tissue sarcomas. These tumors often present with fixation to the soft tissues of the wall of the pelvis and can be resected with the abdominoinguinal incision. Some patients may require abdominobiinguinal incision, that is, bilateral extension of the midline incision to the groins. Tumors involving the innominate bone, with the exception of the medial portion of the pubic bone, are best resected with the use of techniques of internal hemipelvectomy and, if necessary, hemipelvectomy.
- The abdominoinguinal incision renders resectable the majority of pelvic tumors with lateral fixation to the soft tissues of the pelvis and, through improvement in exposure, allows for a safe, deliberate dissection. It is the counterpart of the thoracoabdominal incision for the upper quadrants of the abdomen. The results from the use of this incision obviously depend on the histologic type and stage of the tumor and the expected margin of resection one can obtain. It should be used when appropriate and in the context of the biology of the tumor, the expected margin, and the possible use of adjuvant treatments.

IV. SPECIAL POSTOPERATIVE CARE

- The abdominoinguinal incision heals well without complications. In the event of a previous transverse incision in the lower quadrant, which may have interrupted the vascular connection to the superior epigastric vessels and the distal portion of the intercostal and lumbar branches, a small area of necrosis at the junction of the midline and transverse portions of the incision may occur because this incision divides the inferior epigastric vessels. If a small area of necrosis develops, it is debrided and allowed to heal by second intention.
- Early mobilization is encouraged, and prophylactic heparin is administered to prevent thromboembolism.
- Good pain control can be obtained with use of epidural and/or patient-controlled analgesia. In some cases, intravenous ketorolac may be necessary to allow sparing of narcotic drugs.

SUGGESTED READINGS

Karakousis CP: The abdominoinguinal incision in limb salvage and resection of pelvic tumors, *Cancer* 54:2543–2548, 1984.
Karakousis CP: The abdominoinguinal incision: the equivalent of thoracoabdominal incision for the lower quadrants of the abdomen, *J Surg Oncol* 69:249–257, 1998.

CHAPTER 91

External Hemipelvectomy

Ademar Lopes, MD, PhD, and José Carlos Marques de Faria, MD, PhD

I. SPECIAL PREOPERATIVE PREPARATION

- The term *external hemipelvectomy* (EH) or interilioabdominal amputation is used to designate the complete removal of a lower extremity and the entire innominate bone or part of it. The operative wound can be closed with posterior or anterior myocutaneous flaps.
- EH can be extended by en bloc resection of the rectum, a segment of the bladder, elements of the cord and testicles, and part of the sacrum. The tumor determines the extension of the resection, and the surgeon always tries to obtain free margins.
- Advances in chemotherapy for the treatment of osteosarcoma and Ewing tumor since the 1970s, the use of vascular grafts, advances in the rotation of flaps, and free microvascular flaps have reduced its indication, but the EH procedure is still indicated for tumors that are not resectable by more conservative methods.
- In tumors that respond to chemotherapy and radiotherapy, the procedure can only be indicated in cases where neoadjuvant treatment does not allow free-edge limb-salvage surgery.

Indications

- Indications for EH include the following:
  - ▲ Malignant bone tumors of the hemipelvis or proximal tumors of the thigh with invasion of the iliofemoral vascular-nervous bundle
  - ▲ Primary malignant soft tissue tumors of the hemipelvis or proximal third of the thigh with invasion of the hip joint articulation and or vascular-nervous bundle
  - ▲ Large sarcomas of the proximal thigh with invasion of multiple compartments, which can require immediate amputation to prevent ulceration, hemorrhage, and secondary infection
  - ▲ Bone tumors of soft parts compromising the gluteal region and the sciatic nerve that cannot be dealt with by buttockectomy
  - ▲ Primary malignant skin tumors with extensive involvement of soft parts, coxofemoral articulation, and vascular-nervous bundle
  - ▲ Palliative cases with a hygienic (Fig. 91-1) or antalgic goal due to involvement of the lumbosacral plexus and the sciatic and femoral nerves

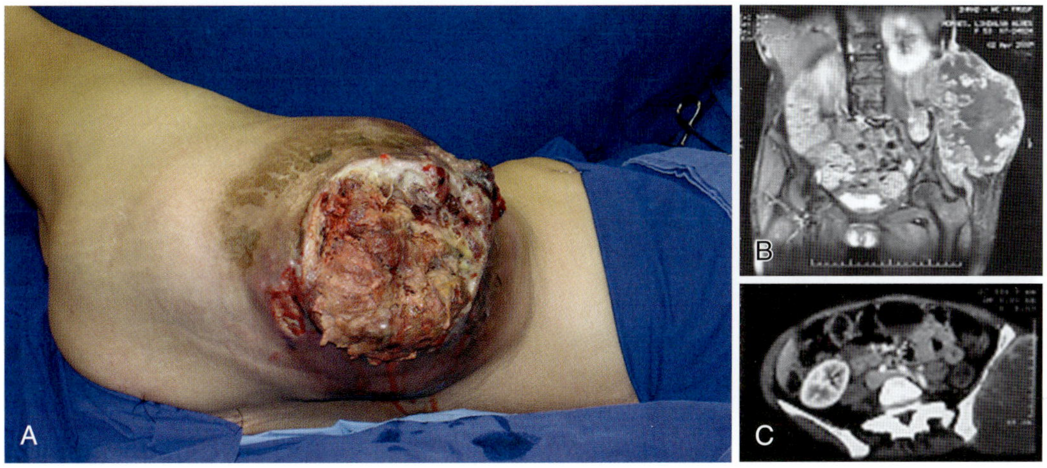

Figure 91-1.

- Bone immaturity can also be an indication for EH in tumors of the proximal femur because of the great difference in limb size caused by conservative surgery.
- Eventually, some patients with extensive metastases to the innominate bone or with important compromise of the vascular-nervous bundle can benefit from this procedure.
- The procedure may also be necessary to save the lives of patients with massive pelvic trauma or those with sepsis deriving from the inferior extremity that cannot be controlled with clinical procedures.
- Relapses of soft tissue sarcomas of the hemipelvic and/or proximal thigh after treatment with surgery, radiotherapy, and hemotherapy not eligible for limb-sparing surgery constitute one of the main indications for EH.
- Good knowledge of anatomy, an expert surgical team, hospital infrastructure represented by a good anesthesia service, intensive therapy, hemotherapy, and physical and psychologic rehabilitation are mandatory conditions for the success of this procedure.
- Although there is currently no consensus among psychologists and psychiatrists, in our personal experience, promoting contact between a patient eligible for EH and one who has already submitted to the procedure has helped with acceptance, in physical and psychologic rehabilitation, and in social and family relationships.
- Figure 91-2 shows some aspects of the anatomy of the region, including the superior and inferior iliac crest, iliacus muscle, femoral nerve, quadratus lumborum muscle, large psoas, femorocutaneous nerve,

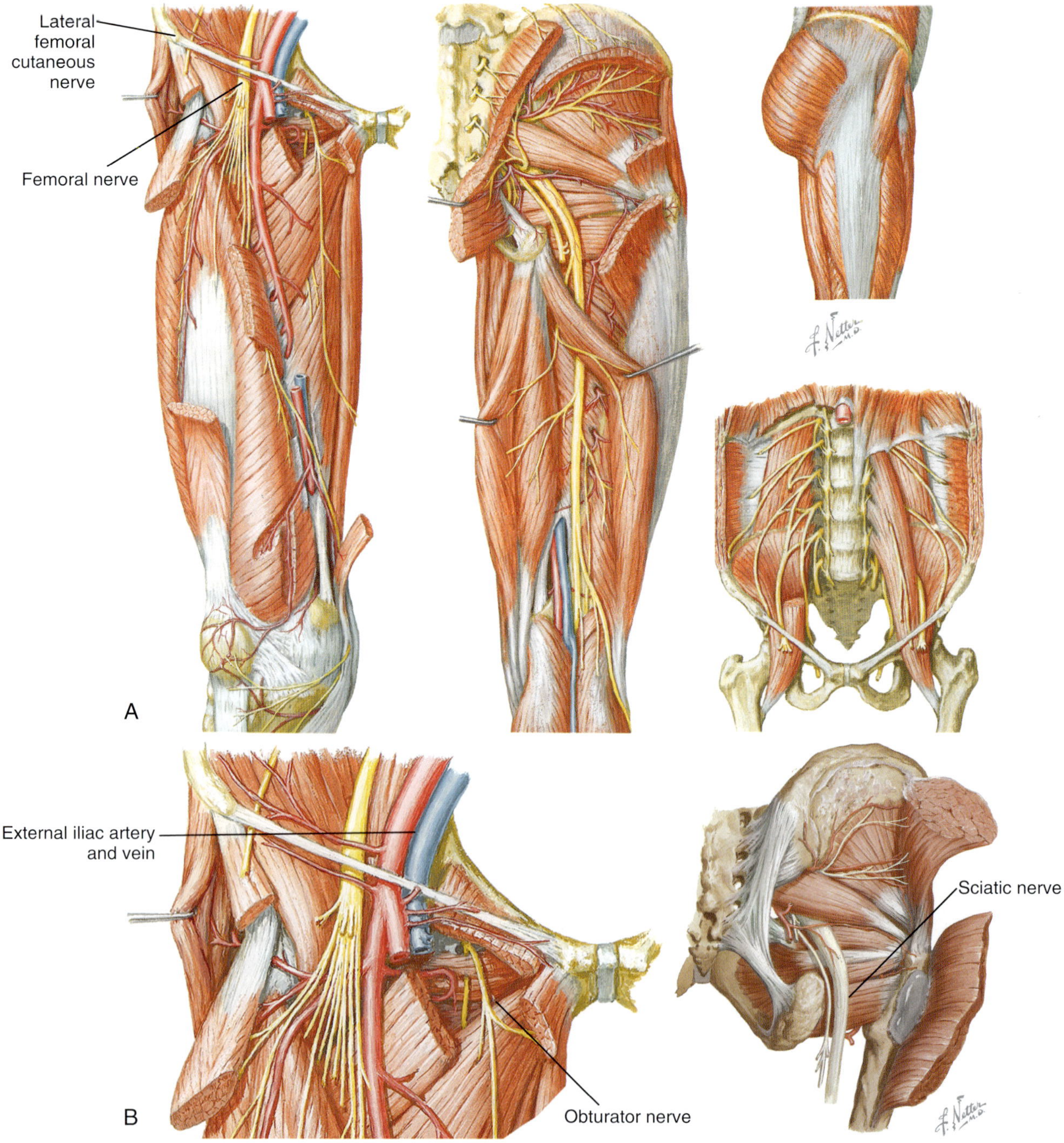

Figure 91-2. **A**, Anatomy of the pelvis, hip, and thigh. **B**, Arteries of the pelvis. *Netter illustrations from* www.netterimages.com. *© Elsevier Inc. All rights reserved.*

small psoas, spermatic cord, ureter, genitofemoral nerve, primitive iliac vessels, external iliac vessels, internal iliac vessels, obturator nerve, and lumbosacral spine.

II. OPERATIVE TECHNIQUE

Position

- The patient is placed in the prone position, a bladder Foley catheter is inserted, and the scrotum is fixed to the opposite side with separated cotton stitches. To prevent possible contamination of the operative wound due to rectal compression during dissection maneuvers, the anus is sutured shut (Fig. 91-3).
- A cushion is placed beneath the scapular-vertebral area up to the 12th rib, resulting in a more or less accentuated inclination of the patient to the side opposite the tumor. The arm on the tumor side is flexed and maintained on an arm rest by straps. The surgical table is flexed to open the angle between the iliac crest and the last rib.
- After antisepsis, the foot and leg are draped, leaving the entire lower extremity to be amputated inside the operative field free for ample movement during the operative procedure, allowing good access to all operative phases. A complete lateral decubitus to the side opposite the tumor can be an option for patient positioning on the surgical table.

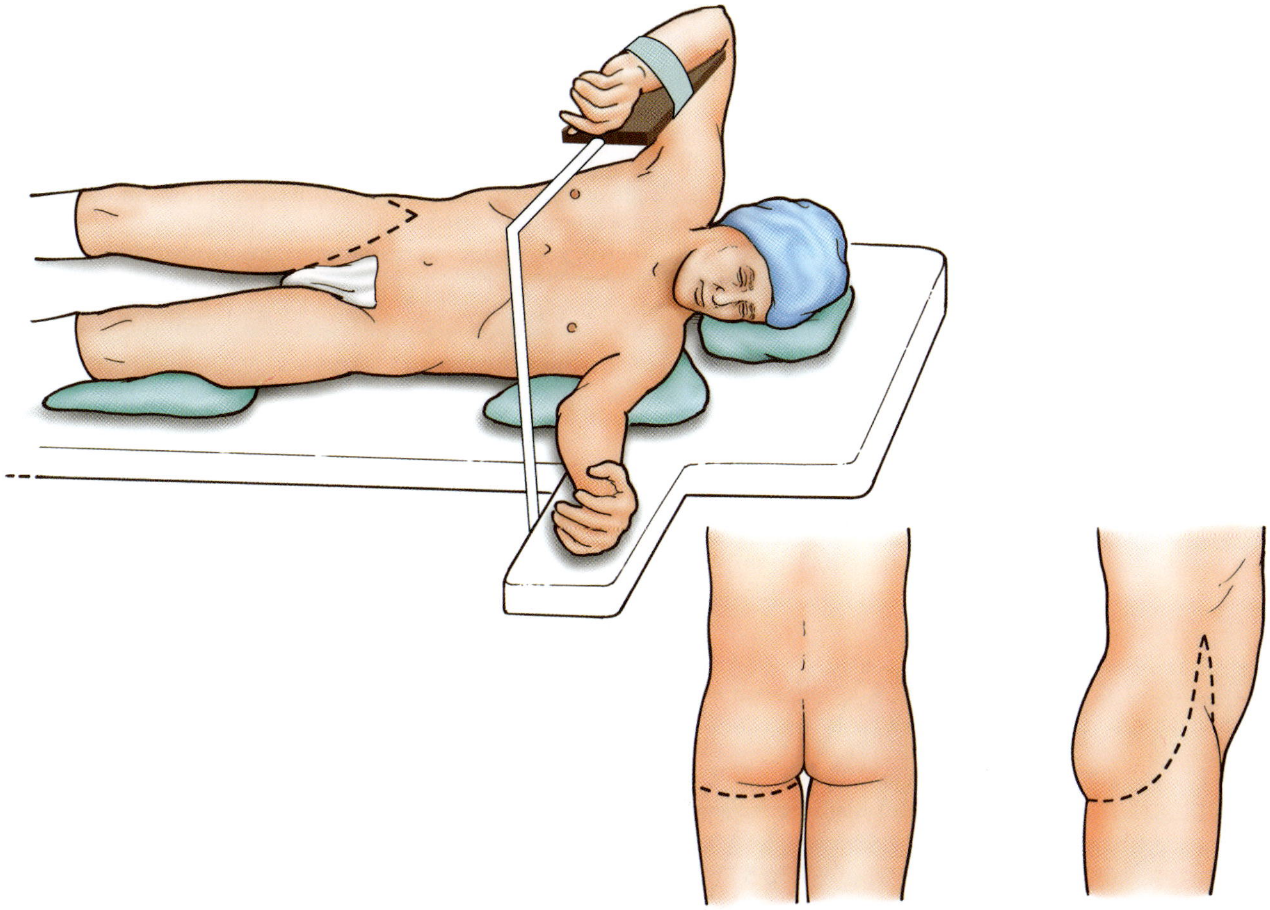

Figure 91-3.

Incision

- Figure 91-4 shows a schematic representation of the incision path, composed of three branches: anteromedial, anterolateral, and posterior.
- For the anteromedial branch, the incision should reach the skin and cellular subcutaneous tissue. It starts at a point situated at the anterior part of the abdomen, about 5 cm above and 2 cm medial to the anterosuperior iliac spine, descending parallel to the inguinal arcade, then passing 2 cm lateral to the pubic crest, where it curves and goes to the proximal third of the thigh, 2 cm lateral to the genitocrural ridge. The dashed line shows the deepness of the section in the muscular-aponeurotic layer of the anterolateral abdominal wall. The spermatic cord is seen penetrating the superficial inguinal orifice.
- After muscular-aponeurotic section, the incision penetrates the retroperitoneal space by blunt dissection, displacing the peritoneum and its contents medially and cranially up to the midline of the sacrum. As the peritoneum is retracted up to the midline and contained by appropriate pushers, the iliac fossa is widely exposed. The iliac vessels are seen covered by the surrounding areolar tissue (Fig. 91-5).
- In cases in which lymphadenectomy is indicated, such as for carcinoma and melanoma, the procedure begins at the origin of the primitive iliac vessels. The external iliac artery is dissected and tractioned. This maneuver facilitates dissection of the external iliac vein and access to the obturator nerve.

Main Dissection

Ligature and Division of Iliac Vessels and Femoral Nerve

- The external iliac artery is ligated immediately below the iliac bifurcation. The artery is held on its posterior wall by a clamp and sectioned between the second and the third ligatures, as shown by the dashed line. The same procedure is applied to the external iliac vein. Alternatively, the vessels can be transected with a linear stapling device. Figure 91-5 shows the stumps of the iliac vessels, highlighting the double proximal ligatures.
- The psoas muscle is then medially pushed away, and the sulcus between it and the iliac muscle is opened, exposing the femoral nerve for ligature with absorbable wire and section by a scalpel. Figure 91-5 shows the femoral nerve stumps already ligated and divided.
- Over the major psoas in the mediolateral direction, one sees the femoral and femorocutaneous stumps, iliac vessels, iliac nerves, and obturator vessels already ligated and divided. The dashed lines show the division levels of the major psoas muscle and the interpubic disarticulation (see Fig. 91-5).
- The quadratus lumborum, major psoas, and anterior rectus abdominis muscles are divided, followed by the interpubic disarticulation. Quadratus lumborum division is followed by iliolumbar ligament division.

Anterior Lateral Dissection

- The incision in the skin and subcutaneous tissue begins at the lateral edge of the quadratus lumborum muscle, extends to the incision that rounds the iliac crest, progresses in the direction of the major

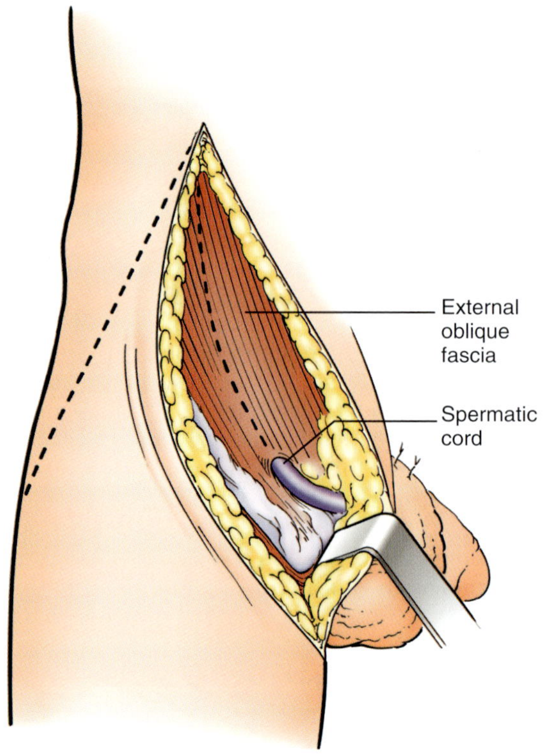

Figure 91-4.

trochanter, and crosses it in its more salient portion. It goes to the posterior part of the thigh, passing 2 cm below of the gluteal fold, and joins the medial portion of the first incision branch (see Fig. 91-3). The small dermal fatty patches of the medial and posterior portion of this incision are dissected over the ischial branches until reaching its tuberosity.

- Figure 91-6 shows the gluteus maximus muscle divided next to its femoral insertion and retracted, forming the great posterior myocutaneous flaps. The dashed line shows the section level of the pyriformis muscle tendon, exposing the sciatic nerve beneath.

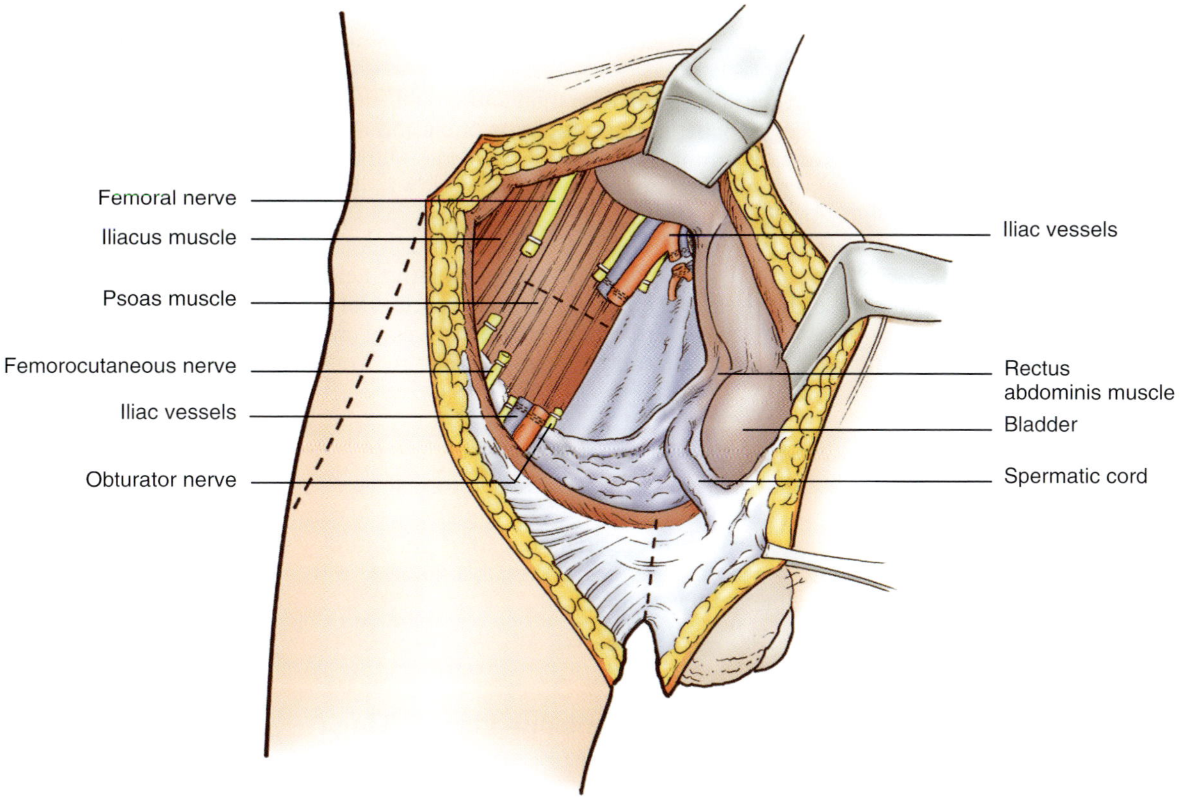

Figure 91-5.

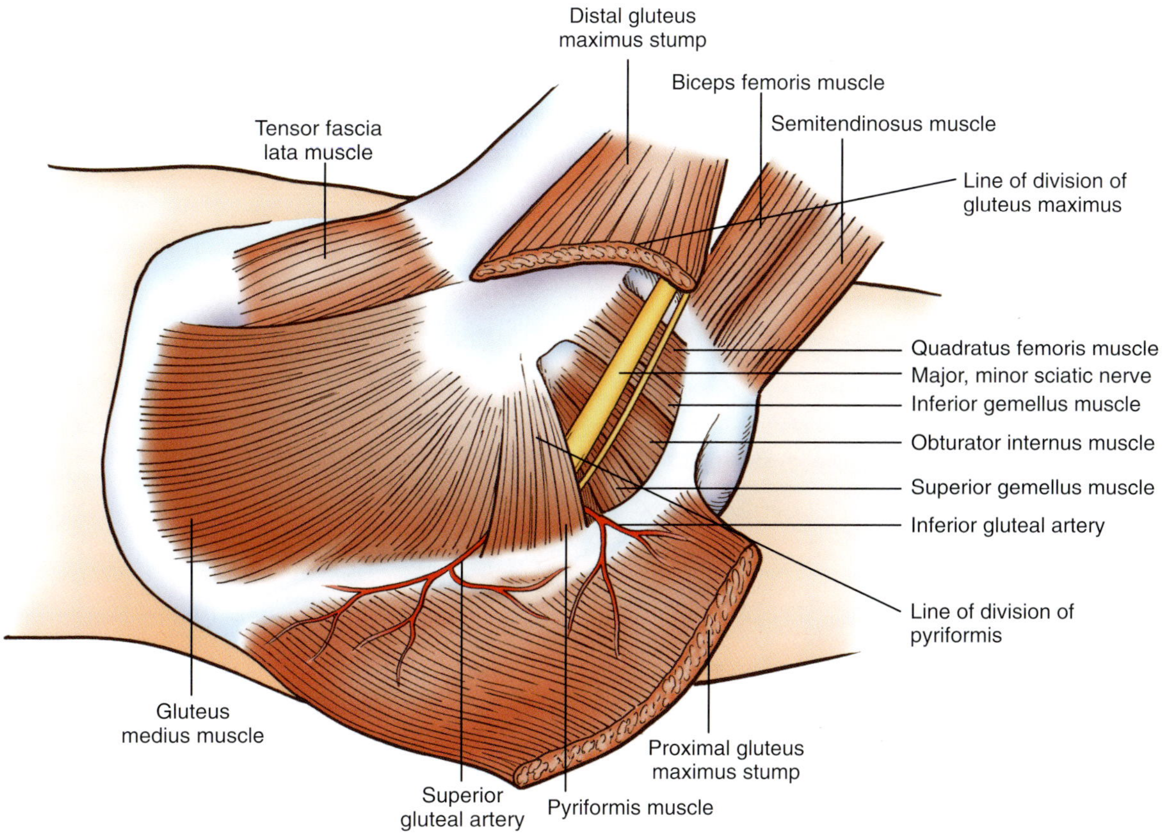

Figure 91-6.

- The piriformis muscle is divided and pushed away to the deep face of the gluteus maximus, displaying the sciatic nerve for posterior ligature and division. This nerve must be sectioned at the highest point possible to keep the stump from staying in the cicatrization line. If there is involvement of the extra-pelvic portion of this nerve, an intrapelvic division should be performed.
- The piriform muscle is pushed away to the deep face of the gluteus maximus, as well as the sciatic nerve stumps, with preservation of the branches that go to the gluteus maximus. Distally, the stumps of this nerve are seen over the superior gemellus, the internal obturator, the inferior gemellus, and the quadratus femoris muscles.
- The dashed line in Figure 91-7 shows the bony portion at the sacroiliac joint, between the insertions of the great and the middle gluteal muscles where division will be done with a Gigli saw, and the gluteus maximus myocutaneous flap. In this phase, care is taken to avoid injury to the trunk of the superior gluteal artery.
- Next, interpubic disarticulation is completed by applying cranial and lateral traction. The pelvic floor muscles and ligament are divided. Dissection starts in the symphysis pubis and is directed to the ischial tuberosity. Great care must be taken to avoid injury to the urethra, bladder, and rectum.
- Once the pelvic floor musculature is sectioned, the operative specimen is held only by the sacrospinal and sacrotuberous ligaments, which are divided.
- After removal of the specimen, one observes a perfect vascularization and innervation of the gluteus maximus that is part of the large posterior myocutaneous flap. The operative field will also show the surface of the iliac bone section, the proximal stump of the psoas muscle, the external iliac vessel stumps, the hypogastric vessel stumps with their branches, the obturator vessel and nerve stumps, the ureter attached to the peritoneum, and the bladder and the surface of the interpubic disarticulation.

Closure

- After rigorous hemostasis, always keeping the blood pressure at its normal level, two Jackson-Pratt drains are placed, and the operative wound is closed by suturing the gluteus maximus muscle to the anterolateral wall muscles of the abdomen. Next, the gluteus maximus aponeurosis is approximated with that of the anterior abdominal wall, with separate nonabsorbable sutures, and finally the skin is approximated with separate nonabsorbable sutures (Fig. 91-8).

III. ALTERNATIVE TECHNICAL APPROACHES

External Hemipelvectomy Using Anterior Myocutaneous Flap of Thigh

- Patients with primary bone tumors of the innominate bone, sarcomas of soft parts, or, eventually, metastatic tumors to this area, with involvement of the gluteal and sciatic muscles, should not be submitted to EH using a posterior myocutaneous gluteal flap, as previously described.
- These patients require EH using an anterior myocutaneous flap of the thigh. This type of flap allows resection of all the skin and soft tissue of the gluteal area up to the midline en bloc with the hemipelvis and the entire lower limb.
- Because of the size of this type of flap, a large operative defect can be closed. Because of its good vascularization, such a flap presents a low risk of necrosis when compared with the former posterior

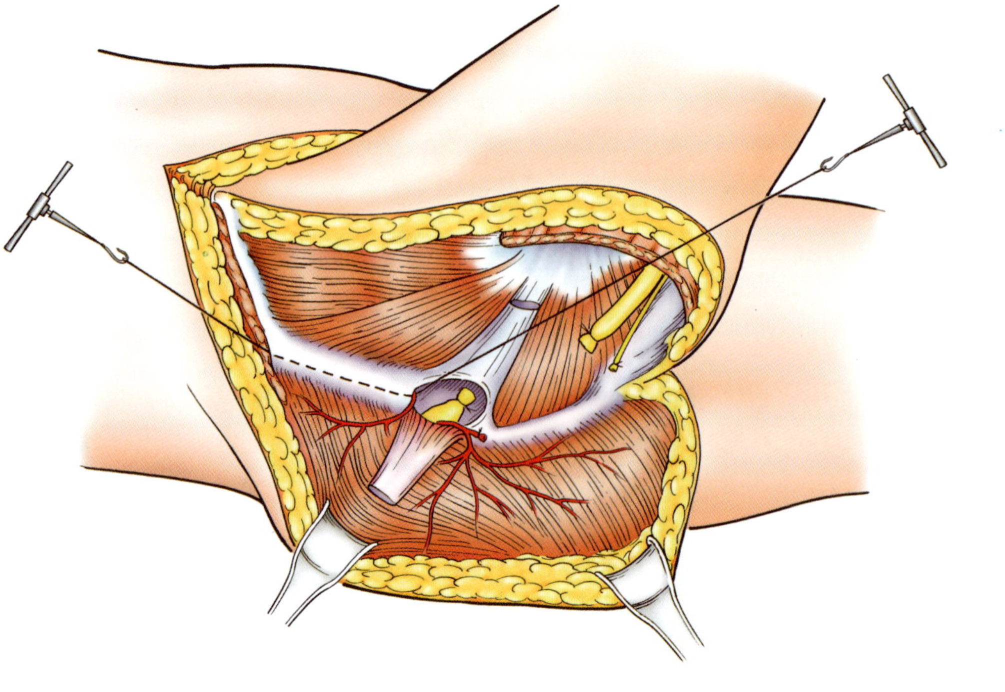

Figure 91-7.

fasciocutaneous flap. In the anterior flap of the thigh, the iliofemoral vascular-nervous bundle and the musculature of the anteromedial portion of the thigh must be free of neoplasia.

- In patients with carcinomas or other tumors, we use this flap only in the absence of lymph node metastases in the ilioinguinal area.
- Figure 91-9, *A* and *B*, shows a massive low-grade chondrosarcoma, primarily of the iliac bone, with extension to the gluteal area and ulceration of the skin.
- Figure 91-9, *C*, shows the anteromedial myocutaneous flap of the thigh after the removal of the surgical specimen comprising the skin, subcutaneous tissue, and quadriceps musculature. Irrigation and venous draining of this flap are done by the superficial femoral artery and vein, respectively, and its innervation by the crural nerve. Figure 91-9, *D*, shows the flap covering the operative defect well (the patient died of another disease 13 years after EH). The potential for rehabilitation with this procedure is generally better than in EH using a posterior flap, because the muscular mass of the quadriceps produces an adequate tissue cushion over the sacrum, where the prosthesis can be held without injuring the tissues.

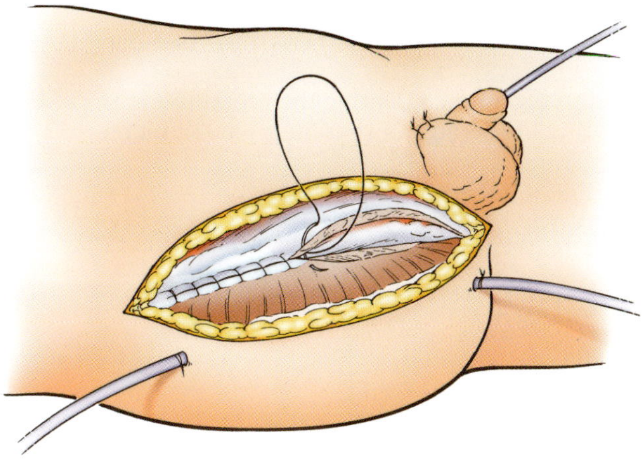

Figure 91-8.

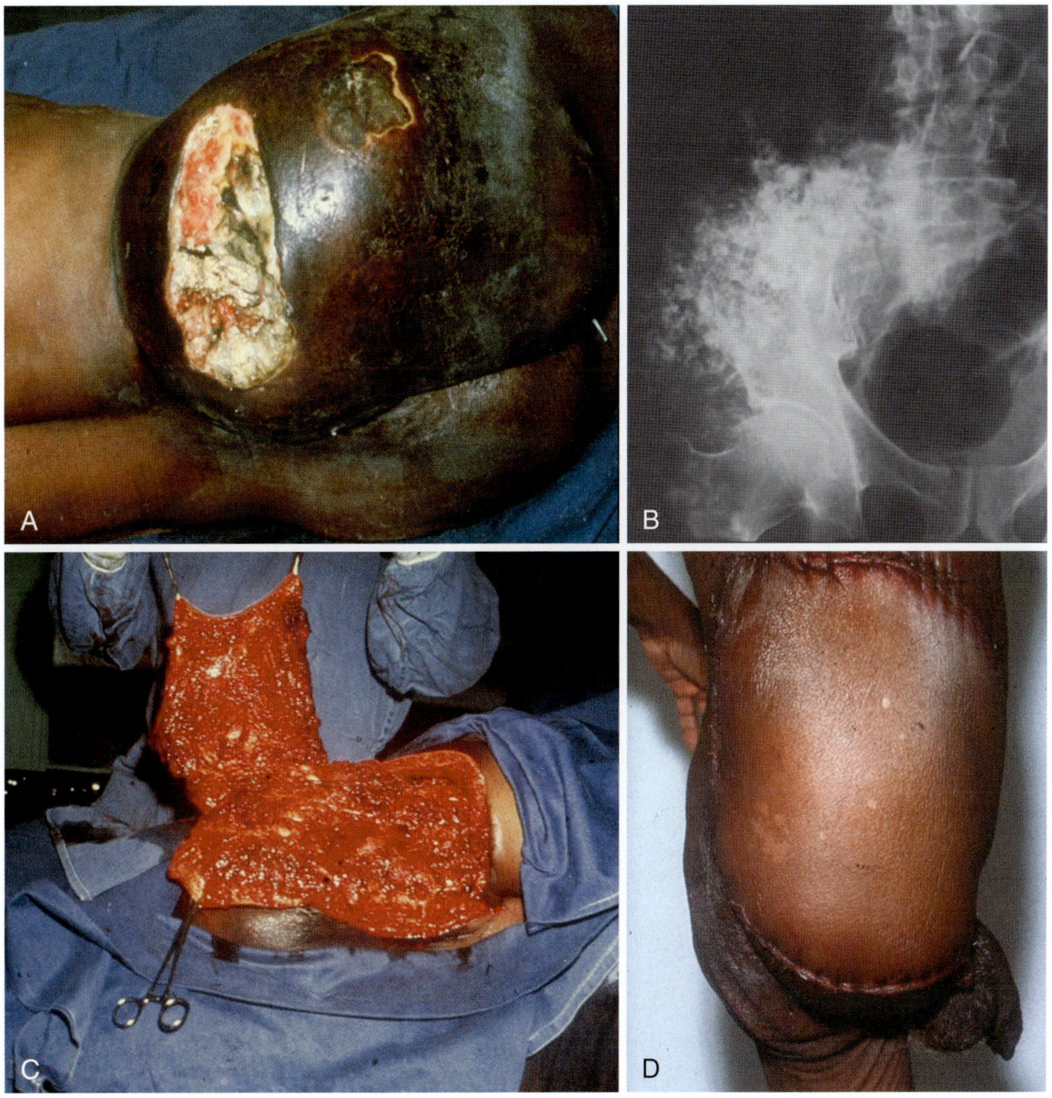

Figure 91-9.

External Hemipelvectomy with Transference of Free Myocutaneous Flap of Leg

- Eventually, a tumor of the hemipelvis can extend massively to the gluteal area (Fig. 91-10, *A*) and anteriorly, with involvement of the iliofemoral vascular-nervous bundle. The use of the posterior or anterior flap is not possible.
- A free myocutaneous flap of the leg to be amputated, with all its dermal fatty tissue and compartments pediculated in popliteal vessels, can later be transferred to the gluteal area. The posterior establishment of its vascularization by anastomosis of the popliteal vessels with the common iliac vessels is a good way to close this operative wound.
- In this procedure, we perform all steps of EH, keeping the hemipelvis attached by the sacroiliac joint, interpubic joint, and sacrotuberous and sacrospinous ligaments and the common iliac vessels.
- The myocutaneous flap of the leg is then prepared, keeping its vascularization by the popliteal vessels and repositioning it in its original place (see Fig. 91-10, *B*, *C*, and *D*).
- Proceeding to the EH, we leave the stumps of the common iliac vessels prepared after removing the operative specimen. The popliteal vessels are divided, and the flap is transferred to the hemipelvic area. The anastomosis of the popliteal vessels with the common iliac vessels is performed (see Fig. 91-10, *E*, *F*, and *G*).
- In this way, the duration of ischemia to the flap is reduced to a minimum. During the procedure, it is impossible to perform simultaneous preparation of the flap and EH because of continuous mobilization of the extremity.

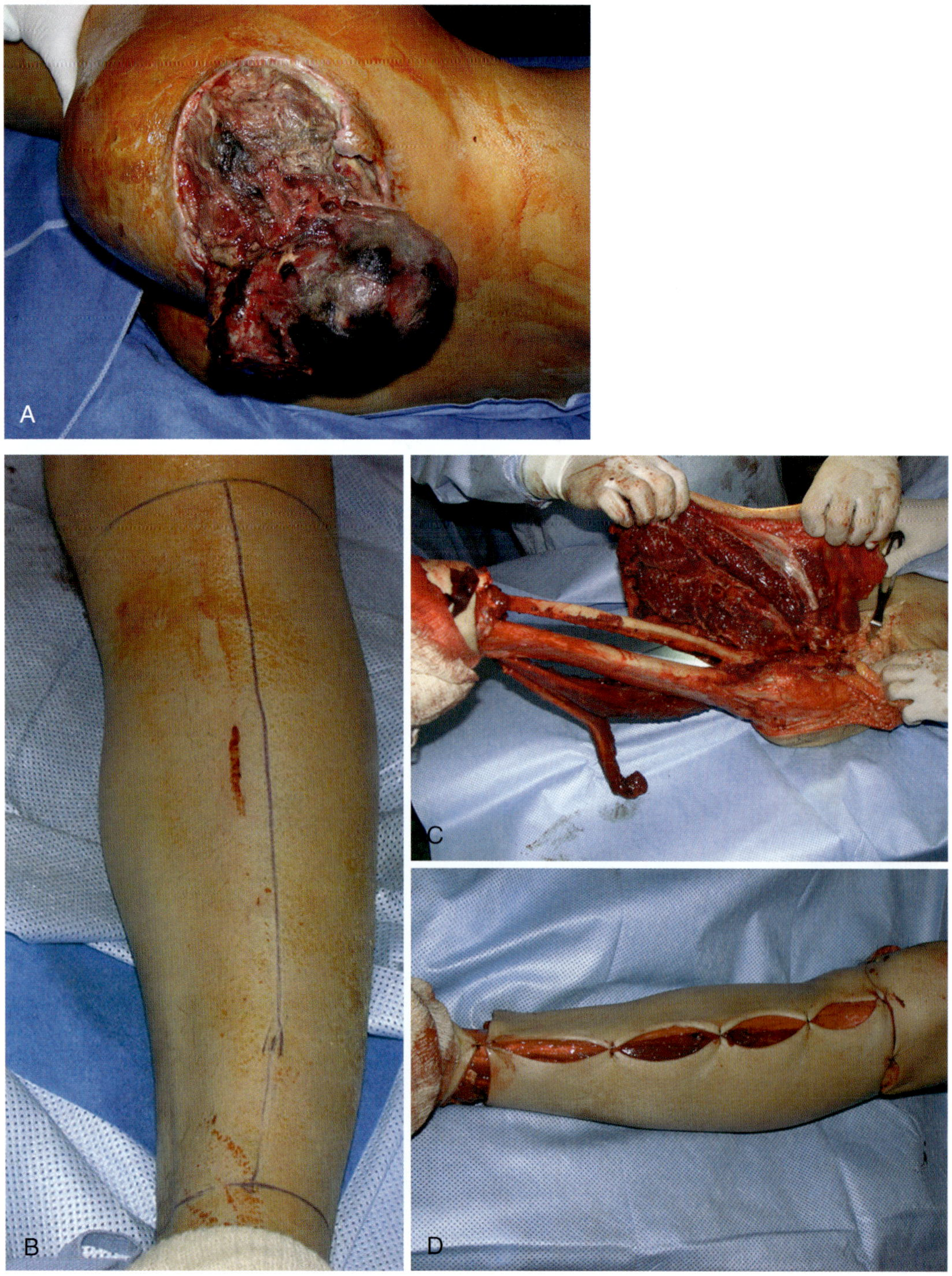

Figure 91-10. *A, C, F, G from Faria JC, Aguiar S Jr, Ferreira Fde O, Lopes A: Fillet flap for reconstruction after hemipelvectomy: report of three cases,* J Plast Reconstr Aesthet Surg *62:e110–1, 2009, Figs. 1 and 2.*

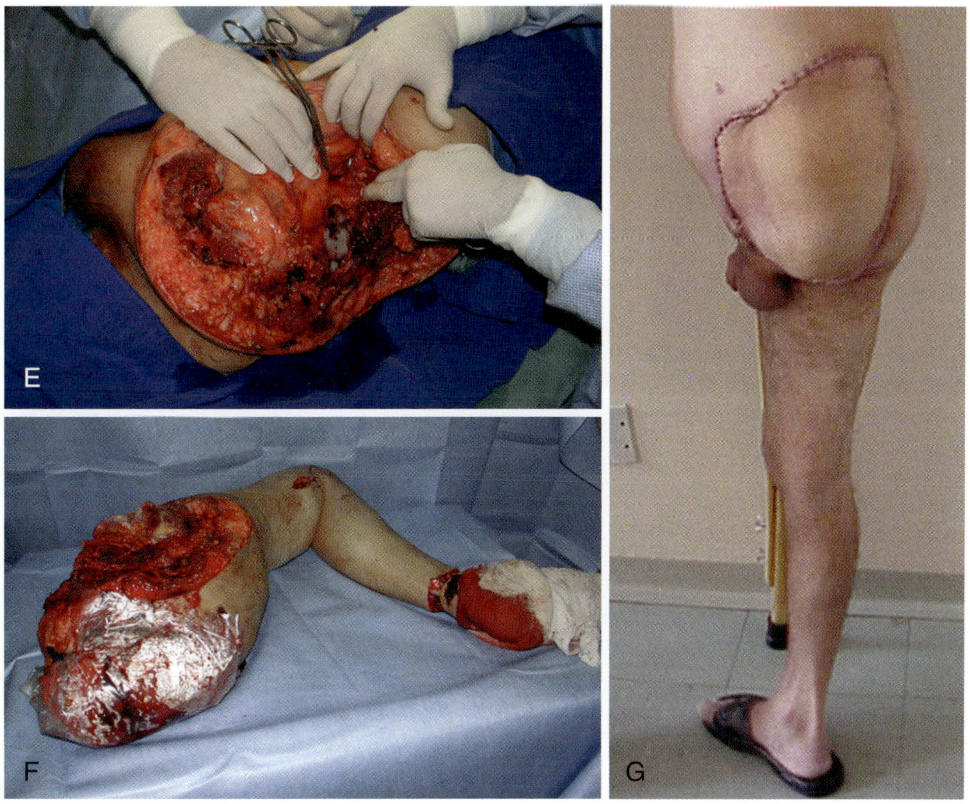

Figure 91-10, cont'd. See legend on opposite page.

- In this flap, the cylindrical conformation of the soft tissue of the leg is changed to an almost flat structure that is large enough to repair great defects, such as the one caused by EH. Moreover, it has the advantage of not causing other aesthetic and functional defects.

IV. SPECIAL POSTOPERATIVE CARE

- Intra- and postoperative mortality in EH is negligible when the procedure is done by an experienced team and in good infrastructural hospital conditions.
- The anterior myocutaneous flap of the thigh and, eventually, the free myocutaneous flap of the leg are efficient alternatives to prevent the frequent necrosis of the fasciocutaneous gluteal flap, which was often used in the past.
- Rigorous antisepsis, the use of broad-spectrum antibiotics, mechanical and biological preparation of the intestines, and good drainage contribute to reduced infection rates.
- Flap ischemia followed by necrosis generally requires debridement and dressings for a long period of time.
- Postoperative heparinization is controversial because of the risk of hematoma in the operative bed. In our practice we use this prophylaxis infrequently. On the other hand, we advise early movement of the remaining extremity to prevent deep vein thrombosis.
- Pain and the sensation of a phantom limb occur in most patients, but gradually disappear. Clinical treatment with anticonvulsive and neuroleptic antidepressant drugs and physical rehabilitation are of great value in this phase.
- In general, in postoperative days 1 to 4, patients feel better in bed. From then on, they must grasp a bar and use other special devices to prevent accidental falls. The rehabilitation team must teach the patient to walk with crutches.
- Discharge is possible when the patient is clinically well, able to walk, and can perform self-care, usually between postoperative days 10 and 14.
- Around 8 weeks after the amputation, the possibility of prosthesis use must be discussed with the patient. The patient must be well informed as to the potential benefits and the imperfections of the device. It is imperative that the patient be the one who wants the prosthesis and not a member of the family or of the team.
- One of the great obstacles to physical recovery is obesity, and patients must be warned to prevent it.

SUGGESTED READINGS

Lampert MH, Sugarbaker PH: Reabilitação de pacientes com sarcomas de extremidades. In Lopes A, editor: *Sarcoma de artes moles*, Rio de Janeiro, 1999, Médsi Editora Médica e Científica Ltda., pp 129–150.

Malawer M, Henshaw R: Posterior flap hemipelvectomy. In Malawer MM, Sugarbaker PH, editors: *Musculoskeletal cancer surgery*, Dordrecht, The Netherlands, 2001, Kluwer Academic Publishers, pp 320–336.

Malawer M, Sugarbaker PH, Henshaw R: In Malawer MM, Sugarbaker PH, editors: *Musculoskeletal cancer surgery*, Dordrecht, The Netherlands, 2001, Kluwer Academic Publishers, pp 306–317.

CHAPTER 92

Total Internal Hemipelvectomy

Ademar Lopes, MD, PhD

I. SPECIAL PREOPERATIVE PREPARATION

Concept

- Until about 1975, patients with Ewing tumor and primary osteosarcoma of the innominate bone were treated by external hemipelvectomy with disappointing esthetic, functional, and psychologic results. The appearance of new effective drugs allowed tumor shrinking and en bloc resection with limb salvage and a significant improvement in survival and quality of life.
- Internal hemipelvectomy means the total or partial removal of the innominate bone en bloc with the tumor, with or without the head of the femur and the soft tissue surrounding it, preserving the ipsilateral extremity.
- Innominate bone tumor localization and extension determine the extent of resection, always with the aim of obtaining free margins.
- Total internal hemipelvectomy (TIH), the subject of this chapter, involves complete resection of the innominate bone with or without the head of the femur. Type I involves the iliac wing, type II involves the periacetabular region with or without the head of the femur, and type III involves the ischium and the pubis. Combining these partial hemipelvectomies, for instance, I plus II or II plus III, is a common procedure.

Indications

- Indications include primary malignant bone tumors such as chondrosarcoma, Ewing tumor, osteosarcoma, and other tumors without extension or with minimal or moderate extension into soft tissue, allowing an en bloc resection with free margins.
- Evaluation for this procedure for Ewing tumor and osteosarcoma, or other chemo- or radiation-responsive tumors, must be done only after neoadjuvant treatment (Fig. 92-1).
- Invasion of the iliofemoral neurovascular bundle and the sciatic nerve must be absent. In exceptional cases, the femoral or sciatic nerve may be resected, although with very poor functional results, and in these cases it is advisable to discuss with the patient the indication for external hemipelvectomy.
- Indications also include tumors of soft tissue with extension to the bone, without invasion of the neurovascular bundle, allowing en bloc resection with free margins and an adequate closing of the surgical wound without significant compromise of function.
- TIH may also be indicated for metastasis to innominate bone, with a controlled primary tumor, without other detected metastases, and in the absence of other, better treatment options.
- Bone immaturity can be a contraindication for internal hemipelvectomy, because resecting the head of the femur removes the proximal bone growth area, causing a significant change in limb size.
- TIH as described here is indicated for patients with large tumors of the innominate bone, involving almost all its segments, which are thus not treatable by partial hemipelvectomies.

Preparation

- History, general clinical examination, imaging, and anatomopathologic tests are vital for diagnosing and staging of bone and soft tissue tumors. Digital rectal examination can be useful for intrapelvic evaluation of bone tumors.

- Bone scintigraphy is important for detecting possible distant metastases and the tumor's bone marrow extension (Fig. 92-2).
- Computed tomography scans are efficient for evaluating the cortical and, mainly, the periacetabular bone regions and are mandatory for detecting possible metastases to the lungs.
- Magnetic resonance imaging is better than computed tomography for evaluating tumor size and its relations with soft tissue, joints, and the neurovascular bundle (Fig. 92-3). Magnetic resonance angiography, arteriography, and venography can be useful to better evaluate the tumor's relations with vessels.
- A well-planned biopsy is mandatory for accurate diagnosis and is important for a future surgery. When badly planned or performed, biopsy can make limb-sparing surgery or the use of flaps for covering the surgical wound impossible.
- Soft tissue tumors or bone tumors with extension to soft tissue are examined with computed tomography–guided core biopsy. Intraosseous lesions are biopsied using a trephine.

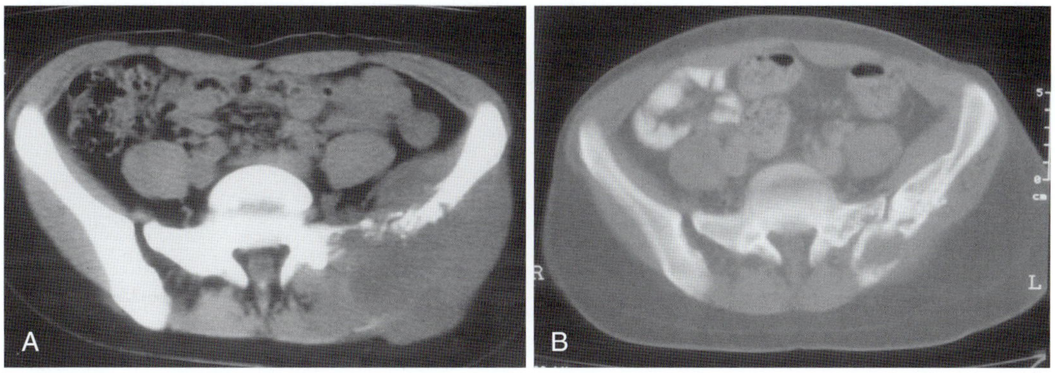

Figure 92-1. Computed tomography scan of Ewing tumor. A, Before neoadjuvant chemotherapy. **B,** After chemotherapy.

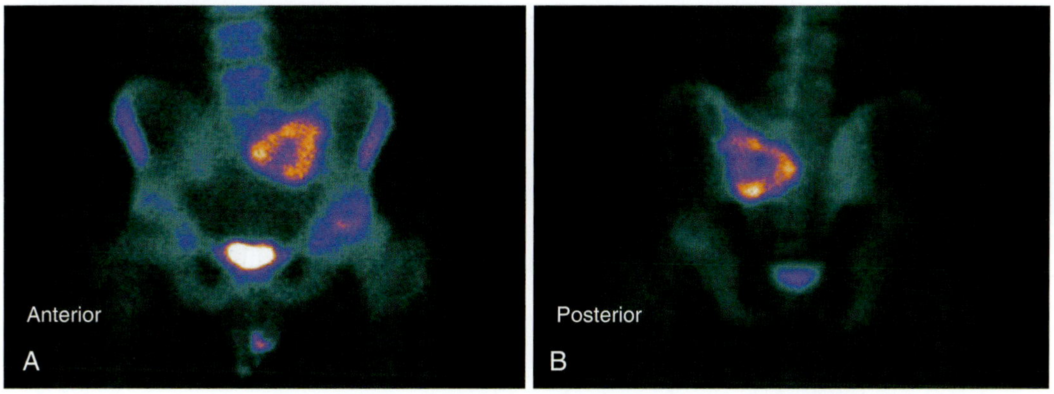

Figure 92-2. Radiotracer hyperconcentration in a patient with osteosarcoma, showing an expansive tumor involving diffusely the right iliac bone, with extension to the sacroiliac joint and a large soft tissue component.

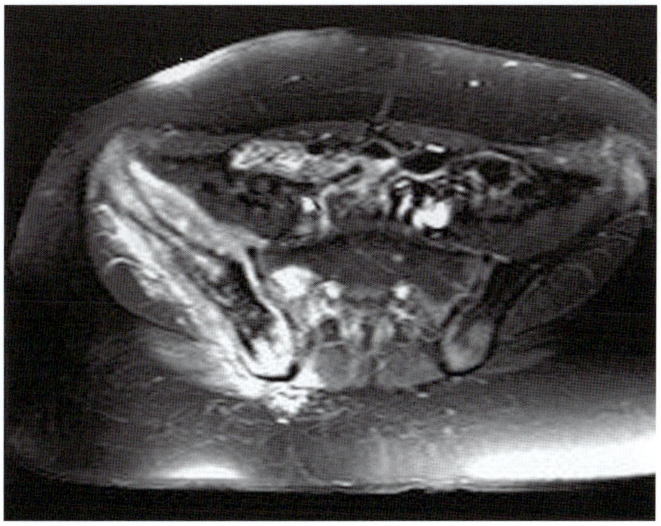

Figure 92-3. Magnetic resonance imaging of a patient with Ewing tumor, extending to soft tissue and the sacroiliac joint.

- Open biopsy is performed only in the absence of adequate material with most conservative methods. In most pelvic bone tumors, biopsy must be made of tissue from a point along the future incision track, so that it is possible to remove the scars en bloc with the tumor in the final surgery.
- Expertise and knowledge of anatomy are crucial for the surgical procedure to succeed (Fig. 92-4).

II. OPERATIVE TECHNIQUE

Position

- The patient is placed in supine position. A bladder Foley catheter is placed, and the scrotum is fixed to the opposite side with separated cotton stitches. A cushion is placed beneath the scapular-vertebral region up to the 12th rib, resulting in an accentuated inclination to the side opposite the compromised hemipelvis. The arm of the tumor side is flexed and maintained on an arm rest by straps. The surgical table is flexed to allow better exposure of the angle between the iliac crest and the costal edge. After rigorous antisepsis, the foot and leg are draped. The lower limb is placed inside the operative field and free for ample maneuvers during surgery, easing the approach to the various phases of the procedure (Fig. 92-5).

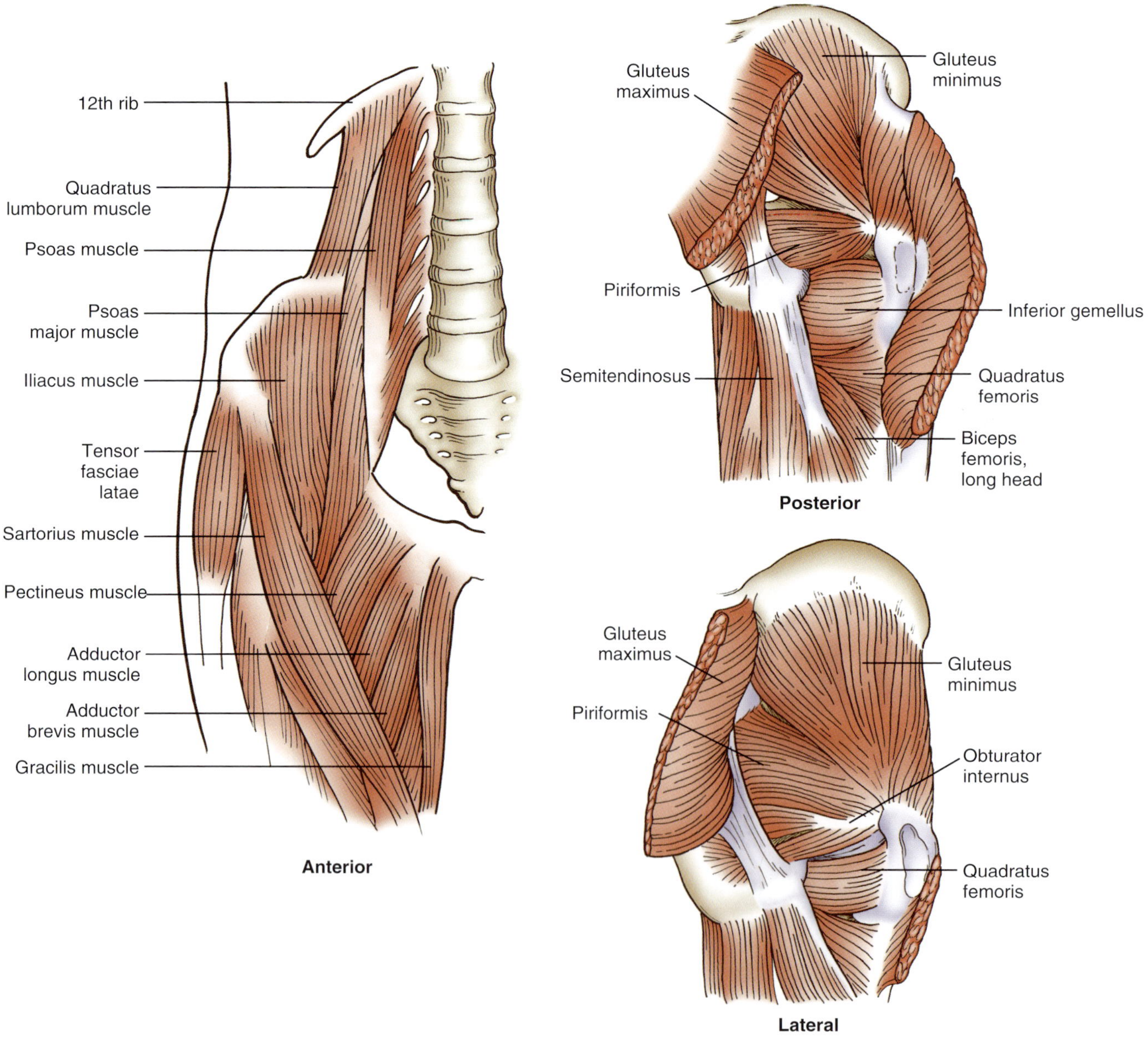

Figure 92-4.

Incision

- The incision should permit ample approach to the sacroiliac joint, pubic symphysis, and sacrotuberous and sacrospinous ligaments, as well as good exposure for the dissection and sparing of the iliofemoral neurovascular bundle and the sciatic nerve. The incision is made from the anterior superior iliac spine and carried along the iliac crest to the posterior inferior iliac spine. Anteriorly, the incision reaches the pubic tubercle, passing 2 cm below the inguinal ligament, and curves medially, passing 2 cm above the genitofemoral crease. Posteriorly, the incision reaches the ischial tuberosity, passing 2 cm below the posterior gluteal crease. Another incision, from the anterior superior iliac crest to about 2 cm behind the major trochanter, allows development of the gluteal myocutaneous flap and the extrapelvic exposure of the sciatic nerve (see Fig. 92-5).

Main Dissection

Approaches to Psoas Muscle, Iliofemoral Neurovascular Bundle, and Pubic Symphysis

- The skin and subcutaneous flap are mobilized away, allowing exposure of the inguinal ligament. The curvilinear incision is deepened over the iliac crest, and the musculature of the anterolateral wall of the abdomen is divided just over it until preperitoneal fat is exposed.
- The inguinal ligament is detached from the anterior superior iliac spine, and upward traction is applied to it. The inferior epigastric vessels are then dissected, ligated, and divided. The inguinal ligament is detached from the pubic tubercle, and blunt dissection mobilizes the peritoneum medially and cranially to the midline.
- The iliac vessels are exposed, and a tape is passed around them. The same is done to the femoral nerve after it is traced lying in the groove between the psoas and iliacus muscles. Lateral and medial branches from the common femoral vessels are ligated and divided, and a tape is passed around them to allow

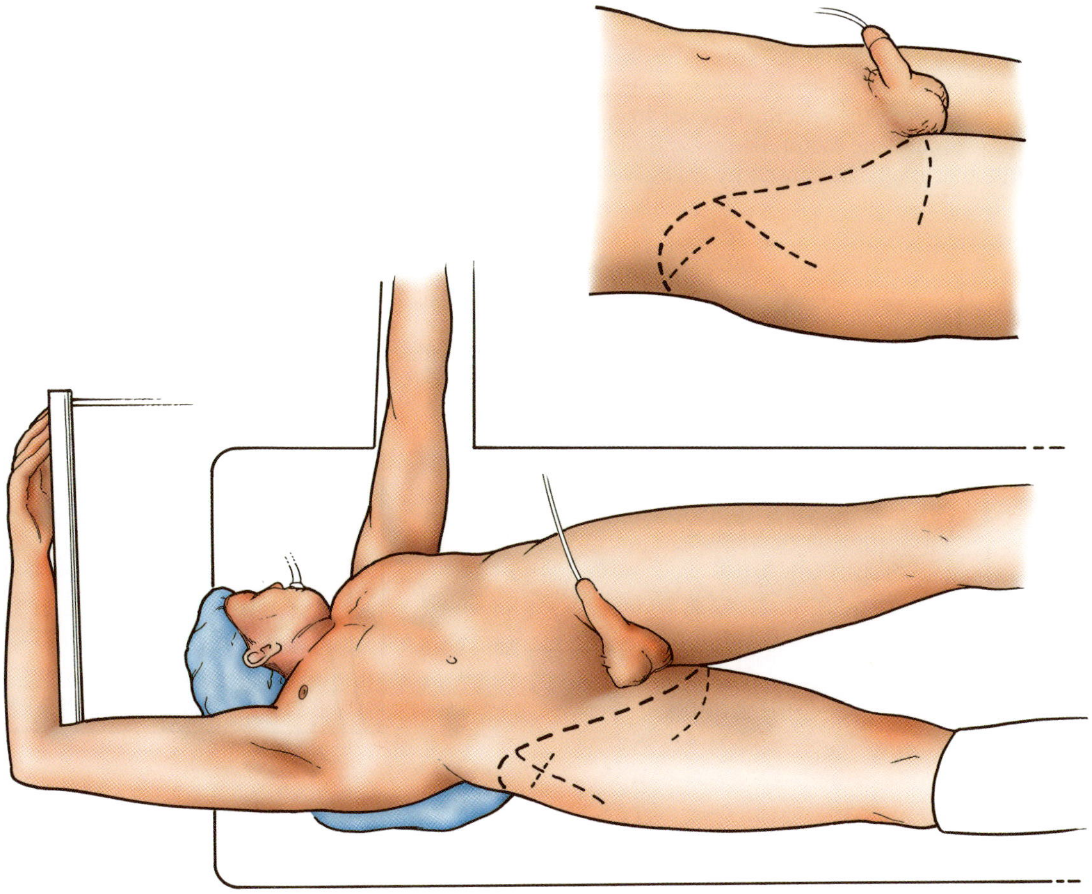

Figure 92-5.

their ample mobilization at the floor of the femoral trigone. The femoral nerve is also dissected, and a tape is passed around it (Fig. 92-6).

- The iliac muscle is removed en bloc with the specimen. The psoas muscle may be retained when it is not involved. If the pelvic portion has been invaded, it may be divided to be removed en bloc with the specimen (see Fig. 92-6). The quadratus lumborum muscle is divided, and then the iliolumbar ligament, allowing the exposure of the anterior surface of the sacroiliac joint.
- The rectus abdominis muscle is detached from its pubic insertion, and the midline is exposed. With blunt dissection of the posterior surface of the pubic symphysis, its posterior arch is exposed. With sharp dissection, the anterior surface of the symphysis is exposed. A right-angle clamp is passed around the symphysis, and then a Gigli saw, with which the symphysis is later divided.

Approach and Section of Posteromedial Musculature of Thigh and Obturator Nerve

- With the thigh flexed and abducted, the adductor muscles are divided at their origin, and the anterior and posterior branches of the vessels and the obturator nerve are tied and divided. The pelvic part of this nerve has already been divided. The obturator externus muscle is left on the specimen.
- With this position maintained, the tendinous muscles (both semitendinosus and semimembranosus) and femoral biceps are divided mediolaterally at the ischial tuberosity (Fig. 92-7, *A* and *B*).

Gluteal Myocutaneous Flap Development, Approaches to Coxofemoral and Sacroiliac Joints and Sciatic Nerve

- The inferolateral incision is deepened, having as landmark the major trochanter, until the fascia lata, which is divided anteriorly to the major trochanter. A gluteal myocutaneous flap is mobilized away and remains attached to its origin at the lateral edge of the sacrum near the sacroiliac joint. The piriformis muscle is divided and mobilized away over the deep surface of the gluteus maximus muscle, exposing the sciatic nerve.
- With the neurovascular bundle medially mobilized away, the sartorius and tensor fascia lata muscles are divided below their origin, and the heads of the rectus femoris muscle are divided at their origin. The tendon of the iliopsoas muscle is divided at the floor of the femoral trigone when part of it is being removed (Fig. 92-8).
- In intra-articular resection, the capsule is circularly incised for a later osteotomy of the neck of the femur. In extra-articular resection, the osteotomy is performed without opening the capsule (the tumor determines the extension of resection and osteotomy).
- Up to this point, the specimen is not free, but is held by the hip joint and sacroiliac joints, the pubic symphysis, and the sacrotuberous and sacrospinous ligaments, avoiding damage to the neurovascular bundle that might be caused by excessive traction during dissection maneuvers.

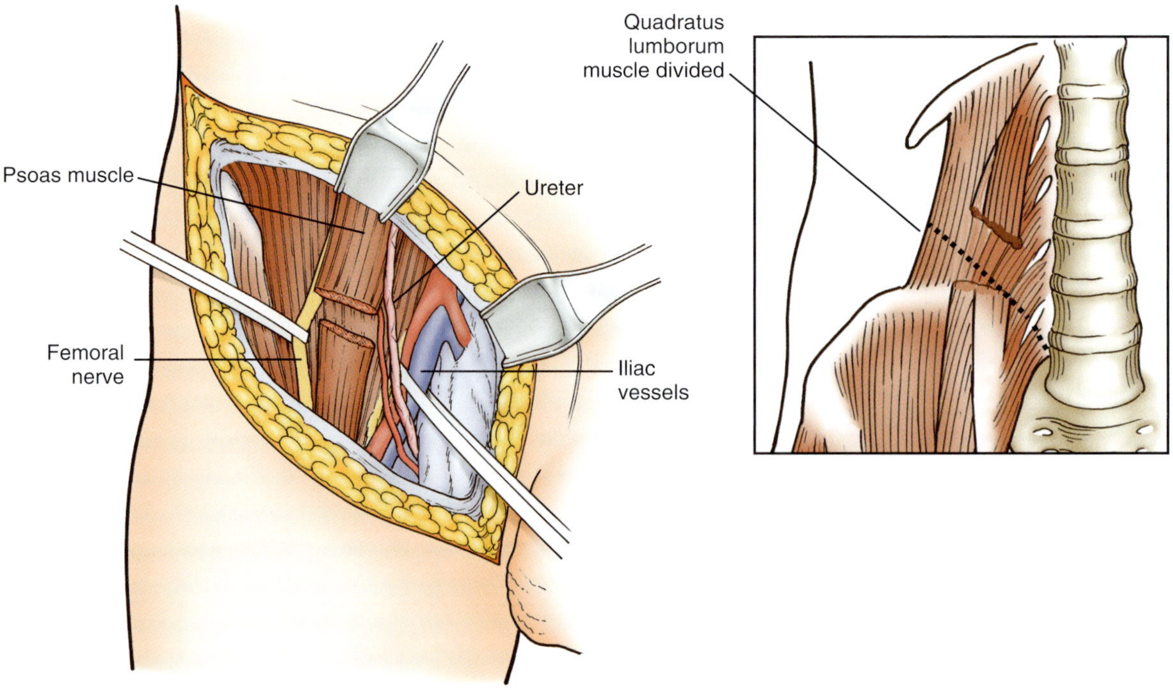

Figure 92-6.

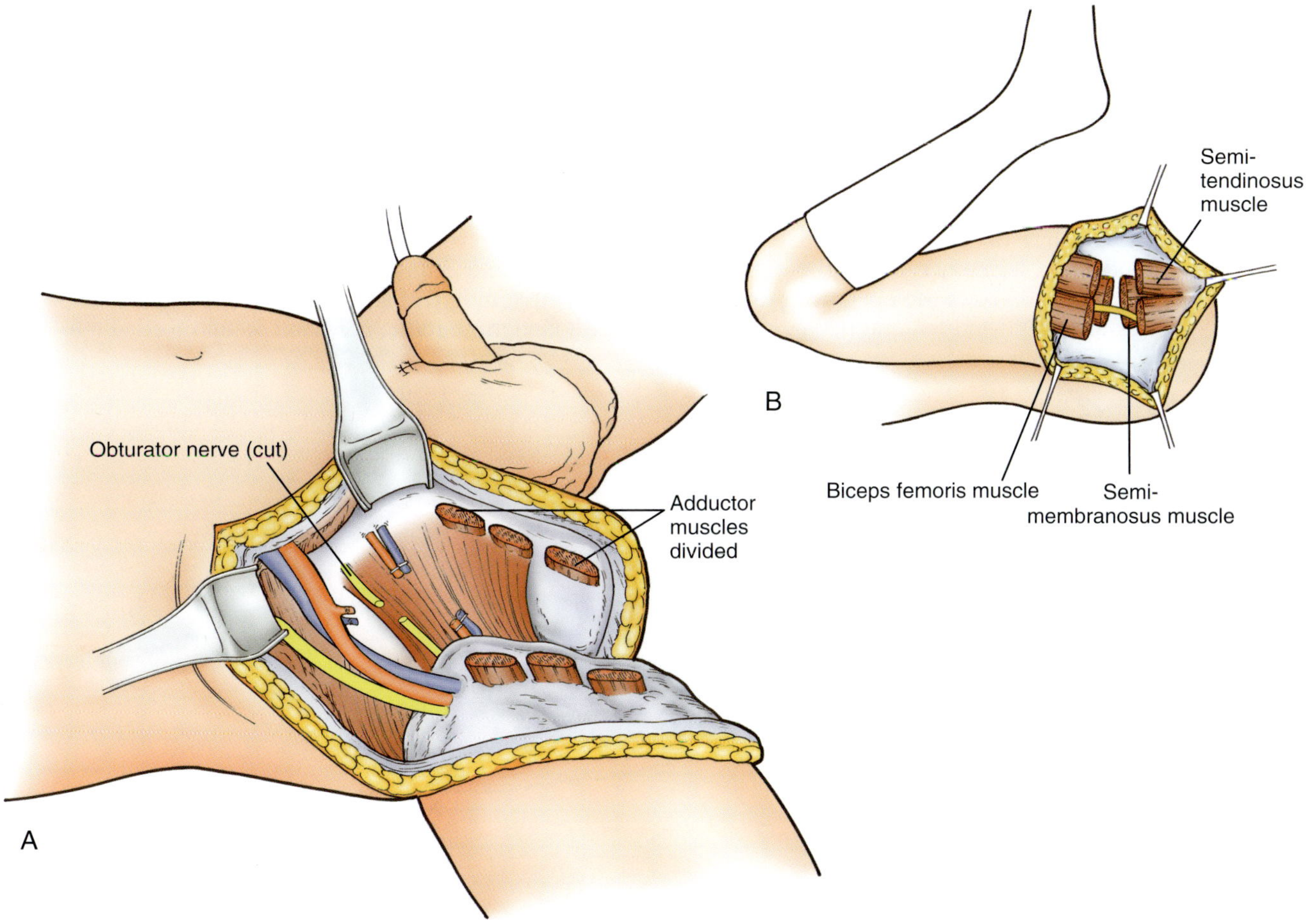

Figure 92-7.

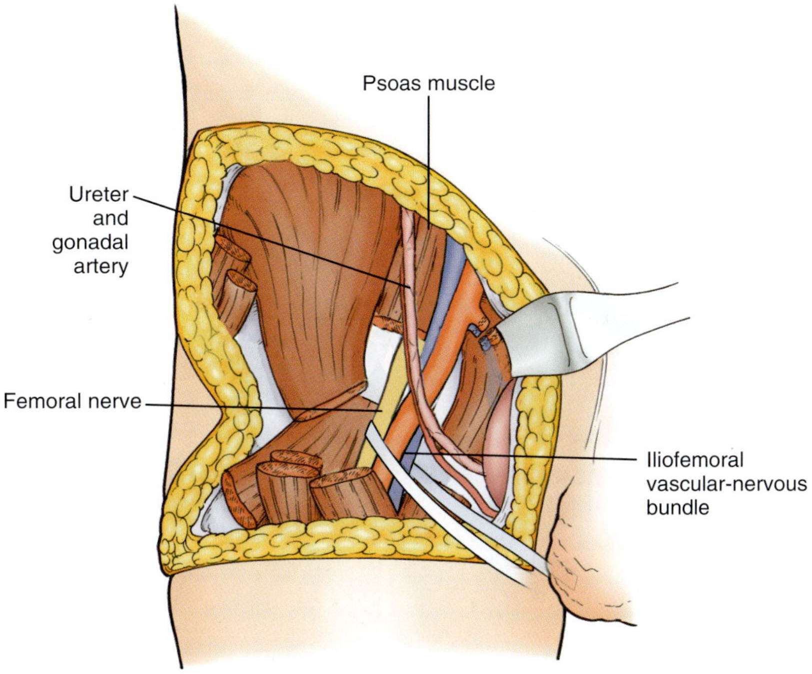

Figure 92-8.

- Intra- or extra-articular osteotomy of the femur is performed, and the sacroiliac joint is divided as well as the pubic symphysis (using a Gigli saw or a chisel). Care must be taken not to damage the trunk of the superior gluteal artery and the pelvic portion of the sciatic nerve (Fig. 92-9, *A*).
- Lateral traction is applied to the specimen. The pelvic floor musculature is divided from the symphysis to the ischial tuberosity, with care not to damage the urethra, bladder, or rectum.
- Once the pelvic floor musculature is divided, the specimen is attached only to the sacrotuberous and sacrospinous ligaments and some pelvic-trochanteric muscles. Once these are divided, the specimen is freed.
- After removal of the specimen, the lower limb is attached to the trunk by the neurovascular iliofemoral bundle, the sciatic nerve, and the preserved portion of skin and cellular subcutaneous tissue.
- Figure 92-10 shows the operative bed after TIH for Ewing tumor. In Figure 92-10, *A* through *D*, one sees the sciatic and femoral nerves and the vascular iliofemoral bundle; the bone section medially to

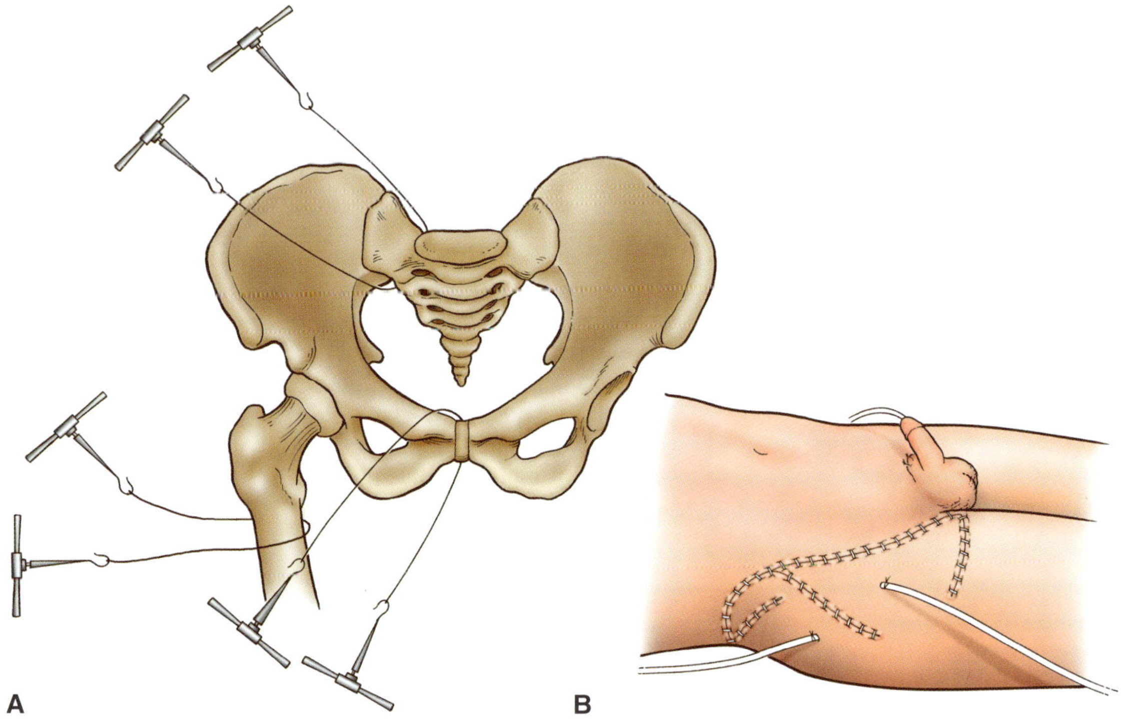

Figure 92-9.

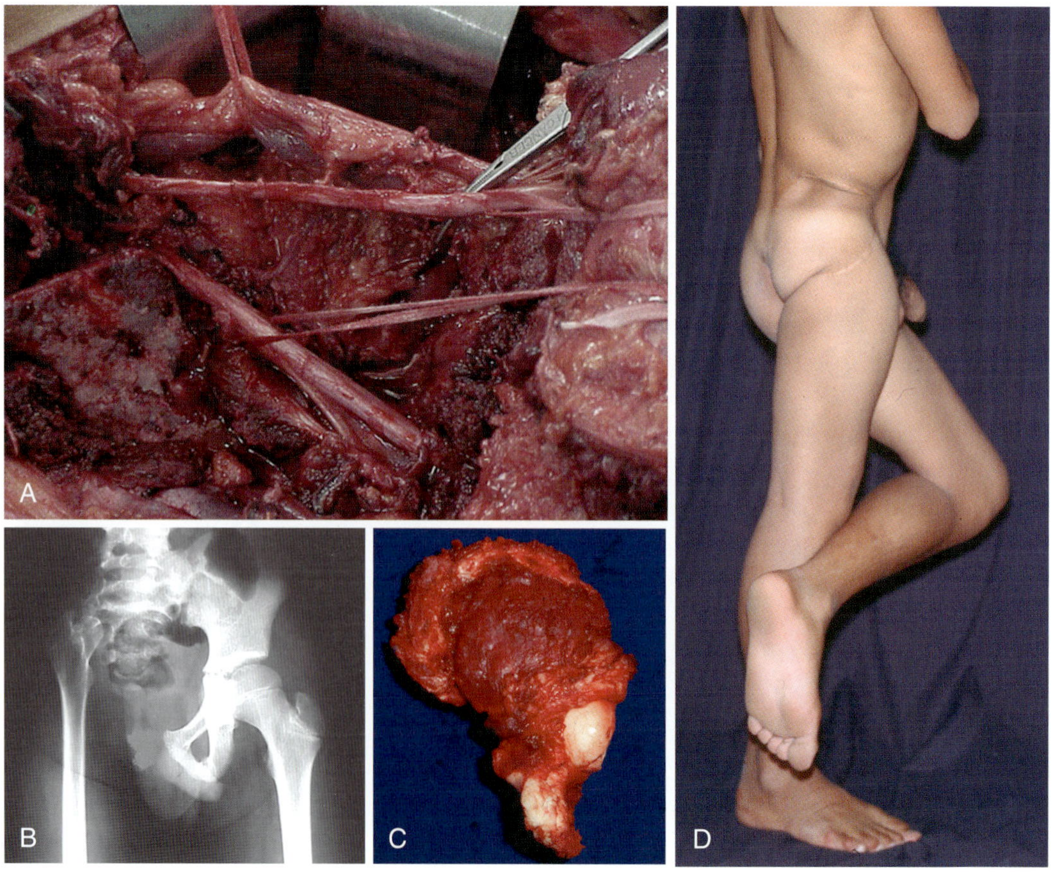

Figure 92-10.

the sacroiliac joint; the specimen; and the patient standing, with full weight bearing on the operated side, 12 months after the procedure.

Closure

- After rigorous hemostasis, two suction drains are placed. The operative wound is closed if possible, approximating the muscles of the anterior abdominal wall to the gluteal muscle with absorbable suture. The fascia is approximated with separate unresorbable stitches. Cellular subcutaneous tissue and dermis are approximated with absorbable suture, and the skin is closed with separate unresorbable stitches (see Fig. 92-9, *B*).

III. ALTERNATIVE TECHNICAL APPROACHES (PRO/CON) AND PEARLS

- In some cases the patient may be treated with partial internal hemipelvectomies. Some examples are shown in Figures 92-11 and 92-12.

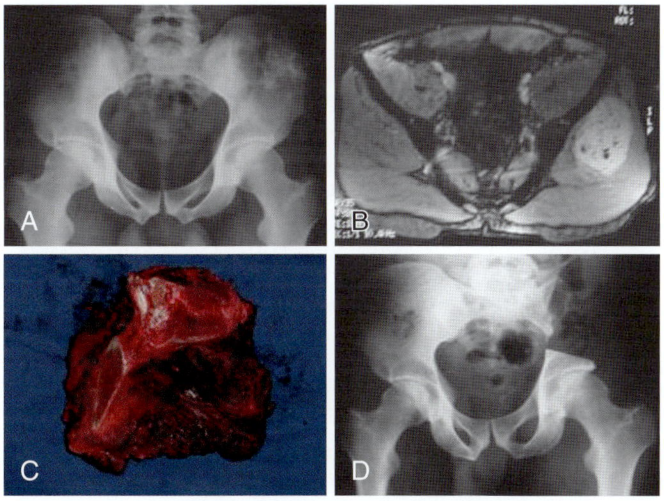

Figure 92-11. **A patient with chondrosarcoma of the iliac wing who underwent type I internal hemipelvectomy. A,** Radiograph. **B,** Computed tomography showing the extension of the lesion. **C,** Specimen. **D,** Radiograph showing bone loss.

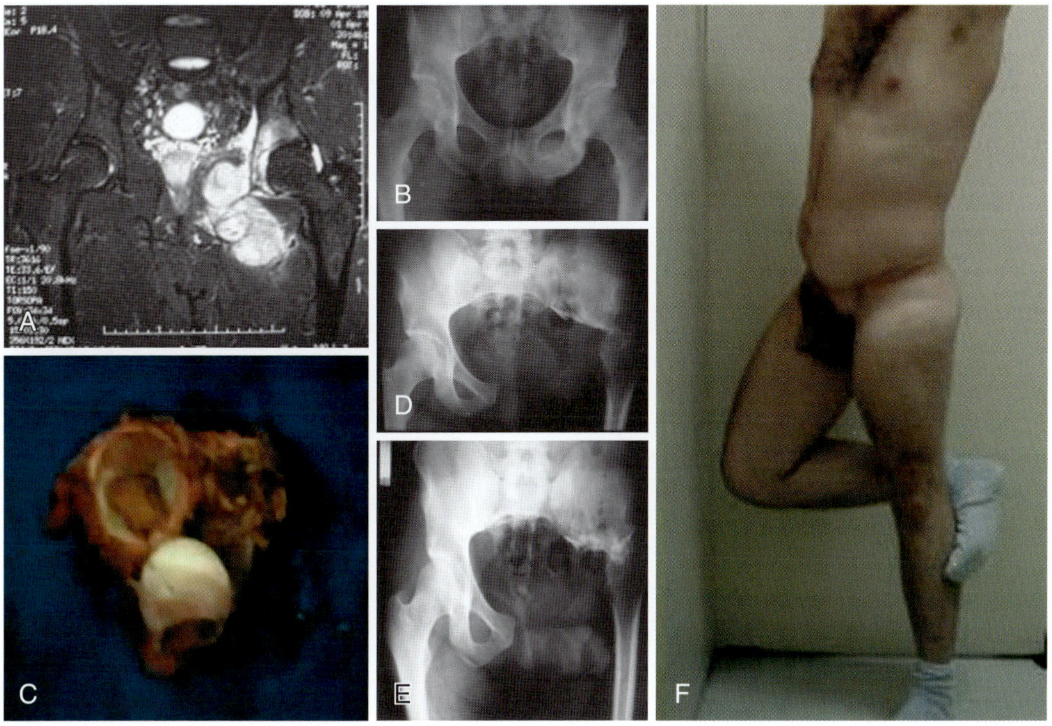

Figure 92-12. **A patient with osteosarcoma involving the anterior arch, acetabulum, and soft tissue, who underwent internal hemipelvectomy type II plus III. A,** Magnetic resonance imaging showing the lesion extent before chemotherapy. **B,** Radiograph after chemotherapy. **C,** Specimen. **D** and **E,** Radiographs showing bone loss. **F,** Patient standing, 14 months after surgery, bearing all weight on the operated side.

- Patients with disease restricted to the anterior arch (ischial and iliopubic branches) are treated by type III hemipelvectomy, and those with disease restricted to the periacetabular region are treated by type II hemipelvectomy.
- When the tumor extends to the acetabulum and anterior arch, a combination of type II and type III is necessary, as seen in Figure 92-12.
- In cases such as this one, even the head of the femur is removed to produce better oncologic margins. The bone division facilitates pseudarthrosis with better functional results.
- As seen in Figure 91-12, we do not use reconstruction, and functional results are good without major risks of complications such as infection and loosening of the prosthesis.

IV. SPECIAL POSTOPERATIVE CARE

- The patient remains on bed rest for 1 to 2 weeks after this operation.
- Prophylactic heparinization may be advisable in reducing the incidence of deep venous thrombosis, although there is no consensus.
- The patient is allowed non–weight-bearing ambulation at 2 weeks, partial weight bearing at 2 to 3 months, and unlimited weight bearing with crutches or a cane on the operated side at 4 to 6 months.
- Hygienic care must be observed, and measures for preventing pressure sores must be taken. Physical therapy must be started immediately with muscle-strengthening exercises for the arms.
- Our team does not use prostheses after TIH. Functional evaluation must be done at 6 to 12 months after surgery. Usually in this period, a fibrosis is formed between the stump of the femur and the soft tissue, appearing as a pseudarthrosis, and 65% of children and young adults on whom we have operated are able to walk without support with full weight bearing on the operated side.
- The stump of the femur migrates cephalad after TIH, shortening the limb. This must be corrected with a shoe lift.
- In 49 patients on whom we performed internal hemipelvectomy, two (4%) presented with necrosis of the external third of the gluteal myocutaneous flap, requiring debridement, antibiotic therapy, and resuture. In these cases, resection extended medially to the sacroiliac joint, and the gluteal artery was ligated. In similar cases, slicing the distal extremity of the flap to ensure its vascularization is necessary before closure.
- Reconstruction after resection involving the acetabulum is usually a challenge, as it is complex and associated with complications.
- Internal hemipelvectomy involving the resection of the acetabulum is more complex than external hemipelvectomy. This is a good example of the progress in surgical oncology in recent decades in improving technical and functional aspects without reducing surgical radicality.

SUGGESTED READINGS

Bickels J, Malawer M: Overview of pelvic resections: surgical considerations and classification. In Malawer MM, Sugarbaker PH, editors: *Musculoskeletal cancer surgery*, Dordrecht, The Netherlands, 2001, Kluwer Academic, pp 203–213.

Karakousis CP: Internal hemipelvectomy. In Sugarbaker PH, Malawer MM, editors: *Musculoskeletal surgery for cancer*, New York, 1992, Thieme Medical Publishers, pp 150–163.

Steel HH: Partial or complete resection of the hemipelvis. An alternative to hindquarter amputation for periacetabular chondrosarcoma of the pelvis, *J Bone Joint Surg* 60A:719–730, 1978.

SECTION XVII

Vascular Surgery

CHAPTER 93

Carotid Endarterectomy/ Stent Placement

Christopher K. Zarins, MD, and Bruce L. Gewertz, MD

I. SPECIAL PREOPERATIVE PREPARATION

- Carotid endarterectomy is effective in preventing stroke in both symptomatic and asymptomatic patients with severe carotid stenosis. Preoperative preparation includes determination of the symptom status of the patient and the degree of carotid stenosis.
- Careful history and physical examination will determine whether the patient has had a transient ischemic attack, prior stroke, amaurosis fugax, vertebrobasilar ischemia, or global ischemic symptoms.
- The most widely used imaging study for carotid stenosis is duplex ultrasound imaging, which can determine the degree of internal carotid stenosis as well as detect plaque ulceration, intraluminal thrombus, dissection channels, and tortuosity. Further imaging may be performed using contrast computed tomography scanning and magnetic resonance angiography. These modalities provide important information about the aortic arch and intracranial vessels, as well as cerebral pathology, in addition to providing details about the carotid bifurcation plaque. Three-dimensional reconstruction of computed tomography and magnetic resonance images is very useful in planning therapy. Contrast angiography has been the gold standard in selecting patients for carotid endarterectomy in prospective randomized clinical trials, but it is invasive and carries a small risk of stroke. Catheter-based angiography is necessary when patients are considered for potential treatment with carotid stenting.
- Patients selected for therapy include symptomatic patients (transient ischemic attack, amaurosis fugax, or prior stroke) with more than 50% stenosis of the ipsilateral internal carotid artery and asymptomatic patients with more than 70% stenosis of the internal carotid artery, especially if the plaque is complex or highly irregular.
- Each patient should also be carefully evaluated for overall perioperative risk, including cardiopulmonary risk for anesthesia, recent myocardial infarction, congestive heart failure and coronary artery disease, significant medical comorbidities, prior neck surgery or radiation, and the presence of significant proximal carotid or intracranial tandem lesions. Patient age is not a specific contraindication to surgery for either symptomatic or asymptomatic patients, but overall life expectancy is an important consideration, particularly in asymptomatic patients. The risk of perioperative stroke and death following carotid endarterectomy (1% for asymptomatic patients) should be weighed against the benefit of annual stroke-risk reduction following carotid endarterectomy (risk of stroke is reduced from 2% per year to 1% per year for severe asymptomatic stenosis). Symptomatic patients with severe carotid stenosis have a significantly higher risk of stroke if left untreated and should be considered for endarterectomy if the degree of stenosis exceeds 50% to 70%, provided perioperative stroke/death risk is less than 6%.

II. OPERATIVE TECHNIQUE

Position

- The patient is placed supine on the operating table with a shoulder roll. The neck is extended and the head is rotated 45 degrees to the opposite side.

Incision

- A small oblique skin incision is made over the anterior border of the sternocleidomastoid muscle, and the underlying platysma muscle is divided.

Main Dissection

- Dissection deep to the anterior border of the sternocleidomastoid muscle reveals the internal jugular vein and facial vein as it crosses over the carotid bifurcation. The facial vein is ligated and divided to expose the underlying carotid artery. The carotid sheath is opened longitudinally to expose the carotid artery, taking care to avoid the vagus nerve, which usually lies posterior to the common carotid artery. The superior thyroid artery and external carotid arteries are mobilized and controlled, and the carotid sinus nerve, coursing between the external and internal carotid arteries, is infiltrated with 1% lidocaine. The internal carotid artery is then mobilized and controlled. Care is taken to avoid manipulation of the carotid bulb, which might case embolization. The hypoglossal nerve is identified and protected from injury as it crosses the internal carotid artery superior to the bifurcation. The ansa hypoglossi (ansa cervicalis), which arises from the hypoglossal nerve, is mobilized and preserved; small branches of the ansa may be divided for better exposure. The small muscular branch of the external carotid artery that crosses the hypoglossal nerve may be ligated and divided in order to mobilize the hypoglossal nerve medially and improve exposure of the distal internal carotid artery. If the plaque extends well beyond the bifurcation, division of the digastric muscle allows exposure of the distal internal carotid artery to the level of the styloid process. Figure 93-1 shows the regional anatomy.
- After systemic heparinization (100 IU/kg), clamps are applied to the distal internal carotid artery, external carotid artery, superior thyroid artery, and common carotid artery. An arteriotomy is made in the common carotid artery and extended along the lateral wall of the carotid bifurcation into the internal carotid artery, past the plaque. An intraluminal shunt is placed in the distal internal carotid

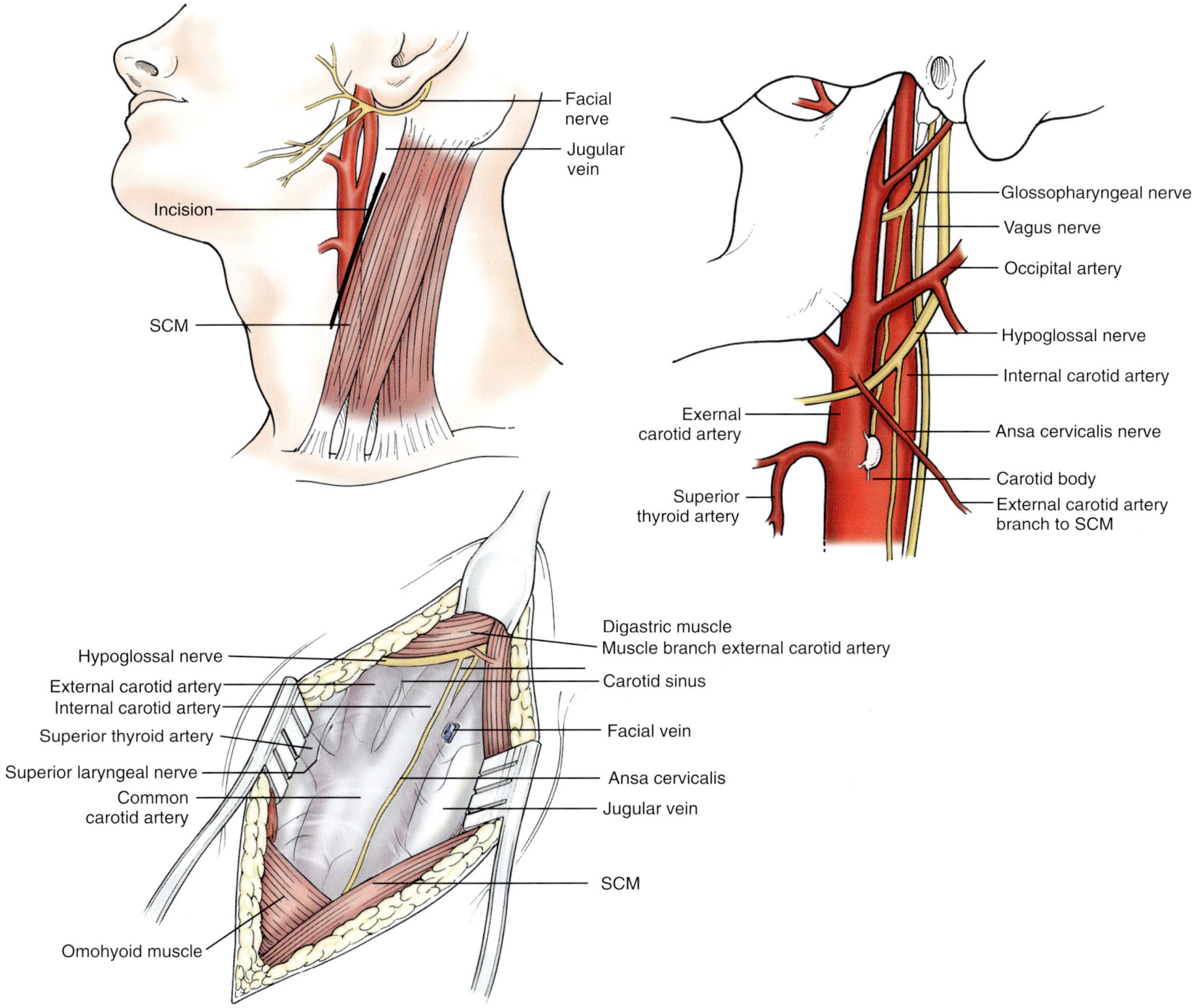

Figure 93-1. *SCM,* Sternocleidomastoid. *Redrawn from Zarins CK, Gewertz BL:* Atlas of vascular surgery, *ed 2, Philadelphia, 2005, Churchill Livingstone, pp 7–23.*

artery and allowed to back bleed. The shunt is then placed in the common carotid artery, and flow is restored to the brain (Fig. 93-2).

- The carotid bifurcation plaque is then removed with an endarterectomy plane just below the external elastic lamina. The proper plane is usually most evident in the thickest portion of the plaque. The proximal common carotid plaque usually requires transection, whereas the distal end of the plaque usually tapers and feathers out in the internal carotid artery. Plaque extension into the external carotid is removed by eversion endarterectomy. The endarterectomized surface is inspected, and residual shreds of circumferentially oriented medial smooth muscle are removed (Fig. 93-3). The distal internal carotid endpoint is carefully inspected, and 7-0 polypropylene tacking sutures are placed to avoid subintimal dissection and development of a distal intimal flap. Tacking sutures may also be necessary

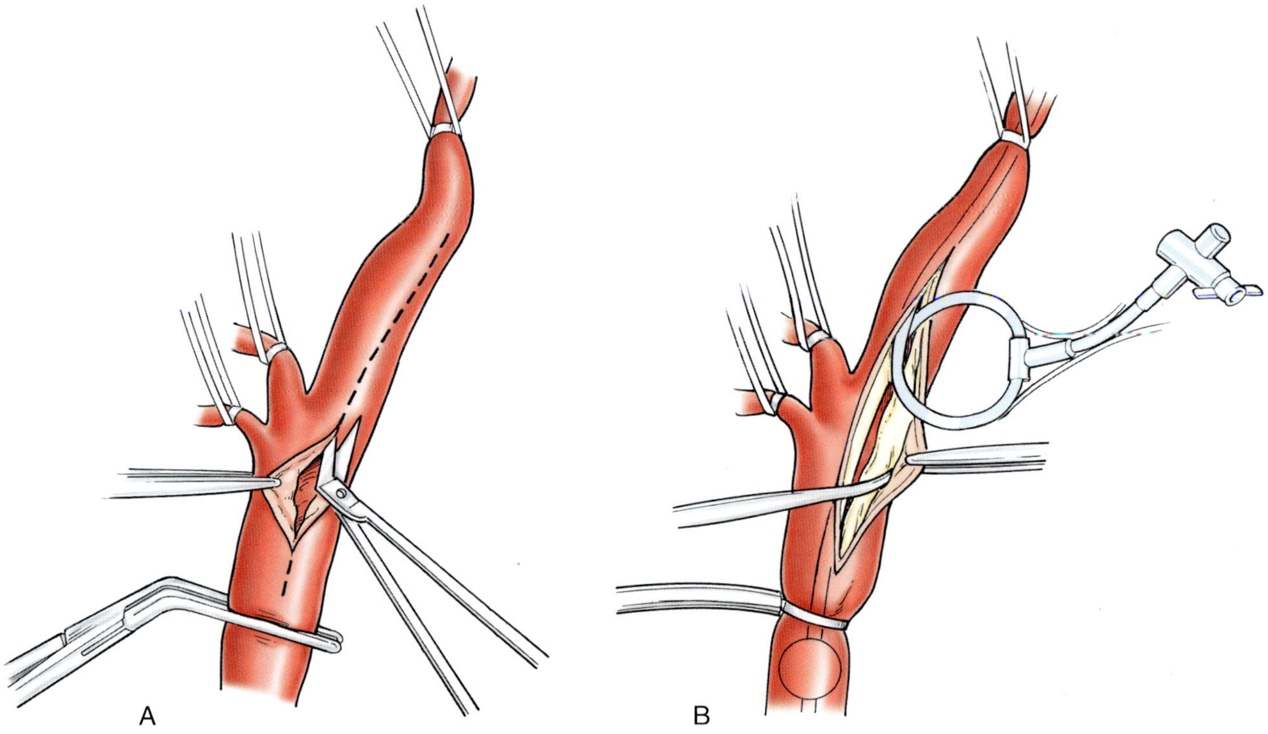

Figure 93-2. *Redrawn from Zarins CK, Gewertz BL: Atlas of vascular surgery, ed 2, Philadelphia, 2005, Churchill Livingstone, pp 7–23.*

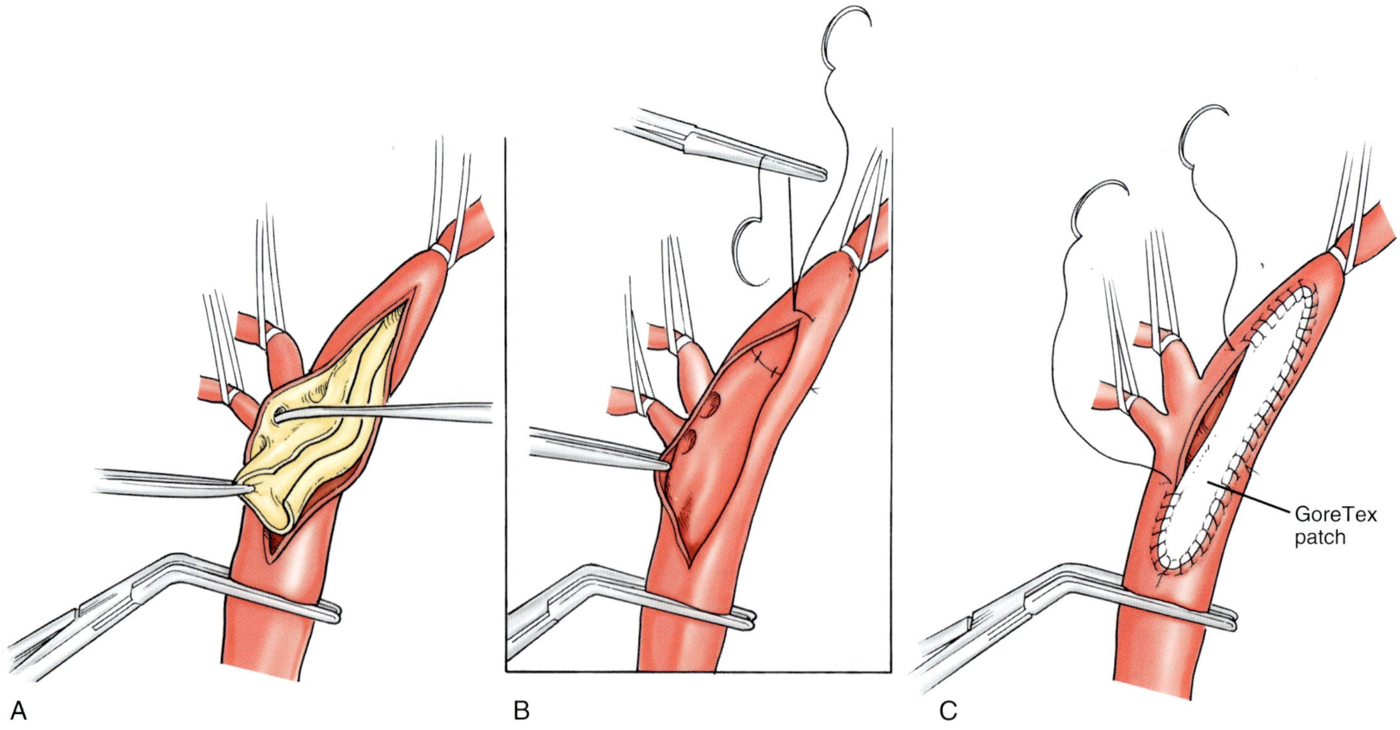

Figure 93-3. *Redrawn from Zarins CK, Gewertz BL: Atlas of vascular surgery, ed 2, Philadelphia, 2005, Churchill Livingstone, pp 7–23.*

to secure the divided proximal common carotid artery intima in order to avoid proximal restenosis, because retrograde and oscillating flow occurs in the carotid bifurcation. The arteriotomy is closed using continuous 6-0 monofilament suture using a prosthetic or vein patch or as a primary closure (see Fig. 93-3). A patch closure is used in most cases. Patch closure is particularly important if the carotid artery is small and in cases where the plaque extends past the carotid bulb into the normal-caliber distal internal carotid artery. Before completion of the suture line, the intraluminal shunt is removed, the carotid branches are allowed to back bleed, and clamps are reapplied to allow completion of the closure. Flow is first restored to the external carotid and then the internal carotid to minimize the risk of embolization.

Closure

- Flow is assessed in the internal and external carotid arteries using Doppler ultrasound, and the suture line and wound are carefully inspected for hemostasis. The platysma muscle is reapproximated, and the skin is closed with subcuticular monofilament suture. Blood pressure is closely monitored to avoid hypertension as the patient wakes from anesthesia.

III. ALTERNATIVE TECHNICAL APPROACHES (PRO/CON) AND PEARLS

Eversion Endarterectomy

- A number of alternative technical approaches to carotid endarterectomy may be used to deal with variations in anatomy and pathology. The primary alternative surgical approach is *eversion endarterectomy*, which involves transection of the proximal carotid bulb and placement of the arteriotomy on the medial rather than lateral aspect of the internal carotid artery. This procedure is particularly useful when there is elongation and coiling of the distal internal carotid artery. The internal carotid arteriotomy is extended past the plaque for a suitable distance, so that when the internal carotid is brought down and anastomosed to the common carotid artery, the internal carotid coil or kink is eliminated (Fig. 93-4).
- After endarterectomy of the carotid plaque using an eversion technique, the distal plaque break point is inspected and the distal intima is tacked with 7-0 suture. The divided internal carotid is

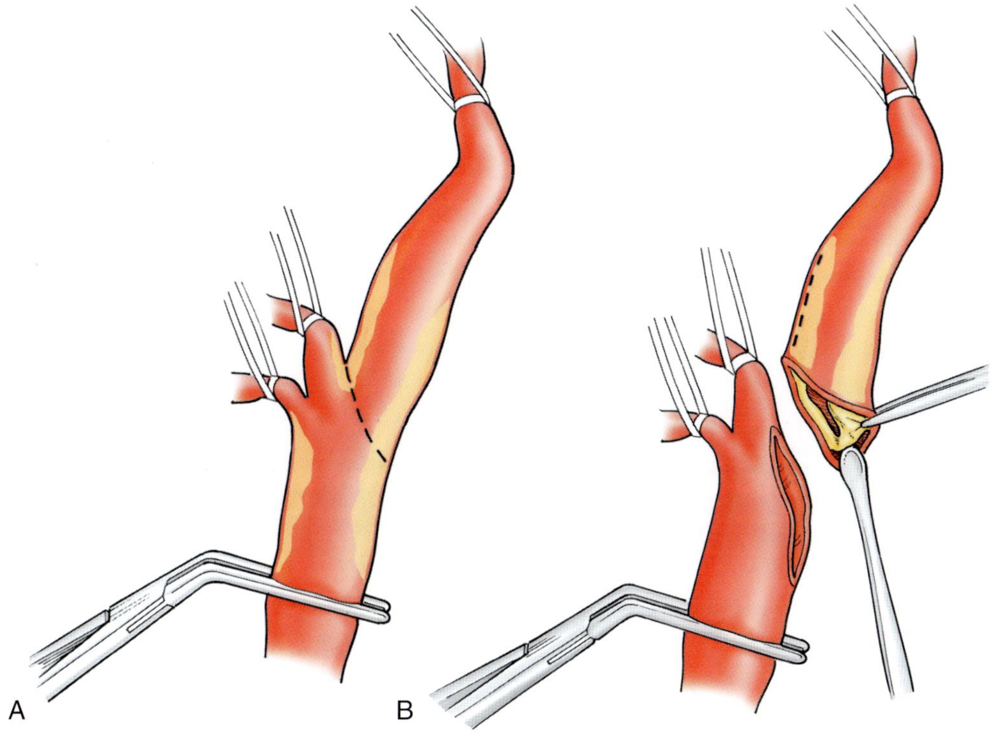

Figure 93-4. *Redrawn from Zarins CK, Gewertz BL:* Atlas of vascular surgery, *ed 2, Philadelphia, 2005, Churchill Livingstone, pp 7–23.*

then anastomosed to the common carotid arteriotomy (Fig. 93-5). No patch is needed, because the endarterectomized carotid bulb serves as a large patch closure of the common carotid. Eversion endarterectomy can readily be performed using an intraluminal shunt, which is inserted as previously described.

Carotid Stenting

- The primary alternative nonsurgical approach to patients with severe carotid stenosis is carotid stenting. Carotid stenting is particularly useful for patients with prior carotid endarterectomy and recurrent carotid stenosis, prior neck radiation or radical neck dissection, hostile neck anatomy, or carotid lesions that are out of reach in the usual operative field. Carotid stenting may result in embolization of plaque material to the brain during manipulation of the plaque with catheters or wires and during balloon angioplasty or stent placement. Therefore distal cerebral protection devices are used during the procedure to trap embolic debris and prevent it from reaching the brain. Carotid stenting with distal cerebral protection is a good alternative for high-risk patients with severe carotid plaque who are not good candidates for surgical treatment (Figs. 93-6 and 93-7).

Pearls

- Technical precision is the key to achieving a low perioperative stroke/death rate. There is no margin for error. The surgeon should not hurry—if needed, a shunt should be used, and adequate time should be taken. The distal intima should be tacked so there is no chance of a distal flap. A patch closure should be used, particularly in women with small carotid arteries. Blood pressure should be monitored—postoperative hypertension can result in reperfusion injury to the brain. Carotid stenting should be considered in patients with scarred or radiated necks, recurrent lesions, or high surgical risk.

IV. SPECIAL POSTOPERATIVE CARE

- Patients should be carefully monitored, with continuous blood pressure and neurologic monitoring. A patient who wakes from anesthesia with a neurologic deficit should be reanesthetized, and patency of the carotid artery should be confirmed with intraoperative duplex ultrasound, intraoperative angiography, or reexploration of the carotid endarterectomy and revision if an abnormality is found.
- Wound hematomas may occur occasionally, especially in patients treated with antiplatelet agents perioperatively. To minimize the incidence of this complication, small suction drains may be placed at the time of wound closure and maintained for the first 24 hours.
- Most patients are discharged from the hospital in 24 to 48 hours.

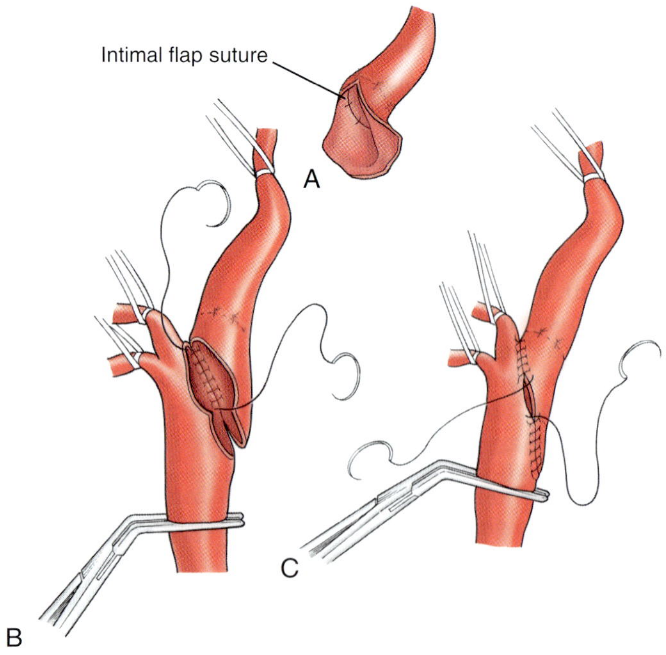

Figure 93-5. *Redrawn from Zarins CK, Gewertz BL:* Atlas of vascular surgery, *ed 2, Philadelphia, 2005, Churchill Livingstone, pp 7–23.*

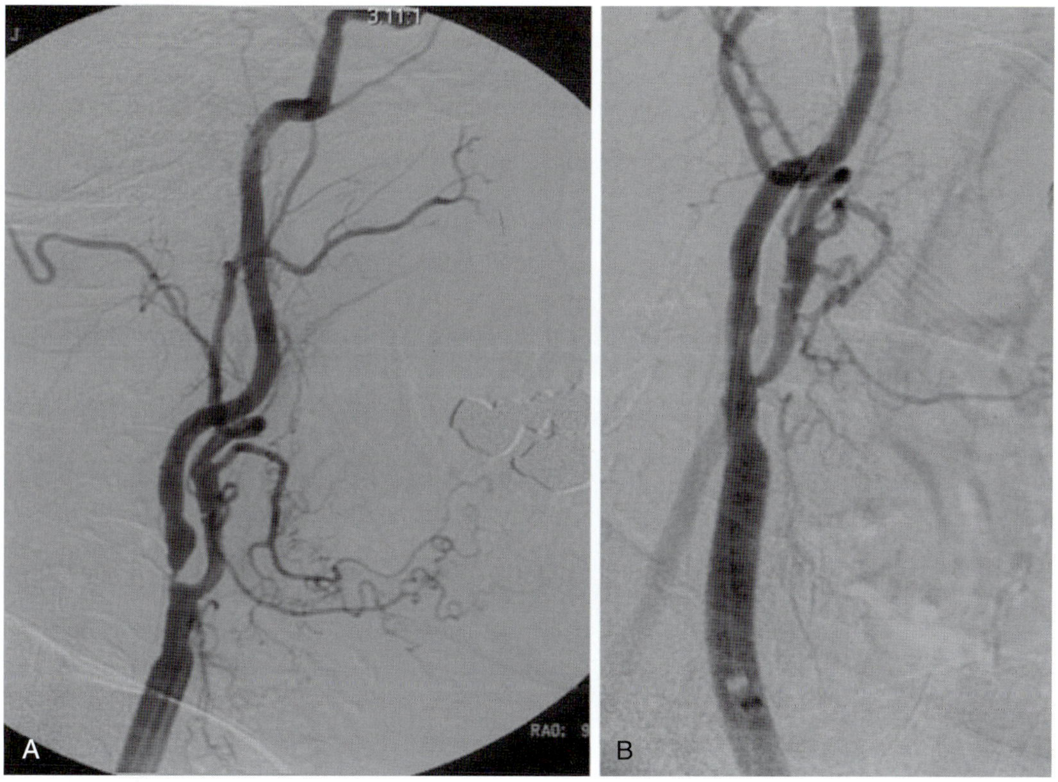

Figure 93-6.

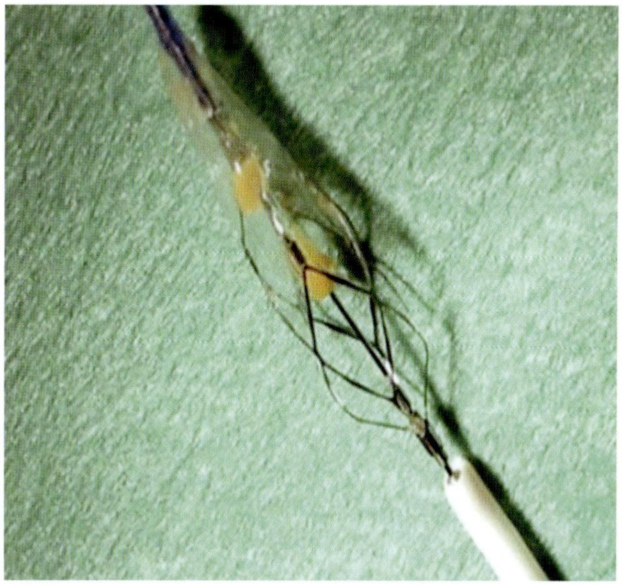

Figure 93-7.

SUGGESTED READINGS

Barrett KM, Brott TG: Carotid artery stenting versus carotid endarterectomy: current status, *Neurol Clin* 24:681–695, 2006.

Biller J, Feinberg WM, Castaldo JE, et al: Guidelines for carotid endarterectomy: a statement for healthcare professionals from a special writing group of the Stroke Council, American Heart Association, *Stroke* 29:554–562, 1998.

Sacco RL, Adams R, Albers G, et al: Guidelines for prevention of stroke in patients with ischemic stroke or transient ischemic attack: a statement for healthcare professionals from the American Heart Association/American Stroke Association Council on Stroke, *Stroke* 37:577–617, 2006.

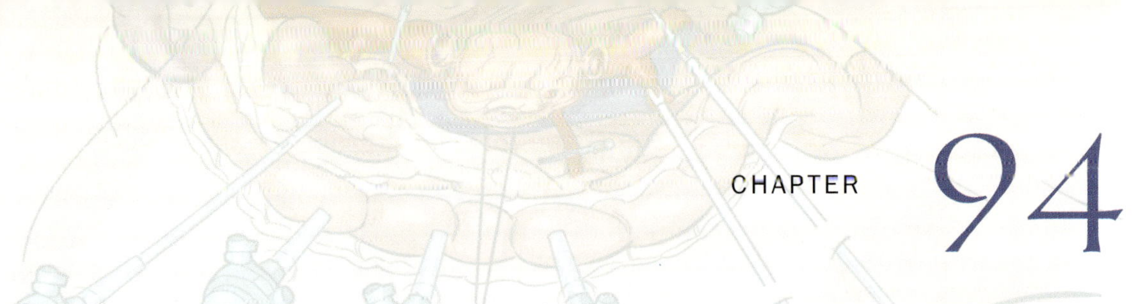

CHAPTER 94

Endovascular Repair of Abdominal Aortic Aneurysms

Jan D. Blankensteijn, MD, PhD, and Leo J. Schultze Kool, MD, PhD

I. SPECIAL PREOPERATIVE PREPARATION

Imaging

- In order to determine whether endovascular repair of an abdominal aortic aneurysm (AAA) is an option, preoperative imaging is essential. Computed tomography (CT) in the form of computed tomography angiography (CTA) is mainly used for this purpose. The scan needs to cover the abdominal aorta and the pelvis (from the level of the diaphragm to the level of the common femoral artery). Contrast agents should be administered with a high flow rate (at least 4 mL/sec) in order to obtain high-contrast visualization of the vessels.
- Multislice spiral CT with 1-mm slices at the level of the renal arteries is recommended.

Measurements

- Dedicated three-dimensional (3D) software programs are now available to ensure precise measurement, which otherwise is not possible. These programs can perform various reconstructions (multiplanar reformats, 3D volume rendering) and include dedicated vessel measurement software with automated central luminal line determination. The following measurements should be made: neck length, angulation, and size; distance of renal artery to aortic bifurcation; diameter of aorta above the aortic bifurcation; length, tortuosity, and diameter of the iliac arteries; and extent of thrombus and calcification at the level of the proximal and distal landing zones (Fig. 94-1).

Device Selection

- The device should be chosen according to the device characteristics and criteria set out in the manufacturer's instructions for use (IFU) for the specific stent-graft system. In case of angulation or a relatively short neck, a system with a suprarenal fixation is recommended.

Training

- The surgeon should become familiar with the system selected for the procedure. He or she should be trained to deal with unexpected problems and should have sufficient extra materials available during the procedure (graft extensions, balloons, stents, etc.).

Patient Preparation

- The patient's clinical condition should be optimized as if an open procedure were planned. Although this is rare, unexpected conversion from an endovascular to an open procedure may be required.
- Because a significant volume of contrast may need to be administered during an endovascular procedure, prehydration and acetylcysteine should be considered in case of renal function impairment.

II. OPERATIVE TECHNIQUE

Position

- The patient is positioned on a radiolucent operating table in either an operating suite that is equipped for angiography (mobile or ceiling-mounted unit) or in an angiography suite that complies with institutional regulations on aseptic environments. At least a 12-inch image intensifier (II) with digital subtraction angiography is required.
- The column of the operating table should be positioned at the feet of the patient to allow freedom of movement of the II from the aortic arch down to the popliteal arteries.
- A urinary catheter is advised. The patient will receive a large amount of fluids to protect the kidneys from contrast nephropathy, and procedures can sometimes take several hours.
- Both groins and abdomen are prepped and draped for full midline laparotomy to allow for unanticipated conversion to conventional open aneurysm surgery.
- Two intravenous lines are placed in the sterile field to act as flush lines.

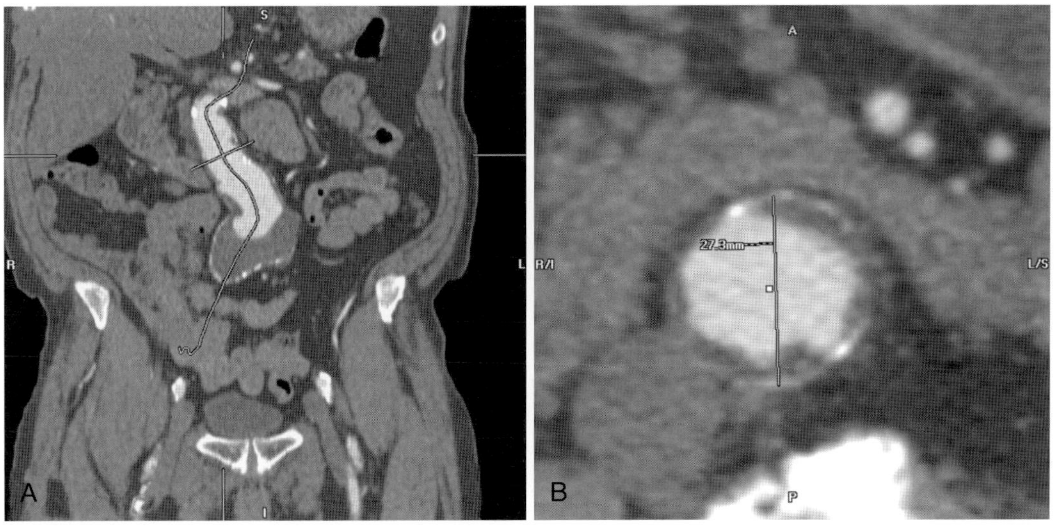

Figure 94-1. **A**, Sagittal multiplanar reconstruction (MPR) with central luminal line. **B**, Corresponding MPR perpendicular to the central luminal line.

- Operating table, instrument tables, image intensifier, surgeon, assistants, scrub nurse, and radiology technician are positioned as shown in Figure 94-2.

Incision

- According to the surgeon's preference, access to both groins is achieved by percutaneous techniques (using closure devices) or conventional open femoral exposure (using a double purse-string suture around the arterial puncture site).
- Systemic heparinization is performed (50 international units of heparin per kilogram).
- A 5-Fr sheath is introduced bilaterally.
- On the ipsilateral side, a 5-Fr Cobra catheter (or similar) loaded with a hydrophilic-coated 0.035-inch guidewire (i.e., Terumo Glidewire) is introduced under fluoroscopy, well into the thoracic aorta.
- The Glidewire is subsequently exchanged with a super-stiff or extra-stiff 0.035-inch guidewire (i.e., Lunderquist) whose tip is then carefully placed in the ascending aorta. To prevent arrhythmia, care should be taken not to enter the left ventricle.
- On the contralateral side, a 5-Fr angiography flush catheter (i.e., pigtail) also loaded with a Glidewire is positioned at the level of the upper edge of lumbar vertebra 1 (L1).
- The introducer system of the selected main endograft body is prepared according to the IFU of the endograft system.

Main Dissection

- After removal of the 5-Fr femoral sheath on the ipsilateral side and digital control of the femoral puncture hole, the introducer system of the main endograft body is advanced over the superstiff guidewire into the ipsilateral iliac artery under careful fluoroscopic control. Care should be taken to maintain traction on the guidewire.
- The superior end of the endograft, still enclosed in the introducer system, is then positioned at the approximate level of the renal arteries, aiming at the position of the pigtail.
- The C-arm is focused on this area, and the II unit is set to maximal magnification. As determined by preoperative 3D-CTA imaging, the C-arm is also angulated (Fig. 94-3) and rotated (Fig. 94-4) to achieve the best projection of the lowermost renal artery and landing zone.

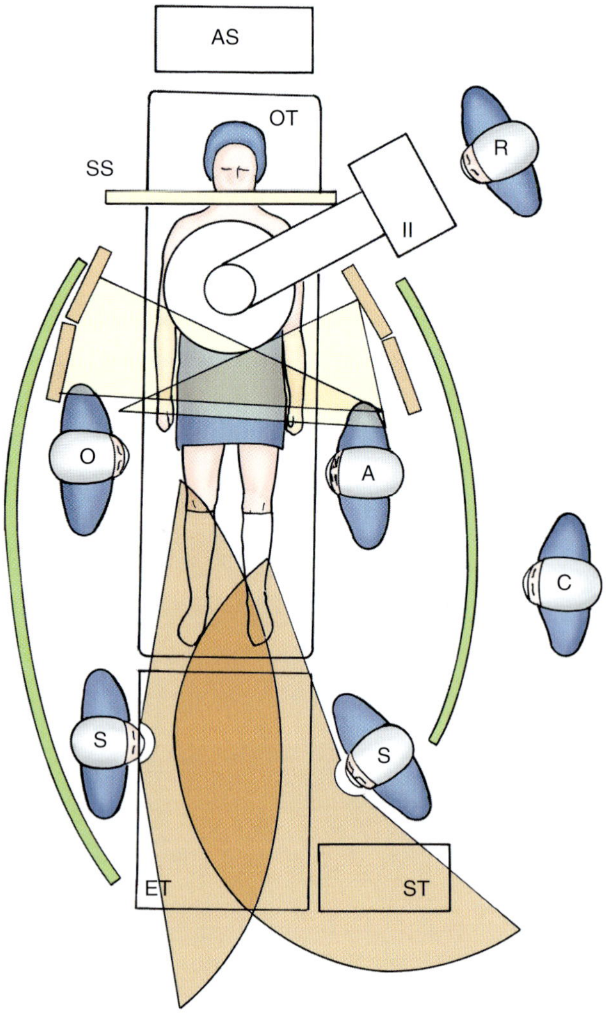

Figure 94-2. *A,* Assistant; *AS,* anesthesiology; *C,* camera operator; *ET,* extension table; *II,* image intensifier; *O,* operator (surgeon); *S,* scrub nurse; *OT,* operating table; *R,* radiology technician; *ST,* surgical instrument table.

- A first aortic-neck subtraction angiogram is performed using 15 to 20 mL of contrast over the pigtail catheter from a pressure injector at an approximate rate of 10 to 15 mL/sec.
- The position of the lower margin of the lowermost renal artery is marked on the II monitor, and the superior edge of the endograft is positioned at the desired landing level using fluoroscopy with optional use of roadmapping (Fig. 94-5).

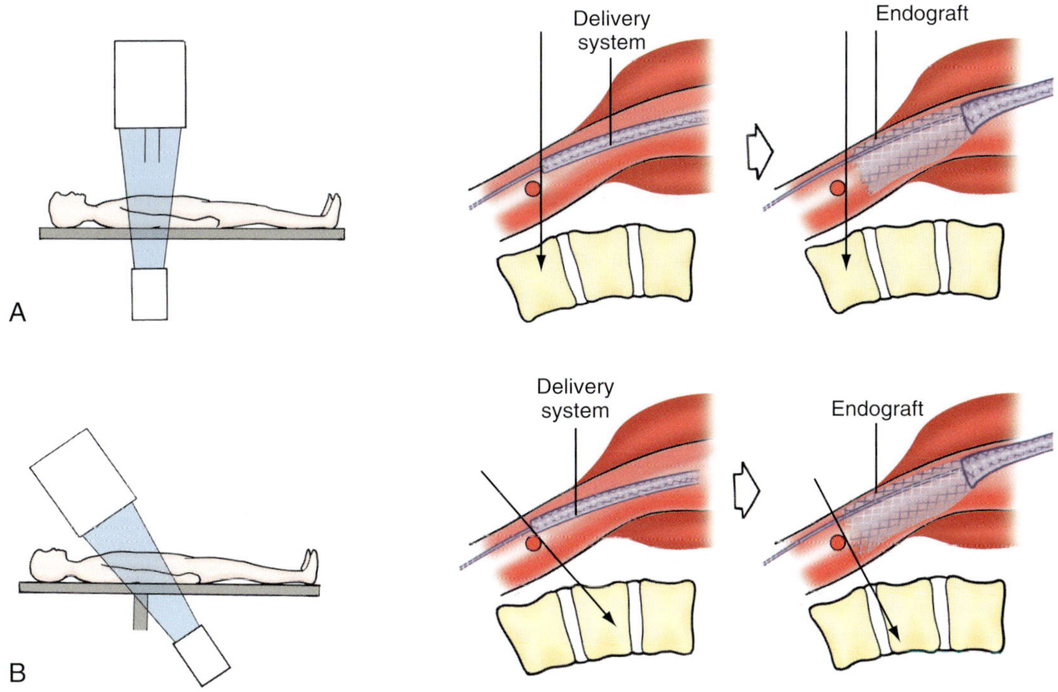

Figure 94-3. *Redrawn from Broeders IA, Blankensteijn JD: A simple technique to improve the accuracy of proximal AAA endograft deployment,* J Endovasc Ther *7:389–393, 2000, Fig. 3.*

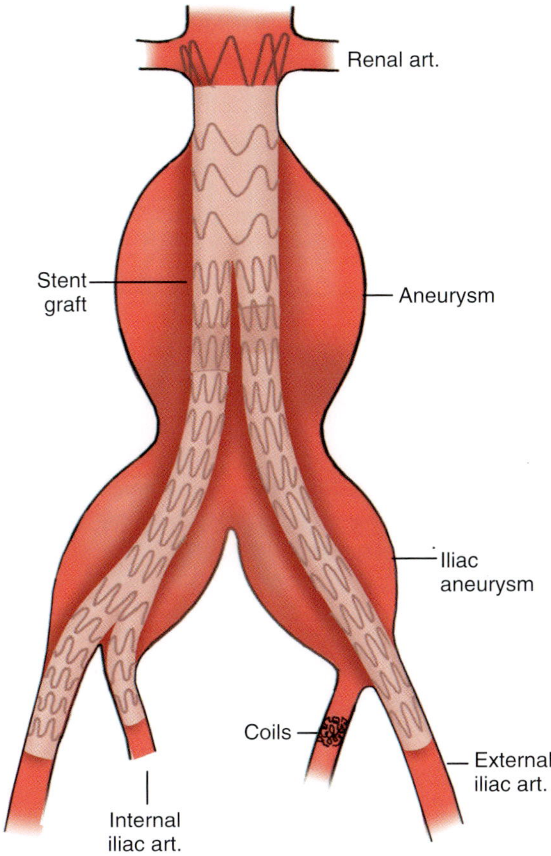

Figure 94-4. *Redrawn from Broeders IA, Blankensteijn JD: A simple technique to improve the accuracy of proximal AAA endograft deployment,* J Endovasc Ther *7:389–393, 2000, Fig. 4.*

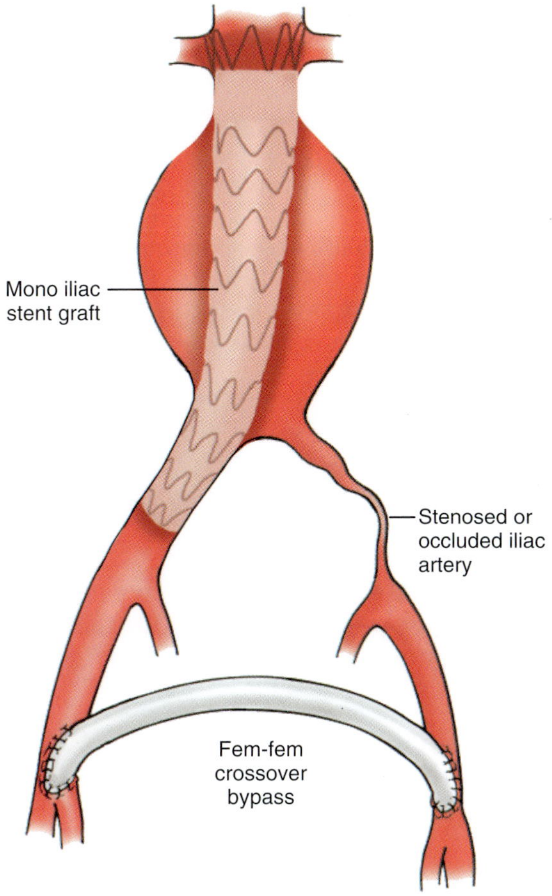

Figure 94-5. Aortic-neck subtraction angiogram showing the position of the lower margin of the lowermost renal artery (*horizontal line*) and the superior edge of the endograft (*E*) at the desired landing level using plain fluoroscopy and roadmap overlay.

- The superior part of the endograft is deployed according to the IFU of the endograft system. Some endograft systems allow for repositioning and/or retrieval of the endograft after an initial, tentative deployment. A second neck angiogram may be appropriate when using these systems.
- After final deployment of the superior end of the endograft, another neck angiogram is performed for a final check of the position of the endograft relative to the renal arteries (Fig. 94-6). At this stage, repositioning is generally not possible, although some tricks, depending on the type of endograft, can correct a few millimeters downstream.
- Deployment of the entire body of the endograft releases the short, contralateral limb, which is subsequently accessed from the contralateral groin using a catheter and Glidewire.
- A radiopaque pigtail catheter is positioned over the newly acquired access to the contralateral limb into the body of the endograft at the level of the infrarenal sealing area. Unrestricted rotation of the pigtail catheter confirms the intraluminal position of the contralateral guidewire.
- A retrograde flush angiogram from the contralateral groin (through the side port of the femoral sheath) is made to find the position of the contralateral internal iliac artery. The position of the C-arm should be adapted to the plane of the iliac bifurcation (usually angulation caudally and rotation to the right for the left iliac arteries and vice versa).
- After confirmation of the required length of the contralateral endograft limb, it is introduced and deployed according to the IFU, with its inferior end as close as possible to the takeoff of the internal iliac artery.
- The remaining portion of the main body and ipsilateral long limb is deployed, and the introducer system is removed from the ipsilateral side.
- A retrograde flush angiogram from the ipsilateral groin (through the side port of the femoral sheath) is made to find the position of the ipsilateral internal iliac artery. The position of the C-arm should again be adapted to the plane of the iliac bifurcation.
- After confirmation of the required length of the ipsilateral endograft limb, it is introduced and deployed according to the IFU, with its inferior ending as close as possible to the takeoff of the internal iliac artery.
- At this stage, the large ipsilateral introducer sheath for the main body can be replaced by a smaller sheath, using the purse-string sutures to maintain hemostasis. This will allow reperfusion of the ipsilateral extremity, perfusion of which may have been limited by the large ipsilateral introducer system. This also increases flow through the ipsilateral endograft limb.
- According to the IFU, balloon dilatation of the sealing zones is performed from both sides, and a completion angiogram is performed (Fig. 94-7). Attention should be focused on the sealing zones, looking for type I endoleaks.

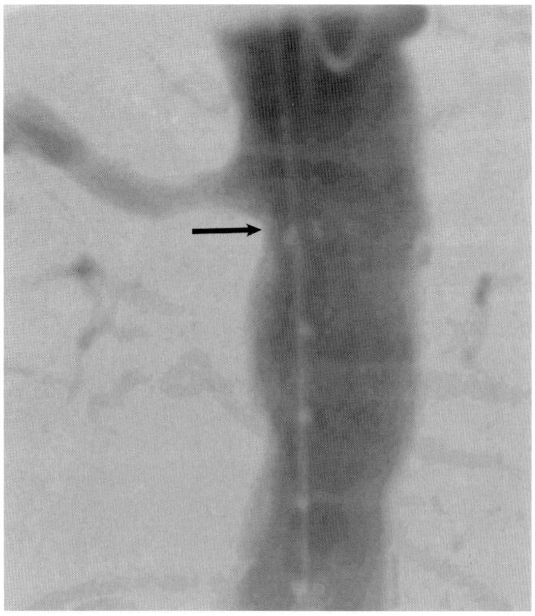

Figure 94-6. Neck angiogram after final deployment of the proximal endograft to show the position of the endograft relative to the renal arteries (*arrow*).

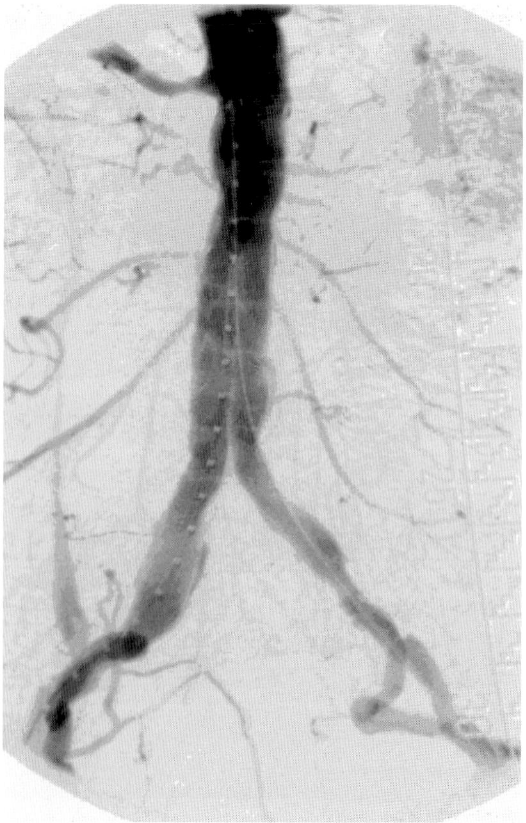

Figure 94-7. Completion angiogram.

Closure

- In case of a percutaneous procedure, the closure devices are deployed according to the IFU. In case of open femoral exposure, the double purse-strings are tied at removal of the sheaths. After rigorous control for hemostasis and unobstructed femoral flow, the fascia and the dermis are carefully approximated in two layers with 2-0 absorbable suture, and the skin is closed with intracutaneous absorbable 4-0 suture. Drains are not placed.

III. ALTERNATIVE TECHNICAL APPROACHES (PRO/CON) AND PEARLS

Unsuitable Anatomy

- If only a small length of neck or no neck is present and the patient is considered unfit for open surgery, the option may exist for fenestrated or branched stent grafts (Zenith; Cook Inc., Bloomington, Ind.). The potential for these techniques is strongly dictated by anatomic issues such as angulation of the neck, quality of access vessels, and location of the renal arteries, mesenteric artery, and celiac trunk. Because both measuring and placement are often technically challenging, the use of these stent grafts should be limited to centers experienced with these techniques.
- If the iliac arteries are also dilated and no landing zone exists, the following endovascular options are available:
  - ▲ If only one common iliac artery is dilated, the surgeon should consider extending the stent graft into the external iliac. To avoid a retrograde leak from the internal iliac artery, this vessel must be occluded preoperatively. Occlusion can be achieved in different ways, by means of coils, glue, or an Amplatzer device. To lower the risk of buttock claudication, it is critical that the occlusion be chosen as proximal as possible to allow good collateral development. In addition, the internal iliac artery occlusion and the stent-graft placement are generally performed in two separate sessions, with an interval of several weeks (staged procedure) (Fig. 94-8, *left*).
  - ▲ If both common iliacs are dilated, the use of an iliac bifurcated stent graft (Zenith) on one side and an extension into the external iliac artery on the other side (see Fig. 94-8, *right*) should be considered.

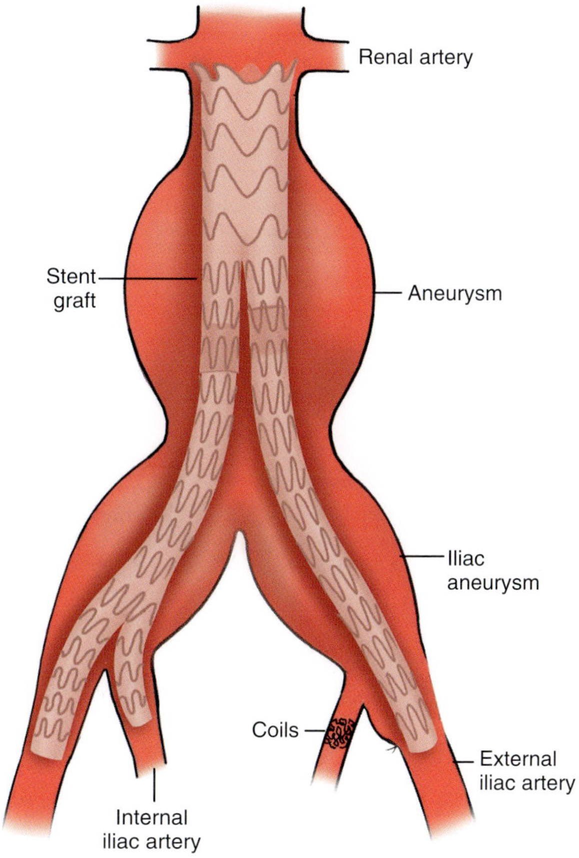

Figure 94-8.

Access

- If the diameter of the access vessels (external iliac or common iliac) is less than the outer diameter of the delivery sheath of the stent graft, several options are available:
  - ▲ Percutaneous transluminal angioplasty of the stenosis can be performed before introduction of the main device.
  - ▲ If stenting is necessary, a self-expandable stent with a closed cell design can be selected to allow smooth passage of the stent graft. Applying stents with an open-cell design may result in struts protruding into the lumen at vessel curvature, causing inability to advance the stent graft.
  - ▲ If the vessel is stenosed and heavily calcified and therefore not amenable to percutaneous transluminal angioplasty and/or stent placement, the contralateral iliac artery may be used for introduction of the main device.
  - ▲ Ultimately, introduction of the main device might be performed through a conduit sutured onto the iliac bifurcation, if the common iliac is of sufficient diameter. After placement of the stent graft, the conduit can be removed or connected distally as a bypass to the common femoral artery. In this case, the conduit can also be used as a landing area for the distal limb of the stent graft.
  - ▲ If one common iliac artery is occluded or severely stenosed and therefore unsuitable, the surgeon should consider using a monoiliac stent graft with a crossover bypass and, if necessary, an occlusion device for the common iliac artery on the contralateral side (Fig. 94-9).

Deployment Issues

- If tortuous vessels are present, it can be difficult or even impossible to advance the stent graft over the stiff wire. This problem could be solved by fixating the guidewire at its proximal end. To do this, a transbrachial or transaxillary puncture is performed, and a 5-Fr sheath is placed. After introduction of a snare wire into the aorta, the super-stiff guidewire is snared and either fixed or pulled out of the sheath (through-and-through wire). Care must be taken not to damage the ostium of the subclavian artery when straightening the wire (femoral and brachial) while introducing the stent graft. A protective catheter introduced over the wire from the proximal end (brachial or axillary) will afford additional protection.

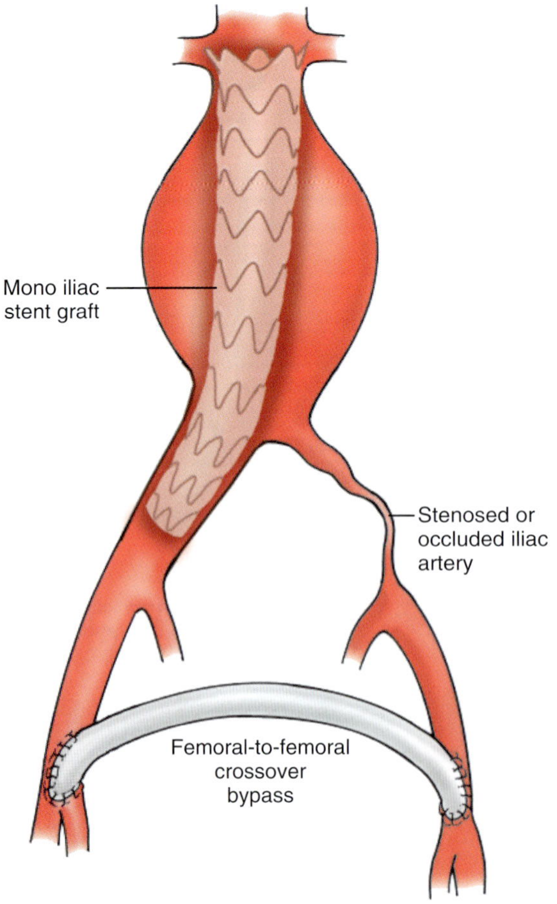

Figure 94-9.

- If the contralateral limb of the main body of a device cannot be catheterized, an option is to use the ipsilateral limb to place a guidewire over the bifurcation of the main body, using a reverse curved catheter or a pigtail catheter. Subsequently, the guidewire is snared from the contralateral side and brought out by the contralateral sheath. Next, a catheter is advanced over the wire into the contralateral leg. The wire is then exchanged for a stiffer wire for introduction of the stent-graft leg.

Postdeployment Issues

- If a proximal endoleak is noted on the completion angiogram, the following actions can be taken. If the stent graft has been placed too low, placement of an additional cuff (see IFU for correct sizing) is advised. If the position is correct, placement of a giant bare balloon-expandable stent (Palmaz) is advised to try to force the stent graft against the aortic wall.
- If covering of the renals is noted on the completion angiogram, one option is to pull down the stent graft by means of a crossover wire over the stent-graft bifurcation. This maneuver should be performed with great care in order to avoid dislodging the stent graft. The other option is to insert stents into the renal arteries. Catheterization of the renal arteries alongside the stent graft is easiest from a brachial or axillary approach.
- If a kink in a stent-graft leg is noted on the completion angiogram, consider placing a stent within the graft to straighten out the leg in order to prevent early thrombosis.

IV. SPECIAL POSTOPERATIVE CARE

- Specific intraoperative complications that may be encountered with endovascular AAA repair are injury to access arteries, particularly the common femoral artery and the external iliac artery; occlusion of side branches, particularly the renal artery and the internal iliac arteries; and distal embolization. Type I (attachment site) and type III (modular connection) endoleaks should be dealt with before completing the procedure.
- Specific immediate postoperative complications that may be encountered with endovascular AAA repair are infection, hematoma, neuropathic pain, and wound disruption. With the percutaneous approach, infection of the closure device (and its sutures), hematoma, and neuropathic pain have also been described. Renal function should be checked, because contrast nephropathy may follow the administration of large amounts of contrast material or in cases of preexisting renal dysfunction.
- Specific delayed postoperative complications that may be encountered with endovascular AAA repair are stent-graft migration with or without type I endoleak, side-branch (type II) endoleak with or without aneurysm growth, component separation (type III endoleak), structural failure (metal failure or graft material tears), and endograft infection.
- There is no objection to immediate mobilization and early ambulation.
- Venous access is maintained until the postoperative CT scan is done, usually on the first postoperative day when renal function is normal. Otherwise, the postoperative CT scan can be postponed until after 3 to 4 weeks.

SUGGESTED READINGS

Broeders IA, Blankensteijn JD: A simple technique to improve the accuracy of proximal AAA endograft deployment, *J Endovasc Ther* 7:389–393, 2000.

Greenhalgh RM, Brown LC, Kwong GP, et al: EVAR trial participants: Comparison of endovascular aneurysm repair with open repair in patients with abdominal aortic aneurysm (EVAR trial 1), 30-day operative mortality results: randomised controlled trial, *Lancet* 364:843–848, 2004.

Prinssen M, Verhoeven EL, Buth J, et al; Dutch Randomized Endovascular Aneurysm Management (DREAM) Trial Group: A randomized trial comparing conventional and endovascular repair of abdominal aortic aneurysms, *N Engl J Med* 351:1607–1618, 2004.

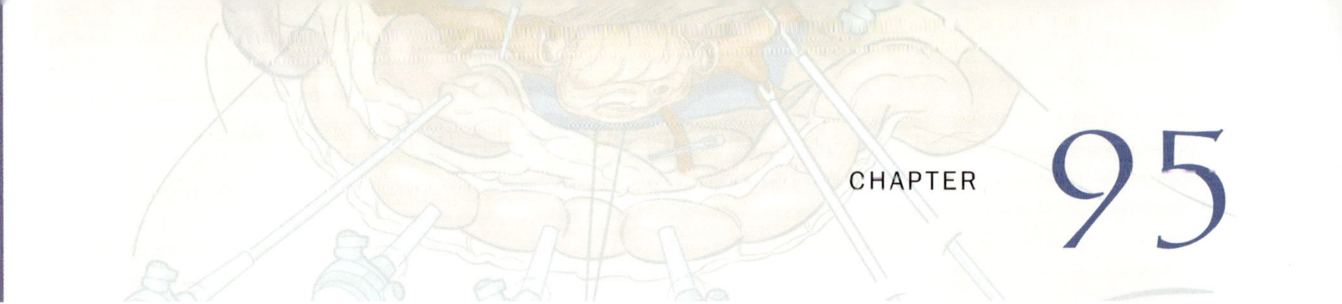

CHAPTER 95

Laparoscopic Abdominal Aortic Aneurysm Repair

Marc Coggia, MD, and Olivier Goëau-Brissonnière, MD, PhD

- Open direct repair (ODR) is still considered the most reliable and durable technique to treat severe aortoiliac occlusive disease (AIOD) and abdominal aortic aneurysms (AAAs). Postoperative mortality is less than 5%, and long-term results are excellent. However, systemic morbidity of ODR remains substantial. Complications are related to the surgical approach in about 30% of cases. The concept of minimally invasive techniques, either endovascular or laparoscopic, is to decrease the operative trauma of ODR. Endovascular techniques have been increasingly used since 1990. Their benefits in terms of postoperative morbidity and mortality have been demonstrated, and they are now considered the treatment of choice for the majority of AIOD. For AAA, uncertainties remain as to the mid- and long-term benefit of endovascular repair in patients suitable for ODR.
- Laparoscopy recently entered the field of vascular surgery. As in other specialties, its concept is to decrease operative trauma, avoiding large abdominal or lumbar incisions. Potential benefits of laparoscopy are faster recovery, reduced complaint of pain, and decreased incidence of abdominal, intestinal, and pulmonary complications. In the field of minimally invasive aortic surgery, laparoscopy has a major advantage over endovascular techniques, which is the performance of a proven and durable surgical technique. In addition, we can expect excellent long-term results similar to those for ODR. However, other than some pioneers, few vascular teams have entered this new field for aortic surgery, especially for AAA repair. The specific difficulties of aortic surgery have discouraged vascular surgeons because most of them lack laparoscopy skills. Laparoscopic aortic surgery is in fact feasible with excellent results, once training and the learning curve are overcome.

I. SPECIAL PREOPERATIVE PREPARATION

Laparoscopic Training

- Training to gain laparoscopic skills is of particular importance for vascular surgeons because they lack education and experience in laparoscopic surgery. It is important to remember that performing anastomosis under videoscopy is probably the most difficult step during general, urologic, or vascular surgery. An additional challenge in vascular surgery is that the time required for laparoscopic anastomosis increases aortic clamping time, with subsequent lower limb ischemia and increased cardiac afterload. Moreover, aortoprosthetic anastomosis requires the application of strict technical principles to avoid immediate leakage and to ensure strength, patency, and durability. This technical challenge has discouraged the majority of vascular surgeons. Some of them are expecting the development of anastomotic devices with either clips or staples. Use of such devices is still under evaluation, with limits according to the properties of aortic walls, either brittle or calcified. Moreover, anastomotic devices are useful only for the performance of laparoscopic anastomosis. It is important to remember that a laparoscopic aortic procedure cannot be confined to aortoprosthetic anastomosis. Other important steps require laparoscopic skills, especially exposure of the aorta and preparation of anastomotic sites.

- Training in laparoscopic sutures consists of a thorough training in all laparoscopic skills. The materials needed are listed in Box 95-1.
- Training consists of performing end-to-end and/or end-to-side anastomoses similar to those for human procedures and with the same preparation of stitches. Such training is possible in the office, in the operating room, or at home. We recommend daily training for at least 3 months before the first human procedure. Once expertise is gained, it is possible to proceed with discontinuous training, but this depends on the surgeon's skills. Long-term training is essential because vascular surgeons do not perform simple weekly procedures such as cholecystectomy to maintain their level of expertise.
- Training on animals or cadavers is also important to gain expertise in all steps of laparoscopic aortic procedures. Such training is usually organized during courses and workshops. We encourage vascular surgeons to attend such courses.

Laparoscopic Approaches to the Abdominal Aorta

- Laparoscopic approaches to the abdominal aorta use the same anatomic landmarks and surgical dissection planes as open surgery. These approaches, either transperitoneal or retroperitoneal, are well known by vascular surgeons. Four different laparoscopic approaches have been described: transperitoneal retrocolic (TPRC), transperitoneal retrorenal (TPRR), transperitoneal direct (TPD), and retroperitoneal (RP). The main differences among the approaches consist of the technical tools used to achieve and maintain a stable aortic exposure.

II. OPERATIVE TECHNIQUE: TRANSPERITONEAL APPROACHES

Position

- For transperitoneal approaches, we use always the 80-degree right lateral decubitus (RLD) position. The patient is placed in the dorsal decubitus position with an inflatable pillow (Pelvic-Tilt, O.R. Comfort, Glen Ridge, N.J.) placed behind the left flank. Insufflation of the pillow gives a 50- to 60-degree rotation of the abdomen. A maximal right rotation of the operating table affords an

BOX 95-1. Materials Needed for Training in Laparoscopic Surgery

- Laparoscope, camera, monitor, and light; a compact system is manufactured by Karl Storz (Medi Pack), and a homemade video system with a simple camcorder is also usable.
- Needle holder, grasping forceps, and scissors
- Pelvitrainer with the same ergonomics as in human aortic procedures
- Prostheses and stitches

abdominal slope of 80 degrees (Figs. 95-1 and 95-2, *A* and *B*). The surgeon faces the patient's abdomen and is not bothered by orientation of surgical instruments. The camera assistant stands in front of the surgeon, and the second assistant stands to the surgeon's right (see Fig. 95-1).

Trocar Placement

- We usually use a blind technique to create the pneumoperitoneum. A Veress needle is introduced 3 cm below the costal margin on the left midclavicular line, and pneumoperitoneum is insufflated up to 14 mm Hg. If there are previous abdominal scars, the first port is positioned using an open technique on the left anterior axillary line just below the costal margin. This port is used to create the pneumoperitoneum and to introduce the endoscope (Storz-France SA, Paris). A drawback of the open technique is that the port site moves downward and medially during insufflation of the pneumoperitoneum.

Main Dissection

Transperitoneal Retrocolic Approach

- Positioning of ports depends on the type of lesion. We use only 10-mm ports because of the need for large instruments. For AIOD, port 1 is positioned 3 cm below the costal margin on the anterior axillary

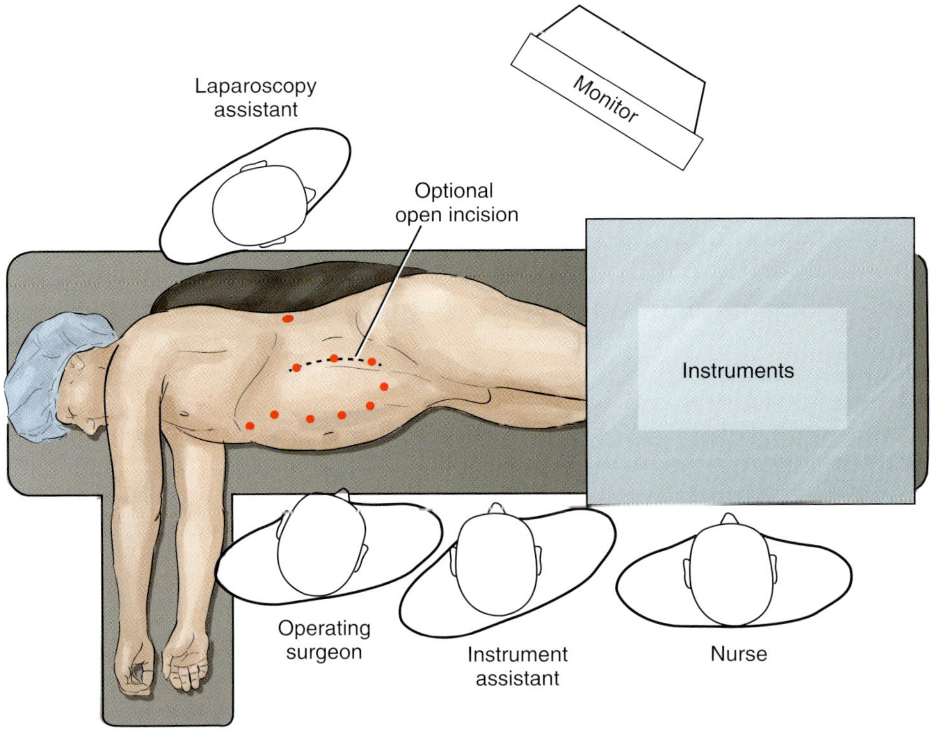

Figure 95-1.

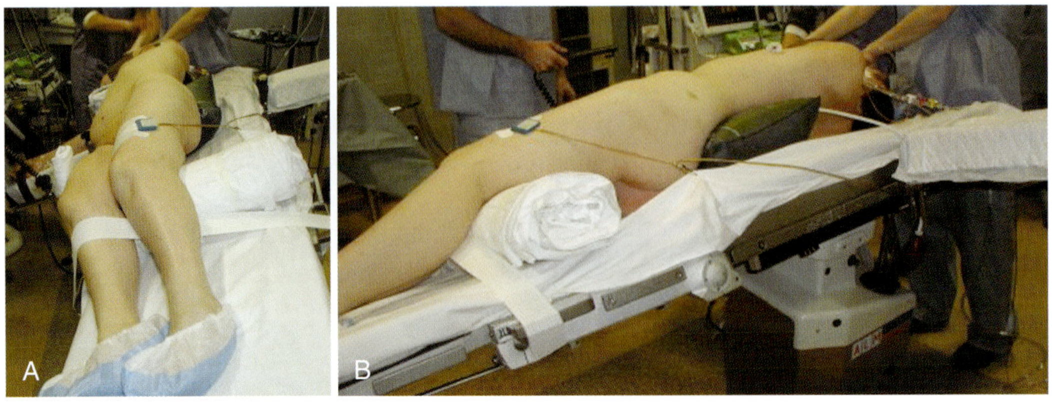

Figure 95-2. Operative views showing the positioning of the patient in right lateral decubitus position with the use of an inflatable pillow.

line. Ports 2 and 3, about 8 cm distant, are placed at the supraumbilical and left paramedian level to insert surgical instruments. Port 4 is positioned below the navel to introduce assistant instruments and the distal aortic clamp. Port 5 is placed in the left lower abdomen to insert assistant instruments. Finally, port 6 is placed under the xiphoid. It has two functions: (1) at the beginning of the procedure, an endoretractor (Endoretract II, Autosuture, Elancourt, France) is introduced through this port to maintain the left mesocolon; and (2) during aortic repair, this port is used to introduce the proximal aortic clamp. For AAA repair, port 1 is placed just below the costal margin, especially if the aortic neck is short or angulated. Just before this port is introduced, abdominal pressure is increased to 20 mm Hg in order to increase parietal strength and avoid aortic injury. Once the first port is placed, pneumoperitoneum pressure is decreased to 14 mm Hg. An additional port (port 7) is introduced between ports 1 and 5 to insert instruments and/or an endoscope, especially if distal aortic or common iliac anastomoses are needed.

- A peritoneal incision is made in the left paracolic gutter up to the splenic flexure (Fig. 95-3). By elevating and displacing the left colon, the avascular plane of the Toldt fascia is entered and developed medially to reach the internal edge of the kidney. The left genital vein provides an interesting landmark and leads to the left renal vein.
- Once the left renal vein is visualized, we always perform two steps to maintain the exposure: (1) an endoretractor (Endoretract II) is positioned through port 7 to maintain the left mesocolon and (2) we place a stitch in the Gerota fascia and pull it out through the left abdominal wall. Traction on this stitch allows retraction of the kidney and opens the operative field in front of the preaortic ganglia (Fig. 95-4). Because of the RLD position, the small bowel and left mesocolon drop to the right part of the abdomen. Dissection of the aorta is then conducted cranially to the left renal artery

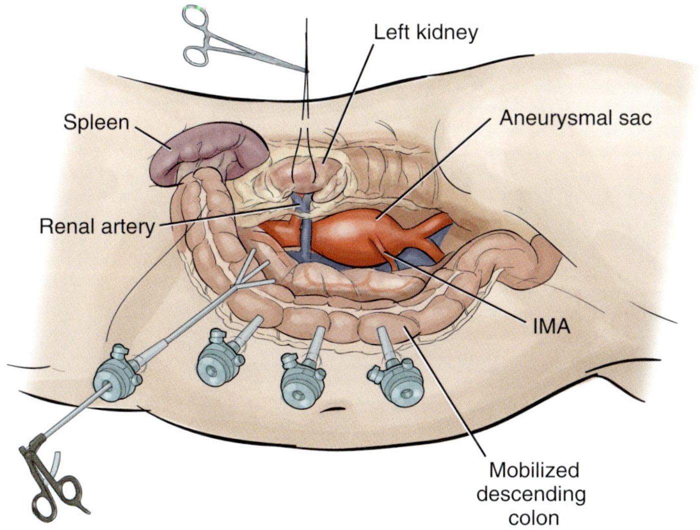

Figure 95-3. *IMA,* Inferior mesenteric artery.

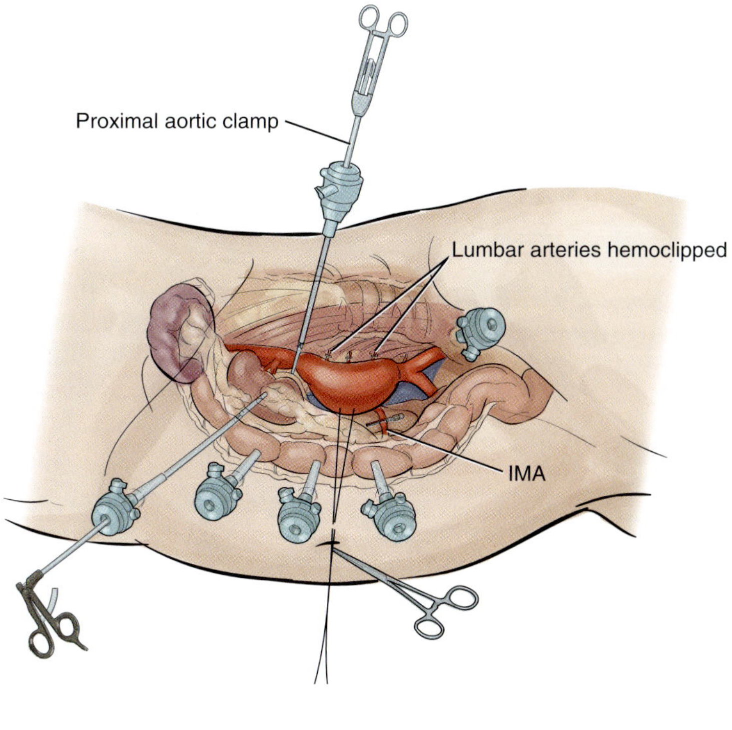

Figure 95-4. *IMA,* Inferior mesenteric artery.

and caudally to the left iliac artery. The inferior mesenteric artery (IMA) is dissected and leads toward the mesocolon.

- The last step is exposure of the right common iliac artery, either to prepare the tunneling of a graft limb or to perform an anastomosis. For this step, we always perform the same motions. The assistant introduces the endoretractor through port 4 and the suction device through port 5, then points these two instruments toward the common iliac artery and retracts the left mesocolon. The surgeon conducts the dissection as far as possible with this help, if possible until crossing the right ureter. Once dissection is completed, exposure of the aorta is maintained by traction on additional stitches placed in the paraaortic fat (Fig. 95-5).
- After exposure is achieved, the patient is returned to the dorsal decubitus position. The pillow is deflated, and the operating table is rotated to the left, which allows a conventional approach to the iliac or femoral arteries if needed (Fig. 95-6).

Transperitoneal Retrorenal Approach

- Positioning of ports is quite similar to the TPRC approach (Fig. 95-7). Port 1 is positioned 2 cm medially from the line of the anterosuperior iliac spine. Other ports are positioned as in the TPRC approach,

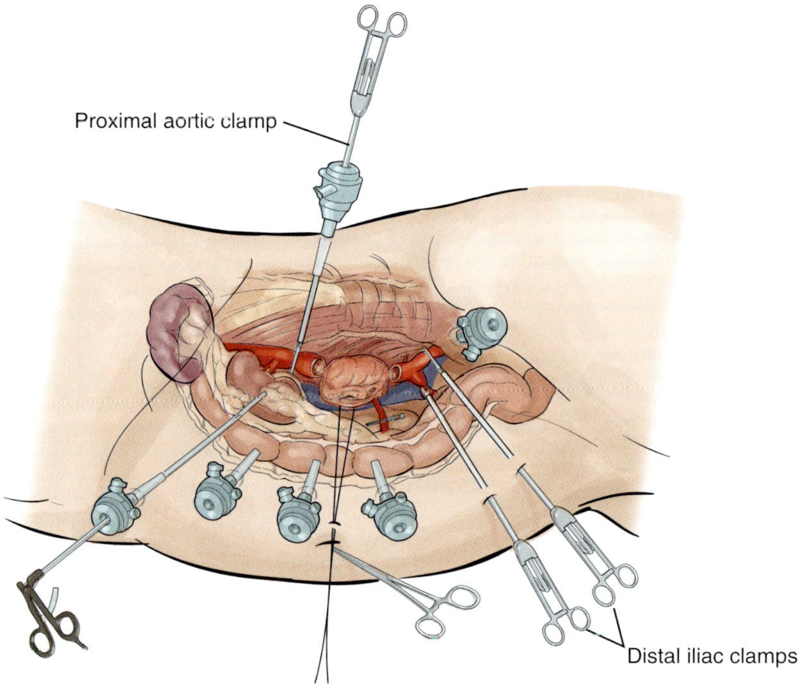

Figure 95-5.

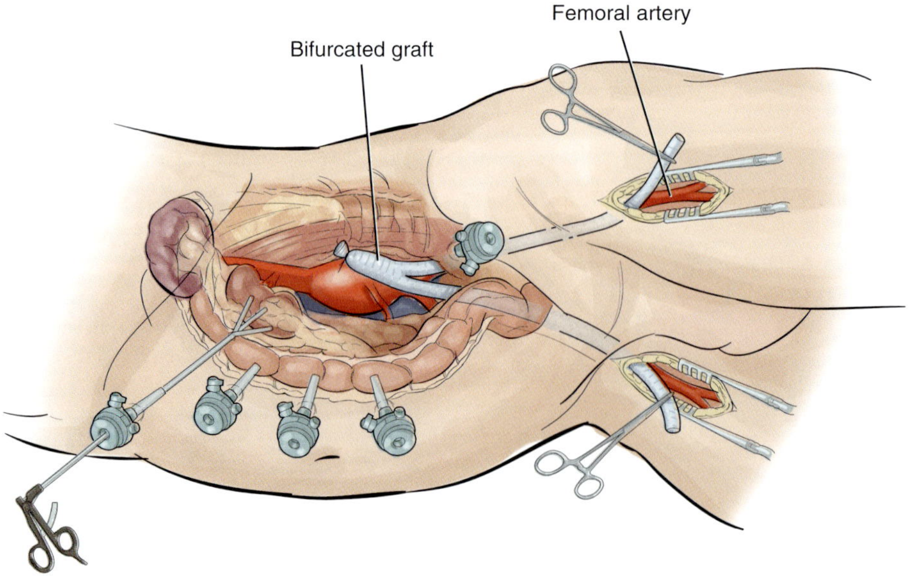

Figure 95-6.

but slightly translated laterally. We do not place port 6 at the beginning of the procedure, because we wait for positioning of the spleen after completion of the medioviscera rotation.

- A peritoneal incision is made in the left paracolic gutter up to the diaphragm (see Fig. 95-7). We enter the retroperitoneal plane in the iliac fossa until the left ureter and iliac artery are visualized.
- Left retrorenal dissection is conducted cranially and medially from the psoas muscle after incision of the retrorenal fascia. We perform a complete rather than a partial right medial visceral rotation in order to avoid effraction of the spleen during the retraction of viscera. Moreover, it allows a larger working space. Because of the RLD, the small bowel, left mesocolon, left kidney, and spleen drop into the right side of the abdomen. We place a stitch in the left perirenal fat and pull it out through the right abdominal wall. This allows the viscera to be maintained.
- Dissection of the aorta is conducted cranially from the left iliac to the left renal artery. We section the left lumbar splanchnic nerve, which lies over the left side of the aorta. Just below the left renal artery, the venous reno-azygo-lumbar trunk often crosses the left side of the aorta. Section of this trunk provides (1) complete retraction of the kidney without risk of bleeding and (2) dissection of the juxtarenal aorta. If necessary, we develop the dissection cranially beyond the left renal artery up to the left crus of the diaphragm. This section exposes the aortic visceral segment. Exposure of the right iliac artery is conducted as in a TPRC approach.
- After the dissection is achieved, subcostal port 6 is placed, taking care to avoid injuring the spleen. We introduce an endoretractor (Endoretract II) through this port to maintain the left kidney. The tip of the retractor is placed just below the left renal artery and allows a stable exposure of the juxtarenal aorta.

Transperitoneal Direct Approach

- Positioning of ports is similar to that in the TPRC approach. After abdominal exploration, the transverse mesocolon is elevated with a stitch pulled out through the left subcostal abdominal wall. A longitudinal incision of the retroperitoneum overlying the aortic anterior wall is made, just to the left of the mesentery. This incision is conducted down to the iliac arteries. Another stitch is placed on the posterior peritoneum, near the duodenum, and pulled out through the right abdominal wall. If needed, an additional port is used to maintain the small bowel with a retractor (Endoretract II) introduced in the left flank or in the pelvis, on the right paramedian line. Intestinal retractors could also be used to maintain the small bowel. The aortic periadventitial plane is freed, and circumferential aortic dissection is obtained from iliac arteries up to the left renal vein.
- After aortoiliac dissection is achieved, the pillow is deflated and the operating table is rotated to the left, which enables conventional approaches to the femoral arteries. The patient is then returned to the RLD position for aortoiliac laparoscopic reconstruction.

III. OPERATIVE TECHNIQUE: RETROPERITONEOSCOPIC APPROACH

Position

- The patient is under general anesthesia and placed in a dorsal decubitus position with an inflatable pillow (Pelvic-Tilt) behind the left flank, which gives a 30-degree rotation of the abdomen. The surgeon stands at the patient's left side, and the video monitor is viewed distally on the right side.

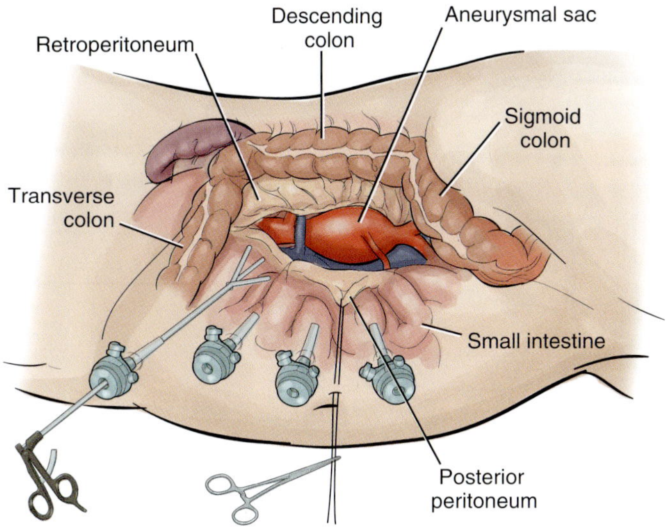

Figure 95-7.

Trocar Placement

- The port used to introduce the 45-degree endoscope (Storz-France) is positioned using an open technique halfway between the costal margin and the anterosuperior iliac spine. A retroperitoneal blunt dissection is first performed to prepare the working space. After insufflation, the dissection is started with the endoscope. The psoas muscle is the first anatomic landmark. The left kidney is identified. Two operator ports are placed in the left flank, between the iliac crest and the rib cage. Two 10-mm ports are inserted in the left iliac fossa for assistant instrumentation and a retractor (Fig. 95-8).

Main Dissection

- Dissection is conducted after incision of the left retrorenal fascia. The kidney is freed on its lower pole and retracted cephalad and medially. The left common iliac artery is visualized. The infrarenal aorta is then cranially dissected until the left renal artery. The venous reno-azygo-lumbar trunk is sectioned, which provides exposure of the juxtarenal aorta. The peritoneal sac and left kidney are maintained with a retractor (Endoretract II). The anterior side of the right common iliac artery is dissected over 3 to 5 cm if needed. As in conventional surgery, ligation of an occluded IMA can expand the exposure of the right common iliac artery. After the dissection is achieved, the pillow is deflated, which allows a conventional approach to the femoral arteries if needed.

IV. OPERATIVE TECHNIQUE: LAPAROSCOPIC AORTIC REPAIR

- Laparoscopic aortic repair is the second step of the procedure. Two main challenges during this step are aortic clamping time and blood loss. We describe AAA repair through a TPRR approach, with tube graft implantation as the gold standard technique. We then discuss specific technical tips and tricks using other laparoscopic approaches.
- Before aortic repair, we prepare specific stitches for anastomoses. We prepare two types of stitches using 3-0 or 4-0 Prolene. Stitches for running sutures are between 18 cm and 22 cm in length and knotted on 10 × 10 mm Teflon or prosthetic pledgets. Stitches for single sutures are between 8 cm and 12 cm and knotted on small pledgets.

Main Dissection

Tube Graft Implantation

- Once the aortic approach is stable, three steps are prepared before clamping: (1) A stitch is placed through the right abdominal wall and the needle is left free in the iliac fossa. It will be used for

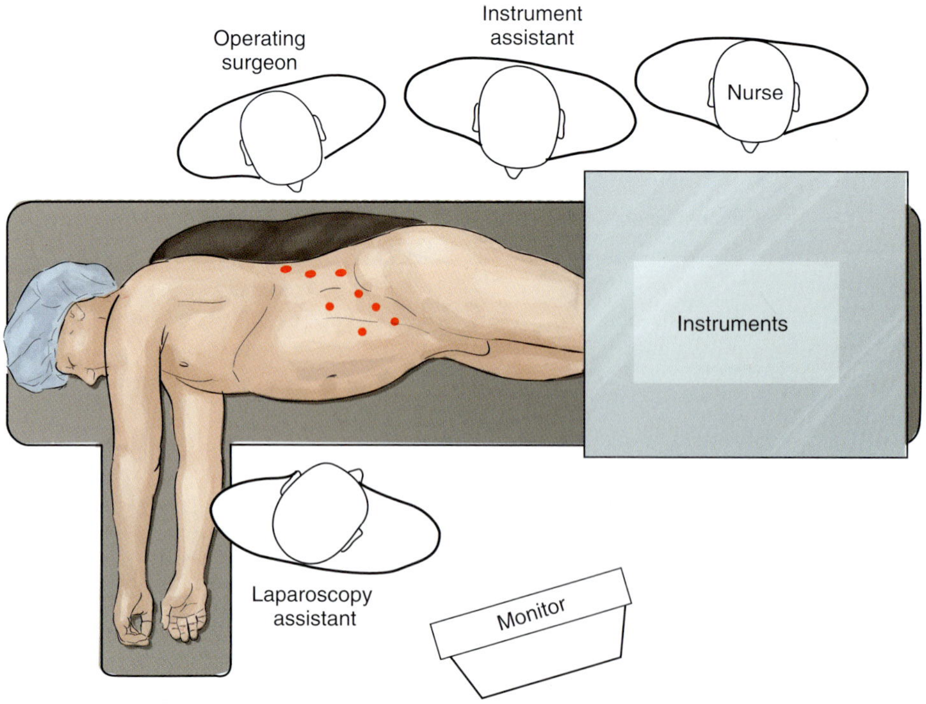

Figure 95-8. Basic operating room setup for retroperitoneoscopic approach of the abdominal aorta.

retraction of the aneurysmal sac. (2) Iliac clamps are introduced percutaneously in the left iliac fossa. Finally, (3) a conventional Dacron graft (Gelweave or Gelsoft Plus, Vascutek-Terumo, Inchinnan, Scotland) is prepared for an end-to-end anastomosis, and the body of the graft is secured at its distal extremity with a stitch.

- Once these steps are achieved, a proximal laparoscopic clamp (Storz-France) is positioned through either subcostal port 6 or an additional port placed in the left flank (see Fig. 95-5).
- We place the stitch into the aneurysmal sac and pull it out through the right abdominal wall. Traction on this stitch allows retraction of the aneurysmal sac on the right for the dissection of the left and posterior side of the aorta. We control the lumbar and medial sacral arteries with hemoclips (Ligaclip ERCA, Ethicon Endo-Surgery, Brussels) before opening the aneurysmal sac (see Fig. 95-5). A clip or a bulldog clamp occludes the IMA. Iliac clamping is performed with the laparoscopic clamps previously placed in the left iliac fossa. Laparoscopic detachable clamps (Storz-France) could also be used, but they do not allow simple maneuvers for clamping and unclamping, especially during retrograde flushes. Moreover, unlike detachable clamps, straight clamps stabilize the left mesocolon into position and allow a stable exposure during the performance of endoaneurysmorrhaphy and anastomoses.
- A longitudinal aortotomy is performed on the left side on the aorta. Traction on the stitch that was previously placed in the aortic wall allows opening the aneurysmal sac (see Fig. 95-5). The mural thrombus is removed and placed temporarily in the left hypochondrium. It will be removed at the end of the procedure with a container. In cases of residual bleeding in the aneurysmal sac, lumbar arteries are controlled either externally with clips or internally with staples (EMS, Ethicon Endo-Surgery) or polypropylene stitches. As in the Creech technique, the proximal aortic neck is usually sectioned circumferentially. Whenever possible, the distal aorta is also sectioned circumferentially for tube graft implantation.
- In cases of close adhesions between distal aorta and the inferior vena cava, we keep the right aortic wall to avoid injury to the inferior vena cava during its dissection. The prosthesis is introduced into the abdomen through one of the ports. Proximal and distal anastomoses are performed with hemicircumferential running sutures previously knotted on pledgets. At the end of each anastomosis, both ends of the thread are tied together intracorporally (Fig. 95-9, *A* and *B*). Retrograde flush from the common iliac arteries is checked before the suture line is closed.

Bifurcated Graft Implantation

- When a bifurcated graft is indicated, specific steps are performed. After achieving laparoscopic exposure, the patient is returned to the dorsal decubitus position. The pillow is deflated, and the operating table is rotated on the left, which allows a conventional approach to the iliac and femoral arteries. A knot is placed as a landmark on the left prosthetic limb. We always proceed methodically for the next steps. A right tunnel is initiated right away from the groin/iliac incision. At the abdominal level, the assistant exposes the right common iliac artery with an endoretractor in the left hand (port 4) and a suction device in the right hand (port 5). The surgeon introduces an aortic clamp from the groin and conducts its tip over the right common iliac artery under abdominal laparoscopic control. Once the clamp is positioned, the vascular prosthesis is introduced into the abdomen through one of the ports, and its right limb is easily brought to the groin incision. The left prosthetic limb is also brought down with the help of an aortic clamp introduced through the left groin. Unlike the right side, the left tunnel is short and wide open because the organs have dropped toward the right. Care must be taken to avoid a large tunnel because of the risk of gas leakage.

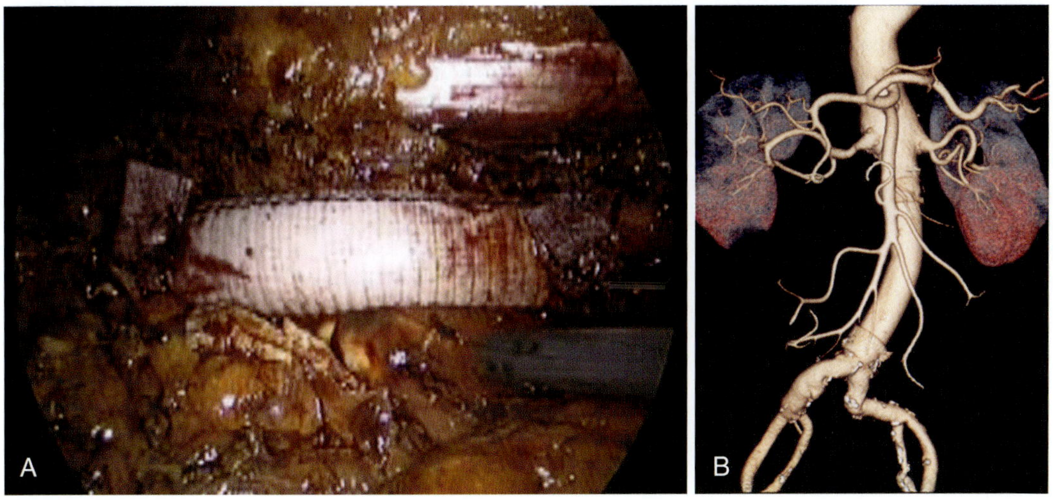

Figure 95-9. Operative (**A**) and computed tomography scan (**B**) views showing a tube graft after laparoscopic abdominal aortic aneurysm repair.

- Some technical steps are different for bifurcated grafts. If distal anastomoses are feasible on common iliac arteries, the entire procedure is performed through the abdominal route. In cases of external iliac anastomoses, we prefer to perform a separate RP approach in the iliac fossa, especially on the right side. Blood flow to the internal iliac arteries is ensured by either retrograde perfusion or reimplantation. In such cases, we use videoscopy for the left side but an open approach for the right side. The main technical point for bifurcated grafts is in fact the strategy used to decrease clamping time. Whenever possible, once the graft limbs are tunneled, the distal iliac and/or femoral anastomoses are performed first (see Fig. 95-6). With such a strategy, total aortic clamping time is required only for aneurysmorrhaphy and proximal anastomosis.

Juxtarenal AAA

- Juxtarenal AAA does not contraindicate laparoscopic repair. Whenever possible, the laparoscopic approach is TPRR (see Fig. 95-5). Laparoscopic juxtarenal AAA aneurysmorrhaphy follows steps similar to those in inflammatory AAA repair. When we need suprarenal clamping, we use sequential steps to decrease the duration of renal ischemia. When the juxtarenal aorta is unusable for clamping, aneurysmorrhaphy and proximal anastomosis are performed as quickly as possible under suprarenal clamping. The duration of renal ischemia is the time needed for aneurysmorrhaphy and proximal anastomosis. When preparation of the juxtarenal aorta allows enough length for infrarenal clamping and suture, we move the proximal clamp below the renal arteries before we perform the proximal anastomosis. The duration of renal ischemia is then the time needed for aneurysmorrhaphy alone. Finally, when the juxtarenal aorta is large but free of thrombus, we perform infrarenal clamping whenever possible in order to carry out the aneurysmorrhaphy. If the target zone for proximal anastomosis is too short, we move the clamp above the renal arteries. The duration of renal ischemia is then the time needed for the proximal anastomosis.

Closure

- At the end of the procedure, we perform a laparoscopic inspection of the left colon to assess its viability. Back bleeding from the IMA and preoperative Doppler ultrasound (Ultrasonic Doppler Flow Detector, Parks Medical Electronics, Aloha, Ore.) are used to assess the adequacy of collateral blood flow to the left mesocolon. If reimplantation of the IMA is needed, it can be performed laparoscopically or via a minilaparotomy. Hemostasis is checked, especially in the aneurysmal sac to detect back bleeding from lumbar arteries after unclamping of the iliac arteries. On closure, a suction drain is positioned near the prosthesis. There is no need to reattach viscera, because they fall back into place once the patient is returned to a dorsal decubitus position. The aneurysmal wall covers the graft when the kidney falls into place. Ports are removed under laparoscopic control to check that there is no parietal bleeding. The abdominal fascia at port holes is closed with absorbable sutures.

V. ALTERNATIVE TECHNICAL APPROACHES (PRO/CON) AND PEARLS

Choice of Laparoscopic Approach

- Indications of approaches depend on patient conditions. The TPRR approach is now our first choice. It allows a large exposure, especially when control of the juxtarenal aorta is needed. Dissection of the suprarenal or celiac aorta is conducted in line with the left side of the aorta after section of the crus of the diaphragm. Unlike the TPRC or TPD approaches, neither the kidney nor the mesocolon blinds exposure of the left side of the aorta. This is of particular importance for control of lumbar arteries during AAA repair. At the end of the procedure, the viscera fall back into place and allow optimal covering of the prosthesis.
- The TPRR approach is contraindicated in cases of perisplenic adhesions and/or a retroaortic left renal vein. In such cases, we use the TPRC approach, which is also indicated for concomitant left renal or superior mesenteric laparoscopic bypass.
- In cases of very hostile abdomen, we use the RP approach. However, working space with this approach is reduced, either externally for placement of ports or internally behind the peritoneal sac. For AAA repair, the RP approach is feasible but is quite difficult. In such cases, conversion to open repair is often necessary. For these reasons, the RP approach is rarely indicated. Even in cases of previous abdominal scars, we often try to enter the peritoneal cavity in order to perform a transperitoneal approach.
- Finally, in a few cases we use the TPD approach. This approach is theoretically the simplest, using common landmarks for vascular surgeons. However, the TPD approach requires careful dissection close to the intestine. Upward retraction of the transverse mesocolon is not always simple and requires two or more stitches. Exposure of the juxtarenal aorta is then difficult, especially for AAAs with short or angulated necks. The use of various tools is essential to keep bowel loops from frequently falling into the operative field. The main drawback of the TPD approach is in fact the covering of the prosthesis,

especially when the patient is thin. For these reasons, we use the TPD approach only in cases of previous left nephrectomy when retrorenal and retrocolic dissection planes are blocked.

Technical Variations in Laparoscopic Aortic Repair

Aortic Repair through TPRC and TPD Approaches

- Aortic repair through TPRC and TPD approaches uses the same steps as in the TPRR approach. The main differences are positioning of clamps and tunneling of graft limbs. Positioning of the proximal aortic clamp uses the subxiphoid port (port 6) after removal of the endoretractor. This clamp stabilizes the left mesocolon (see Fig. 95-5). Tunneling of graft limbs for aortobifemoral bypass grafts is very much the same for the TPRC and TPRR approaches. For the right side, there are no differences. For the left side, through the TPRC approach, the surgeon moves clamps from the groin toward the aorta under laparoscopic control. The tip is conducted behind the ureter, which lies over the iliac artery. Through the TPD approach, left tunneling is more demanding. Laparoscopic dissection along the anterior side of the left iliac artery is blinded by the left mesocolon and does not allow enough exposure to be sure that tunnel is strictly behind the ureter. We recommend a short peritoneal incision in the left iliac fossa with retroperitoneal dissection and exposure of the distal common iliac artery. With such exposure, tunneling is simple, and the surgeon moves the clamp behind the ureter under strict laparoscopic control.

Aortic Repair through the RP Approach

- The proximal clamp is introduced through a sixth port placed above the left 12th rib. The distal clamp is positioned through a seventh port placed in the left iliac fossa. For AAA repair, right iliac clamping can be performed with a detachable clamp or with an additional clamp introduced 3 cm below the navel, which stabilizes the peritoneal sac into position. Aortoprosthetic anastomoses use the same principles but are in reverse compared to transperitoneal exposures.

Conversion to Open Direct Repair

- Conversion to ODR through a short incision is not a failure; it is a safe and reasonable strategy when difficulties arise during total laparoscopic procedures. Such a decision is sometimes difficult for surgeons, especially at the beginning of their experience. Discussion with anesthesiologists is essential to deciding conversion time. Usual indications are (1) difficult reconstruction with prolonged aortic clamping time; (2) extensive calcifications with an unclampable aorta; (3) difficult or unstable exposure of the abdominal aorta, especially with a retroperitoneoscopic approach, small abdominal cavities, unexpected adhesions, or extensive dilatation of the small bowel; and (4) injury to structures adjacent to the aorta such as the small bowel, inferior vena cava, or iliac veins. Relative indications are (1) the need for IMA reimplantation; (2) difficult control of endpoint endarterectomy in iliac or visceral arteries; and (3) insufficient accuracy and visibility for bleeding control.
- The technique for conversion is relatively simple. The patient is still in the RLD position. We conduct a short vertical laparotomy between the laparoscope and assistant's ports (ports 1 and 5) (Fig. 95-10;

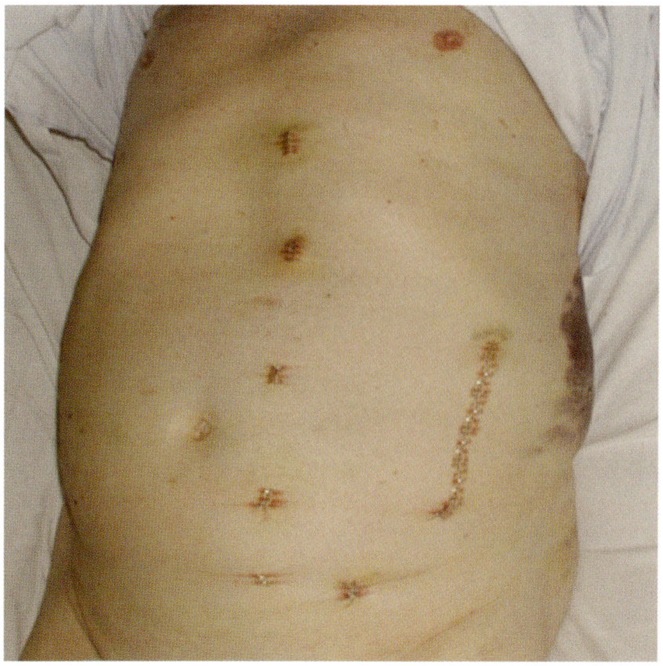

Figure 95-10. Postoperative view showing a patient after conversion to open repair.

see also Fig. 95-1). If necessary, this laparotomy can be extended. Exposure through the initial direct, retrocolic, or retrorenal route is maintained with autostatic retractors or valves. Completion of the procedure uses the same principles as conventional ODR. Sometimes it is useful to use laparoscopic clamps, which are less cumbersome than conventional aortic clamps. Another useful tool is the percutaneous introduction of conventional or laparoscopic clamps.

VI. SPECIAL POSTOPERATIVE CARE

- It is important to provide adequate postoperative pain control, which can be achieved with patient-controlled analgesia or an epidural.
- Patients undergoing aortic aneurysm repair are at moderate to high risk of developing deep vein thrombosis. An intermittent pneumatic compression device and early ambulation therefore seem appropriate. Patients considered to be at high risk (e.g., history of deep vein thrombosis or pulmonary embolism, obesity [body mass index over 25], limited mobility status, malignancy, hypercoagulable state) should receive either low–molecular-weight heparin or unfractionated heparin. Any electrocardiographic changes must be investigated with serum troponin levels for early diagnosis of myocardial infarction.
- If there is any postoperative evidence of troublesome ileus, placement of a nasogastric tube for decompression should be considered.

SUGGESTED READINGS

Coggia M, Javerliat I, Di Centa I, et al: Total laparoscopic bypass for aortoiliac occlusive lesions: 93-case experience, *J Vasc Surg* 40:899–906, 2004.

Javerliat I, Coggia M, Bourriez A, et al: Total laparoscopic aortomesenteric bypass, *Vascular* 12:126–129, 2004.

Javerliat I, Coggia M, Di Centa I, et al: Total laparoscopic aortic surgery: left retroperitoneoscopic approach, *Eur J Vasc Endovasc Surg* 29:244–246, 2005.

CHAPTER 96

Axillofemoral Bypass

Christopher K. Zarins, MD, and Bruce L. Gewertz, MD

I. SPECIAL PREOPERATIVE PREPARATION

- Axillofemoral bypass grafts are used to provide blood flow to the lower extremities in instances where standard aortofemoral or aortoiliac bypass grafts cannot be used. The indications include revascularization before or after removal of an infected abdominal aortic graft and bypass of the aortoiliac segment in patients who are too ill to withstand a direct operative approach to the aorta.
- Preoperative preparation includes evaluation of the upper and lower extremities with physical examination, ankle-brachial index (ABI) measurement, and duplex ultrasound imaging. Most importantly, vascular imaging should be performed with contrast angiography and computed tomography angiography or magnetic resonance angiography in order to evaluate the aortoiliac and femoral vessels as well as the aortic arch and axillosubclavian vessels. These studies will allow proper preoperative planning.

II. OPERATIVE TECHNIQUE

Position

- The patient is placed supine on the operating table with the arm extended on an arm board. This positioning elevates the distal portion of the clavicle, allowing easy exposure of the subclavian artery. Either the right or left subclavian artery may be used as a donor vessel, and the least diseased should be selected.

Incision

- Three incisions are made: one fingerbreadth below the clavicle from the level of the coracoid process to the sternoclavicular joint, and over both femoral arteries just below the inguinal ligament (Fig. 96-1).

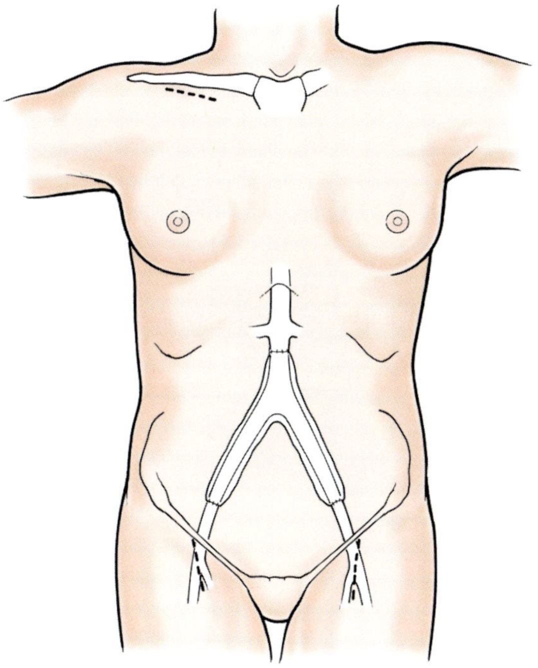

Figure 96-1.

Main Dissection

- The subclavicular incision is deepened, and the clavipectoral fascia is divided. The cephalic vein may be seen penetrating the clavipectoral fascia to join the subclavian vein. The fibers of the pectoralis major muscle are split to expose the subclavian vein, which is retracted inferiorly to expose the subclavian artery exiting the thoracic outlet. The subclavian artery is mobilized laterally to the level of the pectoralis minor muscle. The highest thoracic artery in the proximal portion of the subclavian artery is divided to permit complete mobilization of the proximal portion of the subclavian artery (Fig. 96-2).
- The common femoral, superficial femoral, and deep femoral arteries are mobilized and controlled in each groin incision. A tunnel is then created between the subclavian artery and femoral artery using a long tunneling instrument. This tunnel passes along the chest wall deep to the pectoralis minor muscle and passes through the serratus anterior muscle to a subcutaneous plane in the midaxillary line. It then courses anterior to the anterior superior iliac spine and across the inguinal ligament into the femoral incision. If a sufficiently long tunneler is not available, a counterincision may be made in the midaxillary line to facilitate tunneling. The bypass graft is then fixed to the tunneling instrument and withdrawn from the groin to the subclavicular incision. Polytetrafluoroethylene or Dacron grafts may be used. The diameter selected is based on the diameter of the donor subclavian artery and usually measures 8 to 10 mm in diameter. Externally ring-supported grafts are preferred because they resist extrinsic compression of the graft against the chest wall and costal margin.
- Following systemic heparinization, vascular clamps are applied to the subclavian artery to allow a 90-degree torque to the artery. A longitudinal arteriotomy is then made on the inferior side of the artery, just anterior to the highest thoracic artery, which is used as a guide for orientation. The length of the arteriotomy must be same as the diameter of the graft opening in order to avoid kinking the subclavian artery when the soft artery is anastomosed to the noncompliant graft material. The anastomosis is performed with 5-0 or 6-0 monofilament nonabsorbable suture. It is begun in the middle of the back wall and is run in both directions. Most often the graft lies behind the subclavian vein against the chest wall, thus avoiding the possibility of extrinsic compression of the subclavian vein. On some occasions, however, the graft may be anastomosed to the anterior portion of the artery and may then pass over the subclavian vein (Fig. 96-3).
- After completion of the proximal anastomosis, an atraumatic clamp is placed on the graft, and the vascular clamps are released. This allows reperfusion of the right upper extremity and rotation of the artery back to its normal alignment (Fig. 96-4).
- Vascular clamps are placed on the common femoral, superficial femoral, and deep femoral vessels. A longitudinal arteriotomy is made in the common femoral artery and extended onto the deep or superficial femoral artery as needed to correct orifice stenoses. If necessary, a femoral endarterectomy may be performed. The graft is tailored to the arteriotomy and anastomosed using 5-0 monofilament nonabsorbable suture in a running fashion (Fig. 96-5).
- After completion of the femoral anastomosis and before allowing blood to enter the graft, a window of graft is removed from the hood of the femoral anastomosis, and a ring-supported bypass graft is sutured to the hood of the graft in an end-to-side fashion. The proximal and distal clamps are sequentially released to flush the graft and evacuate all air from it through the open end of the cross-femoral bypass. The femorofemoral crossover limb is then passed through a suprapubic subcutaneous tunnel to the left groin and anastomosed to the femoral artery. Care must be taken to ensure a good alignment

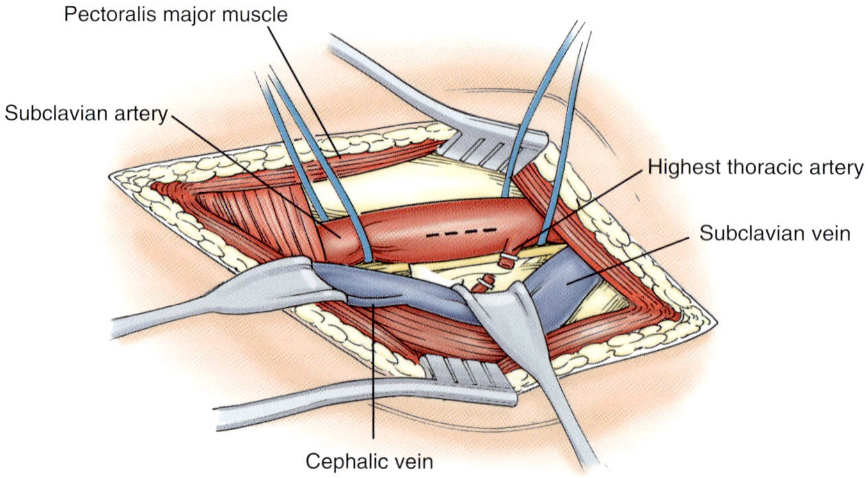

Figure 96-2.

and to avoid kinking of the graft or artery. The bypass is carefully flushed before completion of the anastomosis (Fig. 96-6).

- The completed axillofemoral bypass graft is in place. The infected aortic graft has been removed, and the infrarenal aorta and iliac arteries oversewn. Infected grafts may be removed before or after placement of the axillofemoral bypass graft. Removal of the infected aortic graft first has the theoretic advantage of reducing the risk for subsequent infection in the axillofemoral bypass graft. However, this increases the length and complexity of the operation and ensures a period of ischemia after removal of the aortic graft and before completion of the axillofemoral bypass. We usually prefer to place the

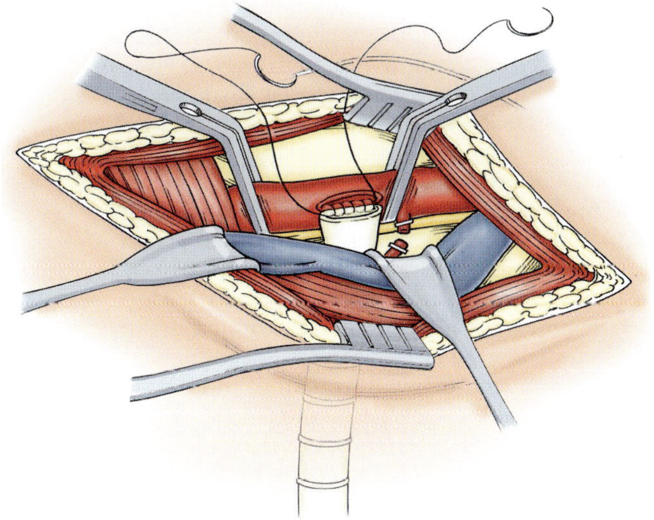

Figure 96-3.

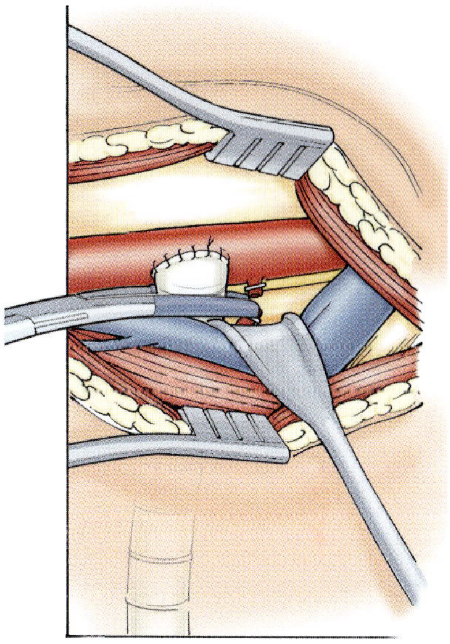

Figure 96-4.

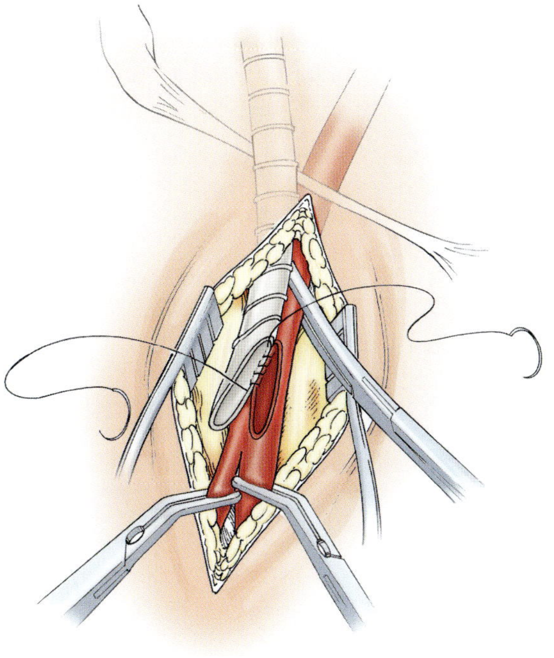

Figure 96-5.

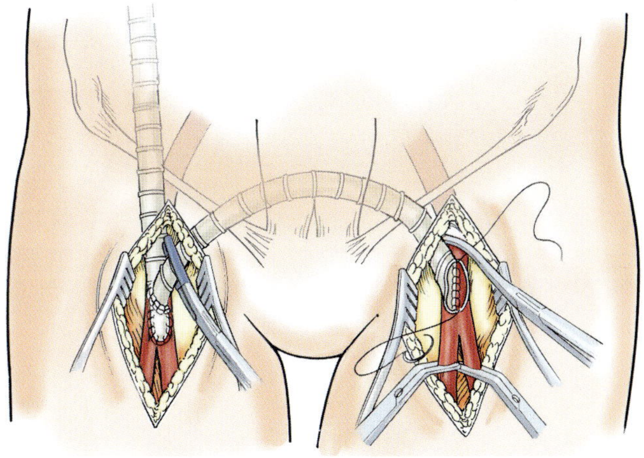

Figure 96-6.

axillofemoral bypass first and then remove the infected graft, either during the same operation or as a secondary staged procedure (Fig. 96-7).

Closure

- The incisions are meticulously closed in layers. The skin is approximated with staples.

III. ALTERNATIVE TECHNICAL APPROACHES (PRO/CON) AND PEARLS

- Alternative technical approaches to revascularization of aortoiliac occlusive disease include a variety of catheter-based endovascular strategies including balloon angioplasty, stenting, thrombolysis, endoluminal atherectomy, cryoplasty, and endoluminal laser recanalization. Iliac balloon angioplasty and stenting are now widely used to treat lower extremity occlusive disease with very good results in treating focal iliac lesions. Results of endovascular treatment of extensive aortoiliac disease are not as favorable, but should be considered in high-risk surgical patients. However, if endovascular therapies are not possible, are ineffective, or result in complications, axillofemoral bypasses should be considered in patients who are high risk for open abdominal surgery.
- For patients with infected aortic grafts, endoluminal strategies are not an option. In these patients, alternative technical approaches include excision of the infected aortic graft and in situ replacement using autologous superficial femoral vein, harvested from both legs in order to obtain sufficient length. Alternatively, cryopreserved aortic homografts or venous homografts can be used for aortofemoral revascularization. Such cryopreserved homografts withstand infection well but may require late secondary procedures to maintain long-term function. Finally, in some patients, partial excision of the graft and prosthetic extra-anatomic bypass through a noninfected field may be performed. For example, if one limb of an aortofemoral bypass is infected, that limb can be excised with ligation of the femoral artery and a crossover femorofemoral bypass used to revascularize the lower extremity.
- *Note:* Although the operation discussed in this chapter is called an axillofemoral bypass, in fact, the subclavian artery, below the clavicle and medial to the pectoralis minor muscle, is the inflow vessel. Therefore, strictly speaking, it should be called a subclavian-femoral bypass. However, common usage and all of the published literature refers to this operation as an axillofemoral bypass.
- *Note:* Although this operation is referred to as an "extra-anatomic bypass," in fact the bypass does not extend outside of the anatomy; rather, it courses through a different anatomic plane within the body.

IV. SPECIAL POSTOPERATIVE CARE

- Postoperative care involves monitoring of graft patency and assessment of adequacy of lower extremity perfusion. This can be most readily be performed by clinical evaluation of the perfusion status of the

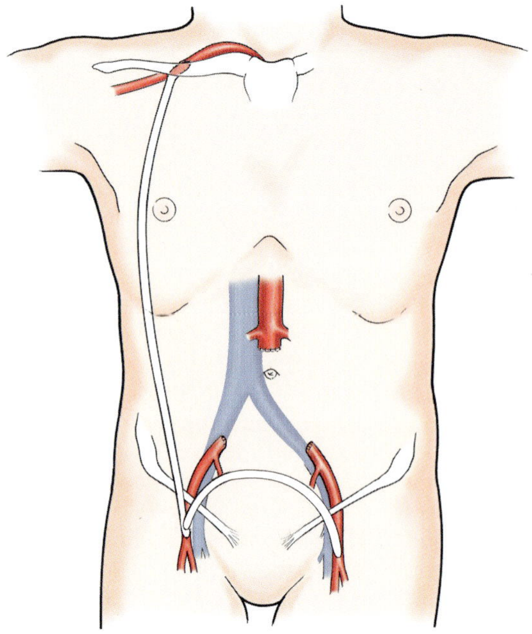

Figure 96-7.

feet and by measurement of ankle-brachial indices (ABI) using a blood pressure cuff and Doppler ultrasound probe. Preoperative ABIs should be compared to postoperative ABIs.

- If the proximal anastomosis is made to the subclavian artery and the graft is tunneled under the pectoralis minor muscle, there is no need for immobilization or limitation of motion of the upper extremity. If, however, the proximal anastomosis is made more laterally to the axillary artery, or tunneled over the pectoralis minor muscle, movement of the upper extremity may place tension on the anastomosis and disrupt it. This may result in acute hemorrhage or anastomotic pseudoaneurysm formation. Restriction of upper extremity motion is necessary in the perioperative period to avoid such complications.
- Graft patency is largely dependent on adequacy of outflow from the distal anastomosis. Good flow through the deep femoral artery is usually sufficient to maintain graft patency, even in the face of superficial femoral artery obstruction. Therefore, particular attention should be made to making sure there is no stenosis at the orifice of the deep femoral artery at the time of femoral anastomosis. If flow through the deep femoral artery is compromised and the superficial femoral artery is diseased, an additional femoral-popliteal bypass may be required.

SUGGESTED READINGS

Angle N, Dorafshar AH, Farooq MM, et al: The evolution of the axillofemoral bypass over two decades, *Ann Vasc Surg* 16:742–745, 2002.

Blaisdell FW, Hall AD: Axillary femoral artery bypass for lower extremity ischemia, *Surgery* 54:563–568, 1963.

Rutherford RB, Patt, A, Pearce WH: Extra-anatomic bypass: a closer view, *J Vasc Surg* 5:437–446, 1987.

CHAPTER 97

Renal Artery Revascularization

Bruce L. Gewertz, MD, and Christopher K. Zarins, MD

I. SPECIAL PREOPERATIVE PREPARATION

- Renovascular disease in the elderly is caused primarily by atherosclerotic narrowing of the renal arteries and may result in both progressive hypertension and diminished renal function. In younger patients, especially children and women between 20 and 35 years of age, renovascular disease is most commonly caused by fibromuscular dysplasia.
- Clinical features associated with renovascular hypertension include new onset of hypertension, rapid progression of previously stable hypertension, and hypertension associated with renal function impairment.
- Currently accepted indications for renal revascularization include the presence of a hemodynamically significant renal artery stenosis (>60% diameter reduction) in patients with refractory hypertension or hypertension associated with renal functional impairment.
- Renal duplex scanning has evolved into the principal noninvasive screening test for both the presence of renal arterial disease and its hemodynamic significance. The modality combines B-mode ultrasound imaging with pulsed Doppler ultrasound determinations of blood flow velocity. The ratio of renal artery peak systolic velocity to aortic peak systolic velocity (RAR) has been used to define hemodynamically significant lesions. Lesions of 60% or greater are associated with RAR of greater than 3.5.
- Arteriography is still the accepted standard for diagnosis of renovascular disease. Multiple views of the renal vessels are obtained, including, at least, anteroposterior and oblique views. The measurement of renal vein renin levels has been used as an adjunct to arteriography to help identify functionally significant renal arterial stenoses. Such values can be expressed as renal vein renin ratios, which compare one kidney with the other (ratios > 1.5 are considered diagnostic), or renal/systemic renin indices, which quantify the contribution of each kidney to the total systemic renin level.
- Percutaneous renal angioplasty has been a prominent form of modern therapy in both atherosclerotic and fibromuscular lesions of the renal artery, aided by the continued development of self-expanding and balloon-expandable stents. That said, operative repair remains an important option in these patients, especially those who have lesions that are not amenable to angioplasty because they involve the distal portion of the renal artery or its bifurcation. Furthermore, open-surgical intervention may be a better option in patients with recurrent disease after angioplasty or ischemic nephropathy in which salvage of renal parenchyma is the primary indication.
- Surgical options include endarterectomy and aortorenal or hepatorenal bypass. Endarterectomy through a transaortic route is most useful in bilateral orificial disease, but it requires suprarenal aortic exposure and clamping with resultant greater cardiac risk. Aortorenal bypass from a relatively disease-free area of the infrarenal aorta has been the most widely used technique in the past, although hepatorenal and splenorenal bypasses are currently used more frequently. The latter procedures avoid manipulation of the often diseased aorta and obviate any need for aortic occlusion. Irrespective of the origin of these bypass grafts, long-term patency is excellent, approaching 95% over 5 years if autologous vein is used.

II. OPERATIVE TECHNIQUE: LEFT RENAL REVASCULARIZATION

Position

- The patient is placed in the supine position. A bean bag is used to position the patient with the left shoulder at a 45-degree angle and the left arm suspended in a sling (Fig. 97-1).

Incision

- A supraumbilical transverse incision is made and extended to the tip of the 12th rib (see Fig. 97-1). The internal and external oblique muscles and left rectus muscle are divided. The fibers of the transversus abdominis are split, and the peritoneum is mobilized from the costal margin to the iliac crest.

Main Dissection

- The peritoneum is retracted to the right, and the ureter and iliopsoas muscles are identified. The retroperitoneal plane between the left colon and kidney is developed to expose the testicular vein and left renal vein. The left renal vein is mobilized, and control is obtained of the infrarenal abdominal aorta between the level of the renal arteries and inferior mesenteric artery. The kidney is not mobilized or removed from the Gerota capsule so that collateral blood supply is preserved (Figs. 97-2 and 97-3).

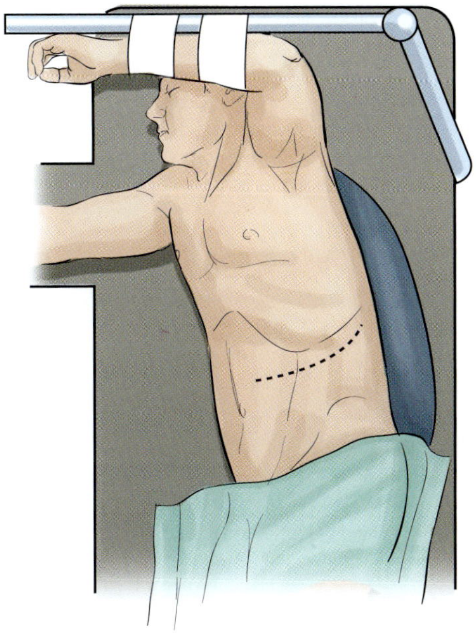

Figure 97-1.

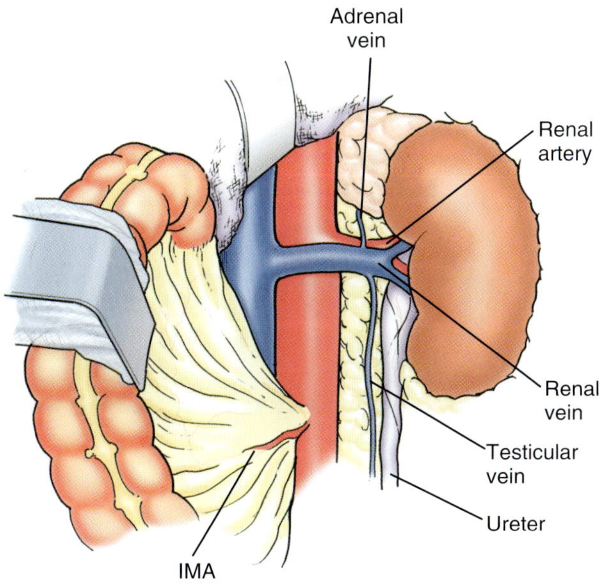

Figure 97-2. *IMA,* Inferior mesenteric artery.

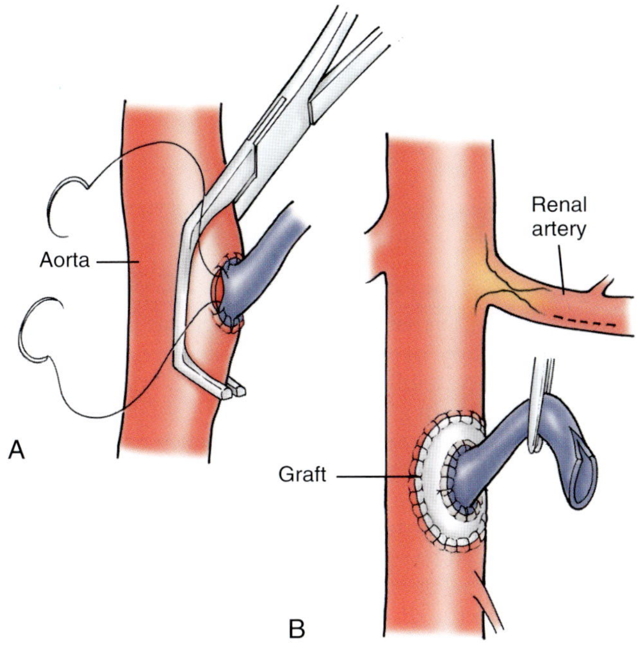

Figure 97-3. *Redrawn from Zarins C, Gewertz B: Mesenteric revascularization. In Zarins C, Gewertz B, editors:* Atlas of vascular surgery, *ed 2, Philadelphia, 2005, Churchill Livingstone, p 151, Figs. E and F.*

- The left renal vein is retracted superiorly, exposing the underlying left renal artery. The testicular vein is divided and ligated to facilitate exposure. Control is obtained of the renal artery distal to the obstructing lesion (see Fig. 97-3, *A*; Fig. 97-4).
- To minimize the duration of renal ischemia, the saphenous vein bypass is first anastomosed to the infrarenal aorta. After systemic heparinization, the aorta is clamped. If the aorta is soft and does not have significant atherosclerosis, a partial occlusion clamp is used so that flow is maintained to the lower extremities. If the aorta is severely diseased, cross-clamping the aorta with two vascular clamps will provide better exposure of the aorta for anastomosis and the opportunity to perform local aortic endarterectomy. The aorta is opened with a longitudinal aortotomy.
- The saphenous vein, previously harvested from the thigh, is reversed and anastomosed to the infrarenal aorta using 5-0 or 6-0 continuous monofilament suture. The vein is spatulated to prevent anastomotic stenosis. The aortic clamp is released to flush out any atherosclerotic debris before completion of the suture line. The aorta is unclamped, the graft is flushed, and a Heifetz vascular clamp is applied to the vein graft for hemostasis during the distal anastomosis (see Fig. 97-4, *A* and *B*).
- An atraumatic vascular clamp is placed on the distal renal artery, and the proximal renal artery is clamped and transected distal to the obstructing lesion. The distal renal artery is flushed with cold, heparinized balanced salt solution. The proximal renal artery stump is suture ligated. The distal renal artery is cut longitudinally on its anterior surface for at least the length of the vessel diameter. The clamp on the saphenous vein is released, and the distal vein graft is pinched to ascertain proper length and orientation of the vein relative to the renal artery.
- The saphenous vein is cut to appropriate length and spatulated to match the renal artery. The anastomosis is begun by placing 6-0 monofilament suture at the 6- and 12-o'clock positions using loupe magnification to ensure precision. Both sutures are tied, and care is taken to avoid undue tension that may tear the renal artery. One side of the anastomosis is then completed with continuous suture running from the vein to the artery (see Fig. 97-3, *B*).
- The anastomosis is rotated, and the other side is completed. Before completion of the anastomosis, the proximal and distal clamps are temporarily released to flush out air and debris. Satisfactory flow through the vein graft is confirmed by palpation of the pulse and Doppler ultrasound signals in the graft and distal renal artery.

Closure

- The muscles are then closed in layers with 1-0 nonabsorbable monofilament suture. Skin is approximated with staples.

III. OPERATIVE TECHNIQUE: RIGHT RENAL REVASCULARIZATION

Position

- The patient is placed in the supine position. A bean bag is used to position the patient with the left shoulder at a 45-degree angle and the left arm suspended in a sling.

Incision

- Exposure of the right renal artery is obtained through a transverse supraumbilical incision extending from the midline to the right flank.

Main Dissection

- The duodenum and right colon are mobilized to the midline, exposing the right renal vein and vena cava. Care should be taken to avoid avulsion of the gonadal vein, which enters the anterior surface of the inferior vena cava. The right renal vein and right side of the inferior vena cava are mobilized (Fig. 97-5). The right renal artery lies behind and superior to the renal vein and is mobilized and encircled with Silastic tapes. The inferior vena cava is dissected free of the infrarenal aorta, and a segment of soft infrarenal aorta is exposed. The vena cava is mobilized posteriorly between the aorta and renal artery along the course of the aortorenal bypass. Lumbar veins are carefully identified, ligated, and divided, if necessary, for mobilization of the vena cava. The saphenous vein is harvested from the thigh.
- After systemic heparinization, the proximal renal artery is clamped and transected. The distal renal artery is flushed with cold, heparinized balanced salt solution, and the distal renal artery is occluded with a Heifetz clip. If the main renal artery is extensively diseased, it may be necessary to individually control and clamp the branches of the renal artery. The proximal renal artery is suture ligated. The distal renal artery is opened longitudinally on its anterior surface and is spatulated to enlarge the anastomotic area and to ensure that there is no residual occlusive disease at or distal to the anastomotic location. The reversed saphenous vein is anastomosed end-to-end to the distal renal artery using two 6-0 monofilament vascular sutures placed under loupe magnification. The saphenous vein is carefully tunneled underneath the vena cava for anastomosis to the aorta (Fig. 97-6, *A* and *B*).

- The aorta is usually soft and may be clamped using a partial occluding clamp. If the aorta has significant atherosclerosis, total occlusion of the aortic segment using two vascular clamps provides better exposure for the anastomosis. The aortotomy is performed on the anterolateral right side of the aorta to achieve the best lie of the graft.
- The saphenous vein is cut to appropriate length and tailored to match the size of the aortotomy. The anastomosis is performed using a single continuous monofilament suture. The suture is begun in the center of the back wall and is run in both directions. Before completion of the suture line on the anterior wall, the aorta is flushed, and the distal renal artery clamp is removed to permit back bleeding. Flow in the graft and distal renal artery is checked by palpation of the pulse and Doppler ultrasound.

Closure

- The muscles are then closed in layers with 1-0 nonabsorbable monofilament suture. Skin is approximated with staples.

IV. ALTERNATIVE TECHNICAL APPROACHES (PRO/CON) AND PEARLS

Hepatorenal and Splenorenal Bypass for Left and Right Renal Bypass, Respectively

- In patients with previous aortic surgery or with advanced aortoiliac disease, hepatorenal bypass offers the possibility of successful revascularization of the kidney without the difficulties of repeat aortic

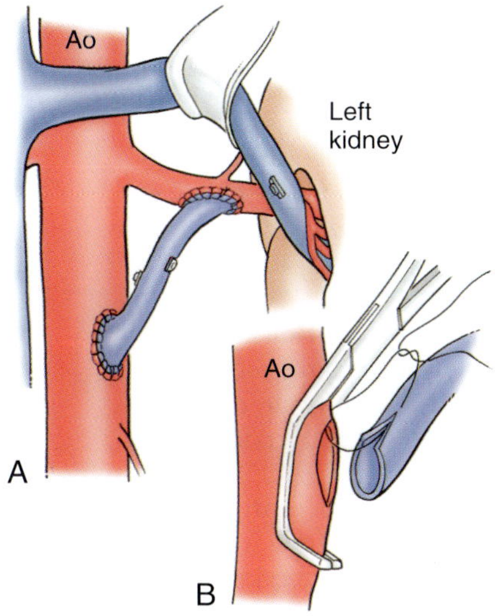

Figure 97-4. *Ao,* Aorta.

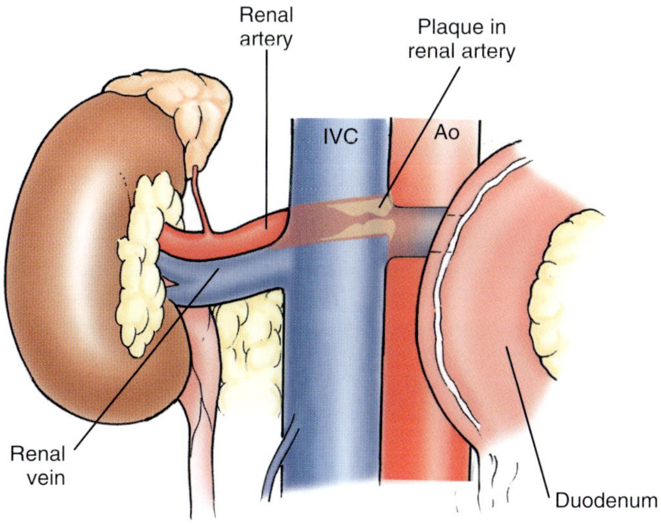

Figure 97-5. *Ao,* Aorta; *IVC,* inferior vena cava.

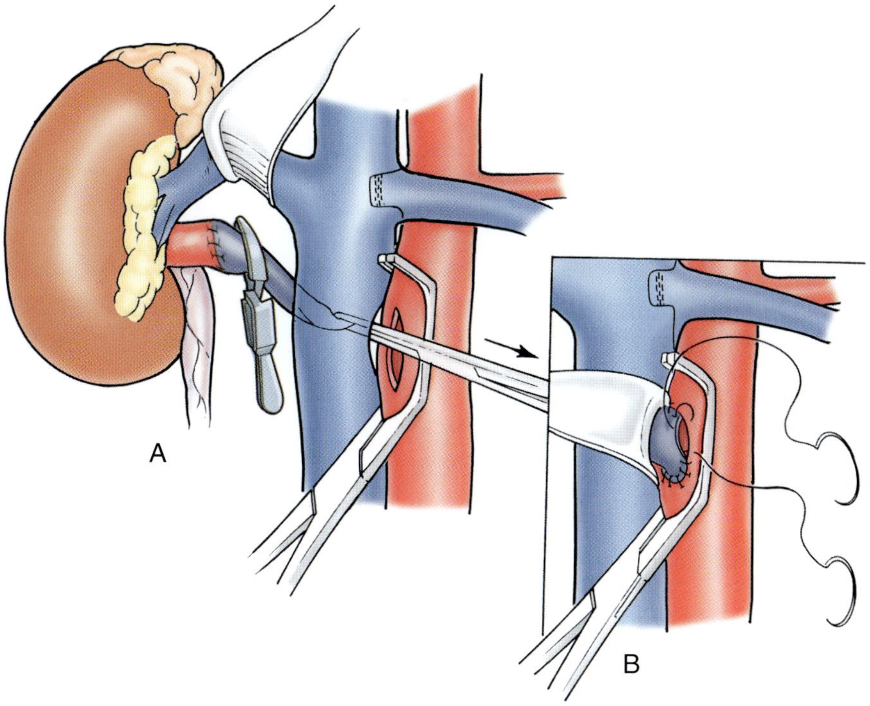

Figure 97-6. *Redrawn from Zarins C, Gewertz B: Mesenteric revascularization. In Zarins C, Gewertz B, editors:* Atlas of vascular surgery, *ed 2, Philadelphia, 2005, Churchill Livingstone, p 157, Figs. B and C.*

exposure or the stress of aortic occlusion. Attention must be directed to the lateral views of the celiac axis and its branches on the aortogram to ensure that there is no inflow lesion of the celiac artery.

- After a generous Kocher maneuver, the hepatic artery is exposed. The preferred site of a proximal anastomosis is distal to the origin of the gastroduodenal artery. A vein graft or the hypogastric artery is the ideal conduit. Proximal anastomosis is performed in an end-to-side fashion to the hepatic artery, and a relatively short graft is placed to the more distal aspect of the right renal artery (Fig. 97-7).
- Alternatively, if the gastroduodenal artery is of large caliber (>3 mm), the artery can be transected at its most distal point and sewn to the right renal artery in an end-to-end fashion. If there is a size discrepancy between the gastroduodenal and renal artery, or if transection of the renal artery would make exposure and stabilization of the distal anastomotic site more difficult, an end-to-side anastomosis can be carried out.
- For left renal revascularization, similar surgical techniques can be used with the splenic artery as an inflow vessel. Multiple branches of the splenic artery are ligated, allowing mobilization of the transected splenic artery to the left renal artery. As shown here, an end-to-end anastomosis can be performed. Similarly, an end-to-side anastomosis can also be used. In general, splenorenal bypasses are more difficult than hepatorenal bypass because the splenic artery can be more fragile and has multiple branches requiring some mobilization from the pancreas (Fig. 97-8).

Bench Surgery for Renal Artery Stenosis

- Renal artery stenoses involving the branch renal arteries in the hilum of the kidney may be difficult to visualize and to repair in situ. In these unusual circumstances, it may be best to temporarily remove the kidney from the abdomen so that the lesions can be better visualized and more precisely corrected.
- A vascular clamp is placed on the proximal renal vein, and the proximal renal artery is suture ligated. The renal artery and vein are transected, and the kidney is gently lifted from its fossa, leaving the ureter intact. The renal artery is flushed with cold, heparinized balanced salt solution until the venous effluent is clear.
- The kidney is placed on a plastic sheet in a basin filled with ice. The renal artery branches in the hilum of the kidney are carefully dissected under magnification, and lesions are identified. Renal artery branches are opened as necessary to expose all lesions.
- The reversed-saphenous vein is then tailored for the anastomosis to the renal artery branches. The anastomosis is performed using continuous 6-0 or 7-0 monofilament suture under magnification. The kidney is replaced into the renal fossa, and the saphenous vein is anastomosed to the infrarenal aorta. A Heifetz clip is maintained on the saphenous vein, and the kidney is not perfused until completion of the venous anastomosis.
- The left renal vein is anastomosed using three 6-0 sutures tied at 10-, 2-, and 6-o'clock (triangulation) positions to avoid "purse-string" stenosis. After completion of the venous anastomosis, flow is restored to the renal artery. Patency of the bypass is confirmed by immediate return of color to the kidney, fill of the renal vein, and Doppler flow signals in the branch renal arteries.

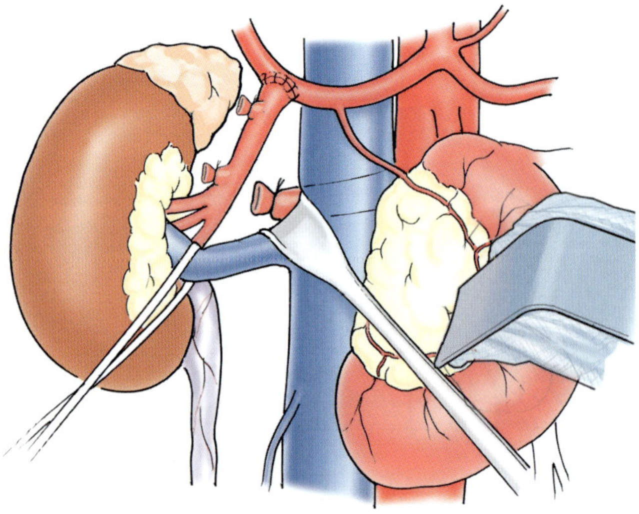

Figure 97-7. *Redrawn from Zarins C, Gewertz B: Mesenteric revascularization. In Zarins C, Gewertz B, editors:* Atlas of vascular surgery, *ed 2, Philadelphia, 2005, Churchill Livingstone, p 159, Fig. A.*

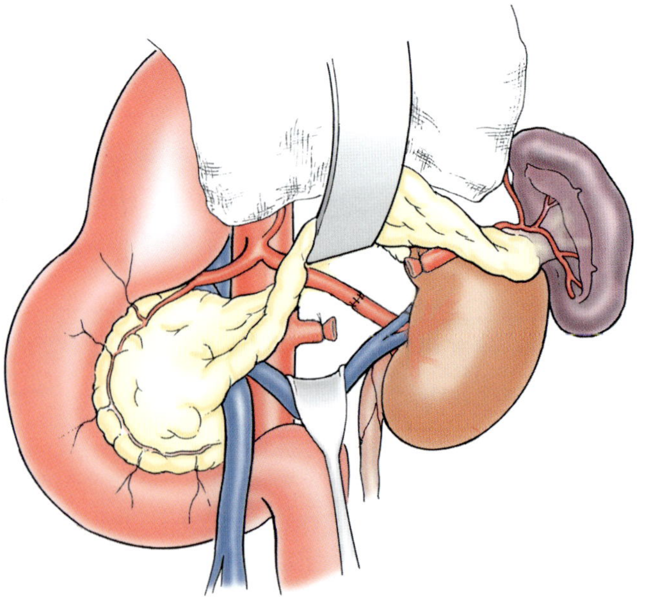

Figure 97-8. *Redrawn from Zarins C, Gewertz B: Mesenteric revascularization. In Zarins C, Gewertz B, editors:* Atlas of vascular surgery, *ed 2, Philadelphia, 2005, Churchill Livingstone, p 163, Fig. D.*

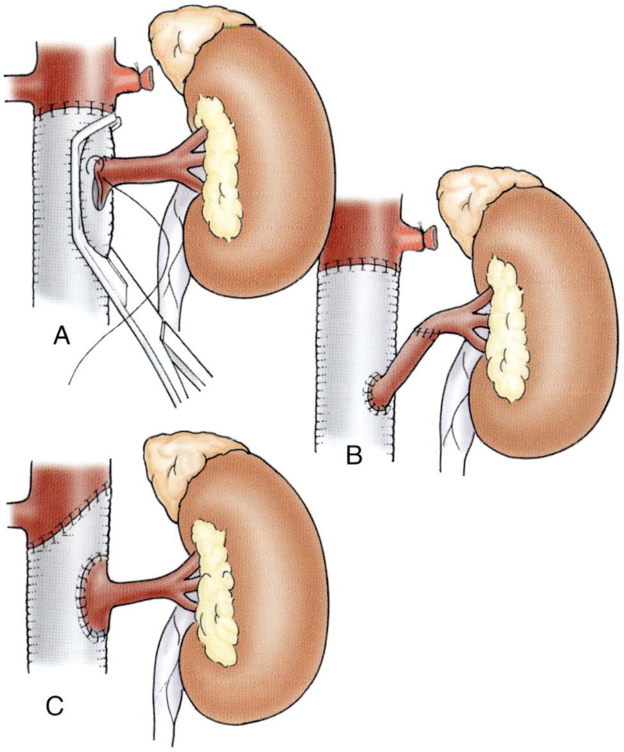

Figure 97-9. *Redrawn from Zarins C, Gewertz B: Mesenteric revascularization. In Zarins C, Gewertz B, editors:* Atlas of vascular surgery, *ed 2, Philadelphia, 2005, Churchill Livingstone, p 169, Figs. A, B, and C.*

Renal Revascularization in Association with Aortic Procedures

- Patients with severe hypertension or deteriorating renal function, or both, who have severe renal artery stenosis may benefit from renal revascularization in association with aortic reconstruction.
- If the renal artery stenosis is limited to the orifice and there is a sufficiently long renal artery, it may be possible to reimplant the vessel directly into the aortic graft. After completion of the aortic procedure, the left renal artery is suture ligated and transected. The distal renal artery is flushed with cold, heparinized balanced salt solution and clamped with a Heifetz clip. The renal artery is mobilized, and a suitable location on the aortic graft is identified. The aortic graft is partially occluded with a vascular clamp, and a window is excised from the graft. The renal artery is anastomosed to the aortic graft using a 6-0 continuous suture (Fig. 97-9, *A*, *B*, and *C*).
- If the renal artery is too short for direct implantation into the aortic graft, an interposition graft is sutured end-to-end to the distal renal artery and anastomosed end-to-side to the body of the aortic graft. Saphenous vein or a short-length (6-mm) prosthetic graft may be used.
- As an alternative technique, one renal artery can be excised with a cuff of aorta, as shown here. The proximal anastomosis is then carried obliquely above the level of the left renal artery. The left renal artery and aortic patch are then reimplanted into the side of the aortic graft. The suprarenal clamp is removed as soon as the proximal anastomoses are completed and replaced below the renal arteries.

V. SPECIAL POSTOPERATIVE CARE

- Careful attention to fluid management is critical. Replacement should be guided by pulmonary capillary wedge pressure measurements along with attention to urine outputs. Urine output should be maintained at 0.5 mL/kg/hr.
- In the very rare instance of dramatic reduction in urine output in patients with a solitary kidney, ultrasound assessment of the patency of the graft should be done after the urinary catheter patency is assured.

SUGGESTED READINGS

Dean RH, Benjamin ME, Hansen KJ: Surgical management of renovascular hypertension, *Curr Probl Surg* 34:209–308, 1997.

Fergany A, Kotettis P, Novick AL: The contemporary role of extra-anatomic surgical renal revascularization in patients with atherosclerotic renal artery disease, *J Urol* 153:1798–1802, 1995.

Hansen KJ, Edwards MS, Craven TE, et al: Prevalence of renovascular disease in the elderly: a population-based study, *J Vasc Surg* 36:443–451, 2002.

CHAPTER 98

Celiac and Mesenteric Artery Revascularization

Bruce L. Gewertz, MD, and Christopher K. Zarins, MD

Acute Intestinal Ischemia

I. SPECIAL PREOPERATIVE PREPARATION

- Acute mesenteric ischemia usually occurs in patients older than 70 years who may also have other systemic illnesses, especially gastrointestinal, peripheral vascular, and coronary artery disease. These concomitant factors may color the presentation of the problem and contribute to the frequent delays in diagnosis. Such serious comorbidity also decreases the likelihood of successful treatment.
- The classic presentation of *acute* mesenteric ischemia is abdominal pain out of proportion to physical findings. The pain is usually steady, severe, and midabdominal. If peritoneal signs are elicited, it is likely that intestinal infarction has already occurred. The occurrence of bowel infarction greatly increases mortality and morbidity. In some series, infarction is associated with a greater than 80% mortality rate. This fact underscores the importance of early diagnosis and treatment of acute ischemia and of expeditious arterial reconstructions in chronic ischemia before acute ischemia supervenes.
- One of the most frequently encountered causes of acute ischemia is *embolism*, which accounts for about one third of all mesenteric vascular catastrophes. Most emboli occur in association with cardiac arrhythmias (especially atrial tachyarrhythmias) or myocardial infarctions. The superior mesenteric artery (SMA) is the site of most embolic occlusions because of its near parallel course to the abdominal aorta.
- *Acute thrombosis* of an already compromised vessel lumen occurs in another one third of cases. Such preexisting atherosclerotic lesions are often associated with prodromal symptoms. In fact, more than 50% of patients with acute SMA thrombosis have a history of postprandial abdominal pain and weight loss. Intestinal angina typically occurs 15 to 60 minutes after meals and is more closely correlated with the volume of food consumed rather than any specific type of food. In situ thrombosis typically occurs at the origin of the SMA, resulting in gut infarction from the proximal jejunum to the midtransverse colon.
- Other causes of mesenteric ischemia are *nonocclusive vasospasm* and mesenteric *venous thrombosis*. These entities are usually not treated surgically other than for resection of nonviable bowel.
- The clinician's single greatest tool for the successful diagnosis of an acute mesenteric vascular event is a high index of suspicion in patients with multiple risk factors. Although many laboratory abnormalities occur with mesenteric ischemia and infarction, most are nonspecific and therefore not diagnostic. These abnormalities include hemoconcentration, leukocytosis with a "left shift," metabolic acidosis, hyperamylasemia, and hyperphosphatemia.
- Abdominal radiography is useful in excluding other causes of abdominal pain, such as mechanical small-bowel obstruction, perforation of a hollow viscus, or appendicitis with fecalith. That said, the single most important diagnostic test is arteriography, which can generally differentiate embolic from thrombotic occlusions. Emboli to the SMA usually lodge just proximal or distal to the origin of the middle colic artery. Thrombotic occlusions of preexistent stenotic lesions more often occur at the SMA origin and are associated with both generalized atherosclerosis of the aorta and the presence of extensive collaterals.
- All patients with suspected embolic or thrombotic occlusions should undergo urgent laparotomy. Fluid resuscitation and administration of both heparin and antibiotics are indicated before surgery.

II. OPERATIVE TECHNIQUE

SUPERIOR MESENTERIC ARTERY EMBOLECTOMY

Position

- Patients are positioned supine (Fig. 98-1). The entire abdomen and lower chest is draped along with both thighs for potential saphenous vein harvest.

Incision

- Surgical exposure is obtained through a vertical midline incision, allowing thorough abdominal exploration and determination of intestinal viability (see Fig. 98-1).

Main Dissection

- The omentum and transverse colon are retracted superiorly, and the small bowel and mesentery are lifted and gently retracted to the patient's right. The SMA is identified at the junction of the small bowel mesentery and transverse mesocolon as it crosses the duodenum. The peritoneum covering the

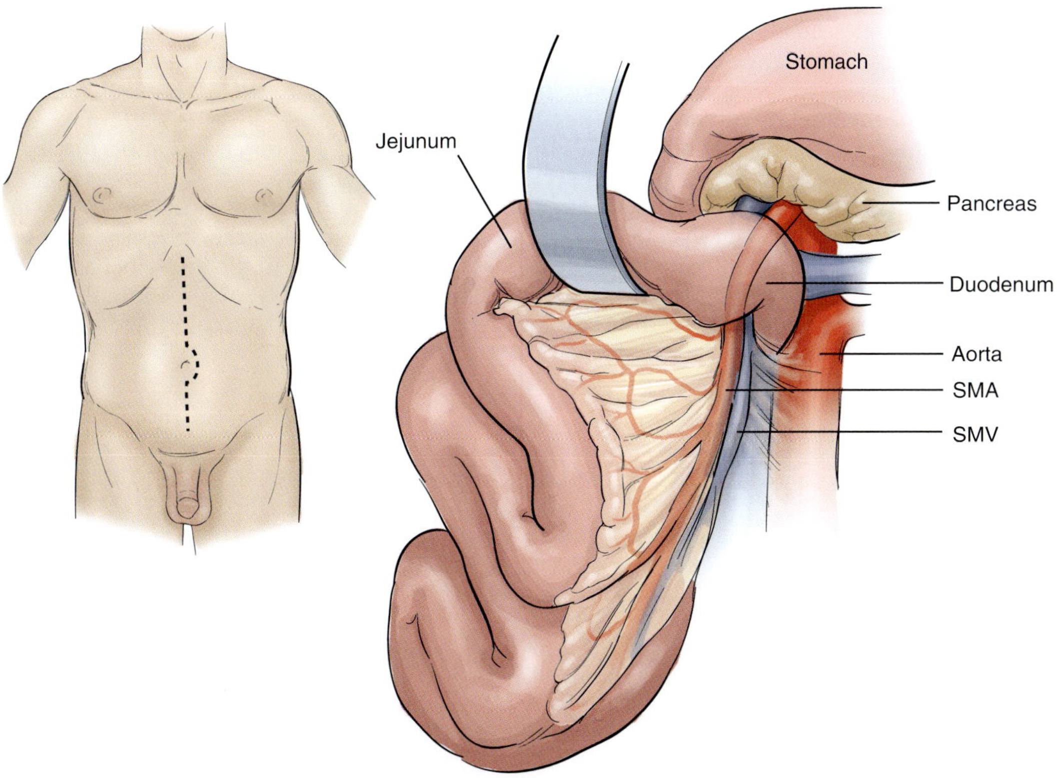

Figure 98-1. *SMA,* Superior mesenteric artery; *SMV,* superior mesenteric vein. *Redrawn from Zarins C, Gewertz B: Mesenteric revascularization. In Zarins C, Gewertz B, editors:* Atlas of vascular surgery, *ed 2, Philadelphia, 2005, Churchill Livingstone, p 175, Figs. A and B.*

mesentery is incised, and the SMA is gently dissected, taking care to avoid injury to the superior mesenteric vein (see Fig. 98-1; Fig. 98-2).

- The superior mesenteric artery is encircled with Silastic tapes. After systemic heparinization, a transverse arteriotomy is performed, and a balloon embolectomy catheter is gently advanced proximally, inflated, and withdrawn to remove the thromboembolus. The catheter is then passed distally to extract distal thrombus. If the clinical history and nature of the clot are consistent with embolus rather than in situ thrombosis of an occlusive lesion, and if excellent pulsatile inflow is obtained, bypass of the superior mesenteric artery may not be necessary.
- The transverse arteriotomy may be closed with precise interrupted sutures. If the artery is small, a vein patch may be necessary to avoid narrowing of the lumen.
- After restoration of blood flow in the superior mesenteric artery, the bowel is carefully inspected to determine viability. Pulsations in the mesentery, the return of color and peristalsis, and the presence of Doppler ultrasound signals on the antimesenteric border of the intestine are signs of intestinal viability. However, the gross visual appearance of the bowel after revascularization does not always guarantee long-term viability.

Closure

- The linea alba is closed with 1-0 nonabsorbable monofilament suture. The skin is approximated with staples.

III. ALTERNATIVE TECHNICAL APPROACHES (PRO/CON) AND PEARLS

Retrograde Celiac and Superior Mesenteric Bypass

- Aortosuperior mesenteric artery bypass is useful in patients with acute mesenteric ischemia and in those in whom superior mesenteric embolectomy/thrombectomy has been unsuccessful in restoring blood flow. A reversed saphenous vein may be sutured end-to-side to the superior mesenteric artery at the site of the arteriotomy used for the embolectomy. This anastomosis is performed using 6-0 continuous monofilament suture. The graft is anastomosed to the aorta at a location that provides a satisfactory lie of the graft without kinking (Fig. 98-3).
- Proper length of the saphenous vein bypass and location of the aortic anastomosis are critical in avoiding kinking of the graft when the small-bowel mesentery is returned to the abdomen. The tendency of grafts in this location to kink limits the usefulness of anastomoses to the infrarenal aorta.
- Revascularization of the celiac axis can be accomplished using a bypass from the infrarenal aorta to a branch of the celiac axis such as the common hepatic artery. The right colon and duodenum are

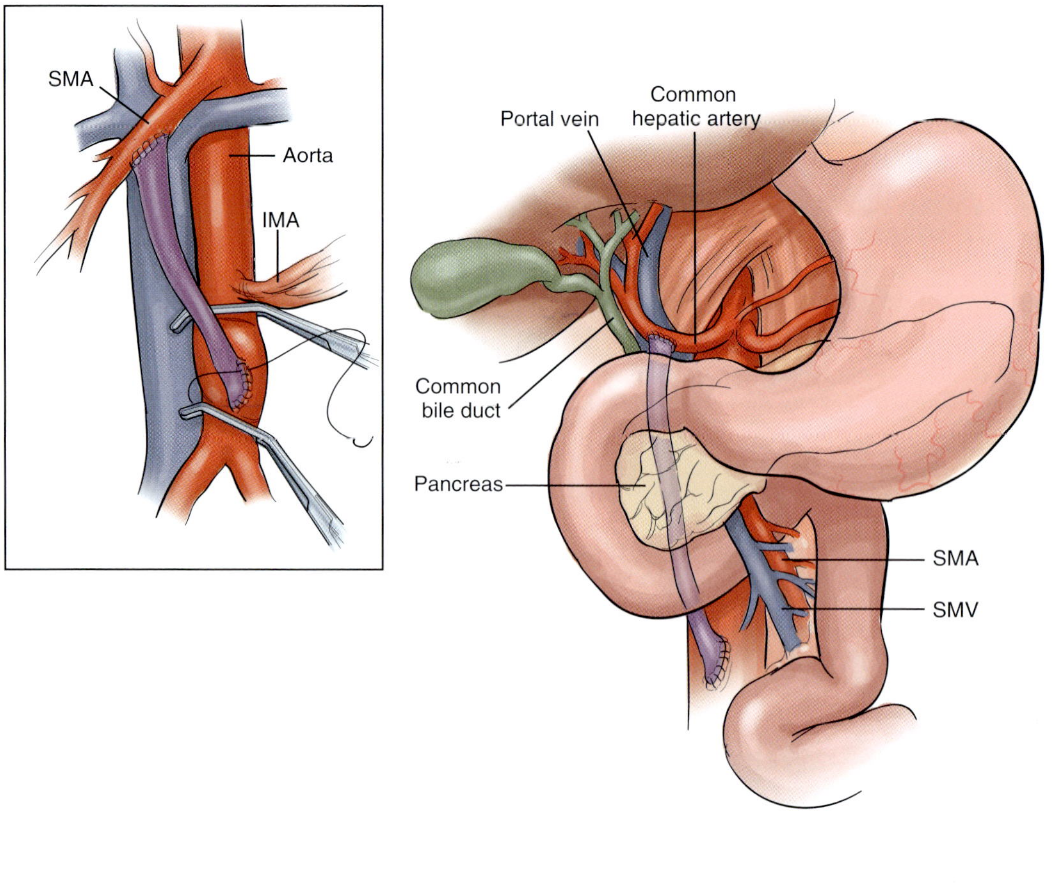

Figure 98-2. *IMA,* Inferior mesenteric artery; *SMA,* superior mesenteric artery; *SMV,* superior mesenteric vein. *Redrawn from Zarins C, Gewertz B: Mesenteric revascularization. In Zarins C, Gewertz B, editors.* Atlas of vascular surgery, *ed 2, Philadelphia, 2005, Churchill Livingstone, p 179, Figs. B and C.*

mobilized to the left past the inferior vena cava to expose the infrarenal abdominal aorta. The common hepatic artery is identified in the portal triad and dissected free. A saphenous vein or prosthetic bypass is sutured end-to-side to the infrarenal aorta. The bypass is passed retrograde behind the duodenum and head of the pancreas and anastomosed end-to-side to the hepatic artery using 6-0 monofilament suture (see Fig. 98-2).

IV. SPECIAL POSTOPERATIVE CARE

- The surgeon treating acute intestinal ischemia should consider a “second look” operation after 24 hours to confirm intestinal viability. The only exceptions to this course would be very short periods of ischemia (<4 hr) with excellent appearance of all bowel after revascularization. If any bowel resection was required at first operation, reexploration at 24 hours is highly recommended.

Chronic Intestinal Ischemia

I. SPECIAL PREOPERATIVE PREPARATION

- Chronic mesenteric ischemia is most frequently associated with atherosclerotic occlusions or stenoses. Because of the abundant collateral network, multiple vessel involvement is usually required before classic postprandial symptoms occur.
- The presentation of chronic ischemia depends on the region of the gut affected. The most common syndromes involve the midgut (jejunum, ileum, and right colon) and reflect vascular insufficiency of the distribution of the SMA caused by atherosclerosis or midaortic developmental abnormalities. Because consumption of a meal predictably induces severe incapacitating pain, eating is dramatically curtailed (“food fear”) and patients invariably lose weight. Weight loss is usually substantial and may exceed 25% of body mass.
- Ischemia of the foregut (stomach and liver) is much less common and may be irregular in its symptomatology. Patients frequently describe nonspecific symptoms such as bloating and early satiety; food fear and weight loss are often absent.

Figure 98-3.

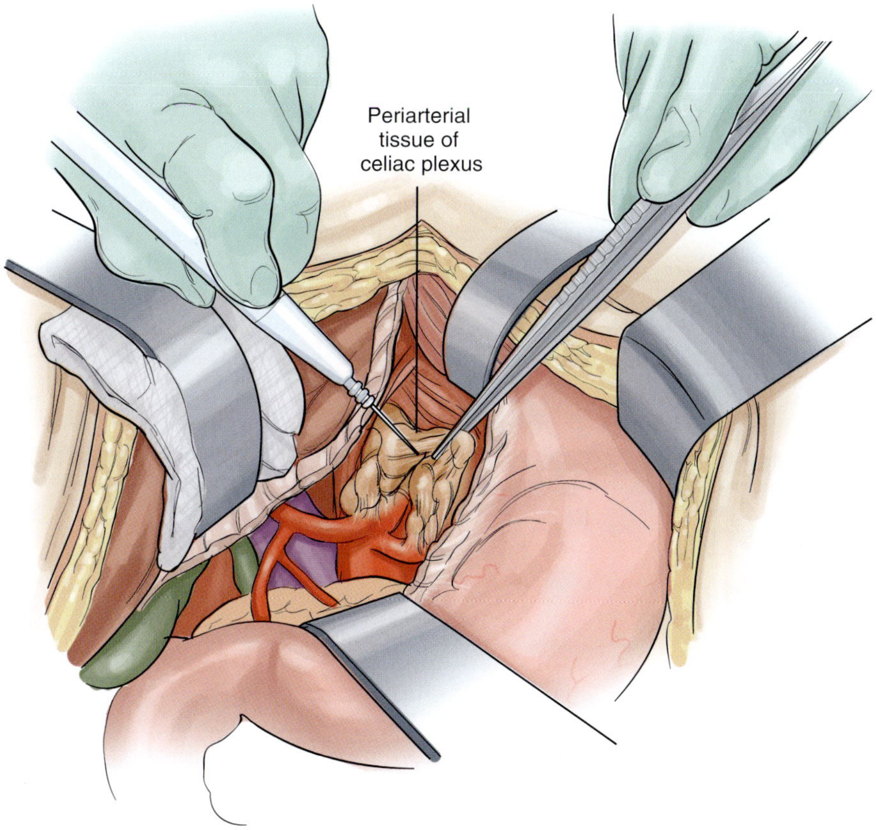

- Ischemia of the hindgut (left colon and rectum) rarely presents with postprandial pain or weight loss. Patients present with Hemoccult-positive diarrhea and chronic strictures caused by mucosal ischemia. These syndromes reflect insufficiency of the inferior mesenteric artery distribution, usually due to atherosclerosis of the origin of the vessel that is associated with disease of the internal iliac arteries. Colonic ischemia may infrequently follow vascular reconstructions of the infrarenal aorta, which may inadvertently compromise collateral blood flow.
- The definitive diagnosis of chronic intestinal ischemia is based on several factors, including (1) symptoms consistent with the arterial obstructions, (2) exclusion of the other gastrointestinal pathology, and (3) arteriographic demonstration of appropriate occlusive lesions and collateral development. Selective arterial catheterizations are usually required, together with oblique or lateral views to adequately image the origins of the three main visceral vessels.
- Recently, angioplasty with stent placement has been shown to be effective in treating these lesions. This approach is most attractive in higher-risk patients with severe malnutrition and hypoalbuminemia or limiting cardiac reserve. Although initial relief of symptoms is very acceptable, sustained success is approximately 60% at 3 years in comparison with 80% in patients treated operatively. Vascular reconstruction for chronic foregut and midgut ischemia can be accomplished by endarterectomy or aortomesenteric bypass. In our practice, antegrade bypasses from the supraceliac aorta to the celiac axis and SMA are currently the most frequently used techniques and are described in detail in this chapter.

II. OPERATIVE TECHNIQUE

ANTEGRADE CELIAC AND SUPERIOR MESENTERIC BYPASS

Position

- Patients are positioned supine. The entire abdomen and lower chest is draped along with both thighs for potential saphenous vein harvest.

Incision

- Excellent operative exposure is afforded through an upper midline incision. Most patients requiring revascularization are thin or even emaciated.

Main Dissection

- After the "lesser space" is entered through the gastrohepatic omentum, the left lobe of the liver is carefully reflected laterally, with care to avoid injury to the hepatic veins.
- The esophagus is identified after placement of a large nasogastric tube or bougie. The diaphragmatic crus is divided layer by layer using electrocautery, exposing the dense periarterial tissue of the celiac plexus. The supraceliac aorta and the entire celiac trunk are exposed (Fig. 98-4).
- After heparinization and reduction in systemic systolic blood pressure to 90 to 110 mm Hg, aortic occlusion is obtained by placement of a partially occlusive Lemole clamp (as shown in Fig. 98-5) or two aortic clamps above and below the supraceliac segment. In the technique illustrated, a single limb graft is anastomosed to the aorta with a 3-0 monofilament suture. A suitable opening is made in the graft, allowing for end-to-side anastomosis of the cut end of the main celiac trunk. After removal of the proximal clamp, the graft is passed behind the pancreas and to the left of the aorta in a tunnel

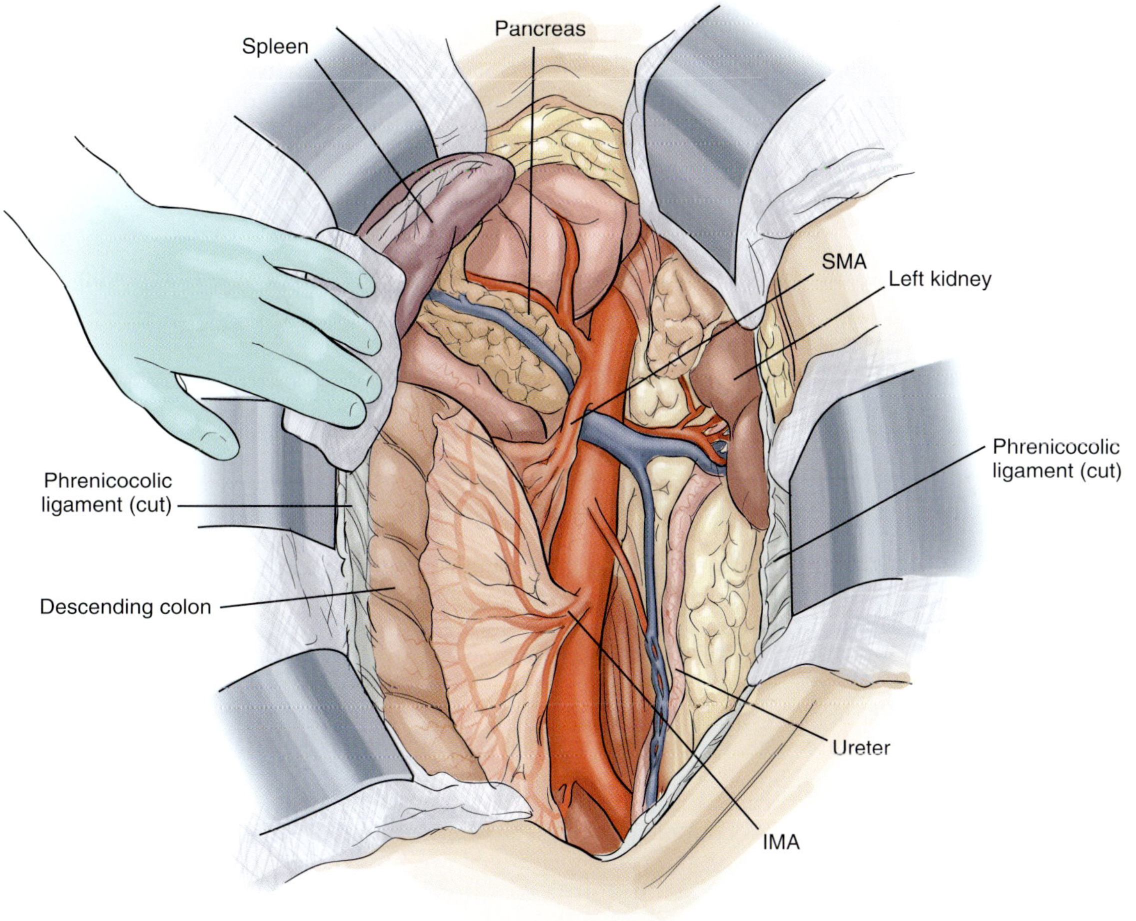

Figure 98-4. *IMA,* Inferior mesenteric artery; *SMA,* superior mesenteric artery. *Redrawn from Zarins C, Gewertz B: Mesenteric revascularization. In Zarins C, Gewertz B, editors:* Atlas of vascular surgery, *ed 2, Philadelphia, 2005, Churchill Livingstone, p 185, Fig. C.*

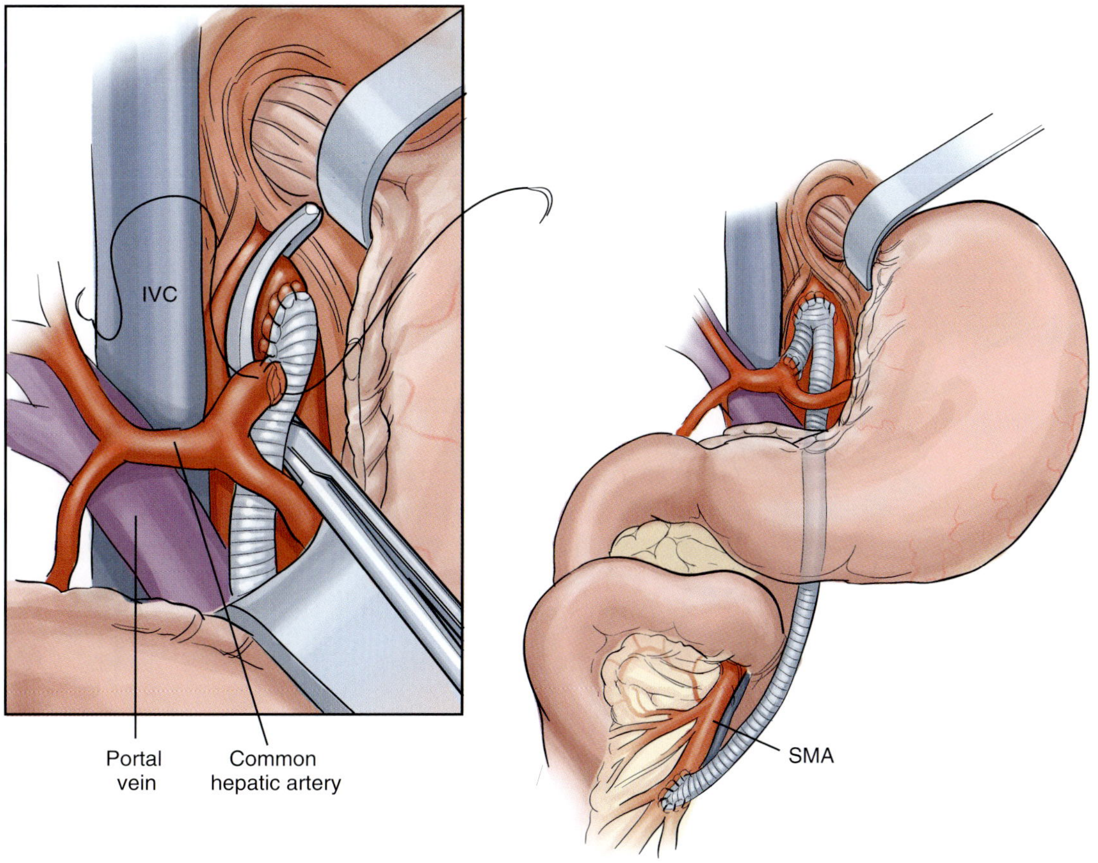

Figure 98-5. *IVC,* Inferior vena cava; *SMA,* superior mesenteric artery. *Redrawn from Zarins C, Gewertz B: Mesenteric revascularization. In Zarins C, Gewertz B, editors:* Atlas of vascular surgery, *ed 2, Philadelphia, 2005, Churchill Livingstone, p 183, Figs. D and E.*

previously created using blunt finger dissection. An end to side anastomosis is performed to the SMA distal to the occlusive lesion (not shown) (Fig. 98-6).

- An alternative reconstruction employs similar intraoperative exposure, but uses a bifurcated 12 × 6 mm graft. The limbs are then anastomosed to the celiac artery end-to-end, and the superior mesenteric artery end-to-side. Note the direct route of both graft limbs, which minimizes kinking.

Closure

- The linea alba is closed with 1-0 nonabsorbable monofilament suture. The skin is approximated with staples.

III. ALTERNATIVE TECHNICAL APPROACHES (PRO/CON) AND PEARLS

Transaortic Visceral Artery Endarterectomy

- Occlusive orificial lesions involving both the celiac and superior mesenteric arteries are usually best endarterectomized through a transaortic approach. This approach has the advantage of removing atheroma from the aorta and visceral-branch orifices during the same procedure. This may be accomplished through a transperitoneal medial visceral rotation or retroperitoneal approach to the perivisceral aorta (see Fig. 98-4).
- An incision is made along the retroperitoneum, posterior to the left colon and spleen, to allow atraumatic medial visceral rotation. The spleen, pancreas, stomach, and colon are reflected anteriorly and medially, exposing the origins of the celiac and superior mesenteric arteries. Continuous exposure of the aorta from the supraceliac region to the iliac bifurcations can be obtained.
- After dissection and control of both renal arteries, an arteriotomy is made in the aorta anterior to the left renal artery. The incision is continued superiorly above the celiac axis. Transverse arteriotomies that fashion a "trap door" incision are then made in the aorta.
- The aortic atheroma is removed. Plaque extensions into the orifices of the celiac artery, superior mesenteric artery, and both renal arteries are removed by the eversion technique. If satisfactory distal endpoints are not obtained on all vessels, the distal endpoint must be exposed and intimal tacking sutures placed to avoid postoperative thrombosis (see Fig. 98-6).
- The arteriotomy is closed with continuous 4-0 monofilament suture. Distal blood flow in all four vessels should be critically assessed by palpation and Doppler examination. Any abnormalities must be

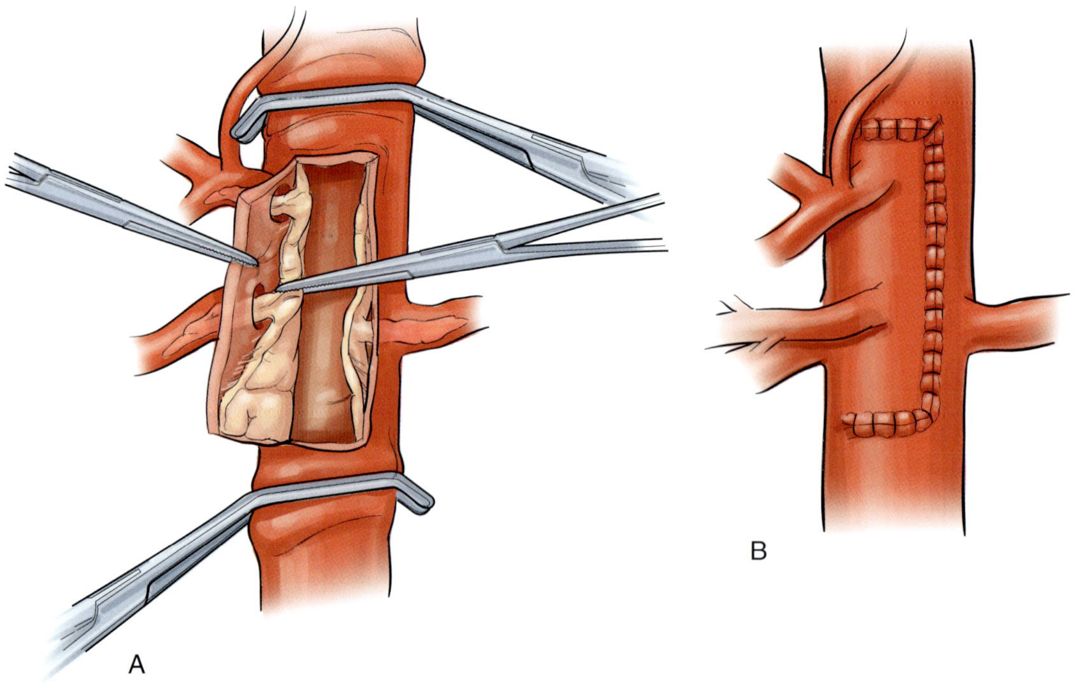

Figure 98-6. *Redrawn from Zarins C, Gewertz B: Mesenteric revascularization. In Zarins C, Gewertz B, editors:* Atlas of vascular surgery, *ed 2, Philadelphia, 2005, Churchill Livingstone, p 189, Figs. F and G.*

evaluated by intraoperative angiogram. This can be performed by clamping the aorta above the celiac axis and below the renal arteries and injecting contrast into the isolated aortic segment, or by selective transfemoral intraoperative arteriography.

IV. SPECIAL POSTOPERATIVE CARE

- In rare instances, postoperative vasospasm can occur. This may result from large blood flow volumes and pressures suddenly infusing the previously "protected" low-flow, low-pressure circulatory bed distal to multiple mesenteric stenoses. The best treatment is calcium channel blockers perioperatively. In persistent cases, angiography and infusion of priscoline or papaverine may be needed.
- The timing of postoperative "refeeding" should be carefully weighed. In patients with long histories of symptoms, it is prudent to begin with small amounts of food in frequency, not bulk.
- Duplex scan is the preferred method of postoperative follow-up for graft patency.

SUGGESTED READINGS

Kasirajan, K, O'Hara PJ, Gray BH, et al: Chronic mesenteric ischemia: open surgery versus percutaneous angioplasty and stenting, *J Vasc Surg* 33:63–71, 2001.

Moawad, J, McKinsey JF, Wyble CW, et al: Current results of surgical therapy for chronic mesenteric ischemia, *Arch Surg* 132:613–619, 1997.

Park WM, Cherry KJ Jr., Chua HK, et al: Current results of open revascularization for chronic mesenteric ischemia: a standard for comparison, *J Vasc Surg* 35:853–859, 2002.

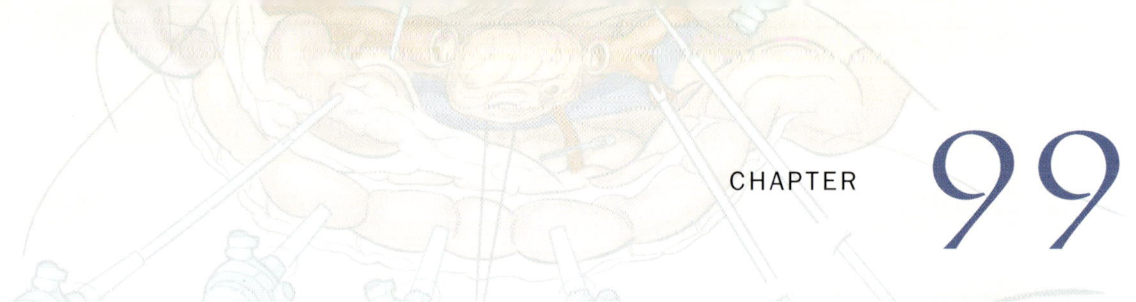

CHAPTER 99

Thoracoscopic First Rib Resection for Thoracic Outlet Syndrome

Randall K. Wolf, MD, FACS, FACC, and Alvin H. Crawford, MD, FACS

I. SPECIAL PREOPERATIVE PREPARATION

- Resection of the first rib is performed for surgical treatment of thoracic outlet syndrome (TOS). TOS refers to compression of the subclavian vessels and/or the brachial plexus by the first rib and adjacent structures at the superior aperture of the chest. Paget in 1875 and von Schroetter in 1884 reported thrombosis of the subclavian vein caused by TOS. This vascular form of TOS is known as Paget-von Schroetter syndrome. However, the most common symptoms are neurologic and are related to compression of the brachial plexus in the distribution of the ulnar nerve.
- Diagnostic evaluation should include history, physical examination, chest radiograph, cervical spine films, electromyogram, and ulnar nerve conduction velocities.
- Arterial and venous compression in thoracic outlet require additional contrast studies.
- Complete cardiologic workup is necessary in selected patients, as is complete neurologic workup in some patients. Once other disease processes have been eliminated and appropriate medical therapy has proved ineffective or is deemed inappropriate, surgical therapy may be considered.
- Chest radiography should be performed in all cases to rule out a superior sulcus tumor of the chest. Superior sulcus or Pancoast tumors can mimic symptoms of TOS.
- Computed tomography is also helpful in determining the rib anatomy and to rule out a congenital cervical rib or fused ribs 1 and 2 (Fig. 99-1).
- If a vascular form of TOS is suspected, noninvasive upper extremity venous and/or arterial testing is recommended.
- If a neurologic form of TOS is suspected, nerve conduction studies can be obtained.
- The anatomy, clinical presentation, and evaluation of the patient with TOS have been extensively reviewed by Urschel, and the reader is referred to textbook chapters by Urschel for clear, concise, and exhaustive information concerning the history, anatomy, presentation, testing, and accepted management of TOS that is beyond the scope of this presentation (Fig. 99-2). This chapter presents a minimally invasive thoracoscopic surgical technique for excision of the first rib for treatment of TOS. The spectrum of thoracic outlet compression symptoms ranges from mild to disabling, and the specific symptoms can be divided by the structure most compressed, whether artery, vein, or nerve. The etiology can be congenital, traumatic, or acquired. Brachial plexus compression accounts for the majority of cases that are evaluated surgically. Presenting symptoms may include pain, paresthesias, and motor weakness, usually in the distribution of the ulnar nerve. Subclavian artery compression can present as arm claudication, pulselessness, or arterial thrombosis. Subclavian vein compression may present with acute pain and edema of the arm secondary to venous thrombosis, or more chronically as Paget-von Schroetter syndrome.
- The most effective single surgical procedure is probably resection of the first thoracic rib. The most successful approach reported is the transaxillary approach initially described by Atkins, reported by Roos, and popularized by Urschel. Urschel has reported 85% good results with the use of complete first rib resection in properly selected patients.

II. OPERATIVE TECHNIQUE

Position

- The surgeon stands on the anterior or posterior side of the patient. The patient is placed in the lateral position after induction of general anesthesia with a double-lumen tube. The kidney rest is raised to slightly open the ribs, and selective ventilation is initiated.

Incision

- Three 10-mm thoracic ports are used for the operation: the two higher ports in the anterior third or fourth and lateral fifth intercostal spaces for the working instruments, and a lower port on the lateral wall in the sixth intercostal space for a rigid 30-degree scope. Three 10-mm ports are placed, two being flexible ports (Flexipath, Ethicon Endo-Surgery, Cincinnati) and one a rigid port. A 10-mm

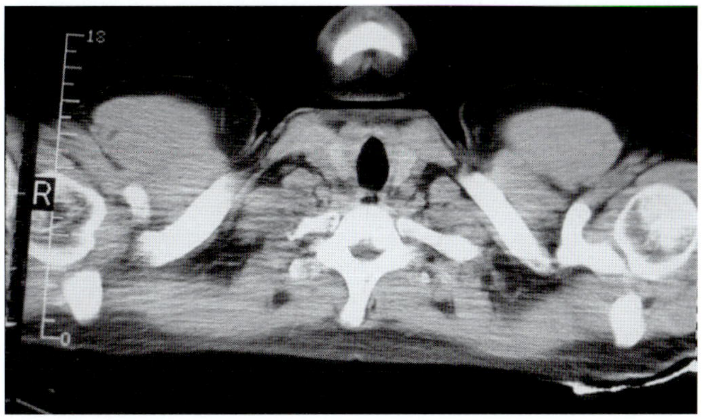

Figure 99-1.

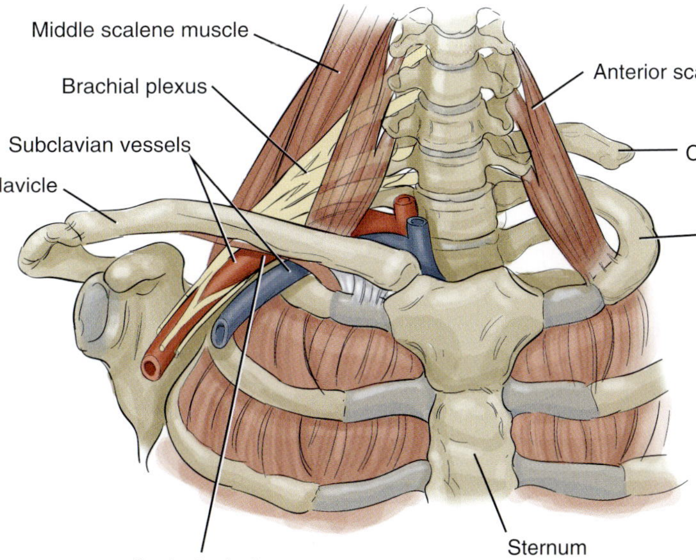

Figure 99-2.

30-degree endoscope with a three-chip camera is placed through the rigid inferior port. The anatomy is carefully evaluated (Fig. 99-3).

- We focus on the forces that can cause compression on the thoracic outlet and the anatomy as seen from inside the thorax. The subclavian vessels and brachial plexus drape over the first rib as they transverse the cervicoaxillary canal and exit to the upper extremity. Compression of the contents in this canal can be caused by the muscles, ligaments or bony structures that comprise the borders. These include the anterior scalene and middle scalene muscles, subclavius muscle, costocoracoid ligament, cervical rib, first rib, and anomalies of the first rib or clavicle. This anatomy can be best appreciated and the first rib clearly visualized from inside the thoracic cavity.
- On thoracoscopic examination, the first rib can be easily identified in the "roof" of the thorax. The first rib is a wide flat rib that forms a C in the apex of the chest cavity (Fig. 99-4, *A*). It can be "palpated" indirectly using an endoscopic Kittner and can be clearly visualized. Care should be taken to note the relationship of the internal mammary artery anteriorly and the sympathetic chain posteriorly to the borders of the first rib. On the left, the subclavian artery is also easily visualized on thoracoscopic examination (see Fig. 99-4, *B*).
- The flexible ports are used for placement of the orthopedic instruments. The thoracoscopic approach to first rib resection has been presented by Wolf and colleagues.

Main Dissection

- The thoracoscopic rib resection begins by dissecting the parietal pleura as well as intercostal muscles from the costal edge of the first rib using the Harmonic scalpel (Ethicon Endo Surgery). Endoscopic instruments including endoscopic elevators, curettes, and rongeurs (Medtronic Sofamor Danek, Memphis) have been altered from the regular orthopedic tools by extension and modification to pass through 10-mm endoscopic ports. In the initial report, an endoscopic drill (Midas Rex, Midas Rex Pneumatic Tools, Fort Worth, Texas) capable of pulverizing bone through ports with a coarse ball tip revolving at high speed was initially used. The Harmonic scalpel, which operates with ultrasonic energy and produces less smoke and lower heat than regular electrocautery, facilitates endoscopic dissection of the first rib (Fig. 99-5, *A*).
- The subclavian vein, artery, and brachial plexus, lying from anterior to posterior in each groove of the first rib, are freed from the bone bluntly using an endoscopic Cobb elevator and endoscopic curettes (see Fig. 99-5, *B*).

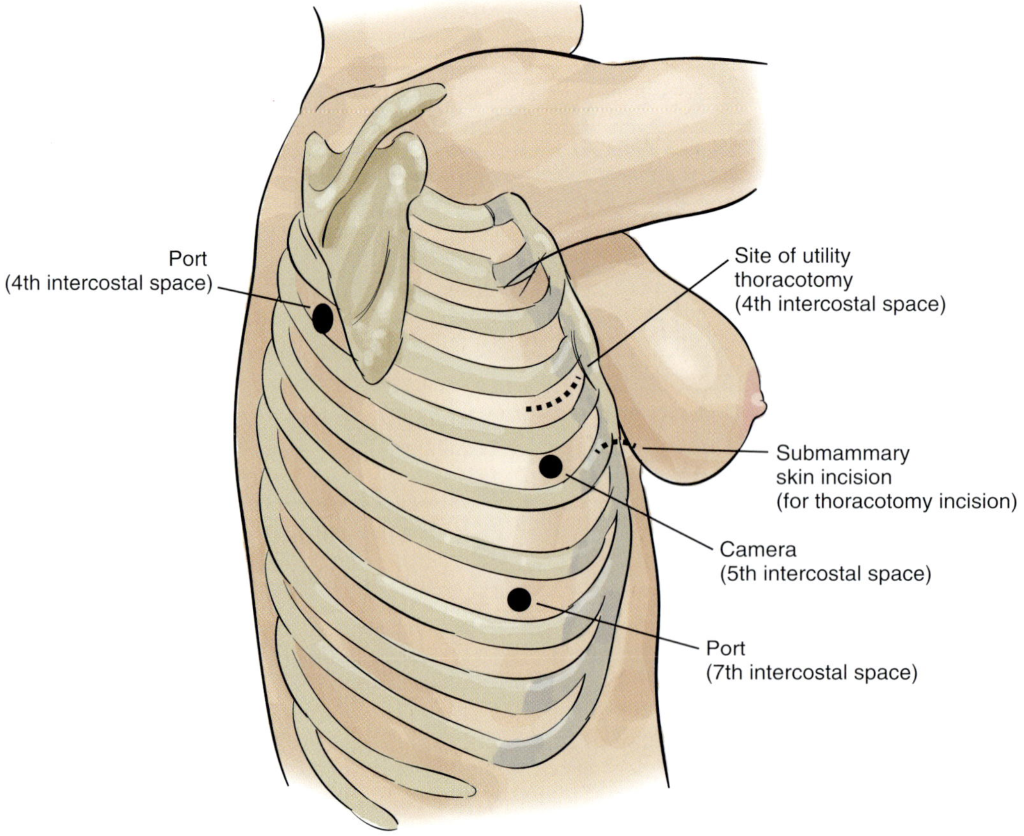

Figure 99-3.

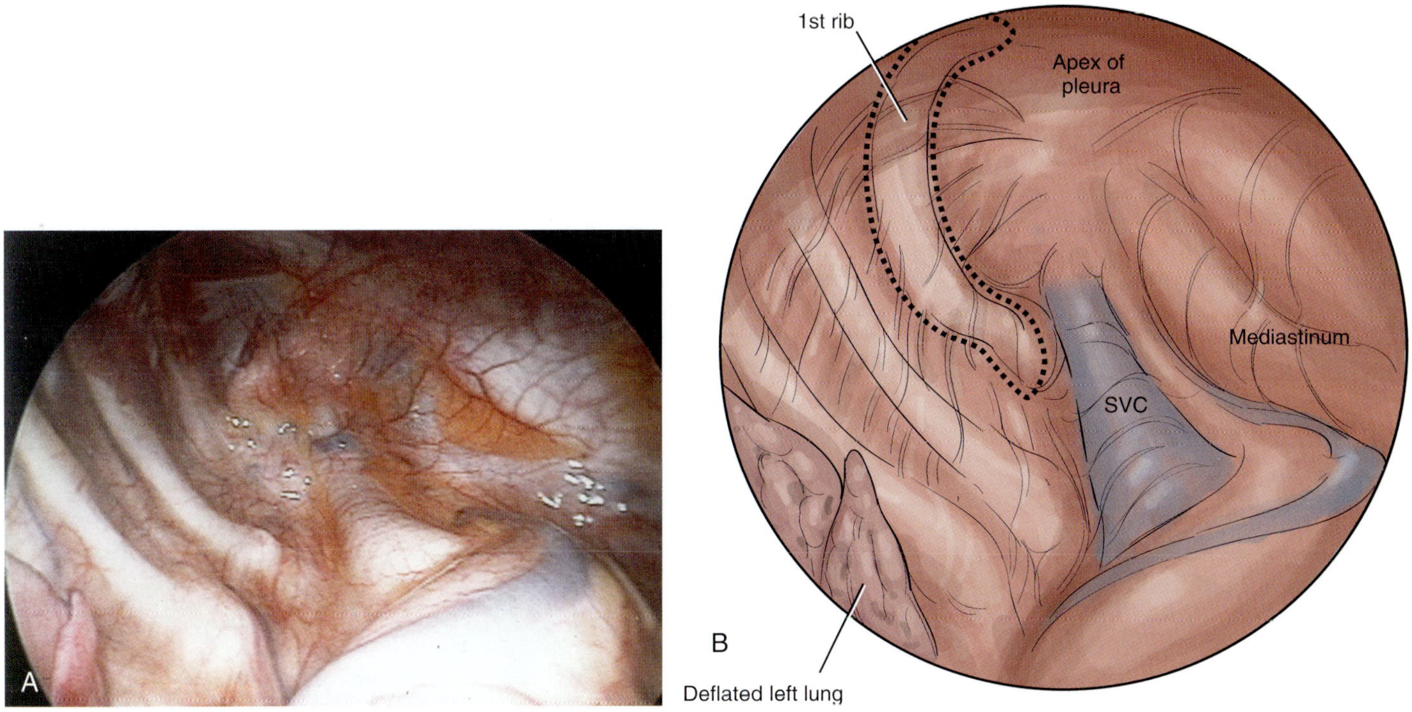

Figure 99-4. *SVC*, Superior vena cava.

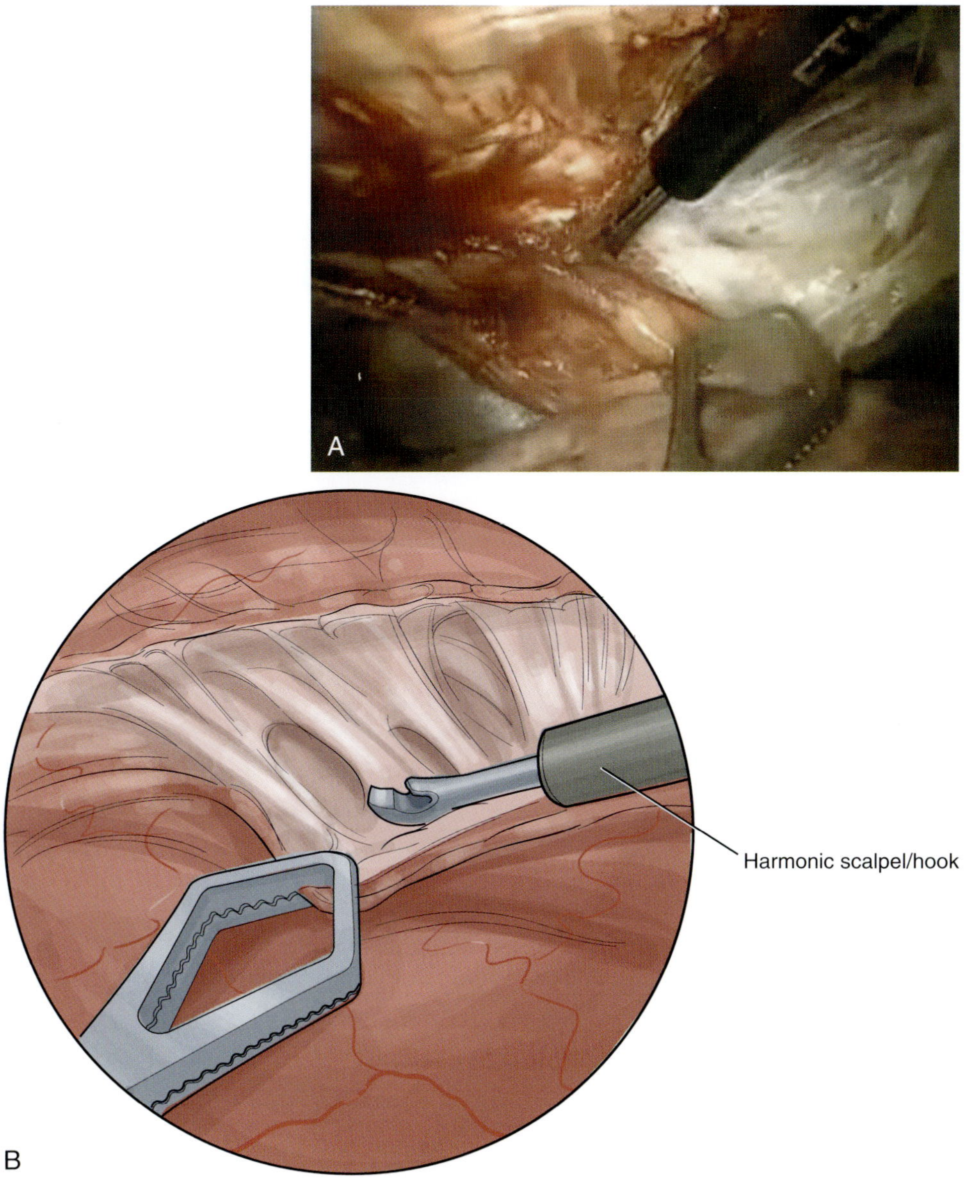

Figure 99-5.

- Next, cautious dissection with a spinous process elevator frees the ribs circumferentially (Fig. 99-6). Recently, special angled elevators have been manufactured to facilitate this maneuver (Fig. 99-7, *A* and *B*). To divide the rib, an endoscopic drill can also be used (Fig. 99-8). The vessels and nerve are protected from the revolving drill by placing an endoscopic elevator behind the rib. The powdered tissue is evacuated by suction. Currently, the drill has been replaced by an endoscopic rib cutter.
- The endoscopic rib cutter is simpler, easier to use, and safer than the drill. The endoscopic rib cutter is employed to divide the first rib both anteriorly and posteriorly in its midportion. The divided rib is then removed through one of the port incisions (Fig. 99-9).
- Endoscopic orthopedic rongeurs are then used to trim the resected ends of the rib back to the transverse process posteriorly, and anteriorly to the manubrium (Fig. 99-10).
- Final assessment should include palpation of the transverse process posteriorly, as well as the costochondral junction anteriorly. This allows for complete excision of the first rib, a point emphasized by Urschel.

Closure

- The inferior port site is used for a 19-Fr Blake-type chest tube. The port sites are closed with absorbable suture and skin glue.

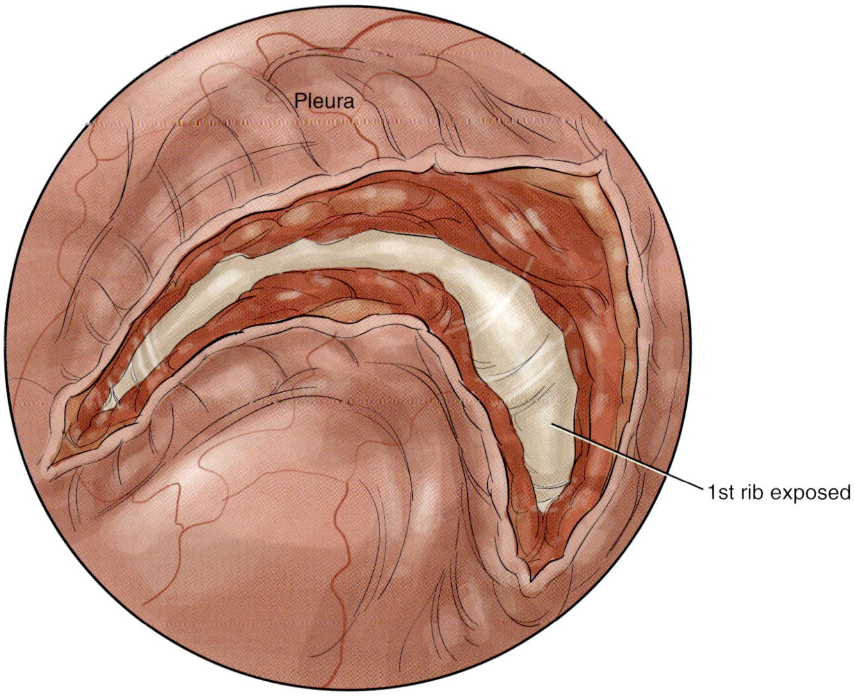

Figure 99-6.

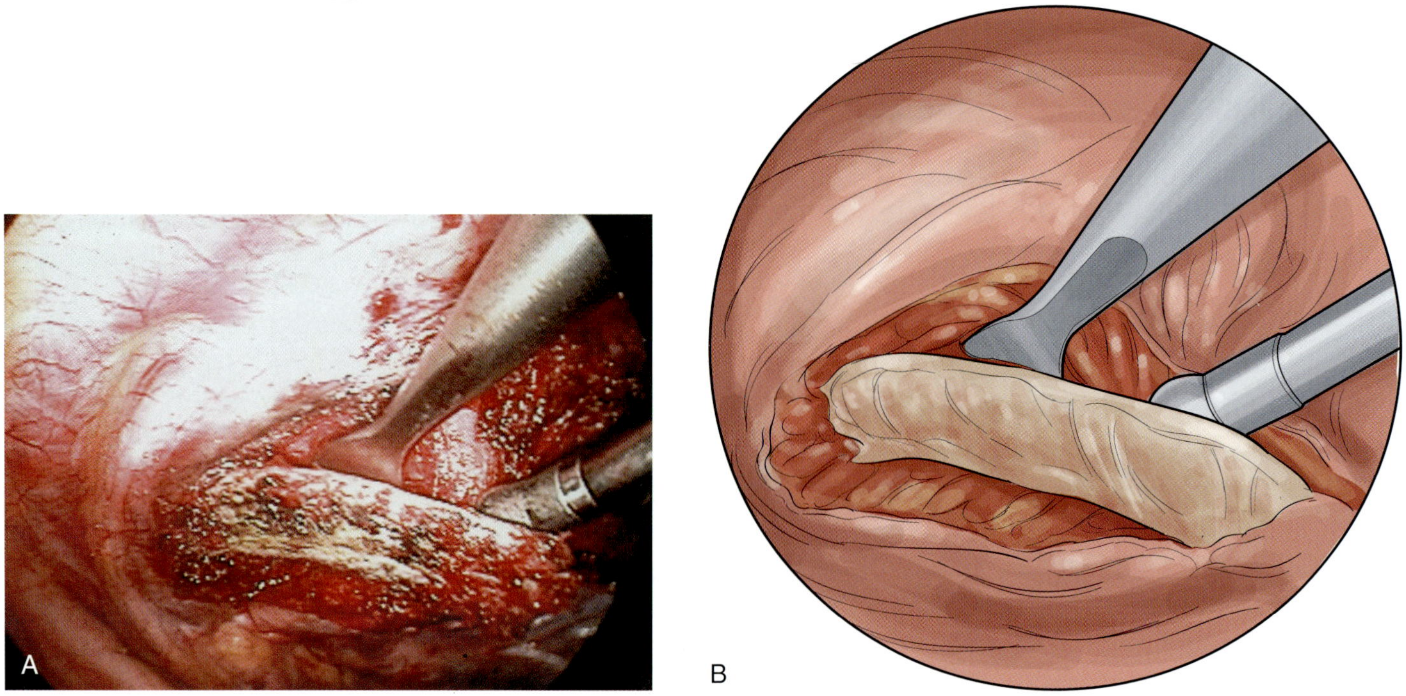

Figure 99-7.

III. ALTERNATE TECHNICAL APPROACHES (PRO/CON) AND PEARLS

- A few technical points of the thoracoscopic first rib resection are worth emphasizing. Care must be taken in developing the plane of dissection, and it is recommended to dissect anterior to the vein initially.
- After transection of the rib, any additional muscle attachments, such as anterior or middle scalene, can be divided under direct vision. The rib can be delivered easily through one of the port sites after the port is removed.
- During this dissection, the mammary artery anteriorly and the sympathetic chain posteriorly are clearly observed and preserved.
- Port sites are best placed at some distance from the target to allow adequate manipulation of the instruments in a comfortable arc.
- As noted earlier, to divide the rib, an endoscopic rib cutter is favored over a bone drill, as the cutter is easier to control. The endoscopic rib cutter appears to add safety to the division maneuver and is relatively easy to use compared to the drill. Excellent visualization of the thoracic outlet is the main advantage of the thoracoscopic approach. It is quite dramatic to observe the contents of the thoracic outlet drape gently across the superior thorax after the first rib has been successfully resected thoracoscopically. Thoracoscopic first rib resection is feasible and reproducible using endoscopic instruments. The entire first rib can be resected with a clear view of the subclavian artery and vein and brachial plexus. There is no possibility of intercostal brachialis cutaneous nerve injury.
- Complete excision of the first rib is possible using this thoracoscopic technique. Urschel stated that thoracoscopy expedites the transaxillary approach and helps teach the procedure. With the totally

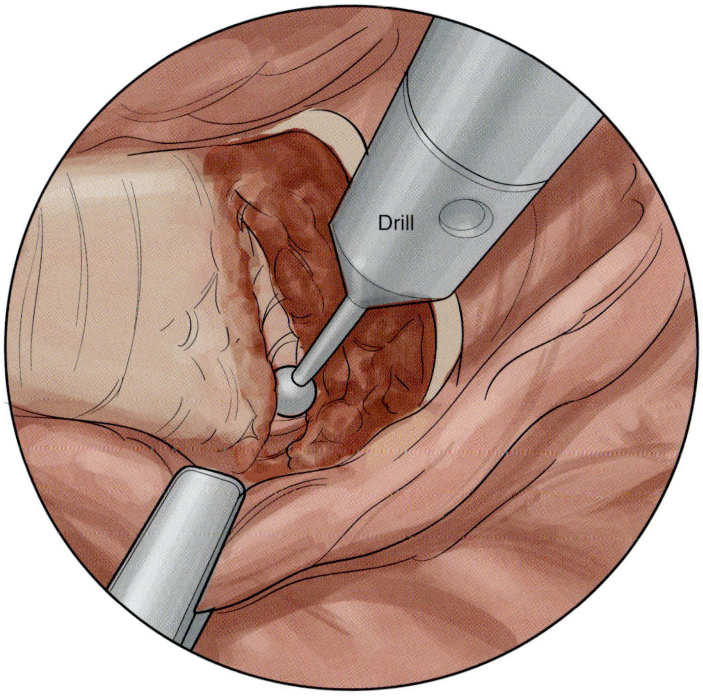

Figure 99-8.

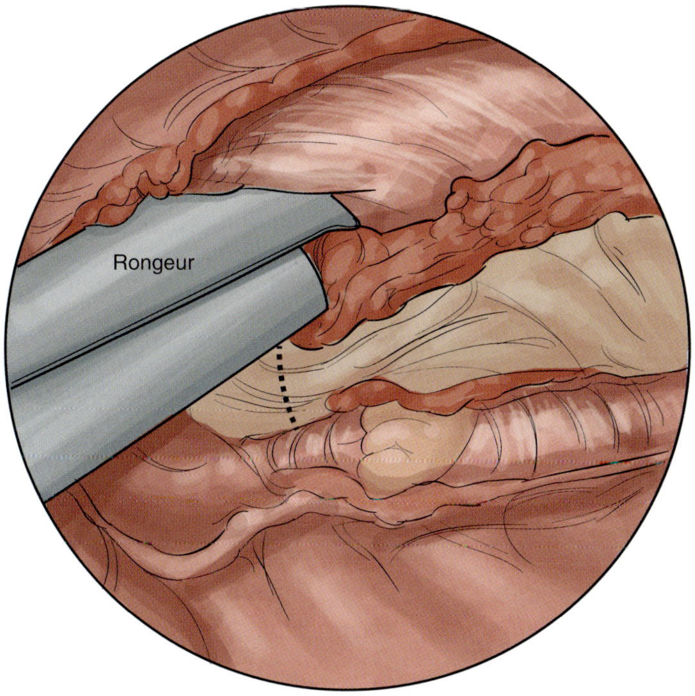

Figure 99-9.

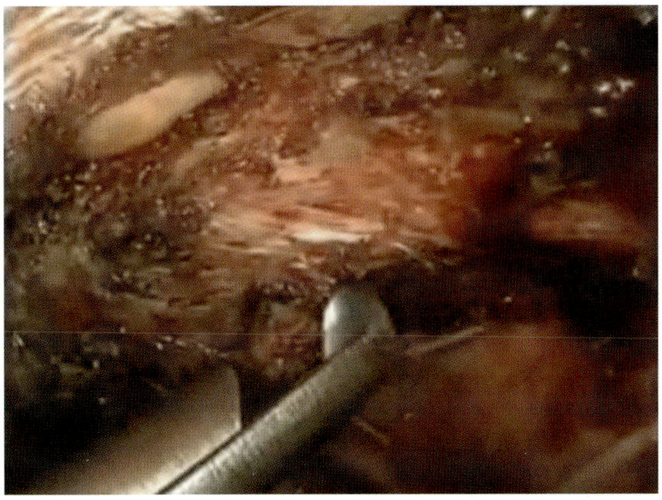

Figure 99-10.

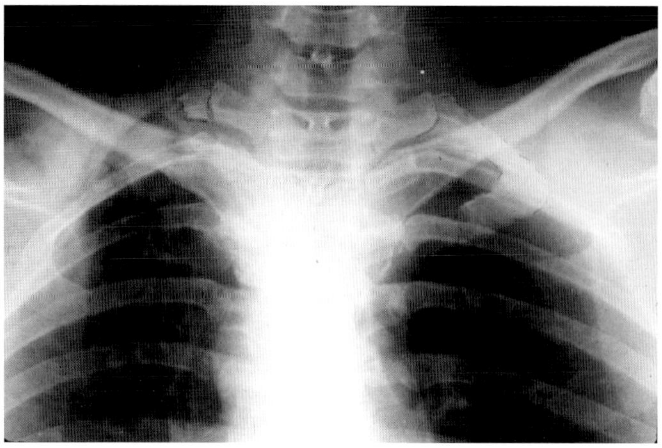

Figure 99-11.

thoracoscopic approach, the pleural side of the first rib is visualized in its entirety, and the anatomic relationship of the first rib to the adjacent structures is clearly identified. The extent of rib-resection and its immediate effect on the structures of the thoracic outlet are clearly visualized.

- In seven cases performed by Wolf and co-workers, the first rib was removed by this technique to decompress the subclavian vessels and brachial plexus lying on the first rib. In the first patient, who presented with right subclavian vein thrombosis, the symptoms on the right side resolved completely after the procedure. He subsequently developed symptoms in the left arm and underwent the same procedure on the left side. The duration of the initial operation was 110 minutes. However, the operation times were reduced with experience to 100 minutes for the second case and 75 minutes for the third. Blood loss was minimal in each case, and the hospital stays were 3, 2, and 1 day in the first, second, and third cases, respectively. Currently, a 1-day stay in the hospital is routine. Ten years after surgery, the patient with Paget-Schroetter syndrome remained asymptomatic.
- Surgical treatment for neurologic TOS has a long history going back to the last century but is still controversial. Patients with neurologic or vascular symptoms can be treated successfully by resecting the first rib, usually through a transaxillary approach. The transaxillary resection of the first rib has been detailed by Urschel.
- Advantages of this open technique are that it can be accomplished without major muscle division, without brachial plexus retraction, and with a very acceptable cosmetic result.
- The disadvantages of the open transaxillary approach include limited visualization of the important structures and the possibility of injury to the intercostobrachialis cutaneous nerve.
- Described here is an alternative approach for resection of the first rib using new tools developed for endoscopic orthopedic surgery. A thoracoscopic rib-cutter allows thoracoscopic division of the first rib through ports, and the Harmonic scalpel facilitates thoracoscopic dissection and exposure of the first rib, providing smokeless views.
- Additional specialized elevators have been employed to facilitate clearing of the ribs from the muscular attachments.

IV. SPECIAL POSTOPERATIVE CARE

- The patient goes from the recovery room to a room on the floor for an overnight stay. The chest tube is removed on postoperative day 1, and the patient is discharged, to be seen in the office in 1 week. A chest radiograph is obtained (Fig. 99-11).
- There are no restrictions.
- Although we do not have any experience with intraoperative complications using this thoracoscopic technique, the surgical team should be prepared to perform a more standard thoracotomy, in the third or fourth intercostal space, if a vascular injury occurs during the procedure.
- Finally, the thoracoscopic first rib resection technique lends itself to teaching quite naturally, because the anatomy is clearly visualized. With future instrumental and technical progress, this approach is expected to become a reproducible, minimally invasive technique for resection of the first rib.

SUGGESTED READINGS

Ohtsuka T, Wolf RK, Wurnig P, Dunsker SB: Port-access first rib resection with new instruments: a report of two cases, *J Endosc Surg* Jan. 1998.

Urschel HC: Thoracic outlet syndrome. In Sabiston DC, Spencer FC, editors: *Surgery of the chest*, ed 5, Philadelphia, 1990, Saunders.

Wolf RK, Crawford AH, Hahn BY: Thoracoscopic first rib resection for thoracic outlet syndrome. In Yim AP, Hazler SR, Izzat MB, et al, editors: *Minimal access cardiothoracic surgery*, Philadelphia, 2000, Saunders.

CHAPTER 100

Femorodistal (Peroneal/ Dorsalis Pedis) Bypass for Occlusive Disease

Mauri Lepäntalo, MD, PhD, and Anders Albäck, MD, PhD

I. SPECIAL PREOPERATIVE PREPARATION

- Distal bypass surgery is indicated only in the treatment of critically ischemic leg or in cases with complicated neuroischemic diabetic foot not amenable to an endovascular approach.
- As an increasing number of legs with critical ischemia can be revascularized by endovascular means, remaining candidates for distal bypass surgery often have long occluded segments, poor runoff, ischemic skin lesions, and fragile tissues, as well as many concurrent diseases.
- There are no universally accepted criteria for critical ischemia, but ankle pressure below 50 to 70 mm Hg and toe pressure or transcutaneous oxygen tension ($tcpO_2$) on the dorsum of the foot below 30 to 50 mm Hg are used as definitions; higher values are expected in the presence of diabetes and tissue lesions.
- The arterial tree can be visualized by duplex, magnetic resonance, computed tomography, or digital subtraction angiography. The last is most precise for outflow assessment, especially when performed in four planes (Fig. 100-1). In multisegmental disease, the use of selective antegrade arteriography through the ipsilateral common femoral artery improves visualization. However, the pedal outflow bed may not always be properly visualized. Duplex should be used as a complementary method, and

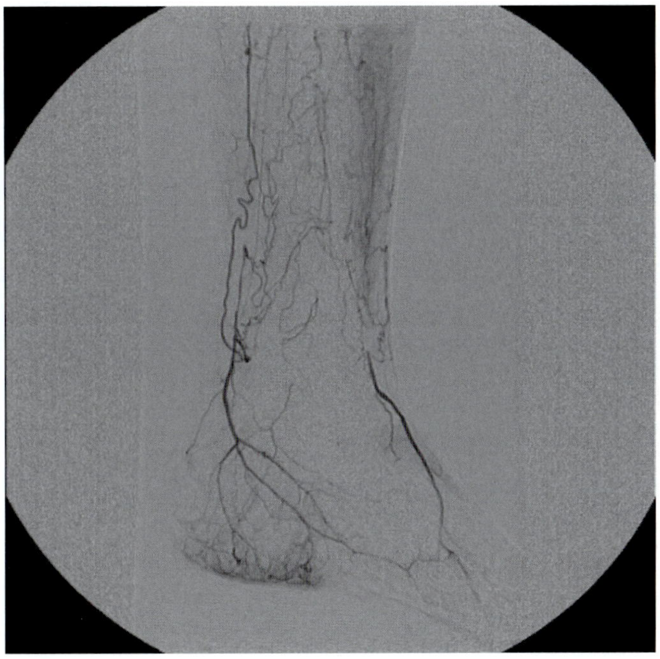

Figure 100-1.

sometimes the outflow tract may be explored and bypass performed based on evidence from duplex rather than arteriography (Fig. 100-2, *A* and *B*).

- Vein mapping should be done by duplex to optimize vein harvesting. The great saphenous vein, its anterior branch, and arm veins are often more useful than the small saphenous vein, because the harvest area for the small saphenous vein, especially in the target leg, may be vulnerable to wound problems.
- Because patients in need of long distal bypass are vulnerable and at great risk for wound complications, careful preoperative planning of skin incisions and graft routing is helpful in preventing postoperative skin problems. Special attention should be paid to this, especially if the patient has infected ischemic lesions in the lower extremity.
- A common postoperative complication and cause of death in patients with critical limb ischemia is myocardial infarction. All patients should undergo preoperative evaluation by an internist and/or anesthesiologist to minimize peri- and postoperative cardiac complications. There is clear evidence for the benefits of using beta-blockers and statins.
- Diabetic patients need special attention, because perioperative hyperglycemia and large fluctuations in plasma glucose levels increase postoperative mortality and morbidity. Careful measures must be taken to minimize these effects.

II. OPERATIVE TECHNIQUE

Position

- The patient is placed in the supine position (Fig. 100-3) and should be kept warm. However, the ischemic leg or a leg in which arteries are cross-clamped should not be externally heated. Locoregional anesthesia is preferred and supplemented by epidural anesthesia to decrease the need for opiates postoperatively and potentially to increase postoperative graft flow.

Incision

- An atraumatic surgical technique is important: sharp dissection of tissue planes, preferably by cutting diathermy to maintain hemostasis. Wound edges should not be grasped with forceps, and retractors should be spread only to the extent that provides necessary visualization. Especially in the groin, care should be taken not to tear the skin and subcutaneous tissue from the fascia. Bridges of intact skin should always be left between incisions when possible.
- The femoral bifurcation is exposed using a longitudinal incision just laterally to the lymphatics of the groin and to the artery. Sharp dissection extends directly downward to the fascia lata, continuing medially to cut the fascia sharply over the superficial femoral artery (see Fig. 100-3).

Main Dissection

Femoroperoneal Bypass

- Dissection continues in the midline over the artery upward to the inguinal ligament. If the artery is heavily calcified, dissection should proceed upward below the ligament, cutting the inferior epigastric

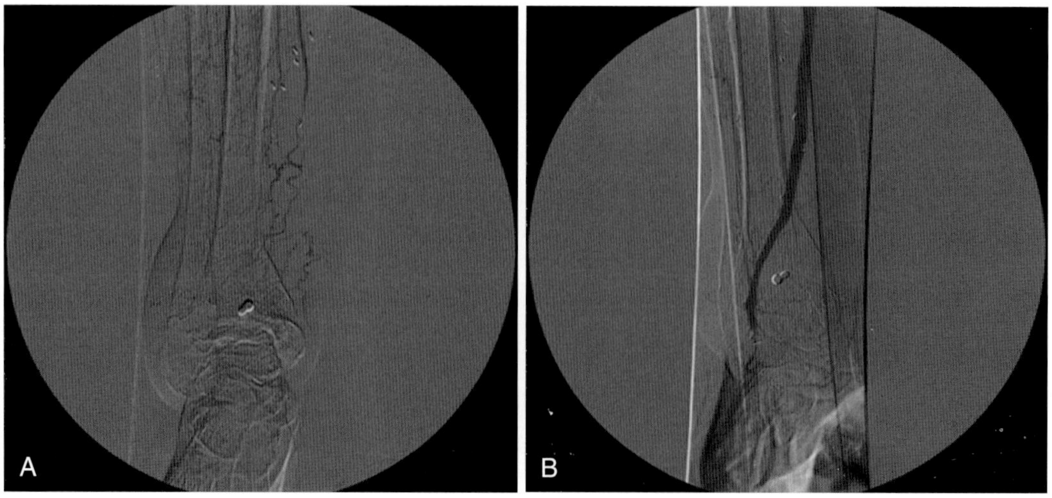

Figure 100-2.

and deep circumflex iliac veins between vascular clips to expose the distal external iliac artery, which can be palpated and clamped well above the ligament without dividing it. The deep femoral artery should be exposed distal to any ostial calcification, dividing the lateral femoral circumflex vein if necessary (Fig. 100-4).

- The peroneal artery is exposed (Fig. 100-5) through a longitudinal medial skin incision placed over the anterior edge of the medial belly of the gastrocnemius muscle. (*Note:* If the vein is to be harvested from the medial calf, the incision should follow the course of the vein instead.)

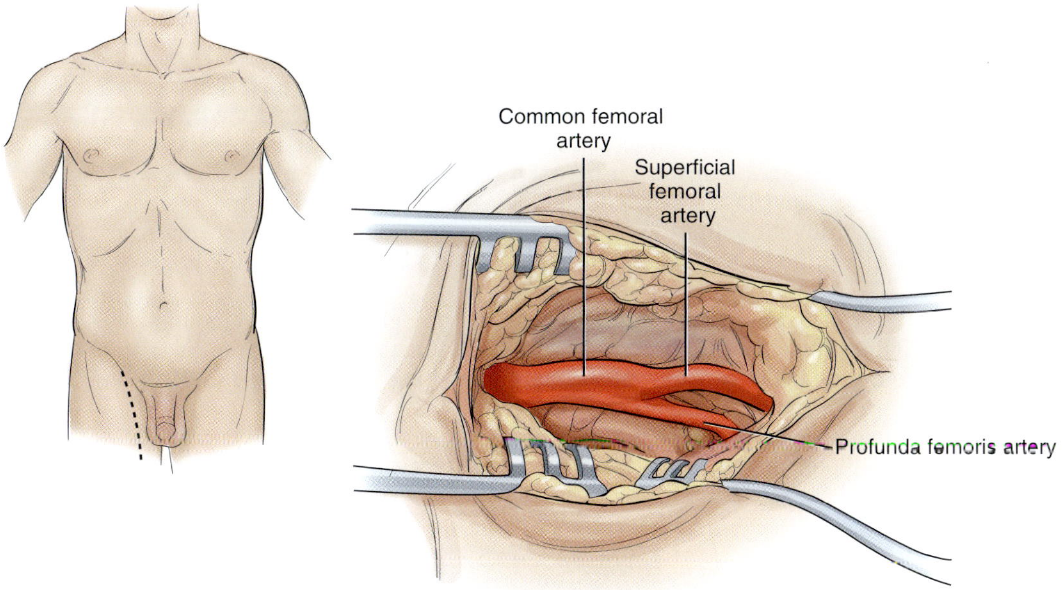

Figure 100-3.

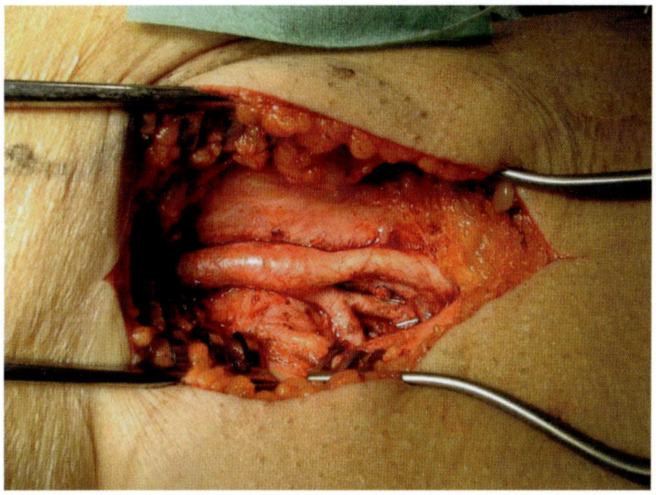

Figure 100-4.

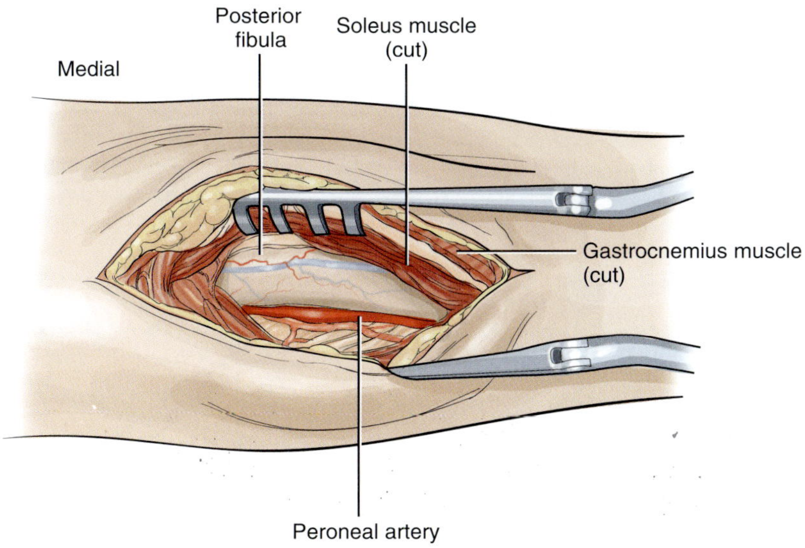

Figure 100-5.

- The superficial posterior compartment is entered by cutting the fascia. The edge of the gastrocnemius muscle is mobilized, and dissection continues sharply by cautery through the soleus muscle, ligating perforating vessels as they are encountered (Fig. 100-6). Care should be taken not to damage the posterior tibial vessels, which are left anteriorly (Fig. 100-7).
- The dissection is continued toward the fibular bone, dividing the fascia of the deep posterior compartment and separating the deep flexor muscles to expose the peroneal vessels just posteriorly to the palpable medial rim of fibular bone. The artery should be dissected free only to uncover its medial aspect, making arteriotomy possible (Fig. 100-8). We prefer not to dissect it for branches, nor is the artery mobilized or surrounded with vessel loops. Care should be taken not to stretch or crack a mediasclerotic artery.
- It is our preference to harvest the mapped vein through several small incisions, dividing the branches under direct vision using vascular clips. Spliced vein grafts of optimal segments are preferred over a one-piece graft with segments of inferior quality. We do not believe that size matching, made by interrupted sutures and end-to-end intervenous anastomoses, will decrease graft patency. The vein is commonly used unreversed to avoid anastomotic mismatch between vein graft and recipient artery, and the valves are destroyed by valve cutters. Because wound problems are common, it is preferable to tunnel the graft deep by a route entering the subsartorial plane in the groin and down below the muscle along the thigh, anatomically behind the knee joint and down the calf under the edge of the gastrocnemius muscle.
- In situ versus ex situ is not an issue. The most important issue is to optimize graft quality and minimize risk of wound problems, avoiding dissecting for the saphenofemoral junction through the incision exposing the arteries, and avoiding parallel incisions at the calf. Liberal use of contralateral leg vein can minimize wound problems in the revascularized leg.
- Reconstruction of the arterial anastomosis necessitates a bloodless field, which may be obtained with delicate clamps or intraluminal balloon closure (Fig. 100-9). Because at least one half of patients have

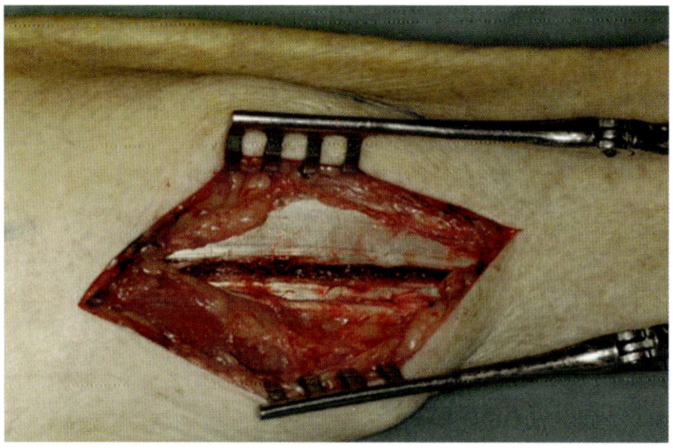

Figure 100-6.

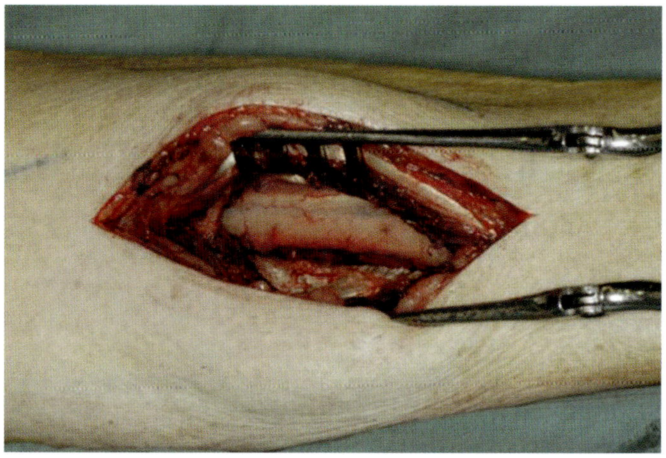

Figure 100-7.

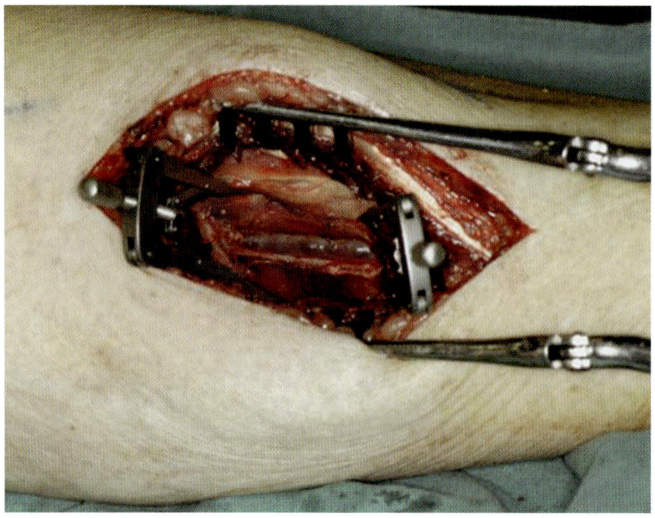

Figure 100-8.

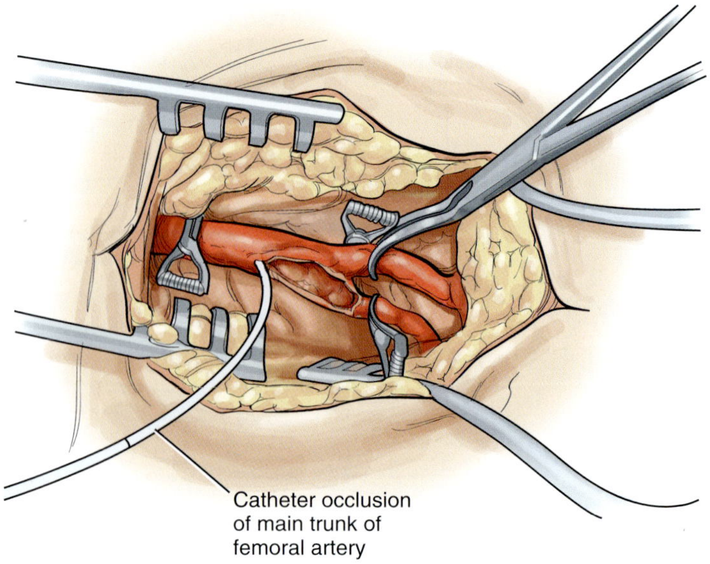

Figure 100-9.

diabetes, medial sclerosis and incompressible arteries are encountered frequently; a bloodless field for distal anastomosis may necessitate the use of tourniquet ischemia. This is achieved most often with a distal thigh cuff, emptying the distal vessels with elastic bandaging or merely elevating the leg and filling the tourniquet with suprasystolic pressure.

- Proximal anastomosis is placed on the anterolateral aspect of the common femoral artery (Fig. 100-10). Patching any deep femoral artery ostial stenonis is preferred as it will keep the anastomosed vein deep (enabling fascial closure over the anastomosis) and will direct the vein graft nicely into the subsartorial space (Fig. 100-11, *A*, *B*, and *C*).

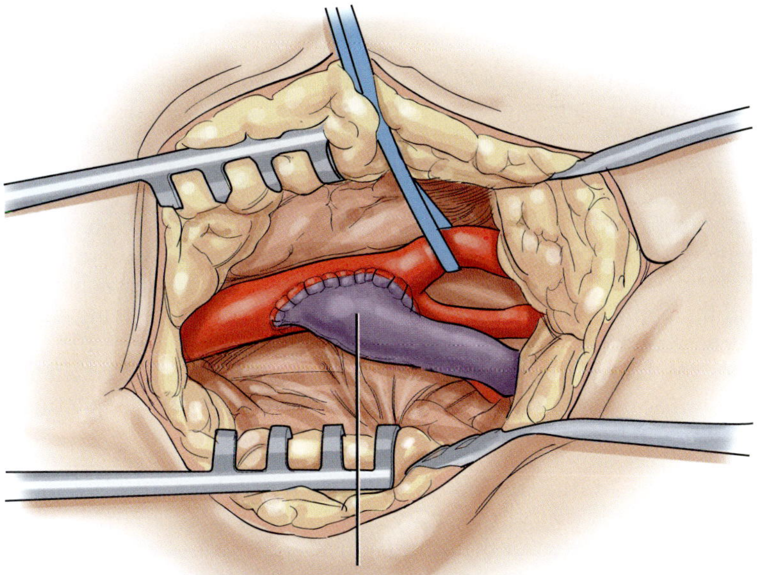

Figure 100-10.

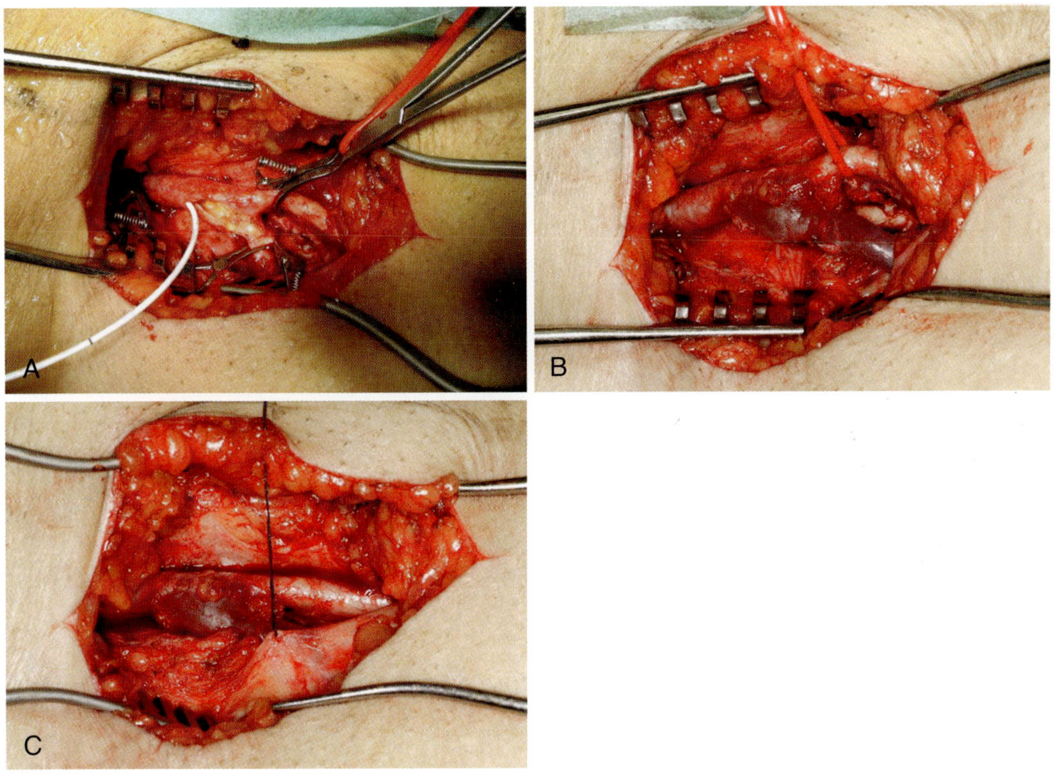

Figure 100-11.

- Distal anastomosis is done using a tourniquet with continuous 7-0 uninterrupted sutures, avoiding cracking of mediasclerotic vessels. The toe of the anastomosis is placed at a soft spot of the artery (Fig. 100-12). The use of small atraumatic retractors, a head light, and a carbon dioxide blower may facilitate the reconstruction. Elevation of the leg will decrease arterial back bleeding, which will, however, quickly decrease as the isolated leg exsanguinates. The inflow artery is usually cross-clamped while using a tourniquet to decrease the pressure needed for hemostatic control. Soft arterial probes can be used to check the patency of the anastomosis and the distal artery. Before the sutures are tied, the tourniquet should be released, and back flow as well as unobstructed graft flow should be observed.
- Graft volume flow and intraoperative duplex are used routinely as completion investigations. Intraoperative angiography is reserved for cases with unexpected runoff problems or for adjunctive inflow procedures.

Femoro- and Popliteopedal Bypass

- The exposition of the femoral bifurcation is done as outlined earlier. If the superficial femoral artery is patent, and especially if there is a lack of good-quality vein, more distal inflow is preferable even if the superficial femoral artery is not entirely free from disease, as long as there are no significant stenoses that cannot be treated endovascularly. Data indicate that shorter popliteopedal bypasses may fare at least as well as long ones with femoral inflow.
- For exposition of the distal popliteal artery, a medial longitudinal incision should be made, along the mapped saphenous vein if it is to be harvested from the same area. After the vein has been secured to one side, the muscular fascia is incised, the medial head of the gastrocnemius muscle is retracted posteriorly, and the popliteal artery is dissected free from its adjacent veins. Care should be taken not to stretch or bend a calcified artery. It is usually not necessary to control the easily accessible artery with vessel loops. We have not used a tourniquet on an inflow artery during anastomosis of a calcified artery. Rather, the proximal artery is controlled by an intraluminal balloon and the distal artery clamped.
- We prefer to do a duplex scan on the dorsalis pedis artery preoperatively to look for its exact position and a good landing zone for the anastomosis, keeping the incision to a minimum. If the exposition is to be made to the proximal part of the artery close to the ankle joint, the artery will be found deep between the tendons of the extensor digitorum longus and extensor hallucis longus muscles, but more distally between the hallucis longus tendon and the extensor hallucis brevis muscle. A longitudinal skin incision is made along the artery. The skin edges must not be touched with any forceps, and delicate adjustable retractors should be used carefully so as not to cause too much tension to the skin. The inferior extensor retinaculum is cut to expose the anterior surface of the artery, which is dissected

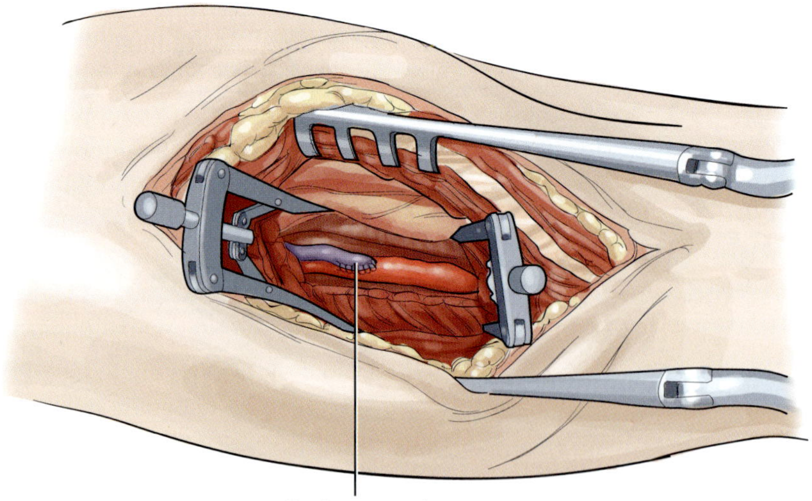

Figure 100-12.

free just to enable an arteriotomy, as a tourniquet is preferably used over the calf for making the anastomosis (Figs. 100-13 and 100-14, *A* and *B*).

- The vein is harvested according to the principles outlined earlier. For a long femoropedal bypass using ipsilateral saphenous vein, mapping must be exact. The surgeon must strive to make the skin bridge between the sites of vein harvesting and dorsalis pedis artery exposure as short and as wide as possible (the vein-harvesting wound should always be closed with a free skin transplant if the tension at the two incisions tends to be large). It is preferable to avoid this situation by moving the inflow to the superficial femoral artery if possible. If the vein is to be upgraded because of segments of inferior quality, enough vein should be harvested elsewhere to leave the saphenous vein at the foot in place. When doing shorter popliteopedal bypasses, we always harvest an optimal-size vein from the leg, leaving the saphenous vein of the most distal calf, ankle, and foot in place (it is optimal to harvest the vein from the thigh, leaving the whole calf untouched). The contralateral saphenous vein should be used liberally when there are vein quality problems and when the condition of the skin in the distal leg is poor because of ischemia and infection.
- There are two options for graft tunneling. In cases with no skin problems over the distal leg and foot and where the skin of the calf is intact (vein having been harvested elsewhere), it is preferable to make a subcutaneous tunnel over the medial aspect of the calf, curving toward the dorsalis pedis artery at

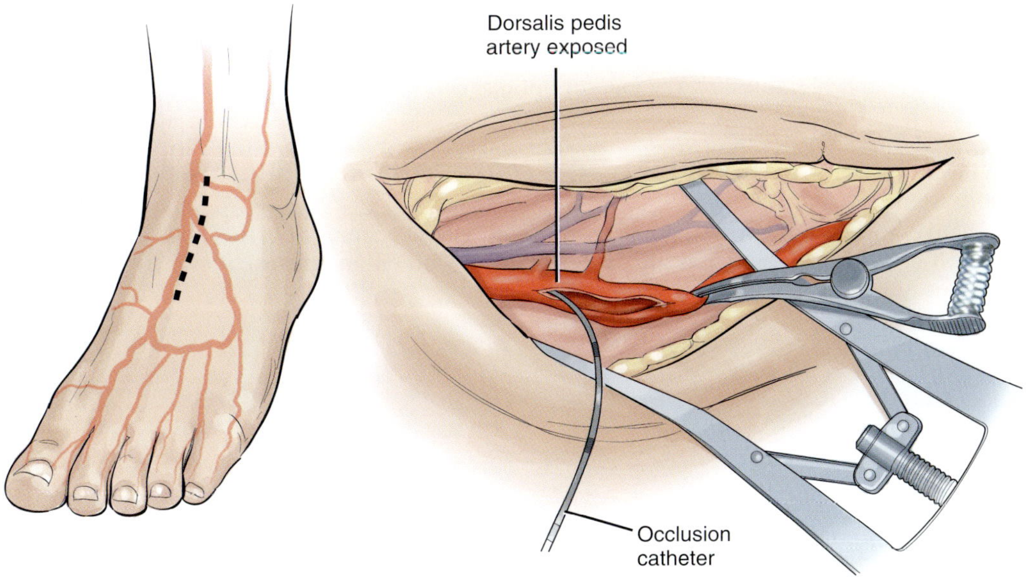

Figure 100-13.

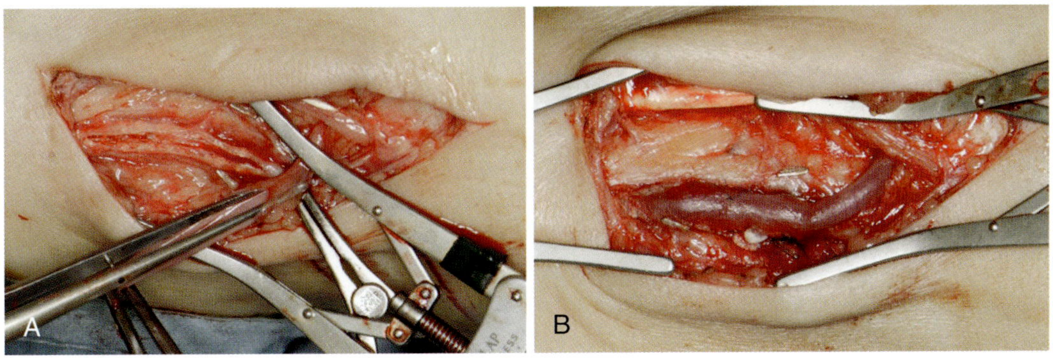

Figure 100-14.

foot level (avoiding tunneling the vein over the tibial bone margin) (Fig. 100-15). When the skin of the distal leg is in poor condition, or when there are ischemic lesions at the medial calf, it is preferable to cut the interosseous membrane under direct vision using a small lateral incision. The vein can thereafter be tunneled "anatomically" (cutting the fascia and the extensor retinaculum structures at the ankle joint level to avoid compression of the graft) or subcutaneously down the lateral calf. Especially when the anastomosis is placed at or just below the ankle joint, lateral tunneling is recommended (Fig. 100-16).

- The arteriotomy for the proximal anastomosis is usually made anteromedially on the popliteal artery. However, if the graft is to be tunneled laterally, it is wise to make the arteriotomy more anterior (by slightly twisting a soft artery) or by directing the arteriotomy slightly obliquely to the lateral side. This minimizes the risk for kinking after tunneling. An ordinary anastomosis using continuous 6-0 unabsorbable suture is made.
- The dorsalis pedis artery is vulnerable to any hard instrumentation and often mediasclerotic in patients with diabetes. A bloodless field may be achieved with tourniquet ischemia or catheter occlusion (Fig. 100-17). Distal anastomosis is done using continuous 7-0 uninterrupted sutures, avoiding damage to the sclerotic artery and again placing the toe of the anastomosis at a soft spot of the artery if possible. Soft arterial probes can be used to check the patency of the anastomosis and distal artery. The tourniquet should be released, and back-flow as well as unobstructed graft-flow should be observed before the sutures are tied to complete the anastomosis.

Closure

- Wound closure of the foot must be done with care, striving to appose some vital subcutaneous tissue over the anastomosis with a few 5-0 absorbable interrupted sutures. We prefer to use interrupted skin sutures (not surgical staples) on the foot for optimal control of apposition and tension of wound edges.

III. ALTERNATIVE TECHNICAL APPROACHES (PRO/CON) AND PEARLS

- Alternative approaches to the peroneal artery are lateral, either with the knee hyperflexed or with resection of the fibula, but veins are easily damaged with either approach.

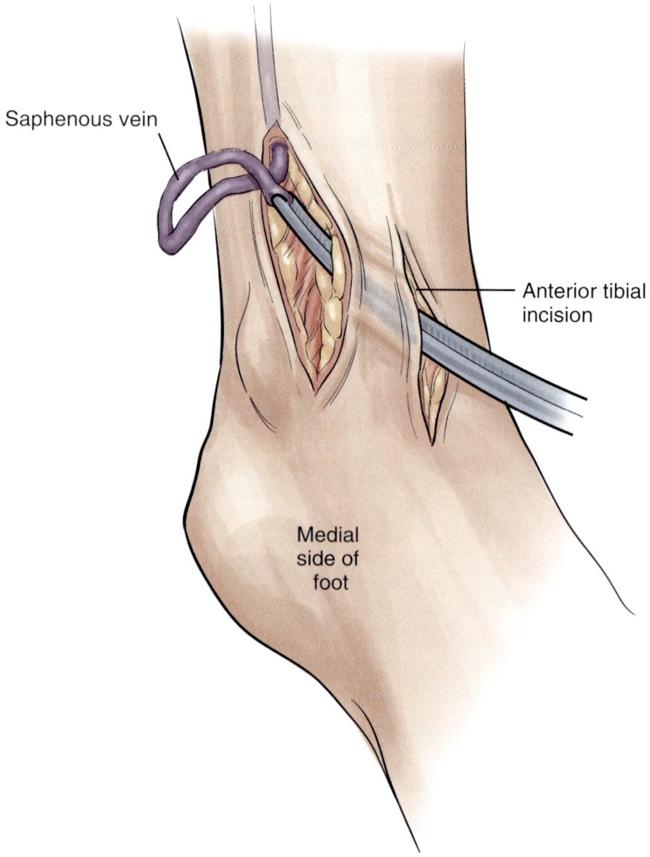

Figure 100-15.

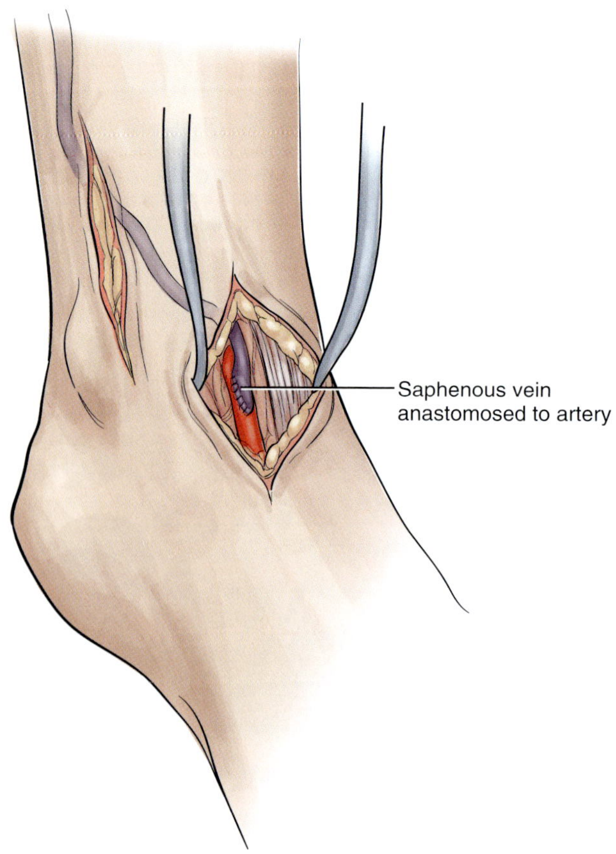

Figure 100-16.

- When using medial approach, the leg should be externally rotated. Because the peroneal artery lies deep in the wound, veins could be mobilized with adjacent tissue, which all can be fixed en bloc with a stay suture using a long straight needle through the leg. This allows better visualization of the target artery (Fig. 100-18, *A* and *B*).
- When using spliced veins as a conduit, the vein-to-vein anastomosis should be made using hold sutures and interrupted 7-0 sutures. Care should be taken not to lose anastomotic circumference. The tension on each side of the anastomosis should be kept equal (Fig. 100-19).
- Needle hole bleeding occasionally appears from very thin vessel walls. This may stop spontaneously, but it can be controlled with a new delicate suture including a small piece of fat or fascia taken from the tissue adjacent to the operative field (see Fig. 100-11, *B*).

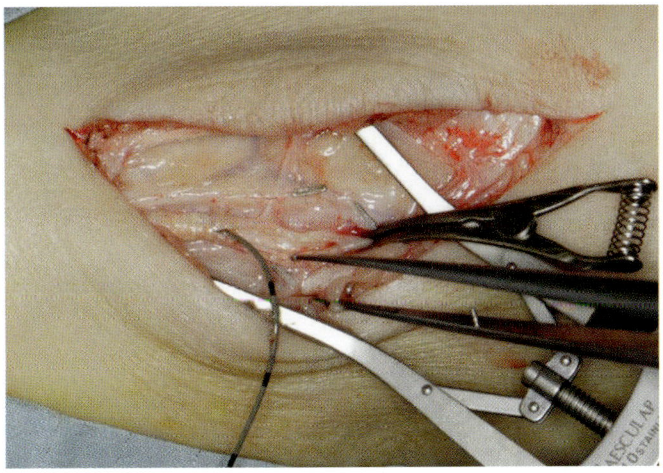

Figure 100-17.

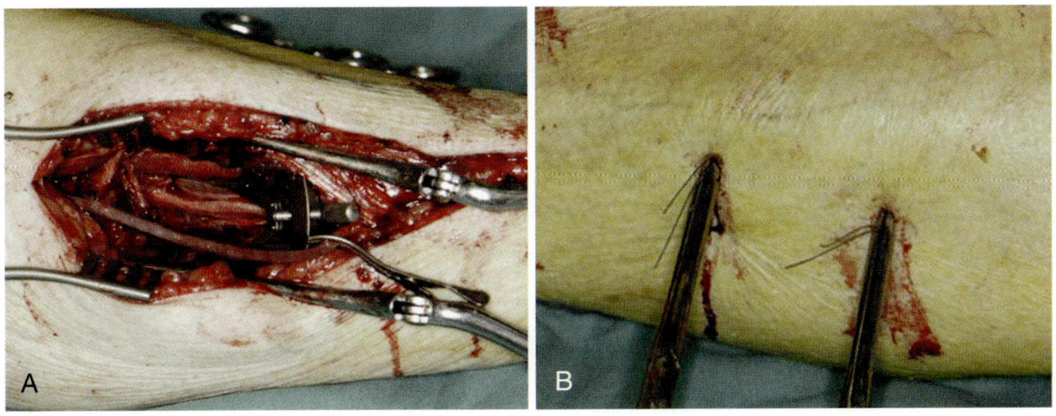

Figure 100-18.

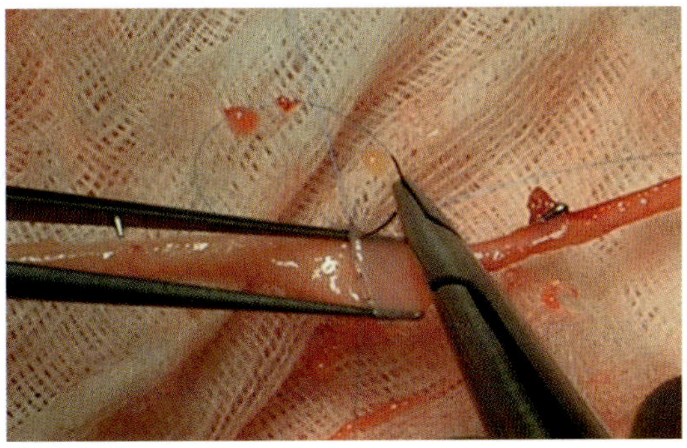

Figure 100-19.

- Inflow should be ensured with endovascular intervention or surgical reconstruction. Typically, endarterectomy of the common femoral and the diseased origin and first part of the deep femoral artery may be needed (see Fig. 100-11, *A* and *B*).
- Remember the possibility of using a microvascular free flap transfer in conjunction with distal bypass in cases with large tissue defects.

IV. SPECIAL POSTOPERATIVE CARE

- Postoperative antithrombotic medication must be carefully used. Antiplatelet therapy should be started preoperatively and continued infinitely after the operation if not subsequently contraindicated. We prefer to use acetylsalicylic acid instead of warfarin even after venous bypass because of the risk of hemorrhage in elderly patients. Low–molecular-weight heparin is administered while the patient is hospitalized.
- Ensure the patency of the graft with duplex or ankle-brachial index postoperatively. Remember that any graft occluded by a pressure cuff gives ankle-brachial index values around 1 if open (stump pressure of the graft).
- Clinical surveillance programs are recommended for up to 2 years. The risk of myointimal hyperplasia is of minor importance thereafter.

SUGGESTED READINGS

Bandyk DF: Infrainguinal vein bypass graft surveillance: how to do it, when to intervene, and is it cost-effective? *J Am Coll Surg* 194:S40–S52, 2002.

Hingorani A, Ascher E, Marks N: Preprocedural imaging: new options to reduce need for contrast angiography, *Semin Vasc Surg* 20:15–28, 2007.

Tukiainen E, Kallio M, Lepäntalo M: Advanced leg salvage of the critically ischemic leg with major tissue loss by vascular and plastic surgeon teamwork: long-term outcome, *Ann Surg* 244:949–957, 2006.

Index

Page numbers followed by *f* indicate figures; *t*, tables; *b*, boxes.

D

I

O

P

Q

R

U

V